Gastrointestinal Diseases

ATLAS OF NONTUMOR PATHOLOGY

AMERICAN REGISTRY OF PATHOLOGY 1976

ARMED FORCES INSTITUTE OF PATHOLOGY
founded as ARMY MEDICAL MUSEUM 1862
1949

Editorial Director: Kelley S. Hahn
Production Editor: Dian S. Thomas
Editorial Assistant/Scanning Technician: Mirlinda Q. Caton
Copyeditor: Audrey Kahn

ATLAS OF NONTUMOR PATHOLOGY

First Series
Fascicle 5

Gastrointestinal Diseases

Amy Noffsinger, MD

Cecilia M. Fenoglio-Preiser, MD

Dipen Maru, MD

Norman Gilinsky, MD

Published by the
American Registry of Pathology
Washington, DC
in collaboration with the
Armed Forces Institute of Pathology
Washington, DC

2007

ATLAS OF NONTUMOR PATHOLOGY

Manuscript Reviewed by:
Leslie H. Sobin, MD
Harvey Goldman, MD

Available from the American Registry of Pathology
Armed Forces Institute of Pathology
Washington, DC 20306-6000
www.afip.org
ISBN: 1-933477-03-2
978-1-933477-03-9

INTRODUCTION TO SERIES

This is the fourth Fascicle of the Atlas of Nontumor Pathology, a complementary series to the Armed Forces Institute of Pathology (AFIP) Atlas of Tumor Pathology, first published in 1949.

For several years, various individuals in the pathology community have suggested the formation of a new series of monographs concentrating on this particular area. In 1998, an Editorial Board was appointed and outstanding authors chosen shortly thereafter.

The purpose of the atlas is to provide surgical pathologists with ready expert reference material most helpful in their daily practice. The lesions described relate principally to medical non-neoplastic conditions. Many of these lesions represent complex entities and, when appropriate, we have included contributions from internists, radiologists, and surgeons. This has led to some increase in the size of the monographs but the emphasis remains on diagnosis by the surgical pathologist.

Previously, the Fascicles have been available on CD-ROM format as well as in print. In order to provide the widest possible advantages of both modalities, we have formatted the print Fascicle on the World Wide Web. Use of the Internet allows cross-indexing within the Fascicles as well as linkage to PubMed.

Our goal is to continue to provide expert information at the lowest possible cost. Therefore, marked reductions in pricing are available to residents and fellows as well as to pathology faculty and other staff members purchasing the Fascicles on a subscription basis.

We believe that the Atlas of Nontumor Pathology will serve as an outstanding reference for surgical pathologists as well as an important contribution to the literature of other medical specialties.

Donald West King, MD
Leslie H. Sobin, MD
J. Thomas Stocker, MD
Bernard Wagner, MD

PREFACE

This Fascicle is devoted to benign gastrointestinal diseases and provides an in-depth discussion of many lesions, both common and uncommon. This volume is, for the most part, organized by category of disease rather than by anatomic site. This approach allows us to cover each entity comprehensively and avoids redundant descriptions of lesions that occur in multiple regions of the gastrointestinal tract. Each disease entity is discussed from the point of view of its demographics, pathophysiology, clinical features, gross and microscopic pathology, and treatment. The text is heavily illustrated with diagrams and gross and microscopic photographs. Numerous tables have been included in order to facilitate comparison of diseases and generation of differential diagnoses. Because of the extreme importance of clinical and endoscopic correlation with interpretation of gastrointestinal pathologic specimens, we have included an actively practicing gastroenterologist among the authors. He has added endoscopic pictures and provided clinical insights critical to the understanding of gastrointestinal diseases.

In many areas we have provided text and references related to animal models of disease since these have become very powerful tools for understanding gastrointestinal diseases, particularly inflammatory bowel disease, motility disorders, and benign polyposis syndromes. Where it is most relevant, we provide a discussion of some of the molecular alterations that are present since these provide an understanding of the pathophysiology of the disease. We also provide some discussion of the genetic predispositions to gastrointestinal diseases that occur as a result of genetic loss, mutation, overexpression of genes, or genetic polymorphisms.

A text such as this would not have been possible without the close working relationships we have been privileged to have had with other pathologists and gastroenterologists. Such relationships are most rewarding when there is a continuing dialogue that provides increased understanding of disease processes in individual patients. This book would also not have been possible without the numerous consults we have received over the years from our colleagues in both pathology and gastroenterology. This has enabled us to illustrate the majority of the entities we discuss. Finally, the many residents and fellows that we have worked with over the years have unknowingly contributed to this work by taking gross photographs, calling our attention to interesting cases that we might not have seen otherwise, and continuing to send us cases after they have left our training programs to practice. We hope that readers will find that this book provides information not otherwise available in a single reference.

Amy Noffsinger, MD
Cecilia M. Fenoglio-Preiser, MD
Dipen Maru, MD
Norman Gilinsky, MD

Permission to use copyrighted illustrations has been granted by:

American Roentgen Ray Society
American Journal of Roentgenology 1993;160:59-61. For figure 10-14.

Armed Forces Institute of Pathology
Atlas of Gastrointestinal Endoscopy & Endoscopic Biopsies, 2000. For figures 4-14, 5-1, 6-34, 7-17, 7-18, 8-4, 10-17, 10-18, 10-44, 10-58, 11-23, and 11-24.

Blackwell Publishing
Aliment Pharmacol Ther 2004;19:1051-61. For figure 8-5.

Lippincott Williams & Wilkins
Gastrointestinal Pathology, An Atlas and Text, 2nd ed., 1999;312. For figure 2-9.

Radiological Society of North America
Radiology 1975;117:519-21. For figure 4-5.

CONTENTS

1 GENERAL FEATURES OF THE GASTROINTESTINAL TRACT AND ITS EVALUATION

INTRODUCTION

The gastrointestinal (GI) tract is a remarkable organ with many functions and several distinct functional regions: esophagus, stomach, small intestine, colon, and anus. Although the cell types in these various areas have many similarities, important regional histologic differences allow specific physiologic functions to be carried out in each area. The cellular rearrangements and migrations that accompany early embryogenesis play a critical role in organizing the eventual adult GI tract. Interactions between cell populations regulate subsequent patterns of gene expression and organ development (1).

The GI tract serves as the digestive organ of the body, taking in everything that is swallowed, converting it into nutrients, and discarding what is left over as waste. These processes begin in the mouth and terminate at the anus. While digesting everything to which it is exposed and breaking it down into smaller, absorbable chemical substances, the gut is itself able to withstand these processes and avoid autodigestion. Complex neuromuscular interactions move food and liquids from one section of the GI tract to the next, while at the same time controlling the passage of food in such a way that allows maximum digestion and absorption.

Not everything that enters the GI tract is healthy for the patient. The GI tract serves as a major interface between the outside world and other portions of the body. It is continuously exposed to toxins and infectious organisms, yet is often capable of eliminating these agents without any harm coming to the body. Not surprisingly, breakdown in these defense mechanisms often results in disease. This generally occurs when the integrity of the bowel wall becomes compromised, as is discussed in many of the following chapters. As a part of this mucosal defense, the GI tract serves as a major immune organ. It is the major site of the generation of mucosal immunity; hence the utility of oral vaccines.

GASTROINTESTINAL STRUCTURE

In general, the gut consists of four concentric layers as one progresses outward from the lumen: the mucosa, submucosa, muscularis propria, and serosa or adventitia (fig. 1-1). The mucosal features differ significantly from one region of the GI tract to another. The other layers share many of the same characteristics throughout the length of the gut, although some differences do occur.

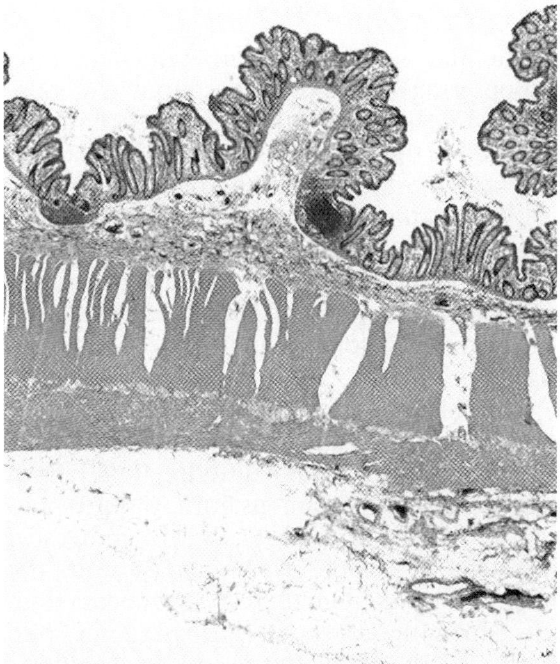

Figure 1-1

FOUR TISSUE LAYERS OF COLON

Uppermost in the photograph is the mucosa, which is composed of the epithelium, a supporting lamina propria, and the muscularis mucosae. Deep to this layer is the submucosa, composed of connective tissue, vessels, and nerves. Next is the muscularis propria. The outermost layer in this case is the subserosa. This layer contains abundant adipose tissue underlying a mesothelial covering, the serosa.

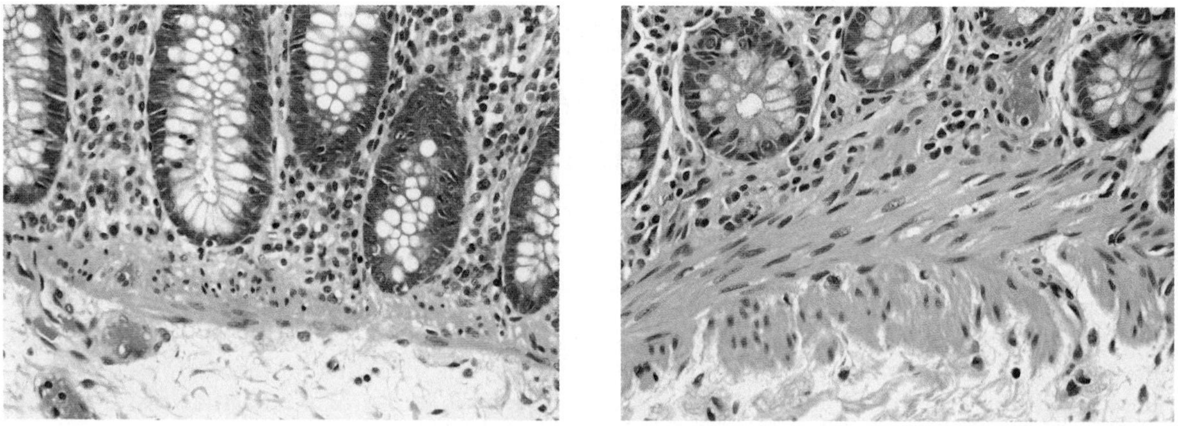

Figure 1-2

MUSCULARIS MUCOSAE

Left: Like the muscularis propria, the muscularis mucosae is comprised of two distinct muscle layers, an inner circular layer and an outer longitudinal layer.

Right: Higher-power view shows the two muscle layers more distinctly.

Mucosa

The mucosa consists of an epithelial lining, a supporting lamina propria composed of loose connective tissue rich in immune cells and capillaries, and the muscularis mucosae. The lamina propria is most visible in the stomach, large and small intestines, and appendix, and least visible in the esophagus and anus. The smooth muscle cells in the muscularis mucosae are predominantly arranged in a circular orientation, although some longitudinal muscle fibers are also present (fig. 1-2).

The character of the epithelium differs substantially in various regions of the GI tract, with differences reflecting the differing functions of each region. The squamous lining of the esophagus protects it from the passage of undigested food over its surface. Likewise, in the anus, the squamous epithelium protects the mucosa from the damaging effects of the passage of solid waste. In the stomach, the mucosa facilitates digestion by secreting acid. The epithelial lining of the small intestine is uniquely suited to the further digestion and absorption of nutrients along a gradient from the duodenum to the ileum. The colon predominantly reabsorbs water. The specific features of the various portions of the gut are discussed below.

The lamina propria represents the interglandular tissue of the mucosa. It consists of delicate, loose connective tissue containing lymphocytes, plasma cells (fig. 1-3), eosinophils, and mast cells. Most of the cells are plasma cells and lymphocytes. The majority of plasma cells secrete immunoglobulin (Ig)A; however, IgM-, IgG-, and IgE-secreting cells are also present. The lamina propria also contains large numbers of macrophages (55), which play an important role in mucosal immunity and immunoregulation (5,26,32, 45,52). Macrophages also engulf and remove apoptotic epithelial cells that are shed normally from the mucosal surface. As a result, lamina propria macrophages are sometimes immunoreactive with antibodies against epithelial-associated antigens, including carcinoembryonic antigen, BerEp4, and cytokeratin (34). The highest number of lamina propria macrophages is present in the colon and rectum (42).

Gut-associated lymphoid tissue (GALT) primarily lies within the lamina propria. It is distributed diffusely or appears as solitary (fig. 1-4) or aggregated nodules, which in the ileum and appendix are called Peyer patches. Larger aggregates contain germinal centers (fig. 1-4). Peyer patches often span the muscularis mucosae (fig. 1-5), creating gaps in this muscular layer. Solitary lymphoid nodules occur in the esophagus, gastric pylorus, and along the small and large intestines.

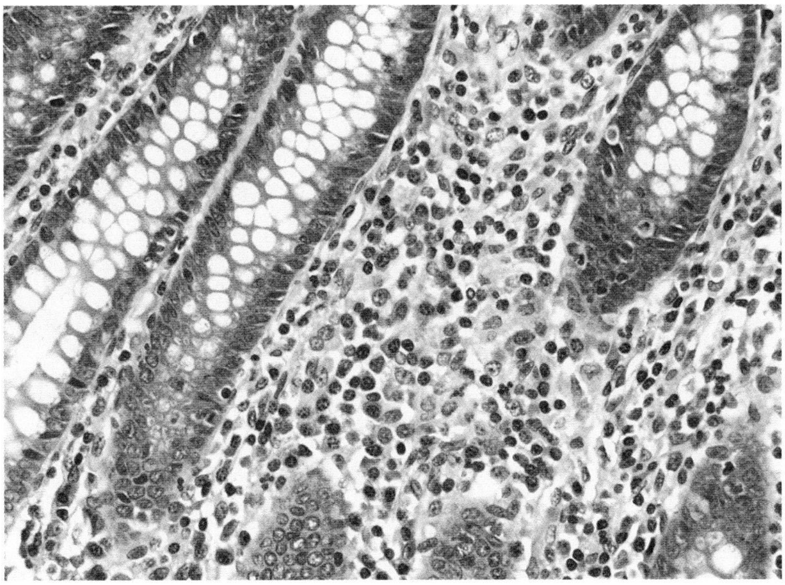

Figure 1-3

LAMINA PROPRIA

The lamina propria contains numerous immunocytes including lymphocytes, plasma cells, and eosinophils, which lie within a connective tissue background.

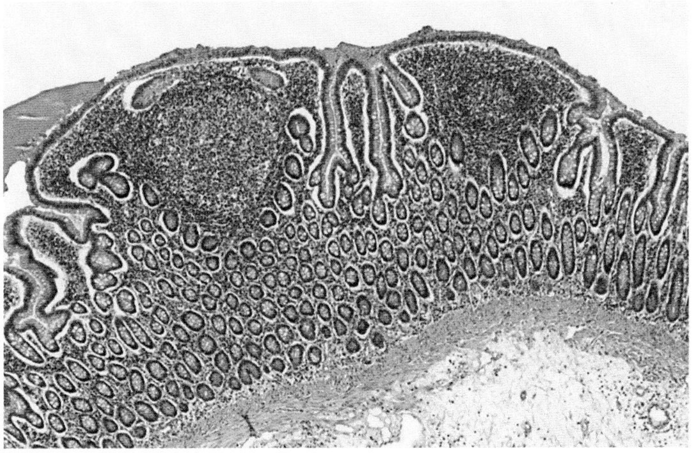

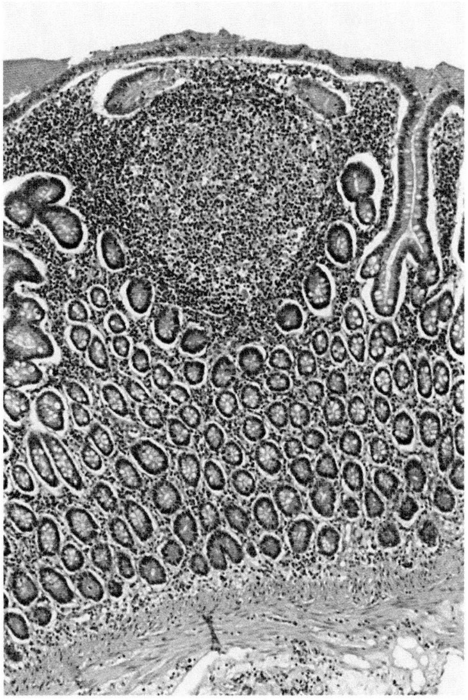

Figure 1-4

PEYER PATCH

Above: Low-power view of the ileum of a 6-year-old child shows prominent Peyer patches. The large lymphoid aggregate distorts the overlying mucosa causing a loss of the normal villous architecture.

Right: Higher-power view shows a lymphoid aggregate with a well-formed germinal center.

Mast Cells

Mast cells are an important, but heterogeneous, component of the lamina propria and submucosa. Mast cells are mononuclear and contain numerous cytoplasmic granules (fig. 1-6). The granules contain various mediators, including peptides, proteins, proteoglycans, and amines. The cytoplasmic granules stain with dyes, such as toluidine blue and Alcian blue. In addition, mast cells stain immunohistochemically with antibodies to CD117 (c-kit) and tryptase (fig. 1-7).

The relative proportion of mast cells differs between anatomic sites, and their recognition may be sensitive to formaldehyde fixation in

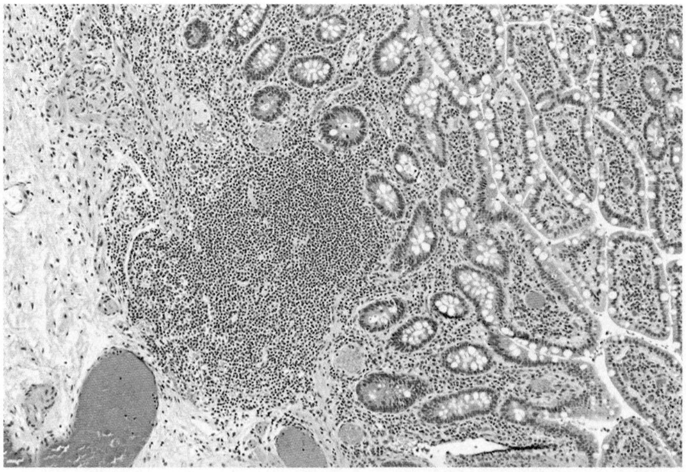

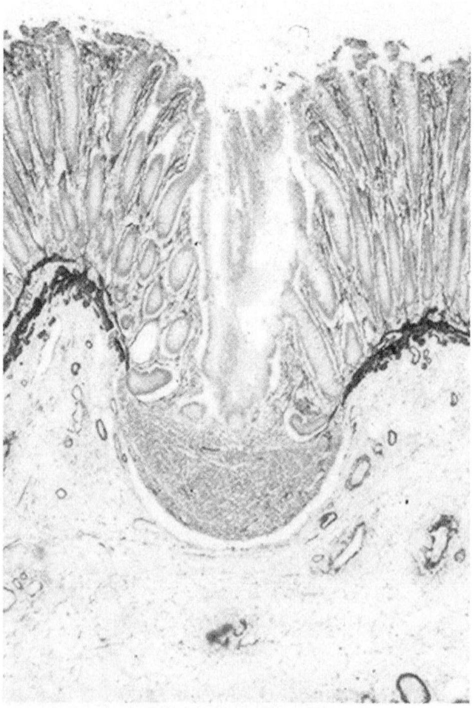

Figure 1-5

PEYER PATCH

Above: Hematoxylin and eosin (H&E)-stained section shows a lymphoid aggregate that extends from the submucosa across the muscularis mucosae and into the mucosa.

Right: Immunohistochemical staining for actin demonstrates that the muscularis mucosae in this area is disrupted.

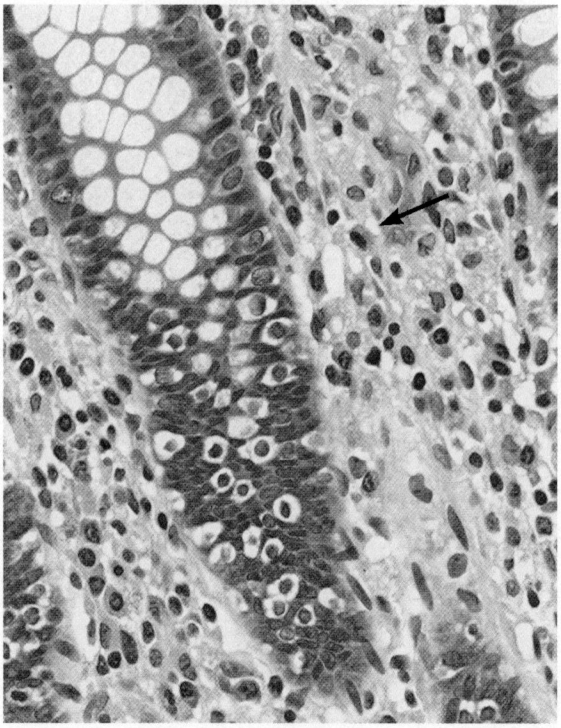

Figure 1-6

LAMINA PROPRIA

On routine H&E-stained sections, mast cells appear eosinophilic and have prominent cytoplasmic granules (arrow). The nucleus is not lobated like that of an eosinophil.

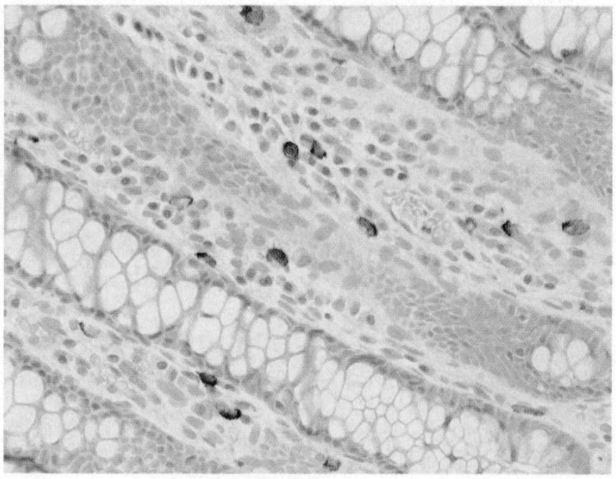

Figure 1-7

LAMINA PROPRIA

Mast cells in the lamina propria are easily recognized with the CD117 immunostain.

the intestinal mucosa (11,35,46). Mast cells are often adjacent to blood or lymphatic vessels, near or within nerves, and beneath epithelial surfaces, particularly those exposed to environmental antigens (3,19,33). Mast cell infiltrates are often associated with increased numbers of eosinophils. They degranulate after IgE-mediated stimulation. Following immunologic

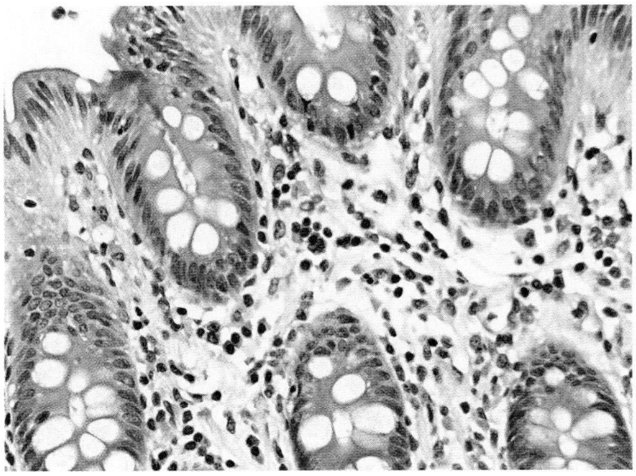

Figure 1-8

LAMINA PROPRIA

Eosinophils appear as red granular cells with bilobed nuclei.

activation via the IgE receptor, mast cells release cytokines, lipid-derived mediators, amines, proteases, and proteoglycans, all of which regulate adjacent cells and the metabolism of the extracellular matrix.

By virtue of their location and number, mast cells play a role in a wide variety of gastrointestinal abnormalities. The most important include food allergies, eosinophilic diseases, immunodeficiency syndromes, immediate hypersensitivity reactions, host responses to parasites and neoplasms, and immunologically nonspecific inflammatory and fibrotic conditions (4,30). Mast cells are also important in angiogenesis, wound healing, peptic ulcer disease, reactions to neoplasms, and other chronic inflammatory conditions, including graft versus host disease and inflammatory bowel disease (3,19,33).

Eosinophils

Eosinophils are commonly present within the lamina propria (fig. 1-8). Their brightly eosinophilic cytoplasmic granules and bilobed nucleus are characteristic identifying features. The cytoplasmic granules contain lysosomal hydrolases as well as many of the cationic proteins unique to eosinophils, including major basic protein (7,21) and eosinophil peroxidase. Eosinophils express receptors for IgG, IgE, and IgA on their plasma membranes (2,8,22,53). They also have receptors for complement components (9,20,23) and cytokines (29).

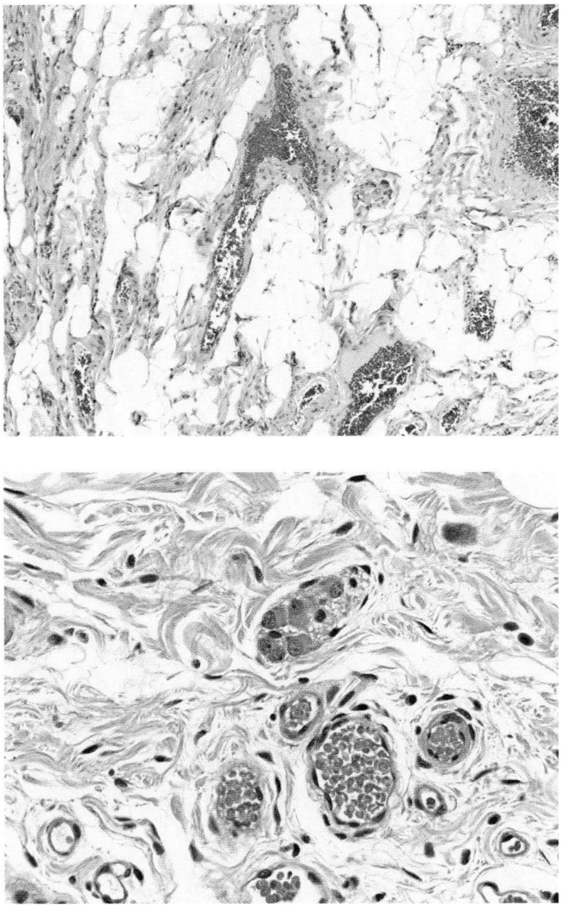

Figure 1-9

SUBMUCOSA

Top: The submucosa is composed of loose connective tissue containing nerves, clusters of ganglion cells, and vessels. Adipose tissue is also commonly present.

Bottom: Higher-power view shows a submucosal ganglion, vessels, and bundles of collagen fibers.

Eosinophils have both beneficial and detrimental roles in the host. They function in host defense, including phagocytosis and killing of bacteria and other microbes. They also mediate allergic reactions, however, and the oxidative products of eosinophils can damage cells. The eosinophilic products that are most damaging are the cationic proteins (53).

Submucosa

The submucosa is a more densely collagenous and less cellular layer than the mucosa (fig. 1-9). Major blood vessels, lymphatics, nerves, ganglia, and occasionally lymphoid collections are

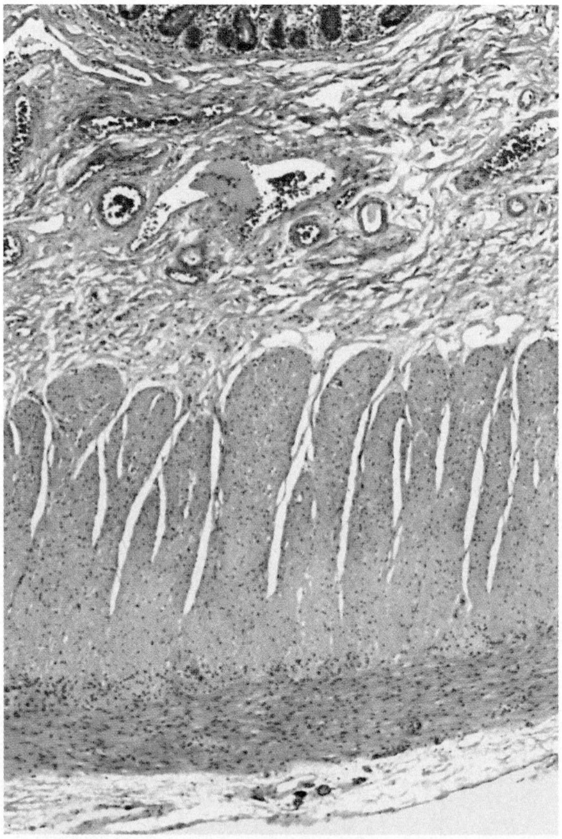

Figure 1-10

MUSCULARIS PROPRIA

Low-power view shows a distinct inner circular muscle layer and an outer longitudinal layer. The myenteric plexus contains nerve fibers and ganglion cells, and lies between the two layers of smooth muscle.

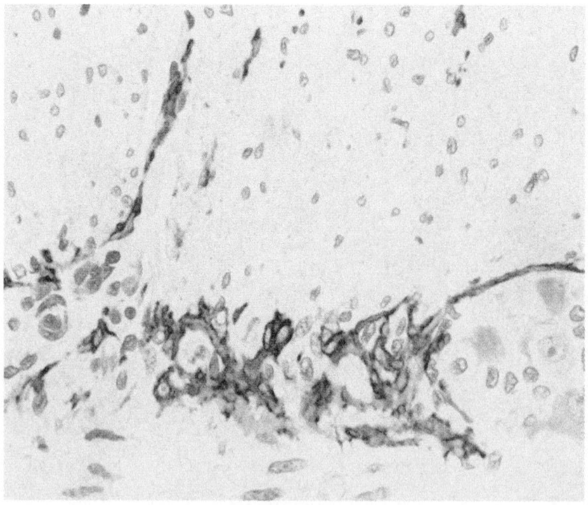

Figure 1-11

INTERSTITIAL CELLS OF CAJAL

Although difficult to identify on routine H&E-stained sections, immunostaining for CD117 highlights the interstitial cells of Cajal. The cells are associated with the myenteric plexus, appear somewhat spindled, and have scant cytoplasm. (Fig. 1-9A from Fascicle 32, 3rd Series.)

located here. The submucosa may also contain adipose tissue in variable amounts.

Muscularis Propria

The muscularis propria is a continuous structure made up of two smooth muscle layers that extend from the upper esophagus to the anal canal (fig. 1-10). The only exception to this occurs in the stomach, where three layers are present. At the junctions between adjacent regions of the GI tract, the muscular coat rearranges to form sphincters (pharyngoesophageal, esophagogastric, pyloric, ileocecal, and anal sphincters). In the upper esophageal and anal sphincters, skeletal muscle fibers may be admixed with smooth muscle fibers (10). In the portion of the muscularis propria comprised of two layers, the inner muscular layer is arranged in a concentric circular fashion, while the outer muscle fibers are arranged longitudinally. In the cecum and in parts of the colon, the longitudinal muscle is attenuated except in the areas where it forms thick cords, the taeniae coli.

In the stomach, the arrangement of the musculature is more complex because in some areas there are three muscle layers. In the small intestine, the innermost portion of the circular layer consists of specialized muscle cells that are much smaller and more electron dense than the bulk of the circular muscle. A large number of nerve fibers run between the muscle layers, and it has been suggested that some of these are sensory fibers working in conjunction with the smooth muscle cells to function as stretch receptors (17,18).

The musculature also contains the interstitial cells of Cajal (ICCs), which share ultrastructural features with fibroblasts (38–40). ICCs are large, oval cells with light-staining nuclei and scant cytoplasm. They have two to five, long ramifying primary cell processes, giving them a spindled or stellate shape (fig. 1-11). They form a three-dimensional network and are closely associated with ganglion nerve bundles; they also extend

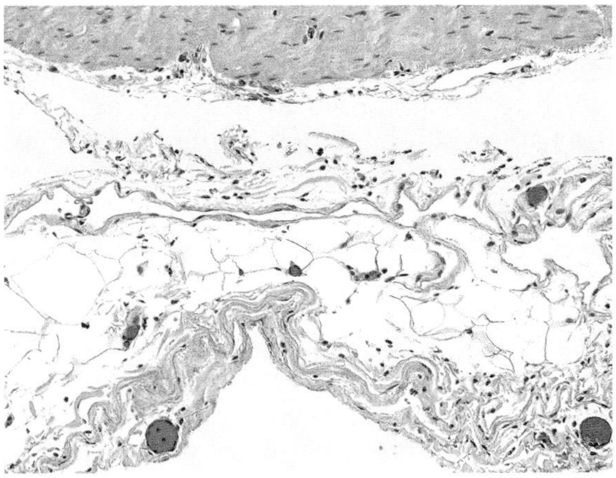

Figure 1-12

SUBSEROSA/ADVENTITIA

The subserosa of the gastrointestinal tract contains loose connective tissue, fat, blood vessels, and nerves. The outermost aspect is covered by mesothelium, the serosa.

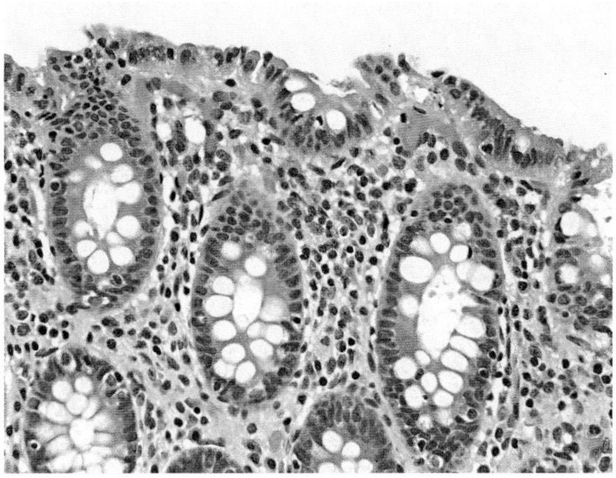

Figure 1-13

MUCOSAL VASCULATURE

A network of capillaries underlies the mucosal surface.

over the smooth muscle cells. The ICCs connect to both the circular and longitudinal cells via gap junctions, creating a network of interstitial cells that conduct electrical signals (27,28). ICCs have three major functions: they act as pacemakers for the gastrointestinal muscle (13–15,48); they facilitate active propagation of electrical events; and they mediate neurotransmission (15). They may also act as mechanoreceptors (13–15,48). These unique cells appear to require the *c-kit* gene or stem cell factor in order to develop (41), as well as to elicit their pacemaker activity (24).

The cells of the muscularis propria contain numerous receptors that allow them to respond to neural as well as other stimulatory and inhibitory signals during the digestive process. Contraction of the circular layer constricts the lumen; contraction of the longitudinal layer shortens the digestive tube.

Adventitia or Serosa

The adventitia is the outermost layer of the GI tract, and consists of loose connective tissue containing fat, collagen, and elastic tissue (fig. 1-12). If it is covered by mesothelium, the serosa, it is called the subserosa. A serosa and subserosa are present on the stomach, those parts of the small intestine that are not retroperitoneal, the appendix, and the large intestine above the peritoneal reflection.

Vasculature

The intestinal mucosa is a highly perfused organ. The largest arteries pass through the wall of the GI tract and are arranged longitudinally in a submucosal plexus. The submucosal plexus sends arterioles and capillaries into the mucosa, muscularis propria, and adventitia or serosa. The mucosa contains an irregular capillary plexus, often with its most terminal branches underlying the luminal surface epithelium (fig. 1-13). Veins arising in the mucosa anastomose in the submucosa and course with the arteries out of the intestine. Valves are present in the adventitia or subserosa.

The gut is richly supplied with lymphatic vessels, but their distribution, particularly in the mucosa, varies with the site within the GI tract. The richest lymphatic distribution occurs in the small intestine, where these vessels are intimately involved in nutrient absorption (fig. 1-14). Larger submucosal lymphatics branch freely and contain numerous valves. Smaller mucosal and submucosal lymphatics may be difficult to detect because they are often collapsed and blend in with the surrounding connective tissue. They are often difficult to distinguish from small capillaries.

Innervation

The enteric nervous system is the most complex portion of the peripheral nervous system. Three divisions of the nervous system

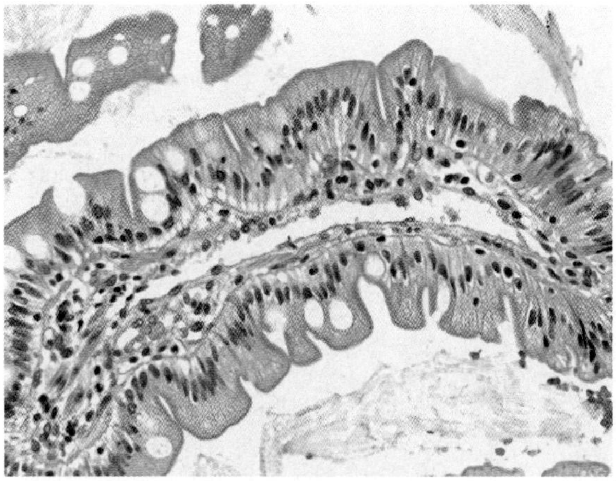

Figure 1-14

SMALL INTESTINAL LYMPHATICS

A central lymphatic vessel (lacteal) lies within the core of this villus. The lacteals are often difficult to see unless there is some degree of lymphangiectasia.

(sympathetic, parasympathetic, and enteric) contribute to the neural control of at least four physiologic effector systems: 1) the visceral smooth muscle responsible for motility and sphincteric functions; 2) the mucosa responsible for gastric acid secretion and homeostasis of intestinal fluid and electrolytes; 3) the immune cells responsible for mucosal immunity; and 4) the vasculature. Complex reflex activities involving gastrointestinal motility, ion transport, and mucosal blood flow all occur in the absence of extrinsic autonomic and sensory input.

Functionally, the neurons of the enteric nervous system fall into five types: 1) motor neurons controlling smooth muscle tone in the wall of the gut; 2) vasomotor neurons controlling vascular muscle tone; 3) secretory neurons regulating exocrine and endocrine secretion; 4) sensory neurons carrying sensory information to the central nervous system; and 5) interneurons that provide communication between neurons and the gut wall (16). The interneurons intermingle in the myenteric and submucosal ganglia, making their identification difficult.

Gastrointestinal Endocrine System

Endocrine cells are widely distributed within the epithelium of the stomach, small and large intestines, the distal esophageal glands, and anus. Some are also present in the lamina propria in the stomach and the appendix. Endocrine/paracrine cells differ in various parts of the gut in their overall density, contents, and structure. They are sensitive to chemical and mechanical stimuli, to which they respond by releasing extracellular mediators. The composition of enteroendocrine cells depends on their position along both the vertical and horizontal axes of the GI tract. At least 16 types of endocrine/paracrine cells inhabit the mucosa of the GI tract (Table 1-1).

Gastrointestinal endocrine cells have endocrine, paracrine, and neurotransmitter functions, constituting a complex system that regulates many functions of the GI tract. Some substances produced by enteroendocrine cells act as true peptide hormones. For example, gastrin, secretin, and cholecystokinin are secreted into the blood to reach their target organs (stomach, pancreas, and gallbladder) and soon after are metabolized and eliminated. Some peptides, such as somatostatin, are released from enteroendocrine cells into the local subepithelial connective tissue or directly on other types of cells via long basal cytoplasmic processes. This influences cells and tissues in the immediate vicinity via a paracrine mechanism.

Interactions exist between different components of the neuroendocrine system and the neural system. Neurons interact with endocrine cells, endocrine cells interact with other endocrine cells, and endocrine cells may influence neurons (47). In addition, many gastrointestinal hormones interact with the hypothalamic-pituitary axis to orchestrate the secretory activity and motility necessary for effective digestion (25,36,47). Gastrointestinal hormones and paracrine messengers control digestive processes such as acid secretion, bicarbonate secretion, enzyme secretion, and local blood flow. They also influence the immune system, metabolism, and gastrointestinal growth (49).

The circulating levels of the gastrointestinal peptides are influenced by numerous factors. For endocrine cells that lie in contact with the gastrointestinal lumen, such as gastrin cells (44), gastric inhibitory polypeptide cells (6), and secretin-producing cells (43,51), direct contact with, and absorption of, nutrients and secretions are the most important stimuli. In contrast, peptides like pancreatic polypeptide and insulin, produced in cells outside of the GI tract,

Table 1-1

GASTROINTESTINAL ENDOCRINE CELLS

Cell	Location	Product(s)	Action
CCK[a]	Small intestine	Cholecystokinin	Stimulates pancreatic and biliary enzyme secretion
D	Stomach Small intestine Colon	Somatostatin Vasoactive intestinal polypeptide	Inhibit secretion and motility
EC	Stomach Small intestine Appendix Colon	Serotonin Motilin Substance P	Stimulate motility
ECL	Stomach	Histamine	Stimulates acid secretion
G	Pylorus Duodenum	Gastrin	Gastric acid secretion
GIP	Small intestine	Gastric inhibitory polypeptide Xenin	Inhibits gastric acid secretion
L	Small intestine Colon	Glucagon-like peptides Peptide YY	Stimulate hepatic glycogenolysis
M	Small intestine	Motilin	Stimulates motility
N	Small intestine	Neurotensin	
P/D_1	Stomach	Ghrelin	
S	Small intestine	Secretin Serotonin	Stimulates pancreatic and biliary secretion

[a]CCK = cholecystokinin cell; EC = enterochromaffin cell; ECL = enterochromaffin-like cell; GIP = gastric inhibitory polypeptide cell.

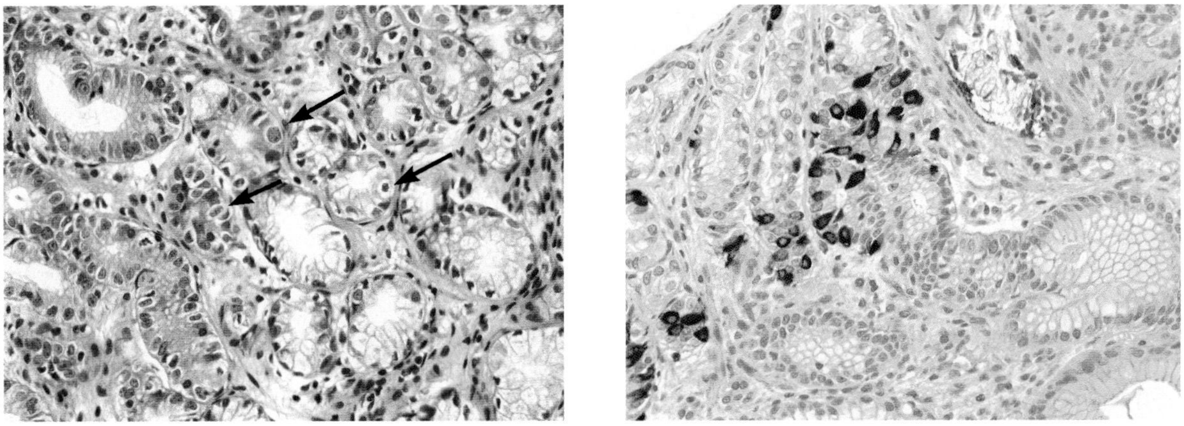

Figure 1-15

ENDOCRINE CELLS

Left: Gastric endocrine cells are difficult to visualize on routine H&E-stained slides. They are located in the neck of the gastric gland, and often have relatively clear cytoplasm and round, regular nuclei (arrows).

Right: A chromogranin stain highlights the endocrine cells.

depend on absorbed nutrients and stimulation by other peptides in the nervous system. Endocrine cells are also influenced by the nature of the intraluminal microflora (50).

Endocrine cells occur singly (fig. 1-15) or in discontinuous clusters. They appear as small, clear cells with a broad basal cytoplasm that contains electron-dense granules. Some endocrine

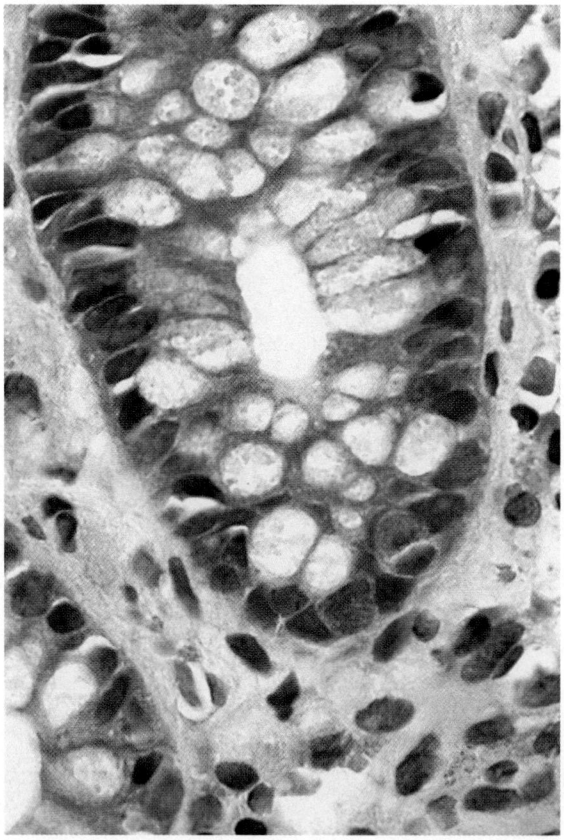

Figure 1-16

ENDOCRINE CELL

An H&E-stained section demonstrates an endocrine cell in the base of a colonic crypt. The cell contains prominent subnuclear eosinophilic granules.

cells, particularly those in the colon, contain prominent eosinophilic granules (fig. 1-16). Endocrine cells may be identified histochemically using Grimelius or Fontana-Masson stains. Other markers of neuroendocrine differentiation include antibodies to neuron-specific enolase, protein gene product 9.5, synaptophysin, and chromogranin (fig. 1-17) (12,31,37,54). Specific peptide hormones can also be identified immunohistochemically.

NORMAL FEATURES OF INDIVIDUAL GASTROINTESTINAL SITES

Esophagus

The normal esophageal mucosa is readily recognizable by its squamous epithelial lining and submucosal glands (fig. 1-18). The basal layer of the squamous epithelium consists of cuboidal or columnar cells with central basophilic nuclei. This layer typically comprises no more than 10 to 15 percent of the total epithelial thickness, although distally the basal cell layer can be somewhat thicker, probably in response to physiologic reflux. Melanocytic or endocrine cells may be scattered among the basal cells (58). Cells in the basal layer give rise to daughter cells that migrate upward, differentiating as they approach the luminal surface. The most superficial layers may contain basophilic granules. The cells of the superficial or functional zone appear flattened, with their long axis parallel to the mucosal surface. Papillae, which are invaginations of vascularized lamina propria, extend into the epithelium. These usually do not penetrate more than two thirds of the way into the overlying mucosa (fig. 1-18). The height of a papilla (or rete ridge) is measured from the basal lamina of the surrounding squamous epithelium to the basal lamina at the top of the papilla. Nonepithelial elements include lymphocytes and antigen-presenting cells (56,57).

Submucosal glands lie in straight rows that extend outward from the esophageal lumen toward the muscularis propria (fig. 1-19). The glands lie both within the mucosa and the submucosa. The glandular lobules connect to the lumen via a straight duct. Mucous cells within the submucosal glands often have a pyramidal shape and contain numerous large, pale secretory granules. Myoepithelial cells lie between the secretory cells and the underlying basement membrane.

Although the esophageal mucosa is repeatedly exposed to potentially injurious materials that are ingested or that reflux into the distal esophagus, it is rare for injury to occur because preepithelial, epithelial, and postepithelial defenses protect against injury. Preepithelial defenses rely on intact neuromuscular function to maintain lower esophageal sphincter pressure and normal esophageal motility, thus minimizing gastroesophageal reflux and promoting clearance of esophageal luminal contents. Gravity and normal peristalsis move the intraluminal contents distally, thereby preventing prolonged mucosal contact and protecting against mucosal damage. The multilayered squamous epithelium also protects against damage from substances

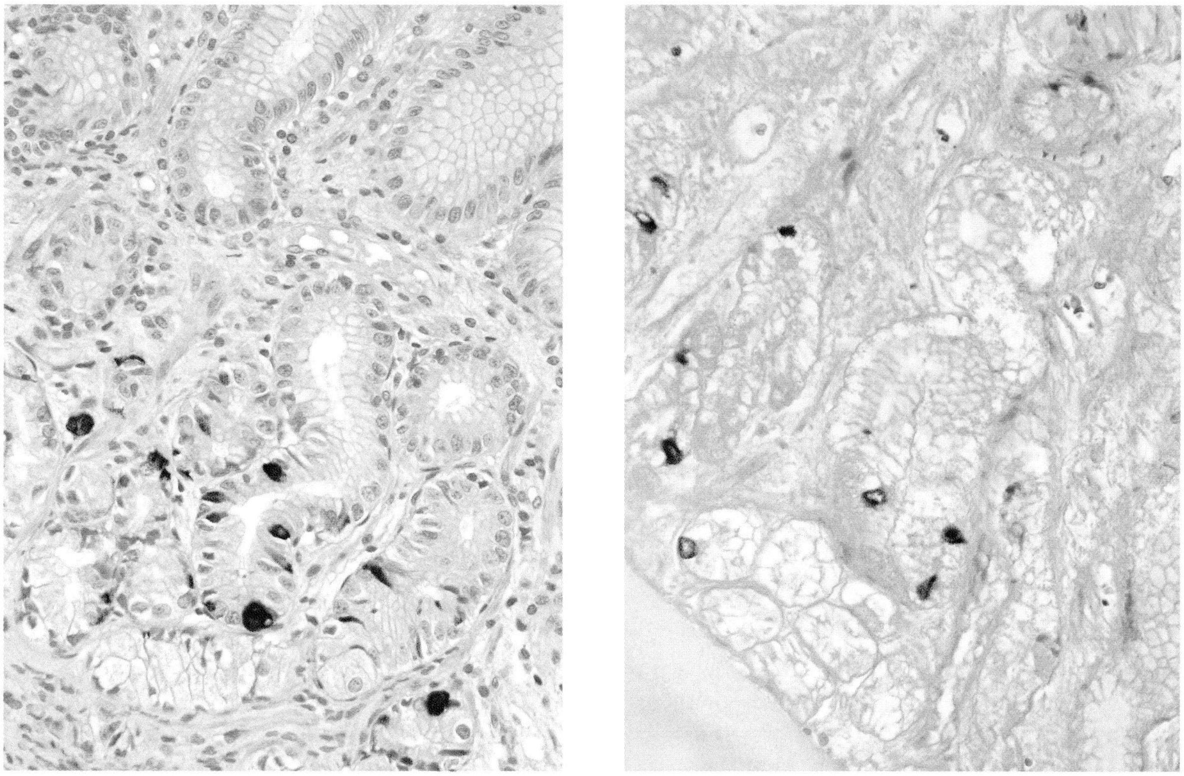

Figure 1-17

GASTRIC ENDOCRINE CELLS

Left: Endocrine cells within the neck region of the gastric glands are highlighted with the chromogranin immunostain. Right: Antral glands contain scattered G cells, as demonstrated with this gastrin immunostain.

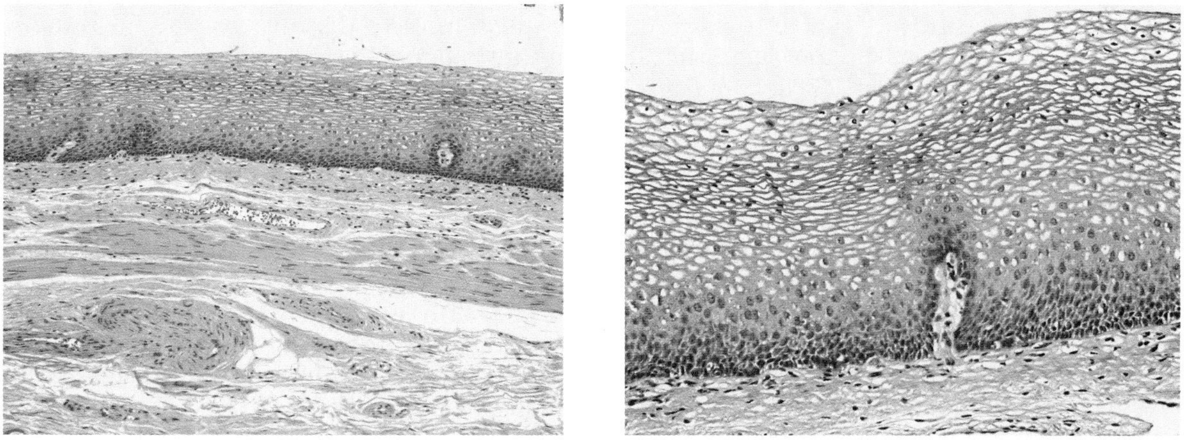

Figure 1-18

NORMAL ESOPHAGEAL HISTOLOGY

Left: The basal layer is only a few cells thick, and the papillae extend approximately to one third to half the thickness of the epithelium. The underlying muscularis mucosae is thicker in the esophagus than in other parts of the gastrointestinal tract.

Right: Higher-power view shows a basal cell layer composed of only a few layers of cells and short papillae. Only rare intraepithelial lymphocytes lie in the deep portion of the mucosa.

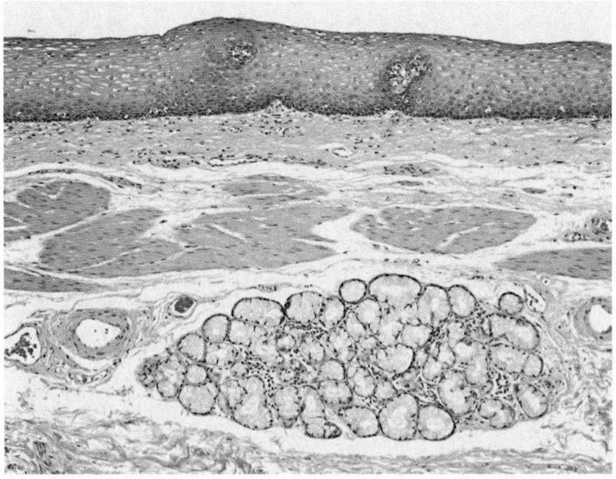

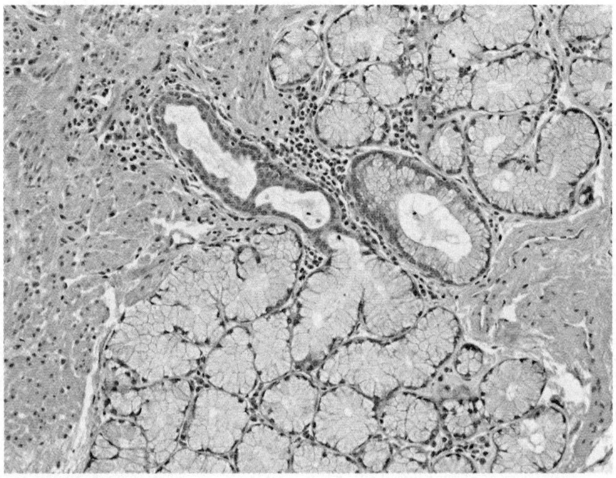

Figure 1-19

SUBMUCOSAL GLANDS

Left: Small lobules of glandular tissue are seen within the submucosa of the distal esophagus.

Right: Higher-power view shows glands with abundant intracytoplasmic mucin. The duct is lined by cuboidal to columnar cells.

passing over it. When the protective mechanisms are overwhelmed, epithelial erosions or ulcers develop. Four general situations predispose to esophageal injury: 1) motility disturbances, 2) the presence of esophageal reflux, 3) infection, and 4) drug- or chemical-induced injury. Increased cell proliferation and secondary basal cell hyperplasia compensate for cells lost to injury.

Stomach

The stomach has three major histologic compartments: the gastric pits and surface lining, the mucous neck region, and the glands (fig. 1-20). Additionally, the stomach has four anatomic regions: the cardia, fundus, body, and antropyloric region (fig. 1-21). The cardia, a narrow, ill-defined region, is not grossly distinctive and is histologically identified by the presence of cardiac glands. The fundus, the most superior part of the stomach, protrudes above a horizontal line drawn from the esophagogastric junction. It blends imperceptibly into the major portion of the stomach, called the body. Oxyntic mucosa lines the body and fundus. The antrum comprises the distal third of the stomach just proximal to the pyloric sphincter. It is a triangular zone that extends further along the lesser curvature than along the greater curvature.

Surface, or foveolar, cells line the surface and gastric pits; they are histologically identical throughout the stomach. Foveolar epithelium consists of tall, columnar, mucus-secreting cells (fig. 1-20) that form an integral part of the mucosal barrier. These cells have irregular, basally situated nuclei and apically, mucin-filled cytoplasm. The cardiac pits appear shorter than those in other regions of the stomach. The pits are deepest in the antrum. Mucous neck cells reside in the neck and isthmus in the middle and upper parts of the gastric glands. They merge with both the glandular epithelium below and the foveolar epithelium above.

In contrast to the foveolar and pit regions, the histology of the gastric glands, which empty into the base of the gastric pits, differs in different regions of the stomach. Cardiac glands share histologic features with esophageal submucosal glands (fig. 1-22) and with pyloric and antral glands. Oxyntic glands contain four cell types: mucous neck cells, endocrine cells, parietal (oxyntic) cells, and chief (zymogenic) cells (fig. 1-22). Parietal cells constitute approximately one third of the cells in the oxyntic mucosa and tend to be more numerous distally than proximally. This contrasts with chief cells, which are found in greater numbers in the proximal rather than the distal oxyntic mucosa. Parietal cells chiefly localize to the midportion of the oxyntic glands, whereas chief cells lie at the glandular bases. Some parietal cells are found in the antrum. The acid-secreting parietal cells are easily identified by their large size,

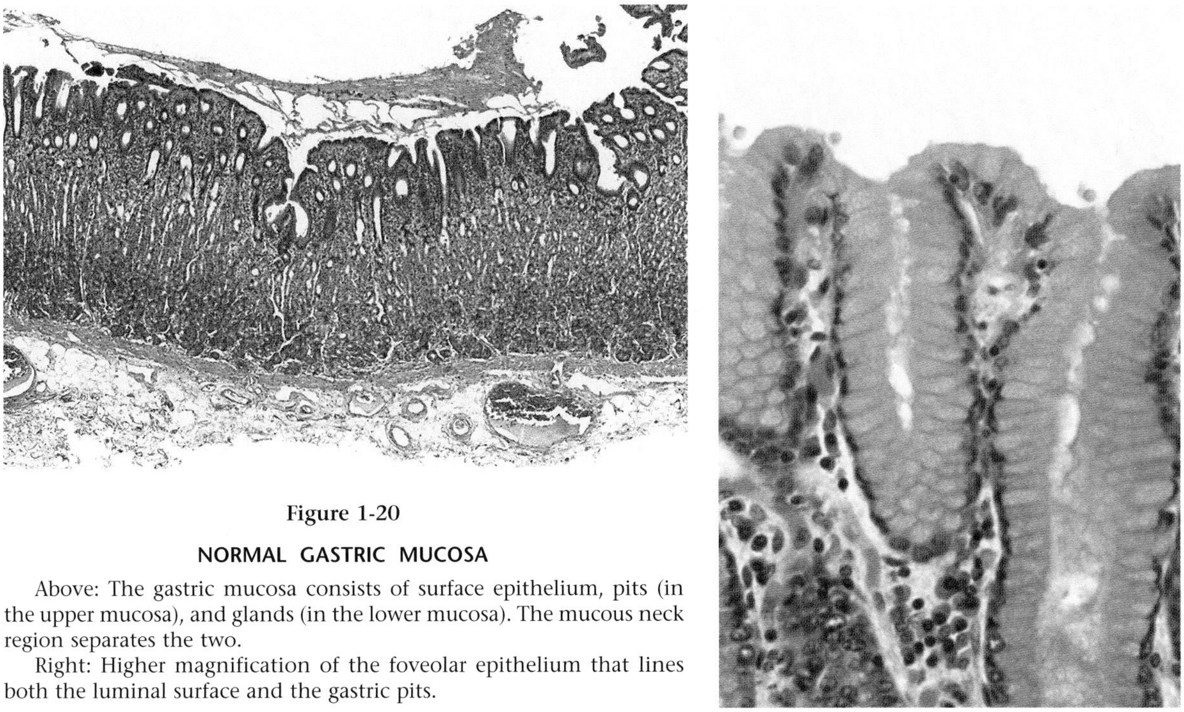

Figure 1-20

NORMAL GASTRIC MUCOSA

Above: The gastric mucosa consists of surface epithelium, pits (in the upper mucosa), and glands (in the lower mucosa). The mucous neck region separates the two.

Right: Higher magnification of the foveolar epithelium that lines both the luminal surface and the gastric pits.

pyramidal shape, large central nuclei, and intensely eosinophilic cytoplasm (fig. 1-22). Chief cells, which make pepsinogen (fig. 1-22) and lipase, appear as triangular, low columnar cells containing a coarse, granular, pale, gray-blue, basophilic cytoplasm. The nucleus contains one or more small nucleoli.

The stomach contains a diverse population of endocrine cells. These are widely distributed in various regions of the gastric mucosa. At least seven distinct endocrine cell types exist: enterochromaffin, G, enterochromaffin-like (ECL), D, D1, P, and X cells. The predominant antral endocrine cell, the gastrin-producing G cell, causes ECL cell, parietal cell, and gastric mucosal growth. Somatostatin-secreting D cells are distributed uniformly throughout the antral and oxyntic mucosa. They inhibit the release of gastric acid, gastrin, intrinsic factor, and acetylcholine. ECL cells, the major endocrine cells of the oxyntic mucosa, are usually found in the fundus but they can occur more distally. They play a pivotal role in mediating gastrin-induced parietal cell secretion.

Small Intestine

The major functions of the small intestine are terminal digestion and absorption of nutrients. The anatomy of this region of the GI tract

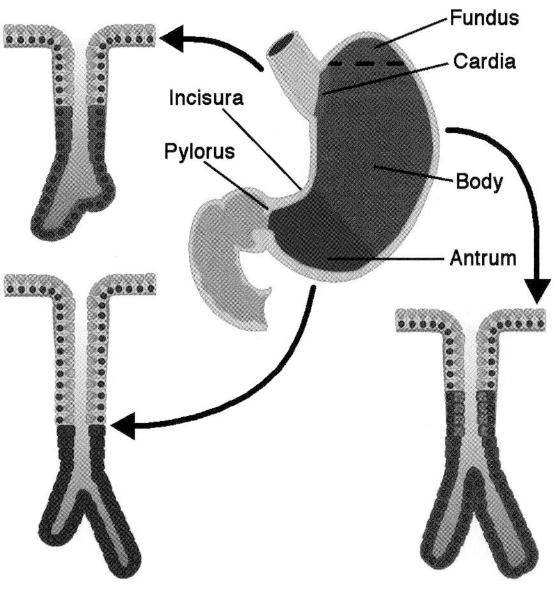

Figure 1-21

DIAGRAM OF THE NORMAL ANATOMY OF THE STOMACH

The stomach is divided into different histologic regions. The major feature differentiating them is the nature of the glandular epithelium (see text).

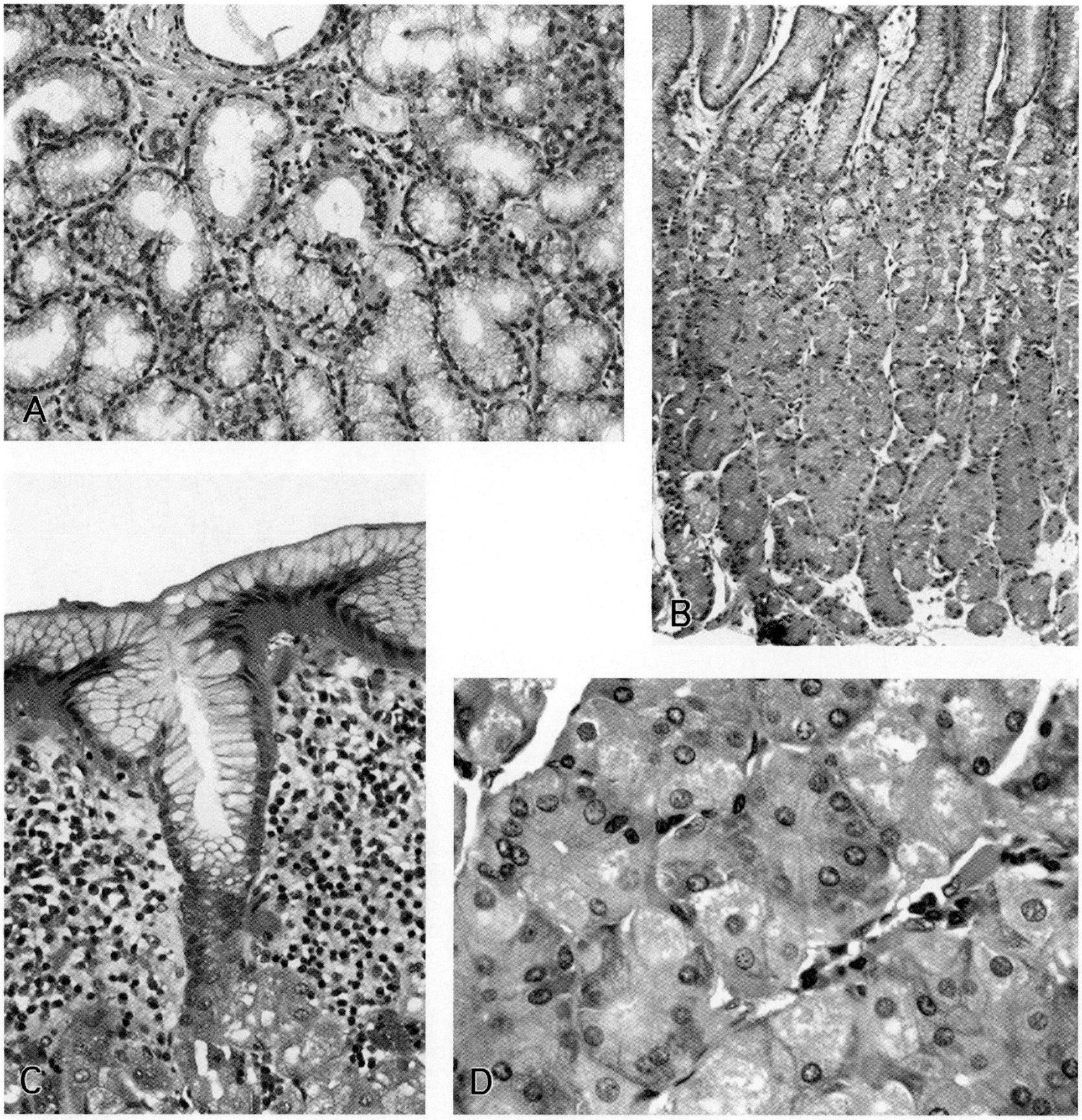

Figure 1-22

HISTOLOGY OF CARDIAC AND OXYNTIC MUCOSAE

A: Cardiac glands include mucin-filled glands and, occasionally, cystically dilated glands.
B: Pits and glands of the oxyntic mucosa.
C: Higher magnification of the junction of the pit and mucous neck region.
D: Oxyntic glands with parietal cells and chief cells.

reflects these functions. Intestinal folds, known as plicae circulares, increase the surface area available for absorption. Innumerable villi stud the intestinal surface, further increasing the absorptive surface (fig. 1-23). The villi are unique to the small intestine, and are finger- or leaf-like mucosal evaginations. They are lined by epithelium overlying a connective tissue core that contains a highly cellular lamina propria, a capillary network, lacteals, and nerves. Simple

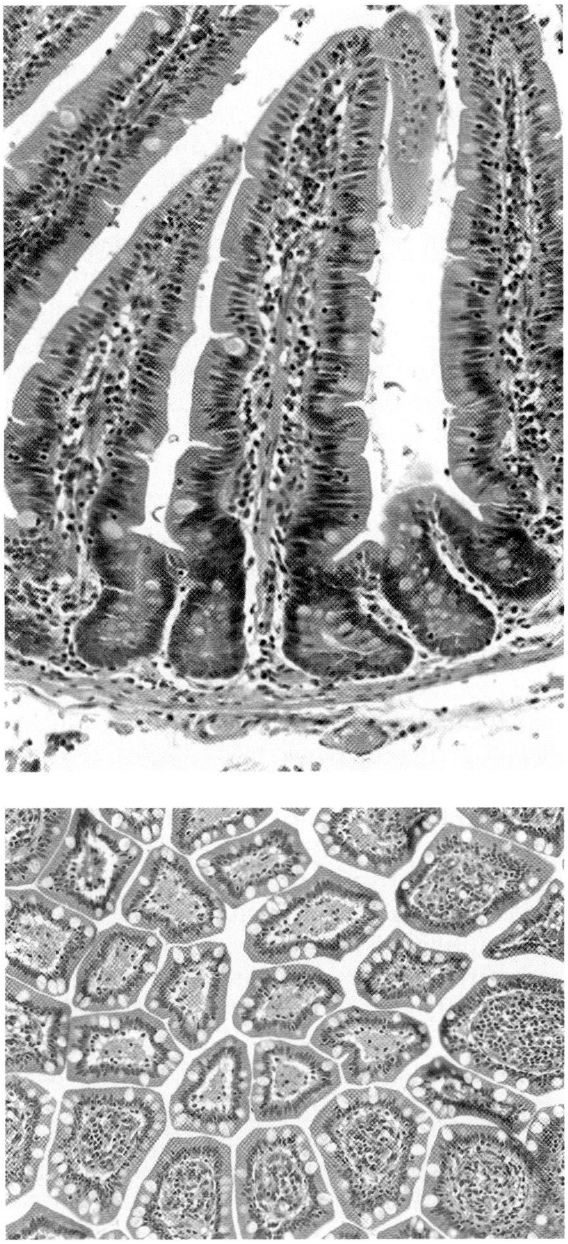

Figure 1-23

SMALL INTESTINAL VILLI

Top: Long finger-like villi project upward into the lumen of the small intestine.

Bottom: Tangential sectioning demonstrates uniform, slender villous structures.

tubular invaginations (crypts of Lieberkuhn) at the bases of the villi (fig. 1-24) extend downward toward the muscularis mucosae but do not penetrate it. The openings to several crypts empty into the intervillous basin.

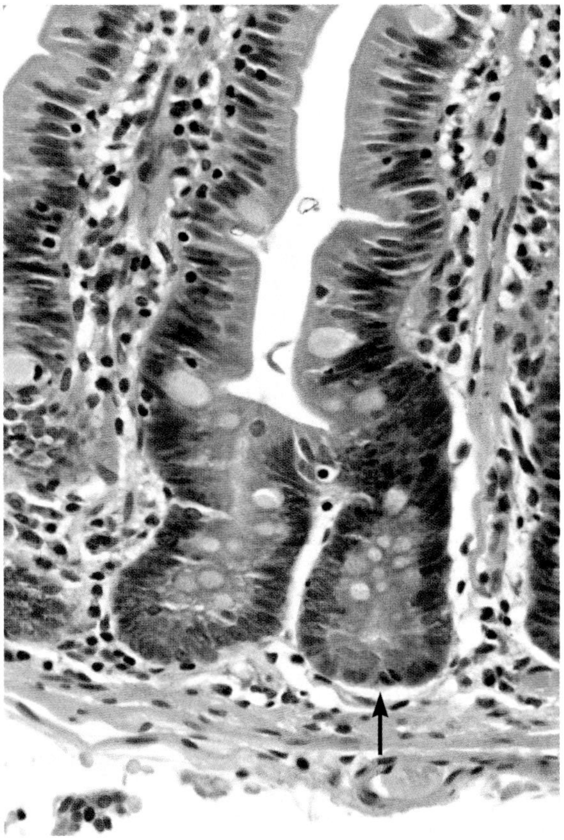

Figure 1-24

CRYPTS OF LIEBERKUHN

Straight crypts project downward from the base of the villi. In this case, two crypts empty into the intervillous space. Paneth cells are present in the crypt bases (arrow).

Villi vary in height and form in different regions of the small intestine. The duodenum has the greatest villous variability. The villi in the proximal duodenum are shorter and broader than elsewhere; jejunal villi show little variation in their width from their base to their apex; and in the ileum, the villi are broader and shorter than in the jejunum.

Measurement of the ratio of villous height to crypt length is often required for the assessment of small intestinal absorptive function. Well-oriented sections allow optimal examination of the villous architecture. In adults, the villous height is approximately three or more times the depth of the crypts, whereas in children this ratio is lower, more typically 2 to 1 (fig. 1-25). The villous height is also lower in elderly patients (76). Villi are often stubby or

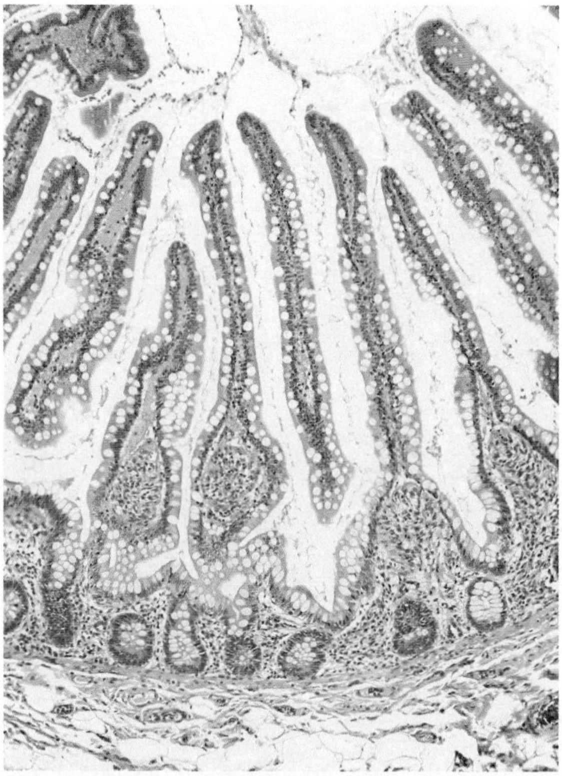

Figure 1-25

NORMAL VILLUS IN AN ADULT

A section from the distal small intestine shows a villus to crypt ratio of greater than 4 to 1.

absent overlying lymphoid areas, and frequently contain increased numbers of intraepithelial lymphocytes.

The small intestinal crypts and villi represent two morphologically and functionally distinct compartments. Each crypt consists of a single clone of cells and several crypts contribute cells to each villus. The epithelial lining harbors a heterogeneous cell population, including absorptive cells (enterocytes), goblet cells, Paneth cells, undifferentiated crypt cells, endocrine cells, cup cells, tuft cells, and M cells.

Enterocytes are highly polarized cells with an apical microvillous or brush border. The mature brush border, which covers the cell apex, consists of closely packed microvilli and the terminal web (fig. 1-26). Microvilli vary in length depending on the maturity of the cell, increasing in height as one migrates up the crypt villus axis (60,73,82). The microvillus brush border is periodic acid–Schiff (PAS) positive (fig. 1-26).

Goblet cells occur in both the crypts (fig. 1-27) and among the surface enterocytes, but they progressively decrease in number as one progresses toward the villus tip (fig. 1-27). Goblet cells increase in frequency along the length of the small intestine, being most numerous in the lower ileum. These cells are primarily columnar in shape and contain large numbers of mucin droplets in the supranuclear portion of the cell. Goblet cells secrete mucin, ions, and water into the overlying mucous gel that lines and protects the mucosal surface.

Paneth cells populate the bases of the small intestinal crypts. Paneth cells are also seen in the right colon. These strongly eosinophilic, pyramidal cells have the cytologic characteristics of secretory cells (fig. 1-28). Irregular microvilli cover their apical surfaces. Paneth cells play an important role in maintaining the relatively sterile state of the small intestine because they produce many substances with antimicrobial properties (64,65,67–69,71,72,74). They are also phagocytic and secrete cytoplasmic granules into the intestinal crypt lumen after bacterial entry. In addition, Paneth cells contain IgA and IgE, possibly from phagocytosis of immunoglobulin-coated microorganisms (77).

Lymphoid Tissues. Small intestinal lymphoid aggregates split the muscularis mucosae; they are partially mucosal and partially submucosal, and often have a central germinal center (see figs. 1-4, 1-5). Lymphoid aggregates increase in number along the length of the small intestine, becoming confluent in the ileum where they are known as Peyer patches. The duodenum may also contain well-formed lymphoid nodules that extend from the surface to the base of the mucosa. A lymphoid aggregate is composed of a follicular B-cell area, a parafollicular T-cell area, and the follicle-associated epithelium. The follicle-associated epithelium consists of enterocytes, M cells, rare mucus-secreting goblet cells, occasional tuft cells, and abundant intraepithelial lymphocytes (61,70,78).

Intraepithelial lymphocytes (IELs) constitute a distinct population of intestinal lymphocytes (81). IELs are T cells and are typically found in the basal portion of the epithelium. They possess small dense nuclei, contrasting with the paler,

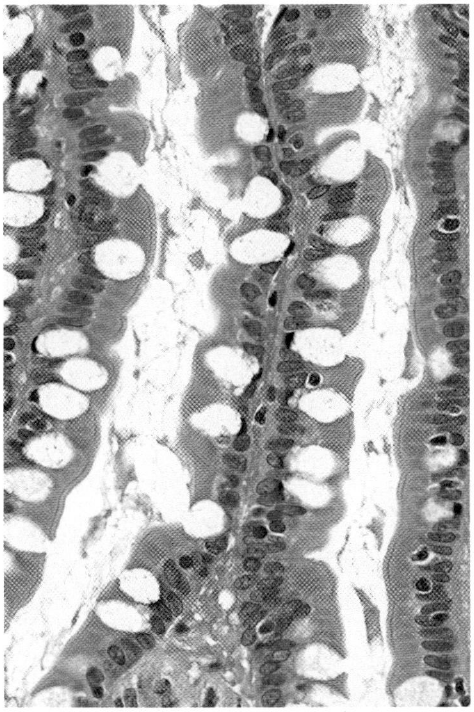

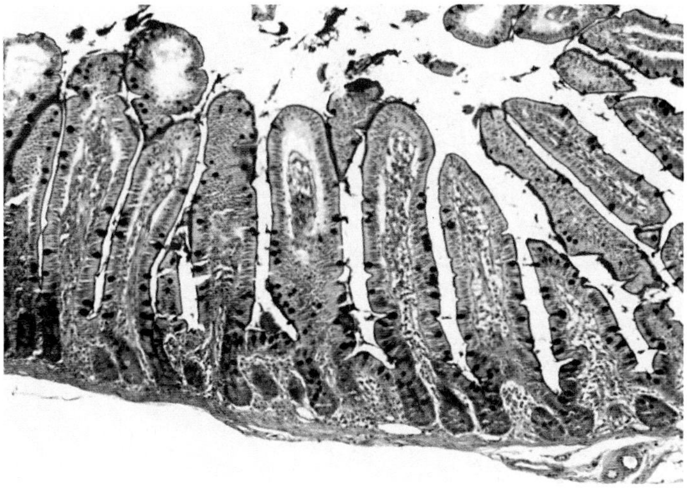

Figure 1-26

SMALL INTESTINAL BRUSH BORDER

Left: On H&E-stained sections, the brush border is visible as a slightly refractile layer on the epithelial surface.

Above: A periodic acid–Schiff (PAS) stain highlights the brush border of the small intestine. The goblet cells are also PAS positive.

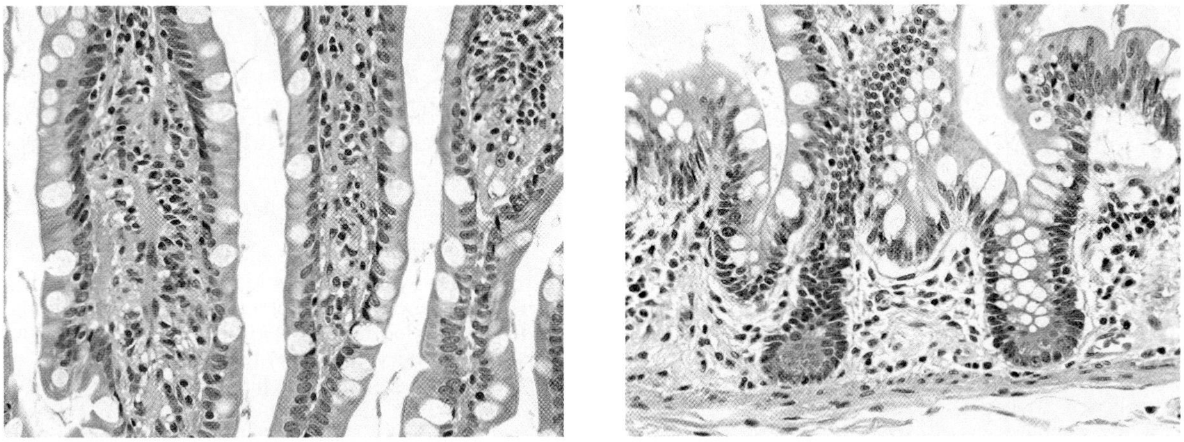

Figure 1-27

GOBLET CELLS

Left: A section from the intestinal villi shows scattered plump, pale-staining goblet cells among the columnar enterocytes. The nuclei of the goblet cells are displaced to the basal portion of the cells by the abundant mucin contained within the cytoplasm.

Right: Goblet cells are also present within the intestinal crypts.

more vesicular enterocyte nuclei (fig. 1-29). The human small intestine contains a large number of IELs, estimated to be approximately 1 IEL for every 6 to 10 epithelial cells (63,66,75). Lymphocytes account for up to 30 percent of the total cell population of the mucosal surface. In contrast to the IELs in the villi, IELs overlying lymphoid follicles are predominantly of B-cell derivation (79).

Lamina Propria. The jejunal lamina propria is estimated to contain several thousand cells per mm^2 (66,75). Most are located in the region

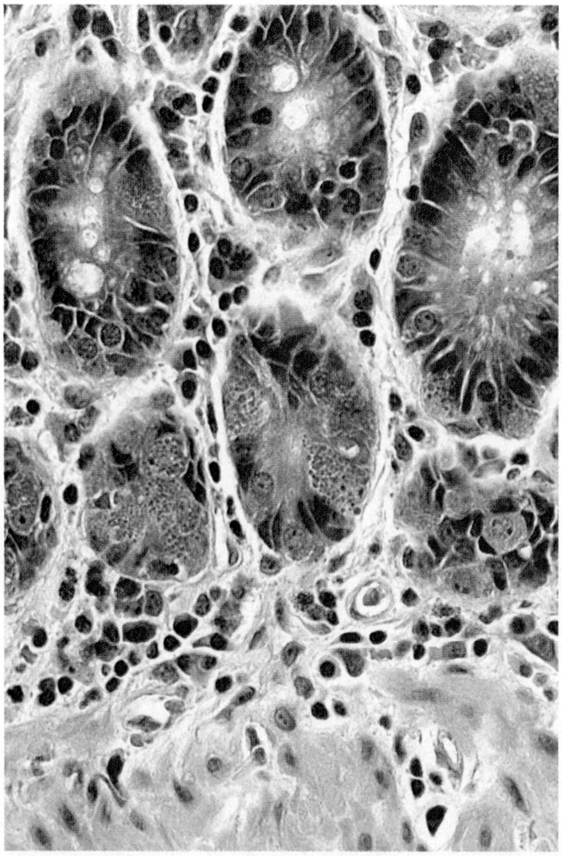

Figure 1-28

PANETH CELLS

Paneth cells are present in the bases of the intestinal crypts. They contain characteristic coarse, eosinophilic cytoplasmic granules (see also fig. 1-27, right).

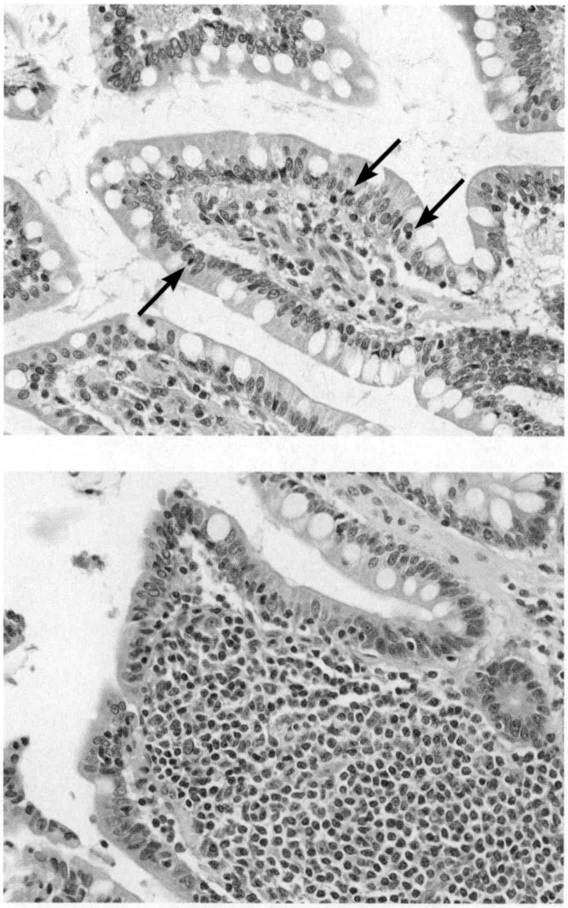

Figure 1-29

INTRAEPITHELIAL LYMPHOCYTES

Top: Scattered dark-staining lymphocyte nuclei are interspersed among the small intestinal epithelial cells (arrows). Lymphocytes are relatively few in number (less than one lymphocyte for every five or six enterocytes).

Bottom: Larger numbers of intraepithelial lymphocytes are normally seen in the epithelium overlying lymphoid follicles. A diagnosis of intraepithelial lymphocytosis should not be made on the basis of lymphocyte counts from areas such as this.

of the crypts rather than in the villi. These cells consist of immunocytes, particularly plasma cells and lymphocytes (fig. 1-30). The majority are IgA-containing plasma cells, although IgM-, IgD-, IgG-, and IgE-containing cells are also present. Eosinophils are commonly found within the lamina propria, but should not be present within the epithelium. Neutrophils are not present within the lamina propria under normal circumstances.

The lamina propria of the villus contains a central, blind-ending lacteal that is usually collapsed. It also contains blood and lymphatic vessels, nerve fibers, and smooth muscle cells (fig. 1-31).

Brunner Glands. Brunner glands are a continuous series of branched or coiled tubular glands in the submucosa of the first part of the duodenum. Morphologically, Brunner glands resemble gastric antral glands. They are found mainly in the submucosa but can extend focally into the basal portion of the mucosa (fig. 1-32). In the first portion of the duodenum, where Brunner glands are relatively large, bands of smooth muscle from the muscularis mucosae occasionally lie between the acinar lobules (fig. 1-32).

The glands produce a neutral glycoprotein that stains with PAS, but not mucicarmine

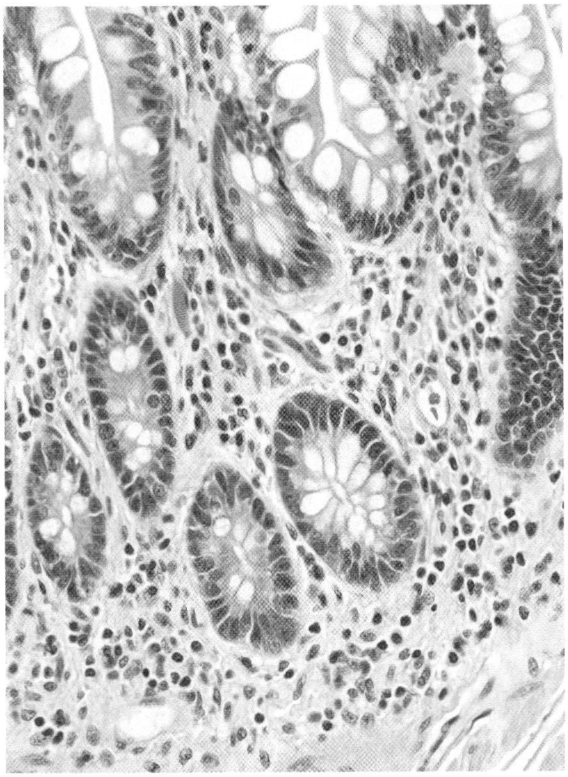

Figure 1-30

SMALL BOWEL LAMINA PROPRIA

Scattered plasma cells, lymphocytes, and eosinophils are present. No neutrophils are seen.

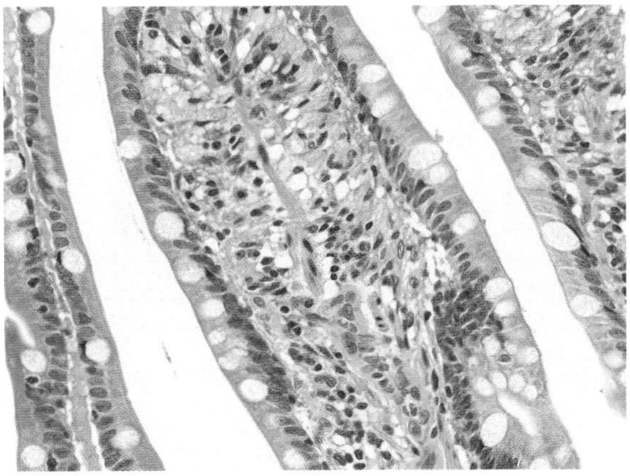

Figure 1-31

SMALL BOWEL LAMINA PROPRIA

The lamina propria of the villi contains inflammatory cells, smooth muscle fibers, capillaries, lymphatics, and nerves.

(62,80). In addition, they stain with antibodies directed against lysozyme (fig. 1-33). Brunner glands also contain endocrine cells that store somatostatin, gastrin, cholecystokinin, and peptide YY. Peptidergic nerves containing vasoactive intestinal peptide (VIP), substance P, neuropeptide Y, and gastrin-releasing peptide are also present (59).

Ampulla of Vater. The ampulla of Vater is located in the second portion of the duodenum and is the site where the common bile duct and major pancreatic duct reach the intestinal lumen. The mucosa overlying this area is highly variable in appearance. A complex network of glands arranged in a lobular configuration can be seen in the submucosa and passing through the muscularis mucosae into the overlying mucosa. These glands are surrounded by smooth muscle cells and a loose stroma (fig. 1-34).

Colon

The mucosa of the large intestine is relatively smooth (fig. 1-35) except distally in the rectum where more prominent folds occur. No villi are present. The surface of the colon is arranged in a regular geometric way (83,85), with the flat large intestinal mucosa regularly punctuated by the openings of the colonic crypts (fig. 1-36). Normal colonic epithelium consists of absorptive cells (colonocytes), undifferentiated cells, mature goblet cells, tuft cells, and endocrine cells. In addition, M cells occur in the epithelium overlying lymphoid follicles, and intraepithelial T lymphocytes lie scattered within the epithelium.

Mature absorptive cells have numerous short, regularly spaced microvilli and function in absorption of water and electrolytes. The nuclei are small, round, and basally located (fig. 1-37).

Goblet cells are numerous in the crypt epithelium, with approximately one goblet cell for every four absorptive cells (fig. 1-38). Their broad shape creates the false impression that they constitute the majority of the cells. As they differentiate, they migrate toward the mucosal surface, becoming progressively filled with mucus droplets. The nucleus is compressed into a small dense structure in the basal region of the cell.

The colon has the least number of endocrine cells of any region of the GI tract. Colonic endocrine cells are primarily located in the proximal

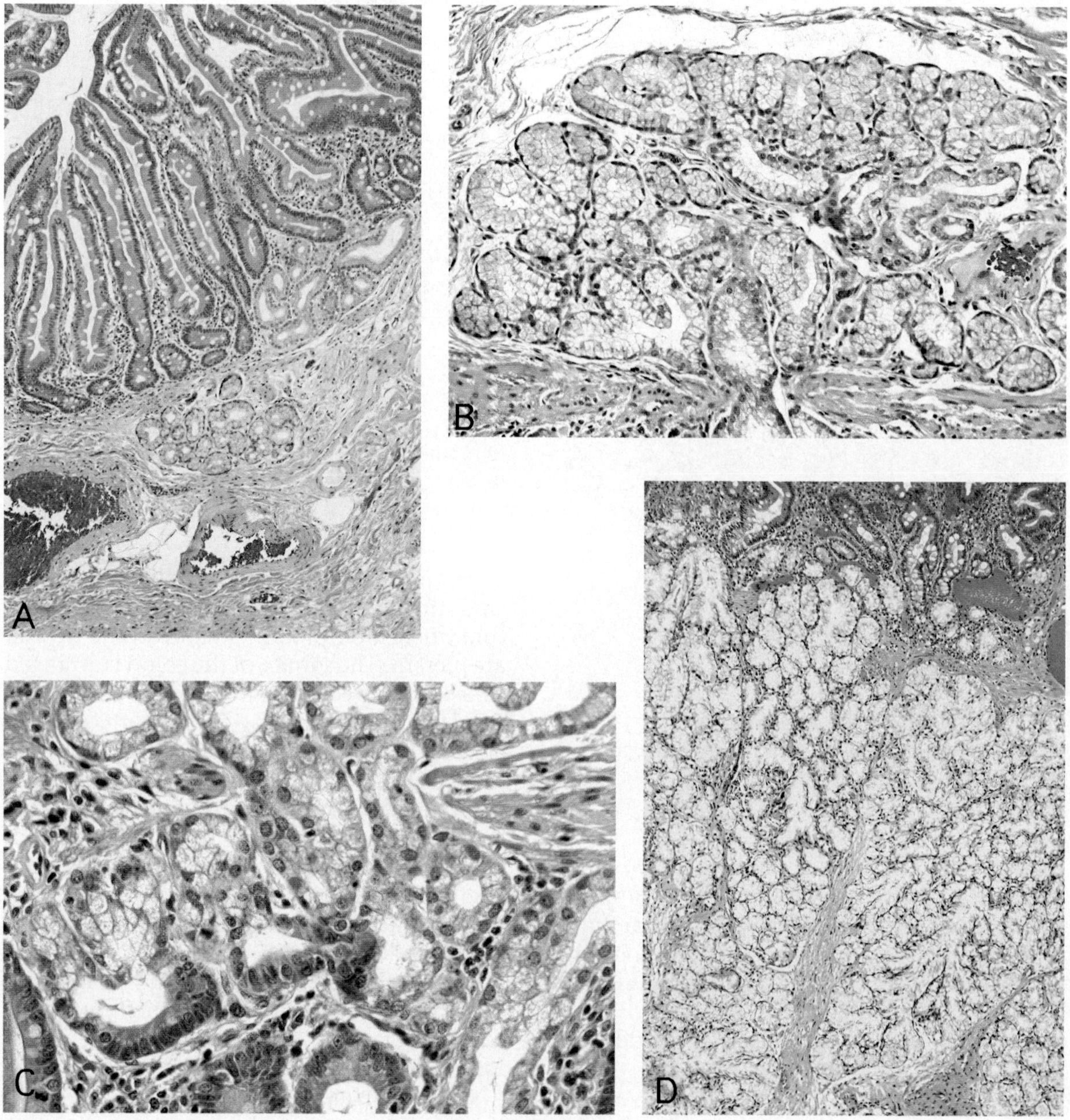

Figure 1-32

BRUNNER GLANDS

A: Glands resembling those of the gastric antrum lie within the submucosa of the duodenum. To the left and slightly above this group of glands, another cluster lies in the deep mucosa.

B: Higher-power view shows the pale, vacuolated, mucin-containing cytoplasm of Brunner glands.

C: High-power view of the Brunner glands within the deep mucosa. The epithelium of the glands merges with that of the deep portion of the intestinal crypts.

D: Brunner glands in the proximal duodenum often contain strands of smooth muscle, which extend between lobules from the muscularis mucosae.

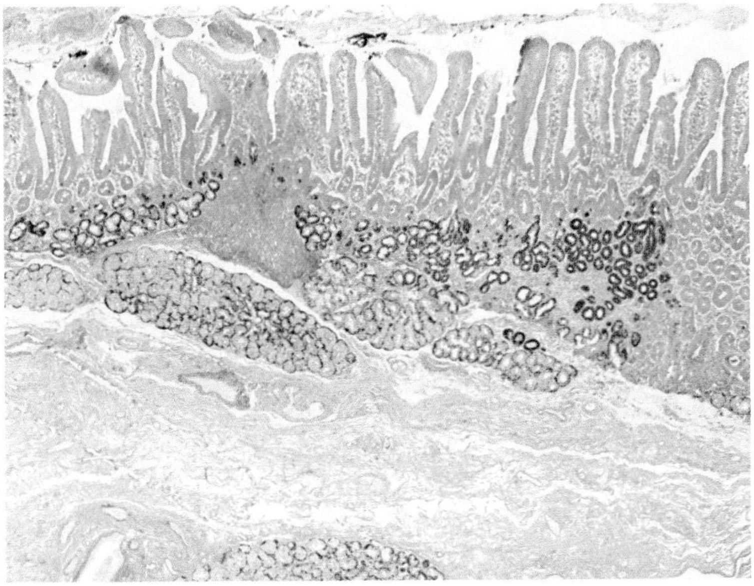

Figure 1-33

BRUNNER GLANDS

Immunohistochemical stain for lysozyme shows diffuse immunoreactivity in the Brunner glands.

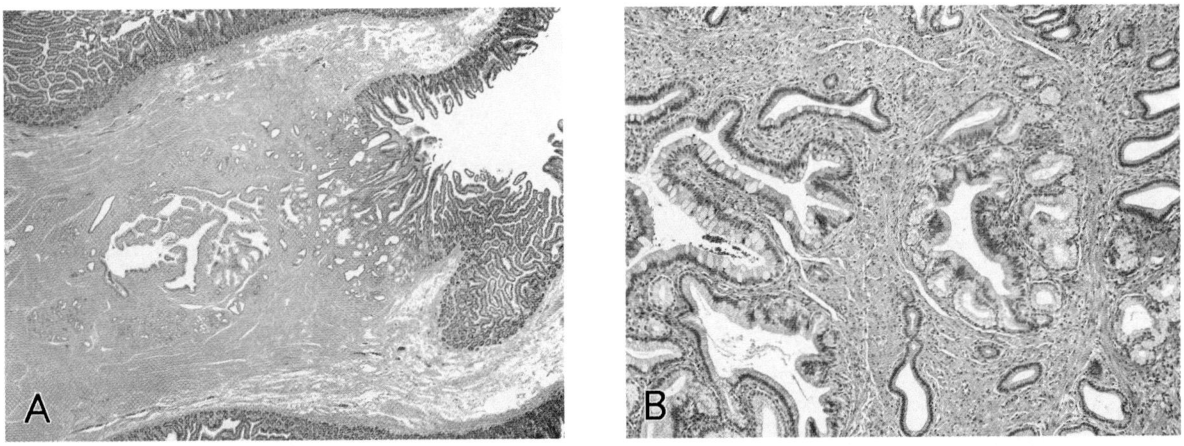

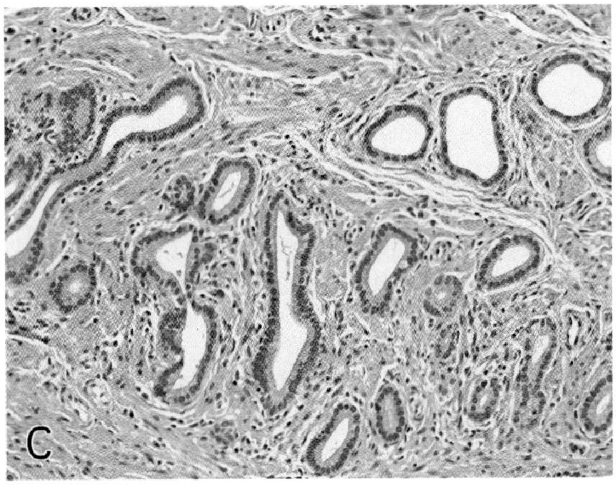

Figure 1-34

AMPULLA OF VATER

A: Numerous ducts enter the area through the submucosa. These ducts are surrounded by smooth muscle.

B: Higher-power view shows the presence of small glands lined by epithelium resembling the biliary or pancreatic ductal lining and intestinal type glandular epithelium.

C: Higher-power view of the small ductules entering the ampulla. The cells lining them are cuboidal and do not contain mucin.

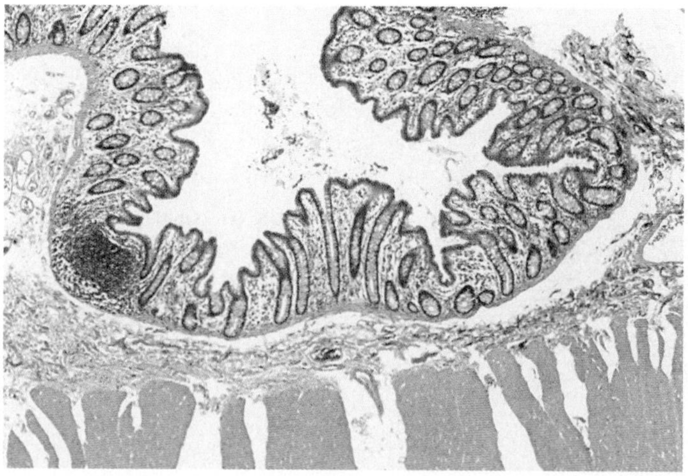

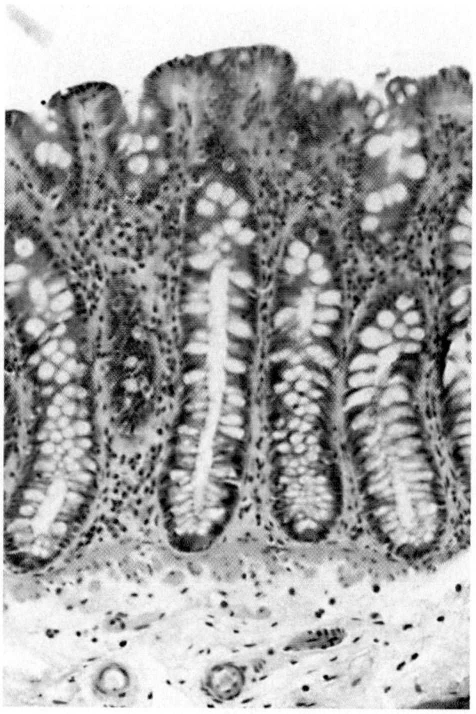

Figure 1-35

COLONIC MUCOSA

Above: The mucosal surface is relatively smooth and without villi. The crypts are composed of straight, tubular glands. A lymphoid aggregate is on the left.

Right: Higher-power view of nonbranching, regularly spaced crypts lined by absorptive and goblet cells.

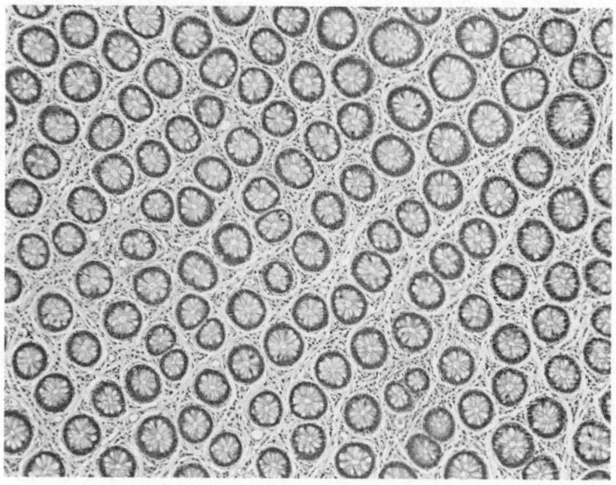

Figure 1-36

COLONIC MUCOSA

An en face section shows evenly distributed, straight glands.

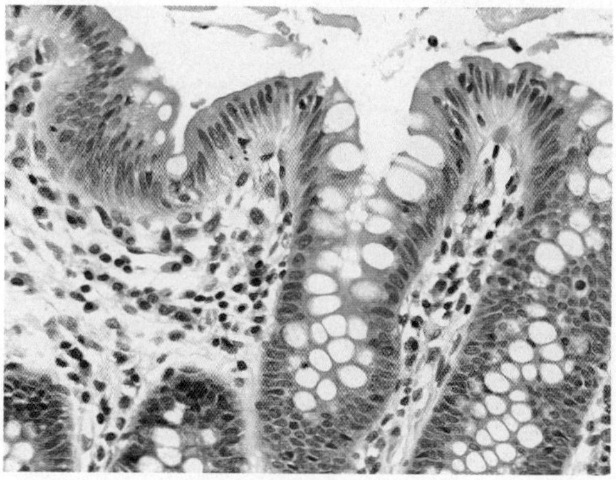

Figure 1-37

COLON

Absorptive cells outnumber goblet cells, although this is difficult to appreciate in histologic sections. The absorptive cells, best seen at the luminal surface, are columnar with basally situated nuclei, slightly eosinophilic cytoplasm, and no mucin.

and distal colon, particularly the rectum (84,86). They are most prominent in the deep portions of the crypts (fig. 1-39). Colonic endocrine cells appear as small, round or pyramidal cells scattered among the nonendocrine epithelial cells. The broad basal cytoplasm appears clear or eosinophilic and contains basal granules.

Scattered Paneth cells are usually present in the cecum and the proximal ascending colon (fig. 1-40). They are absent from the remainder of the normal large intestine.

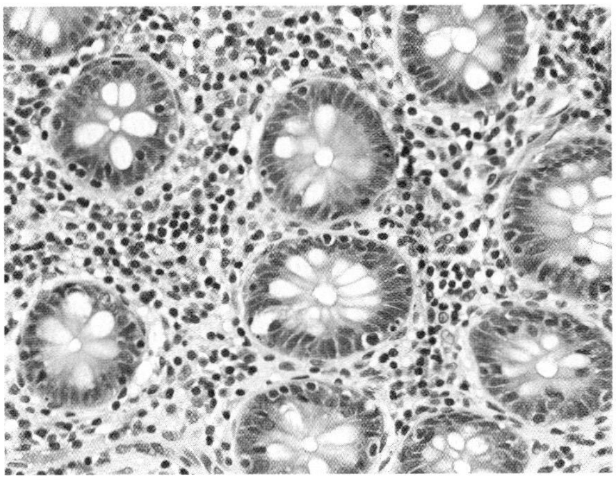

Figure 1-38

COLONIC CRYPTS

Goblet cells are numerous and appear identical to those in the small intestine.

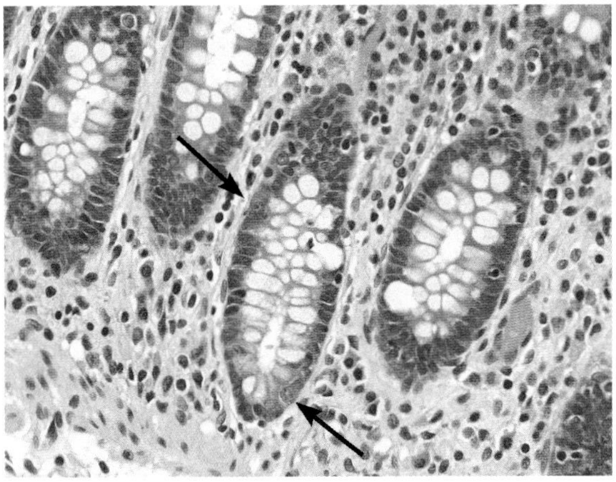

Figure 1-39

COLONIC ENDOCRINE CELLS

The cells often appear eosinophilic, with fine, generally basal, cytoplasmic granules (arrows).

Lamina Propria. The lamina propria of the colon consists of loose, reticular connective tissue that contains fibroblasts, capillaries, and mononuclear cells, including macrophages, plasma cells, lymphocytes, and scattered mast cells. Eosinophils may also be seen. The area immediately under the epithelium primarily contains fibroblasts, myofibroblasts, and macrophages. Isolated smooth muscle fibers may also be seen in the lamina propria.

The lamina propria contains solitary lymphoid nodules that may be sufficiently large to displace the crypts and extend into the submucosa. These follicles may additionally splay apart the fibers of the muscularis mucosae, or the underlying muscularis mucosae may be discontinuous (fig. 1-41). They increase in number as one approaches the rectum.

Appendix

The appendiceal mucosa resembles that of the large intestine, except for the presence of a prominent lymphoid component. Straight, unbranched crypts are lined by absorptive cells and mucus-secreting goblet cells. As in the colon, the proliferative zone lies in the basal portion of the crypts. Immature cells migrate upward to the luminal surface, differentiating into absorptive and goblet cells along the way. The crypts also contain endocrine cells, Paneth cells, and IELs (fig. 1-42).

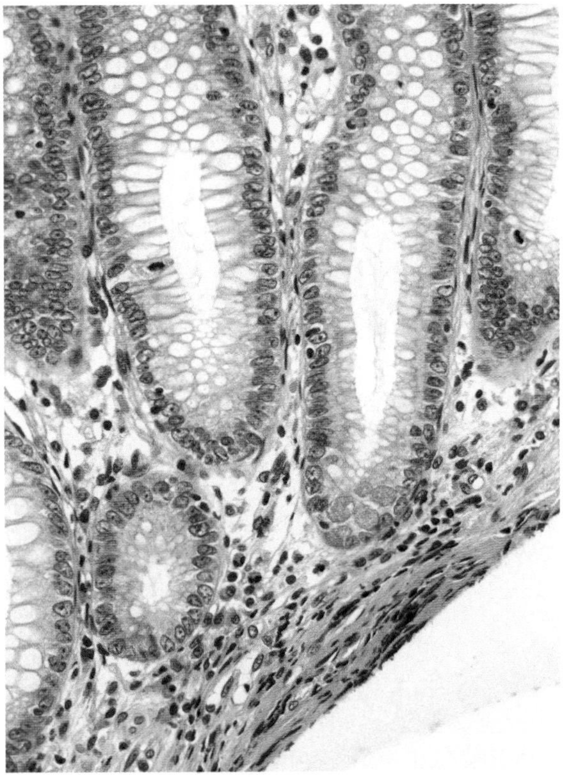

Figure 1-40

COLONIC PANETH CELLS

Paneth cells are often seen in the bases of the colonic crypts of the cecum and ascending colon. They are not normally present in other parts of the colon.

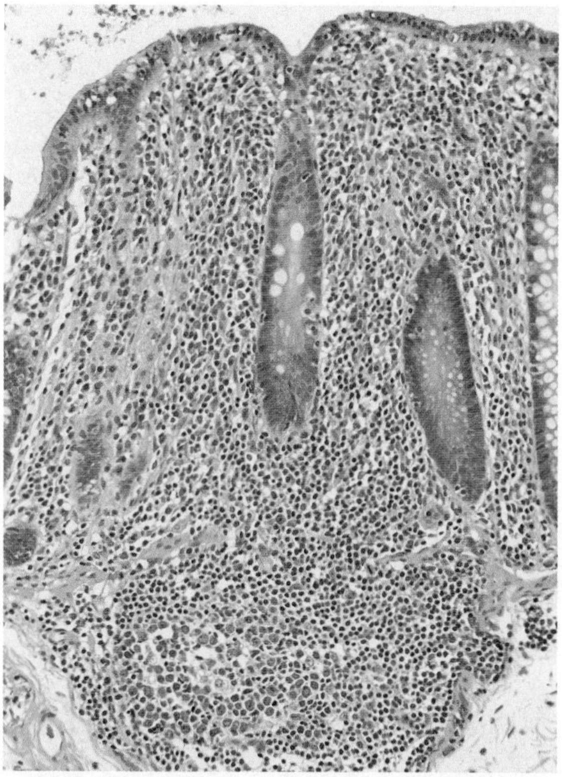

Figure 1-41

COLON

A lymphoid follicle lies within both the mucosa and submucosa. The smooth muscle of the muscularis mucosae is discontinuous in the region where it is traversed by the lymphoid follicle.

Like the ileum, the appendix contains numerous lymphoid follicles. The appendiceal epithelium is modified over the dome of each lymphoid follicle with a structure similar to that seen in the small intestine. The lymphoid follicles of the appendix are regularly arranged at the junction of the mucosa and submucosa (fig. 1-43). A well-defined lymphatic sinus surrounds both the lateral and basal parts of the follicle and empties into a system of fine collecting lymphatics in the submucosa.

The appendix contains two populations of endocrine cells: those in the crypts and those in the lamina propria. Crypt endocrine cells tend to lie near the base of the crypts, and occur singly or in small clusters (fig. 1-44). More endocrine cells populate the distal than the proximal appendix. Lamina propria endocrine cells lie scattered near the crypt bases, apparently unattached to crypt epithelium; they are highlighted with silver stains or antibodies such as chromogranin (fig. 1-44). Both crypt and lamina propria endocrine cells contain serotonin, somatostatin, VIP, and substance P. Subepithelial endocrine cells also contain cytokeratin, as do the endocrine cells of the crypts, supporting an origin from endocrine cells or their progenitors in the intestinal crypts.

The histologic features of the appendix change with age. The appendix in the elderly appears small, with loss of its lymphoid tissue and an increase in the amount of fat and fibrous

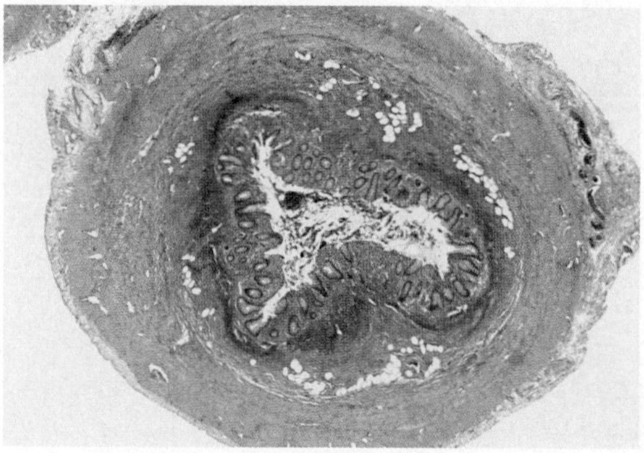

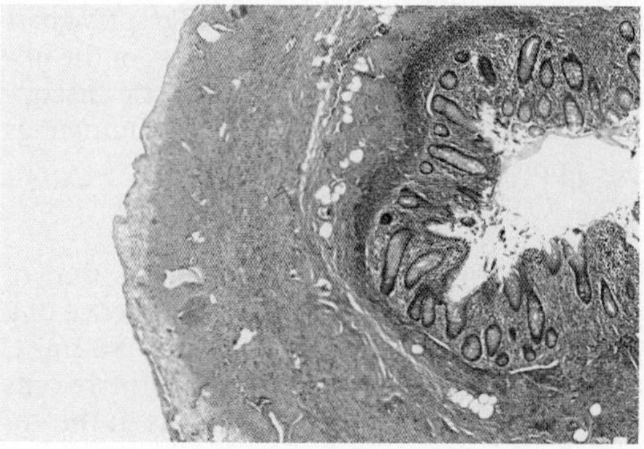

Figure 1-42

NORMAL ADULT APPENDIX

Left: Dark blue staining lymphoid cells are present diffusely in the deep mucosa and superficial submucosa. Like most of the remainder of the GI tract, the muscularis propria is comprised of two layers of smooth muscle.

Right: Higher-power view shows that the mucosa resembles that of the normal colon.

tissue. This occurs particularly at the distal tip (see chapter 13). It is unclear whether atrophy represents a physiologic change or a reaction to previous disease.

Anus

The mucosa of the anal canal contains a complex mixture of epithelial cell types. The mucosa of the upper portion of the anal canal resembles rectal mucosa except that the crypts may appear shorter and more irregular (fig. 1-45). The anal transitional zone (ATZ) contains many epithelial cell types. The cells comprising the basal epithelial layer in this region frequently appear small and contain nuclei arranged perpendicularly to the basement membrane. The surface cells may appear columnar, cuboidal, or flattened (fig. 1-46) (87–89). Mature goblet cells are present (93). Surface cells may acquire an umbrella shape, with distinct cell borders superficially resembling urothelium.

Anal glands originate in the ATZ from anal crypts. Four to eight anal ducts lie in the anal canal of the adult. Each has a short tubular submucosal portion that branches into a sparsely ramifying glandular pattern. Anal ducts follow a tortuous course through the lamina propria before penetrating the internal sphincter musculature and extending into the fat. The lining of the anal glands is variable in appearance (fig. 1-47). Squamous type cells are commonly seen

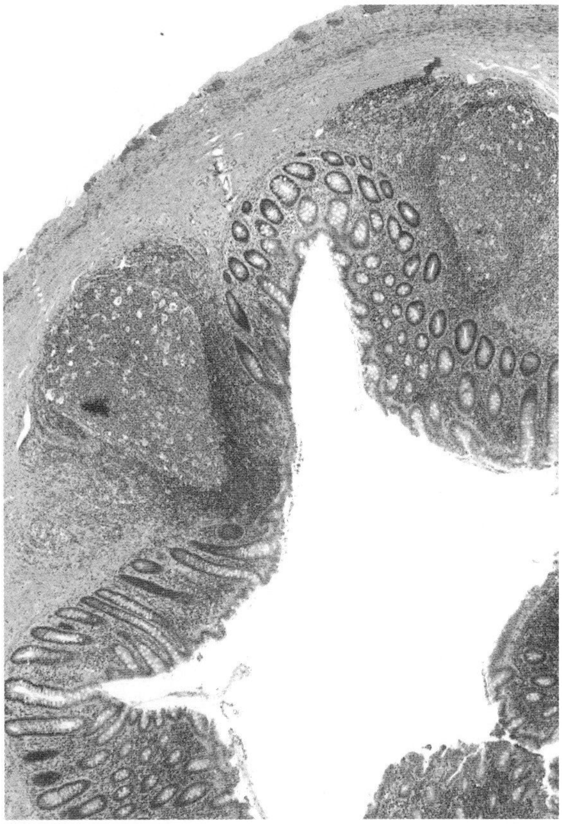

Figure 1-43

APPENDIX

This appendix from a 1-year-old child has prominent lymphoid follicles with germinal centers.

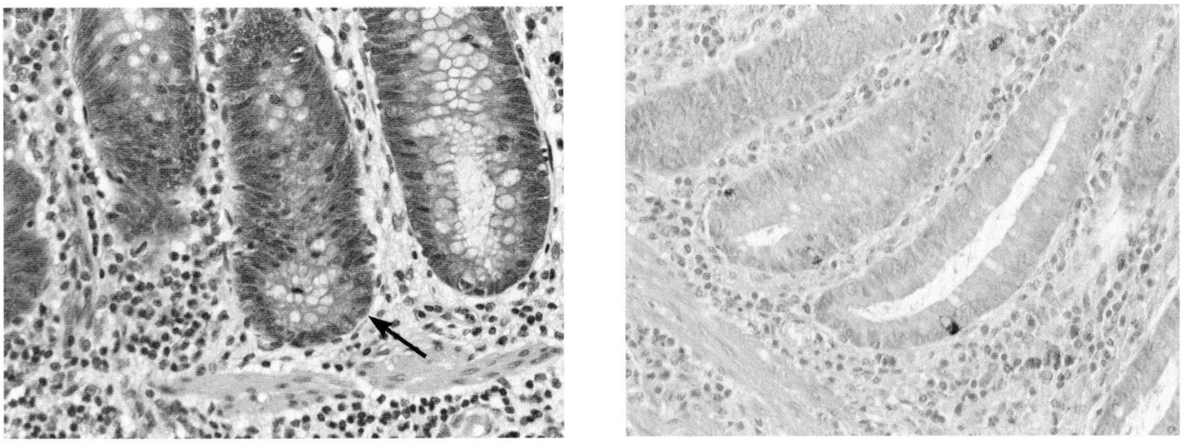

Figure 1-44

APPENDICEAL ENDOCRINE CELLS

Left: An H&E-stained section shows an endocrine cell within an appendiceal crypt. The cytoplasm contains numerous reddish secretory granules (arrow).

Right: Chromogranin highlights the endocrine cells in the basal portion of the crypts.

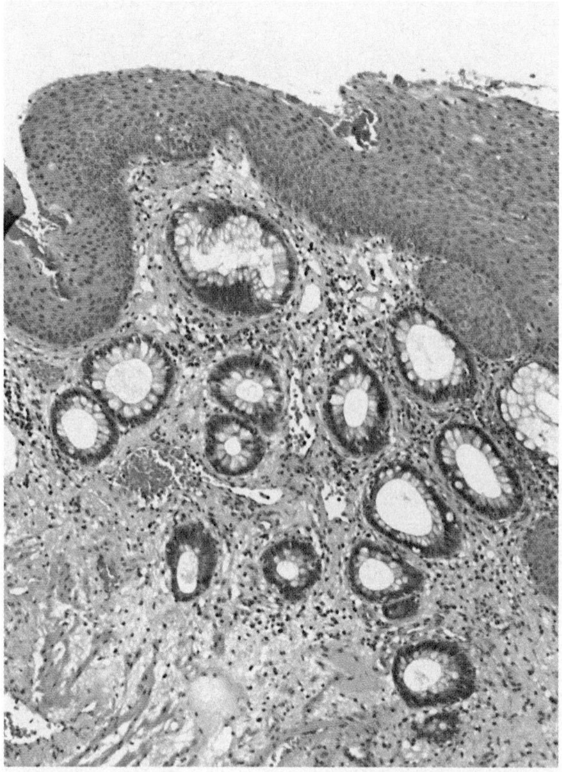

Figure 1-45

UPPER ANAL CANAL

The colonic type glands in the transition area of rectal mucosa to anal canal have a more irregular appearance than those of the more proximal colon. The overlying epithelium is squamous or transitional in appearance.

at the gland opening, transitional epithelium is seen in the middle, and simple columnar cells are present in its deepest part. Goblet cells occur in large numbers within the anal ducts, particularly at their terminal portions. A characteristic feature of the anal glands is the presence of intraepithelial microcysts.

The nonkeratinized squamous epithelium of the anal canal changes into keratinized stratified squamous epithelium at the anus proper (fig. 1-48). Melanocytes regularly populate the squamous epithelium below the dentate line and increase in number as one approaches the anal margin (fig. 1-48). In addition, there may be melanin-containing cells above the dentate line (90).

Endocrine cells lie above the dentate line in the colorectal mucosa, in the transitional mucosa, in anal ducts and glands, in crypts, and in perianal sweat glands (91,92). Like endocrine cells elsewhere in the GI tract, those in the anal region lie close to the basement membrane.

GENERAL INTERPRETATION OF PATHOLOGIC SPECIMENS

Gastrointestinal pathology specimens fall into three major categories: biopsy specimens, resection specimens, and cytology specimens. Biopsies are taken to establish a specific diagnosis or to follow the evolution of a disease. They are also taken to determine disease extent

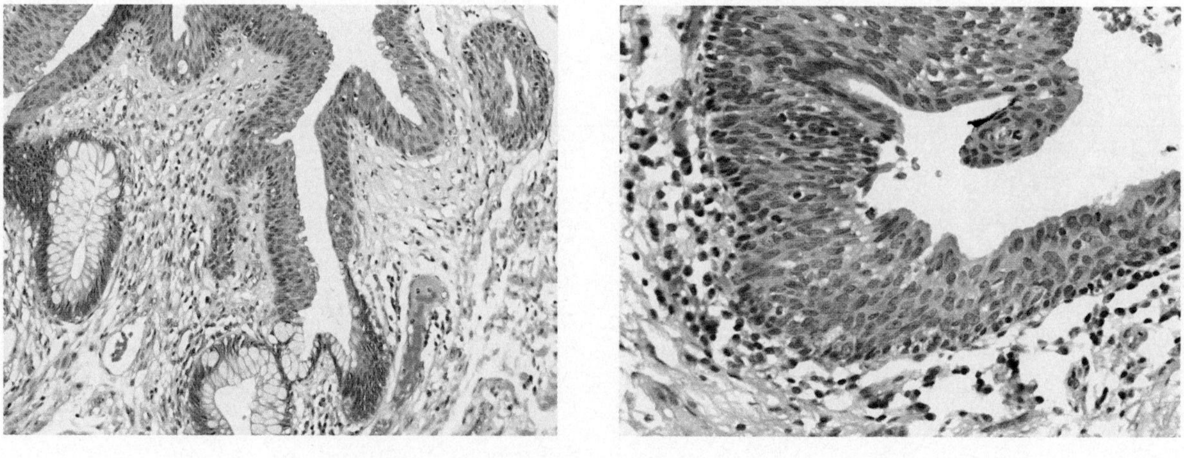

Figure 1-46

ANAL TRANSITION ZONE

Left: Transition from rectal type mucosa to anal mucosa.

Right: Higher-power view of the anal transitional mucosa. The basal cells are small and slightly darker than those in the upper portions of the epithelium. The surface cells are cuboidal, and resemble the umbrella cells of urothelium.

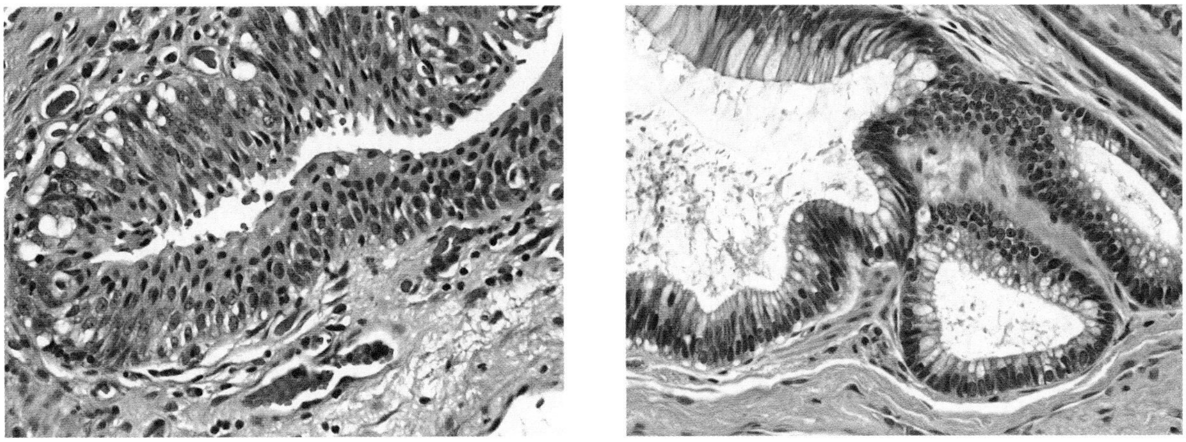

Figure 1-47

ANAL GLANDS

Left: The proximal portion of an anal duct is lined by transitional type epithelium.
Right: The more distal portions of the ducts are lined by simple columnar, mucin-producing epithelium.

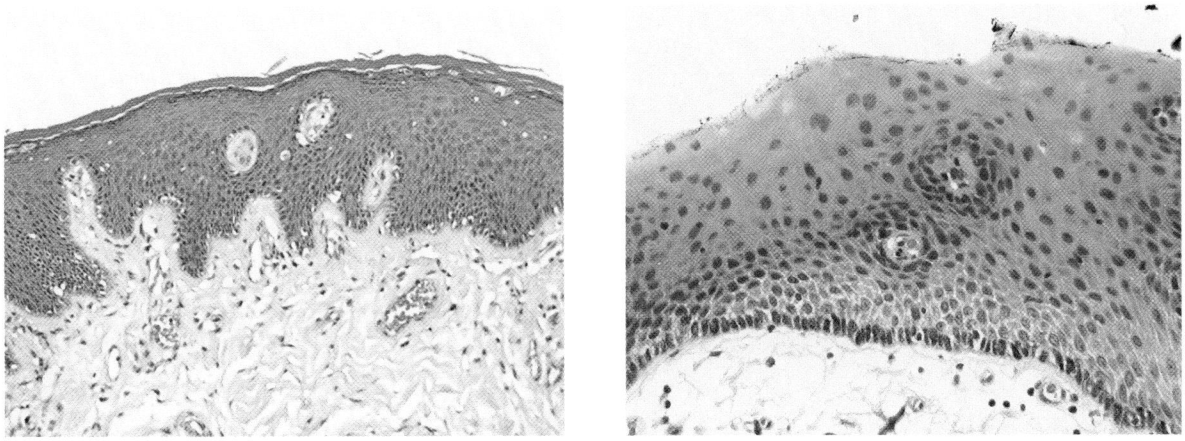

Figure 1-48

ANUS

Left: The anus proper is lined by keratinizing, stratified squamous epithelium.
Right: Melanin pigment is frequently seen within the basal layer of the epithelium.

(as in inflammatory bowel disease) or to judge its severity, determine response to therapy, or detect neoplasia. Biopsies are also taken to acquire tissues for other purposes, including microbial culture, biochemical examination, ultrastructural examination, or evaluation of molecular markers. Biopsy interpretation is always enhanced by an effective dialogue between the pathologist and the clinician.

Resections are performed to surgically treat cancer or precancerous lesions, life-threatening ischemia, severe ulcerating diseases, obstructions, and pseudoobstructions, as well as various other conditions. Resection specimens received in the fresh state should be examined as soon as possible to determine whether or not the specimen requires special handling for procedures such as microbial cultures, ultrastructural examination, biochemical analysis, imprints, cytogenetic studies, or molecular studies prior to fixation. Additionally, the specimen should be photographed if it contains an obvious lesion.

When the specimen is photographed, it should be properly oriented and should include some normal tissue for orientation. The specimen should also be cleaned to remove blood, stool, and other substances present that may interfere with obtaining information from the specimen.

Ten percent buffered formalin is the most commonly used fixative in histology laboratories because it is stable and allows staining with most of the histochemical and immunohistochemical stains currently in use. It does, however, induce substantial tissue shrinkage. In circumstances in which a more accurate rendering of the cytologic features is required, additional fixatives can be used that contain heavy metals, such as Bouin, B5, or Hollande solution. These fixatives cause less tissue shrinkage and permit analysis of nuclei that appear less distorted. The latter fixatives, however, interfere with the ability to isolate high-quality nucleic acids from the biopsy specimens should this be intended later. In addition, some immunohistochemical studies are difficult to perform on tissues fixed by these methods.

The specimen should be placed in a fixative volume that is at least ten times that of the tissue. Resection specimens should be opened longitudinally and pinned out. If a specimen is pinned to a cork board, gauze or paper towels can be placed beneath the specimen to serve as a wick for the fixative. Tissues should be adequately fixed prior to sectioning. Specimens submitted to the histology laboratory should be no more than 3-mm thick because they do not fit appropriately into the cassettes and they fail to become adequately infiltrated during processing.

Histologic sections, whether from biopsy or resection specimens, should be made with the proper orientation. Optimally, the sections should be made in a plane perpendicular to the mucosal surface. This allows for the evaluation of mucosal height and component parts. Care must be taken with orienting small intestinal biopsies because an interpretation of many diseases involves an analysis of the crypt/villus ratio. Gastrointestinal biopsies are usually small and multiple levels should be examined in order to adequately assess the histologic features, especially in biopsies that are not well oriented. This approach allows for the detection of focal lesions, such as microorganisms and granulomas.

REFERENCES

Introduction

1. Ettensohn CA. The regulation of primary mesenchyme cell patterning. Dev Biol 1990;140:261–71.

Gastrointestinal Structure

2. Abu-Ghazaleh RI, Fujisawa T, Mestecky J, Kyle RA, Gleich GJ. IgA-induced eosinophil degranulation. J Immunol 1989;142:2393–400.
3. Barrett KE, Metcalfe DD. The histological and functional characterization of enzymatically dispersed intestinal mast cells of non-human primates: effects of secretagogues and anti-allergic drugs on histamine secretion. J Immunol 1985; 135:2020–6.
4. Befus AD, Pearce FL, Gauldie J, Horsewood P, Bienenstock J. Mucosal mast cells. I. Isolation and functional characteristics of rat intestinal mast cells. J Immunol 1982;128:2475–80.
5. Bland PW, Kambarage DM. Antigen handling by the epithelium and lamina propria macrophages. Gastroenterol Clin North Am 1991;20:577–96.
6. Buchan AM, Polak JM, Capella C, Solcia E, Pearse AG. Electron immunocytochemical evidence for the K cell localization of gastric inhibitory polypeptide (GIP) in man. Histochemistry 1978;56:37–44.
7. Butterworth AE, Wassom DL, Gleich GJ, Loegering DA, David JR. Damage to schistosomula of *Schistosoma mansoni* induced directly by eosinophil major basic protein. J Immunol 1979;122: 221–9.
8. Capron M, Prin L. The IgE receptor of eosinophils. Springer Semin Immunopathol 1990;12:327–48.
9. Changelian PS, Fearon DT. Tissue-specific phosphorylation of complement receptors CR1 and CR2. J Exp Med 1986;163:101–15.
10. Christensen J. The controls of gastrointestinal movements: some old and new views. N Engl J Med 1971;285:85–98.

11. Enerback L. Mast cells in the gastrointestinal mucosa. I. Effects of fixation. Acta Pathol Microbiol Scand 1966;66:289–302.
12. Facer P, Bishop AE, Lloyd RV, Wilson BS, Hennessy RJ, Polak JM. Chromogranin: a newly recognized marker for endocrine cells of the human gastrointestinal tract. Gastroenterology 1985;89:1366–73.
13. Faussone-Pellegrini MS. Histogenesis, structure, and relationships of interstitial cells of Cajal (ICC): from morphology to functional interpretation. Eur J Morphol 1992;30:137–48.
14. Faussone-Pellegrini MS. Morphogenesis of special circular muscle layer and of the interstitial cells of Cajal related to the plexus muscularis profundus of mouse intestinal muscle coat. An EM study. Anat Embryol 1984;169:151–8.
15. Faussone-Pellegrini MS, Cortesini C. Ultrastructural peculiarities of the inner portion of the circular layer of colon. I. Research in the human. Acta Anat 1984;120:185–9.
16. Furness JB, Costa M. Types of nerves in the enteric nervous system. Neuroscience 1980;5:1–20.
17. Gabella G. Hypertrophic smooth muscle I. Size and shape of cells, occurrence of mitoses. Cell Tissue Res 1979;201:63–78.
18. Gabella G. Special muscle cells and their innervation in the mammalian small intestine. Cell Tissue Res 1974;153:63–77.
19. Galli SJ, Dvorak AM, Dvorak HF. Basophils and mast cells: morphologic insights into their biology, secretory patterns, and function. Prog Allergy 1984;34:1–141.
20. Gerard NP, Hodges MK, Drazen JM, Weller PF, Gerard C. Characterization of a receptor for C5a anaphylatoxin on human eosinophils. J Biol Chem 1989;264:1760–6.
21. Gleich GJ, Adolphson CR. The eosinophilic leukocyte: structure and function. Adv Immunol 1986;39:177–253.
22. Graziano RF, Looney RJ, Shen L, Fanger MW. Fc gamma R-mediated killing by eosinophils. J Immunol 1989;142:230–5.
23. Hamada A, Greene BM. C1q enhancement of IgG-dependent eosinophil-mediated killing of *Schistosoma* in vitro. J Immunol 1987;138:1240–5.
24. Huizinga JD, Thuneberg L, Kluppel M, Malysz J, Mikkelsen HB, Bernstein A. W/kit gene required for interstitial cells of Cajal and for intestinal pacemaker activity. Nature 1995;373:347–9.
25. Jacoby HI, Bonfilio AC, Raffa RB. Central and peripheral administration of serotonin produces opposite effects on mouse colonic propulsive motility. Neuroscience Lett 1991;122:122–6.
26. Janossy G, Bofill M, Poulter LW, et al. Separate ontogeny of two macrophage-like accessory cell populations in the human fetus. J Immunol 1986;136:4354–61.
27. Komuro T. The interstitial cells in the colon of rabbit. Scanning and transmission electron microscopy. Cell Tissue Res 1982;222:41–51.
28. Komuro T. Three-dimensional observation of the fibroblast-like cells associated with the rat myenteric plexus, with special reference to the interstitial cells of Cajal. Cell Tissue Res 1989;255:343–51.
29. Kroegel C, Yukawa T, Westwick J, Barnes PJ. Evidence for two platelet activating factor receptors on eosinophils: dissociation between PAF-induced intracellular calcium mobilization degranulation and superoxide anion generation in eosinophils. Biochem Biophys Res Commun 1989;162:511–21.
30. Lemanske RF Jr, Atkins FM, Metcalfe DD. Gastrointestinal mast cells in health and disease. Part II. J Pediatrics 1983;103:343–51.
31. Lloyd RV, Mervak T, Schmidt K, Warner TF, Wilson BS. Immunohistochemical detection of chromogranin and neuron specific enolase in pancreatic endocrine neoplasms. Am J Surg Pathol 1984;8:607–14.
32. Mahida YR, Wu KC, Jewell DP. Characterization of antigen-presenting activity of intestinal mononuclear cells isolated from normal and inflammatory bowel disease colon and ileum. Immunology 1988;65:543–9.
33. Metcalfe DD, Kaliner M, Donlon MA. The mast cell. CRC Crit Rev Immunol 1981;2:23–74.
34. Nagashima R, Maeda K, Imai Y, Takahashi T. Lamina propria macrophages in the human gastrointestinal mucosa: their distribution, immunohistological phenotype, and function. J Histochem Cytochem 1996;44:721–31.
35. Otsuka H, Denberg J, Dolovich J, et al. Heterogeneity of metachromatic cells in human nose: significance of mucosal mast cells. J Allergy Clin Immunol 1985;76:695–702.
36. Pineiro-Carrero VM, Clench MH, Davis RH, Andres JM, Franzini DA, Mathias JR. Intestinal motility changes in rats after enteric serotonergic neuron destruction. Am J Physiol 1991;260: G232–9.
37. Rindi G, Buffa R, Sessa F, Tortora O, Solcia E. Chromogranin A, B and C immunoreactivities of mammalian endocrine cells. Distribution, distinction from costored hormones/prohormones and relationship with the argyrophil component of secretory granules. Histochemistry 1986;85:19–28.
38. Rumessen JJ, Mikkelsen HB, Qvortrup K, Thuneberg L. Ultrastructure of interstitial cells of Cajal (ICC) in the circular muscle of human small intestine. Gastroenterology 1993;104:343–50.

39. Rumessen JJ, Mikkelsen HB, Thuneberg L. Ultrastructure of interstitial cells of Cajal (ICC) associated with deep muscular plexus of the human small intestine. Gastroenterology 1992;102:56–68.
40. Rumessen JJ, Thuneberg L. Interstitial cells of Cajal in human small intestine. Ultrastructural identification and organization between the main smooth muscle layers. Gastroenterology 1991;100:1417–31.
41. Sanders KM. A case for interstitial cells of Cajal as pacemakers and mediators of neurotransmission in the gastrointestinal tract. Gastroenterology 1996;111:492–515.
42. Sminia T, Jeurissen SH. The macrophage population of the gastrointestinal tract of the rat. Immunobiology 1986;172:72–80.
43. Solcia E, Capella C, Vezzadini P, Barbara L, Bussolati G. Immunohistochemical and ultrastructural detection of the secretin cell in the pig intestinal mucosa. Experientia 1972;28:549–50.
44. Solcia E, Vassallo G, Capella C. Studies on the G cells of the pyloric mucosa, the probable site of gastrin secretion. Gut 1969;10:379–88.
45. Sperber K, Ogata S, Sylvester C, et al. A novel human macrophage-derived intestinal mucin secretagogue: implications for the pathogenesis of inflammatory bowel disease. Gastroenterology 1993;104:1302–9.
46. Strobel S, Miller HR, Ferguson A. Human intestinal mucosal mast cells: evaluation of fixation and staining techniques. J Clin Pathol 1981;34:851–8.
47. Sundler F, Bottcher G, Ekblad E, Hakanson R. The neuroendocrine system of the gut. Acta Oncologica 1989;28:303–14.
48. Thuneberg L. Interstitial cells of Cajal: intestinal pacemaker cells? Adv Anat Embryol Cell Biol 1982;7:1–130.
49. Tutton PJ. The influence of serotonin on epithelial cell proliferation in the jejunum of the rat. Virchows Arch B Cell Pathol 1974;16:79–87.
50. Uribe A, Alam M, Johansson O, Midtvedt T, Theodorsson E. Microflora modulates endocrine cells in the gastrointestinal mucosa of the rat. Gastroenterology 1994;107:1259–69.
51. Usellini L, Capella C, Frigerio B, Rindi G, Solcia E. Ultrastructural localization of secretin in endocrine cells of the dog duodenum by the immunogold technique. Comparison with ultrastructurally characterized S cells of various mammals. Histochemistry 1984;80:435–41.
52. Verspaget HW, Pena AS, Weterman IT, Lamers CB. Disordered regulation of the in vitro immunoglobulin synthesis by intestinal mononuclear cells in Crohn's disease. Gut 1988;29:503–10.
53. Weller PF. The immunobiology of eosinophils. N Engl J Med 1991;324:1110–8.
54. Wilson BS, Lloyd RV. Detection of chromogranin in neuroendocrine cells with a monoclonal antibody. Am J Pathol 1984;115:458–68.
55. Yunis E, Sherman FE. Macrophages of the rectal lamina propria in children. Am J Clin Pathol 1970;53:580–91.

Normal Esophagus

56. Geboes K, DeWolf-Peeters C, Rutgeerts P, et al. Lymphocytes and Langerhans cells in the human esophageal epithelium. Virchows Arch A Pathol Anat 1983;401:45–55.
57. Seefeld U, Krejs GJ, Siebenmann RE, Blum AL. Esophageal histology in gastroesophageal reflux. Morphometric findings in suction biopsies. Am J Dig Dis 1977;22:956–64.
58. Tateishi R, Taniguchi H, Wada A, et al. Argyrophil cells and melanocytes in esophageal mucosa. Arch Pathol Lab Med 1974;98:87–9.

Normal Small Intestine

59. Bosshard A, Chery-Croze S, Cuber JC, Dechelette MA, Berger F, Chayvialle JA. Immunocytochemical study of peptidergic structures in Brunner's glands. Gastroenterology 1989;97:1382–8.
60. Boyle JT, Celano P, Koldovsky O. Demonstration of a difference in expression of maximal lactase and sucrase activity along the villus in the adult rat jejunum. Gastroenterology 1980;79:503–7.
61. Braegger CP, Spencer J, MacDonald TT. Ontogenetic aspects of the intestinal immune system in man. Int J Clin Lab Res 1992;22:1–4.
62. Crescenzi A, Barsotti P, Anemona L, Marinozzi V. Carbohydrate histochemistry of human Brunner's glands. Histochemistry 1988;90:47–9.
63. Crowe PT, Marsh MN. Morphometric analysis of intestinal mucosa. VI. Principles in enumerating intra-epithelial lymphocytes. Virchows Arch 1994;424:301–6.
64. Eisenhauer PB, Harwig SS, Lehrer RI. Cryptidins: antimicrobial defensins of the murine small intestine. Infect Immun 1992;50:3556–65.
65. Erlandsen SL, Parsons JA. Taylor TD. Ultrastructural immunocytochemical localization of lysozyme in the Paneth cells of man. J Histochem Cytochem 1974;22:401–13.
66. Ferguson A, Murray D. Quantitation of intraepithelial lymphocytes in human jejunum. Gut 1971;12:988–94.
67. Geboes K, Ray MB, Rutgeerts P, Callea F, Desmet VJ, Vantrappen G. Morphological identification of alpha-1-antitrypsin in the human small intestine. Histopathology 1982;6:55–60.
68. Huttner KM, Ouellette AJ. A family of defensin-like genes codes for diverse cysteine-rich peptides in mouse Paneth cells. Genomics 1994;24:99–109.

69. Jones DE, Bevins CL. Paneth cells of the human small intestine express an antimicrobial peptide gene. J Biol Chem 1992;267:23216–25.
70. Keren DF, Holt PS, Collins HH, Gemski P, Formal SB. The role of Peyer's patches in the local immune response of rabbit ileum to live bacteria. J Immunol 1978;120:1892–6.
71. Keshav S, Lawson L, Chung LP, Stein M, Perry VH, Gordon S. Tumor necrosis factor and mRNA localized to Paneth cells of normal murine intestinal epithelium by in situ hybridization. J Exp Med 1990;171:327–32.
72. Molmenti EP, Perlmutter DH, Rubin DC. Cell-specific expression of alpha 1-antitrypsin in human intestinal epithelium. J Clin Invest 1993;92: 2022–34.
73. Mooseker MS. Organization, chemistry and assembly of the cytoskeletal apparatus of the intestinal brush border. Annu Rev Cell Biol 1985;1:209–41.
74. Ouellette AJ, Hsieh MM, Nosek MT, et al. Mouse Paneth cell defensins: primary structures and antibacterial activities of numerous cryptidin isoforms. Infect Immun 1994;62:5040–7.
75. Phillips AD, Rice SJ, France NE, Walker-Smith JA. Small intestinal intraepithelial lymphocyte levels in cow's milk protein intolerance. Gut 1979;20:509–12.
76. Potten CS, Loeffler M. Stem cells: attributes, cycles, spirals, pitfalls and uncertainties. Lessons for and from the crypt. Development 1990; 110: 1001–20.
77. Rodning CB, Wilson ID, Erlandsen SL. Immunoglobulins within human small intestinal Paneth cells. Lancet 1976;1:984–7.
78. Rosner AJ, Keren DF. Demonstration of M-cells in the specialized follicle-associated epithelium overlying isolated follicles in the gut. J Leukocyte Biol 1984;35:397–404.
79. Selby WS, Janossy G, Bofill M, Jewell DP. Lymphocyte subpopulations in the human small intestine. The findings in normal mucosa and in the mucosa of patients with coeliac disease. Clin Exp Immunol 1983;52:219–28.
80. Skutelsky E, Moore RP, Alroy J. Lectin histochemistry of mammalian Brunner's glands. Histochemistry 1989;90:383–90.
81. Trejdosiewicz LK. Intestinal intraepithelial lymphocytes and lymphoepithelial interactions in the human gastrointestinal mucosa. Immunol Lett 1992;32:13–9.
82. West AB, Isaac CA, Carboni JM, Morrow JS, Mooseker MS, Barwick KW. Localization of villin, a cytoskeletal protein specific to microvilli, in human ileum and colon and in colonic neoplasms. Gastroenterology 1988;94:343–52.

Normal Colon

83. Balcerzak SP, Lane WC, Bullard JW. Surface structure of intestinal epithelium. Gastroenterology 1970;58:49–55.
84. Buffa R, Capella C, Fontana P, Usellini L, Solcia E. Types of endocrine cells in the human colon and rectum. Cell Tissue Res 1978;192:227–40.
85. Fenoglio CM, Richart RM, Kaye GI. Comparative ultrastructural features of normal, hyperplastic, and adenomatous human colonic epithelium. Gastroenterology 1975;69:100–9.
86. Sjolund K, Sanden G, Hakanson R, Sundler F. Endocrine cells in human intestine: an immunocytochemical study. Gastroenterology 1983;85: 1120–30.

Normal Anus

87. Fenger C. The anal transitional zone. A method for macroscopic demonstration. Acta Pathol Microbiol Scand A 1978;86:225–30.
88. Fenger C. The anal transitional zone. Location and extent. Acta Pathol Microbiol Scand A 1979;87:379–86.
89. Fenger C, Knoth M. The anal transitional zone: a scanning and transmission electron microscopic investigation of the surface epithelium. Ultrastruct Pathol 1981;2:163–73.
90. Fenger C, Lyon H. Endocrine cells and melanin-containing cells in the anal canal epithelium. Histochem J 1982;14:631–9.
91. Fetissof F, Dubois MP, Assan R, et al. Endocrine cells in the anal canal. Virchows Arch A Pathol Anat 1984;404:39–47.
92. Horsch D, Weihe E, Muller S, Hancke E. Distribution and coexistence of chromogranin A-, serotonin- and pancreastatin-like immunoreactivity in endocrine-like cells of the human anal canal. Cell Tissue Res 1992;268:109–16.
93. McColl I. The comparative anatomy and pathology of anal glands. Ann R Coll Surg Engl 1967;40:36–67.

2 CONGENITAL GASTROINTESTINAL ABNORMALITIES

EMBRYOLOGY

Gastrulation, which occurs 2 weeks after fertilization, induces a massive rearrangement of the embryo, transforming a relatively uniform cell ball into a multilayered organism with recognizable body plans. Cells stream across the embryo in a precise pattern that is maintained across multiple species. A number of genetic signaling cascades link molecules that affect the movement of gastrulation to mechanisms that cause cells to stick together and promote embryonic movement. Certain cells divide faster than others, resulting in a change in embryonic shape. Cells converge on the embryonic midline in a process of convergent extension. As these cells crowd together, they push each other toward the future head and tail, and the embryo lengthens. Paraxial protocadherin helps determine these motions (18).

There are two major steps in gastrointestinal development: formation of the gut tube and formation of individual organs, each with their own specialized cell types (12). These events are regulated by homeobox-containing genes. Each homeobox gene has a distinct rostrocaudal expression pattern in many tissues, including the gastrointestinal tract. Two homeotic genes, *Cdx1* and *Cdx2*, are expressed only in the intestine whereas the remainder are expressed in many sites.

Gastrulation gives rise to three germ layers, one of which, the endoderm, is the precursor to the gastrointestinal epithelial lining. Endodermal development requires the expression of the homeotic genes *MIXER, SOX17 α,* and *SOX17 β* (8). Multiple interactions occur between the endoderm, mesoderm, and ectoderm during development. The endoderm induces the mesoderm to develop, conferring on it a dorsal-ventral pattern. Endoderm and ectoderm contact one another in the 2- to 4-week embryo; the endoderm forms the yolk sac roof.

The primitive gut forms in the 3rd to 8th weeks as a result of the cephalocaudal and lateral embryonic folding that incorporates the dorsal endodermally lined yolk sac cavity. The amnion and yolk sac communicate through the neurenteric canal (fig. 2-1). The neurenteric canal closes and the notochord grows forward, becoming intercalated within the endoderm. The neural tube then separates from the ectoderm. Mesoderm surrounds the notochord, separating the ectoderm and endoderm (10). Gastrointestinal duplications associated with a defective spinal cord and/or vertebra develop if mesodermal ingrowth does not occur and neural and gastrointestinal elements fail to separate. Splanchnic mesoderm surrounding the primitive gut forms the muscular and connective tissue layers.

The former yolk sac elongates out under the developing nervous system to form the primitive foregut anteriorly and the primitive hindgut posteriorly. The central portion develops into the midgut, which freely communicates with the yolk sac (the vitellointestinal duct) (fig. 2-1). The anterior abdominal wall develops by simultaneous cranial, caudal, and lateral infolding, which attenuates the yolk sac. As a result, the yolk sac becomes intracoelomic (fig. 2-1). The foregut is short at first, lying closely apposed to the developing vertebrae from which it becomes suspended by a short mesentery. It gives rise to the esophagus, stomach, duodenum as far as the ampulla of Vater, liver, pancreas, and respiratory system, and it has its own arterial blood supply deriving from the celiac axis (13).

Esophagus

The esophagus develops from the cranial end of the primitive foregut, appearing at the 2.5-mm developmental stage (approximately the 3rd gestational week) (Table 2-1) as an annular constriction lying between the stomach and the pharynx (3). As the esophagus elongates, it

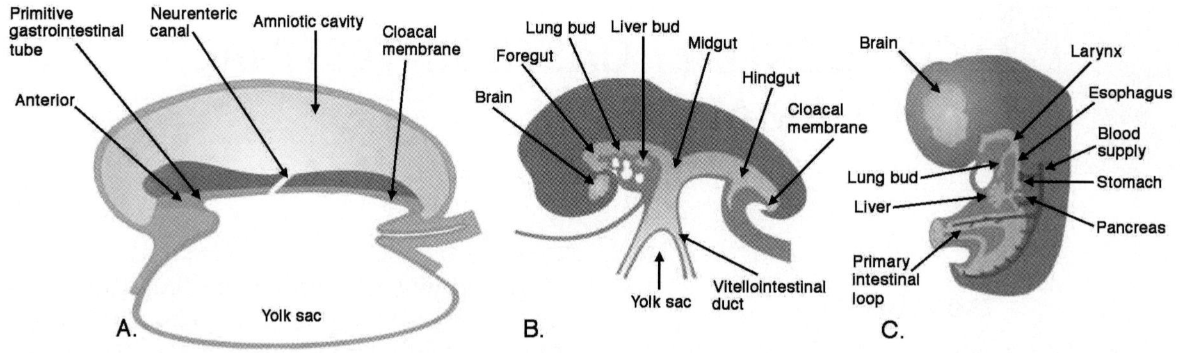

Figure 2-1

EMBRYONIC DEVELOPMENT WITH PROGRESSIVE GASTROINTESTINAL FORMATION

A: The gastrointestinal tract develops early as a primitive endodermal tube closely related to primitive neural tissue. The neural and endodermal tissues communicate through the neurenteric canal.

B: With further embryonic development, the vitellointestinal duct begins to differentiate and the primitive gut divides into a foregut, midgut, and hindgut. Diverticula start to develop that will eventually give rise to the lung and the liver.

C: Embryo viewed from the side and with detail of the umbilical cord. This diagrammatic representation is slightly later in development than the embryo illustrated in B.

Table 2-1

APPROXIMATE RELATIONSHIP BETWEEN FETAL AGE AND EMBRYO LENGTH

Postfertilization (days)	Embryo Length (mm)
22	1.5–2.0
25	2.5–3.5
30	6.0–7.5
35	1–15
40	20–23
45	24–28
50	29–34
55	35–41
60	42–50
70	53–67
84	80–95
98	110–130
112	130–150
126	155–180
140	175–205

becomes increasingly tubular. At approximately 4 weeks, a small outgrowth appears in the ventral wall of the foregut, termed the respiratory or laryngotracheal diverticulum (fig. 2-2). Initially, the cephalad esophagus and trachea lie within a common tube. Later, however, lateral epithelial ridges develop in the upper segment, dividing the lumen into anterior and posterior compartments. Mesenchymal tissue grows into the ridges to form a septum that completely separates the esophagus and trachea (3,5). The esophagus lies dorsally; the trachea and lung buds lie ventrally.

The initially round esophageal lumen flattens. Later, extensive longitudinal folding of the wall begins. During the 7th and 8th weeks, the esophageal epithelium proliferates and nearly fills the lumen, although complete occlusion does not occur. The esophageal mucosal lining progresses through a sequence of epithelial changes before becoming stratified squamous epithelium (figs. 2-3, 2-4). Squamous epithelium appears at 20 to 25 weeks, beginning in the midesophagus and proceeding both caudally and cephalad. Nests of embryonic esophageal epithelial cells that persist in adults give rise to some congenital abnormalities.

Stomach and Duodenum

The stomach develops from a fusiform, primitive foregut swelling at approximately 4 weeks gestation (7 mm). It originates in the neck, descending into the abdomen during the next 8 weeks. The dorsal gastric wall grows more rapidly than the ventral wall, leading to the development of the greater curvature. As the stomach rotates to the left, the esophagus deviates slightly to the left and the duodenum deviates

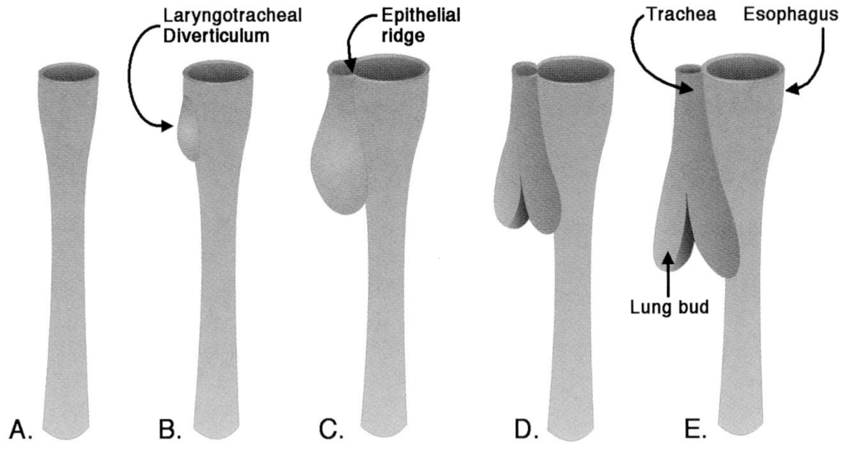

Figure 2-2

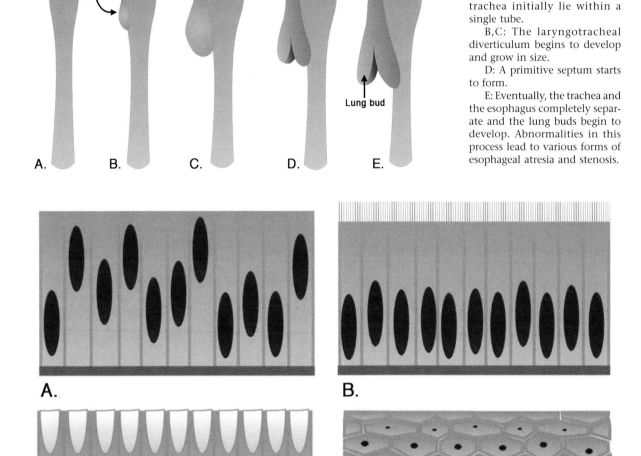

ESOPHAGEAL DEVELOPMENT

A: The esophagus and early trachea initially lie within a single tube.

B,C: The laryngotracheal diverticulum begins to develop and grow in size.

D: A primitive septum starts to form.

E: Eventually, the trachea and the esophagus completely separate and the lung buds begin to develop. Abnormalities in this process lead to various forms of esophageal atresia and stenosis.

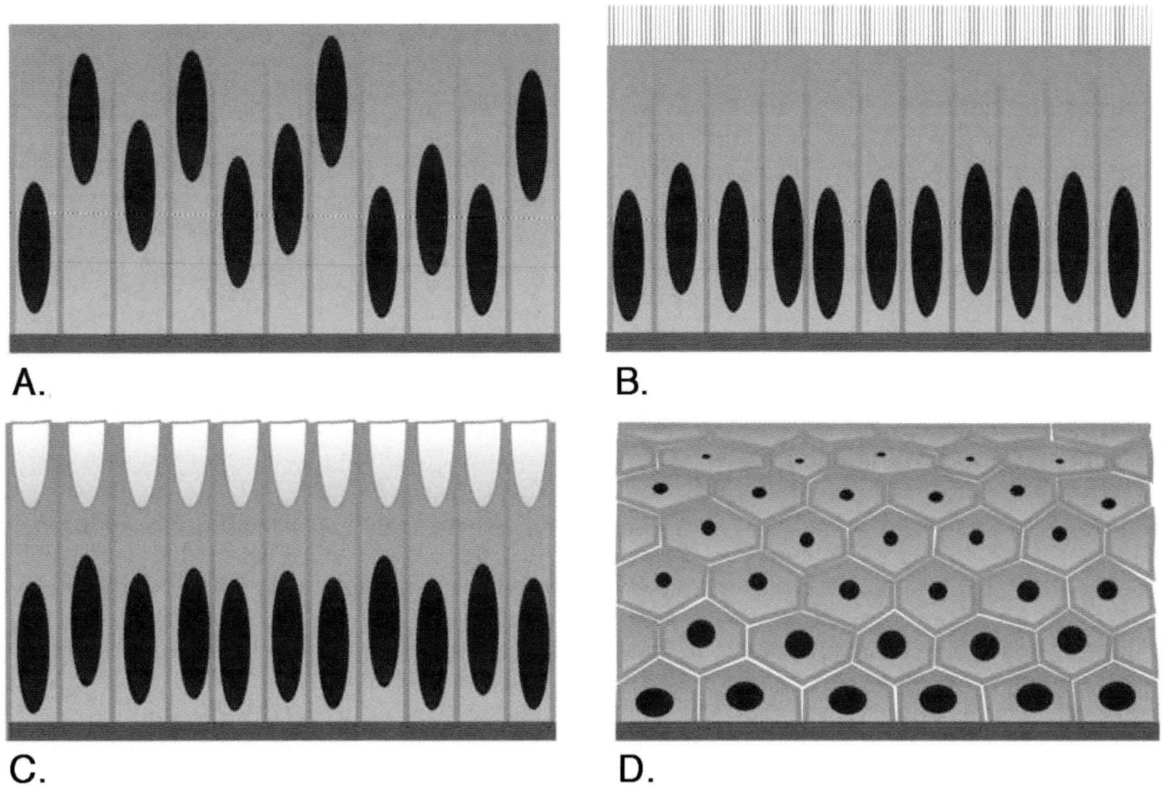

Figure 2-3

CHANGES IN THE ESOPHAGEAL LINING EPITHELIUM DURING FETAL DEVELOPMENT

The epithelial lining changes from a pseudostratified epithelium (A) to one in which the cells are less stratified (B). They become columnar with mucinous secretion (C). Eventually, squamous epithelium develops (D).

slightly to the right. Duodenal diverticula give rise to the subsequent pancreas and biliary system. By the time the embryo reaches the 15-mm stage, gastric dorsal expansion has created the mature stomach. The enlarging thoracic contents push the stomach and duodenum caudally. Initially the stomach attaches to the back of the abdomen by the dorsal mesogastrium and

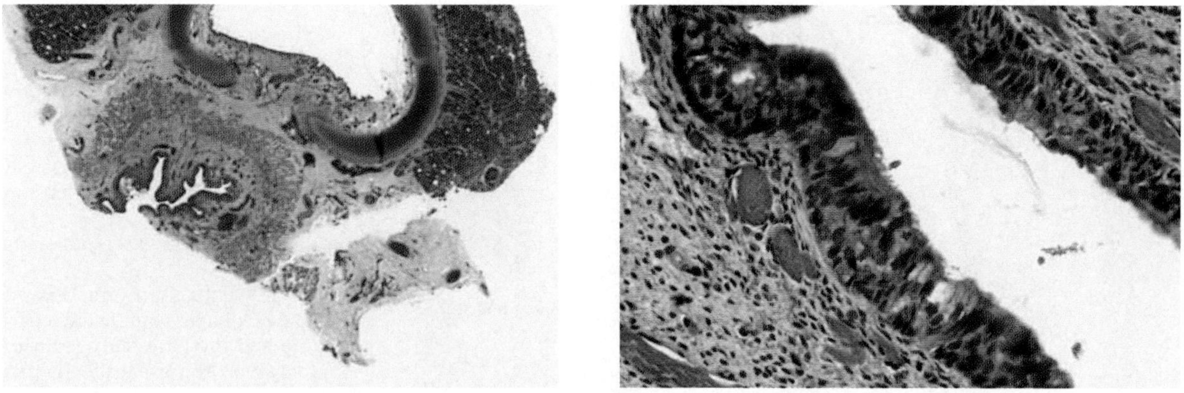

Figure 2-4

FETAL ESOPHAGUS

Left: The esophagus and trachea have separated from one another. In this photograph the esophagus lies below the trachea. Right: High magnification of the esophageal lining shows that it consists of pseudostratified epithelium.

to the septum transversum (the diaphragm) by the ventral mesogastrium. As the stomach enlarges, the dorsal mesogastrium becomes the greater omentum and the ventral mesogastrium becomes the lesser omentum. Characteristic gastric anatomic features (greater curvature, lesser curvature, fundus, body, and pylorus) can be identified by 14 weeks (12).

Early glandular differentiation of the gastric lining occurs at the 80-mm stage of fetal development. The stomach is initially lined by stratified or pseudostratified epithelium; later, cuboidal cells appear. The first differentiated cell types to appear are the mucous neck cells. These act as progenitors for other cell types. Gastric pits are well developed by 5 to 7 weeks. Parietal cells appear by 9 to 11 weeks. Gastric glands begin to develop at 11 to 14 weeks; they grow by progressive branching, a process that continues until birth. Acid is found in the fetal stomach at 19 weeks (15). By term, 20 percent of neonates exhibit the adult pattern of parietal cell distribution (11). Mesoderm surrounding the stomach differentiates into the gastric connective tissue and the muscularis propria by the end of the 2nd fetal month.

Intestine

The duodenum distal to the bile duct as well as the jejunum, ileum, cecum, ascending colon, and proximal half to two thirds of the transverse colon derive from the midgut and are supplied by the superior mesenteric artery. At the 5- to 12-mm stage, the midgut lengthens, becoming tubular and growing away from the vertebral axis. It then coils, inducing dorsal mesenteric development. During the 5th fetal week, the midgut is U-shaped and suspended by a dorsal mesentery distributed around the superior mesenteric artery. The apex of the intestinal loop communicates with the vitellin duct, which rapidly decreases in size. During the 5th to 6th fetal weeks, increases in intestinal length, along with the disproportionate amount of abdominal space occupied by the fetal liver, cause intestinal herniation into a mesothelial-lined sac within the umbilical cord (13). The cecum develops on the caudal limb and the vitellointestinal duct lies at the apex. A small portion of the caudal limb, between the attachment of the vitellointestinal duct and cecum, forms the terminal ileum. The appendix develops as a cecal diverticulum.

The midgut starts sliding back into the abdomen between the 10th and 12th weeks, a process accomplished in three phases (fig. 2-5). The first is a 90° counterclockwise rotation around the superior mesenteric artery. The second phase occurs at about the 10th week when there is enough room for the bowel to return to the abdominal cavity. The cranial loop of small bowel reenters the abdomen, first passing to the right of the superior mesenteric artery and rotating a further 180°, thereby making the total rotation of 270°. Small intestinal loops fill the central abdomen. The colon then returns, with

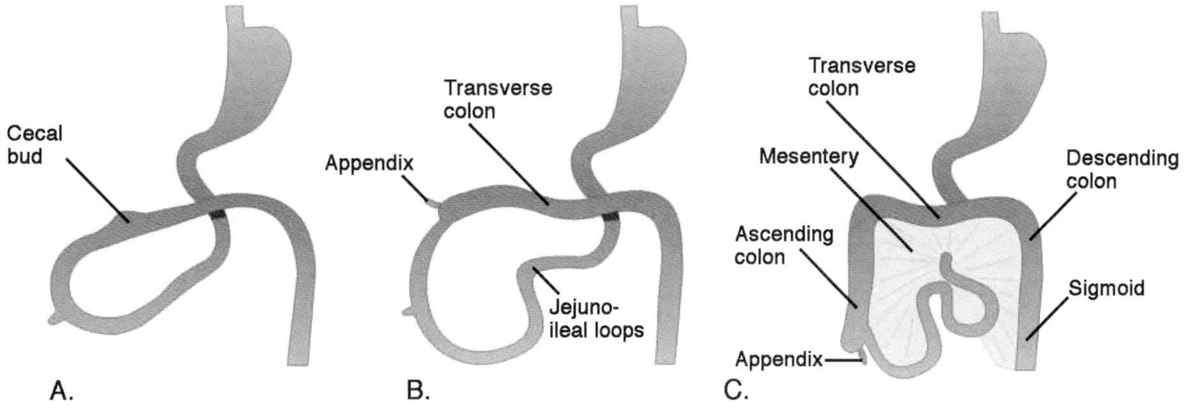

Figure 2-5

DEVELOPMENT OF THE INTESTINAL TRACT

A: Schematic diagram of the primitive intestinal loop after a 180° counterclockwise rotation. The transverse colon passes in front of the duodenum.

B: Intestinal loop after a 270° counterclockwise rotation.

C: Intestinal loops in their final position with the development of the mesenteries.

the cecum being the last to return to the right iliac fossa anterior to the duodenum and the superior mesenteric artery and below the liver (fig. 2-6). Later, the colon angulates as it crosses the duodenum to form the hepatic flexure. The distal transverse, descending, and sigmoid colon (hindgut derivatives) are supplied by the inferior mesenteric artery and occupy the left abdominal periphery, completing the colonic distribution around the small bowel.

The final phase is the fixation phase. The mesenteries of the cecum, ascending and descending colon shorten and are absorbed, thereby attaching the large bowel to the posterior abdominal wall. The transverse and sigmoid portions of the colon retain a full mesentery (6).

Although an anatomically distinguishable intestinal tract develops early in embryonic life, functional absorptive cells do not appear until later in gestation. A solid epithelial core fills the fetal gut during the 8th and 9th weeks. This core then vacuolates, creating the intestinal lumen. Apoptosis probably plays a role in the process. Intestinal differentiation occurs along a proximal to distal gradient. The epithelium develops from simple endodermal tubules early in embryogenesis, appearing as a multilayered sheet of undifferentiated endodermal cells with short microvilli. Deeper cells do not demonstrate any polarity; mitoses occur throughout

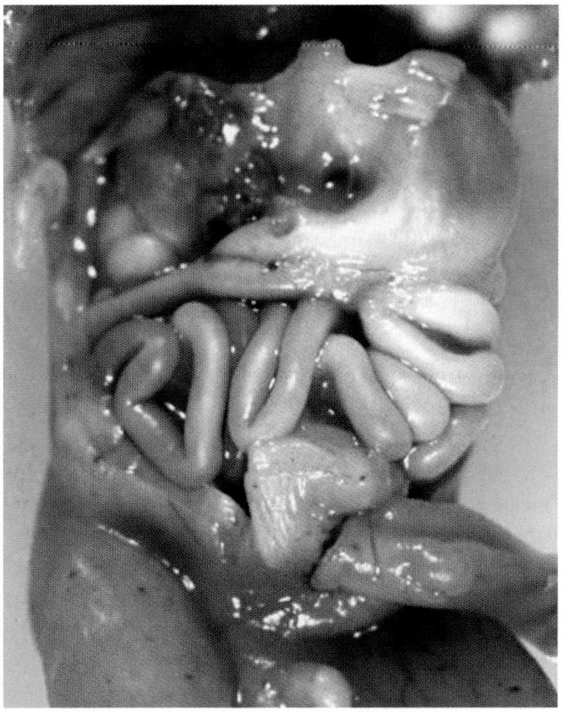

Figure 2-6

DEVELOPMENT OF THE INTESTINAL TRACT

Fourteen-week fetus shows the small intestine lying to the right side of the abdomen and the colon bunched on the left side. The fetus had not developed sufficiently for the rotation to have been complete. As a result, the intestines have not reached their final positions in the abdominal cavity.

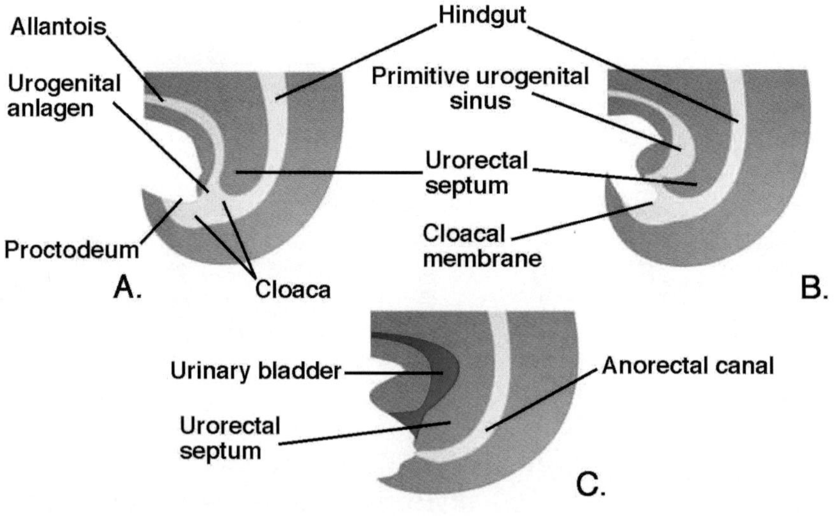

Figure 2-7

DEVELOPMENT OF THE ANORECTAL REGION

Figures A through C show the progressive development of the cloaca and its determination. At the 6th fetal week, the hindgut and urogenital sinus open to a common cloaca. The cloaca continues into the allantois. The inferior boundary is the cloacal membrane. The urogenital septum grows caudally toward the cloacal membrane, separating the posterior anorectum from the anterior genital sinus (B,C). The urogenital sinus forms the future urethra and urinary bladder.

the epithelium. Villus formation, with mesenchymal infiltration into the villous core, begins at the 9th gestational week. Between 9 and 10 weeks, the stratified epithelium converts to simple columnar epithelium (5). The progenitor cell region, which gives rise to the crypts, localizes to the intervillous area (4). Villi are long and tapering by 20 weeks; the muscle coats are obvious at this time. Enterocyte proliferation occurs along the entire villous length until several days before birth. The epithelium finishes its morphologic differentiation in the 4 to 5 days prior to birth (7).

Distal Colon, Rectum, and Anus

Hindgut development follows that of the midgut. The hindgut develops into the left transverse colon, descending colon, sigmoid colon, rectum, and upper anal canal. The descending colon becomes fixed. The sigmoid retains a mesocolon that reduces in length as other hindgut derivatives become fixed in the abdomen.

The complex development of the anal canal depends on the coordinated development of the proctodeum and the urorectal septum. It also depends on regression of the tail and tailgut and on the development of the sacrococcygeal vertebrae and lower spinal cord (2). The area must also maintain the relational positions of the uterus, adnexa, genitourinary tract, spinal sacrococcygeal region (1), and external genitalia.

A cloaca is identifiable by the 4th gestational week; major development of the anorectal canal occurs between the 5th and 6th weeks (fig. 2-7) (17). The fetal anal canal has two components: the cloacal component contributes to its upper two thirds; the proctodeal component forms its lower third. In adults, the junction of the cloacal and proctodeal components (the site of the former anal membrane) is defined by the pectinate line and anal valves. Coincident with the development of the urorectal septum, the mesenchyme around the cloacal membrane proliferates, leading to the development of the genital tubercles and the anal pit, on the floor of which is the cloacal membrane. The deep anal pit produces the proctodeal canal, and its development is accompanied by the shrinkage and ultimate disappearance of the tailfold and tailgut.

The cloacal membrane is divided into an anal membrane posteriorly and the larger urogenital membrane anteriorly. The anal membrane covers the terminal rectum, separating it from the external environment until the end of the 7th week when it ruptures. When the urogenital membrane disintegrates, it is incorporated into the urethral floor in the male and into the hymen in the female. After rupture of the anal membrane, squamous epithelium begins to extend cranially from the dorsal cloaca to reach the anal sinuses at about 180 mm of crown-rump length (9,17). At this time the characteristic epithelium of the anal transitional zone is present. The anal cushions are also present early in fetal life (14).

The tailgut is a blind hindgut extension into the tailfold, just distal to the cloacal membrane. As it grows, the proctodeum develops and the tailgut progressively resolves and is taken up into the lower cloaca. This process is completed by 56 days of gestation (16,17).

Developmental abnormalities of the urorectal septum result in a malpositioned rectum, imperforate anus, and abnormal connections between the rectum and the genitourinary tract. All developmental anomalies that are associated with fistulas between the gastrointestinal and genitourinary systems relate to the defective formation of the urorectal septum. Aberrant development of the lower spine or persistence of the tailgut and vestigial tail-like appendages are associated with anal or rectal malformations.

POSITIONAL ABNORMALITIES

An anatomic left-right asymmetry is established during embryogenesis. Variation from normal organ position (situs solitus) results in heterotaxy, expressed either as a randomization (situs ambiguous) or complete reversal (situs inversus) of normal organ position. The term heterotaxy refers to "other arrangements." Familial heterotaxy occurs with autosomal dominant, autosomal recessive, and X-linked inheritance (25).

Situs Inversus

Definition. In *situs inversus*, the organs lie in locations that are the mirror images of their normal positions. When complete, it affects both thoracic and abdominal organs. When incomplete, it affects the abdominal organs. Limited situs inversus affects only the stomach and duodenum.

Demography. Situs inversus affects 1/1,400 live births and it forms part of Kartagener's syndrome.

Associated Findings. In 80 percent of cases, partial situs inversus is associated with other malformations, including asplenia and duodenal stenosis, and may have a genetic basis. Complete situs inversus is nearly always sporadic and not accompanied by other abnormalities.

Etiology. Complete situs inversus is the most common chemically-induced congenital abnormality. Several chemical teratogens cause symmetric body defects. Many children with situs inversus and a neural tube defect have mothers with insulin-dependent diabetes mellitus.

Clinical Features. Significant mortality is associated with situs inversus because most patients (95 percent) have associated cardiac defects. Major associated gastrointestinal anomalies include annular pancreas, midgut volvulus, duodenal atresia, and mucosal duodenal diaphragm. Patients present in the neonatal period with bilious vomiting and upper abdominal distension. Duodenal atresia may cause a "double bubble" sign with absent distal gas on plain abdominal radiographs. Upper barium contrast films are usually diagnostic. Jaundice is common.

Gross Findings. See definition.

Microscopic Findings. Situs inversus does not change organ function or histology.

Treatment and Prognosis. The prognosis in individuals with complete situs inversus is usually excellent. Prognosis is most adversely affected by the presence of associated abnormalities. The prognosis of these patients is generally reflected in the severity of the upper respiratory problems. Patients may also be infertile. Patients with Kartagener's syndrome may have a worse prognosis. These patients have abnormal cilia and as a result produce thick, tenacious bronchial and sinus secretions that lead to chronic sinusitis and bronchiectasis. Common gastric disorders may present in atypical ways in these patients, possibly delaying diagnosis.

Dextrogastria

Definition. *Dextrogastria* exists when the stomach and esophageal diaphragmatic hiatus lie to the right of the midline and the first part of the duodenum lies to the left.

Demography. Dextrogastria affects approximately 1/6,000 to 8,000 births (24). As an isolated anomaly, it affects less than 1/100,000 births.

Clinical Features. No specific clinical features result from dextrogastria. When the stomach lies in an abnormal position, however, other typical gastric diseases may present in atypical ways. The endoscopist may experience some difficulty in orientation if the anomaly is not appreciated.

Gross Findings. Dextrogastria occurs in three forms: 1) associated with total situs inversus, 2) associated with dextrocardia but with no other transposition, and 3) as an isolated abnormality.

Microscopic Findings. There are no histologic abnormalities associated with this condition.

Malrotations/Nonrotations

Definition. Intestinal malrotations or nonrotations are those conditions in which various gastrointestinal organs lie in an abnormal position due to a failure to complete normal fetal rotational events or retention of their nonrotated location. *Nonrotation* occurs when the midgut fails to rotate as it returns to the abdomen, so that the duodenal-jejunal loop remains in the right abdomen. *Malrotation* presents as a 180° anti-clockwise extra-abdominal rotation in which the cecum fails to descend into its normal position in the right iliac fossa. *Mixed* or *incomplete rotation* occurs when only the caudal limb of the midgut loop rotates an additional 90° beyond the first counterclockwise 90° rotation of both limbs of the midgut. As a result, the subpyloric cecum is partially fixed to the posterior wall by fibrous bands that pass over the duodenum, occasionally causing extrinsic compression. *Reversed rotation* occurs when the midgut loop rotates an additional 180° in a counterclockwise fashion. The duodenum and superior mesenteric arteries lie anterior to the transverse colon.

Demography. Intestinal malrotations affect approximately 1/6,000 live births (22). Some cases show a familial distribution with both autosomal recessive and autosomal dominant inheritance patterns.

Associated Findings. Three percent of patients have associated abnormalities (Table 2-2) (20,21,26–28). Intestinal rotational abnormalities are particularly common in patients with polysplenia (left isomerism) and asplenia (right isomerism) syndromes.

Table 2-2

ABNORMALITIES ASSOCIATED WITH SMALL INTESTINAL MALROTATION

Prune-belly syndrome
Natal teeth with intestinal pseudoobstruction
Delayed gastric emptying
Duodenal dilatation
Patent ductus arteriosus
Annular pancreas
Midgut volvulus and facial anomalies
Omphalocele
Gastroschisis
Craniofacial anomalies (especially in infants with intrauterine opiate or heroin exposure)
Trisomy 13, 18, and 21
Situs inversus
Atresias
Esophageal atresia
Biliary atresia or stenosis
Intestinal atresia or stenosis
Hernias
Diaphragmatic
Paraduodenal
Internal
OIES complex
Omphalocele
Exstrophy of the cloaca
Imperforate anus
Spinal defects
Sirenomelia
Unseparated lower limbs
Absent genital structures
Lower colonic agenesis
Renal agenesis

Etiology. Intestinal malrotations or nonrotations result from disordered or interrupted embryonic intestinal counterclockwise rotations around the superior mesenteric artery.

Clinical Features. Malrotations frequently cause symptoms in the neonatal period, due in part to the presence of other associated malformations. Patients with intestinal malrotation present with signs and symptoms of duodenal obstruction, intermittent volvulus, or intussusception. Patients develop bilious vomiting, abdominal distension, and rectal bleeding. Infants may develop malabsorption with steatorrhea and protein-losing enteropathy due to mesenteric lymphatic obstruction.

Adults with intestinal malrotations often have a lifelong history of nonspecific abdominal complaints, including acute symptoms when they were children. The most common symptoms are vomiting and chronic intermittent crampy abdominal pain from torsion, obstruction, peritoneal bands, volvulus, or intussusception (23). The incidence of volvulus is greater in the sigmoid colon than elsewhere in the large intestine, perhaps reflecting the solid nature of its luminal contents. Occasionally, a malrotation becomes evident during pregnancy. Patients often have a history of constipation and intermittent abdominal distension. The clinical presentation may be as an acute bowel obstruction. Plain abdominal films are often diagnostic.

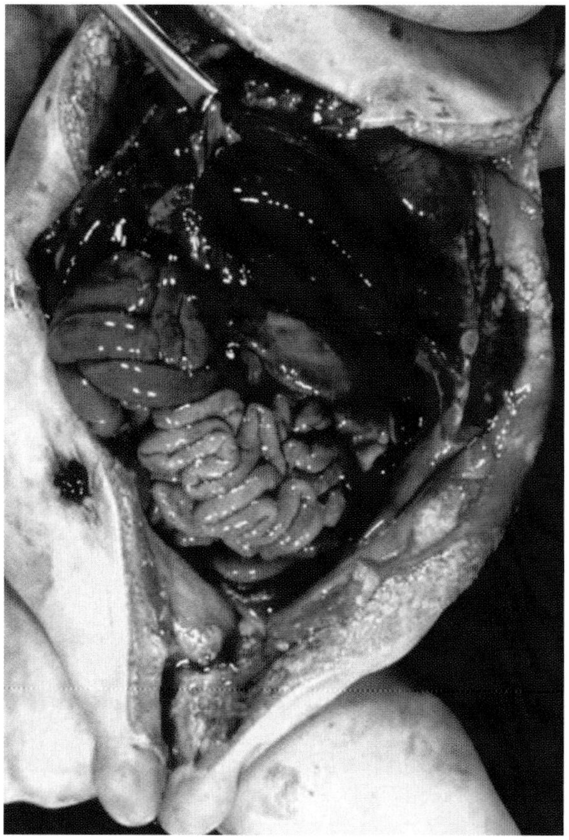

Figure 2-8

INTESTINAL MALROTATION

The small intestine in this term infant lies as a mass of coiled bowel loops in the lower portion of the abdominal cavity. The large intestine lies as a mass of coiled loops just beneath the liver.

Gross Findings. There is obvious intestinal misplacement within the abdominal cavity with malrotation. The intestines often lie to one side, appearing as a large mass of nonrotated bowel (fig. 2-8). The duodenum lacks the normal C-shaped configuration, lying vertically downward and to the right of the superior mesenteric vessels. The cecum lies in various locations, depending on the extent to which it failed to rotate: in the left iliac fossa, in the midline of the pelvis, or in a subhepatic location. The ascending colon retains its mesentery and runs upward, just to the left of the midline, lying below the gastric curvature where a loop of transverse colon connects to a normally situated descending colon. The transverse colon and splenic flexure may lie posterior to the stomach and anterior to all, or part, of the pancreas, in a location known as pancreatico-interposition. They may also lie in a retrosplenic location. The entire malpositioned bowel, from the duodenum to the splenic flexure, remains unanchored, supported by a single mesentery with a very narrow base, predisposing it to undergo intestinal volvulus. The body attempts to correct the unstable state of the malpositioned intestine by forming fibrous bands or adhesions between abdominal structures. These bands and adhesions may cause future obstruction or volvulus.

Microscopic Findings. The histology of the abnormally placed organs is normal unless there is a coexisting abnormality, such as an atresia or stenosis.

Treatment and Prognosis. Positional abnormalities in and of themselves require no treatment. Infants presenting with obstruction without mucosal compromise (as in acute volvulus), may undergo a laparoscopic Ladd procedure to correct the malrotation, bypassing the need for open abdominal surgery (19). Unknown rotational anomalies, however, may pose serious risks to patients. This typically occurs when organs lying in an unusual location cause symptoms. Thus, appendicitis developing in an unusual location is often clinically diagnosed as some other disorder. Subhepatic appendicitis may mimic pancreatitis or cholecystitis, resulting in a delayed diagnosis. Many of these complications may only be diagnosed during the course of a laparotomy for peritonitis.

ABDOMINAL WALL DEFECTS

The most common anomalies of the fetal ventral abdominal wall are omphalocele, gastroschisis, and umbilical cord hernia.

Gastroschisis

Definition. *Gastroschisis* is the persistent herniation of abdominal viscera through an abdominal wall defect at the base of the umbilicus. The abdominal organs remain outside the abdominal cavity. No peritoneal sac or amniotic remnant covers the eviscerated abdominal contents.

Demography. The incidence of gastroschisis has risen, increasing from 0.48/10,000 births in 1980 to 3.16/10,000 in 1993 (41,42). Young (15 to 19 years), socially disadvantaged women

Table 2-3
ABNORMALITIES ASSOCIATED WITH GASTROSCHISIS
Gastrointestinal
Intestinal atresia
Gastric heterotopia
Intestinal nonrotation
Pancreatic heterotopia
Abnormal intestinal fixation
Misplaced gallbladder
Ventricular septal defect
Cryptorchidism

have the highest risk of having a child with gastroschisis (43). An increased risk of gastroschisis also is associated with the intrapartum use of recreational drugs or smoking (41), exposure to salicylates, and exposure to radiation (34). Gastroschisis predominates among male infants.

Associated Findings. Gastroschisis is an isolated malformation in up to 79 percent of cases (31). Associated congenital malformations are seen in 16 to 20 percent of infants (Table 2-3) (30,40,41).

Etiology. Gastroschisis probably results from vascular injury and ischemia of the abdominal wall during the 5th to 11th fetal weeks, leading to defective somatopleural mesenchymal differentiation (40). The ischemia results from intrauterine disruption of the right omphalomesenteric artery.

Clinical Features. There is a strong association with preterm delivery, low birth weight, and perceived fetal distress as reflected by an increased rate of emergency cesarean section (41). The average birth weight and gestational age of infants with gastroschisis are low, especially for those with multiple anomalies (31). The degree of growth failure correlates with the level of prematurity. Exposure of the bowel to amniotic fluid leads to perivisceritis and premature birth. The damaged bowel frequently develops secondary motility problems and malabsorption, which may present even following surgical repair. Other complications include obstruction due to coexisting malrotation, diverticulitis, ischemia, and perforation. Patients with ectopic gastric mucosa in the exteriorized bowel may present with a gastrointestinal hemorrhage. Gastroschisis is associated with increased

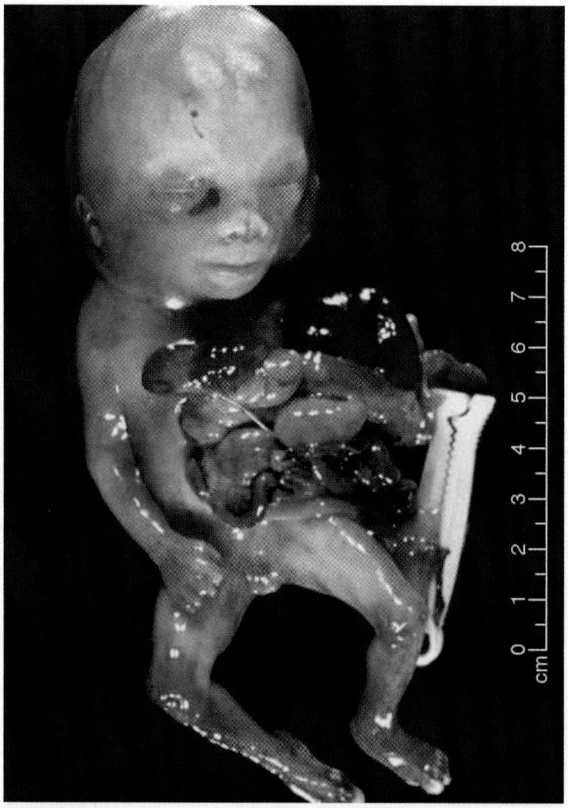

Figure 2-9

GASTROSCHISIS

The mass of abdominal organs remains outside the abdominal wall in this premature infant. This includes the intestines as well as the liver, spleen, and stomach. (Fig. 9.4 from Fenoglio-Preiser C. Gastrointestinal pathology, an atlas and text, 2nd ed. Philadelphia: Lippincott-Raven; 1999:312.)

maternal serum and amniotic fluid alpha-fetoprotein (AFP) levels because the exposed membrane surfaces allow AFP to transude. Nearly all patients with gastroschisis have AFP elevations, and acetyl cholinesterase is nearly always detectable in amniotic fluid, albeit at much lower concentrations than for open neural tube defects (32).

Radiologic Findings. Antenatal ultrasound often allows an accurate diagnosis of gastroschisis.

Gross Findings. Gastroschisis may involve only the intestines or it may affect many other organs. Parts of the stomach, small intestine, and colon herniate through an abdominal wall defect, usually to the right of the umbilical cord (fig. 2-9). All infants with gastroschisis have coexisting intestinal nonrotation and abnormal intestinal fixations.

Microscopic Findings. The histology of the various organs may be normal or changes may be present reflecting the presence of associated congenital abnormalities, heterotopias, atresia, meconium peritonitis, or perivisceritis. The last two entities lead to gastrointestinal wall thickening, serosal edema, fibrinous exudates, and fibrosis. The intestinal muscularis propria may become hypertrophic. Acute inflammation, consisting predominantly of neutrophils and mononuclear cells, may be present and may lead to postnatal bowel dysfunction.

Treatment and Prognosis. Long-term outcome in the absence of major chromosomal and structural abnormalities is excellent (37). Patient prognosis depends in part on whether the gastroschisis is an isolated lesion or whether there are associated abnormalities. The goal of the surgeon is to accomplish abdominal wall closure in a single stage. An alternate approach is to perform a staged closure using prosthetic materials while maintaining adequate nutritional support. Other considerations include prevention and control of sepsis, maintenance of respiratory status, and risk of dysfunction of the kidneys, liver, and intestine because of increased abdominal pressure. Necrotizing enterocolitis may affect as many as 20 percent of infants following repair of gastroschisis and is responsible for significant morbidity (36). Other complications of the repair include motility disorders and abdominal wall hernias.

Animal Models. Gastroschisis occurs with a high frequency in the HLG inbred mouse strain. The risk of gastroschisis increases significantly after exposure to irradiation with X rays during preimplantation and its development involves a recessively inherited HLG susceptibility allele. There is a possible locus responsible for radiation-induced gastroschisis (Rigs1) in a region of mouse chromosome 7 (34).

Omphalocele

Definition. *Omphalocele* is an external mass of abdominal contents covered by a variably translucent peritoneal and/or amniotic membrane. Synonyms include *exomphalos* and *exomphalocele*.

Demography. Omphaloceles affect 2.5/60,000 to 2.0/3,000 live births. Significant heterogeneity exists in the prevalence rates among different geographic regions, with especially high rates occurring throughout the British Isles (31). The male to female incidence is 3 to 1; however, a significant female excess exists among the cases of omphalocele associated with neural tube defects. The rare OEIS (omphalocele, cloacal exstrophy, imperforate anus, spinal defects) complex affects 1/200,000 to 400,000 pregnancies. In the United Kingdom and Ireland, there is a tendency for omphaloceles to be associated with anencephaly and spina bifida.

Table 2-4

ABNORMALITIES ASSOCIATED WITH OMPHALOCELES
Heart anomalies
Intestinal atresia
Chromosomal defects
Genitourinary anomalies (cloacal or bladder exstrophy)
Craniofacial defects
Diaphragmatic abnormalities
Liver and bile duct abnormalities
Single umbilical artery
Syndromes
OEIS complex
Major changes
Omphalocele
Cloacal exstrophy
Imperforate anus
Spinal defects
Possible associated changes
Meningomyeloceles
Lower limb defects
Colonic duplication
Duodenal webs
Malrotation
Short bowel syndrome
Cryptorchidism

Associated Findings. Up to 54 percent of infants with omphaloceles have associated anomalies (Table 2-4) compared with only 5 percent of those with gastroschisis (29,31). Omphaloceles complicate several syndromes (Table 2-4). Many fetuses with an omphalocele have an abnormal karyotype.

Etiology. OEIS complex occurs sporadically or it affects twins or siblings, suggesting that some cases have a genetic basis. There is often a history of maternal diabetes mellitus or hydantoin or diazepam administration (35,38). The OEIS complex arises from a single, localized

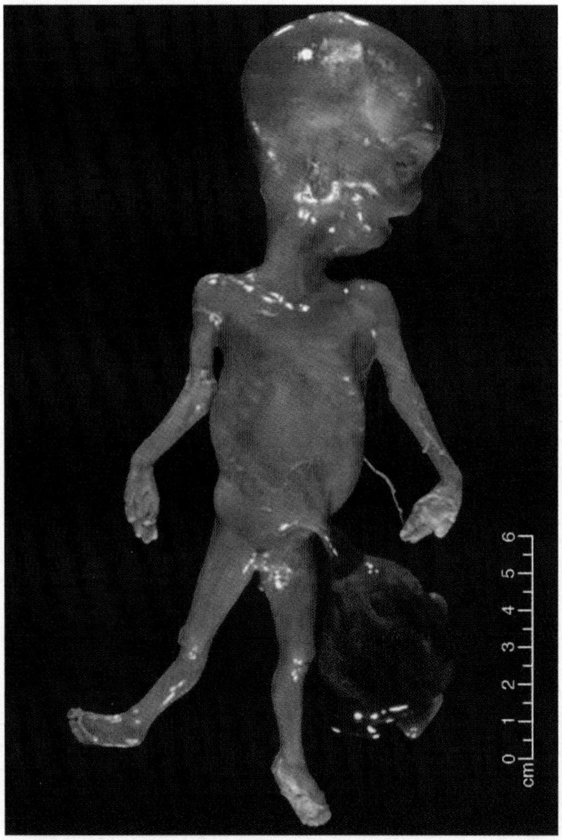

Figure 2-10
OMPHALOCELE
The viscera within the omphalocele had twisted, leading to infarction of the contents.

mesodermal defect early in development that contributes to infraumbilical mesenchymal, cloacal septum, and caudal vertebral abnormalities. Some patients with omphalocele and the Miller-Dieker syndrome have a deletion at chromosome 17p13.3, suggesting that a gene(s) in this region plays a major role in lateral fold closure or the return of the midgut from the body stalk to the abdomen. Trisomy 18 affects some patients.

Pathophysiology. Four somatic folds (a cephalic fold, two lateral folds, and a caudal fold) define the anterior thoracic and abdominal walls during the 3rd gestational week. These folds migrate centrally to fuse at the umbilical ring, usually by the 18th week. Arrested fold migration or development results in anterior wall defects and a widening of the umbilical ring.

Clinical Features. The average birth weight and gestational age of infants with omphalocele are low. The amniotic membrane and peritoneum protect the developing intestinal loops from the damaging effects of exposure to amniotic fluid seen in gastroschisis. This may be important, since it has been suggested that amniotic fluid may be toxic to myenteric neurons.

Gross Findings. Omphaloceles range in size from only a few centimeters to lesions that involve almost the entire anterior abdominal wall. The abdominal viscera lie within a sac (fig. 2-10) that initially is moist and transparent but with time becomes dry, fibrotic, opaque, friable, and prone to rupture, resulting in secondary evisceration. Abdominal skin may cover the sac base and the umbilical cord is usually attached to its apex or slightly to the side. Giant omphaloceles, measuring 5 cm or more in greatest dimension, may contain the stomach, liver, spleen, pancreas, and intestines. Smaller omphaloceles usually only contain the intestines.

Microscopic Findings. The histology of the displaced organs tends to be normal unless there is a coexisting congenital abnormality. The lining of the sac that covers the eviscerated organs consists of peritoneum internally and amnion externally (fig. 2-11).

Differential Diagnosis. The major entity in the differential diagnosis of omphalocele is umbilical hernia. The presence of an amniotic membrane or peritoneal membrane serves to distinguish the two lesions, since these are only present in patients with omphaloceles.

Treatment and Prognosis. Patient prognosis depends on the associated anomaly(ies). Omphalocele repair is similar to that for gastroschisis. Formerly, most infants with the OEIS complex died. Today, long-term survival of such patients can be achieved by successful corrective surgery but the associated structural anomalies, including meningomyelocele and severe limb aplasia or hypoplasia, influence the patient's quality of life. The current treatment includes closure of the omphalocele, separation of the gastrointestinal tract from the hemibladders, and closure of the two hemibladders as a single viscus. The colon can be pulled through in some cases either immediately or later. The bladder is augmented, sometimes using the stomach. Although two thirds of patients are

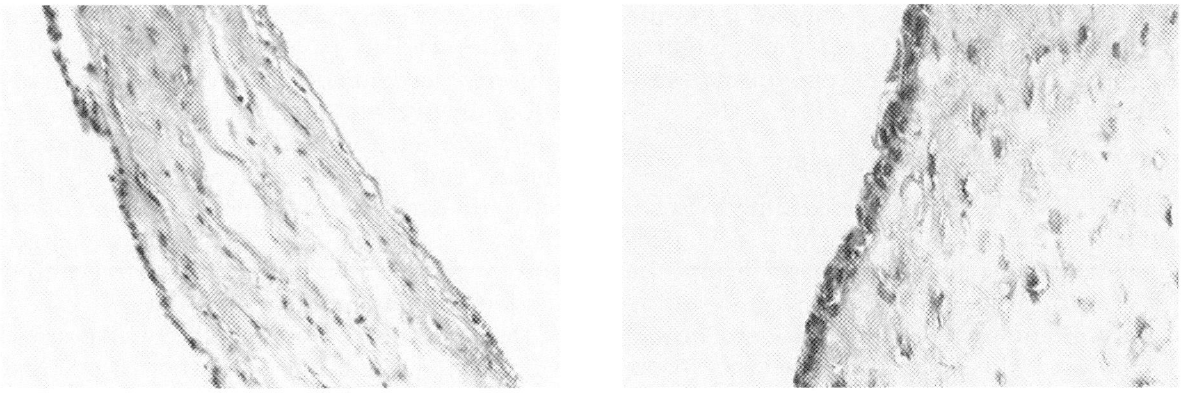

Figure 2-11

SAC COVERING THE ORGANS IN THE OMPHALOCELE

Left: Histologically, the sac consists of amnion externally (left) peritoneum internally (right). Right: The amnion is shown at higher magnification.

genetic males, some advocate that they should be raised as females because they lack adequate tissues to construct a phallus (39). Magnetic resonance imaging (MRI) of the spine shows tethering of the spinal cord in all patients, which can be released neurosurgically (39).

Umbilical Hernia

Definition. An *umbilical hernia* is a protrusion of the umbilicus that is more pronounced when the infant strains and reduces when the infant is supine and at rest.

Demography. Umbilical hernias occur in 10 to 30 percent of term infants and the incidence increases to as high as 75 percent in premature children who weigh between 1.0 and 1.5 kg at birth (33). A fascial defect in the abdominal wall allows intestinal contents to protrude through the opening. Umbilical hernia is 6 to 10 times more likely to develop in African-American infants than in white infants (33). Birth weight is a predisposing factor. More than 80 percent of infants weighing less than 1,200 g have an umbilical hernia compared with 21 percent of infants weighing more than 2,500 g.

Etiology. An umbilical hernia develops when the umbilical ring fails to close after cord separation.

Clinical Features. The diagnosis is made by the presence of a bulge in the umbilicus coupled with an easily palpable fascial defect. The bulge becomes more apparent with crying, straining, or during defecation (33). It is rarely painful and the risk of incarceration or strangulation is negligible. Most close spontaneously during the first 24 months of life.

Gross Findings. The diameter of the defect is rarely more than 2 cm.

Microscopic Findings. The defect is covered posteriorly by peritoneum and anteriorly by skin. There is no amnion as there is in an omphalocele.

Differential Diagnosis. The differential diagnosis of umbilical hernia includes epigastric hernia, omphalocele, and diastasis recti. Epigastric hernias are small, midline bulges between the umbilicus and the xiphoid process that result from preperitoneal fat that protrudes through a small fascial defect. Omphaloceles are discussed in a previous section and represent a defect in the center of the abdomen with exteriorization of the viscera. These are covered with a translucent membrane and require surgery for treatment. Diastasis recti is a longitudinal separation of the rectus abdominal muscle. It is most commonly found in a supraumbilical position but can also be suprapubic.

Treatment and Prognosis. Most umbilical hernias undergo spontaneous closure and surgery is not recommended unless the hernia persists beyond the age of 4 to 6 years or unless the fascial defect is bigger than 1.5 to 2.0 cm by 2 years of age. The size of the fascial defect rather than the amount of reducible omentum or protruding bowel should be considered in any decision regarding surgical repair. If the fascial ring is not completely intact, spontaneous closure is unlikely. Referral to a pediatric surgeon is appropriate. The risk of incarceration and strangulation increases with age.

MESOCOLIC HERNIAS

Definition. When the descending mesocolon fails to adhere to the posterior parietal peritoneum, the small bowel can herniate into the sac that forms between these layers, resulting in what is known as a left *paraduodenal hernia*. Similarly, a right paraduodenal hernia can occur in a sac formed by a nonadherent descending mesocolon in the posterior parietal peritoneum. When a defect occurs in the transverse mesocolon, a *transmesocolic* or *omentomesenteric parietal hernia* occurs. The term *mesenterico-parietal hernia* is also used.

Etiology. Mesocolic hernias result from the abnormal return of the midgut after its physiological herniation into a defective mesenteric attachment, with formation of a retroperitoneal sac. Additional hernias can occur around the ileocecal valve, the bladder, and at the foramen of Winslow.

Clinical Features. Patients present with nausea, vomiting, abdominal pain, distension, and dehydration. They may become obstipated, with or without passage of either feces or gas. The pain most typically occurs in the periumbilical region. Closed loop obstructions may occur. Mesocolic hernias may present as an acute abdominal emergency should the bowel become incarcerated. Conventional radiology may suggest the diagnosis. Occasionally, computerized tomography (CT) (with contrast) or barium studies are required.

Gross Findings. The inferior mesenteric arteries run near the orifice of left paraduodenal hernias whereas the superior mesenteric vessels course near the orifice of right hernia sacs. The transmesocolic hernia has a middle colic artery coursing on the right side of the orifice.

CONGENITAL DIAPHRAGMATIC HERNIA

Definition. *Congenital diaphragmatic hernia* is the presence of abdominal contents in the thoracic cavity secondary to a congenital diaphragmatic defect. There are four types of diaphragmatic hernia: 1) left posterolateral through the left Bochdalek canal. In this situation, the stomach, intestines, and spleen herniate into the thoracic cavity; 2) right posterolateral (through the right Bochdalek canal). In this situation, the liver and intestines herniate into the thorax; 3) retrosternal through the Morgagni canals. This form occurs less commonly and only the liver and intestines herniate; and 4) hiatal hernia. The esophageal hiatus enlarges and the stomach herniates. Rarely, the central tendon of the diaphragm is absent.

Demography. Diaphragmatic hernias affect 1/2,000 to 5,000 births (44). The left posterolateral hernia is the most common type of congenital diaphragmatic hernia.

Associated Findings. Patients often have coexisting malformations, especially midgut malrotation. Urinary tract abnormalities and Wiedemann-Beckwith syndrome affect patients with congenital posterolateral diaphragmatic defects. Patients with the autosomal recessive Fryns syndrome often have a lateral diaphragmatic hernia and a number of associated abnormalities.

Etiology. There are four components contributing to the diaphragm: 1) the pleural peritoneal membrane, 2) the septum transversum, 3) the dorsal mesentery of the esophagus, and 4) the body wall; these fuse by the 6th developmental week. Defective development of one or more of these units results in diaphragmatic hernias. The ventral part of the diaphragm derives from the septum transversum, which separates the embryonic heart from the abdominal contents. Normally it fuses with the sternum and rib cage leaving small canals known as the foramina of Morgagni lying laterally on either side of the sternum. The dorsal diaphragm forms from the dorsal mesentery, but posterolateral communications, known as the canals of Bochdalek, persist on either side between the pleural and peritoneal cavities. At first, only the pleural and peritoneal membranes fuse. Later, muscle grows into them from the body wall. The thoracic and abdominal cavities are separate from one another by the 8th to 9th weeks of gestation. Diaphragmatic hernias result when there is agenesis of one or both diaphragmatic leaflets, muscle aplasia with eventration, or defective formation with herniation. A gap results which, depending on its size and location, allows abdominal organs to herniate through it into the thoracic cavity.

Clinical Features. Large diaphragmatic hernias are frequently associated with both gastrointestinal and respiratory symptoms, mainly due to compressive effects. The mediastinal contents (heart and thymus) may shift, compressing the contralateral lung. Cyanosis and dyspnea are the earliest neonatal manifestations, as well as gasping and vomiting. Clinically, respiratory movements and breath sounds are decreased or absent with audible peristaltic sounds in the affected hemithorax. Patients with right posterolateral hernias usually develop fewer pulmonary complications because of the presence of the liver. Torsion or volvulus of the gastrointestinal contents within the hernia can lead to obstruction and ischemia if not corrected. A chest radiograph should suggest the diagnosis.

Gross Findings. The hernia wall consists of peritoneum and pleura, and the hernias may contain the stomach and various portions of small bowel and possibly liver. Diaphragmatic hernias tend to be smaller than diaphragmatic eventrations.

Microscopic Findings. The histology of the herniated bowel is normal unless a complication such as obstruction or ulceration has occurred. Then, the histology reflects the complication.

Differential Diagnosis. Congenital hernias differ from acquired hiatal hernias in that the diaphragmatic defect does not usually involve the hiatal orifice.

Treatment and Prognosis. Congenital diaphragmatic hernias require surgical repair. Patient outcome depends on the presence of associated malformations and chromosomal anomalies, as well as on the volume of the contralateral lung and the degree of coexisting pulmonary hypoplasia. Most untreated symptomatic patients die, often due to severe pulmonary hypoplasia.

ATRESIA AND STENOSIS

Definition. *Atresia* means "not perforated"; the term is applied to congenital anomalies in which there is complete discontinuity of the gastrointestinal lumen. *Stenosis* refers to a narrowing of the gastrointestinal lumen without complete obliteration. *Tracheoesophageal* (TE) *fistula* is an anomalous connection between a portion of the esophagus and the tracheobronchial tree. TE fistulas frequently complicate esophageal atresia and stenosis.

Apple peel atresia is a form of atresia in which the bowel demonstrates a spiral configuration in addition to the area of the atresia. *Complex atresia* is an atresia with additional complications, such as secondary ischemia.

Demography. Overall, atresia occurs more often than stenosis, ranging in incidence from 1/2,000 to 6,000 live births (75,89). It represents the most common abdominal surgical disorder of infants. Esophageal atresia is the most frequent gastrointestinal atresia, followed by anal, duodenal, jejunal, ileal, and colonic atresias. Esophageal atresia with a common TE fistula affects 1/800 to 1,500 live births. Complete esophageal atresia affects 1/3,000 live births.

Infantile hypertrophic pyloric stenosis (IHPS) ranges in incidence from 0.28 to 6.80 percent of live births. The incidence depends on the patient population studied (45). White race and male gender are associated with a higher incidence of IHPS; high birth order, older maternal age, higher maternal education, and low birth weight are associated with a lower incidence. The disorder usually affects the firstborn child, with a male to female ratio of approximately 4 to 1. IHPS commonly affects whites; it rarely affects Latin Americans, blacks, or Asians (75).

Pyloric atresia is extremely rare, with an incidence of 0.0001 to 0.0003 percent of live births (52); it accounts for less than 1 percent of all gastrointestinal atresias, as does the rare gastric atresia. Duodenal atresia is less common than duodenal stenosis. Jejunoileal atresia affects 1/500 to 2,000 live births.

Large intestinal atresia accounts for less than 10 percent of all gastrointestinal atresias (54). Atresias of the ascending and transverse colon develop more commonly than distal large intestinal atresias. Colonic atresia unassociated with atresia at other sites is uncommon and accounts for 1.8 to 15.0 percent of all intestinal atresias. The incidence of colonic atresia is 1/20,000 to 50,000 live births, and affects both sexes equally. Low birth weight premature babies and monozygotic twins have a higher risk of intestinal atresia than other infants. Multiple atresias occur in 4.7 percent of infants. Intestinal atresias may be more common in blacks. Patients with VATER (vertebral defects, anal atresia, TE fistula, and renal dysplasia) or VACTERL (vertebral or vascular defects, anal atresia, cardiac anomalies, TE fistula with esophageal atresia, renal agenesis, and radial or other limb defects) syndrome are most likely to be male (78).

Associated Findings. Patients with all gastrointestinal atresias frequently have other congenital anomalies.

Esophagus. Approximately one third of patients with esophageal atresia have associated congenital anomalies involving the cardiovascular (29 to 37 percent), gastrointestinal (8 to 17 percent), neurologic (12 to 20 percent), genitourinary (11 to 28 percent), or orthopedic (10 to 49 percent) systems (Tables 2-5, 2-6) (49,51, 62). Infants with the VACTERL syndrome are significantly more likely to have other defects, including diaphragmatic defects, oral clefts, bladder exstrophy, omphalocele, and neural tube defects (48).

Stomach. Associated anomalies affect 6 to 12 percent of infants with IHPS (50,51), especially intestinal malrotation, obstructive urinary tract defects, and esophageal atresia (45). Pyloric stenosis is associated with several chromosomal aneuploid syndromes (Table 2-7) (96).

Intestine. Duodenal atresia frequently is associated with other anomalies (Table 2-8) (59,84). Familial jejunal atresia may be associated with renal dysplasia and there is an increased frequency of cystic fibrosis among infants with jejunoileal atresia (79). The apple peel atresia has the highest rate of associated anomalies (82). Colonic atresia may coexist with other gastrointestinal or laryngeal atresias, gastroschisis (95), and Hirschsprung's disease (64).

Multiple Atresias. Hereditary multiple gastrointestinal atresias affect the gut from the pylorus to the rectum. Patients with multiple intestinal atresias may also have biliary atresia (95) or an immunodeficiency syndrome (80). Cardiovascular and other gastrointestinal malformations are the most common associated major abnormalities; these are a major cause of morbidity and mortality. Skeletal and limb defects are the most frequent minor anomalies. Epidermolysis bullosa is associated with pyloric, esophageal, and anal atresia.

Etiology. Esophageal atresia and TE fistulas result from the failure of the tracheal bud to develop normally from the primitive foregut (see fig. 2-2). Intestinal atresia occurs as both a sporadic and a familial disorder. Esophageal atresia may have a polygenic basis with environmental influences. There is no consistent cause, although prenatal exposure to lead, thalidomide (72), cafergot (60), or alcohol (87); young maternal age (less than 20 years); and maternal shock, hypotension, and diabetes may represent risk factors. Thalidomide is a teratogen with antiangiogenic properties that causes stunted limb growth. Thalidomide may exert its antiangiogenic properties via the generation of toxic hydroxyl radicals which impair vasculogenesis and angiogenesis during embryoid body development (81). This compound also inhibits the angiogenesis induced by basic fibroblast growth factor (55,63,74,94). Most intestinal atresias follow some form of ischemic injury (68). Small intestinal atresia may complicate midtrimester amniocentesis (89), intrauterine intussusception due to a Meckel diverticulum, or fetal infections.

Twins have a higher rate of small intestinal atresia than single birth infants, possibly due to vascular disruption in monozygotic twins (53). Chromosomal abnormalities occur in 5.2

Table 2-5

NONSYNDROMIC ANOMALIES ASSOCIATED WITH ESOPHAGEAL ATRESIA

Sacral dimple
Abnormal palmar creases
Congenital ptosis
Numerous ear abnormalities
Macrotia
Bat ears
Pharyngeal pouch
High arches
Undescended testes
Clicking hip
Down's syndrome
Antley-Bixler syndrome
Cardiac anomalies
Gastrointestinal anomalies
Hiatal hernia
Pyloric stenosis
Meckel diverticulum
Anorectal agenesis
Imperforate anus
Duodenal atresia
Annular pancreas

Table 2-6

ATRESIA AND STENOSIS: MULTIPLE ANOMALY SYNDROMES

Syndrome	Prominent Features
VATER syndrome	Vertebral defects, anal atresia, tracheoesophageal defects, renal dysplasia
VATER association	3 of the 5 anomalies seen in VATER syndrome
VACTERL anomaly (incidence 1.6/10,000 live births	VATER syndrome + cardiac anomalies, vascular defects, radial or limb defects, single umbilical artery
VACTERL-H syndrome (David-O'Callighan syndrome)	VACTERL + hydrocephaly
VACTERL-X	X-linked form of VACTERL-H syndrome with the absence of cardiac defects
Feingold's syndrome	Hand and foot anomalies, microcephaly, esophageal/duodenal atresia, short palpebral fissures, learning disabilities
Bartsocas-Papas syndrome	Bilateral renal agenesis, esophageal atresia, hypoplastic diaphragm, unilateral renal agenesis, agenesis of the penile shaft, anal atresia
MODED syndrome (Frydman)	Microcephaly, type A brachydactyly, variable learning disabilities, short stature, duodenal atresia, patent ductus arteriosus, hallux valgus, restricted elbow and finger movements, mesophalangy, syndactyly of toes
CHARGE syndrome	Coloboma, heart disease, choanal atresia, growth and development retardation, genital hypoplasia, ear anomalies, micrognathia, cleft lip, cleft palate, renal anomalies
OEIS	Omphalocele, exstrophy of the bladder, imperforate anus, spinal defects
Facio-auriculo-vertebral syndrome	Asymmetric hypoplasia of malar, maxillary, and mandibular areas; microtia; deafness; hemivertebrae; epibulbar dermoid; macrostomia; microphthalmia; cleft lip/palate, cardiac defects, hypoplastic lung; renal anomalies; rib defects
DiGeorge's syndrome	Absent or hypoplastic thymus, absent or hypoplastic parathyroids, aortic arch defects, conotruncal defects, unusual facies, mental deficiency
Down's syndrome	Hypotonia, protuberant tongue, mental deficiency, brachycephaly, upslanting palpebral fissures, small ears, Brushfield spots, short incurved fifth fingers, cardiac defects, loose skin at posterior neck
Trisomy 18	Severe mental deficiency, prominent occiput, short palpebral fissures, camptodactyly, low arch dermal ridges, short sternum, congenital heart defects
Dyskeratosis congenita	Irregular hyperpigmentation and patchy atrophic hypopigmentation of skin, leukoplakia, nail dystrophy, pancytopenia, osteoporosis, mental deficiency
Maternal phenylketonuria	Microcephaly, mental retardation, growth deficiency, congenital heart disease
Opitz syndrome	Genital anomaly in males, hypertelorism, widow's peak, hernias, cardiac defects, cleft lip/palate

percent of patients with esophageal atresia. Rare cases of esophageal atresia are associated with a microdeletion of chromosome 22q11 (56). Chromosome 22q11 deletion is also associated with multiple jejunal atresias, including the apple peel deformity (97). Some patients with anal atresia have an A→G mutation at nucleotide position 3243 of mtDNA (58).

Patients with IHPS may have an autosomal recessive pattern of inheritance. The disorder is disproportionately common in monozygotic twins. IHPS is more frequent in first-born children and is more common in males than females. Factors affecting the expression of IHPS include blood group type, time of birth (peaks in the spring and autumn), and a history of breast feeding. Coexisting epidermolysis bullosa and pyloric atresia have a characteristic integrin mutation (76). The familial pattern is compatible with a multifactorial threshold of inheritance or the effects of multiple interacting loci. Patients with apple peel atresia probably have an autosomal recessive inheritance.

Pathophysiology. *Esophagus.* The failure of the esophagus and trachea to separate completely during embryologic development gives rise to a number of closely related congenital anomalies, broadly classified together as TE fistulas (fig. 2-12). Unequal esophageal-tracheal division leads to an absent esophagus, or an esophagus consisting of only a thin fibrous cord without a lumen or only a fistulous communication to

Table 2-7

SYNDROMES ASSOCIATED WITH PYLORIC STENOSIS

Associated Syndrome	Prominent Features
Deletion 11q	Trigonocephaly, upslanting palpebral fissures, ptosis, epicanthal folds, short nose, anteverted nares, clinodactyly of 5th finger, cardiac defects, hydronephrosis, polydactyly
Duplication 1q	Mild growth deficiency, relative megalencephaly, profound mental deficiency, hypertelorism, downslanting palpebral fissures, small malformed and low-set pinnae, long fingers, cardiac defects, inguinal hernia
Duplication 9q	Growth deficiency, cleft lip, cleft palate, cardiac defects, clubbed feet, camptodactyly, mental deficiency
Marden-Walker syndrome	Mental deficiency, failure to thrive, microcephaly, immobility of facial muscles, absent reflexes, blepharophimosis, strabismus, joint contractures, arachnodactyly, kyphoscoliosis, altered palmar creases
Ring 12	Growth deficiency, microcephaly, moderate mental deficiency, clinodactyly of 5th finger, camptodactyly
Trisomy 18	Prenatal onset growth deficiency, profound mental deficiency, prominent occiput, narrow bifrontal diameter, low-set and malformed pinnae, micrognathia, camptodactyly, short and dorsiflexed halux, short sternum, predominance of low arch dermal patterns, cardiac defects
Trisomy 21	Hypotonia, mental deficiency, brachycephaly, flat nasal bridge, epicanthal folds, Brushfield spots, small and overfolded pinnae, short neck, 5th finger clinodactyly, single transverse palmar crease, wide space between toes I and II, cardiac defects
Occasional Accompaniment of the Following	
Apert's syndrome	Irregular craniosynostosis, short anteroposterior cranial diameter, flat face, shallow orbits, hypertelorism, strabismus, osseous and/or cutaneous syndactyly, cardiac defects
de Lange's syndrome	Profound growth and mental deficiency, low-pitched cry, microbrachycephaly, synophrys, small nose, anteverted nares, micrognathia, hirsutism, micromelia, phocomelia, oligodactyly
Opitz FG syndrome	Mental deficiency, hypotonia, affable personality, short stature, prominent forehead, frontal hair upsweep, hypertelorism, small ears, imperforate anus, broad thumbs and great toes, cryptorchidism
Smith-Lemli-Opitz syndrome	Growth deficiency, moderate to severe mental deficiency, microcephaly, narrow forehead, ptosis, epicanthal folds, strabismus, syndactyly of toes II and III, altered dermal ridge patterning, cryptorchidism, hypospadias, cardiac anomaly
Zellweger's (cerebrohepato-renal) syndrome	Hypotonia, high forehead, flattened occiput, epicanthal folds, anteverted nares, loose skin at back of neck, cataracts, cloudy corneas, hepatomegaly, lissencephaly, micropachygyria, multiple cortical renal cysts

the trachea. Tracheal dominance with esophageal stenosis or atresia represents the most prevalent form of unequal division; it is usually associated with a fistula.

Stomach. The muscular hypertrophy that characterizes IHPS is usually absent at birth. It develops during the first few weeks of life; pyloric growth continues into the third month. Excessive gastrin production (90,92), abnormalities in peptidergic innervation (90), and a lack of nitric oxide (NO) synthetase (50) all play a role in its development (69,90,92). Impaired NO and vasoactive intestinal polypeptide levels lead to an excessively contracted, hypertrophied pyloric muscle (66). IHPS patients may also lack gastrointestinal pacemakers, the interstitial cells of Cajal (90).

Patients with pyloric atresia, epidermolysis bullosa, and an integrin gene mutation may develop gastrointestinal atresia secondary to an inflammatory reaction, which leads to massive fibrosis and secondary obstruction of the gastrointestinal lumen. The sequence of events is initiated by bullous separation of the gastrointestinal mucosa (70).

Intestine. There are three major theories to explain intestinal atresias and/or stenoses: 1) failed recanalization during the 12th fetal week; 2) failure of epithelial growth to keep pace with mesenchymal tissue growth during the phase of rapid intestinal elongation, so that epithelial continuity becomes compromised and atresia develops; and 3) the occurrence of intrauterine vascular accidents, intussusceptions, or intrapartum

Table 2-8

ABNORMALITIES ASSOCIATED WITH INTESTINAL ATRESIA

Duodenal atresia	Colonic atresia
Single umbilical artery	Hirschsprung's disease
Down's syndrome	
Annular pancreas	Omphalocele
Malrotation	
Cystic fibrosis	HIPO syndrome
MODED[a] syndrome	Hemihypertrophy
Esophageal atresia	Intestinal web
Tracheoesophageal fistula	Preauricular skin tags
Anorectal anomalies	Coronal opacity
Renal malformations	
Cardiac malformations	OEIS[b]
Tetralogy of Fallot	
Abdominal situs inversus	Sirenomelia
Apple peel atresia	Renal agenesis
Microcephaly and hydrocephaly	
Short stature	Agenesis distal colon
Global developmental delay	
Ocular anomalies	Absent genitalia
Jejunal atresia	Imperforate anus
Gastroschisis	
Umbilical ulceration	Unseparated lower limbs
Volvulus	
Meconium ileus	

[a]MODED = microcephaly oculo-digito-esophageal-duodenal syndrome.
[b]OEIS = omphalocele, exstrophy of bladder, imperforate anus, spinal defects.

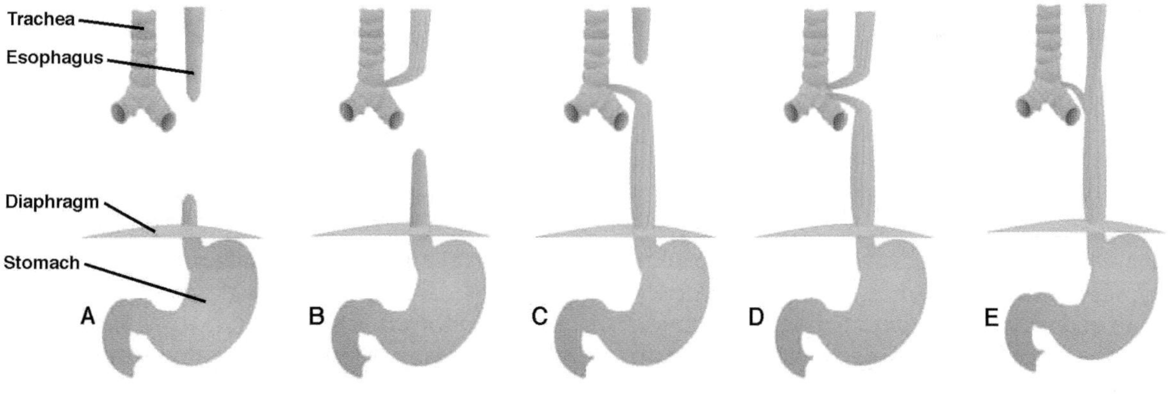

Figure 2-12

ESOPHAGEAL ATRESIAS AND STENOSES

A: In type I atresia, a segment of the esophagus is represented by only a thin, noncanalized cord with formation of an upper blind pouch that connects to the pharynx. The lower pouch leads into the stomach. The atresia usually lies at or near the tracheal bifurcation.

B: Rare type II atresia. The proximal and distal esophageal portions are completely separated from one another. The proximal part connects with the trachea.

C: Type III is the most common anomaly. The lower pouch communicates with the trachea or the mainstem bronchus.

D: In type IV lesions, both the upper and lower pouches connect to the trachea.

E: Esophageal stenosis near the tracheal bifurcation. There is also a tracheoesophageal fistula.

asphyxia leading to segmental intestinal necrosis with subsequent fibrosis or tissue loss (80). The presence of meconium, bile, squamous cells, or lanugo hair in the atretic areas supports intrauterine injury. Apple peel atresia probably results from a narrow mesenteric attachment, volvulus, and occlusion of the superior mesenteric artery distal to its proximal branches (82).

Clinical Features. *Esophagus.* Prenatal ultrasonographic detection of esophageal atresia relies on finding a small or absent fetal stomach bubble associated with maternal polyhydramnios (85) or the presence of a fluid-filled, blind-ending esophagus. Air in the stomach and small bowel indicates the presence of a distal TE fistula. Air confined to the stomach raises the possibility of associated duodenal atresia. Inability to pass a nasogastric tube into the stomach confirms the diagnosis. A plain radiograph shows the tip of the tube lodged in a blind-ending proximal esophagus, usually located at the level of the 2nd to 4th thoracic vertebrae.

Infants with atresia typically present in the first few hours or days of life with regurgitation, excessive drooling, choking, aspiration, cyanosis, and respiratory distress. If a child eats, he or she typically eats hungrily. Coughing, gagging, vomiting, and cyanosis soon follow. Preoperative ventilator dependence and associated major anomalies independently affect survival.

Esophageal stenosis is usually diagnosed much later than atresia. Patients present with dysphagia, regurgitation, and failure to thrive. Milder degrees of stenosis may be asymptomatic. True dysphagia may develop when solid foods are consumed.

Most patients present in the first few days of life with bile-free vomiting, gastroesophageal reflux, abdominal distention, and stools decreasing in quantity. Other signs include regurgitation, excessive drooling, choking, aspiration, cyanosis, and respiratory distress. Perforate diaphragms present later than imperforate ones, depending on the size of the opening. Hypochloremic, hypokalemic metabolic alkalosis may occur.

Stomach. Some infants with IHPS are symptomatic at birth, but most remain well during the first few weeks of life, only to return to the hospital at about a month of age with regurgitation, abdominal distension, and projectile, nonbilious, postprandial vomiting and hypochloremic alkalosis (46). Vomiting is followed by a voracious appetite. There are features of gastric obstruction. As with any patient with chronic gastric outlet obstruction, G-cell hyperplasia develops, possibly contributing to the peptic ulcers that are found in long-standing cases. Some patients become constipated. Physical examination discloses visible peristalsis and the presence of a firm, palpable, ovoid mass corresponding to the hypertrophic pyloric muscle. Occasionally, there is localized hypertrophy of the muscularis propria of the distal esophagus. IHPS is usually diagnosed by ultrasound. An enlarged fetal stomach may herald the presence of gastric outlet obstruction or duodenal atresia. Equivocal cases require endoscopy.

Infants with the simultaneous appearance of epidermolysis bullosa and pyloric atresia (EB-PA) have mixed skin lesions that include blisters and patchy lack of skin. Most have gastrointestinal obstruction due to overproliferation of connective tissue.

Small Intestine. Duodenal atresia can be diagnosed ultrasonographically at 15 weeks of gestation by finding polyhydramnios, and intestinal dilatation proximal to the atretic intestine. Other findings include meconium peritonitis and ascites. Elevated maternal serum AFP levels and polyhydramnios occur in the second trimester of pregnancy in 50 percent of cases (93). Signs of distress or ischemia are frequent. Approximately 50 percent of infants with intestinal atresia are premature. Patients with small intestinal atresias present in the neonatal period with vomiting, unless a coexisting esophageal atresia is also present. The vomitus lacks bile when the obstruction lies proximal to the ampulla of Vater. Duodenal atresia is also suggested radiographically by the presence of a double bubble on a plain abdominal X ray (fig. 2-13), particularly when gas is present in a distended stomach and proximal duodenum.

Some patients with duodenal stenosis remain asymptomatic whereas others have an intermittent or delayed history of duodenal ulcer, symptoms associated with hiatal hernia, gastritis, duodenogastric reflux, motility disturbances, duodenal diverticula, and bezoars (65). The small intestinal loops appear dilated and contain air-fluid levels; colonic gas is absent in complete jejunal or ileal obstruction. The more distal

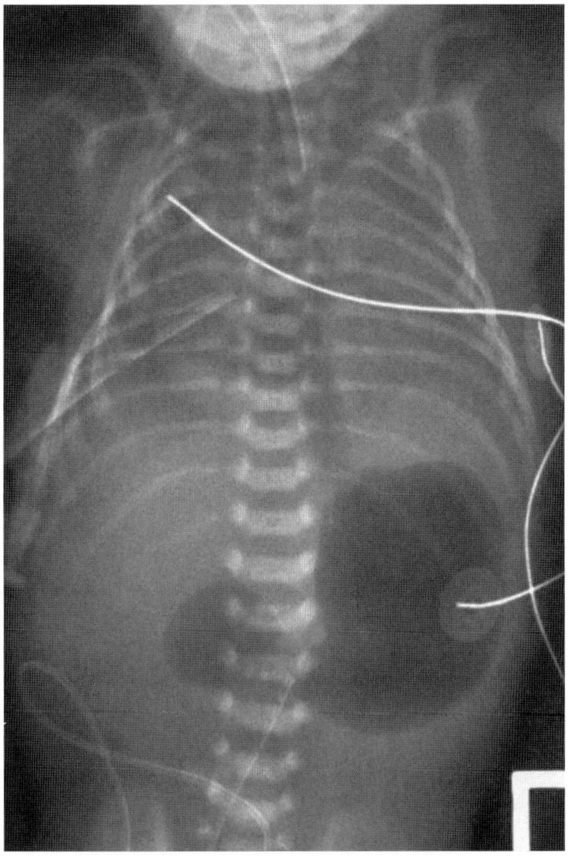

Figure 2-13

RADIOGRAPHIC APPEARANCE OF THE DOUBLE-BUBBLE

The abdomen of the infant is distended. There is a larger bubble in the proximal stomach and a smaller one in the duodenum.

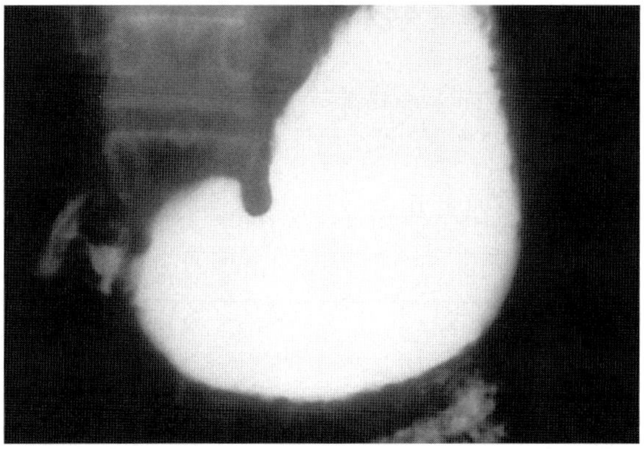

Figure 2-14

ANTRAL MEMBRANE: BARIUM STUDY

The stomach is distended and the site of the membrane is indicated by the defect in the barium within the stomach.

the atresia, the more severe the distension. Microcolon may be present. A barium enema should be performed to rule out Hirschsprung's disease and malrotation.

Gross Findings. Atresia results from a complete occlusion, whereas stenosis is either a narrowed intestinal segment or a luminal diaphragm with a small central aperture. In atresia, a bowel segment is entirely missing, leaving a proximal segment with a blind end separated some distance from the distal segment. Alternately, the proximal and distal segments are united by a solid fibrous cord, or there is an occluding mucosal diaphragm. Some patients have multiple atresias (77).

Esophagus. In esophageal atresia, the esophagus appears normal at the cardia but it progressively narrows as one precedes proximally. The atretic segment varies in length; the gap between the blind upper pouch and the lower end varies from 1 to 5 cm. The five types of congenital esophageal atresias and TE fistulas are illustrated in figure 2-12. The most common form is type C in which the upper esophagus ends as a blind pouch and the lower segment forms a fistula with the trachea, usually communicating with it within 2 cm of its bifurcation. This type accounts for approximately 90 percent of cases (71).

Several types of congenital esophageal stenosis exist: 1) a localized area of muscular and submucosal hypertrophy; 2) the presence of cartilaginous tracheobronchial remnants; and 3) a membranous diaphragm or web arising from the esophageal wall, obstructing the lumen, and containing a small central perforation.

Stomach. Type 1 gastric atresia (the most prevalent form) consists of an internal web or diaphragm completely separating the stomach from the duodenum (61). The diaphragm may be perforate or imperforate. Grossly and radiographically, a large distal antral mucosal fold lies perpendicular to the long axis of the antrum (fig. 2-14). It often contains a central aperture measuring from 1 to 10 mm in diameter. The gastric serosa may appear indented at the level of the diaphragm. Type 2 atresia consists of a thin, fibrous cord which connects a blind gastric pouch to a distal blind small intestinal segment. Type 3 atresia consists of a blind gastric pouch

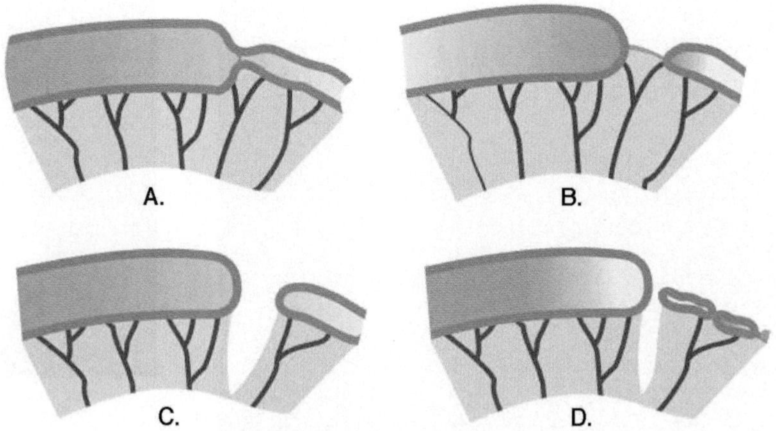

Figure 2-15

DIFFERENT FORMS OF ILEAL ATRESIA

A: Type I: an imperforate septum covered on each side by mucosa stretches across an otherwise continuous bowel.

B: Type II: a thin fibromuscular cord, with or without an associated mesenteric defect, replaces the bowel.

C: Type III: a complete gap and a corresponding mesenteric defect separate the two blind intestinal ends.

D: Type IV: presence of atretic areas with or without a mesenteric gap. Different forms of atresia may coexist and may be single or multiple.

and a blind distal intestinal pouch without intervening tissue.

A concentrically enlarged pylorus characterizes IHPS. The pyloric channel appears two to four times its normal length, and its thickness exceeds 1 cm (normal is 4 to 8 mm). The muscularis propria hypertrophies up to 400 percent of its normal thickness. The hypertrophy of the pyloric canal affects both the muscle and the elastic tissue in the submucosa. The hypertrophy passes through a series of phases, presumably due to the neural abnormalities. The pylorus becomes extremely hard as the hypertrophy increases and a fusiform mass with the consistency of cartilage, measuring 3 to 5 cm, abruptly terminates at the duodenum. The lesion reaches its greatest development between 4 and 9 weeks of age. If surgical intervention is not necessary, the pylorus then begins to relax, becomes smaller and softer, and heals by the time the infant is several months old. The stomach becomes dilated and the antrum hypertrophies. The clinical picture of gastric outlet obstruction occurs when the enlarged pyloric muscle measures more than 3 mm in thickness. Pyloric obstruction can lead to secondary mucosal and submucosal edema and ulceration, further aggravating the distal obstruction. In extreme cases, IHPS distorts the normal anatomy and elevates the pylorus, displacing the duodenum to lie adjacent to or below the gallbladder. Endoscopy demonstrates pyloric narrowing and mucosal thickening.

Intestine. Intestinal atresias may be multiple or single, and are often associated with mesenteric defects (91). Morphologically, there is a discontinuous bowel with an intermediate fibrous cord and a gap that is usually replaced by pancreas or a mucosa-lined membranous atresia (54). Annular pancreas coexists with a duodenal diaphragm or stenosis in 50 percent of cases.

There are four types of ileal atresia (figs. 2-15, 2-16) and two types of intestinal stenosis. The features differ depending on whether or not there is a complete gap in the bowel wall and/or mesentery and on the width of the distal segment. One type of atresia affects the jejunum near the ligament of Treitz. The bowel is short and there is a long defect in the mesentery. The distal small bowel is coiled in an apple peel configuration around the supplying vessel (fig. 2-17).

Microscopic Findings. *Esophagus.* In esophageal atresia, the esophageal and tracheal muscles intimately blend together. The muscle appears hypertrophic and it contains an extra myenteric plexus in the membranous portion of the trachea, a manifestation of the incomplete tracheal-esophageal separation (71).

Distal esophageal stenoses usually contain fibromuscular tissue. One form of esophageal stenosis results from inadequate nitrergic innervation (77,83). Another form results from the presence of intraesophageal cartilaginous tracheobronchial remnants due to esophageal sequestration of a tracheobronchial anlage before embryologic separation. A third form consists of a membranous diaphragm or web arising from the esophageal wall, containing fibromuscular tissue with a small central perforation that obstructs the lumen.

Stomach. Antral cuboidal or squamous epithelium lines both sides of the luminal

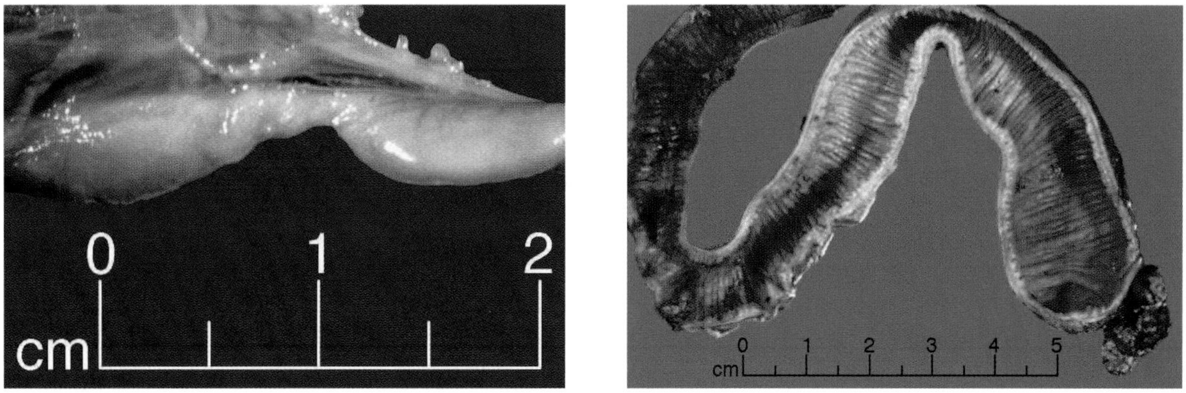

Figure 2-16

SMALL INTESTINAL ATRESIA

Left: Type I jejunal atresia shows an area of narrowing.
Right: Type IV atresia: the intestinal loop ends blindly and there is a small communication with the next segment.

diaphragm in gastric stenosis. The mucosa covers a central submucosal core. The lesion appears variably inflamed. Heterotopic pancreatic tissue sometimes lies within webs and diaphragms. Two thirds of gastric atresias are membranous, consisting of a diaphragm or a web, and usually involve the pylorus.

IHPS usually consists of hypertrophy and hyperplasia of the circular muscle of the muscularis propria of the gastric pylorus and hypertrophic longitudinal muscle fibers. Children also have focal and multinodular variants in addition to the circular form. The submucosal vasculature may appear dilated. Myenteric ganglion cells degenerate and disappear, resulting in reduced or absent nerves. Interstitial cells of Cajal may be decreased in number (90). IHPS is associated with idiopathic focal foveolar hyperplasia secondary to G-cell hyperplasia (90).

Intestine. Normal small intestinal mucosa lines both sides of the atretic or stenotic intestinal segment. The height of the circular folds declines and the muscularis mucosae thickens as one approaches the blind segment. In complex atresia, the proximal bowel appears dilated and gangrenous. The circular folds widen due to stromal edema. The villi may appear shortened or only simple tubular glands are seen. The villi and crypts often appear necrotic or ulcerated, with only a few residual intestinal glands. As a result, the mucosa contains granulation tissue, granulomas, foreign body giant cells, fibroblasts, and hemosiderin-laden macrophages. Dystrophic calcification and inflammation at or near the atretic site suggest previous injury. The blind segment may contain dense fibrosis, meconium, keratinizing squamous cells, lanugo hair, bile pigment, and mucin, also suggesting previous injury. The intervening mucosa between atretic areas is histologically normal. The muscularis propria eventually becomes markedly hypertrophic and the myenteric plexus may show inflammatory or degenerative changes.

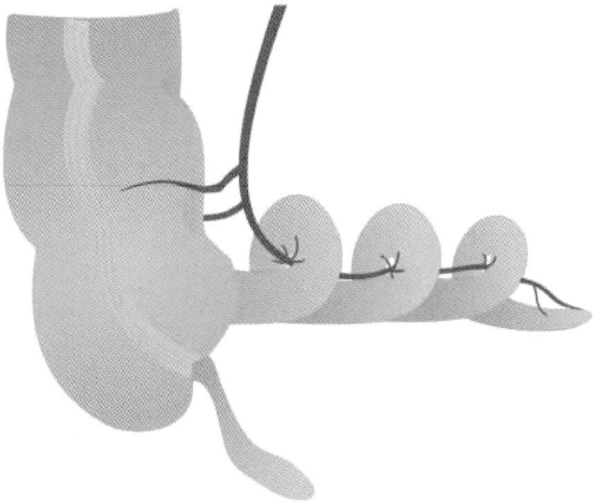

Figure 2-17

APPLE PEEL CONFIGURATION OF INTESTINAL ATRESIA

The distal small bowel spirals around a vascular stalk.

Treatment and Prognosis. Treatment and prognosis depend both on the specific atresia or stenosis, as well as on the presence of associated lesions. Infants with atresia can be evaluated by chest and abdominal X rays and cardiac and renal ultrasonography to detect any associated anomalies. Sweat tests rule out cystic fibrosis in babies with jejunoileal atresia, and a rectal biopsy should be done in patients with a combination of Down's syndrome and duodenal atresia to exclude Hirschsprung's disease.

Esophagus. Neonates with esophageal atresia and/or TE fistula are stratified into prognostic categories based on birth weight, esophageal gap length (49), preoperative ventilator dependence, the presence of pneumonia, and the identification of associated congenital anomalies (49,86). The main therapy is primary anastomosis in infants at 3 months of age (57). Type A (long gap) esophageal atresia without a fistula is treated with native esophageal reconstruction or the missing esophagus is replaced with colon. Morbidity associated with repair of these anomalies is high (88) and there are many complications. These include stricture, leakage, recurrent TE fistulas, pneumonia, wound infection, wound dehiscence, and perforation (88). Many patients develop esophageal reflux after the repair (47) and may need partial wrap fundoplication (67).

Surgical repair is usually feasible in patients with esophageal stenosis, but re-stenosis commonly occurs, leading to aspiration and respiratory infections, secondary strictures, esophagitis, Barrett esophagus, and hiatal hernia (67). Endoscopic dilatation may be necessary but repeated attempts to dilate true congenital esophageal stenosis often fail.

Stomach. Treatment of gastric atresia or stenosis consists of ablation of the diaphragm or resection of the aplastic pylorus with a gastroduodenal anastomosis. Successful endoscopic incision of an antral membrane is possible. Patients often have residual motility problems with consequent gastroesophageal reflux (47) and pulmonary dysfunction.

Patients with IHPS undergo pyloromyotomy without tissue removal. This approach results in an excellent prognosis with few long-term sequelae. Complications include duodenal perforation, postoperative vomiting, and incomplete myotomy.

Intestine. Patients with duodenal obstruction are treated by duodenoduodenostomy, duodenotomy with web excision, or duodenojejunostomy. Patients with jejunoileal atresia are treated with resection (76 percent), temporary ostomy, and web excision. Patients with colonic atresia are managed with initial ostomy and delayed anastomosis. Although apple peel intestinal atresia is rare, it is associated with significant morbidity and a high mortality rate. Such patients can be initially managed with total parenteral nutrition. The dilated proximal bowel is resected and a primary anastomosis performed. Early morbidity is common but excellent long-term outcomes can be achieved. Short bowel syndrome develops in a percentage of patients (54). Ultrashort bowel syndrome (under 40 cm) requires long-term total parenteral nutrition and can be complicated by cholestatic liver disease and gallstones, particularly in patients with jejunoileal atresia. Growth factor therapy and small bowel transplantation may improve long-term outcome (54).

Animal Models. Intraperitoneal injections of adriamycin produce esophageal atresia, TE fistula, and VATER syndrome in animals (73). Intestinal atresia has been produced in chicks by temporarily occluding a branch of the omphalomesenteric artery or in fetal mammals by occluding the superior mesenteric artery (68).

BRONCHOPULMONARY MALFORMATIONS INCLUDING CONGENITAL BRONCHOESOPHAGEAL FISTULAS, BRONCHOGENIC CYSTS, AND PULMONARY SEQUESTRATION

Definitions. *Bronchopulmonary malformations* are collections of pulmonary tissue lying either within the lung substance or separated from the lung by a pleural covering, most commonly maintaining connections to a lobar or segmental bronchus. *Communicating bronchopulmonary foregut malformations* (CBPFMs) are rare tracheobronchial anomalies characterized by a fistula between an isolated portion of respiratory tissue and the esophagus or stomach. If the communication between the pulmonary tissue and the esophagus is lost, the pulmonary tissue appears as a sequestration. In *esophageal bronchus*, the mainstem bronchus originates from the esophagus; this lesion is also called *esophageal lung* (103). The lung receives its arterial supply from the pulmonary artery. The lesion differs from *pulmonary sequestration* in which anomalous systemic arterial blood vessels supply the sequestration.

Demography. Bronchopulmonary foregut malformations are extremely rare and occur much less commonly than tracheoesophageal abnormalities. Approximately equal numbers of girls and boys are affected; patients range in age from newborn to 24 years.

Associated Findings. Bronchopulmonary malformations occur in combination with other anomalies of the upper gastrointestinal tract, diaphragm, and pulmonary and systemic arteriovenous systems (98). These include rib and vertebral abnormalities, congenital diaphragmatic hernias, duodenal stenoses or atresias, multicystic dysplastic kidneys, cardiac anomalies, and gastric duplication cysts (102). Rarely, they are associated with TE fistulas (102) or VATER anomalies.

Etiology. Bronchopulmonary malformations result from the imperfect separation of pulmonary and esophageal anlagen or from an accessory esophageal lung bud. The presence of lung tissue arising from the primitive gastrointestinal tube is a common occurrence in the development of all forms of bronchopulmonary foregut malformations. Three important factors that determine the type of lesion are: 1) the stage of embryologic development at which the accessory lung tissue arises; 2) the direction in which the aberrant pulmonary tissue grows; and 3) retention or involution of the communication between the accessory lung tissue and the parent viscus.

Clinical Features. Patients usually present in infancy with a mediastinal mass or repeated pulmonary infections. Congenital bronchoesophageal fistulas also present in adults (101). The diagnosis is suggested by long-standing, unexplained respiratory symptoms such as coughing, cyanosis, frequent pulmonary infections, or even hemoptysis. Other signs and symptoms include vomiting, the presence of an extrathoracic mass, or chest pain.

Radiologic Findings. Most patients with bronchopulmonary malformations have an abnormal chest radiograph due to the presence of an anterior mediastinal mass, intraparenchymal pulmonary lesion, tracheal deviation, lobar collapse or emphysema, and esophageal dilatation. Radiologic investigation of a suspected bronchopulmonary malformation begins with the injection of contrast material through a feeding tube into the distal third of the esophagus where an ectopic bronchus is most likely to arise. Gastrostomy injection provides distal esophageal opacification by gastroesophageal reflux when passing a feeding tube is contraindicated. When associated with air bronchograms in the same area, absence of a mainstem bronchus during bronchoscopy is diagnostic of an esophageal lung. Esophagoscopy with tracheobronchography is another confirmatory procedure.

Gross Findings. Extralobar sequestrations usually lie in the posterior costodiaphragmatic angle, adjacent to the esophagus; they may communicate with the esophagus, often distally presenting as bronchoesophageal fistulas (100). In a minority of cases, a supernumerary lung bud arises from the lower portion of the foregut and is associated with a congenital diaphragmatic hernia. This form of sequestration generally occurs in the mediastinum along the tracheobronchial tree or within the lung and typically has an anomalous blood supply. A rare type of bronchoesophageal fistula communicates with the normal bronchial tree but it has a systemic arterial blood supply.

Microscopic Findings. The histology of the involved structures is that of normal bronchus or respiratory tract (fig. 2-18).

Microscopic Variants. *Tracheobronchial chondroepithelial hamartoma* is an uncommon related lesion (91) that results from abnormal esophageal-tracheal separation. The hamartoma contains ciliated, mucus-secreting, tracheobronchial lining epithelium; seromucinous minor salivary glands; cartilage; smooth muscle cells; and sometimes ectopic thyroid or pancreatic tissue. Other bronchogenic cysts are lined by respiratory squamous epithelium but they lack cartilage.

Differential Diagnosis. Other cystic lesions in the region of the esophagus fall into several categories, including duplications, bronchogenic cysts, gastric duplication cysts, and neuroenteric cysts. These lesions usually lie in the distal esophagus (99).

Treatment and Prognosis. The majority of patients undergo surgical excision of the lesion.

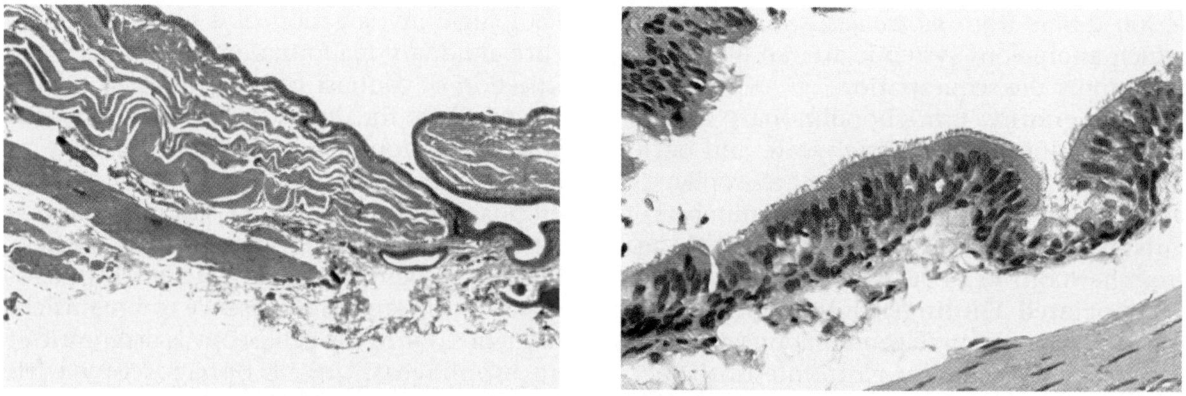

Figure 2-18

BRONCHOGENIC CYST INVOLVING THE WALL OF THE ESOPHAGUS

Left: Low-power magnification shows a cystic structure lined by epithelium, muscle, and loose connective tissue. Right: At higher magnification, the lining resembles that of the normal respiratory tract.

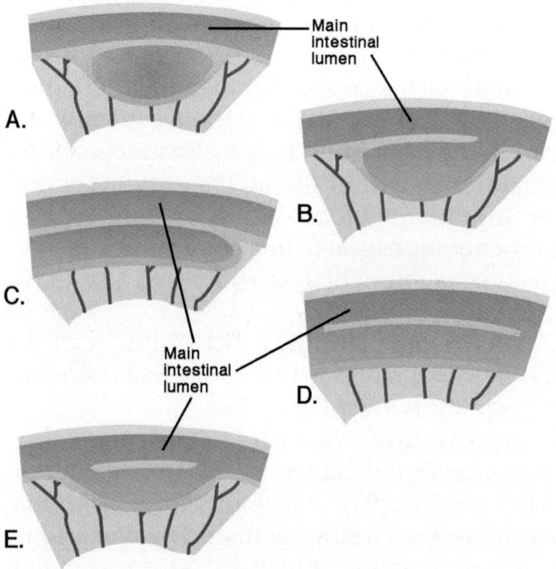

Figure 2-19

DIAGRAMMATIC COMPARISON OF CONGENITAL DIVERTICULA, DUPLICATIONS, AND ENTEROGENOUS CYSTS

A: Cystic duplication that does not communicate with the main intestinal lumen. This lesion is sometimes referred to as an enterogenous cyst.

B: Communicating cystic duplication that communicates at one end. This is sometimes referred to as a congenital diverticulum.

C: Long tubular duplication communicating at one end with the main intestinal lumen.

D: Complete duplication of the intestine without communications.

E: Long tubular duplications with communication at both ends.

DUPLICATIONS, DIVERTICULA, ENTEROGENOUS CYSTS

Congenital diverticula, duplications, and enterogenous cysts are related lesions. The major distinction that separates them is their gross appearance (fig. 2-19).

Duplications and Enterogenous Cysts

Definition. A *duplication* is a complete or partial doubling of a variable length of bowel containing all of the layers of the bowel wall. *Enterogenous cysts* are cysts derived from cells sequestered from the formative gut.

Demography. Thirty-nine percent of gastrointestinal duplications involve the foregut; 61 percent involve the midgut or hindgut. Esophageal duplication cysts are present in approximately 1/8,000 autopsies (118), and account for 10 to 20 percent of all gastrointestinal duplications. Gastric duplications constitute 3.8 to 10.0 percent of all gastrointestinal duplications (104). Intestinal duplications affect 1/4,000 births and are occasionally multiple. Bowel duplications most commonly occur in the small intestine, usually in the ileum (50 percent of duplications affect the ileum), mostly in the area of the ileocecal valve (120); only 8 to 16 percent are in the jejunum. Hindgut tubular duplications are rarer than other gastrointestinal duplications. Approximately 30 percent of intestinal duplications occur in the large intestine. The male to female ratio is 1 to 2.

Table 2-9

LESIONS COEXISTING WITH GASTRIC DUPLICATIONS

Esophageal duplications
Heterotopic pancreas
Gastrointestinal malrotations
Meckel diverticulum
Thoracic vertebral anomalies
Pulmonary sequestration
Accessory spleen
Abnormally shaped spleen
Urinary tract anomalies
Turner's syndrome
Patent ductus arteriosus
Ventricular septal defect
Vertebral anomalies
Esophageal duplications

Associated Findings. Duplications and enterogenous cysts, especially those in the foregut, often coexist with rotational disorders or vertebral body defects. Duplications also are associated with cloacal anomalies and situs inversus (115,124). If a spinal deformity coexists with an alimentary tract duplication, the anomaly probably arose during the 3rd fetal week when the neurenteric canal communicated with the primitive ectodermal plate and yolk sac. Esophageal duplication cysts are associated with pulmonary cystic malformations (121). Thirty-five percent of patients with gastric duplications have associated developmental anomalies (Table 2-9). Anorectal duplications are rare and are almost always associated with abnormalities of the bladder, müllerian structures, and external genitalia (127).

Etiology. Hypotheses to explain duplications include persistence of embryonic diverticula, fusion of embryologic longitudinal folds (the most popular theory) (109), abortive twinning (117), defective luminal vacuolar breakdown (120), intrauterine intestinal ischemia (105,114, 129), endodermal-neurodermal adhesions, and sequestration of embryonic tissues during embryonic movement. The split notochord syndrome postulates that hindgut duplications result from ectodermal-endodermal adhesions during the development of the caudal end of the embryonic disc. These adhesions interfere with notochord development and lead to splitting of the notochord to bypass the adhesion. This notochordal split is associated with defective mesenchyme that allows the endodermal and ectodermal adhesions to persist (105,113, 125). Small diverticula and epithelial islands in the developing small intestinal mesentery may explain the presence of isolated intestinal duplications (123). Extensive intestinal duplications associated with multiple anomalies, including bladder anomalies, presumably result from teratogenic insults that affect several developing organs.

Clinical Features. Duplications and related lesions are usually detected early in life, although a minority remain undetected until adulthood. Most patients present during the first year of life. The size and location of the duplication, and the resultant complications, determine the clinical signs and symptoms. The manifestations may be vague and diverse, usually resulting from compression of normal adjacent bowel. Signs and symptoms include pain, abdominal distension, the presence of a palpable mass, dysphagia, nausea, vomiting, weight loss, anorexia, dyspnea, wheezing or coughing episodes, bleeding, and recurrent pneumonitis. Bleeding or melena results from the presence of ectopic gastric tissue or ischemia. Complications include ulceration, fistula formation, perforation, gastrointestinal obstruction, or carcinoma.

Most gastric duplications present as intrathoracic or extragastric masses. Duodenal duplications may cause portal hypertension or pancreatitis. Ileocecal duplications can act as lead points for chronic or recurrent intussusception or volvulus. Rectal duplications may present as neonatal intestinal obstruction, chronic constipation, a prolapsing rectal polyp, a vulvar growth, acute urinary retention, chronic rectal bleeding, intussusception, volvulus, perforation, or obstruction.

Gross Findings. Gastrointestinal duplications occur anywhere in the gastrointestinal tract and are usually single, but they may be multiple (112), often lying in both the thorax and the abdomen. They can be complete or incomplete, communicating or noncommunicating. Communicating duplications open proximally, distally, or at both ends.

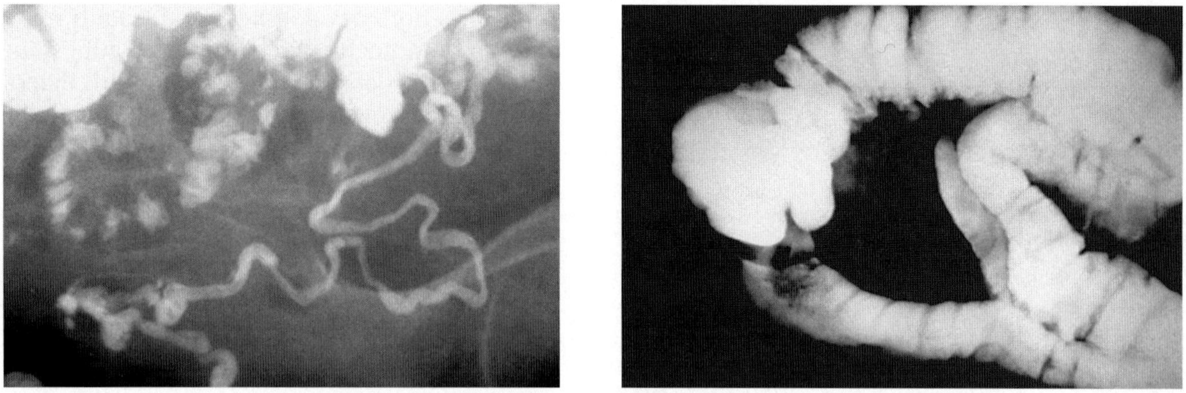

Figure 2-20

RADIOGRAPHIC STUDIES OF COLONIC DUPLICATIONS

Left: The duplicated segments may be the same size as the normal lumen or may be small and malformed. Right: The duplicated segment lies adjacent to the main intestinal lumen.

Grossly, duplications appear as hollow, cylindrical or oval, cystic masses that range in size from a few millimeters to up to 15 cm (116). Duplications tend to be longer in their axial length than enterogenous cysts or diverticula. They appear as tubular reduplications, usually with a common muscular wall between the normal and duplicated segments. They have thick walls and are filled with mucus. Because of their location, duplications may fill with barium during gastrointestinal examination, and vary in length; they can involve long intestinal segments. Bleeding can occur within the duplication or the adjacent mucosa, where a marginal ulcer may develop. Even a triple lumen may be present (110,115).

Sixty percent of esophageal duplication cysts originate in the lower esophagus; the remainder are equally distributed between the upper and middle esophagus. The cysts lie posteriorly in a periesophageal location, protruding into the posterior mediastinum, or they develop within the esophageal wall. Esophageal cysts are unilocular lesions, averaging up to 5 cm in diameter. Their outer surface is tan, smooth, and glistening. The inner lining is smooth and contains thick, clear, mucinous material.

Most gastric duplications lie on the greater curvature or on the anterior or posterior walls; a third affect the distal stomach. Gastric duplications may be intimately related to the gastric wall or may be unattached to the stomach. Some adhere to the pancreas or communicate with aberrant pancreatic ducts or with the main pancreatic duct. Some gastric duplications take the form of a double pylorus, sometimes coexisting with cystic duplication of the duodenal bulb; the two pyloric channels are separated by a septum. Gastric duplications usually fail to communicate with the gastric lumen, appearing as closed spherical cysts (enterogenous cysts). Therefore, ultrasound is the diagnostic modality of choice (124).

Intestinal duplications always lie dorsal to the intestine (fig. 2-20), usually within the mesentery between the spinal cord and the intestine. They are sometimes intramural, lying within the muscularis propria. Rarely, the duplicated segment remains completely isolated from the main intestinal tract, hanging freely on its own mesentery. The blood supply of the normal bowel usually runs in the wall of the duplicated gut so that surgical removal requires removal of the normal segment as well.

Distal large intestinal duplications fall into two categories: those associated with urinary bladder, urethral, or anorectal abnormalities and those that occur alone. Rectal duplications present as presacral, intraspinal, or postsacral enteric cysts or as a fistula between the rectum and the postsacral skin. The structure of these hindgut fistulas varies. Most have a muscular wall that varies in thickness and an epithelial lining that contains colonic, small intestinal, gastric, or mixed epithelium that sometimes includes

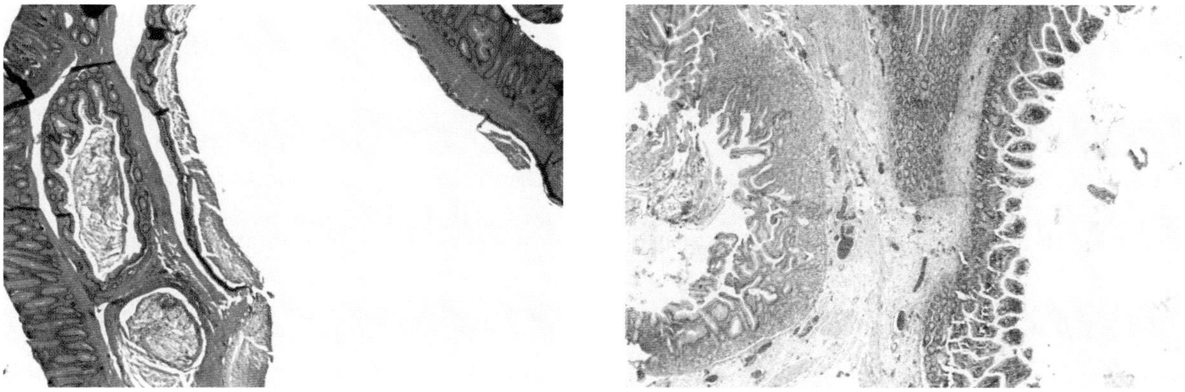

Figure 2-21

GASTROINTESTINAL DUPLICATION

Left: Several intestinal lumens are present within the wall of this sample. Smooth muscle surrounds many of them. Right: Another small intestinal duplication in which the muscular layer is much less obvious.

esophageal and bronchial epithelium. Aberrant cartilaginous nodules may be present (126). Distal intestinal duplications may be associated with presacral teratomas or they may be misdiagnosed as teratomas.

Duplicated ani appear as double perineal ani that open externally, double ani with fistulas of one or both duplicated segments to the genitourinary tract, or as one external anus and one imperforate anus (127). The bladder may be duplicated or septate with double urethral openings and there may be duplication of the uterus and the vagina. There may also be two penes or two clitorides or a combination of the above (127).

Enterogenous cysts may be single or multiple. They appear as rounded, cystic masses that fail to communicate with the intestinal lumen. They are usually filled with clear secretions. Most measure 3 to 6 cm.

Microscopic Findings. Three criteria are required for the diagnosis of a duplication: 1) an intimate attachment to the gastrointestinal tract, 2) the presence of a smooth muscle coat, and 3) an alimentary mucosal lining (fig. 2-21). Of these, only the presence of a smooth muscle coat is absolutely necessary to define the duplication. The absence of a muscle coat is characteristic of an enterogenous cyst. Pressure within a cyst may result in muscular atrophy, causing it to appear incomplete. The lesions are typically lined by glandular mucosa that often contains one or more of the cell types normally present in the gastrointestinal tract, particularly gastric mucosa. Ectopic gastric mucosa is present in a large percentage of duplications (107). As a result, peptic injury often causes mucosal erosions or ulceration and hemorrhage.

Esophagus. Esophageal duplications are lined by stratified squamous, simple pseudostratified ciliated columnar, or gastric cells. The wall contains two layers of smooth muscle fibers, with fibers of the outer layer oriented perpendicularly to those of the inner layer. The muscularis propria of the esophagus is continuous with the muscle layer of the cyst wall. The outermost layer consists of fibrous connective tissue containing small blood vessels, nerve twigs, and ganglion cells. Pancreatic tissue may be present.

Stomach. The epithelial lining of a duplication resembles or differs from that of the normal stomach. Gastric and small intestinal or colonic epithelium may coexist within a single duplication. Pancreatic tissue constitutes a prominent component of the duplication wall in 37 percent of cases (124). Additionally, histologic components of the upper respiratory tract, including respiratory mucosa, cartilage, and ceruminous glands, may be seen. The amount of muscle varies. Peptic ulceration due to the presence of parietal cells can cause cysts to rupture or hemorrhage.

Intestine. Generally, intestinal epithelium lines intestinal duplications (fig. 2-21). They may also contain heterotopic tissues including stratified, squamous, or ciliated epithelium;

thyroid stroma; pancreas and gastric mucosa; lymphoid aggregates resembling Peyer patches; ciliated bronchial epithelium; lung tissue; and cartilage. Ectopic gastric or pancreatic mucosa is found in more than 50 percent of duplications. Peptic ulcers may develop in duplications containing heterotopic gastric tissue. Exceptionally, duplications are lined by benign neoplastic epithelium forming a mucinous adenoma (111). The submucosal inner circular muscle layer and myenteric plexus usually appear normal.

Differential Diagnosis. The types of developmental cysts encountered in the mediastinum are bronchogenic, esophageal, gastroenteric, and pericardial. Distinction among the four is simplified by the fact that gastroenteric cysts are lined by gastric or duodenal type epithelium, whereas pericardial cysts are lined by flattened mesothelium. The distinction between bronchogenic and esophageal cysts is more difficult. Because of the embryologic relationship that exists between the esophagus and the tracheobronchial tree, it may be difficult to distinguish between esophageal duplication cysts and other intrathoracic cystic lesions lined by respiratory columnar, cuboidal enteric, stratified squamous, or gastric epithelium (108). Duplications usually have a duplicated muscularis propria. When ciliated columnar epithelium is seen in the cyst, the presence of cartilage or respiratory glands indicates bronchogenic differentiation. In contrast, a cyst without cartilage, with a double layer of smooth muscle, and an attachment close to the esophagus, probably arose in the esophagus. Since the precise etiology of mediastinal cysts may be difficult to ascertain, some prefer to refer to such lesions as foregut cysts or foregut duplication errors (108).

Other congenital lesions that may be in the differential diagnosis are lymphangioma and malrotation. Lymphangiomas appear as multiloculated cysts and are often manifested by abdominal pain, fever, vomiting, ascites, and a palpable mass. They can become infected and have an enhanced wall on abdominal CT scanning. They are not associated with either enteric fistulas or anemia (122,128). Malrotations manifest with abdominal pain, intermittent obstruction, anemia, and an abnormally positioned jejunum, but do not present as an enteric cystic mass or enteric fistula.

Treatment and Prognosis. Treatment of enteric duplications depends on the age and condition of the patient; the type, location, and extent of the lesion; and the presence or absence of associated abnormalities (104,106,119). Many recommend complete surgical resection when this is feasible. Surgery is especially recommended for symptomatic duplications due to the potential for obstruction, bleeding, and rupture. If the duplications are extensive and do not allow complete excision, partial excision can be performed with internal drainage or removal of the mucosal lining to prevent the possibility of acid secretions.

Congenital Diverticula

Definition. *Congenital diverticula* are outpouchings of the gastrointestinal wall that contain all of the bowel layers. Duplications that widely communicate with the bowel lumen are sometimes termed congenital diverticula.

Demography. Of the three related lesions, duplications, enterogenous cysts, and congenital diverticula, the latter are the rarest except for Meckel diverticula, which are discussed in a subsequent section. Diverticula are rarer in the stomach than anywhere else in the gastrointestinal tract. Approximately 2 percent of all gastrointestinal diverticula are gastric, 9 percent are esophageal, 60 percent are colonic, and the remainder occur in the small intestine. Congenital duodenal diverticula affect 1 to 2 percent of all individuals.

Etiology. Congenital true diverticula arise embryologically, either from the persistence of mucosal diverticula in the embryo or from small blind duplications that subsequently enlarge.

Clinical Features. Patients with congenital diverticula may remain asymptomatic or present with one of the following: 1) abdominal distension, pressure, pain, and possibly perforation due to diverticulitis; 2) ulceration and bleeding, usually from the presence of heterotopic acid-secreting gastric mucosa; and 3) intussusception leading to sudden pain and bleeding. Patients present with dysphagia which results when the diverticula enlarge and fill with food. Gastric diverticula usually do not cause symptoms, but if symptoms develop, they usually consist of epigastric or lower chest pain. Duodenal diverticula may enlarge, causing obstructive jaundice,

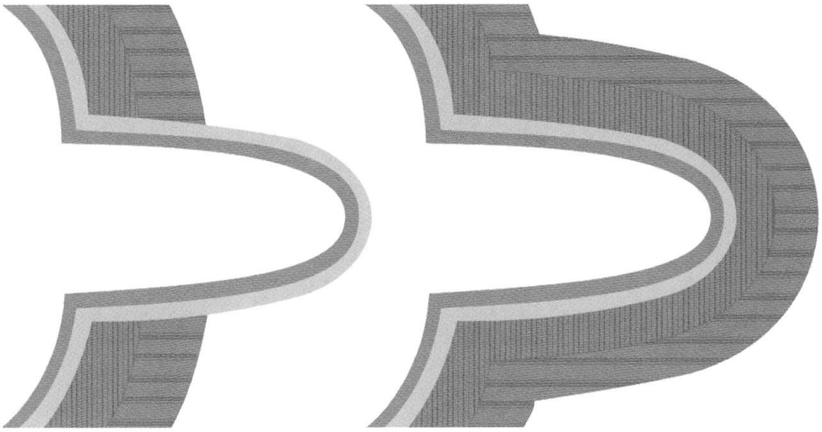

Figure 2-22

COMPARISON OF CONGENITAL AND ACQUIRED LARGE INTESTINAL DIVERTICULA

Left: An acquired diverticulum in which the mucosa and submucosa herniate through the muscularis propria, extending variably out through the bowel lumen. Acquired diverticula often lack the muscularis propria.

Right: In contrast, congenital diverticula are lined by the full thickness of the gastrointestinal wall, including mucosa, submucosa, and muscularis propria.

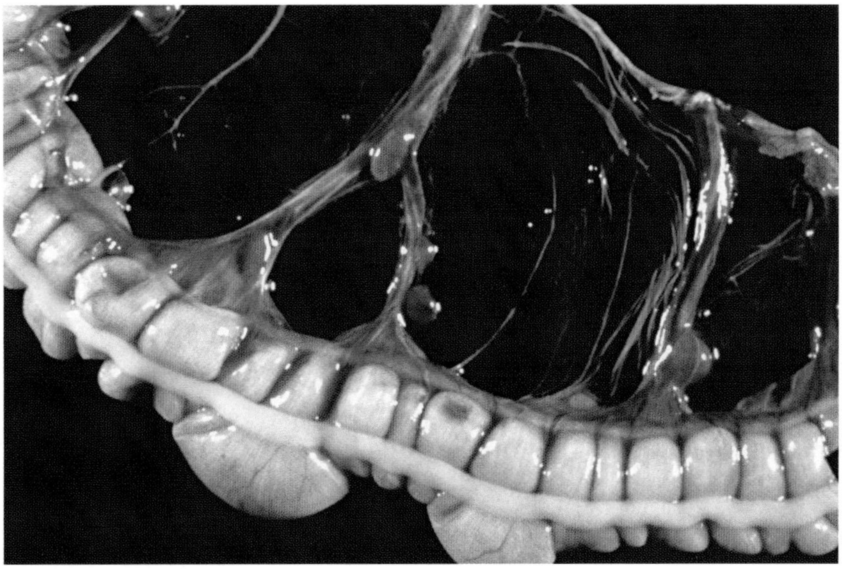

Figure 2-23

CONGENITAL ILEAL DIVERTICULA

Note the outpouchings of the ileal wall. This child had multiple congenital anomalies.

pancreatitis, duodenal obstruction, fistulas, hemorrhage, and perforation (131). Symptomatic patients range in age from 10 to 15 years (133).

Gross Findings. Both congenital and acquired diverticula arise throughout the gastrointestinal tract. The features that distinguish the two lesions are illustrated in figure 2-22. Congenital diverticula appear as solitary, sharply defined, round, oval or pear-shaped pouches that communicate with the gastric lumen via a narrow or broad-based mouth. Some form an intraluminal polyp (130).

Approximately 75 percent of gastric diverticula arise from the posterior wall, in a juxtacardiac position (132). They lie about 2 cm below the junction of the esophagus and stomach, and about 3 cm from the lesser curvature. The remainder originate in the antrum and pylorus. Most measure less than 4 cm in length.

In the intestines, congenital diverticula present as localized outpouchings, and are often multiple (fig. 2-23). Some congenital duodenal diverticula pass upward behind the stomach through a separate opening in the diaphragm to enter the right thoracic cavity where they attach to defective thoracic vertebrae. Eighty percent of solitary congenital cecal diverticula occur within 2.5 cm of the ileocecal valve near the cecal tip. (See next section for Meckel diverticula.)

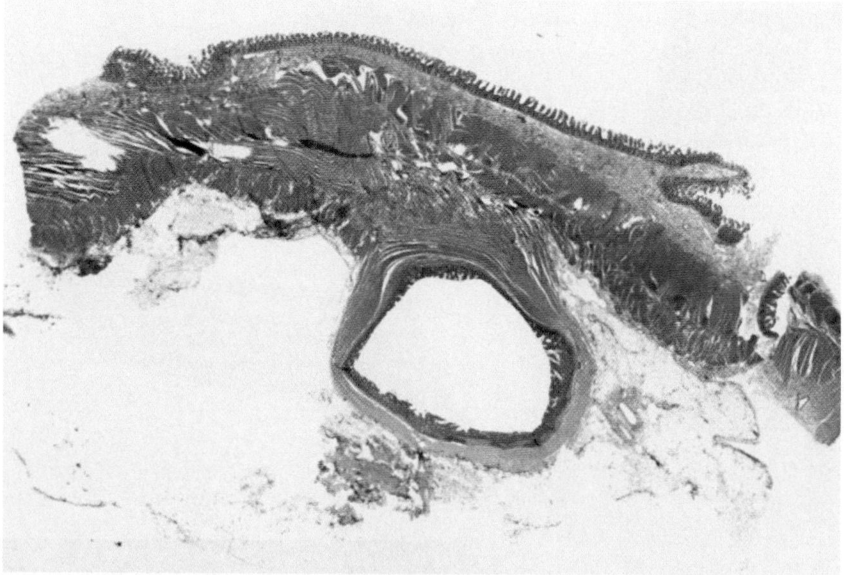

Figure 2-24

CONGENITAL ILEAL DIVERTICULA

Diverticula are lined by the same type of epithelium found within the native lumen. They contain the full thickness of the bowel wall and the lining.

Microscopic Findings. Congenital diverticula consist of all three bowel layers (fig. 2-24). The lining epithelium is usually that of the site of origin. Some diverticula contain heterotopic tissues, similar to those found in duplications and enterogenous cysts. Peptic ulcers may develop within diverticula containing oxyntic mucosa. If the diverticular orifice becomes blocked, diverticulitis develops.

Differential Diagnosis. Esophageal diverticula are of three types: congenital true diverticula, traction diverticula, and pulsion diverticula. Congenital true diverticula are very rare and involve all layers of the esophageal wall. Pulsion diverticula are herniations of the mucosa through intrinsic defects in the muscular wall. Traction diverticula result from adhesions between the esophagus and an external structure leading to stretching of the external wall and diverticulum formation. Acquired diverticula usually herniate through the circular part of the muscularis propria so that the protruding sac is lined by mucosa and covered by submucosa and longitudinal muscle. In contrast, congenital diverticula usually contain a complete muscularis propria.

Treatment and Prognosis. Diverticula usually do not require therapy unless they bleed or become inflamed. Inflamed diverticula may mimic appendicitis, bowel perforation, or intra-abdominal abscess. Symptomatic diverticula require surgical removal.

OMPHALOMESENTERIC REMNANTS

The various abnormalities caused by omphalomesenteric remnants are illustrated in figure 2-25.

Umbilical Fistula

Definition. *Umbilical fistula* is a persistent vitelline duct. The fistula tract communicates from the umbilicus to the small bowel.

Demography. Umbilical fistulas account for 2 percent of vitelline duct anomalies.

Pathophysiology. The umbilical cord represents the fusion of the yolk sac containing the vitelline duct and the body stalk with its paired umbilical arteries, the umbilical vein, and the allantois. It contains primitive mesenchymal tissue (Wharton jelly) and is covered by an outer layer of amnion. Normally, the vitelline duct obliterates between the 5th and 9th weeks of intrauterine life. When it fails to obliterate, an umbilical fistula results.

Clinical Features. Umbilical fistula manifests with persistent umbilical drainage. Its diagnosis may not be apparent on physical examination. A fistulogram to define the abnormality is helpful. A small catheter is inserted into the umbilical opening and a radiopaque dye is injected. The diagnosis is confirmed when the dye is visualized in the lumen of the small bowel.

Gross Findings. See definition.

Differential Diagnosis. When the vitelline duct is only partially obliterated, a vitelline cyst or a vitelline sinus may result. These lesions are illustrated in figure 2-25. Vitelline cysts are rare but can present as umbilical masses. Vitelline sinuses present with persistent umbilical drainage and are usually diagnosed in older children. Injection of contrast material delineates a blind-ending sinus.

Treatment and Prognosis. Persistently draining lesions are resected.

Meckel Diverticulum

Definitions. *Meckel diverticulum* is a partial, proximal, persistent omphalomesenteric or vitellointestinal duct. A Meckel diverticulum strangulated in an external hernia is known as a *Littre hernia*.

Demography. Meckel diverticulum is the most common congenital gastrointestinal anomaly, occurring in 1 to 4 percent of the population. It affects males and females equally. Meckel diverticulum has a higher incidence in patients with trisomy syndromes.

Associated Findings. Approximately 30 percent of patients have other congenital anomalies including TE fistula, microcolon, or duplications.

Etiology. Early in fetal life, the intestinal tract communicates with the yolk sac via the vitelline or omphalomesenteric duct. Typically, this duct detaches from the bowel before its physiologic herniation and then regresses before the bowel returns into the abdominal cavity. By the 7-mm developmental stage, the vitelline duct atrophies, leaving only a residual fibrous cord, which connects the bowel with the umbilicus. Subsequently, this band is absorbed. When the vitelline duct fails to obliterate, various vitelline duct abnormalities develop (fig. 2-25) (138). These include persistent fibrous cord, enteroumbilical fistula, and Meckel diverticulum. The persistent fibrous cord extends from the umbilicus to the bowel wall, the tip of a Meckel diverticulum, or the mesentery.

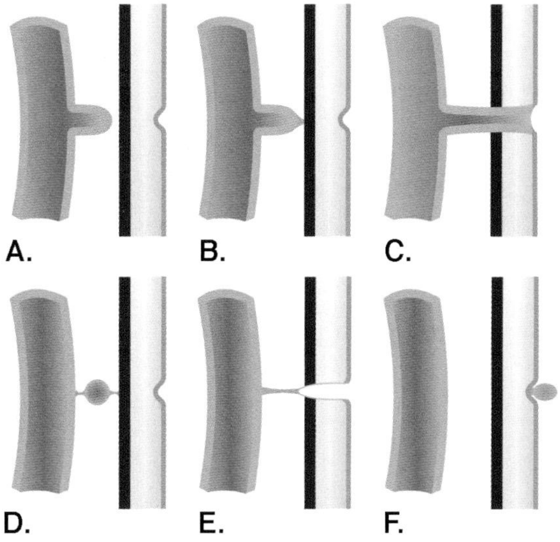

Figure 2-25

VITELLINE DUCT ABNORMALITIES

A: Meckel diverticulum is an outpouching of the bowel (terminal ileum) toward the abdominal wall.

B: A fibrous band attaches a Meckel diverticulum to the abdominal wall. This abnormality differs from A in that there is a residual obliterated fibrous tract from the tip of the Meckel diverticulum to the area of the umbilicus.

C: Umbilical fistula (omphaloileal fistula or patent Meckel diverticulum) in which the entire length of the yolk sac fails to involute and remains patent, connecting the ileum to the umbilicus.

D: Vitelline (umbilical) cysts are cystic structures separated by fibrous bands located between the anterior abdominal wall and the terminal ileum. Vitelline cysts are also called enterocystomas and result from patency of the midportion of the vitellointestinal duct while the proximal ileal or distal umbilical end involutes. The cyst may connect to the ileum or umbilicus with fibrous bands and usually is located at any level between them.

E: Umbilical sinus is a residual sinus tract that communicates from the anterior abdominal wall to the ileum. It extends at a variable depth into the abdominal wall or cavity.

F: Umbilical polyp results from patency of the distal umbilical end of the vitellointestinal duct. The umbilical polyp projects above the abdominal surface, frequently with a central dimple or sinus that may extend to the abdominal wall.

Clinical Features. Only 5 percent of patients with Meckel diverticula are symptomatic. The most frequent manifestations include hemorrhage and pain, usually resulting from peptic ulceration secondary to coexisting heterotopic gastric mucosa. Diverticulitis can develop secondary to peptic ulceration; obstruction of the diverticular orifice can clinically mimic appendicitis. Intestinal obstruction results from intussusception, volvulus, adhesions, compression by a mesodiverticular band, tumor, heterotopic tissue, enteroliths, bezoars, or an incarcerated Littre hernia. Impacted enteroliths cause diverticulitis, gangrene, and perforation. The pathogenesis of the diverticulitis resembles that seen in acute obstructive appendicitis. If the diverticulum ruptures, peritonitis will occur.

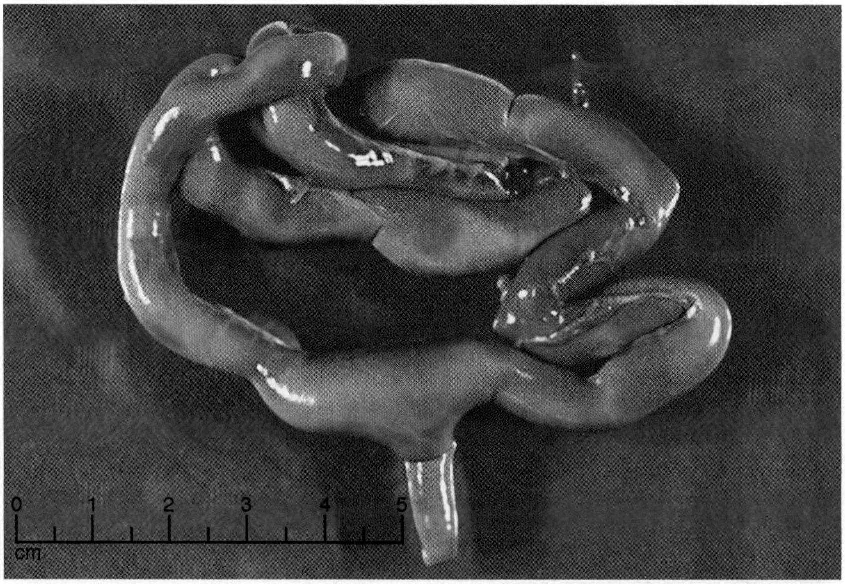

Figure 2-26

MECKEL DIVERTICULUM

The bowel of an infant who died with multiple other abnormalities. The Meckel diverticulum points down toward the 6 o'clock position.

Occasionally, a small bowel barium study demonstrates a Meckel diverticulum.

Gross Findings. A Meckel diverticulum varies in length from 1 to 26 cm. It always lies on the antimesenteric ileal border (fig. 2-26). Variations in size, location, and shape are common. In infants, it usually lies 30 cm proximal to the ileocecal valve; in the adult, it usually lies within 100 cm of the ileocecal valve. An apical fibrous band may connect the diverticulum to the umbilicus. A Meckel diverticulum may also connect to other intestinal loops or mesenteries via a congenital band or via adhesions from previous episodes of diverticulitis.

Sometimes, *a giant Meckel diverticulum* develops, resembling an enterogenous cyst (137). Such lesions are sometimes called *omphalomesenteric cysts*. Table 2-10 lists some of the other conditions that may be associated with Meckel diverticula.

Microscopic Findings. Typically, normal small intestinal epithelium lines the Meckel diverticulum, but heterotopic pancreatic, gastric, duodenal, jejunal, or colonic tissue may also be present. The pancreatic tissue sometimes acts as the lead point of an intussusception or it may cause obstruction. Heterotopic gastric mucosa (fig. 2-27) leads to peptic ulceration, bleeding, or perforation, especially if oxyntic mucosa is present. *Helicobacter pylori* may colonize the foveolar epithelium (135).

Differential Diagnosis. Clinically, acute Meckel diverticulitis mimics acute appendicitis, Crohn's disease, or pelvic inflammatory disease.

Treatment and Prognosis. A Meckel diverticulum has no clinical consequences unless complications develop (Table 2-10). These include perforation, vesicodiverticular fistula, hemorrhage, intussusception, volvulus, intestinal obstruction, and the development of inflammatory pseudotumors and true neoplasms (134,136). The tumors include carcinoid tumors, adenocarcinomas, and stromal tumors. These are more frequently encountered in males. Surgical resection is curative. If surgery is required for hemorrhage, the bleeding ulcer may be near the base of the diverticulum or in the adjacent ileum.

ANNULAR PANCREAS

Definition. *Annular pancreas* is a ring of pancreatic tissue surrounding the second part of the duodenum.

Demography. The incidence of annular pancreas is 1/20,000 births.

Associated Findings. Annular pancreas may be part of a more generalized embryogenic disorder associated with trisomy 21, TE fistulas, or cardiorenal abnormalities (140). When diagnosed in infancy, 80 percent of patients have associated anomalies; anomalies are only found in about 20 percent of adults with annular pancreas.

Etiology. The etiology is unknown.

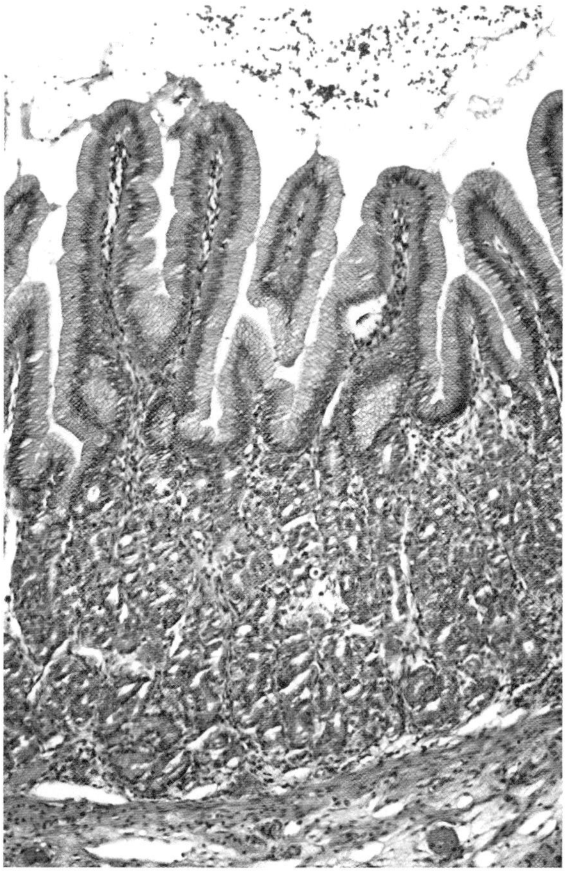

Figure 2-27

HETEROTOPIC GASTRIC MUCOSA IN MECKEL DIVERTICULUM

Table 2-10

ABNORMALITIES ASSOCIATED WITH MECKEL DIVERTICULUM

Ectopias	Complications
Gastric mucosa	Diverticulitis
Pancreas	Bleeding
Colonic tissue	Peptic ulcer
	Obstruction
Tumors	Intussusception
Carcinoid	Volvulus
Smooth muscle	Gangrene
Adenomas	Perforation
Carcinomas	
Lymphomas	

Clinical Features. Annular pancreas either presents in the neonatal period or in the 4th and 5th decades of life (139,140). The clinical presentation may mimic gastric outlet obstruction. The usual neonatal presentation is that of congenital duodenal obstruction. The presentation in adults includes duodenal stenosis, peptic ulcers, upper abdominal pain, and chronic pancreatitis; the lesion may be found incidentally. Peptic symptoms result from gastric stasis and antral overdistension due to the partial duodenal obstruction. The stasis and antral distension lead to hypergastrinemia, hyperchlorhydria, and peptic ulceration.

Gross Findings. Pancreatography may demonstrate pancreatic side-branches encasing the second part of the duodenum. Barium duodenography is remarkable for showing a smooth stenosis in the second part of the duodenum.

Microscopic Findings. Although the location of the pancreas is abnormal, the pancreatic histology appears completely normal. The heterotopic tissue contains ducts, acini, and islets. Secondary inflammatory changes occur if the patient develops duodenal stenosis or peptic ulceration.

Treatment and Prognosis. The prognosis of adults with this lesion is excellent and the lesion is resected when it becomes symptomatic. In children, the prognosis depends on the associated abnormalities.

PERITONEAL ENCAPSULATION

Definition. *Peritoneal encapsulation* is the encasement of the intestines by a peritoneal membrane.

Etiology. Peritoneal encapsulation probably results when an accessory peritoneal membrane forms from the mesocolon during the return of the intestinal loop to the abdomen following its herniation into the umbilical cord (10th fetal week). The dorsal mesentery covers most of the small intestine. It eventrates and moves counterclockwise, fusing with the posterior abdominal wall. Alternatively, the accessory membrane forms from part of the yolk sac peritoneum as it is drawn back into the abdominal cavity with the intestine (141).

Clinical Features. Patients usually remain asymptomatic and the lesion is detected incidentally. Nevertheless, patients may present with cramps, obstruction, abdominal pain, vomiting, and constipation alternating with diarrhea (141,142). Peritoneal encapsulation may mimic left mesocolic hernia.

Gross Findings. The entire intestine may be encapsulated within a thin peritoneal sac. This sac tends to be free and not adherent to the mesentery. The encased intestinal loops often have their own mesenteries.

Microscopic Findings. Peritoneal encapsulations can measure up to 20 cm. A thin peritoneum-like sac encases the entire small bowel. The histology of the encapsulated organs is normal. The histology of the membrane is that of a fibrous band.

Differential Diagnosis. The differential diagnosis includes sclerosing encapsulated peritonitis, usually a complication of peritoneal dialysis or other abdominal interventions. Sclerosing and encapsulating peritonitis is characterized by a thick, grayish white fibrous membrane covering the small intestinal wall. Peritoneal encapsulation must also be differentiated from the abdominal cocoon in which the small bowel is found totally or partially curled up in a concertina-like fashion and encased in a dense white membrane.

Treatment and Prognosis. Symptomatic patients undergo resection of the encapsulated bowel. Prognosis is excellent.

HETEROTOPIAS

Heterotopia, or *ectopia*, is the presence of normal tissue lying in an abnormal location. The term heterotopia derives from the Greek implying "other place." There are many forms of gastrointestinal heterotopia.

Esophageal Inlet Patch

Definition. The term *inlet patch* refers to the presence of ectopic gastric epithelium lying in the subcricoid, upper sphincteric region of the esophagus. Synonyms include *ectopic gastric mucosa* and *heterotopic gastric mucosa*.

Demography. Inlet patch affects from 7.8 to 21.0 percent of the population (145), with the highest incidence in the first year of life. A subsequent decline in incidence with age suggests that the lesions regress with time.

Etiology. Inlet patch represents the persistence of fetal columnar epithelium in the cervical esophagus.

Clinical Features. Inlet patches are usually discovered incidentally at the time of endoscopy for other reasons.

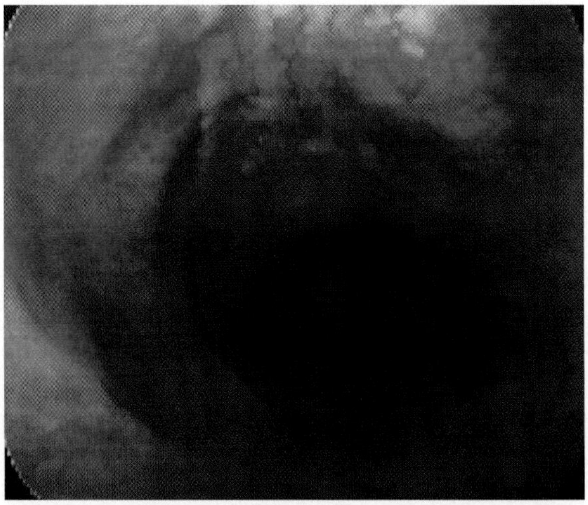

Figure 2-28

ENDOSCOPIC APPEARANCE OF INLET PATCH

There is a flame-shaped area of mucosa that appears red and velvety in contrast to the smooth squamous cell lining.

Gross Findings. Inlet patches lie in the subcricoid, upper sphincteric region, usually within 3 cm of the sphincter. Grossly and endoscopically, inlet patches are easily visualized, well-defined patches of ovoid, velvety, reddish mucosa with distinct borders (fig. 2-28). They vary in diameter from a few millimeters to complete esophageal encirclement (164). Occasionally, the mucosa ulcerates.

The ectopic gastric mucosa is easily detected on full column, single contrast radiologic examination. The typical radiographic finding is a discrete shallow depression surrounded by a subtle rim-like elevation on single contrast images or a pair of small indentations at the level of the thoracic inlet on the same wall on full column single contrast images (163).

Microscopic Findings. Histologically, inlet patches consist of oxyntic mucosa containing chief cells, parietal cells, endocrine cells, and foveolar cells (fig. 2-29). Inflammation, if present, induces secondary proliferative changes and glandular distortion. Large amounts of lymphoid tissue accompany smaller lesions, as compared to larger ones, suggesting that the lymphocytes play a role in lesional regression (164). *H. pylori* may colonize the heterotopic gastric epithelium (146).

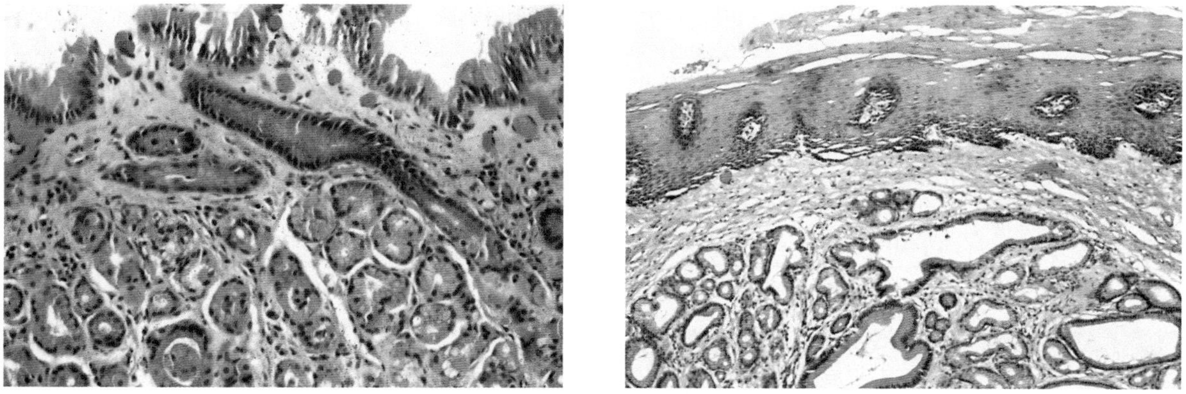

Figure 2-29

HISTOLOGIC APPEARANCE OF INLET PATCH

Left: The tissue resembles normal gastric oxyntic mucosa.
Right: Sometimes the surface glandular epithelium is replaced by squamous epithelium.

Treatment and Prognosis. No treatment is necessary for inlet patches, although complications may require therapy. Postinflammatory changes include the presence of cervical-esophageal webs (147), spontaneous TE fistula, or carcinoma (161).

Heterotopic Gastric Mucosa

Definition. *Heterotopic*, or *ectopic, gastric mucosa* is the presence of gastric mucosa in sites outside the stomach.

Demography. Heterotopic gastric tissue is the most common large intestinal heterotopia (166). It occurs alone or it complicates other congenital malformations, including duplications, Meckel diverticulum, and heterotopic pancreas. Ectopic gastric mucosa is most frequent in the duodenum and in Meckel diverticulum (152), and rarely affects the rectum. Rectal gastric heterotopias are associated with other congenital anomalies, including rectovesicle fistula, incomplete colonic rotation, vertebral body defects, duplication, rectal diverticula, scoliosis, and megacolon (158).

Etiology. Congenital heterotopias result from cellular entrapment during embryonic morphogenetic movement. The congenitally displaced tissues differentiate along the lines of normal organogenesis in response to local environmental factors. Rectal gastric heterotopias result from developmental abnormalities of foregut formation, ectodermal adhesion in the 3- to 4-week-old embryo, a differentiation error of fetal rectal endodermal cells, or proliferation of pluripotential cells.

Clinical Features. Heterotopic gastric epithelium often remains asymptomatic only to be discovered incidentally during endoscopy, at the time of surgery for an unrelated problem, or at the time of autopsy. Heterotopic small intestinal gastric mucosa is most often encountered when patients are evaluated for upper gastrointestinal complaints. Symptoms are usually secondary to peptic ulceration due to the presence of oxyntic mucosa. The lesions cause obstruction, spontaneous fistulas, and intestinal intussusception (148,154). In the rectum, heterotopic gastric mucosa presents as hemorrhoids, fissures, or fistulas, manifested by proctitis, pain, rectal bleeding, and proctalgia.

Gross Findings. Gastric heterotopia may be a single or multifocal lesion. It is most commonly seen in the duodenal bulb because of the frequency of upper endoscopy (fig. 2-30). It typically forms small nodules and polyps measuring less than 1.5 cm in maximum diameter. Giant heterotopic gastric polyps occasionally measure up to 4.5 cm (152). Heterotopic foci are usually surrounded by normal-appearing mucosa. The cut surface of the ectopic tissue may appear solid or cystic. Larger lesions with central depressions may mimic superficial ulcerating cancers (167). Heterotopic gastric tissue in the rectum frequently lies in the posterolateral region, 5 to 8 cm from the anal verge. It may form intrarectal polypoid lesions (162).

Microscopic Findings. Histologically, congenital gastric heterotopias are well-organized structures, more or less recapitulating the normal oxyntic mucosal architecture (fig. 2-31). Thus, they contain chief cells, parietal cells, and mucus-secreting epithelium, sometimes colonized by *H. pylori*. Ulcers, necrosis, and granulation tissue may develop in nearby tissue. Duodenal biopsies typically demonstrate intact duodenal villi and Brunner glands interrupted by discrete masses of gastric glands covered by foveolar epithelium. Rectal heterotopic gastric epithelium may coexist with ectopic respiratory epithelium, presumably representing the equivalent of the heterotopic foregut. Gastric mucosa may line rectal duplications and ectopic salivary gland tissue may also be present. Rarely, the ectopic tissue develops diseases resembling those seen in the native stomach, sometimes manifesting as a gastric hyperplastic polyp in the duodenum.

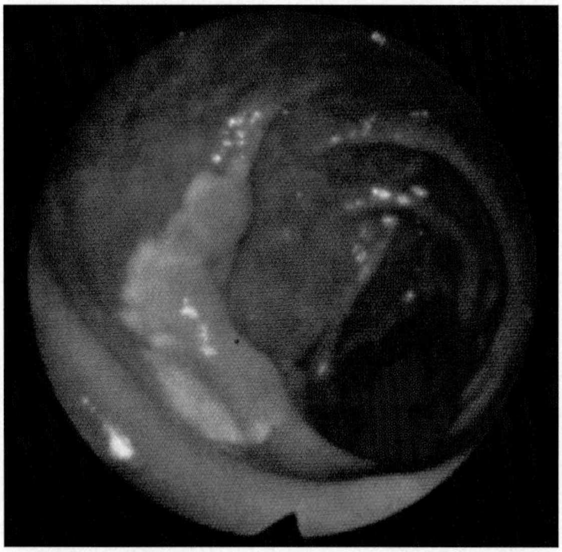

Figure 2-30

HETEROTOPIC GASTRIC MUCOSA IN THE DUODENUM

Endoscopically, the heterotopic tissue presents as a small mucosal nodule.

Differential Diagnosis. The major entity in the differential diagnosis is gastric metaplasia. Distinguishing between the two is relatively easy, since congenital tissue recapitulates normal structures (fig. 2-32). In contrast, metaplastic tissues usually consist of either foveolar epithelium lining the superficial duodenal epithelium or pyloric or antral glands lying in the basal intestinal mucosa. Gastric mucosal components, including surface, mucous neck, and glandular epithelia, are not present in metaplasias.

Treatment and Prognosis. Heterotopic gastric mucosa does not require therapy unless the lesions are large and cause obstruction. The lesion is usually encountered serendipitously during the performance of endoscopic or barium studies. When complications develop from peptic injury, the affected bowel may need to be resected.

Figure 2-31

HETEROTOPIC GASTRIC MUCOSA

The tissue recapitulates normal gastric tissue. Glands, usually of the oxyntic type, lie deep in the mucosa. The surface is covered by foveolar type gastric epithelium.

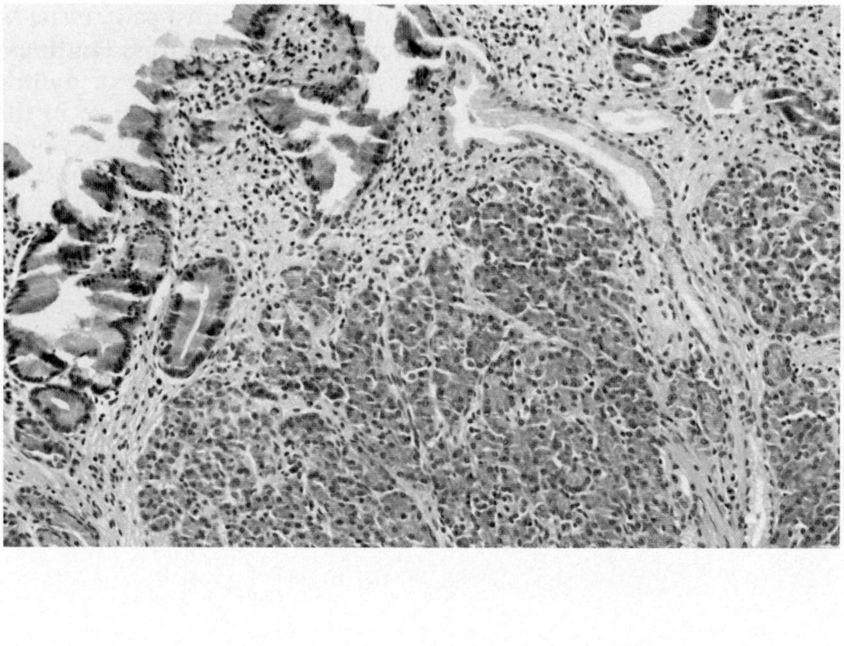

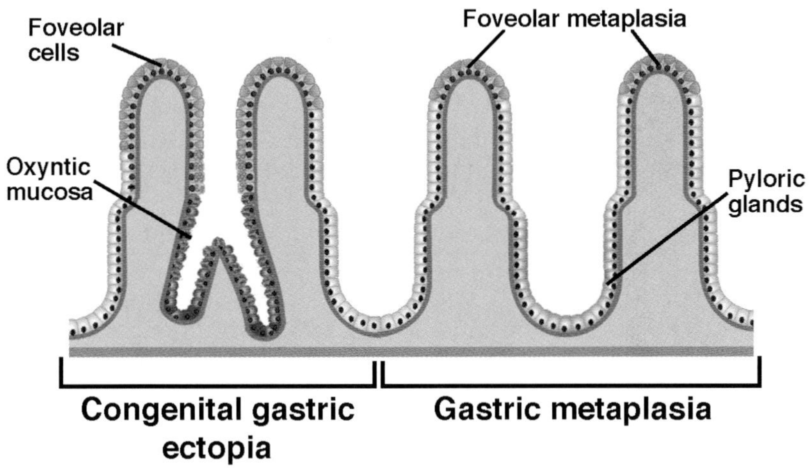

Figure 2-32

COMPARISON OF CONGENITAL GASTRIC HETEROTOPIA WITH ACQUIRED FORMS OF GASTRIC METAPLASIA

Left: In congenital gastric ectopia, intact gastric mucosa is present in the basal portion of the mucosa, complete with parietal and chief cells. Foveolar cells line the surface.

Right: In cases of gastric metaplasia, in contrast, there is either foveolar metaplasia as in peptic duodenitis or antral gland metaplasia as in cases of chronic small intestinal or large intestinal damage. There is no recapitulation of the normal mucosa as there is in congenital gastric ectopia.

Heterotopic Pancreas

Definition. *Heterotopic pancreas* is pancreatic tissue lying outside the pancreatic bed. It lacks any anatomic or vascular connection to the eutopic pancreas.

Demography. Gastric pancreatic heterotopia is seen in 0.25 to 0.50 percent of abdominal procedures and in 0.55 to 13.00 percent of autopsies (144,153). It is particularly common in patients with autosomal trisomy, especially involving chromosomes 13 and 18. It is also associated with gastrointestinal atresias, duplications, and other congenital malformations. Heterotopic pancreas is most frequent in the stomach, duodenum, jejunum, or Meckel diverticulum; it is the most common congenital anomaly seen in the gastric antrum. Esophageal involvement is uncommon, and when it occurs, it usually affects the distal end.

Etiology. Similar to gastric heterotopia.

Clinical Features. Most patients with heterotopic pancreas remain asymptomatic; the lesion is found incidentally at the time of endoscopy, surgery, or autopsy. Symptomatic patients develop crampy abdominal or epigastric pain or fullness. Weight loss, hemorrhage, and intussusception also occur. Secondary lesions, including pancreatitis or tumor development, may lead to obstruction, bleeding, epigastric pain, pseudocysts, mucoceles, or pseudotumors (155). Pancreatitis may be precipitated by biopsy or manipulation of the heterotopic tissue.

Gross Findings. Heterotopic pancreas is usually a well-demarcated, solitary, solid or cystic, tan, lobular, submucosal mass. The lesion typically measures 0.2 to 4.0 cm in diameter. Entry of single or multiple ducts into the gastric lumen produces a symmetric cone or nipple-like projection (fig. 2-33) or a central umbilication. Less commonly, multiple, polypoid or pedunculated pancreatic heterotopias are seen. Approximately 75 percent of heterotopic pancreatic tissue lies in the submucosa; the remainder involves the muscularis propria.

Microscopic Findings. The histologic features of heterotopic pancreas vary considerably. In its most classic form, it consists of lobulated pancreatic acini and ducts surrounded by concentric layers of longitudinal and circular muscle fibers (fig. 2-34). Islets are present in only approximately 33 percent of cases. Deeper lesions tend to appear more disorderly. Blockage of the ducts causes secondary cysts, pancreatitis, bleeding, pseudocyst formation, fat necrosis, abscess formation, and fibrosis secondary to leakage of proteolytic enzymes and acinar damage. Secondary changes may completely distort the histology of the heterotopic tissue (fig. 2-35).

Microscopic Variants. Heterotopic Brunner glands and/or gastric glands can accompany heterotopic pancreas.

Differential Diagnosis. If only pancreatic acini are present, the lesion may represent foci of pancreatic metaplasia, especially if the cells

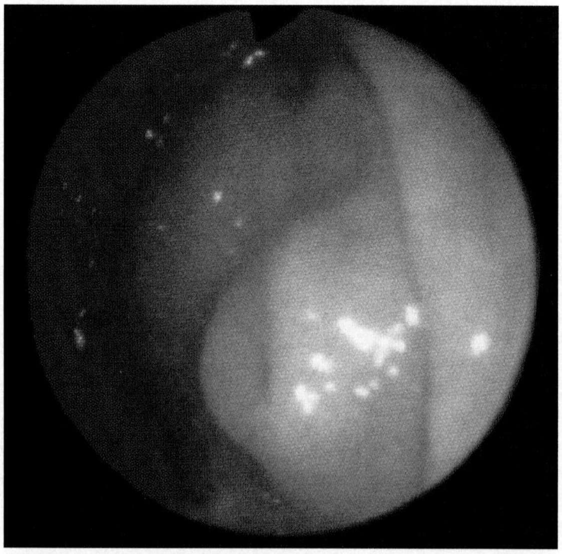

Figure 2-33

ENDOSCOPIC APPEARANCE OF HETEROTOPIC PANCREAS

The lesion presents as a submucosal nodule, often covered by intact gastric mucosa.

lie near the gastroesophageal junction. Lesions containing only ducts surrounded by the circular and longitudinal muscle layers are sometimes erroneously referred to as adenomyomas. The orderly arrangement of the two muscle layers around the ducts, however, serves to separate the two lesions.

Mucinous pools without obvious adjacent pancreatic tissue are sometimes identified and may suggest a diagnosis of colloid carcinoma. In contrast to mucinous carcinoma, the mucinous extravasation associated with heterotopic pancreas shows significant inflammation and fibrosis without overt cellular anaplasia. A diagnosis of invasive cancer should not be made in the absence of significant cytologic atypia and evidence of stromal desmoplasia.

Treatment and Prognosis. Heterotopic pancreas does not require treatment unless complications develop. The lesions are usually treated by local resection. Endocrine or glandular neoplasms may develop in ectopic pancreas

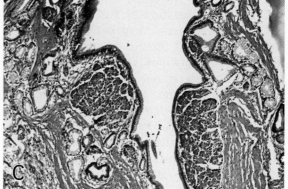

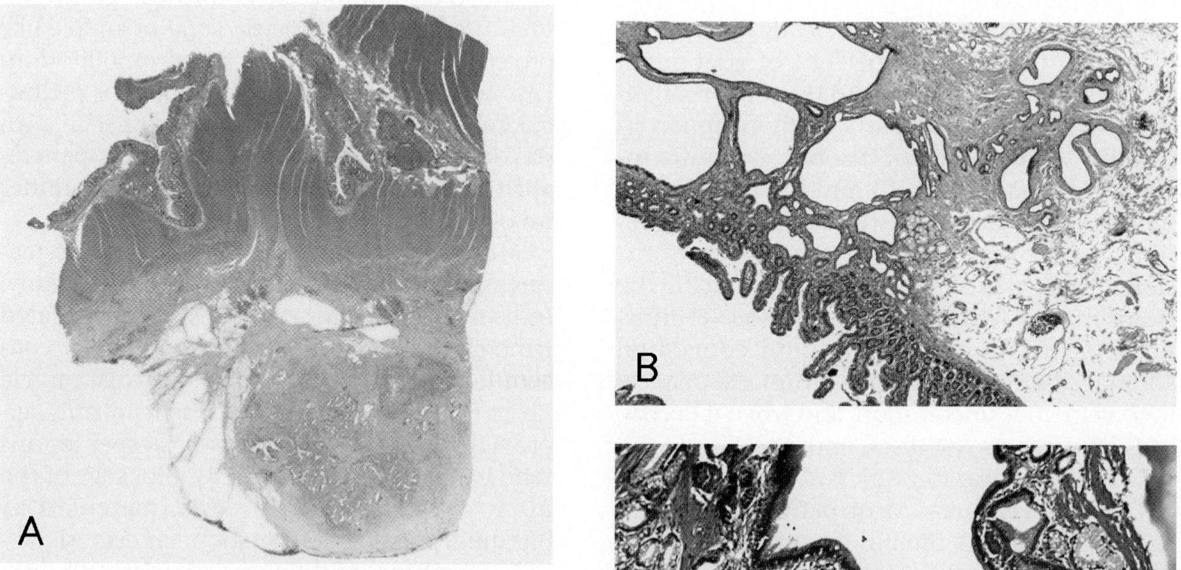

Figure 2-34

HETEROTOPIC PANCREAS

A: The heterotopic pancreas lies external to the bowel wall on the serosal surface of the jejunum.

B: Small intestinal heterotopic pancreas consists mostly of smooth muscle fibers and ductal epithelium. This lesion lies close to the surface and represents one variant of heterotopic pancreas.

C: Higher magnification of the heterotopic pancreatic tissue found in the stomach illustrated in figure 2-33.

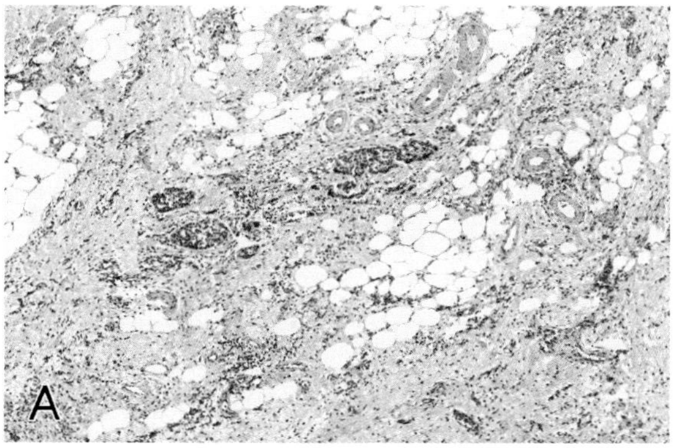

Figure 2-35

HETEROTOPIC PANCREAS IN THE DISTAL ESOPHAGUS

A: The tissue is markedly inflamed and fibrotic. Ductal structures are present, as are areas of inflammation and hemorrhage.

B: In some areas, the tissue is so inflamed that the histologic identity of the tissue is obscured.

C: In some areas, all that is left of the heterotopic pancreatic tissue are residual islets.

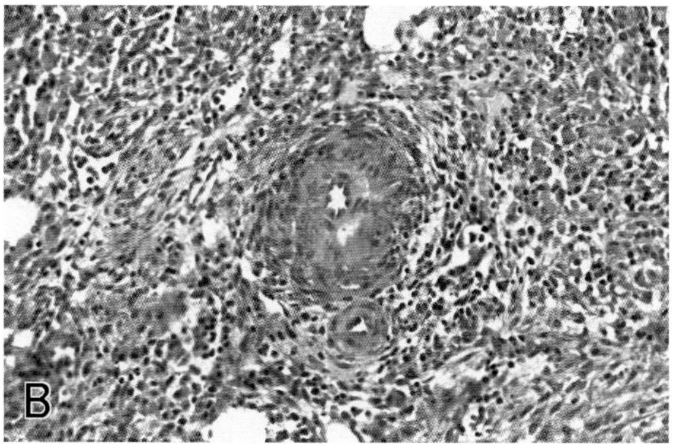

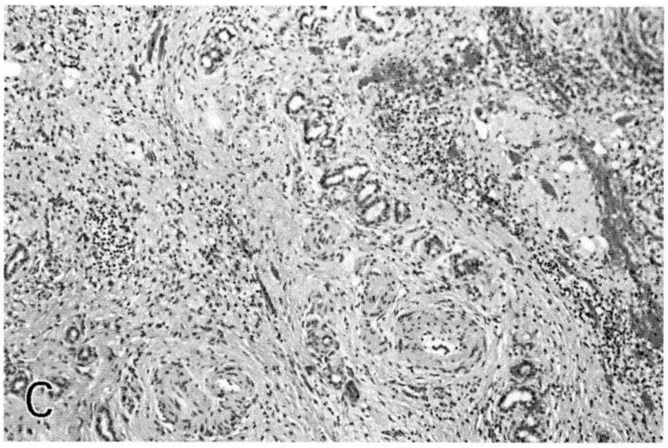

(143,150,151). Neoplastic transformation is rare. If carcinoma develops, it usually forms an intramural mass with relatively late mucosal invasion. As a result, the malignancy may be difficult to diagnose by endoscopic biopsy (150).

Heterotopic Brunner Glands

Heterotopic Brunner glands are Brunner glands lying in locations other than their normal location. Heterotopic Brunner glands are often associated with heterotopic pancreas or heterotopic gastric mucosa.

Heterotopic lesions occur in the pylorus and gastric antrum, and resemble heterotopic gastric or pancreatic tissue. Microscopically, the heterotopia may contain Brunner glands alone or the glands may coexist with smooth muscle fibers and heterotopic gastric or pancreatic tissue. Histologically, the heterotopia resembles duodenal Brunner gland hyperplasia. The lesion has no clinical significance.

Heterotopic Sebaceous Glands

Heterotopic sebaceous glands are sebaceous glands located at sites other than the surface of the skin. The lesion is a developmental abnormality.

Heterotopic sebaceous glands are normally found incidentally at the time of endoscopy. They present as multiple, small, yellowish mucosal plaques, typically affecting the middle or distal esophagus. Histologically, normal mature sebaceous glands underlie a normal squamous mucosa (fig. 2-36). This lesion has no clinical significance.

Heterotopic Salivary Glands

Heterotopic salivary glands are salivary glands in sites other than their normal location. They represent a congenital abnormality. The lesions may arise from vestiges of the postanal gut.

Seromucinous tissue resembling salivary glands can occur in the rectal submucosa, either alone or associated with retrorectal cystic hamartomas or gastric mucosa (159,160,165). Rarely, heterotopic salivary glands present as a perianal fibroepithelial polyp. The lesions often contain both serous and mucinous glands, although pure mucinous lesions occur. The lesion has no clinical significance.

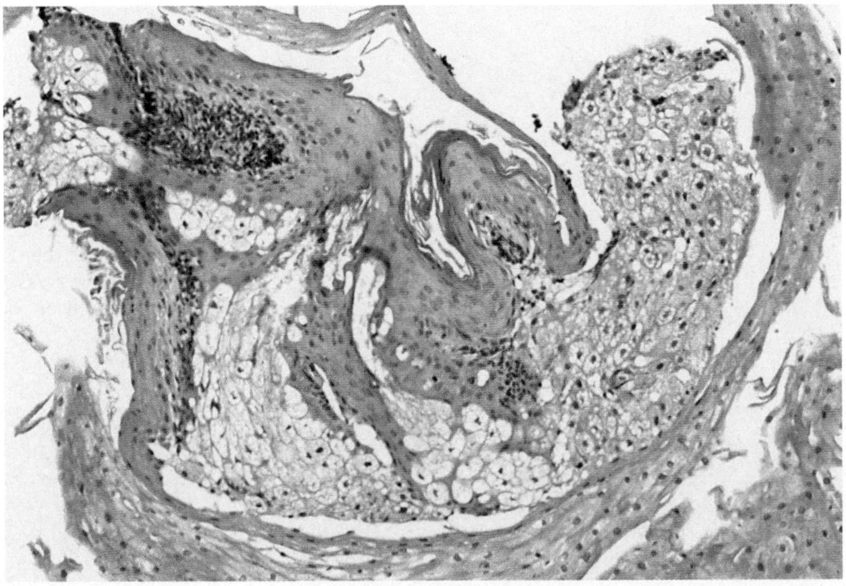

Figure 2-36

HETEROTOPIC SEBACEOUS GLANDS IN THE ESOPHAGUS

Biopsy of squamous lining epithelium shows prominent nests of sebaceous cells that appear histologically normal. The only abnormality is their location.

Heterotopic Prostate

Heterotopic prostate is prostatic tissue in sites other than the normal prostate. This ectopic tissue may represent a metaplasia from endogenous urothelial epithelium (149) or it may result from faulty embryogenesis. The presence of aberrant mesenchymal prostatic rests may induce the prostatic epithelium.

The tissue consists of prostatic glands, usually lying in the submucosa of the anal canal. This lesion has no clinical significance.

Heterotopic Thyroid

Heterotopic thyroid tissue is thyroid tissue located outside the normal thyroid gland. Ectopic thyroid tissue may occur in the esophagus. It has the appearance of normal thyroid tissue and has no clinical significance.

Ectopic Renal Tissue

Ectopic renal tissue lies in the colonic wall encroaching on the colonic surface epithelium of patients with caudal regression syndromes. Ectopic tissue demonstrates a full developmental range of renal differentiation, from undifferentiated blastema to primitive or well-formed glomeruli and tubules (157).

Ectopic Uterus

A single patient was reported to have an intramural ileal mass that had features of the uterine fundus and two smaller contiguous nodules resembling fallopian tube. It is unclear whether this lesion represents a heterotopia or a monodermal teratoma (156).

MÜLLERIAN AND MESONEPHRIC DUCT REMNANTS

Müllerian duct remnants are embryologic remnants of the müllerian system that lie in sites where müllerian tissue is not normally present after birth. Müllerian remnants fail to involute following fetal development.

Usually these lesions are clinically silent. They may become symptomatic when secondary changes, such as abscesses, develop in them (168). Small glands consisting of primitive müllerian or mesonephric tissue are embedded in other tissues, often in the muscular wall of the rectum or anus. They occur in patients with associated congenital abnormalities or in the absence of other changes. These morphologic curiosities have no clinical significance.

MICROGASTRIA

Definition. *Microgastria* is a smaller than normal stomach. Synonyms include *tubular* or *fetal stomach* and *gastric hypoplasia*.

Demography. Microgastria occurs alone or it coexists with other anomalies.

Associated Abnormalities. The many abnormalities that complicate microgastria are shown in Table 2-11 (170,171).

Etiology. The lesion probably results from the failed development of the dorsomesogastrium or lack of differential growth of the primitive foregut. One theory suggests that the origin of the microgastria-limb reduction complex relates to the process of twinning (170). The presence of holoprosencephaly indicates a severe defect of gastrulation/blastogenesis predominantly affecting the cephalad structures.

Clinical Features. Symptoms usually appear in infancy and include failure to thrive, frequent vomiting, and recurrent aspiration pneumonia due to the presence of an incompetent lower esophageal sphincter.

Gross Findings. The stomach appears small, tubular, and often nonrotated. As a result, the stomach lies in the midline and the greater and lesser curvature do not develop. The esophagus may appear grossly dilated (169).

Microscopic Findings. The entire gastric wall appears hypoplastic, making it difficult to distinguish between the cardia, body, and antrum.

Differential Diagnosis. The differential diagnosis includes the CAVE (cerebroacrovisceral-Early) lethality phenotype and the Pallister-Hall syndrome.

Treatment and Prognosis. The underdeveloped lower esophageal sphincter becomes incompetent and gastroesophageal reflux, with all its attendant complications (see chapter 3), develops.

Table 2-11

ABNORMALITIES ASSOCIATED WITH MICROGASTRIA

Atresia
Esophageal
Anal
Intestinal
Intestinal malrotation
Cardiac anomalies
Pulmonary anomalies
Skeletal anomalies
Central nervous system anomalies
Asplenia
Growth hormone deficiencies
Diabetes insipidus
Diaphragmatic hernias
Multicystic, dysplastic kidneys
Psychomotor retardation
Holoprosencephaly sequence
VACTERL[a] association
Ivemark syndrome

[a]VACTERL = vertebral defects, anal atresia, cardiac anomalies, tracheoesophageal defects, renal dysplasia, limb defects.

ANORECTAL ANOMALIES (MALFORMATIONS)

There is a broad spectrum of anorectal anomalies. Typically both the rectum and anal canal are affected. The Santuli International Classification system, commonly used to classify anorectal malformations, is based on the location of the termination of the rectum in relation to the levator ani muscles and the pubococcygeal or ischial lines (Table 2-12) (196). Malformations are classified as high (supralevator), intermediate, or low (translevator) (fig. 2-37), based on the position of the air-filled rectum in the lateral projection with the infant held upside down. This radiograph is referred to as the Wangensteen-Rice invertogram. Seventy-five percent of low anomalies are associated with a fistula from the rectal pouch to the perineal skin just anterior to a covered anal dimple.

Imperforate anus and *anorectal malformation* are terms for anorectal anomaly. The term anorectal anomaly is generally a better term than the term imperforate anus because of the wide range of malformations present in this region, all of which result from abnormal urorectal septal development.

Demography. Anorectal anomalies are common congenital, occasionally familial, malformations with an incidence of approximately 1/3,000 to 5,000 births. Males outnumber females 1.3 to 1.0 and are more likely to have high lesions (178). Intermediate anomalies are rare and include anal agenesis, anorectal stenosis, and the rare anorectal membrane situated above the cloacal membrane. In one study, high-type deformities accounted for 26 percent of cases; intermediate, 10.7 percent; and low, 57.2 percent. The most frequent deformity is male anocutaneous fistula followed by male rectoureteral fistula, and female anovestibular fistula (180).

Associated Findings. Most patients exhibit associated developmental anomalies affecting multiple systems, including the vertebrae,

Table 2-12

INTERNATIONAL CLASSIFICATION OF ANORECTAL ANOMALIES

Anomaly	Female	Male
Low (translevator)	1. Normal anal site a) Anal stenosis b) Covered anus complete 2. Perineal site a) Anocutaneous fistula (covered anus incomplete) b) Anterior perineal anus 3. Vulvar site a) Anovulvar fistula b) Anovestibular fistula c) Vestibular anus	1. Normal anal site a) Anal stenosis b) Covered anus complete 2. Perineal site a) Anocutaneous fistula (covered anus incomplete) b) Anterior perineal anus
Intermediate	1. Anal agenesis a) Without fistula b) Rectovestibular fistula c) Rectovaginal fistula (low) 2. Anorectal stenosis	1. Anal agenesis a) Without fistula b) Rectobulbar fistula 2. Anorectal stenosis
High (supralevator)	1. Anorectal agenesis a) Without fistula b) With rectovaginal fistula (high) c) Rectocloacal fistula 2. Rectal atresia	1. Anorectal agenesis a) Without fistula b) With rectourethral fistula (high) c) Rectovesicle fistula 2. Rectal atresia
Miscellaneous Imperforate anal membrane Cloacal exstrophy Others		

intestines, urologic system, and genital system (182, 191). Congenital heart disease and esophageal atresia with tracheoesophageal fistula occur in about a third of patients. Intestinal atresias, malrotations, duplications, annular pancreas, bicornuate uterus, vaginal atresia, septate vagina, absence of the rectus abdominal muscle, omphalocele, and bladder exstrophy occur. Less commonly, anorectal anomalies are part of a multiple complex malformation syndrome (Table 2-13). An association with VACTERL should be considered in any infant with an anorectal anomaly. Some congenital anorectal malformations have a strong association with sacrococcygeal teratomas, lesions sometimes referred to as "hereditary presacral teratomas" (173,188).

Etiology. Mutations in the putative zinc finger transcription factor gene *SALL1* cause the Townes-Brock syndrome (183), an autosomal dominantly inherited malformation syndrome characterized by anal, renal, limb, and ear anomalies.

Treatment and Prognosis. Mortality in children with anorectal malformations usually relates to concurrent disease and not to the malformation itself. Renal and cardiac abnormalities account for most deaths. The type of reconstructive surgery performed and the resultant sphincteric function is determined by the status of the levator ani muscle (194). Because anal sphincter function is normal in low anomalies, infants with these have less morbidity and better surgical results than those with other anorectal abnormalities (186). Higher lesions require a colostomy followed by anorectal reconstruction and subsequent colostomy closure. Lesions not requiring a colostomy can be repaired in the newborn period with good functional results.

Low Abnormalities

Definition. Low malformations are those that occur below the level of the levator ani musculature. They include the ectopic (perineal, vestibular, or vulvar) anus, covered anus, imperforate anus, anal atresia, and cloacal exstrophy. The designation of lesions as being "covered" indicates that no opening is seen. They are characterized by the confluence of the rectum, vagina, and bladder in a urogenital sinus.

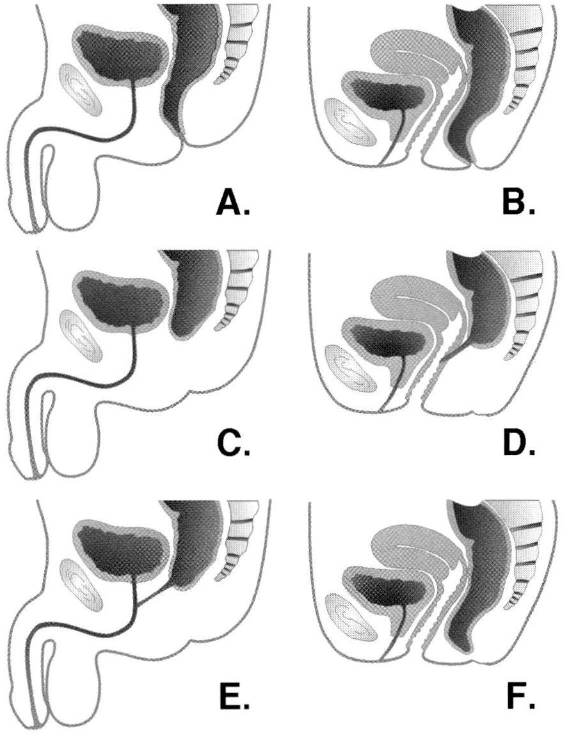

Figure 2-37

ANORECTAL ABNORMALITIES

Figures A, C, and E represent alterations in the male, while B, D, and F represent those in the female.

A,B: In anal stenosis, the anal canal narrows but there is a functional opening to the external environment. This contrasts with the situation that occurs with complete atresia in the female in which there is no visible opening to the distal portion of the gastrointestinal tract.

C: Anorectal agenesis without fistula.

D: Anorectal agenesis with fistula to the female genital tract.

E: Anorectal agenesis with fistula to the genitourinary system.

F: In contrast to B, there is no external opening of the anorectal region to the external environment.

Table 2-13

SYNDROMES ASSOCIATED WITH ANAL ATRESIA

Ritscher-Schinzel syndrome (cranio-cerebello-cardiac syndrome)
Pallister-Hall syndrome
Autosomal inheritance
Hypothalamic hamartoma
Polydactyly
Imperforate anus
Laryngeal clefting
Other abnormalities
Currarino triad
Anorectal stenosis or other low type anorectal malformations
Anterior sacral defect
Presacral mass (teratomas, meningoceles, dermoids, enteric cysts)
Opitz syndrome (midline defects)
Hypertelorism
Hypospadia
Lip-palate-laryngeal clefts
Imperforate anus
Townes-Brocks syndrome
Anal malformation (imperforate anus, anteriorly placed anus or anal stenosis)
Hand malformation (preaxial polydactyly, broad bifid thumb or triphalangeal thumb)
External ear malformation (microtia, "satyr" or "lop" ear, preauricular tags or pits)
Sensorineural hearing loss
Additional features may include urinary tract malformations, mental retardation, and pericentric inversion of chromosome 16
VACTERL association
Vertebral defects
Anal atresia
Tracheoesophageal defects
Renal dysplasia
Radial or limb defects

Demography. Low malformations more often affect males than females. Rarely, the abnormalities affect families (193). A true imperforate anus or membranous anal atresia with the persistence of the anal membrane is rare (184,186) and a significant association exists between anal atresia and parental consanguinity. Cloaca exstrophy is the most severe degree of imperforate anus, affecting approximately 1/50,000 births.

Associated Lesions. Patients with imperforate anus may have an associated neuropathic bladder (189), deafness (185), and rectal and sigmoid atresias (179).

Etiology. Low anomalies result from incomplete or inappropriate development of the anal canal and anal membrane coupled with prominent genital folds that contribute to the covered appearance of the anus. Imperforate anus results from failure of the cloacal membrane to perforate. The anomaly originates during the 6th to 8th week of embryonic development and results from detained ingrowth or an inadequate migration in the rectal segment of hindgut. There is often a history of maternal drug use and a paternal history of exposure to an occupational hazard. Chromosomal abnormalities

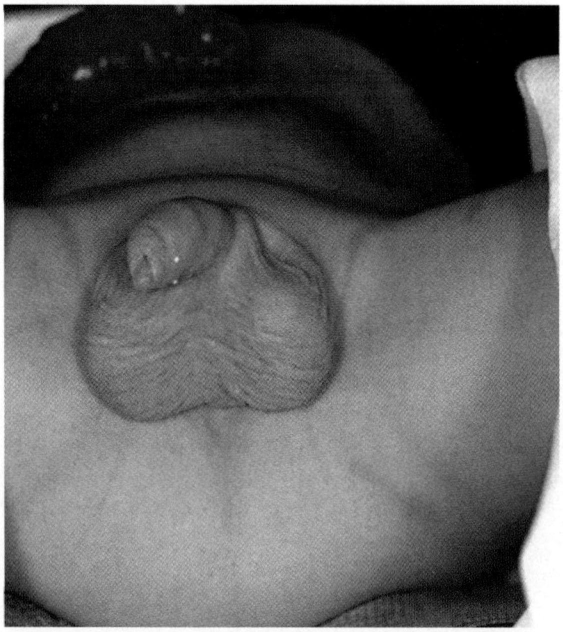

Figure 2-38

IMPERFORATE ANUS

The anal orifice is completely covered. There is no evidence of an anal opening.

associated with imperforate anus include small deletions of chromosome 13 (q32.2qter) and 13 (q32q34) (174), partial monosomy 10q, and partial trisomy 9q (195).

Clinical Features. Mothers of children with anal atresia are more often likely to have threatened abortion, oligohydramnios, and polyhydramnios than other women. Cloacal exstrophy is a complex spectrum of malformations and in the past was uniformly fatal. In addition to imperforate anus, these babies have an omphalocele, two exotropic bladders between which there is an open cecum, and a blindly-ending colon hanging down in the pelvis from the cecum. The genitalia are ambiguous and most of these children are raised as females. The urinary and gastrointestinal systems must be surgically separated to insure survival.

Gross Findings. There are four types of imperforate anus: 1) stenosis alone (11 percent); 2) imperforate anus with only a thin membrane separating the anus and rectum (4 percent); 3) imperforate anus with a widely separated anus and rectum (76 percent) (fig. 2-38); and 4) normal anus with the rectum ending some distance above it (9 percent) (172,173,182,184,188). Fistulas form between the rectum and some part of the urogenital system, especially in type 3 and 4 imperforate anus. In males, the fistulas tend to be urinary (urethra, 25 percent; bladder, 33 percent; or perineal, 42 percent) and in females, rectourinary or rectogenital (vaginal, 84 percent; perineal, 14.5 percent; and urinary bladder, 1.5 percent). Rarely, the rectum opens into the scrotum, the undersurface of the penile shaft, or the prepuce (181).

In some low abnormalities, including ectopic anus, the anus opens anterior to its normal position, sometimes within the vulva. The ectopic anorectum lies below the puborectalis muscle. A congenital rectovestibular or rectovaginal fistula opens into the vagina or the vulva but above the puborectalis muscle (190). In a related anomaly, the covered anus, a bar of skin, derived from the lateral genital folds, covers the anal canal. An anocutaneous fistula passes anteriorly from the anal canal to the exterior at the perineal raphe. A misplaced external sphincter with conjoined fibers inserted behind the elongated, ventrally angulated terminal canal can functionally obstruct fecal passage even in patients with an adequate anal canal and anal orifice.

Microscopic Findings. At first glance, it appears as though organs associated with anorectal atresia are normal; however, careful investigation of the entire thickness of the wall shows that oligoneuronal hypoganglionosis of the myenteric plexus proximal to the anal floor is present in 12 percent of patients and other patients may demonstrate defects in the muscularis propria. The latter are characterized by hypoplasia of the circular muscle layer and/or internal anal sphincter. Intestinal neuronal dysplasia of the submucosal plexus is frequently observed (12 percent) in high type anal atresia. The histologic changes in neuromuscular structure confined to the high type anal atresia are not seen in intermediate or low types. Overall, anomalies of the enteric nervous system are present in 60 percent of anal atresias (187).

Treatment and Prognosis. Females with cloacal anomalies must be recognized at birth so that urologic evaluation can be performed. Hydrocolpos and obstructive uropathy are common and warrant urgent decompression of the urinary tract with a vaginostomy and/or vesicostomy as well as a colostomy. It is also important to recognize precursors to renal insufficiency including renal agenesis, renal dysplasia, and vesicoureteral reflux since their presence mandates early consultation with a pediatric urologist. The morbidity and mortality associated with the renal lesions often exceed that of the imperforate anus. Spinal cord anomalies are also common and can be found in patients who have normal plain films and low defects. Spinal ultrasonography or MRI should be performed in all neonates to rule out occult spinal pathology such as a tethered cord or lipoma of the cord. Early evaluation of patients with imperforate anus leads to the development of a carefully thought out plan which sets the stage for the best possible outcome in later life.

Intermediate Abnormalities

Definition. In intermediate anomalies, the blind segment ends at the level of the levator ani muscle and at the level of a line joining the ischial tuberosities (the ischial line) (194). They include anal agenesis with and without fistula and anorectal stenosis. The fistula can be rectobulbar in males, rectovestibular or rectovaginal in females. The internal sphincter is absent and the external sphincter is poorly formed in both sexes. Anal agenesis, anal stenosis, and anal canal agenesis are types of intermediate anomalies.

Demography. Although intermediate agenesis affects both sexes, most cases occur in males (194).

Etiology. Intermediate anomalies are thought to occur as a result of vascular injury during fetal life.

Gross Findings. Intermediate abnormalities include stenoses in the upper end of the anal canal. The terminal bowel appears ectatic and thickened (175,177), and a shortened anal canal lies within the levator diaphragm.

In males, there is a clear separation between muscle fibers running toward the pubis and others running toward the perineal body and bulbocavernosus muscle ventrally. Striated muscle fibers of the pubococcygeus muscle are associated with the bowel wall. Fibers of the puborectalis may be present dorsally and laterally (176). Girls with a rectovestibular fistula lack the perineal body (central tendon), which normally lies between the rectum and vagina. Fascicles of the pubococcygeus and the external sphincter become displaced laterally.

High (Supralevator) Abnormalities

Definition. High malformations are the most common anomalies seen in males. They are associated with a rectourethral fistula in males and a rectovaginal fistula in females. Sphincteric function is abnormal and there is a high frequency of other malformations. High abnormalities include primitive cloaca, cloacal persistence, rectocloacal fistula, and anorectal agenesis.

Etiology. Anorectal agenesis is a relatively primitive defect reflecting a cloaca that has not yet divided into separate urinary and alimentary canals. Rectal atresia is thought to occur as a result of vascular injury during fetal life. An intact sphincter is usually present (186). Trisomy 4 is found in some fetuses with anal atresia along with other congenital abnormalities.

Gross Findings. In anorectal agenesis, the rectum reaches the upper surface of the pelvic floor, but the musculature of the entire anal canal and pelvic floor is absent and the rectum ends above the levator muscle. There is a single external opening into which a short urethra opens anteriorly and the rectum opens posteriorly. The rectum opens into a posterior urethra or bladder in males and into a posterior vaginal fornix in females. In girls, failure of the müllerian systems to fuse normally creates two uteri that open into the globular cloacal cavity. A fistula enters either the dorsal wall of the cloaca or the caudal end of the septum between the bifid urogenital sinus portion of a double vagina. High rectovaginal fistulas usually near the anterior fornix, may also be present.

Variations of rectocloacal and rectovaginal fistulas of the high type are encountered (192). Confusion centers around rectocloacal fistula formation. In some cases, the cloaca appears to directly communicate with the vagina whereas in others it appears to be a direct continuation of the urethra. If a single peritoneal opening drains all of these viscera, it satisfies the criteria for a cloacal opening and any such pattern is regarded as a rectocloacal fistula. In boys, the orifice of rectourethral fistulas appears quite large and a catheter passed through the urethra usually enters the rectum rather than the bladder. The bowel usually terminates in a fistula to the lower third of the prostate in males, although it may end blindly.

Anal agenesis contrasts with anal atresia in that the rectum ends blindly above the level of the pelvic floor. The anal canal appears anatomically normal.

Microscopic Findings. The histology of the organs is normal.

Treatment and Prognosis. A series of planned surgeries may be required. A diverting colostomy is followed by a pull-through procedure (anorectoplasty). Patients with low anomalies achieve early continence while those with high anomalies seldom do by school age.

THYMIC-RENAL-ANAL-LUNG DYSPLASIA

Thymic-renal-anal-lung dysplasia is a newly described autosomal recessive error of early morphogenesis. The patients present with a syndrome characterized by a unilobed or absent thymus, renal and ureter agenesis/dysgenesis, and intrauterine growth retardation. Patients may also have an imperforate anus and a unilobed lung.

Theories to explain the occurrence of these developmental abnormalities include an autosomal recessive inheritance and an unrecognized chromosomal imbalance. Renal, anal, and lung dysplasia is present in three syndromes: Fraser-Jacquier-Chen (198), Pallister-Hall (199), and Smith-Lemli-Opitz II (197) syndromes.

The disease is detectable prenatally by the presence of progressive oligohydramnios and intrauterine growth retardation. Also seen are a unilateral echogenic cystic mass in the renal fossa and low amniotic fluid disaccharidases in association with an imperforate anus.

CAUDAL DYSPLASIA

Definition. *Caudal dysplasia*, also known as *caudal regression syndrome*, consists of developmental anomalies at the caudal vertebrae, neural tube, urogenital and digestive organs, and hind limbs, the precursors of which derive from the caudal eminence.

Demography. Caudal dysplasia is associated with maternal diabetes or prediabetes (201, 209), suggesting that the syndrome results from the presence of insulin antagonists (214). The disease sometimes affects siblings. A combination of the diabetic trait and unrelated genetic factors that encode skeletal differentiation is required for fully developed caudal dysplasia syndrome; these may both be related to *HLA-DR* genes (206,211,213).

Associated Findings. Associated anomalies include meningomyelocele, anal and genital defects, absent fibula, and short femora. The upper limbs are rarely involved. Congenital anomalies of the heart and great vessels may be present as may TE fistula (210). The most extreme form of caudal dysplasia has associated sirenomelia (203,205,212).

Etiology. The etiology and pathogenetic mechanisms are poorly understood.

Gross Findings. Anal malformations are a prominent component of the constellation of abnormalities in caudal dysplasia, including complete covered anus with or without fistula formation and rectal atresia (205).

Microscopic Findings. Microscopic foci of ectopic renal tissue encroach on the colonic surface epithelium in some patients. The renal tissue demonstrates a full developmental range, from undifferentiated blastema to both primitive and well-formed glomeruli and tubules.

Differential Diagnosis. Some other syndromes that closely resemble caudal dysplasia fall under the general heading of familial sacral dysgenesis. These include the Ashcraft syndrome of familial hemisacrum (200) and the Cohn-Bay-Nielsen syndrome of familial hemisacrum (200,202).

Animal Models. Rumplessness, a condition similar to caudal dysplasia, develops in chick embryos who receive insulin (207). Studies in fetal rats suggest that fetal insulin production may play a role in the genesis of sacral defects (204). Administration of retinoic acid induces the caudal regression syndrome in fetal mice (208).

ANORECTAL CYSTS

Definition. The nature and etiology of developmental *anorectal cysts* remain controversial. Some represent sequestered duplications; others are considered to represent a form of teratoma; still others are thought to arise from embryonic remnants of the postanal segment or tailgut (215a,225). Anorectal cysts include cystic hamartomas, tailgut cysts, enteric cysts, and retrorectal cyst-hamartomas (215a,216,218–220,228).

Demography. Anorectal cysts are uncommon. They affect females more commonly than males, and they often coexist with other congenital abnormalities, particularly spina bifida (209). The age distribution ranges from the neonatal period to 73 years.

Associated Findings. Anorectal cysts may be associated with intraspinal and postsacral cysts.

Etiology. Anorectal cysts result from: 1) remnants of the caudal-postcloacal hindgut located within the embryonic tail, 2) cloacal rests, 3) sequestered rectal duplication, or 4) neuroenteric fistulas associated with sacral anomalies or intraspinal cysts.

Clinical Features. Anorectal cysts present as retrorectal or posterior anal masses in children and young adults. Developmental cysts grow slowly and frequently remain as asymptomatic lesions unless they enlarge, in which case they cause sensations of pressure, fullness, constipation, urinary and/or fecal incontinence, and perineal pain and numbness; they may cause pain in the rectal area or low back and the pain may occur during defecation. In symptomatic patients, the lesion averages 4.6 cm and in the asymptomatic patients, 3.2 cm. When retrorectal developmental cysts become infected, retrorectal abscesses and anal fistulas form (215a). They may also manifest as obstructive extrinsic rectal masses (216,218,221,222,224,227).

Gross Findings. Developmental cysts lie between the coccyx and the rectum. They range in size from 2 to 23 cm, with an average diameter of 3.9 cm. On barium exam they appear as smooth eccentric masses that deform the posterior rectal wall. Approximately half are multicystic and half are unilocular. Cysts that derive from the hindgut are large and unilocular while those derived from tailgut remnants are usually small, multilocular, and associated with satellite cysts (223). The lesions are usually circumscribed but unencapsulated. The cyst fluid varies from clear, thin, and colorless to opaque, brown, and pasty. The cysts do not communicate with the gut and are separated from it by a dense fibrous connective tissue stroma.

Microscopic Findings. Histologically, squamous, transitional, simple, mucinous, and ciliated columnar epithelia line the cystic spaces (fig. 2-39). All gastrointestinal epithelial types (fetal and adult) can be found in these lesions. There is usually some columnar or cloacogenic type epithelium. They are surrounded by a muscle layer of varying thickness and degree of completeness, as seen in duplications. Such lesions also often contain heterotopic tissue such as pancreas or gastric tissue, similar to that seen in duplication cysts. Inflammation is present in approximately half of the lesions.

Anorectal cysts may contain isolated smooth muscle bundles but a clearly defined wall of smooth muscle is usually absent. A double muscle layer (circular and longitudinal) is absent and there is no submucosal or myenteric neural plexus. The cysts may be lined by a variety of epithelial types, including ciliated columnar, mucin-secreting columnar, transitional, and squamous epithelia (223). Squamous epithelium, when present, has been attributed to metaplasia and the presence of inflammation but it may also occur in infants without inflammation (215) suggesting differentiation toward anal epithelium.

Differential Diagnosis. Anal developmental cysts differ from duplication cysts in that the musculature of duplication cysts appears much more orderly than the haphazard muscular orientation seen in anorectal developmental cysts. They differ from retrorectal teratomas in that they lack all three germ cell layers; benign retrorectal cystic teratomas should only be diagnosed when there is evidence of differentiation into all three germ cell layers (225). The differential diagnosis also includes chordoma.

Treatment and Prognosis. Anorectal cysts can give rise to adenocarcinomas (217,225) and neuroendocrine carcinomas (226).

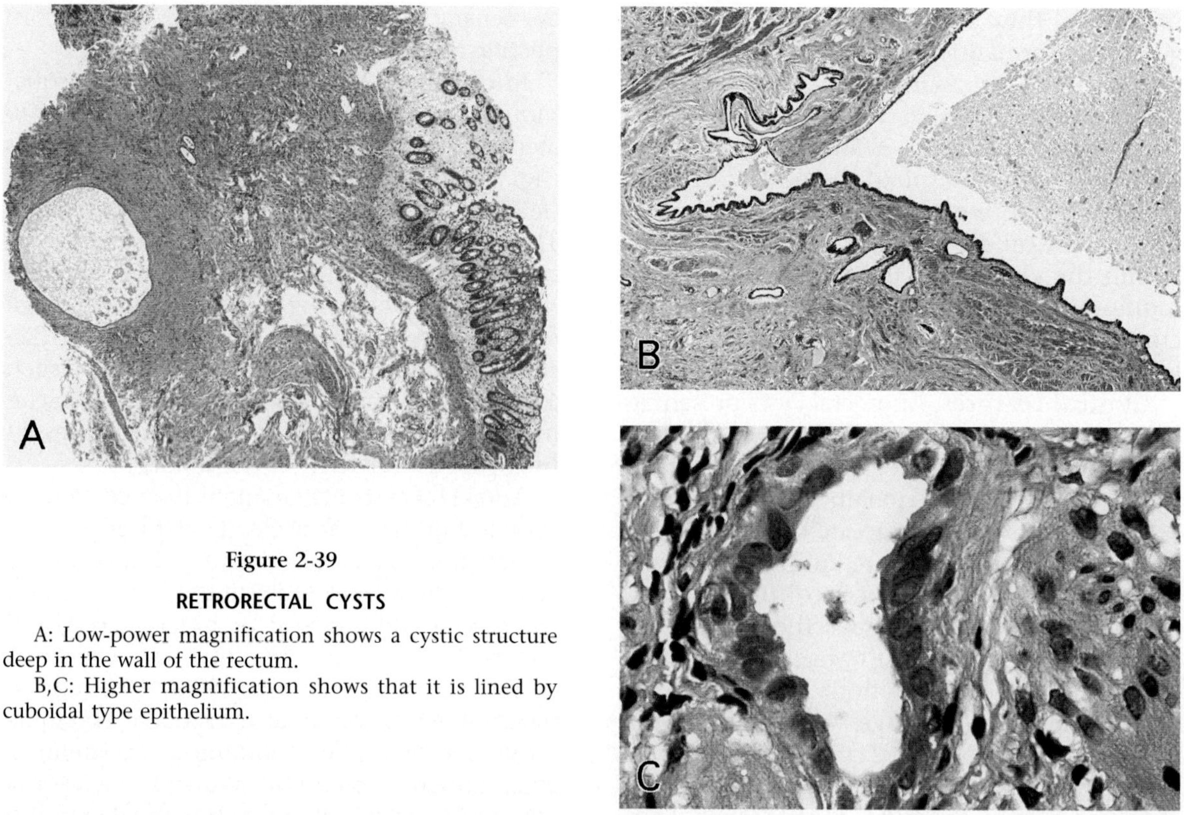

Figure 2-39

RETRORECTAL CYSTS

A: Low-power magnification shows a cystic structure deep in the wall of the rectum.

B,C: Higher magnification shows that it is lined by cuboidal type epithelium.

REFERENCES

Embryology

1. Bale PM. Sacrococcygeal developmental abnormalities and tumours in children. Perspect Pediatr Pathol 1984;8:9–56.
2. Beaulieu JF, Vachon PH, Chartrand S. Immunolocalization of extracellular matrix components during organogenesis in the human small intestine. Anat Embryol 1991;183:363–9.
3. Botha GS. Organogenesis and growth of the gastrointestinal region in man. Anat Rec 1959; 133:219.
4. Calvert R, Pothier P. Migration of fetal intestinal intervillous cells in neonatal mice. Anat Rec 1990;227:199–206.
5. Colony PC. Successive phases of human fetal intestinal development. In: Kretchmer N, Minkows A, eds. Nutritional adaptation of the gastrointestinal tract. Nestle, Vevey: Raven Press; 1983:3–18.
6. Ettensohn CA. The regulation of primary mesenchyme cell patterning. Develop Biol 1990; 140:261–71.
7. Haffen K, Kedinger M, Simon–Assmann P. Cell contact dependent regulation of enterocyte differentiation. In: Lebenthal E, ed. Human gastrointestinal development. New York: Raven Press; 1989:19–26.
8. Henry GL, Melton DA. *Mixer*, a homeobox gene required for endoderm development. Science 1998;281:91–6.
9. Jit I. Prenatal and postnatal structure of the anal canal and development of its sphincters. J Anat Soc India 1974;23:37–56.
10. Kessler DS, Melton DA. Vertebrate embryonic induction: mesodermal and neural patterning. Science 1994;266:596–604.
11. Lucas-Keene MF, Hewer EE. Digestive enzymes in the human foetus. Lancet 1929;1:767–76.
12. Montgomery RK, Mulberg AE, Grand RJ. Development of the human gastrointestinal tract: twenty years of progress. Gastroenterology 1999;116:702–31.

13. Moore TE, Parson. The developing human. In: Clinically oriented embryology, 5th ed. Philadelphia: WB Saunders; 1993:628–44.
14. Morgado PJ, Sùarez JA, Gomez LG, Morgado PJ Jr. Histoclinical basis for a new classification of hemorrhoidal disease. Dis Colon Rectum 1988;31:474–80.
15. Naik KS, Lagopoulos M, Primrose JN. Distribution of antral G-cells in relation to the parietal cells of the stomach and anatomical boundaries. Clin Anat 1990;3:17–20.
16. Partridge JP, Gough MH. Congenital abnormalities of the anus and rectum. Br J Surg 1961;49: 37–50.
17. Van der Putte SC. Normal and abnormal development of the anorectum. J Pediatr Surg 1986; 21:434–40.
18. Vogel G. Tracking the movements that shape an embryo. Science 2000;288:86–7.

Positional Abnormalities

19. Bass KD, Rotherberg SS, Chang JH. Laparoscopic Ladd's procedure in infants with malrotation. J Ped Surg 1998;33:279–81.
20. Carmi R, Abeliovich D, Siplovich L, et al. Familial midgut anomalies: a spectrum of defects due to the same cause. Am J Med Genet 1981;8: 443–6.
21. Dimmick JE, Kalousek DK. Developmental pathology of the embryonal fetus. Philadelphia: JB Lippincott; 1992:526–9.
22. Gary SW, Skandalakis JE. Embryology for surgeons, 1st ed. Philadelphia: WB Saunders; 1972: 135–43.
23. Gilbert HW, Armstrong CP, Thompson MH. The presentation of malrotation of the intestine in adults. Ann R Coll Surg Engl 1990;72:239–42.
24. Hewlett PM. Isolated dextrogastria. Br J Radiol 1982;55:678–81.
25. Kosaki K, Casey B. Genetics of human left-right axis malformations. Sem Cell Develop Bio 1998;9:89–99.
26. Rescorla FJ, Shedd FK, Vane DW, Grosfeld JL, West KW. Anomalies of intestinal rotation in childhood: analysis of 447 cases. Surgery 1990;108:710–5.
27. Smith DW. Recognizable patterns of human malformation. Genetic, embryologic, and clinical aspects. (Major Problems in Clinical Pediatrics, 3rd ed.), Philadelphia: WB Saunders; 1982.
28. Stalker H, Chitayat D. Familial intestinal malrotation with midgut volvulus and facial anomalies: a disorder involving a gene controlling the normal gut rotation? Am J Med Genet 1992;44:46–7.

Abdominal Wall Defects

29. Boyd PA, Bhattacharjee A, Gould S, Manning N, Chamberlain P. Outcome of prenatally diagnosed anterior abdominal wall defects. Arch Dis Child Fetal Neonatal Ed 1998;78:F209–13.
30. Brun M, Grignon A, Guibaud L, Garel L, Saint-Vil D. Gastroschisis: are prenatal ultrasonographic findings useful for assessing the prognosis? Pediatr Radiol 1996;26:723–6.
31. Calzolari E, Bianchi F, Dolk H, Stone D, Milan M and EUROCAT working group. Are omphalocele and neural tube defects related congenital anomalies? Data from 21 registries in Europe (EUROCAT). Am J Med Genet 1997;72:79–84.
32. Elias S, Simpson JL. Maternal serum screening for fetal genetic disorders. New York, Edinburgh: Churchill Livingstone; 1992.
33. Grosfeld JL. Hernias in children. In: Spitz L, Coran AG, eds. Rob & Smith's operative surgery: pediatric surgery, 5th ed. New York: Chapman & Hall; 1995:222–32.
34. Hillebrandt S, Streffer C, Montagutelli X, Balling R. A locus for radiation-induced gastroschisis on mouse chromosome 7. Mamm Genome 1998;9:995–7.
35. Hurwitz RS, Manzoni GA, Ransley PG, Stephens FD. Cloacal exstrophy: a report of 34 cases. J Urol 1987;138:1060–4.
36. Jayanthi S, Seymour P, Puntis JW, Stringer MD. Necrotizing enterocolitis after gastroschisis repair: a preventable complication? J Pediatr Surg 1998;33:705–7.
37. Langer JC. Gastroschisis and omphalocele. Sem Pediatr Surg 1996;5:124–8.
38. Lizcano-Gil LA, Garcia-Cruz D, Sanchez-Corona J. Omphalocele-exstrophy-imperforate-anus-spina bifida (OEIS) complex in a male prenatally exposed to diazepam (letter). Arch Med Res 1995;26:95–6.
39. Lund DP, Hendren WH. Cloacal exstrophy: experience with 20 cases. J Pediatr Surg 1993;28: 1360–9.
40. Moore T, Khalid N. An international survey of gastroschisis and omphalocele (490 cases). Pediatr Surg Int 1986;1:46–55.
41. Nicholls EA, Ford WD, Barnes KH, Furness ME, Hayward C. A decade of gastroschisis in the era of antenatal ultrasound. Aust N Z J Surg 1996;66:366–8.
42. Penman DG, Fisher RM, Noblett HR, Soothill PW. Increase in incidence of gastroschisis in the South West of England in 1995. Br J Obstet Gynecol 1998;105:328–31.
43. Torfs CP, Velie EM, Oechsli FW, Bateson TF, Curry CJ. A population-based study of gastroschisis: demographic, pregnancy, and lifestyle risk factors. Teratology 1994;50:44–53.

Congenital Diaphragmatic Hernia

44. Benjamin DR, Juul S, Siebert JR. Congenital posterolateral diaphragmatic hernia: associated malformations. J Pediatric Surg 1988;23:899–903.

Atresia and Stenosis

45. Applegate MS, Druschel CM. The epidemiology of infantile hypertrophic pyloric stenosis in New York State, 1983 to 1990. Arch Pediatr Adolesc Med 1995;149:1123–9.
46. Bell MJ. Infantile pyloric stenosis. Experience with 305 cases at Louisville Children's Hospital. Surgery 1968;64:983–6.
47. Biller JA, Allen JL, Schuster SR, Treves ST, Winter HS. Longterm evaluation of esophageal and pulmonary function in patients with repaired esophageal atresia and tracheoesophageal fistula. Dig Dis Sci 1987;32:985–90.
48. Botto LD, Khoury MJ, Mastroiacovo P, et al. The spectrum of congenital anomalies of the VATER association: an international study. Am J Med Genet 1997;71:8–15.
49. Brown AK, Tam PK. Measurement of gap length in esophageal atresia: a simple predictor of outcome. J Am Coll Surg 1996;182:41–5.
50. Bult H, Boeckxstaens GE, Pelckmans PA, Jordaens FH, Van Maercke YM, Herman AG. Nitric oxide as an inhibitory non-adrenergic non-cholinergic neurotransmitter. Nature 1990;345:346–7.
51. Canty TG Jr, Boyle EM Jr, Linden B, et al. Aortic arch anomalies associated with long gap esophageal atresia and tracheoesophageal fistula. J Pediatr Surg 1997;32:1587–91.
52. Chang CH, Perrin EV, Bove KE. Pyloric atresia associated with epidermolysis bullosa: special reference to pathogenesis. Pediatr Pathol 1983;1:449–57.
53. Cragan JD, Martin ML, Waters GD, Khoury MJ. Increased risk of small intestinal atresia among twins in the United States. Arch Pediatr Adolesc Med 1994;148:773–9.
54. Dalla Vecchia LK, Grosfeld JL, West KW, Rescorla FJ, Scherer LR, Engum SA. Intestinal atresia and stenosis: a 25-year experience with 277 cases. Arch Surg 1998;133:490–6.
55. D'Amato RJ, Loughnan MS, Flynn E, Folkman J. Thalidomide is an inhibitor of angiogenesis. Proc Natl Acad Sci USA 1994;91:4082–5.
56. Digilio MC, Marino B, Bagolan P, Giannotti A, Dallapiccola B. Microdeletion 22q11 and oesophageal atresia. J Med Genet 1999;36:137–9.
57. Ein SH, Shandling B. Pure esophageal atresia: a 50-year review. J Pediatr Surg 1994;29:1208–11.
58. Feigenbaum A, Chitayat D, Robinson B, et al. The expanding clinical phenotype of the tRNA(Leu(UUR)) A—>G mutation at np 3243 of mitochondrial DNA: diabetic embryopathy associated with mitochondrial cytopathy. Am J Med Genet 1996;62:404–9.
59. Fonkalsrud EW, DeLorimier AA, Hays DM. Congenital atresia and stenosis of the duodenum. A review compiled from the members of the Surgical Section of the American Academy of Pediatrics. Pediatrics 1968;43:70–83.
60. Graham JN, Marin-Padilla N, Hoefnagel D. Jejunal atresia associated with Cafergot ingestion during pregnancy. Clin Pediatr 1983;22:226–8.
61. Haddad V, Macopn WL, Islami MH. Mucosal diaphragms of the gastric antrum in adults. Surg Gynecol Obstet 1981;152:227–33.
62. Jones KL. Smith's recognizable patterns of human malformation, 4th ed. Philadelphia: WB Saunders; 1988:602.
63. Kenyon BM, Browne F, D'Amato RJ. Effects of thalidomide and related metabolites in a mouse corneal model of neovascularization. Exp Eye Res 1997;64:971–8.
64. Kim PC, Superina RA, Ein S. Colonic atresia combines with Hirschsprung's disease: a diagnostic and therapeutic challenge. J Pediatr Surg 1995;30:1216–7.
65. Kokkonen ML, Kalima T, Jaaskelainen J, Louhimo I. Duodenal atresia: late follow-up. J Pediatr Surg 1988;23:216–20.
66. Kusafuka T, Puri P. Altered messenger RNA expression of the neuronal nitric oxide synthase gene in infantile hypertrophic pyloric stenosis. Pediatr Surg Int 1997;12:576–9.
67. Lindahl H, Rintala R, Sariola H. Chronic esophagitis and gastric metaplasia are frequent late complications of esophageal atresia. J Pediatr Surg 1993;28:1178–88.
68. Louw JH. Congenital intestinal atresia and stenosis in the newborn. Observations on pathogenesis and treatment. Ann R Coll Surg Engl 1959;25:109–14.
69. Malmfors G, Sundler F. Peptidergic innervation in infantile hypertrophic pyloric stenosis. J Pediatr Surg 1986;21:303–6.
70. Maman E, Maor E, Kachko L, Carmi R. Epidermolysis bullosa, pyloric atresia, aplasia cutis congenita: histopathological delineation of an autosomal recessive disease. Am J Med Genet 1998;78:127–33.
71. Manning PB, Morgan RA, Coran AG, et al. Fifty years' experience with esophageal atresia and tracheoesophageal fistula. Beginning with Cameron Heights' first operation in 1935. Ann Surg 1986;204:446–53.
72. McBride WG. Thalidomide and congenital abnormalities. Lancet 1961;2:1358–9.
73. Orford JE, Cass DT. Dose response relationship between adriamycin and birth defects in a rat model of VATER association. J Pediatr Surg 1999;34:392–8.

74. Parman T, Wiley MJ, Wells PG. Free radical-mediated oxidative DNA damage in the mechanism of thalidomide teratogenicity. Nat Med 1999;5:582–5.
75. Paterson-Brown S, Stalewski H, Brereton RJ. Neonatal small bowel atresia, stenosis and segmental dilatation. Br J Surg 1991;78:83–6.
76. Pulkkinen L, Kurtz K, Xu Y, Bruckner-Tuderman L, Uitto J. Genomic organization of the integrin beta 4 gene (ITGB4): a homozygous splice-site mutation in a patient with junctional epidermolysis bullosa associated with pyloric atresia. Lab Invest 1997;6:823–33.
77. Puri P, Fujimoto T. New observations on the pathogenesis of multiple intestinal atresias. J Pediatr Surg 1988;23:221–5.
78. Rittler M, Paz JE, Castilla EE. VATERL: an epidemiologic analysis of risk factors. Am J Med Genet 1997;73:162–9.
79. Roberts HE, Cragan JD, Cono J, Khoury MJ, Weatherly MR, Moore CA. Increased frequency of cystic fibrosis among infants with jejunoileal atresia. Am J Med Genet 1998;78:446–9.
80. Santulli TV, Blane WA. Congenital atresia of the intestine. Pathogenesis and treatment. Ann Surg 1961;154:939–41.
81. Sauer H, Günther J, Hescheler J, Wartenberg M. Thalidomide inhibits angiogenesis in embryoid bodies by the generation of hydroxyl radicals. Am J Pathol 2000;156:151–8.
82. Seashore JH, Collins FS, Markowitz RI, Seashore MR. Familial 'apple peel' jejunal atresia: surgical, genetic and radiographic aspects. Pediatrics 1987;80:540–4.
83. Singaram C, Sweet MA, Gaumnitz EA, Cameron AJ, Camilleri M. Peptidergic and nitrinergic denervation in congenital esophageal stenosis. Gastroenterology 1995;109:275–81.
84. Slee J, Goldblatt J. Further evidence for a syndrome of "apple-peel" intestinal atresia, ocular anomalies and microcephaly. Clin Genet 1996;50:260–2.
85. Stringer MD, McKenna KM, Goldstein RB, Filly RA, Adzick NS, Harrison MR. Prenatal diagnosis of esophageal atresia. J Pediatr Surg 1995;30:1258–63.
86. Teich S, Barton DP, Ginn-Pease ME, King DR. Prognostic classification for esophageal atresia and tracheoesophageal fistula: Waterston versus Montreal. J Pediatr Surg 1997;32:1075–9.
87. Tourtet S, Michaud L, Gottrand F, et al. Atrésie de l'intestin grêle et implantation anormale de l'ombilic chez un enfant présentant une foetopathie alcoolique. Arch Pédiatr 1997;4:650–2.
88. Tsai JY, Berkery L, Wasson DE, Redo SF, Spigland NA. Esophageal atresia and tracheoesophageal fistula: surgical experience over two decades. Ann Thorac Surg 1997;64:778–83.
89. van der Pol JG, Wolf H, Boer K, et al. Jejunal atresia related to the use of methylene blue in genetic amniocentesis in twins. Br J Obstet Gynaecol 1992;99:141–3.
90. Vanderwinden JM, Mailleux P, Schiffmann SN, Vanderhaeghen JJ. Nitric oxide synthase activity in infantile hypertrophic pyloric stenosis. N Engl J Med 1992;327:511–5.
91. Walker–Smith J, Wright V. Congenital anatomical abnormalities. In: Booth CC, Neale G, eds. Disorders of the small intestine. London: Blackwell Scientific Publications; 1985.
92. Wattchow DA, Cass DT, Furness JB, Costa M, O'Brien PE, Little KE, Pitkin J. Abnormalities of peptide-containing nerve fibres in infantile hypertrophic pyloric stenosis. Gastroenterology 1987;92:443–8.
93. Weinberg AG, Milunsky A, Harrod MJ. Elevated amniotic fluid alpha-fetoprotein and duodenal atresia. Lancet 1975;2:496.
94. Wells PG, Kim PM, Laposa RR, Nicol CJ, Parman T, Winn L. Oxidative damage in chemical teratogenesis. Mutat Res 1997;396:65–78.
95. Winters WD, Weinberger E, Hatch EI. Atresia of the colon in neonates: radiologic findings. Am J Radiol 1992;159:1273–6.
96. Yamamoto Y, Oguro N, Nara T, Horita H, Niitsu N, Imaizumi S. Duplication of part of 9q due to maternal 12;9 inverted insertion associated with pyloric stenosis. Am J Med Genet 1988;31:379–84.
97. Yamanaka S, Tanaka Y, Kawataki M, Ijiri R, Imaizumi K, Kurahashi H. Chromosome 22q11 deletion complicated by dissecting pulmonary arterial aneurysm and jejunal atresia in an infant. Arch Pathol Lab Med 2000;124:880–2.

Congenital Bronchopulmonary Malformations

98. Gerle RD, Jaretzki A, Ashley CA, Berne AS. Congenital bronchopulmonary foregut malformation: pulmonary sequestration communicating with the gastrointestinal tract. N Engl J Med 1968;278:1413–9.
99. Goldman RL, Ban JL. Chondroepithelial choristoma (tracheobronchial rest) of the esophagus associated with esophageal atresia: report of an unusual case. J Thorac Cardiovasc Surg 1972;63:318–21.
100. Hruban RH, Shumway SJ, Orel SB, Dumler JS, Baker RR, Hutchins GM. Congenital bronchopulmonary foregut malformations. Am J Clin Pathol 1989;91:403–9.
101. Kim JH, Park KH, Sung SW, Rho JR. Congenital bronchoesophageal fistulas in adult patients. Ann Thorac Surg 1995;60:151–5.

102. Leithiser RE Jr, Capitanio MA, Macpherson RI, Wood BP. "Communicating" bronchopulmonary foregut malformations. Am J Roentgenol 1986;146:227–31.
103. Silverman FN, Kuhn JP. Caffey's pediatric x-ray diagnosis. 9th ed. St. Louis: Mosby Year Book; 1993.

Duplications

104. Bartels RJ. Duplication of the stomach: case report and review of the literature. Am Surg 1967;33:747–52.
105. Bentley JF, Smith JR. Developmental posterior enteric remnants and spinal malformations. The split notochord syndrome. Arch Dis Child 1960;35:76–86.
106. Bishop HC, Koop CE. Surgical management of duplications of the alimentary tract. Am J Surg 1964;107:434–42.
107. Bower RJ, Sieber WK, Kiesewetter WB. Alimentary tract duplications in children. Ann Surg 1978;188:669–74.
108. Dahms BB. The gastrointestinal tract. In: Stocker JT, Dehner LP, eds. Pediatric pathology. Philadelphia: JB Lippincott Company 1992: 653–5.
109. Dardik H, Klibanoff E. Retroperitoneal enterogenous cyst: report of a case and mechanisms of embryogenesis. Ann Surg 1965;162:1084–6.
110. De la Torre Mondragon L, Daza DC, Bustamante AP, Fascinetto GV. Gastric triplication and peritoneal melanosis. J Pediatr Surg 1997;32:1773–5.
111. Diaz-Cano SJ, Rivera-Hueto F, Mesa-Navarro A. Double duplication in a nonrotational colon. Study of a case associated with mucinous adenoma. Pathol Res Pract 1995;191:415–9.
112. Fallon M, Gordon ARG, Lendrum AC. Mediastinal cysts of foregut origin associated with vertebral abnormalities. Br J Surg 1954;41:520–33.
113. Faris JC, Crowe JE. The split notochord syndrome. J Pediatr Surg 1975;10:467–72.
114. Favara BE, Franciosi RA, Akers DR. Enteric duplications. Thirty-seven cases: a vascular theory of pathogenesis. Am J Dis Child 1971;122:501–6.
115. Gray AW. Triplication of the large intestine. Arch Pathol 1940;30:121–3.
116. Grosfeld JL, O'Neill JA, Clatworthy HW. Enteric duplications in infancy and childhood: an 18-year review. Ann Surg 1970;172:83–90.
117. Gross RE, Holcomb GM Jr, Farber S. Duplications of the alimentary tract. Pediatrics 1952;9: 449–54.
118. Hocking M, Young DG. Duplications of the alimentary tract. Br J Surg 1981;68:92–6.
119. Holcomb GW III, Gheissari A, O'Neill JA Jr, Shorter NA, Bishop HC. Surgical management of alimentary tract duplications. Ann Surg 1989;209:167–74.
120. Ildstad ST, Tollerud DJ, Weiss RG, et al. Duplications of the alimentary tract. Clinical characteristics, preferred treatment, and associated malformations. Ann Surg 1988;208:184–9.
121. Kitano Y, Iwanaka T, Tsuchida Y, Oka T. Esophageal duplication cyst associated with pulmonary cystic malformations. J Pediatr Surg 1995;30:1724–7.
122. Kosir MA, Sonnino RE, Gauderer MW. Pediatric abdominal lymphangiomas: a plea for early recognition. J Pediatr Surg 1991;26:1309–13.
123. Lewis PL, Holder T, Feldman M. Duplication of the stomach: report of a case and review of the English literature. Arch Surg 1961;82:634–40.
124. McPherson AG, Trapnell JE, Airth G. Duplications of the colon. Br J Surg 1979;56:138–43.
125. Prop N, Frensdorf EL, van der Stadt FR. A postvertebral endodermal cyst associated with axial deformities: a case showing the endodermal-ectodermal adhesion syndrome. Pediatrics 1967;39:555.
126. Rosselet PJ. A rare case of rachischisis with multiple malformations. Am J Roentgenol 1955;73:235–8.
127. Smith ED. Duplication of the anus and genitourinary tracts. Surgery 1969;66:909–21.
128. Takiff H, Calabria R, Yin L, Stabile BE. Mesenteric cysts and intraabdominal cystic lymphangiomas. Arch Surg 1985;120:1266–9.
129. Vaage S, Knutrud O. Congenital duplications of the alimentary tract with special regard to their embryogenesis. Prog Pediatr Surg 1974;7:103.

Diverticula

130. Fleming CR, Newcomer AD, Stephens DH, Carlson HC. Intraluminal duodenal diverticulum. Report of two cases and review of the literature. Mayo Clin Proc 1975;50:244–8.
131. Juler JL, List JW, Stemmer EA, Connolly JE. Duodenal diverticulitis. Arch Surg 1969;99:572–8.
132. Kurgan A, Hoffman J. Aetiology of gastric diverticula—an hypothesis. Med Hypotheses 1981;7:1471–6.
133. Magness LJ, Sanfelippo PM, van Heerden JA, Judd ES. Diverticular disease of the right colon. Surg Gynecol Obstet 1975;140:30–2.

Omphalomesenteric Remnants

134. Eichelberger MR, Anderson KD, Randolph JG. Surgical conditions of the small intestine in infants and children. In: Surgery of the alimentary tract, Vol 5. Shackelford RT, Zuidema GD, eds. Philadelphia: WB Saunders; 1986:364.

135. Hill P, Rode J. *Helicobacter pylori* in ectopic gastric mucosa in Meckel's diverticulum. Pathology 1998;30:7–9.
136. Kusumoto H, Yoshida M, Takahashi I, Anai H, Maehara Y, Sugimachi K. Complications and diagnosis of Meckel's diverticulum in 776 patients. Am J Surg 1992;164:382–3.
137. Michel ML, Field RJ, Ogden WO Jr. Meckel's diverticulum. An analysis of one hundred cases and the report of a giant diverticulum and of four cases occurring within the same immediate family. Ann Surg 1955;141:819–23.
138. Steck WD, Helwig EB. Cutaneous remnants of the omphalomesenteric duct. Arch Dermatol 1964;90:463–70.

Annular Pancreas

139. Kiernan PD, ReMine SG, Kiernan PC, ReMine WH. Annular pancreas—Mayo Clinic experience from 1957 to 1976 with a review of the literature. Arch Surg 1980;115:46–50.
140. Salonen IS. Congenital duodenal obstruction. A review of the literature and a clinical study of 66 patients including a histopathological study of annular pancreas and a follow up of 36 survivors. Acta Paediatr Scand 1978;272:1–87.

Peritoneal Encapsulation

141. Cleland J. On an abnormal arrangement of the peritoneum with remarks on the development of the mesocolon. J Anat Physiol 1868;2:201–3.
142. Sieck JO, Cowgill R, Larkworthy W. Peritoneal encapsulation and abdominal cocoon. Case report and review of the literature. Gastroenterology 1983;84:1597–601.

Heterotopias

143. Ashida K, Eg K, Egashira Y, Tutumi A, et al. Endocrine neoplasm arising from duodenal heterotopic pancreas: a case report. Gastrointest Endosc 1997;46:172–6.
144. Barbosa J, Dockerty MB, Waugh JM. Pancreatic heterotopia: review of the literature and report of 41 authenticated surgical cases of which 25 were clinically significant. Surg Gynecol Obstet 1946;82:527–42.
145. Borhan-Manesh F, Farnum JB. Incidence of heterotopic gastric mucosa in the upper oesophagus. Gut 1991;32:968–72.
146. Borhan-Manesh F, Farnum JB. Study of *Helicobacter pylori* colonization of patches of heterotopic gastric mucosa (HGM) at the upper esophagus. Dig Dis Sci 1993;38:142–6.
147. Buse PE, Zuckerman GR, Balfe DM. Cervical esophageal web associated with a patch of heterotopic gastric mucosa. Abdom Imaging 1993;18:227–8.
148. Galligan ML, Ulich T, Lewin KJ. Heterotopic gastric mucosa in the jejunum causing intussusception. Arch Pathol Lab Med 1983;107:335–6.
149. Gledhill A. Ectopic prostatic tissue. J Urol 1985;133:110–1.
150. Herold G, Kraft K. Adenocarcinoma arising from ectopic gastric pancreas: two case reports with a review of the literature. Z Gastroenterol 1995;33:260–4.
151. Jeng KS, Yang KC, Kuo SH. Malignant degeneration of heterotopic pancreas. Gastrointest Endosc 1991;37:196–8.
152. Kimpton AR, Crane AR. Heterotopic gastric mucosa. N Engl J Med 1938;219:627–9.
153. Monig SP, Selzner M, Raab M, Eidt S. Heterotopic pancreas. A difficult diagnosis. Dig Dis Sci 1996;41:1238–40.
154. Nawaz K, Graham DY, Fechner RE, Eiband JM. Gastric heterotopia in the ileum with ulceration and chronic bleeding. Gastroenterology 1974;66:113–7.
155. Noffsinger AE, Hyams DM, Fenoglio-Preiser CM. Esophageal heterotopic pancreas presenting as an inflammatory mass. Dig Dis Sci 1995;40:2373–9.
156. Peterson CJ, Strickler JG, Gonzalez R, Dehner LP. Uterus-like mass of the small intestine. Heterotopia or monodermal teratoma? Am J Surg Pathol 1999;14:390–4.
157. Potter EL. Pathology of the fetus and the infant. Chicago Year Book Medical Publishers Inc; 1975:469.
158. Santulli TV, Kiesewetter WB, Bill AH Jr. Anorectal anomalies. A suggested international classification. J Pediatr Surg 1970;5:281–7.
159. Schwarzenburg SJ, Whitington PF. Rectal gastric mucosa heterotopia as a cause of hematochezia in an infant. Dig Dis Sci 1983;28:470–2.
160. Shindo K, Bacon HE, Holmes EJ. Ectopic gastric mucosa and glandular tissue of a salivary type in the anal canal concomitant with a diverticulum in hemorrhoidal tissue: report of a case. Dis Colon Rectum 1972;15:57–62.
161. Sperling RM, Grendell JH. Adenocarcinoma arising in an inlet patch of the esophagus. Am J Gastroenterol 1995;90:150–2.
162. Srinivasan R, Loewenstine H, Mayle JE. Sessile polypoid gastric heterotopia of rectum. A report of 2 cases and review of the literature. Arch Path Lab Med 1999;123:222–4.
163. Takeji H, Ueno J, Nishitani H. Ectopic gastric mucosa in the upper esophagus: prevalence and radiologic findings. Am J Roentgenol 1995;164:901–4.

164. Variend S, Howat AJ. Upper oesophageal gastric heterotopia: a prospective necropsy study in children. J Clin Pathol 1988;41:742–5.
165. Weitzner S. Ectopic salivary gland tissue in submucosa of rectum. Dis Colon Rectum 1983;26: 814.
166. Wolff M. Heterotopic gastric epithelium in the rectum: a report of three new cases with a review of 87 cases of gastric heterotopia in the alimentary canal. Am J Clin Pathol 1971;55: 604–6.
167. Yoshimitsu K, Yoshida M, Motooka M, et al. Heterotopic gastric mucosa of the duodenum mimicking a duodenal cancer. Gastrointest Radiol 1989;14:115–7.

Müllerian and Mesonephric Duct Remnants

168. Davis M, Whitley ME, Haque AK, Fenoglio-Preiser C, Waterman R. Xanthogranulomatous abscess of a müllerian duct remnant. A rare lesion of the rectum and anus. Dis Colon Rectum 1986;29:755–9.

Microgastria

169. Gorman B, Shaw DG. Congenital microgastria. Br J Radiol 1984;57:260–2.
170. Lurie IW, Magee CA, Sun CC, Ferencz C. 'Microgastria—limb reduction' complex with congenital heart disease and twinning. Clin Dysmorphol 1995;4:150–5.
171. Rose V, Izukawa T, Moes CA. Syndromes of asplenia and polysplenia. A review of cardiac and non-cardiac malformations in 60 cases with special reference to diagnosis and prognosis. Br Heart J 1975;37:840–52.

Anorectal Malformations

172. Ashcraft KW, Holder TM. Congenital anal stenosis with presacral teratoma. Ann Surg 1964;162:1091–5.
173. Ashcraft KW, Holder TM. Hereditary presacral teratoma. J Pediatr Surg 1974;9:691–7.
174. Bartsch O, Kuhnle U, Wu LL, Schwinger E, Hinkel GK. Evidence for a critical region for penoscrotal inversion hypospadias, and imperforate anus within chromosomal region 13q32.2q34. Am J Med Genet 1996;65:218–21.
175. Brent L, Stephens FD. Primary rectal ectasia: a quantitative study of smooth muscle cells in normal and hypertrophied human bowel. Prog Pediatr Surg 1976;9:41–62.
176. deVries PA, Cox KL. Surgery of anorectal anomalies. Surg Clin N Am 1985;65:1139–69.
177. deVries PA, Pena A. Posterior sagittal anorectoplasty. J Pediatr Surg 1982;17:638–43.
178. Dillon PW, Cilley RE. Newborn surgical emergencies: gastrointestinal anomalies, abdominal wall defects. Pediatr Clin North Am 1993;40: 1289–314.
179. Ein SH. Imperforate anus (anal agenesis) with rectal and sigmoid atresias in a newborn. Pediatr Surg Int 1997;12:449–51.
180. Endo M, Hayashi A, Ishihara M, et al. Analysis of 1,992 patients with anorectal malformations over the past two decades in Japan. J Pediatr Surg 1999;34:435–41.
181. Keith A. Malformation of the hind end of the body. Brit Med J 1908;ii:1736,1804,1857.
182. Kiesewetter WB, Turner CR, Sieber WK. Imperforate anus. Am J Surg 1964;107:412–20.
183. Kohlhase J, Taschner PE, Burfeind P, et al. Molecular analysis of *SALL1* mutations in Townes-Brocks syndrome. Am J Hum Genet 1999;64:435–45.
184. Ladd WE, Gross RE. Congenital malformations of anus and rectum. Am J Surg 1934;23:167–75.
185. Lowe J, Kohn G, Cohen O, Mogilner M, Schiller M. Dominant anorectal malformation nephritis and nerve deafness. Clin Genet 1983;24:191–3.
186. Magnus RV. Rectal atresia as distinguished from rectal agenesis. J Pediatr Surg 1968;3:593–8.
187. Meier-Ruge WA, Holschneider AM. Histopathologic observations of anorectal abnormalities in anal atresia. Pediatr Surg Int 2000;16:2–7.
188. Moazam F, Talbert JL. Congenital anorectal malformations: harbingers of sacrococcygeal teratomas. Arch Surg 1985;120:856–9.
189. Ralph DJ, Woodhouse CR, Ransley PG. The management of the neuropathic bladder in adolescents with imperforate anus. J Urol 1992;148:366–8.
190. Ruiz-Moreno F, Gerdo-Ceballo A, Lozano-Saldivar G. Vaginal anus. Dis Colon Rectum 1980;23:306–7.
191. Smith ED. Urinary anomalies and complications in imperforate anus and rectum. J Pediatr Surg 1968;3:337–49.
192. Snyder WH Jr. Some unusual forms of imperforate anus in female patients. Amer J Surg 1966;111:319–25.
193. Soussou I, Der Daloustian V, Slim M. Familial imperforate anus. Report of a family. Dis Colon Rectum 1974;17:562–4.
194. Stephens FD, Smith ED. Ano-rectal malformations in children. Chicago: Year Book Medical Publishers; 1971.
195. Tsukuda T, Nagata I, Sawada H, et al. Partial monosomy 10q and partial trisomy 9q with anal atresia due to maternal translocation:t(9;10)(q32;q26). Clin Genet 1996;50: 220–2.
196. Van de Geijn EJ, Van Vugt JM, Sounie JE, et al. Ultrasonographic diagnosis and perinatal management of fetal abdominal wall defects. Fetal Diagn Ther 1991;6:2–10.

Thymic-Renal-Anal-Lung Dysplasia

197. Curry CJ, Carey JC, Holland JS, et al. Smith-Lemli-Opitz syndrome-type II: multiple congenital anomalies with male pseudohermaphroditism and frequent early lethality. Am J Med Genet 1987;26:45–57.
198. Fraser FC, Jequier S, Chen MF. Chondrodysplasia, situs inversus totalis, cleft epiglottis and larynx, hexadactyly of hand and feet, pancreatic cystic dysplasia, renal dysplasia/absence, micropenis and ambiguous genitalia, imperforate anus. Am J Med Genet 1989;34:401–5.
199. Hall JG, Pallister PD, Clarren SK, et al. Congenital hypothalmic hamartoblastoma, hypopituitarism, imperforate anus and postaxial polydactyly—a new syndrome? Part I: clinical, causal and pathogenetic considerations. Am J Med Genet 1980;7:47–74.

Caudal Dysplasia

200. Ashcraft KW, Holder TM, Harris DJ. Familial presacral teratomas. Birth defects: Orig Art Ser XV (National Foundation: March of Dimes) 1975;11:143–6.
201. Blumel J, Evans EB, Eggers GW. Partial and complete agenesis or malformation of the sacrum with associated anomalies. J Bone Joint Surg Am 1959;41A:497–518.
202. Cohn J, Bay-Nielsen E. Hereditary defect of the sacrum and coccyx with anterior sacral meningocele. Acta Pediatr Scand 1969;58:268–74.
203. Currarino G, Weinberg A. From small pelvic outlet syndrome to sirenomelia. Pediatr Pathol 1991;11:195–210.
204. Deuchar EM. Experimental evidence relating fetal anomalies to diabetes. In: Sutherland HW, Stowers JM, eds. Pregnancy and the newborn. New York: Springer-Verlag; 1979:21.
205. Duhamel B. From the mermaid to anal imperforation: the syndrome of caudal regression. Arch Dis Child 1961;36:152.
206. Finer NN, Bowen P, Dunbar LG. Caudal regression anomalad (sacral agenesis) in siblings. Clin Genet 1978;13:353–8.
207. Landauer W, Clarke EM. Teratogenic interaction of insulin and 2–deoxy–D–glucose in chick development. J Exp Zool 1962;151:245.
208. Padmanabhan R. Retinoic acid–induced caudal regression syndrome in the mouse fetus. Reprod Toxicol 1998;12:139–51.
209. Passarge E, Lenz W. Syndrome of caudal regression in infants of diabetic mothers: observations of further cases. Pediatrics 1966;37:672–5.
210. Smith ED. Congenital sacral anomalies in children. Aust N Z J Surg 1959;29:165–76.
211. Stewart JM, Stoll S. Familial caudal regression anomalad and maternal diabetes. Lancet 1964;2:1124.
212. Stocker JT, Heifetz SA. Sirenomelia. A morphological study of 33 cases and review of the literature. Perspect Pediatr Pathol 1987;10:7–50.
213. Welch JP, Aterman K. The syndrome of caudal dysplasia: a review including etiologic considerations and evidence of heterogeneity. Pediatr Pathol 1984;2:313–27.
214. Wilson JS, Vallance-Owen J. Congenital deformities and insulin antagonism. Lancet 1966;2:940–1.

Anorectal Cysts

215. Bale PM. Sacrococcygeal developmental abnormalities and tumours in children. Perspect Pediatr Pathol 1984;8:9–56.

215a. Campbell WL, Wolff M. Retrorectal cysts of developmental origin. AJR 1973;117:307–13.

216. Caropreso PR, Wengert Jr PA, Milford EH. Tailgut cyst—a rare retrorectal tumor. Dis Colon Rectum 1975;18:597–600.
217. Colin JF, Branfoot AC, Robinson KP. Malignant change in rectal duplication. J R Soc Med 1979;72:934–7.
218. Edwards M. Multilocular retrorectal cystic disease—cyst hamartoma: report of twelve cases. Dis Colon Rectum 1961;4:103–10.
219. Ferry CL, Merritt Jr JW. Presacral enterogenous cyst. Ann Surg 1949;129:881–9.
220. Gius JA, Stout AP. Perianal cysts of vestigial origin. Arch Surg 1938;37:268.
221. Guillermo C, Grossman IW. Presacral cyst, an uncommon entity: report of a case and review of the literature. Am Surg 1972;38:448–50.
222. Hawkins WJ, Jackman RJ. Developmental cysts as a source of perianal abscesses and fistulas. Am J Surg 1953;86:678–83.
223. Marco V, Autonell J, Farre J, et al. Retrorectal cyst-hamartoma: report of two cases with adenocarcinoma developing in one. Am J Surg Pathol 1982;6:707–14.
224. Mills SE, Walker AN, Stallings RG, et al. Retrorectal cystic hamartoma. Report of three cases, including one with a perirenal component. Arch Pathol Lab Med 1984;108:737–40.
225. Prasad AR, Amin MB, Randolph TL, Lee CS, Ma CK. Retrorectal cystic hamartoma. Report of 5 cases with malignancy arising in 2. Arch Pathol Lab Med 2000;124:725–9.
226. Thomason TH. Cysts and sinuses of the sacrococcygeal region. Ann Surg 1934;99:585.
227. Uhlig BE, Johnson RL. Presacral tumors and cysts in adults. Dis Colon Rectum 1975;18:581–96.

3 DISEASES OF THE ESOPHAGUS

GENERAL PATHOLOGIC FEATURES

Since the esophagus responds to different types of injury in the same way, regardless of the cause, identical histologic features are present in esophagitis of diverse etiologies. Therefore, determination of the specific cause of the esophagitis may be difficult unless there is a specific infection, in which case an etiologic agent is identified. In general, esophagitis causes variable degrees of inflammation, epithelial necrosis, and regeneration. Mild esophageal injury results in mild reversible mucosal changes with transient inflammation, as well as the presence of balloon cells, vascular dilation, and infiltration of the epithelium by inflammatory cells, particularly mononuclear cells and eosinophils. More severe damage results in epithelial destruction, in either the form of erosion, a superficial lesion involving only the mucosa, or an ulcer that extends deeper into the lamina propria or submucosa. Neutrophils may be identified if ulcers or erosions are present. With time, the damaged epithelium becomes hyperplastic, as evidenced by basal cell hyperplasia and papillary elongation. Patients with chronic damage extending into the submucosa or beyond may develop submucosal fibrosis, sometimes with stricture formation. Distal esophagitis in the absence of identifiable microorganisms most likely results from gastroesophageal reflux.

REFLUX ESOPHAGITIS

Definition. The term *gastroesophageal reflux* refers to retrograde flow of gastric and sometimes duodenal contents into the esophagus. The term *gastroesophageal reflux disease* (GERD) describes the spectrum of clinical conditions and histologic alterations resulting from gastroesophageal reflux. *Reflux esophagitis* describes a type of GERD with histopathologic esophageal changes. *Alkaline reflux* refers to reflux of duodenal contents and implies incompetence of both the pyloric and the gastroesophageal sphincters.

Demography. The prevalence of patients with symptoms associated with GERD (heartburn or acid regurgitation) ranges from 40 to 45 percent in the United States and Canada (9, 24,38). Frequent symptoms (at least once per week) are reported by 20 percent of the general population (24). The incidence of GERD is lower in Eastern than in Western countries (7), but is rising (34). Endoscopic evidence of esophagitis, esophageal erosion, or ulceration is present in one third to half of patients with symptoms (7,27,32,43). GERD affects more men than women, and men are more likely to develop extensive erosive esophagitis.

GERD is also common in children and represents a frequent reason for pediatric patients to be referred to a gastroenterologist (6). GERD is particularly common in children with neurologic or psychiatric disorders, or in those with congenital esophageal or gastric abnormalities (10,13,16). Cystic fibrosis predisposes to severe, complicated GERD.

In adults, predisposing conditions include increased intraabdominal or intragastric pressure as a result of pregnancy, ascites, obesity, or motility disorders (23,25). GERD also complicates acquired structural abnormalities, including hiatal hernias. Patients who undergo prolonged periods of recumbency (ventilator dependent, stroke, and immobile nursing home residents) are prone to reflux esophagitis.

Pathophysiology. GERD is a multifactorial process with different abnormalities predominating in different patients (Table 3-1) (4,5,12, 14,20,26). Factors predisposing to GERD include: 1) decreased esophageal sphincter pressure; 2) diminished esophageal clearance secondary to defective esophageal peristalsis; 3) delayed gastric emptying or abnormal gastric contractility; 4) decreased salivary flow; and 5) increased gastric acid production. Transient relaxation of the lower esophageal sphincter (LES) (a physiological occurrence in normal individuals) allows

Table 3-1

CAUSES OF, OR PREDISPOSITION TO, GASTROESOPHAGEAL REFLUX

Abnormal lower esophageal sphincter position or pressure
Hiatus hernia
Certain foods, drinks
Alcohol
Smoking
Smooth muscle medications
Iatrogenic destruction of lower esophageal sphincter
Pregnancy
Motility disorders
Zollinger-Ellison syndrome
Decreased esophageal mucosal resistance secondary to Infections Prior chemotherapy Nasogastric intubation
Gastric outlet obstruction
Refluxed duodenal contents
Esophageal or gastric structural abnormalities

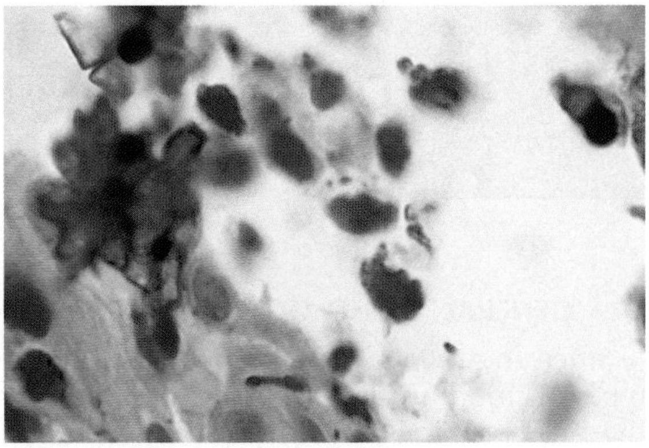

Figure 3-1

REFLUX ESOPHAGITIS

Yellowish bile crystals are present in this biopsy specimen from a patient with reflux of duodenal and gastric contents into the esophagus.

reflux to occur (41). Esophageal dysmotility contributes to poor clearance of the refluxed material, thereby leading to an increased mucosal contact time. With persistent reflux, esophageal motor function becomes increasingly abnormal, leading to further deterioration of LES pressure. Once esophagitis develops, LES pressure becomes further impaired, increasing acid exposure in the distal esophagus.

A mechanically defective LES, increased esophageal acid exposure time, and frequent suboptimal peristaltic esophageal contractions during supine, upright, and meal periods correlate with the severity of the mucosal injury. The nature and amount of refluxed material and the length of time the refluxate remains in contact with the esophageal mucosa also determine whether disease develops. Acid alone causes relatively few changes. When combined with pepsin, bile acids, or trypsin, however, more severe damage results (11,36). Bile acids and trypsin are present if the refluxate contains duodenal contents (fig. 3-1).

During the past three decades, hospital discharges and mortality rates of patients with gastric cancer, gastric ulcer, and duodenal ulcer have declined, while those of patients with esophageal adenocarcinomas and GERD have markedly risen. These opposing time trends suggest that gastritis secondary to *Helicobacter pylori* infection protects against GERD (7,16). This hypothesis is consistent with geographic and ethnic distributions of GERD. Case control studies also indicate that patients with erosive esophagitis are less likely to have active or chronic corpus gastritis than controls without esophagitis (8,32). The mechanism underlying the "protective" effect of *H. pylori* on the esophagus is likely related to its effect on gastric acid output: patients with extensive *H. pylori*-associated corpus gastritis have lower gastric acid outputs than those without gastritis affecting the corpus of the stomach (6). As a result, esophageal acid load is reduced, and patients do not develop GERD (despite the fact that they may still have gastroesophageal reflux) (15).

Clinical Features. *Adults.* Patients with GERD present with diverse symptoms including epigastric pain, pharyngeal burning, nausea, vomiting, heartburn, regurgitation of gastric contents resulting in a bitter tasting fluid into the mouth, dysphagia, hypersalivation, atypical intermittent chest pain, hiccups, odynophagia, and globus sensation (21,29,35). Occasional patients present with angina-like chest pain (39); others present with pulmonary or pharyngeal symptoms, including hoarseness, coughing, asthma, or recurrent pulmonary complaints (33). These symptoms may be experienced daily, weekly, or only several times a month. The frequency and

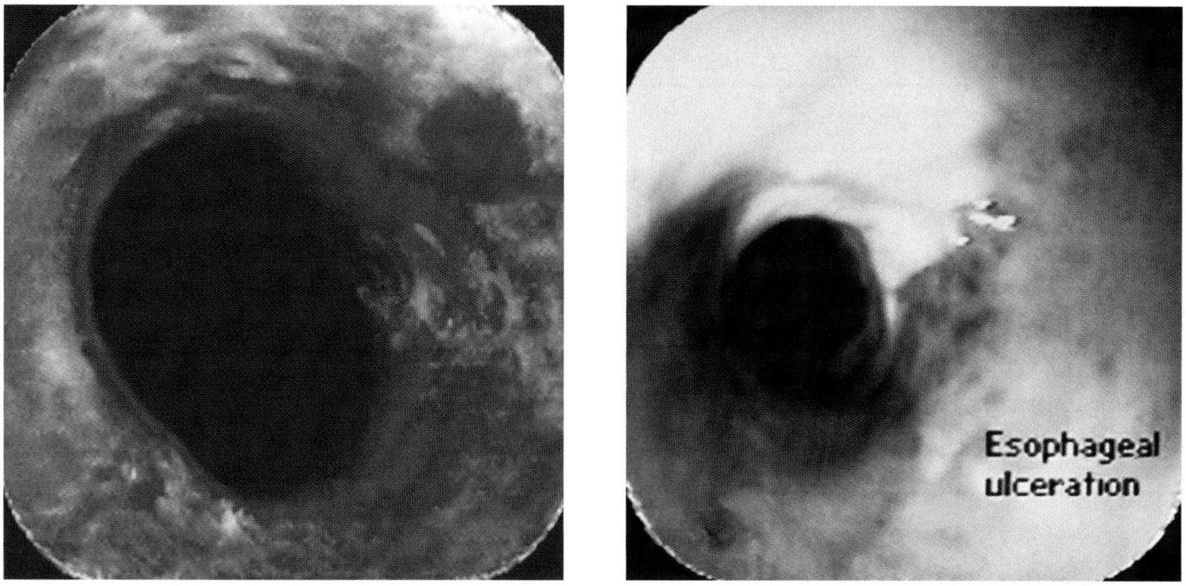

Figure 3-2

REFLUX ESOPHAGITIS: ENDOSCOPIC APPEARANCE

Left: The esophageal mucosa appears diffusely erythematous with foci of hemorrhage. Right: Long-standing reflux esophagitis with ulceration and stricture formation.

severity of symptoms from gastroesophageal reflux do not correlate with the morphologic changes seen in the esophageal mucosa (18,31).

Some patients develop complications, including erosions or ulcers, strictures, Barrett esophagus, and cancer. The symptoms associated with esophageal peptic ulcers resemble those associated with gastric or duodenal peptic ulcers, except that the pain usually localizes to the xiphoid or high substernal region. Peptic stricture or peristaltic dysfunction causes progressive dysphagia (17). Esophagitis may cause massive, but usually limited, hemorrhage.

Children. Gastroesophageal reflux is common in infants, and is probably physiological, usually resolving spontaneously (37). In such preverbal children, the classic adult history of heartburn cannot be elicited. General symptoms include regurgitation, prolonged crying and irritability, vomiting, apnea, asthma, choking, stridor, and respiratory distress. Older children may experience heartburn, dysphagia, odynophagia, night walking, hoarseness, chronic cough, and asthma (3). The most frequent complication of recurrent GERD is failure to thrive, resulting from caloric deprivation and recurrent bronchitis or pneumonia caused by repeated episodes of pulmonary aspiration. Severe dental caries are common. The best test for diagnosing and quantifying GERD in children is 24-hour esophageal pH monitoring.

Gross and Endoscopic Findings. The gross appearance of the esophagus varies with disease severity. Areas of erythema and longitudinal red streaks in the distal esophagus are the first endoscopic abnormalities. In severe reflux, the esophagus appears friable, diffusely reddened, and hemorrhagic (fig. 3-2). Mucosal erosions, ulcerations, intramural thickening, strictures, or Barrett esophagus are characteristic of severe chronic disease. Most erosions and ulcers occur distally, tapering off proximally. Inflammatory polyps may be present at the Z-line margin. Strictures develop close to the gastroesophageal junction or immediately proximal to a hiatus hernia.

Microscopic Findings. There are four stages of reflux esophagitis: 1) acute (necrosis, inflammation, and granulation tissue); 2) repair (basal cell hyperplasia and elongation of the papillae); 3) chronic (fibrosis and formation of Barrett esophagus); and 4) complications (dysplasia and

Table 3-2

HISTOLOGIC FEATURES OF REFLUX ESOPHAGITIS

Balloon cells
Basal zone hyperplasia (>15% to 20% of total epithelial thickness)
Basal layer spongiosis (edema)
Nuclear enlargement
Mitoses in basal cell layer
Elongated papillae (>75% of total epithelial thickness)
Venular dilatation
Intraepithelial eosinophils
Increased intraepithelial lymphocytes
Polymorphonuclear leukocytes
Erosions or ulcers, if severe

adenocarcinoma). Repetitive episodes of tissue destruction and healing produce histologic features that reflect disease activity at the time of examination, superimposed on those from previous injury. Biopsies are performed to confirm the presence of esophagitis, to determine its nature (e.g., peptic- versus drug-induced) and severity, and to rule out the presence of a coexisting infection, such as Candida, cytomegalovirus, or herpesvirus (particularly in immunosuppressed patients); Barrett esophagus; or tumor development. Esophagitis can heal completely or progress to any of the complications discussed below.

Since the histologic features of GERD are not specific, several histologic features must be assessed before a presumptive diagnosis can be made (Table 3-2). In addition, it is important to be aware of the clinical and drug history of the patient.

Balloon Cells. Balloon cells are swollen, pale, globoid, periodic acid–Schiff (PAS)–negative cells with irregular pyknotic nuclei that develop in the epithelial mid-zone (fig. 3-3). They are present in approximately two thirds of GERD cases. Balloon cells develop in any damaged mucosa but in the absence of other more characteristic features of GERD, they may be the only clue that a chemical injury has occurred.

Vascular Changes. Capillary ectasia (sometimes called vascular lakes) consists of dilated and congested venules located high in the lengthened esophageal papillae. Red blood cells frequently extravasate into the surrounding epithelium. Capillary ectasia affects up to 83 percent of GERD patients contrasting with its presence in only 10 percent of control patients (2,13). This change is often present in the absence of any inflammation and corresponds to the endoscopically identified red mucosal streaks.

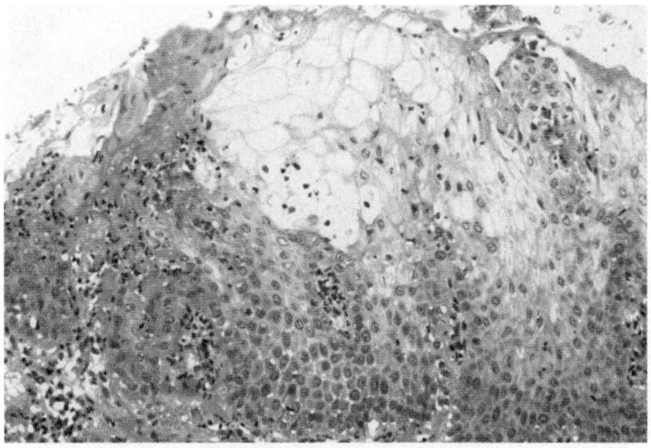

Figure 3-3

REFLUX ESOPHAGITIS

The superficial squamous epithelial cells demonstrate hydropic degeneration in this case of severe gastroesophageal reflux disease.

Intercellular Edema (Spongiosis). Intercellular edema often results from acid reflux. It is usually most prominent in the basal layers, often in the absence of inflammation. The intercellular fluid accumulation may make the intercellular bridges unusually prominent (fig. 3-4).

Epithelial Hyperplasia. Normally, the basal layer is only 1 to 4 cells thick and occupies less than 15 percent of the squamous epithelial thickness. Prolonged bathing of the esophageal mucosa with acid accelerates mucosal cell shedding and results in compensatory basal cell hyperplasia. As a result, the basal cell layers increase in thickness (fig. 3-5). Since normal individuals have mild epithelial hyperplasia 2 to 3 cm proximal to the LES, this feature is not useful in diagnosing GERD if biopsies are taken in this area. In contrast, epithelial hyperplasia occurring 3 cm or more proximal to the Z line is sufficient to suggest the diagnosis of reflux esophagitis (18). Basal cell hyperplasia is most easily appreciated when these layers exceed 25 percent of the mucosal thickness. Stromal papillae lengthen (fig. 3-5). The lamina propria papillae often extend into more than two thirds of the mucosal thickness. Riddell (27) suggests

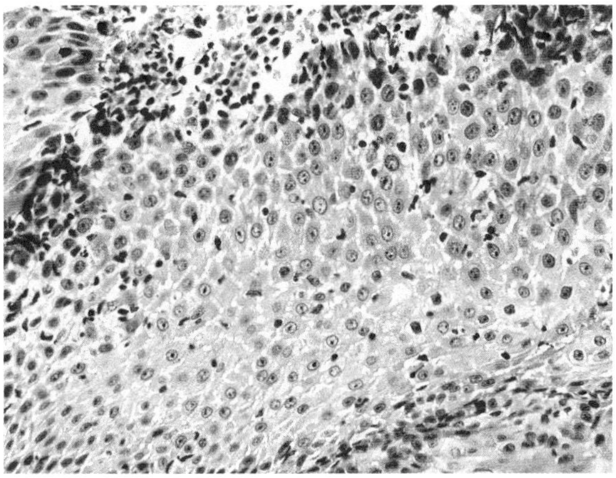

Figure 3-4

REFLUX ESOPHAGITIS

The squamous epithelium shows evidence of spongiosis, making intercellular bridges appear prominent.

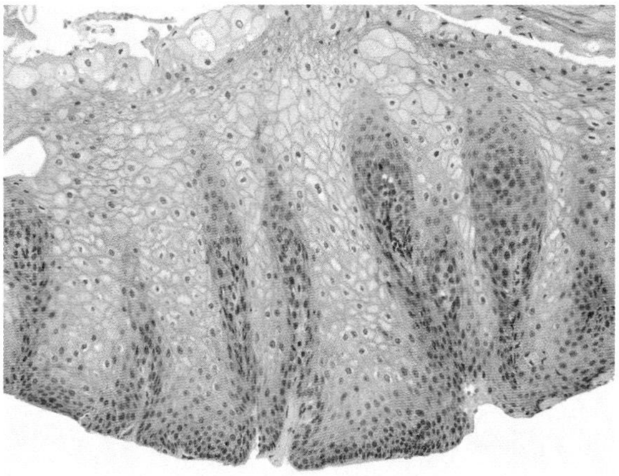

Figure 3-5

REFLUX ESOPHAGITIS

The squamous epithelium shows mild basal hyperplasia and elongation of the papillae. In this case, the papillae reach upward to approximately two thirds the epithelial thickness. The surface squamous cells show ballooning change.

using the rule of thirds to evaluate the mucosa for evidence of hyperplasia. This rule divides the full epithelial thickness into thirds. Papillae should not extend into the upper third. When the lower third is divided in half, the basal cells should be confined to the lower half; extension beyond this is abnormal.

Regenerating basal epithelium is characterized by nuclear enlargement, hyperchromasia, and mitotic figures in the basal cell layers (fig. 3-6). (Mitoses are rare in the normal, noninjured esophageal mucosa.) Nucleoli may also be prominent. The hyperplastic regenerating cells lack the normal glycogenation characteristic of superficial cells. Therefore, PAS stains show expanded PAS-negative areas.

When the epithelium becomes very hyperplastic, the elongated epithelial pegs extend deep into the underlying lamina propria, producing the lesion known as *acanthosis*. Extensive acanthosis, also termed *pseudoepitheliomatous hyperplasia*, may mimic invasive cancer, especially when the cells exhibit severe cytologic atypia. Atypical cells have cytoplasmic basophilia, an increased nuclear to cytoplasmic ratio, glycogen depletion, and increased mitotic activity. The uniformly sized cell nuclei may contain prominent nucleoli. The reactive cells more or less maintain their normal polarity, the nuclei generally do not overlap, and abnormal mitoses are absent. Squamous cell maturation

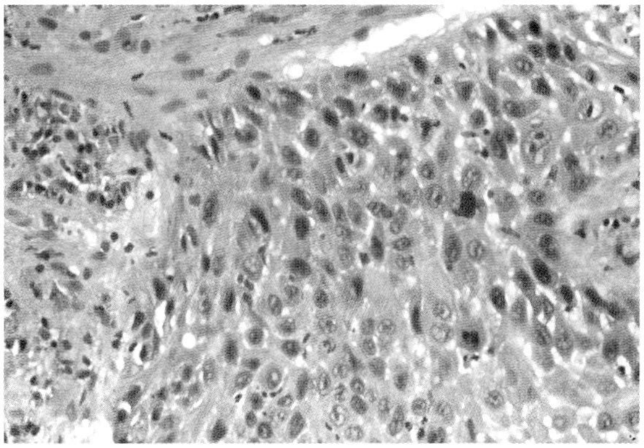

Figure 3-6

REGENERATIVE SQUAMOUS EPITHELIUM IN GASTROESOPHAGEAL REFLUX DISEASE

The squamous cells appear atypical with enlarged, but regular, nuclei and prominent nucleoli. The nuclear to cytoplasmic ratio, however, is not increased to the degree seen in neoplasia, and there is normal maturation of the squamous cells toward the mucosal surface. Despite the cytologic atypia, the nuclei do not overlap, and normal polarity is maintained.

occurs in the more superficial cell layers. The individual cell keratinization characteristic of high-grade dysplasia is absent. The epithelial-stromal boundary appears smooth, with an obvious basement membrane, unless extensive inflammation is present. The lamina propria

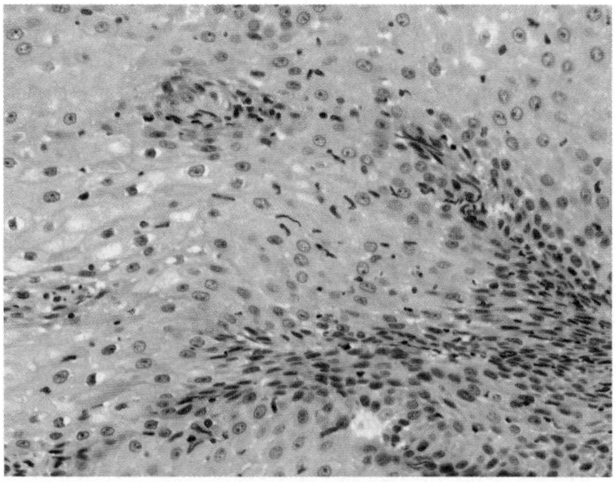

Figure 3-7

REFLUX ESOPHAGITIS

The squamous epithelium contains an increased number of intraepithelial lymphocytes. These appear as elongated "squiggle" cells.

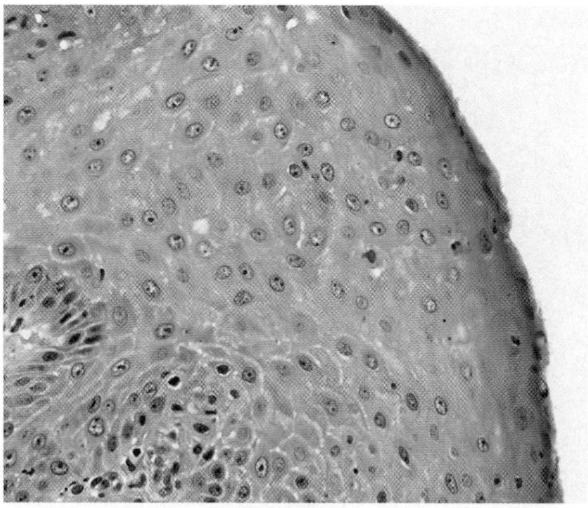

Figure 3-8

REFLUX ESOPHAGITIS

Scattered intraepithelial eosinophils are often seen in reflux esophagitis.

and submucosa may become very inflamed and isolated reactive epithelial cells can drop into a severely inflamed and ulcerated stroma. Desmoplasia, however, should not be seen surrounding the epithelial cells. Antibodies to cytokeratin may help distinguish a truly invasive cancer from reactive endothelial cells in the underlying stroma. Such immunoreactions should be carefully interpreted since reactive stromal cells are occasionally cytokeratin positive.

Very small or poorly oriented biopsies, especially those with significant inflammation and associated reactive atypia, may be impossible to interpret. In this situation, repeat biopsies may be necessary once the reflux has been treated.

Inflammation. Small numbers of lymphocytes and plasma cells typically populate the normal esophageal lamina propria; their presence does not establish a diagnosis of esophagitis. Mucosal lymphocyte numbers (intraepithelial and in the lamina propria) are conspicuously increased, however, in patients with GERD. Intraepithelial lymphocytes have been referred to as "squiggle cells" or "cells with irregular nuclear contours" because of their curved nuclei, which appear to fit between the epithelial cells (fig. 3-7). They have almost no visible cytoplasm. Intraepithelial lymphocytes are present in esophagitis of diverse etiologies, but they are often present in large numbers in reflux esophagitis (42), averaging more than 6 cells per high-power field (22). Most intraepithelial lymphocytes are CD3-positive T cells and a smaller proportion are S-100 protein–positive antigen-presenting cells (42).

Intraepithelial eosinophils are considered by many to be the single most specific diagnostic feature of reflux esophagitis, as shown by esophageal pH monitoring (1,19,43). Their presence is not a sensitive marker, however, since they are seen in only 40 to 50 percent of symptomatic individuals (fig. 3-8), and they can be found in control patients and occasionally in any of the entities listed in Table 3-3. Intraepithelial eosinophils may be focal, necessitating a search for them on serial sections and in multiple levels. There is also a group of patients with eosinophilic esophagitis who have large numbers of eosinophils and no evidence of reflux by pH monitoring studies. It is important to note that in many cases, eosinophils are absent in biopsies with other features of GERD.

Neutrophils, in either the squamous epithelium or in the lamina propria, serve as evidence of acute erosive or ulcerative esophagitis. Large collections of neutrophils suggest that a biopsy comes from an ulcer or an erosion. Although neutrophils provide evidence of erosions or ulcers, they are not specific for GERD-associated esophagitis.

Table 3-3

DIFFERENTIAL DIAGNOSIS OF ESOPHAGEAL EOSINOPHILIA

Primary disorders
Eosinophilic esophagitis
Atopic
Nonatopic
Familial
Secondary eosinophilic disorders
Hypereosinophilic syndrome
Eosinophilic gastroenteritis
Secondary noneosinophilic disorders
Gastroesophageal reflux disease
Parasitic infection
Fungal infection
Recurrent vomiting
Drug-induced injury
Inflammatory bowel disease
Esophageal leiomyomatosis
Allergic vasculitis
Periarteritis nodosa
Scleroderma
Neoplasia

Table 3-4

DIFFERENTIAL DIAGNOSIS OF GASTROESOPHAGEAL REFLUX DISEASE

Infections
Fungal
Viral
Drug effects
Azidothymidine (AZT)
Chemotherapy (mucositis)
Pill esophagitis
Caustic ingestion
Radiotherapy
Systemic diseases
Allergies
Behcet's disease
Graft versus host disease
Crohn's disease
Progressive systemic sclerosis
Other collagen vascular diseases
Eosinophilic gastroenteritis
Uremia
Trauma

Multinucleated Epithelial Giant Cells. Multinucleated giant squamous epithelial cells with histologic features simulating a viral cytopathic effect or dysplasia are seen in patients with many forms of esophagitis, including reflux esophagitis. Typically, the multinucleated cells have a mean of 3 nuclei/cell (ranging from 2 to 9) and there are typically 2 to 11 cells/biopsy. The nuclei may contain a single or multiple eosinophilic nucleoli with a perinuclear halo but the cells lack inclusions, hyperchromasia, or atypical mitoses. The giant cells are generally confined to the basal epithelium, although occasionally they occur more superficially. Following treatment, these cells disappear (30).

Carditis. Biopsies obtained from the cardiac mucosa immediately distal to the Z line in patients with GERD often contain large numbers of acute or chronic inflammatory cells, even in areas appearing endoscopically normal. The inflammation is limited to the gastric cardia in the absence of similar changes in the remaining stomach (27). Carditis may be a more sensitive marker of GERD than inflammation involving the squamous mucosa as judged by pH monitoring studies. This is a controversial subject, however, with some believing that carditis is associated with *H. pylori* infection, especially in those patients with intestinal metaplasia in the cardia and elsewhere in the stomach (14).

Differential Diagnosis. The histologic features discussed in the preceding sections suggest the diagnosis of GERD, especially in the distal esophagus, but none are specific for this entity since they represent the pattern of response of stratified squamous epithelium to diverse injuries. Entities to be considered in the differential diagnosis of GERD include those listed in Table 3-4. Reactive changes in biopsies from patients with GERD may appear so atypical that the differential diagnosis includes malignancy. Similarly, when extensive pseudoepitheliomatous hyperplasia is present, the question of an invasive carcinoma or squamous dysplasia arises. The base of ulcers may contain bizarre cells that mimic an invasive carcinoma. Granulation tissue, if present, may contain prominent capillaries with enlarged endothelial cells that mimic an adenocarcinoma. In patients with acquired immunodeficiency syndrome (AIDS), the lesion may resemble Kaposi's sarcoma. Marked lymphoid hyperplasia may simulate a lymphoma (28).

Immunohistochemical stains using antibodies directed against endothelial and epithelial cells distinguish between the reparative reactions and malignancy. The presence of isolated cytokeratin-positive cells strongly suggests the presence of an invasive cancer, especially if the cytokeratin-positive cells demonstrate significant nuclear atypia and lie within a desmoplastic stroma. It is important to note that reactive mesenchymal cells are sometimes cytokeratin immunoreactive.

The differential diagnosis of GERD with ulcers or erosions includes infection, drug reaction, and many other entities. Patients whose biopsies show significant atypia and irregular epithelial nests, in a setting of severe inflammation, may need to have the diagnosis deferred until the inflammation subsides.

Treatment and Prognosis. Only a small proportion of patients with heartburn see a physician; the majority choose to self medicate with proprietary medications. Investigation is necessary in those with long-standing symptoms (to rule out Barrett esophagus), those with symptoms unresponsive to therapy, or those who have alarming features (dysphagia, vomiting, blood loss, or weight loss). Treatment depends on disease severity. Generally, therapy is aimed at reducing the reflux, enhancing esophageal clearing, and minimizing the aggressive impact of the refluxed material. Mild symptomatic GERD is usually managed by lifestyle and dietary modifications along with treatment with antacids, H2-receptor antagonists, or proton pump inhibitors (40). Antacids, Gaviscon, and motor-stimulating drugs may be sufficient to treat patients without histologic evidence of esophagitis who have occasional low-grade heartburn. Prokinetic drugs are used to increase LES tone, enhance gastric emptying, and improve peristalsis, thereby counteracting some of the abnormalities that lead to esophagitis.

Once erosive or ulcerative lesions have developed, more rigorous medical treatment, including the use of proton pump inhibitors, is mandatory. Patients with intractable symptoms require more intensive pharmacologic therapy, often utilizing combination medications with frequent dosing or antireflux surgery. Mechanical dilatation of strictures may relieve symptoms but if this is not possible, then surgery may become necessary. Prolonged reflux may cause esophageal shortening which may dictate the type of procedure necessary, should surgery be required to control symptoms. When the symptoms are severe in children, gastroesophageal fundoplication and/or pyloroplasty may alleviate the symptoms.

Complications of GERD range from superficial erosion or deeper ulceration to transmural inflammation, circumferential fibrosis with stricture formation and fixation to surrounding structures, development of Barrett esophagus, and cancer.

BARRETT ESOPHAGUS

Definition. *Barrett esophagus* (BE) is defined endoscopically as visible columnar epithelium in the esophagus which, on biopsy, is metaplastic columnar epithelium as defined by the presence of acid mucin–containing (Alcian blue–positive) goblet cells (68). Long segment BE is esophageal columnar mucosa with intestinal metaplasia located 3 cm or more proximal to the esophagogastric junction. Short segment BE is the presence of tongues and/or circumferential columnar-appearing mucosa less than 3 cm above the proximal margin of the gastric folds. A diagnosis of BE cannot be made without the identification of intestinal metaplasia on biopsy specimens obtained from the areas of suspected esophageal columnar mucosa.

Demography. Most cases of BE in the general population are unrecognized. The clinical prevalence is 22.6 cases/100,000 population and is much lower than the autopsy prevalence of 376/100,000 (59). The discrepancy may relate to the fact that up to one third of patients do not have reflux symptoms at the time of diagnosis and many patients do not seek medical advice for their heartburn. Additionally, patients have access to over-the-counter antacid drugs. BE develops in approximately 10 to12 percent of patients with GERD (66,69,71,77). The mean age at which BE is diagnosed is approximately 60 years (56). Disease incidence plateaus by age 70. Children also develop this lesion (53,57). BE preferentially affects white males, and is less common in African-Americans and Asians (49,61,70).

Etiology. BE results from the reflux of gastric acid, bile salts, lysophospholipids, and activated pancreatic enzymes (70,72,77,78). It may also accompany lye ingestion (71) or treatment with some chemotherapeutic agents. There may be a genetic predisposition to developing BE (48,52,59).

Pathophysiology. BE may be viewed as an adaptive response in which stratified squamous epithelium is replaced by potentially acid-resistant columnar epithelium (70). Recurrent ulceration denudes the normal squamous epithelium, which then becomes lined by columnar epithelium. This columnar epithelium arises from multipotential stem cells lying in the basal mucosa. It is presumed that there is a neoplastic progression that occurs in BE which goes from chronic gastroesophageal reflux to esophagitis to the presence of metaplastic columnar epithelium. Dysplasia develops within this, followed eventually, in some cases, by adenocarcinoma.

Clinical Features. The symptoms associated with BE resemble those of the underlying reflux esophagitis: heartburn, regurgitation, and dysphagia. Many patients with BE are asymptomatic (55,67). Strictures causing dysphagia may develop, usually at the junction of the displaced squamocolumnar junction. The advent of dysphagia must be aggressively investigated in order to differentiate between a peptic origin and the onset of neoplasia. Unfortunately, the presenting symptom of BE may be the development of an adenocarcinoma.

Gross and Endoscopic Findings. Beefy red, velvety areas lie proximal to the end of the gastric folds. BE extends proximally in a continuous sheet, as a circumferential lesion, in finger-like or flame-like projections, or as isolated islands in the tubular esophagus (fig. 3-9). These areas contrast with the lighter pink-tan or white, smooth, native squamous epithelium. Distally, BE merges imperceptibly with the native gastric mucosa. The junction with the esophageal squamous epithelium may appear symmetric or asymmetric, or as islands of normal mucosa alternating with BE. Short (less than 2 cm) tongues of BE are most common in short segment BE. Island type BE accompanies less severe epithelial injury than the circumferential type.

Biopsy Evaluation. The combination of endoscopy and biopsy is the gold standard for the diagnosis of BE. The mucosal changes are measured with respect to the gastroesophageal junction, which is usually recognized by the proximal extent of the gastric folds (62,73,74). The columnar segment is described by terms including "salmon-pink tongues" and "flame-like extensions" into the surrounding "pearly white" squamous epithelium. Discrete islands of pink epithelium are sometimes seen. The mucosa may appear somewhat atrophic, similar to that seen in atrophic gastritis, with vessels visible through the columnar lining. A finely nodular or mammillary appearance has also been described (73,74).

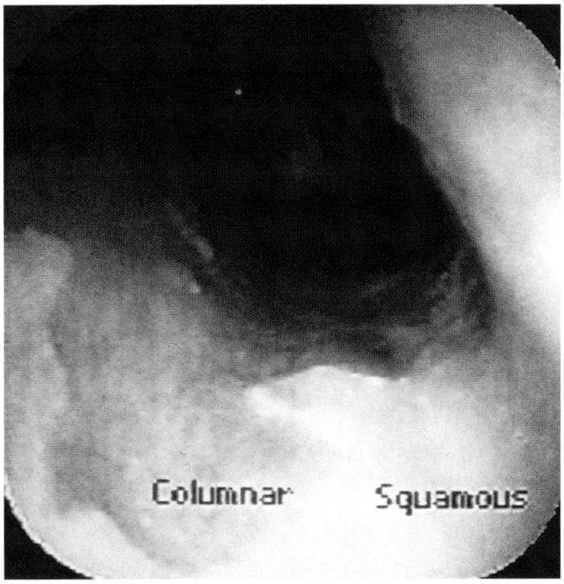

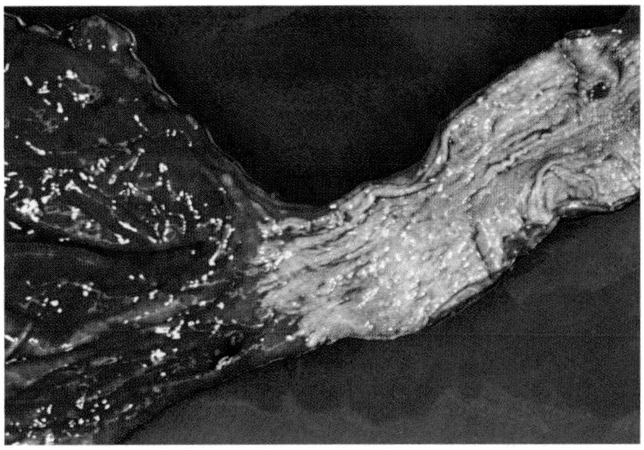

Figure 3-9

BARRETT ESOPHAGUS

Top: Endoscopically, a salmon-colored tongue of Barrett mucosa extends upward into the esophagus. The adjacent squamous epithelium is whitish tan.

Bottom: Resection specimen has a similar appearance. Reddish columnar mucosa extends into the esophagus.

The suggestion of BE on endoscopic examination prompts multiple biopsies to prove the diagnosis and exclude the possibilities of dysplasia and malignancy. The latter are not seen

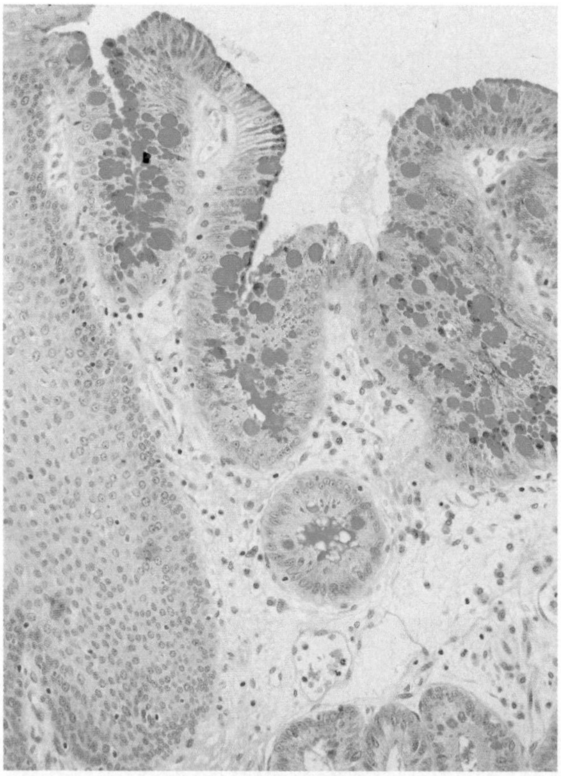

Figure 3-10

BARRETT ESOPHAGUS

The Alcian blue stain (pH 2.5) highlights the intestinal type mucin present in the goblet cells of intestinal metaplasia in Barrett esophagus. Goblet cells stain blue, while the gastric foveolar type mucin stains pink.

endoscopically. Tytgat (74) suggests four-quadrant biopsies be taken every 2 cm of the columnar lining, whereas Nishimaki (63) believes that the area just above the endoscopically obvious columnar segment must always be biopsied carefully because it is a high-risk zone for dysplasia and malignancy. Additional sampling of any associated elevated lesions or strictures must be done. Chromoendoscopy (coating the esophagus with various dyes to identify BE/dysplasia) is also a useful tool.

Microscopic Findings. The current definition of BE requires intestinalized (specialized) mucosa to be present, even if only a single biopsy is examined. Such specialized epithelium is characterized by the presence of goblet and intestinal columnar cells (fig. 3-10). The goblet cells contain acid mucins, predominantly sialomucins, which stain positively with Alcian blue at pH 2.5 (fig. 3-10). The pattern of sulfomucin staining may show a selective association with dysplasia and adenocarcinoma (58,60, 78). The columnar epithelium resembles either small intestinal absorptive cells (complete intestinal metaplasia) or colonic epithelium (incomplete intestinal metaplasia). BE sometimes acquires a villiform surface architecture.

The recent identification of intestinal metaplasia in the cardia, along with the observation that it occurs in an inflamed cardiac mucosa, has led to focus on the type and the condition of the mucosa at the gastroesophageal junction and its relationship to GERD. Specialized intestinal metaplasia at the cardia is only found in inflamed cardiac mucosa and its prevalence increases both with increasing acid exposure and the presence of esophagitis. Intestinal metaplasia in the cardia is histologically indistinguishable from the specialized metaplasia of BE (58). It could be argued that it makes little difference whether the specialized columnar epithelium lies in the gastric cardia or in the distal esophagus, since both conditions predispose patients to tumors arising at the gastroesophageal junction (50). The incidence of adenocarcinoma of both the esophagus and the gastric cardia has increased at a rate far exceeding that of any other cancer (45,46) and short segments of intestinal metaplasia at the gastroesophageal junction may underlie this phenomenon. Since cancer of the cardia and cancer arising in typical BE share some demographic features and predisposing factors, these two diseases may be related (51). Intestinal metaplasia detected in a biopsy, regardless of whether it comes from the cardia or from the esophagus, serves as a marker of a cell population at risk of neoplastic transformation. A conservative approach would suggest that surveillance of patients with intestinal metaplasia arising at this site be undertaken until the controversy surrounding this issue is settled by better data.

Diagnostic problems in BE include the presence of columnar epithelium in the esophagus which may be normal, and the fact that not all goblet-shaped cells are metaplastic as evidenced by Alcian blue positivity, not all Alcian blue–positive cells are metaplastic, and the significance of a few metaplastic epithelial cells is unknown. Although distended gastric foveolar cells may

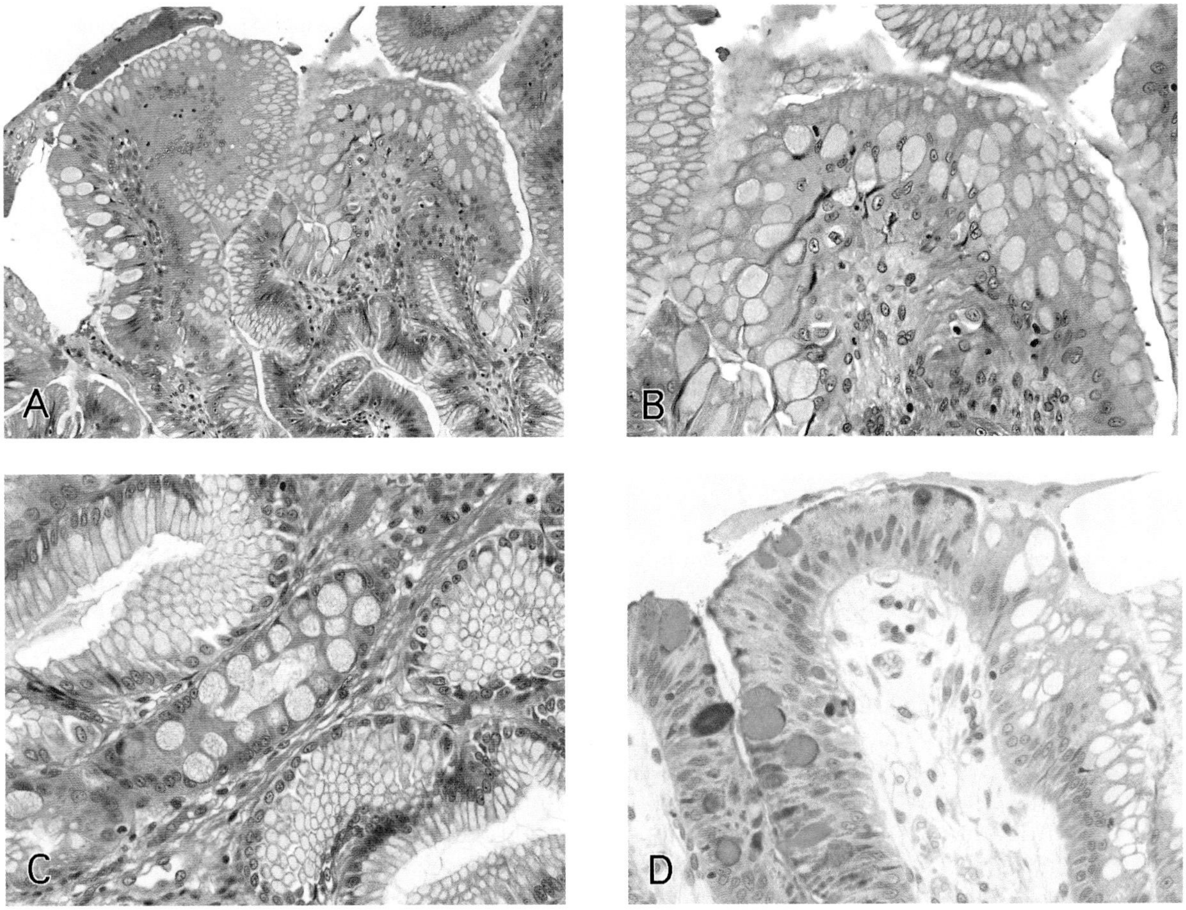

Figure 3-11

BARRETT ESOPHAGUS

A: True intestinal metaplasia is seen on the left, and distended foveolar cells mimicking goblet cells on the right.
B: Higher-power view shows dystrophic foveolar cells. The mucin in the foveolar cells appears eosinophilic.
C: In contrast, the mucin in the goblet cells has a bluish tinge.
D: An Alcian blue stain may aid in differentiating between dystrophic foveolar cells and goblet cells. The goblet cells on the left stain strongly, while the distended foveolar cells on the right appear light pink and unstained.

acquire a goblet cell shape (fig. 3-11), true goblet cells generally have a bluish appearance with routine hematoxylin and eosin (H&E) stains, whereas dystrophic foveolar cells usually are deeply eosinophilic. Such cells are often Alcian blue negative; it is important to note, however, that reactive gastric surface cells may sometimes stain with Alcian blue (fig. 3-12).

Special Techniques. Cytokeratin immunoreactivity patterns may be useful in the diagnosis of short segment BE. Cytokeratins are epithelial structural proteins that comprise the cytoskeleton of human cells. They preferentially stain different types of epithelia. In the context of esophageal disease, a unique pattern of staining for cytokeratins (CK) 7 and 20, designated as the Barrett CK7/20 pattern, is sensitive and specific for the diagnosis of long segment BE when compared to the diagnosis of gastrointestinal metaplasia (64). A strong band of CK20 staining is seen in the superficial portion of the mucosa in BE; CK7 stains the epithelium diffusely. In contrast, gastric intestinal metaplasia shows patchy CK20 staining throughout the full thickness of the mucosa, and an absence of CK7 staining. A Barrett CK7/20 pattern is present in 98 percent of patients with long segment BE (65) and in 82 percent of patients with suspected

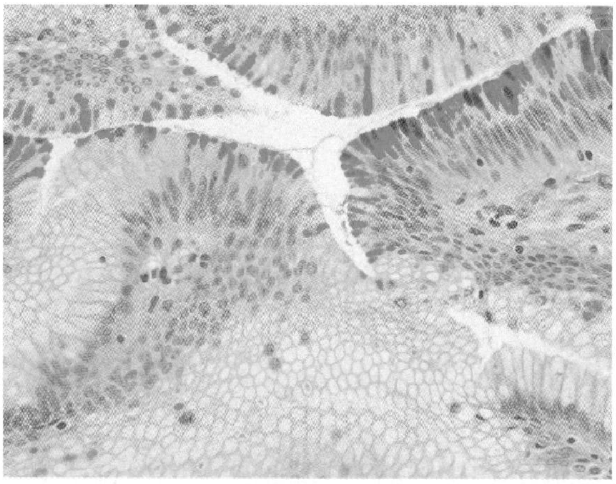

Figure 3-12

BARRETT ESOPHAGUS

Foveolar cells sometimes demonstrate Alcian blue positivity, as illustrated here. Cells that do not morphologically resemble goblet cells should not be interpreted as such on the basis of the Alcian blue stain alone.

Table 3-5

DIFFERENTIAL DIAGNOSIS OF BARRETT MUCOSA

Inadvertently sampled gastric mucosa (especially in hiatal hernias)
Esophageal junctional mucosa Cardiac-like mucosa located in distal 1-2 cm
Esophageal superficial cardiac glands Often located in upper esophagus
Ectopic gastric fundic mucosa Noted in upper esophagus of 4-10% of normal subjects

short segment BE, whereas none of the patients with gastrointestinal metaplasia have this pattern. This suggests that a Barrett CK7/20 pattern is an objective marker of Barrett mucosa in conjunction with appropriate clinical and endoscopic data (65).

Differential Diagnosis. The differential diagnosis of BE is listed in Table 3-5.

Treatment and Prognosis. A major milestone in the management of patients with BE and reflux esophagitis has been medical management with proton pump inhibitors and prokinetics. The proton pump inhibitors reduce gastric acid output and also the volume of the refluxate. Laparoscopic antireflux surgery also may be appropriate for patients with BE (75). Management of BE involves treating the underlying reflux and monitoring the risk of adenocarcinoma. The current standard is to treat all patients with BE with the most potent antisecretory medication available (currently, proton pump inhibitors), even if asymptomatic. In some cases, BE has the potential to revert to normal if the acid reflux is treated (47,54), although this is rare (76). When regression has occurred, squamous epithelium typically overlies the columnar epithelium, especially near the area of the squamocolumnar junction.

Various ablative techniques for eradicating BE are being explored. The aim of these therapeutic strategies is to eliminate the abnormal epithelium and remove the risk of progression to malignancy. Laser photoablation is emerging as a popular treatment method, although strictures or mediastinitis may occur. The most striking patterns of squamous reepithelialization are seen in patients treated with photodynamic therapy. These patients develop extensive squamous metaplasia deep within the Barrett glands, with squamous epithelium overlying the columnar epithelium (44). Unfortunately, a significant discrepancy exists between the endoscopist's assessment of squamous reepithelialization and the histologic findings in the biopsy samples from these cases (44).

EOSINOPHILIC ESOPHAGITIS

Definition. *Eosinophilic esophagitis* is a form of esophagitis characterized by a prominent intraepithelial eosinophilic infiltrate.

Demography. Patients with eosinophilic esophagitis (also referred to as *idiopathic eosinophilic* or *allergic esophagitis*) are typically young males, but the disease affects both sexes and all ages. Symptoms include vomiting, epigastric or chest pain, dysphagia, and respiratory obstructive problems (83,87). Many patients have a history of atopic disease (86).

Etiology. The cause of eosinophilic esophagitis is poorly understood, but is most likely associated with food allergy (84). Most affected patients have clinical evidence of food and airborne allergen hypersensitivity (80). In addition, many patients report seasonal variation in their symptoms (84).

Gross and Microscopic Findings. Histologically, esophageal biopsies demonstrate epithelial hyperplasia and extensive infiltration of the mucosa by eosinophils (fig. 3-13). Eosinophils

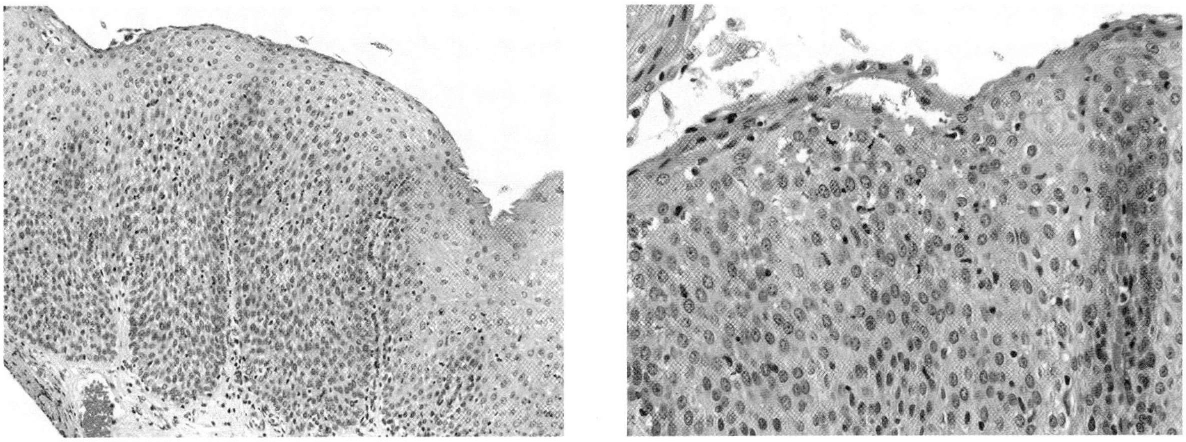

Figure 3-13

EOSINOPHILIC ESOPHAGITIS

Left: Eosinophilic esophagitis with marked basal hyperplasia and papillary elongation.
Right: On higher power, numerous intraepithelial eosinophils are seen (over 20 per high-power field).

Table 3-6

FEATURES DISTINGUISHING EOSINOPHILIC ESOPHAGITIS AND GASTROESOPHAGEAL REFLUX DISEASE (GERD)

Typical Features	Eosinophilic Esophagitis	GERD
Clinical		
Presence of atopy	Very common	Normal (possibly increased)
Sex preference	Male	Slight male
Abdominal pain, vomiting	Common	Common
Food impaction	Common	Uncommon
Endoscopic Findings		
Endoscopic furrowing	Very common	Occasionally
pH probe	Usually normal	Abnormal
Histologic Findings		
Proximal involvement	Yes	No
Distal involvement	Yes	Yes
Epithelial hyperplasia	Markedly increased	Increased
Number of eosinophils	>20/hpf[a]	0-7/hpf
	Eosinophils in clusters	Scattered eosinophils, no clusters

[a]hpf = high-power field.

generally number in excess of 20 to 24 per high-power field (83,85). In contrast, GERD is characterized by lower numbers of intramucosal eosinophils, usually 7 or fewer per high-power field. Seven to 20 eosinophils per high-power field may be indicative of a combination of GERD and food allergy (85,86). The features that are helpful in distinguishing eosinophilic esophagitis and GERD are summarized in Table 3-6.

Differential Diagnosis. Eosinophilic infiltrates of the esophageal wall commonly pose a diagnostic dilemma. The differential diagnosis usually centers around reflux esophagitis, parasitic infection, drug reactions, or eosinophilic esophagitis. The esophagus normally does not contain any eosinophils, and therefore, their identification represents a pathologic accumulation in this site (80,85). Esophageal eosinophilic disorders can be classified as primary or secondary. Primary disorders are further categorized into those that are associated with atopy, those that are unassociated with atopy, and those that are familial. Secondary disorders may occur with or without a coexisting systemic eosinophilic disease. The differential diagnosis of esophageal eosinophilic infiltrates is listed in Table 3-3.

Treatment and Prognosis. The treatment of patients with eosinophilic esophagitis includes avoidance of known specific food and airborne allergens in atopic patients. In cases where dietary changes are ineffective, an elemental diet may improve symptoms (81). Administration of systemic or topical steroids may also be of benefit (79,82). Gastric acid should be neutralized, even in patients without GERD (84). If left untreated, eosinophilic esophagitis may progress, resulting in chronic scarring and esophageal stricture formation. The risk for the development of BE is unknown.

ESOPHAGEAL INFECTIONS

Because of the increased use of steroids, cytotoxic drugs, and other immunosuppressive agents, as well as the increase in human immunodeficiency virus (HIV)-associated disease worldwide, the prevalence of opportunistic infective esophagitis has increased. The presence of underlying GERD or an anatomic abnormality may further predispose a patient to develop infectious esophagitis. As the population ages, host defense mechanisms deteriorate, predisposing elderly patients to infectious diseases. Esophageal infectious diseases are discussed in detail in chapter 10.

Bacterial Esophagitis

Clinical Features. Esophageal bacterial infections are uncommon and generally occur either in profoundly neutropenic patients or as a result of extension of an infection from an adjacent structure. The pathogenesis of *bacterial esophagitis* often involves a previous esophageal injury that damaged the integrity of the squamous mucosal barrier. Such injuries include previous reflux esophagitis, radiation, chemotherapy, or nasogastric intubation. Disruption of the mucosal barrier allows bacteria to easily invade the underlying lamina propria, especially in immunologically deficient individuals. Other predisposing factors include defective peristalsis, mechanical obstruction, ethanol abuse, ulceration from pills sticking in the esophagus, or congenital abnormalities. The most common infecting organisms are normal flora of the mouth and upper respiratory tract.

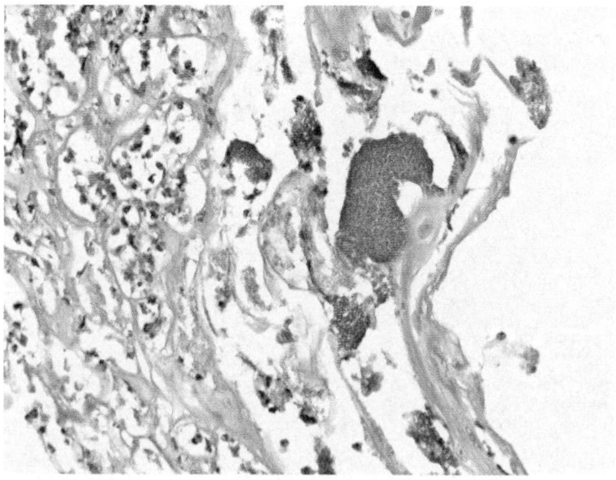

Figure 3-14

BACTERIAL ESOPHAGITIS

Large clusters of bacteria lie in the esophageal lumen and within the squamous epithelium. In addition, scattered organisms invade the underlying tissues.

Gross and Microscopic Findings. Grossly, bacterial esophagitis features nonspecific mucosal friability, plaques, pseudomembranes, and ulcerations. Histologically, bacterial infections produce a diffuse, acute necrotizing process characterized by the presence of an intense neutrophilic exudate, cellular necrosis, and degeneration. Sheets of bacteria (highlighted by Gram stains) invade the underlying tissues (fig. 3-14). Often, several bacterial species are present, supporting the polymicrobial nature of the infections. The total number of bacteria appears to be inversely related to the intensity of the accompanying inflammation (89).

Tuberculosis

Clinical Features. Individuals at risk for developing *esophageal tuberculosis* include immigrants from and natives of underdeveloped countries and immunocompromised patients. Esophageal tuberculosis usually represents a secondary manifestation of the disease in patients with primary pulmonary, intestinal, laryngeal, or mediastinal tuberculosis. Hematogenous spread of miliary tuberculosis occurs less commonly than mediastinal extension. Patients present with dysphagia resulting from extrinsic esophageal

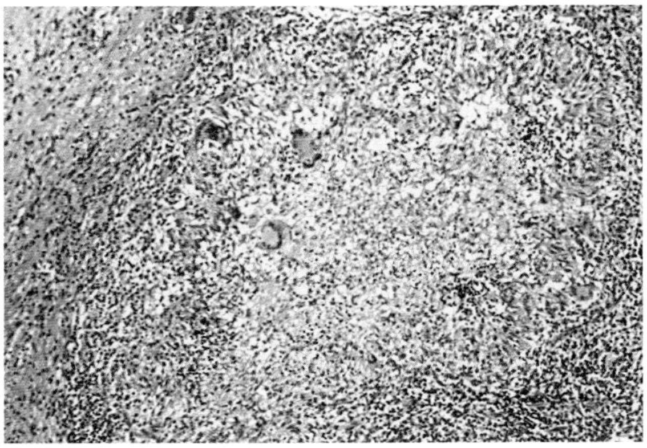

Figure 3-15

TUBERCULOUS ESOPHAGITIS

A typical granuloma with central necrosis is seen. (Courtesy of the Division of Gastrointestinal Pathology, Armed Forces Institute of Pathology, Washington, DC.)

compression by enlarged mediastinal lymph nodes. Rupture of mediastinal disease into the esophagus causes fistula formation between the tracheobronchial tree and the esophagus.

Gross and Microscopic Findings. Grossly, the lesions appear ulcerative, hyperplastic (pseudotumoral), or both (88). An esophageal mucosal biopsy might not yield relevant diagnostic tissue in patients with esophageal tuberculosis because the esophagus is usually involved by direct extension of mediastinal or thoracic disease; therefore, a biopsy may not be deep enough to provide diagnostic material. When the diagnosis is clear, the histologic features of tuberculosis resemble those seen elsewhere in the gastrointestinal tract, with the presence of caseating granulomas containing epithelioid histiocytes, giant cells, and acid-fast bacilli (fig. 3-15).

Viral Esophagitis

Viruses commonly infect the esophageal mucosa, especially in immunocompromised patients. It is important to recognize these infections so that they can be treated appropriately. It is also important not to overdiagnose viral infections so that needless, potentially harmful drugs will not be administered. Pseudoviral inclusions associated with nuclear pyknosis and intranuclear cytoplasmic inclusions develop in degenerating cells. If doubt exists as to the presence of a viral infection, it can be confirmed by an ancillary technique such as immunohistochemistry or in situ hybridization.

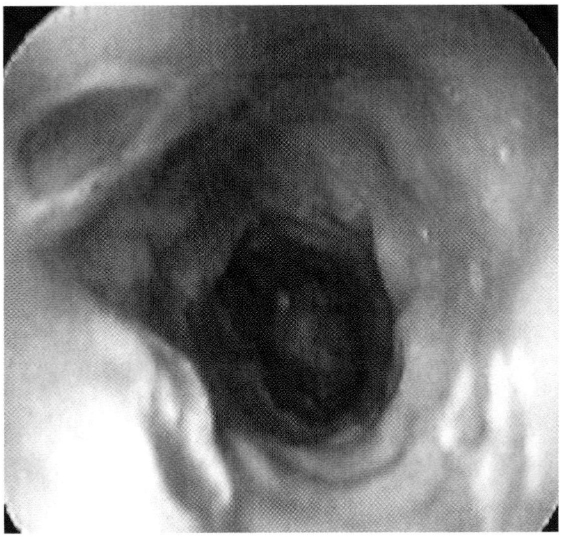

Figure 3-16

HERPES ESOPHAGITIS

Endoscopic view of a well-demarcated area of ulceration.

Herpes Esophagitis. *Clinical Features.* Typical herpetic esophagitis, as seen in the immunocompromised patient, presents with the acute onset of odynophagia, fever, and retrosternal pain. When severe, herpetic esophagitis may cause hemorrhage (91). The disease also develops in immunocompetent individuals, usually as a result of reactivation of latent viral infection. Herpes esophagitis also occurs in children and neonates. In neonates, the disease is acquired as an intrauterine, intrapartum, or postnatal infection (93).

Gross and Microscopic Findings. The esophagus is involved in about 90 percent of patients with visceral herpes; the distal half is the most commonly affected region. Early in the course of herpes infection, vesicular lesions develop on the squamous mucosal surface. Because the vesicles do not last long, the presence of isolated or confluent ulcers is a more common finding. The discrete, "punched-out" ulcers have white exudates covering their bases and erythematous or yellow raised margins (fig. 3-16). Typically, the ulcers appear shallow, even in extensive disease.

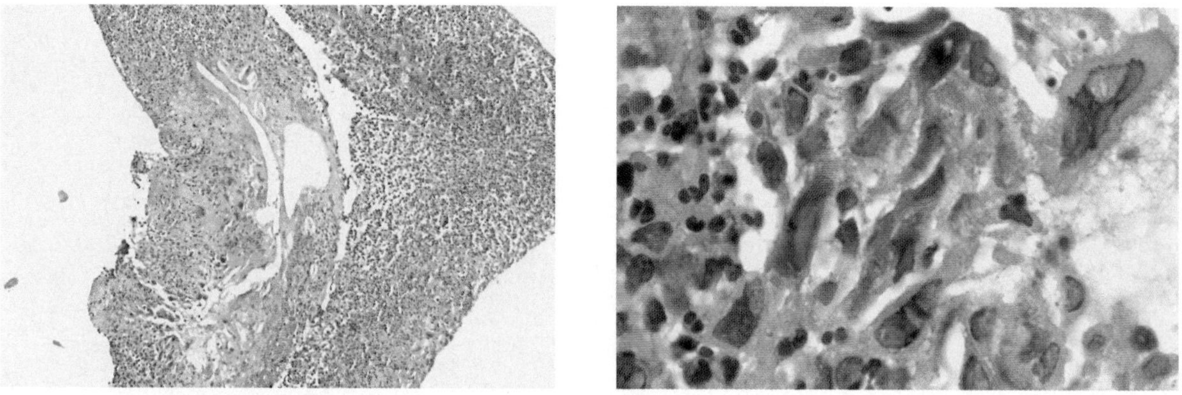

Figure 3-17

HERPES ESOPHAGITIS

Left: Low-power view of reactive-appearing squamous epithelium and granulation tissue adjacent to an ulcer.
Right: Higher-power view of the squamous epithelium shows cells with typical herpesvirus inclusions. Many cells are multinucleated and the nuclei are molded to one another. The nuclei appear glassy with marginated chromatin.

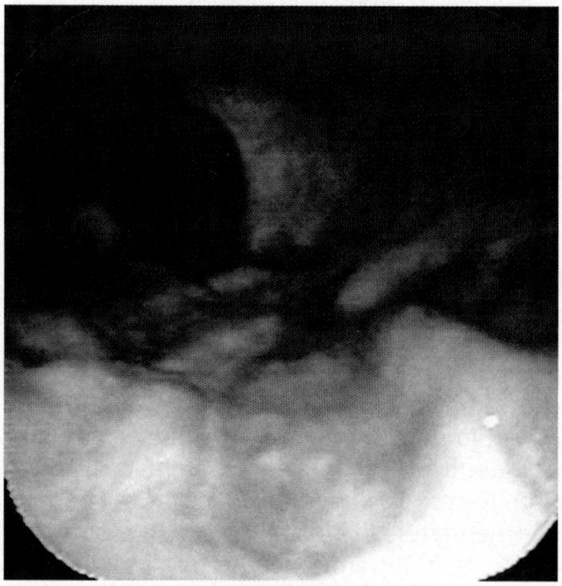

Figure 3-18

CYTOMEGALOVIRUS ESOPHAGITIS

Endoscopic view of an area of ulceration due to cytomegalovirus (CMV) infection.

Herpes esophagitis is usually easy to recognize histologically if a biopsy is taken from the edge of the ulcer (fig. 3-17). The squamous epithelial cells in this region contain Cowdry type A inclusions. A dark margin of condensed chromatin at the nuclear membrane surrounds large, intranuclear, glassy, eosinophilic inclusions. Multinucleate syncytial squamous cells contain molded nuclei and a typical "ground glass" appearance (fig. 3-17). In immunocompetent patients, only a small number of viral inclusions are present, contrasting with the large number present in immunosuppressed patients.

Cytomegalovirus. *Clinical Features.* Cytomegalovirus (CMV) infection is a common cause of viral esophagitis. Like herpes simplex virus, CMV exhibits a tendency to affect debilitated, elderly, or immunocompromised individuals. Symptoms associated with CMV esophagitis are not specific, and include nausea, vomiting, fever, epigastric pain, diarrhea, and weight loss. Dysphagia, odynophagia, and retrosternal pain occur less commonly than in patients with herpes infections (90,92), and symptoms manifest more gradually. CMV affects the entire gastrointestinal tract, and esophageal involvement may be its first manifestation.

Gross and Microscopic Findings. Grossly, CMV esophagitis appears as discrete superficial ulcers in the mid or distal esophagus, similar in appearance to those associated with herpes infection (fig. 3-18). Smaller ulcers may coalesce to form giant ulcers, particularly in the distal esophagus.

The characteristic cytopathic effects of CMV infection include prominent eosinophilic, intranuclear inclusions; cellular enlargement; and occasional, granular basophilic cytoplasmic inclusions (fig. 3-19). The affected cells differ from those seen in herpes infection in that the

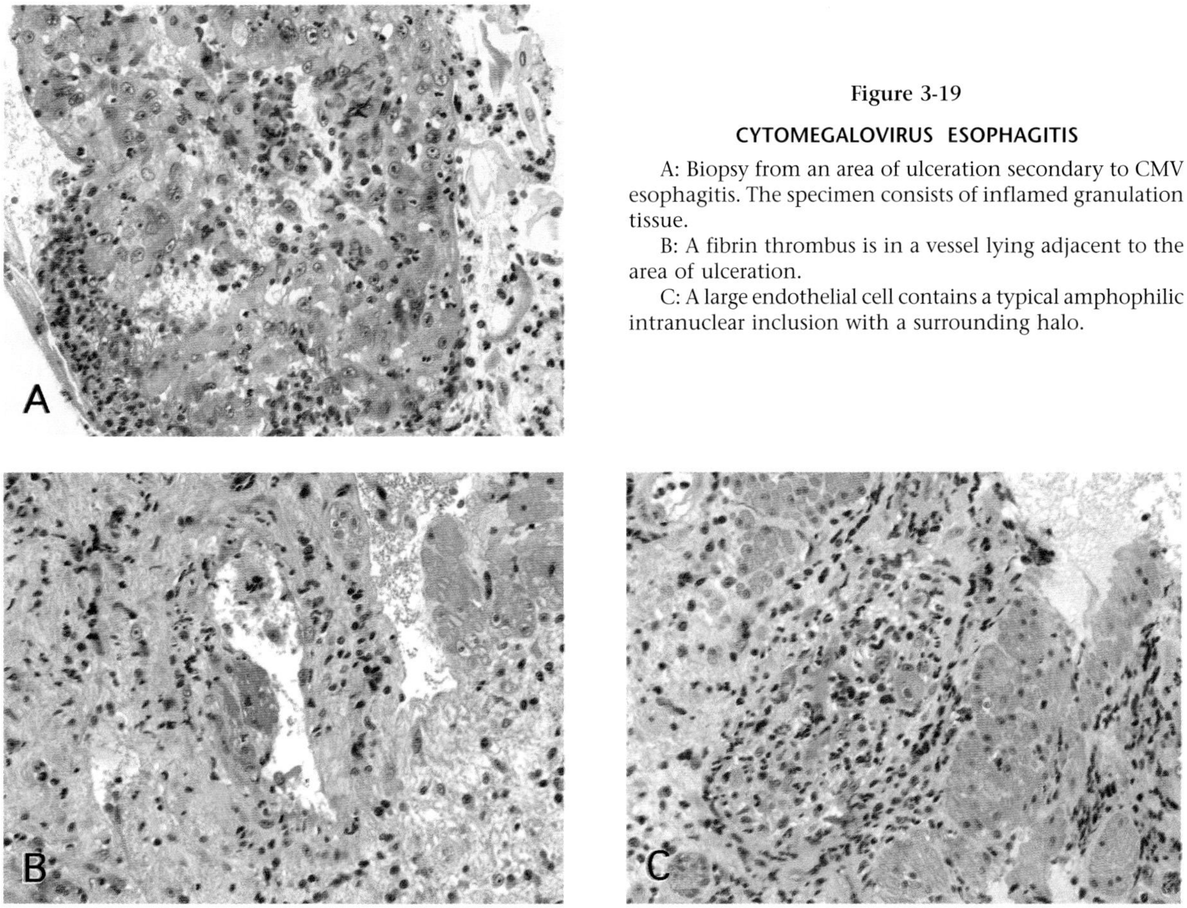

Figure 3-19

CYTOMEGALOVIRUS ESOPHAGITIS

A: Biopsy from an area of ulceration secondary to CMV esophagitis. The specimen consists of inflamed granulation tissue.

B: A fibrin thrombus is in a vessel lying adjacent to the area of ulceration.

C: A large endothelial cell contains a typical amphophilic intranuclear inclusion with a surrounding halo.

cytopathic effects of CMV typically do not affect squamous cells, but are commonly seen in submucosal endothelial cells, macrophages, and fibroblasts in the granulation tissue of the ulcer bases. CMV inclusions may also be seen in the epithelium of submucosal glands (fig. 3-19) or in the glandular cells of BE. As with herpes infection, the use of specific antibodies or genetic probes for the virus may aid in the diagnosis.

Fungal Esophagitis

Like viral esophagitis, fungal esophagitis tends to affect debilitated individuals, such as the elderly, diabetics, patients with cancer, and those that are immunocompromised. Other predisposing factors include a damaged mucosal barrier secondary to previous esophagitis, indwelling nasogastric tubes, chemotherapy, protracted periods of severe neutropenia, and prolonged use of antibiotics and steroids. Esophageal stasis resulting from dysmotility disorders also predisposes patients to fungal infection. Most commonly, fungal esophagitis results from *Candida* infection, although other organisms such as *Histoplasma, Aspergillus, Cryptococcus, Blastomyces,* and *Mucor* also infect the esophagus. Fungal infections may be superimposed on other types of infections.

Candida. *Clinical Features. Candida* infection is the most common cause of infectious esophagitis (95). *Candida albicans*, a yeast found in the normal human oral flora, is the predominant cause of fungal esophagitis. Other *Candida* species such as *C. tropicalis, C. glabrata, C. parapsilosis,* and *C. krusei* are occasionally pathogenic. Patients with *Candida* esophagitis frequently have no symptoms, especially those who are immunologically competent. Such patients have only scattered adherent esophageal plaques. Patients with more severe immune dysfunction develop painful or difficult swallowing as the initial manifestation of their disease. Other symptoms

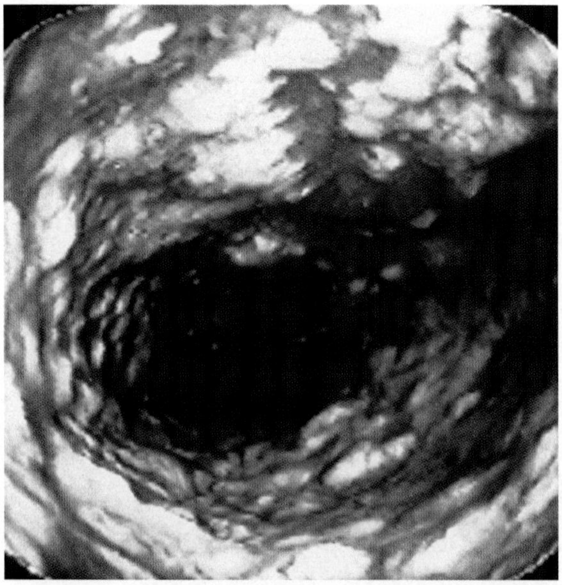

Figure 3-20

ENDOSCOPIC APPEARANCE OF *CANDIDA* ESOPHAGITIS

Numerous whitish plaques are present on the luminal surface of the esophagus.

include chest pain or a globus sensation as food passes through the esophagus.

Gross and Microscopic Findings. The esophagus is the preferential site for *Candida* infection in the gastrointestinal tract. Grossly, the esophagus may show areas of moderate erythema, hyperemia, and friability, or it may become covered by a black membrane. Whitish, raised, longitudinally oriented, discrete or confluent plaques or membranes, measuring less than 1 cm, cover a friable, erythematous, ulcerated mucosa, particularly in the distal esophagus (fig. 3-20). The fungi become densely adherent to the esophageal mucosal surface and are not easily removed. In advanced cases, the esophagus becomes narrowed, with a shaggy or cobblestoned appearance that is easily confused grossly with pseudodiverticulosis, strictures, varices, or carcinoma.

Histologically, the mucosa and lamina propria of the esophagus appear acutely and chronically inflamed; there are also areas of ulceration. The fungal plaque consists of hyphae and budding spores embedded in a fibrinous exudate and necrotic debris (fig. 3-21). Neutrophils and eosinophils lie in the superficial epithelium. When *Candida* becomes pathogenic, it invades the underlying tissues (fig. 3-21). As a result, colonization of the epithelial surface, particularly of devitalized tissue, does not necessarily imply the presence of significant clinical disease.

Aspergillus. *Aspergillus* species are ubiquitous, rapidly growing molds. The most important species involved in human infections are *A. fumigatus* and *A. flavus*. The fungi are characterized by the presence of innumerable, dichotomously branching, 45° septate hyphae with smooth, parallel walls, ranging in size from 2 to 4 µm in diameter (fig. 3-22). Aspergillosis rarely affects the gastrointestinal tract, but when it does, the esophagus is the usual site of involvement. Invasive aspergillosis generally affects severely debilitated individuals.

Histoplasma. *Clinical Features. Histoplasma* is endemic in a broad area centered around the Ohio and Mississippi River valleys in the United States, in the Caribbean, and in Central and South America. Even a brief exposure to this dimorphic fungus may result in infection. The fungi usually gain access to the body through the lungs, with extrapulmonary dissemination occurring particularly frequently in immunosuppressed patients or those with malignancy. The disease may extend to the esophagus from the lungs or from mediastinal lymph nodes that contain large caseating granulomas. Dysphagia results from extrinsic compression of the esophagus by mediastinal lymph nodes or from progressive mediastinal fibrosis. Less common are esophageal bleeding and esophagobronchial fistula formation (94).

Gross and Microscopic Findings. Endoscopic biopsies are unlikely to provide a diagnosis because the esophagus is usually involved from its external aspect inward. As a result, the mucosa is rarely involved by the process. Histologically, the infection results in necrotizing granulomatous inflammation. Organisms are found within the cytoplasm of histiocytes and multinucleated Langerhans type giant cells surrounding foci of caseating necrosis. The organisms appear round to oval, and measure 2 to 4 µm in diameter. Budding forms are commonly seen.

Mucor. *Mucor* mycosis develops in immunosuppressed or malnourished patients. The fungi are ubiquitous in nature and grow as saprophytes

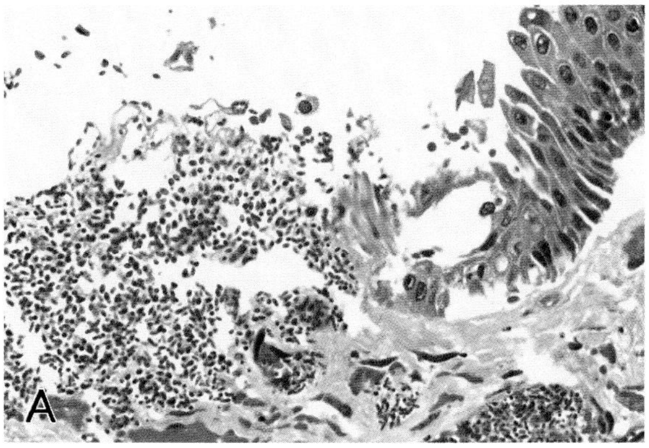

Figure 3-21

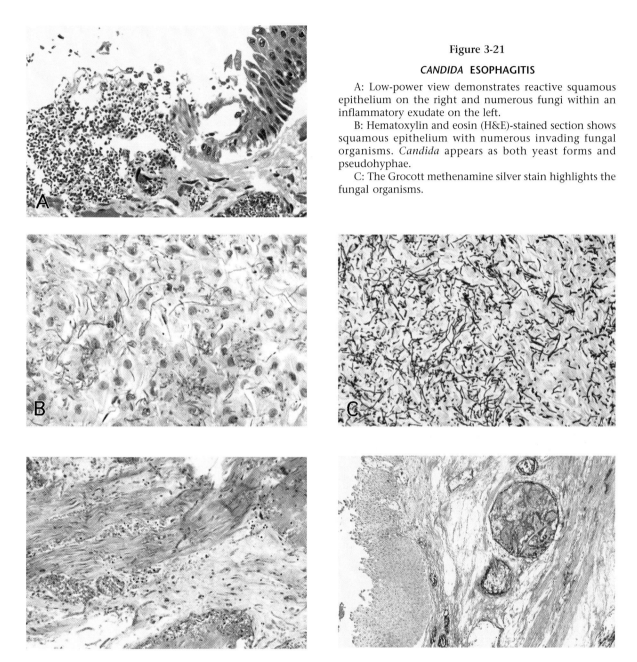

CANDIDA ESOPHAGITIS

A: Low-power view demonstrates reactive squamous epithelium on the right and numerous fungi within an inflammatory exudate on the left.

B: Hematoxylin and eosin (H&E)-stained section shows squamous epithelium with numerous invading fungal organisms. *Candida* appears as both yeast forms and pseudohyphae.

C: The Grocott methenamine silver stain highlights the fungal organisms.

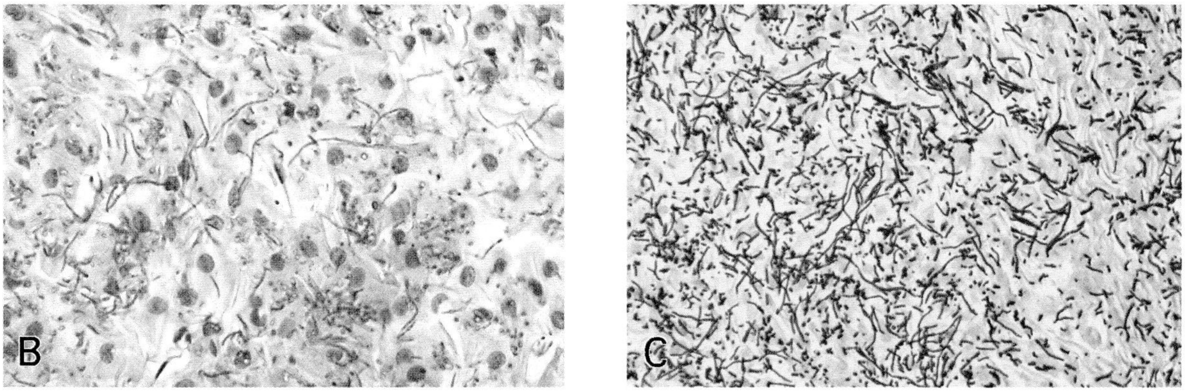

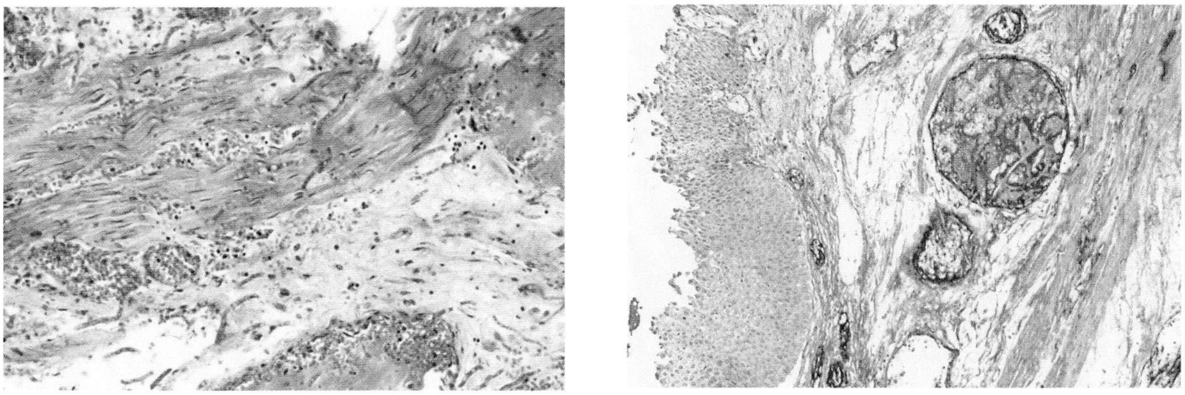

Figure 3-22

ASPERGILLUS ESOPHAGITIS

Left: H&E-stained section shows scattered fungal organisms invading the submucosal tissues of the esophagus. Hyphae are within the smooth muscle of vessel walls.

Right: Factor VIII and periodic acid–Schiff (PAS) dual staining highlights the angioinvasive character of *Aspergillus*.

on fruits and vegetable matter. They have broad, rarely septate, haphazardly branched hyphae that measure 10 to 15 µm in diameter, and characteristically stain deeply with hematoxylin. The fungi have a tendency to penetrate blood vessels thereby causing thrombosis and vascular damage.

Coccidioides. *Coccidioides,* also a dimorphic fungus, can be acquired via the pulmonary tract by travel through an endemic region. Esophageal

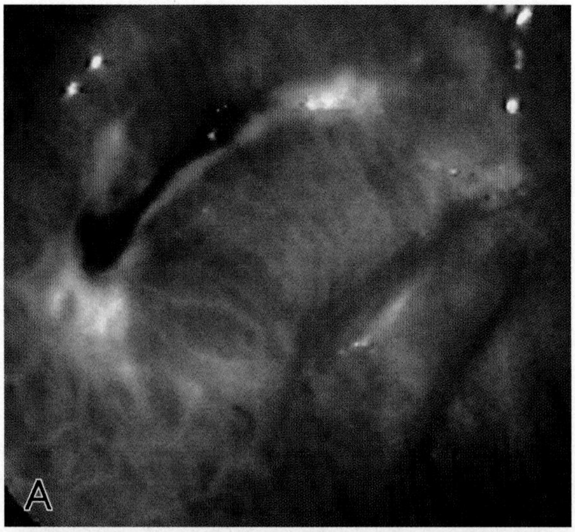

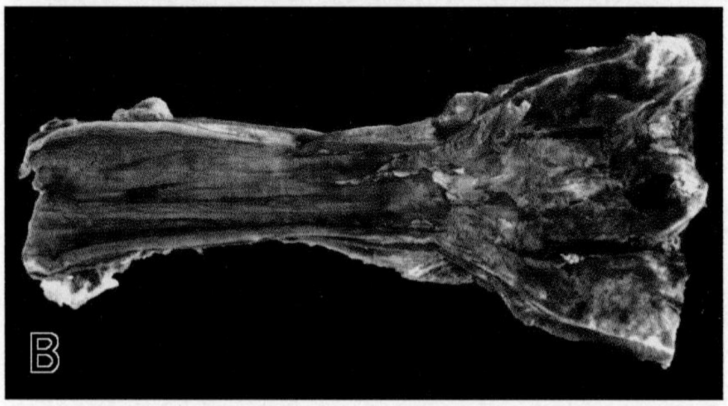

Figure 3-23

CAUSTIC ESOPHAGITIS

A: Endoscopic view shows marked edema and erythema of the mucosa.

B: Another case of corrosive esophagitis. The distal portion of the specimen (right) shows a diffusely erythematous and edematous mucosal surface. Adherent pseudomembranes are seen in some areas. (Courtesy of the Division of Gastrointestinal Pathology, Armed Forces Institute of Pathology, Washington, DC.)

C: There is extensive necrosis of the esophageal lining.

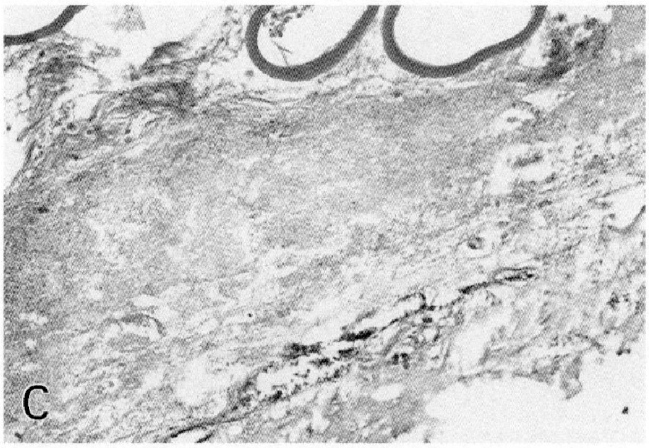

involvement usually represents extension of pulmonary disease. *C. immitis* grows in soil where rainfall is low and summer temperatures are high. In tissue, it is identified by the presence of large globular sporangia measuring 30 to 60 µm or more that contain sporangiospores measuring 1 to 5 µm in diameter. Hyphae can sometimes be seen. The intact sporangia elicit a granulomatous reaction consisting of histiocytes, epithelioid cells, and giant cells of foreign body or Langerhans type.

CORROSIVE ESOPHAGITIS

Definition. Caustic injury results from the ingestion of strong alkaline or acidic agents or very hot liquids.

Clinical Features. The extent of corrosive injury depends on the type of agent ingested, its concentration and quantity, patient physical state, and exposure duration (96,97). Corrosive esophagitis usually follows suicide attempts in adults or accidental ingestion in children. When severe, the injury leads to esophageal hemorrhage, perforation, and death. The acute phase lasts for several days or weeks, with pain as the predominant symptom. Symptoms are unreliable in predicting disease extent or severity.

The most severe injury occurs in areas of luminal narrowing, i.e., those where the aorta or the left main stem bronchus cross the esophagus. Alkalis produce liquefactive necrosis with intense inflammation of the mucosa, submucosa, and muscularis propria. Thrombosis of adjacent vessels leads to ischemic necrosis, followed by bacterial or fungal colonization. Liquid agents tend to produce extensive geographically continuous erosive esophagitis, whereas granular agents produce more localized lesions. Acids produce coagulation necrosis that results in a firm protective eschar.

Microscopic Findings. Histologically, caustic strictures demonstrate dense, uniform, mucosal and submucosal fibrosis throughout the involved esophagus. The overlying surface appears normal, inflamed, ulcerated, hypertrophic, or atrophic, depending on when the tissue is examined relative to the time of the acute event and if recurrent damage has occurred (fig. 3-23). Another change that sometimes follows lye ingestion is the formation of metaplastic epithelium resembling that seen with BE.

RADIATION ESOPHAGITIS

Clinical Features. Patients with *radiation esophagitis* present with dysphagia, odynophagia, or symptoms of dysmotility. Dysphagia during radiation therapy probably results from epithelial damage as well as disordered motility. Whether or not esophagitis develops is related to both the radiation dose and the tissue radiosensitivity. In addition, concomitant administration of chemotherapeutic drugs may produce radiosensitizing effects that increase the degree of esophageal injury. These drugs may also be directly toxic to the mucosa, predisposing it to further damage by radiation. Severe esophagitis, stricture formation, and rare fistulas develop in patients treated with both chemotherapy and radiation therapy.

Gross and Microscopic Findings. Radiation esophagitis may be associated with areas of ulceration, fibrosis, and stricture formation (fig. 3-24) depending on the amount of time that has elapsed following the radiation treatment. Early in the process, the tissues appear edematous, erythematous, and friable, with erosions coalescing to form larger superficial ulcers. Prominent endothelial cells lie in the edematous granulation tissue. Bizarre (radiation) fibroblasts develop and suggest the diagnosis. The regenerating epithelium may show features simulating dysplasia.

Histologic examination in the chronic or late period discloses the presence of acanthosis, parakeratosis, hyalinized blood vessels, submucosal fibrosis, and muscular degeneration (fig. 3-24). These changes result from ischemia due to the underlying vascular lesions. Esophageal strictures and webs develop during the chronic period following large radiation doses.

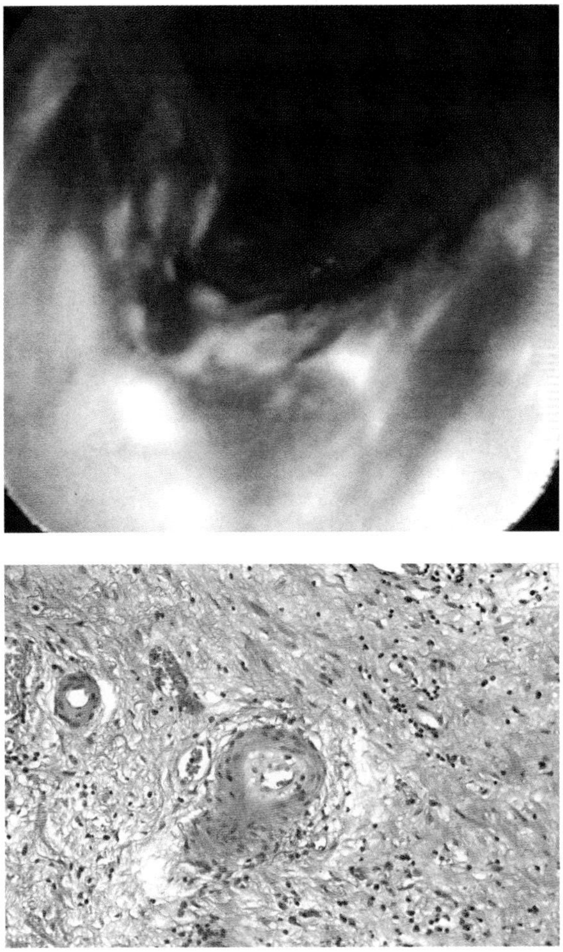

Figure 3-24

RADIATION ESOPHAGITIS

Top: Endoscopic view of an erythematous and eroded epithelium.

Bottom: Microscopically, the submucosa is edematous with scattered enlarged, atypical-appearing stromal cells. A submucosal vessel shows prominent intimal thickening.

DRUG-ASSOCIATED ESOPHAGITIS

No characteristic pathologic findings exist for *drug-induced esophagitis* because different drugs damage the esophagus via different mechanisms. Drugs commonly implicated in drug-induced esophagitis include those listed in Table 3-7. Age, posture, volume of a fluid chaser, and dissolution pH of the medication all influence drug-mediated esophageal injury (98,100). Hiatal hernia, esophageal dysmotility, or stricture predispose to prolonged retention of esophageal medication and enhance the ability of drugs to damage the mucosa.

Some injuries result from physical entrapment of undigested medicines, especially those that contain a hydrophilic swelling agent or fiber that ensures rapid disintegration when the pills contact water (101). These medicines act

Table 3-7

DRUGS ASSOCIATED WITH ESOPHAGITIS

Acetaminophen	Ibuprofen
Antimitotic agents	Indomethacin
Acetylsalicylic acid	Minocycline
Ascorbic acid	Naproxen
Barbiturates	Pantogar
Carbachol	Phenylbutazone
Chemotherapeutic agents	Phenobarbital
Chloral hydrate	Phenoxymethyl penicillin
Clindamycin	Potassium chloride
Clinitest tablets	Prednisone
Cromolyn sodium	Quinidine
Digoxin, digitoxin	Tetracycline
Doxycycline	Theophylline
d-Penicillamine	Tinidazole
Emepronium bromide	Tolectin
Erythromycin	Zidovudine
Ferrous salts	

as foreign bodies impacting in the esophageal lumen, especially if they are taken with a minimum of liquid. As the medication dissolves, localized esophageal damage, ranging from inflammation to severe hemorrhage and even perforation, develops (100).

Other mechanisms of drug-induced esophagitis are allergic in nature, and these may be suspected based on the history or the presence of eosinophilia in the absence of reflux esophagitis. Still other drugs, such as chemotherapeutic agents, directly damage replicating cells. Basal cell hyperplasia, mild atypia, and numerous mitoses, some of which may appear atypical, characterize recovery from chemotherapeutic injury. Antibiotics account for at least half of the reported cases of drug-associated esophagitis, with the tetracyclines, especially doxycycline, being the usual offenders (100).

The most dangerous drug-related esophagitis results from potassium chloride ingestion. Several patients have died of esophagitis directly related to its ingestion. Histologically, there is subepithelial edema, thickening of the stratum corneum, and the presence of balloon cells (99). The presence of balloon cells serves as an early esophageal mucosal marker of chemical injury but is not specific for it.

Table 3-8

CAUSES OF ESOPHAGEAL PERFORATION

Penetrating wounds
Iatrogenic trauma
Iatrogenic intraoperative injury
Iatrogenic endoscopic perforation
Swallowed foreign body
Blast injury
Postemetic (Mallory-Weiss syndrome)
Blunt trauma (such as auto accidents)
Esophageal ulcers regardless of cause
Esophageal diverticula
Esophageal cancer
Ingestion of corrosives
Severe inflammation
Sclerotherapy or other recent esophageal procedure

MUCOSAL LACERATIONS, ULCERATIONS, AND PERFORATIONS

Acquired perforations, whether transmural or intramural, usually result from instrumentation, foreign body impaction, and trauma (Table 3-8).

Mallory-Weiss Syndrome

Definition. The term *Mallory-Weiss syndrome* refers to painless gastrointestinal bleeding that results from esophageal or gastroesophageal mucosal laceration following an episode of vomiting.

Clinical Features. The sequence of events suggests that the increased pressure created by vomiting plays an important etiologic role. Most patients are males with a history of alcohol and/or salicylate abuse or associated hiatal hernia.

Gross and Microscopic Findings. The lacerations lie along the long axis of the distal esophagus, crossing the esophageal-gastric junction or lying in the gastric fundus. The lacerations vary in depth, measuring on average 1.5 cm, often only affecting the mucosa. They are acute in nature, without scarring, unless previous lacerations have occurred.

Boerhaave's Syndrome

Definition. *Boerhaave's syndrome* is spontaneous, full-thickness esophageal rupture.

Clinical Features. The sudden development of a pressure gradient between the internal portion of the viscus and its external supporting tissues is the common pathogenetic denominator in cases of gastrointestinal rupture (102). The antecedent background varies: the viscus may become overdistended by food, drink, gas, or any combination thereof. Forced vomiting is often sufficient to increase the intraluminal pressure. Hiatal hernia, peptic esophagitis, and atrophic gastritis are predisposing factors. In Boerhaave's syndrome the pain is constant. Hematemesis occurs at times, and the clinical features and radiologic findings often point to an intrathoracic catastrophe. Immediate surgical repair must occur if the patient is to survive.

Gross and Microscopic Findings. Characteristically, the laceration is linear, longitudinal, and lies in a left lateral posterior location, 1 to 3 cm above the gastroesophageal junction. This is the weakest part of the esophagus. The tears measure 1 to 20 cm in length, with an average length of 2 cm; the mucosal part of the tear is usually longer than the muscular part.

MELANOSIS

Demography. Melanocytes lie in the epithelial-stromal junction in 4 to 8 percent of normal esophageal specimens examined at autopsy (103), 21 percent of consecutive upper endoscopy specimens, and 29.9 percent of surgical specimens of esophageal melanoma (103,104). There is a higher prevalence of melanocytes in the normal esophageal mucosa in Japanese than in Western populations. They are more common in patients with cancer.

Etiology. The etiology is unknown. Mechanisms postulated to explain an increase in epidermal melanocytes include: 1) proliferation of preexisting melanocytes; 2) activation of resting melanocytes following activation of melanogenesis; 3) migration of dermal melanocytes; and 4) differentiation of peripheral neural cells (103).

Gross Findings. Melanosis appears as single or multiple, discrete, 1- to 3-mm, circular or oval, brown or brownish black mucosal patches. The pigmented areas also appear as linear streaks. These pigmented lesions may lie adjacent to carcinomas. Although pigmentation can affect the middle, upper, and lower esophagus, the distal esophagus is the most common site of involvement.

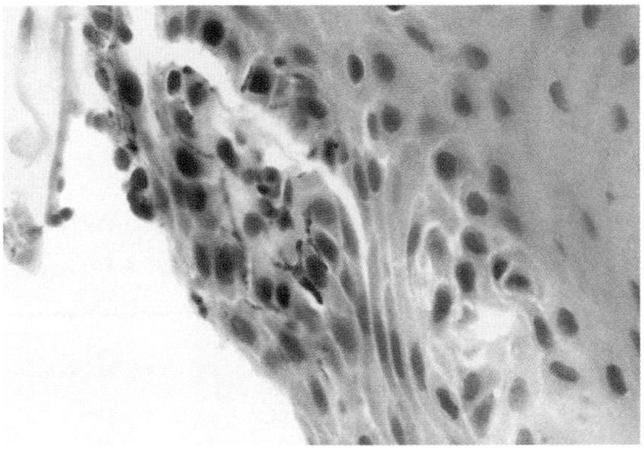

Figure 3-25

ESOPHAGEAL MELANOSIS

Melanin pigment is in the dendritic cells within the basal portion of the squamous epithelium.

Microscopic Findings. Histologically, melanosis consists of increased numbers of melanocytes in the basal part of the mucosa, increased numbers of melanosomes in the melanocytes, and melanosomal transfer to keratinocytes, stromal macrophages, and fibroblasts (fig. 3-25). The pigment is identified with melanin stains.

NEVUS

White sponge nevus, a rare benign disorder of the mucosal membranes with a familial distribution, recently has been reported in the esophagus (105,107). The pattern of inheritance seems to be that of an autosomal dominant disorder.

Most lesions exist at birth or have their onset in infancy, childhood, or adolescence. The condition is usually seen in Caucasians. It is characterized by the presence of a thickened, deeply folded mucosa with a creamy white appearance. The lesions are small and wart-like, or large, moist, and white. Such areas are easily mistaken for *Candida* infections. They increase in size and number after puberty and then stabilize.

Histologically, the lesions are characterized by irregular acanthosis with spongy hydropic squamous cells in all levels except for the uninvolved basal layer, which forms an intact lower rete border. Mitoses may be seen but there is no nuclear atypia (105). The finding of parakeratotic plugs appears to be pathognomonic. Because of surface fragmentation, the superficial squamous cells may appear shaggy. Inflammation is absent.

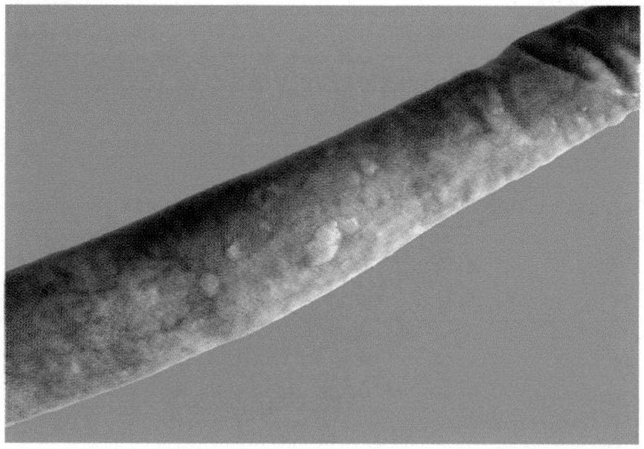
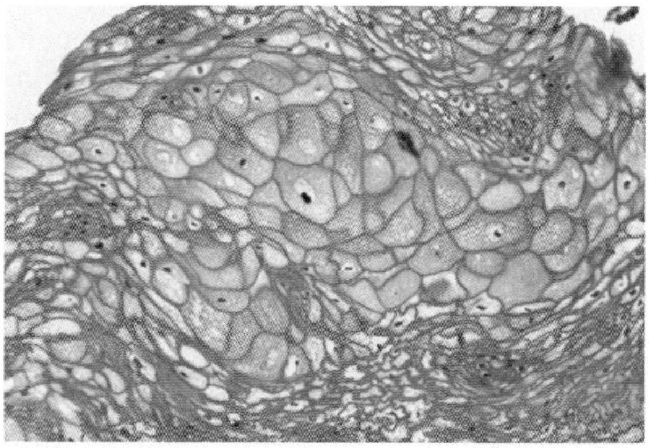

Figure 3-26

GLYCOGEN ACANTHOSIS

Left: An esophagus from a patient with Cowden syndrome. Scattered whitish mucosal plaques representing glycogen acanthosis are in the mid-esophagus.

Right: Microscopically, the squamous cells are enlarged with pale pink cytoplasm.

Blue nevus has also been reported in the esophagus (106).

GLYCOGEN ACANTHOSIS

Demography. *Glycogen acanthosis* is a relatively common condition of unknown etiology that is felt by some to represent a normal variant of esophageal histology. The presence of diffuse esophageal glycogen acanthosis is an endoscopic marker of Cowden's disease (110,111).

Gross Findings. The lesion is most easily recognized grossly. Glycogen acanthosis appears as discrete, raised, white, plaque-like esophageal lesions usually measuring less than 1 cm in diameter (fig. 3-26). When extensive, they coalesce into larger plaques, but they rarely measure more than 3 cm in diameter. A nodular appearance of the esophageal mucosa with double-contrast esophagograms is observed in 25.0 to 28.3 percent of such studies (109). Glycogen acanthosis affects any part of the esophagus but primarily the distal third (108). Clinically, glycogen acanthosis may resemble and be confused endoscopically with fungal infections or leukoplakia.

Microscopic Findings. Histologically, the plaques consist of large clusters of enlarged squamous cells of the prickle cell layer (fig. 3-26). These contain abundant glycogen. Due to the extraction of the glycogen during processing, the cells appear clear. There is no inflammation and no basal cell hyperplasia. The lesion can be accentuated by the use of the PAS stain.

Differential Diagnosis. Histologically, the lesion may resemble the ballooning degeneration seen in reflux esophagitis. PAS stains can distinguish the two lesions, since glycogen acanthosis contains abundant glycogen whereas ballooning degeneration does not.

SYSTEMIC DISORDERS

Amyloidosis

Amyloid forms deposits in the gastrointestinal tract in all forms of generalized amyloidosis. The esophagus is involved in 35 to 100 percent of cases (114,118). Because amyloid deposits randomly in esophageal tissues, the disease presents in unpredictable ways, sometimes primarily resembling a muscular disorder and sometimes resembling a primary neural disturbance (114,118). Patients with esophageal involvement present with motility disorders, dysphagia, and gastroesophageal reflux disease (112,113,115, 116,119). Abnormalities occur in the LES, in the body of the esophagus, or both. Amyloid is deposited in skeletal or smooth muscle, vagus nerve, myenteric plexus, or vasa vasora (fig. 3-27). Patients with esophageal amyloidosis may present with vascular complications. Perforation and hematemesis also occur (117).

Diabetes

Esophageal motility abnormalities commonly affect patients with diabetes mellitus

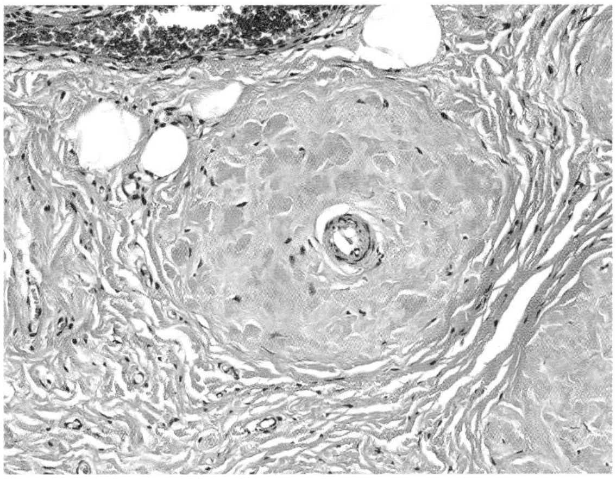

Figure 3-27

AMYLOIDOSIS

A submucosal vessel shows a thick cuff of surrounding eosinophilic, hyaline-appearing amyloid protein.

(120,121). More than half of diabetics with peripheral or autonomic neuropathy have esophageal dysmotility resulting from neuropathic involvement of the vagus nerve. The neuropathy results in a secondary myopathy, eventually leading to atony.

Cystic Fibrosis

Recent attention has focused on the high frequency of gastroesophageal reflux in patients with cystic fibrosis because it increases the risk of lung complications in these patients (122). Gastroesophageal reflux begins during childhood and becomes increasingly more troublesome as the patient ages (123–125). Numerous factors, including chronic persistent cough resulting in an increased pressure gradient between the peritoneal cavity and the thorax and a delay in gastric emptying, play etiologic roles in the reflux.

Autoimmune Diseases

Collagen vascular and rheumatoid diseases affect the esophagus through chronic inflammation, vasculitis, and variable degrees of vascular obliteration. Scleroderma presents with dysphagia and is discussed in detail in chapter 17. Patients with rheumatoid arthritis present with esophageal dysmotility and lowered LES pressure, which results in reflux esophagitis. Rarely, patients with severe rheumatoid arthritis have rheumatoid nodules within the esophageal wall. Patients may also have an associated drug-induced esophagitis from treatment with nonsteroidal antiinflammatory drugs (NSAIDs). Rheumatoid vasculitis may also result in gastrointestinal manifestations. The vasculitis typically occurs in the setting of severe arthritis, rheumatoid nodules, and high titers of rheumatoid factor. Patients with Sjögren's syndrome display esophageal connective tissue abnormalities (127,129,131): 10 percent of patients have upper esophageal webs, 25 percent have hiatal hernias, and 36 percent display motility abnormalities (126,128–131).

Inflammatory Bowel Disease

Crohn's disease may affect the esophagus and when it does, it may be difficult to distinguish from other forms of granulomatous esophagitis. In bona fide cases of Crohn's disease, there may be areas of acute and chronic inflammation, ulcers, sinus tracts, and possibly granulomas in the esophagus. The granulomas are compact and sarcoid-like, without necrosis. They may be infiltrated by inflammatory cells. Muscular hypertrophy and neural hyperplasia are often present. In other cases, only granulomas are seen. Many patients only show a focal nonspecific inflammation deep in the esophageal wall, and it may be impossible to make a definitive diagnosis.

Patients with ulcerative colitis may have coexisting esophagitis and ulcers, but this more than likely reflects coexisting reflux esophagitis.

DERMATOLOGIC CONDITIONS INVOLVING THE ESOPHAGUS

A number of primary dermatologic disorders affect the esophagus (Table 3-9). The esophageal changes resemble those seen in the skin, a reflection of the fact that both sites are lined by squamous epithelium. In some patients, esophageal disease develops in the absence of dermatologic evidence of the disease.

Pemphigus

Pemphigus vulgaris usually affects patients between the ages of 40 and 60 and is characterized by the development of flaccid dermal and mucosal bullae. Involved mucosal surfaces include the oral cavity, pharynx, larynx, conjunctiva, esophagus, nasal mucosa, cervix, and anal canal. Pemphigus may also be induced by drugs, including D-penicillamine and angiotensin-converting enzyme inhibitors (135). If untreated, pemphigus vulgaris may be fatal. Esophageal bleeding, webs, strictures, and formation of epithelial casts may develop.

Histologic examination of esophageal lesions shows the presence of a blister or erosion. The squamous epithelial cells separate from one another in a process known as acantholysis. As a result, the cells lose their cohesive properties and a suprabasal cleft forms. The disorder may also present as eosinophilic spongiosis.

Benign Mucous Membrane Pemphigoid

Bullous pemphigoid affects the esophagus in the form of *benign mucous membrane pemphigoid.* This chronic disease of the elderly is characterized by the presence of tense pruritic skin bullae. Oral bullae develop in 20 percent of cases. Esophageal bullae occur rarely, but cause epithelial sloughing.

Esophageal lesions appear suddenly and may persist for several days. They reappear at the same site, often following mild trauma such as that induced by ingestion of hot foods or food passing over the mucosa. Patients may present with bullae and webs, or later with strictures (131,133). Histologic examination shows the presence of subepithelial bullae.

Erythema Multiforme

Erythema multiforme represents an acute self-limited eruption involving the skin and mucous membranes. Mucosal involvement is referred to as the *Stevens-Johnson syndrome*. Esophageal disease ranges from mild to severe, with the severity of esophageal lesions corresponding to the severity of the dermal disease. Endoscopically, the lesions resemble peptic esophagitis. Keratinocytes become necrotic, containing homogeneous pink cytoplasm and pyknotic nuclei. Biopsies reveal areas of ulceration or inflamed granulation tissue.

Epidermolysis Bullosa Acquisita

Epidermolysis bullosa acquisita, an acquired mechanobullous disease, is characterized by the presence of autoantibodies to type VII collagen. These antibodies localize to the anchoring filaments at the dermal-epidermal junction. The disease primarily affects the skin, but esophageal involvement can occur. Patients with severe disease present with dysphagia resulting from web-like stenosis of the upper esophagus.

Table 3-9

DERMATOLOGIC DISEASES INVOLVING THE ESOPHAGUS

Acanthosis nigricans
Behcet's syndrome
Benign mucous membrane pemphigoid
Darier's disease
Dermatitis herpetiformis
Epidermolysis bullosa
Erythema multiforme
Lichen planus
Pemphigus
Scleroderma
Toxic epidermal necrolysis
Tylosis palmaris et plantaris

Epidermolysis Bullosa Dystrophia

Epidermolysis bullosa dystrophia includes a group of hereditary mechanobullous disorders that affect both the skin and gastrointestinal mucosa. Esophageal problems develop insidiously, often in patients with previous skin lesions. Bullae form in the esophagus, followed by ulceration and edema. This eventually predisposes to severe stricture or web formation (134).

Lichen Planus

Lichen planus is a common disease of unknown etiology that often affects the oral cavity. Esophageal disease is rare and results in esophageal papules and benign strictures. The papules are visible in the lower third of the esophagus in most cases, although occasionally the entire esophagus is involved. Histologically, there are submucosal band-like lymphocytic infiltrates.

Acanthosis Nigricans

Acanthosis nigricans is a distinctive dermatosis characterized by hyperpigmented, velvety plaques with a predilection for the neck and flexural areas. The disease may involve the entire skin, including the palms, soles, and mucous membranes (136). Histologically, the squamous epithelium displays hyperkeratosis, papillomatosis, and slight and irregular acanthosis in the valleys between the papillae. There is usually no associated hyperpigmentation. Acanthosis nigricans serves as a marker of internal disease, and may be associated with malignancy.

Graft Versus Host Disease

Graft versus host disease (GVHD) usually affects the upper third of the esophagus. The lesions are focal or diffuse and characteristically consist of desquamative or bullous esophagitis with web formation (137,138). The diagnosis of GVHD is based on the history and presence of single cell necrosis (apoptosis) as well as the failure to identify specific infectious agents. Often, only nonspecific inflammation is evident. Infections often coexist with GVHD.

INFLAMMATORY FIBROID POLYPS

Inflammatory fibroid polyps (IFPs) commonly arise in the submucosa of the stomach and small intestines, but they also develop in the esophagus. These solitary lesions are raised and sometimes ulcerated, often with a prominent submucosal component. They are often detected endoscopically or radiographically, and since they appear as polypoid lesions, clinically must be differentiated from sarcomatoid carcinoma.

Microscopically, inflammatory fibroid polyps appear variably cellular and edematous. They are often highly vascular, containing fibrous tissue, proliferating blood vessels, inflammatory cells, fibroblasts, myofibroblasts, and histiocytes.

FIBROMUSCULAR HAMARTOMA

Fibromuscular hamartoma presents in infancy with dysphagia due to compression of the cervical esophagus. The lesion consists of atrophic-appearing skeletal muscle fibers, fibrous connective tissue, and hyaline cartilage. The lesion may appear to have infiltrative margins.

REFERENCES

Reflux Esophagitis

1. Brown LF, Goldman H, Antonioli DA. Intraepithelial eosinophils in endoscopic biopsies of adults with reflux esophagitis. Am J Surg Pathol 1984;8:899–905.
2. Collins BJ, Elliott H, Sloan JM, McFarland RJ, Love AH. Oesophageal histology in reflux oesophagitis. J Clin Pathol 1985;38:1265–72.
3. Davidson GP, Omari TI. Reflux in children. Bailliere's Clin Gastroenterol 2000;14:839–55.
4. Dent J, Fendrick AM, Fennerty MB, et al. An evidence-based appraisal of reflux disease—the General Workshop Report. Gut 1999;44(suppl 2):S1–16.
5. Dodds WJ, Dent J, Hogan WJ, et al. Mechanisms of gastroesophageal reflux in patients with reflux esophagitis. N Engl J Med 1982;307:1547–52.
6. El-Omar EM, Oien K, El-Nujumi A, et al. *Helicobacter pylori* infection and chronic gastric hyposecretion. Gastroenterology 1997;113:15–24.
7. El-Serag HB, Sonnenberg A. Opposing time trends of peptic ulcer and reflux disease. Gut 1998;43:327–33.
8. El-Serag HB, Sonnenberg A, Jamal MM, Inadomi JM, Crooks LA, Feddersen RM. Corpus gastritis is protective against reflux oesophagitis. Gut 1999;42:181–5.
9. Fass R. Epidemiology and pathophysiology of symptomatic gastroesophageal reflux disease. Am J Gastroenterol 2003;98(suppl):S2–7.
10. Faubion WA Jr, Zein NN. Gastroesophageal reflux in infants and children. Mayo Clin Proc 1998:73;166–73.
11. Fiorucci S, Santucci L, Chiucchiu S, Morelli A. Gastric acidity and gastroesophageal reflux patterns in patients with esophagitis. Gastroenterology 1992;103:855–61.
12. Fonkalsrud EW, Ament ME. Gastroesophageal reflux in childhood. Curr Probl Surg 1996:33;1–70.
13. Geboes K, Desmet V, Vantrappen G, Mebis J. Vascular changes in the esophageal mucosa: an early histologic sign of esophagitis. Gastrointest Endosc 1980;80:29–32.

14. Goldblum JR, Vicari JJ, Falk GW, et al. Inflammation and intestinal metaplasia of the gastric cardia: the role of gastroesophageal reflux and *H. pylori* infection. Gastroenterology 1998;114:633–9.
15. Graham DY. The changing epidemiology of GERD: geography and *Helicobacter pylori*. Am J Gastroenterol 2003;98:1462–70.
16. Graham DY, Yamaoka Y. *H. pylori* and cagA: relationships with gastric cancer, duodenal ulcer, and reflux esophagitis and its complications. Helicobacter 1998;3:145–51.
17. Jacob P, Kahrilas PJ, Vanagunas A. Peristaltic dysfunction associated with nonobstructive dysphagia in reflux disease. Dig Dis Sci 1990;35: 939–42.
18. Johnston MH, Hammond AS, Laskin W, Jones DM. The prevalence and clinical characteristics of short segments of specialized intestinal metaplasia in the distal esophagus on routine endoscopy. Am J Gastroenterol 1996;91:1507–11.
19. Lee RG. Marked eosinophilia in esophageal mucosal biopsies. Am J Surg Pathol 1985;9:475–9.
20. Lidums I, Holloway R. Motility abnormalities in the columnar-lined esophagus. Gastroenterol Clin North Am 1997:26;519–31.
21. Locke GR 3rd, Talley NJ, Fett SL, Zinsmeister AR, Melton LJ 3rd. Prevalence and clinical spectrum of gastroesophageal reflux: a population based study in Olmsted County, Minnesota. Gastroenterology 1997;112:1448–56.
22. Mangano MM, Antonioli DA, Schnitt SJ, Wang HH. Nature and significance of cells with irregular nuclear contours in esophageal mucosal biopsies. Mod Pathol 1992;5:191–6.
23. Mattox HE 3rd, Richter JE. Prolonged ambulatory esophageal pH monitoring in the evaluation of gastroesophageal reflux disease. Am J Med 1990;89:345–56.
24. McDougall NI, Johnston BT, Collins JS, McFarland RJ, Love AH. Disease progression in gastro-oesophageal reflux disease as determined by repeat oesophageal pH monitoring and endoscopy 3 to 4.5 years after diagnosis. Eur J Gastroenterol Hepatol 1997;9:1161–7.
25. Murray L, Johnston B, Lane A, et al. Relationship between body mass and gastro-oesophageal reflux symptoms: the Bristol *Helicobacter* Project. Int J Epidemiol 2003;32:645–50.
26. Okamoto K, Iwakiri R, Mori M, et al. Clinical symptoms in endoscopic reflux esophagitis: evaluation in 8031 adult subjects. Dig Dis Sci 2003;48:2237–41.
27. Riddell RH. The biopsy diagnosis of gastroesophageal reflux disease, "carditis" and Barrett's esophagus, and sequelae of therapy. Am J Surg Pathol 1996;20:S31–51.
28. Sheahan DG, West AB. Focal lymphoid hyperplasia (pseudolymphoma) of the esophagus. Am J Surg Pathol 1985;9:141–7.
29. Shi G, Bruley des Varannes S, Scarpignato C, Le Rhun M, Galmiche JP. Reflux related symptoms in patients with normal oesophageal exposure to acid. Gut 1995;37:686–95.
30. Singh SP, Odze RD. Multinucleated epithelial giant cell changes in esophagitis: a clinicopathologic study of 14 cases. Am J Surg Pathol 1998;:22:93–9.
31. Smout AJ. Endoscopy-negative acid reflux disease. Aliment Pharmacol Ther 1997;11(suppl):81–5.
32. Sonnenberg A, El-Serag HB. Clinical epidemiology and natural history of gastroesophageal reflux disease. Yale J Biol Med 1999;72:81–92.
33. Sontag SJ. Gastroesophageal reflux and asthma. Am J Med 1997;103:84S–90S.
34. Sung JJ. Westernisation of gastrointestinal diseases in Asia. Gut 2004;53:152.
35. Tougas G, Chen Y, Hwang P, Liu MM, Eggleston A. Prevalence and impact of upper gastrointestinal symptoms in the Canadian population: findings from the DIGEST Study. Am J Gastroenterol 1999;94:2845–54.
36. Vaezi MF, Richer JE. Role of acid and duodenogastroesophageal reflux in gastroesophageal reflux disease. Gastroenterology 1996;111: 1192–9.
37. Vandenplas Y, Belli D, Benhamou PH, et al. Current concepts and issues in the management of regurgitation in infants: a reappraisal: management guidelines from a working party. Acta Paediatr 1996;85:531–4.
38. van Herwaarden MA, Samsom M, Smout AJ. Excess gastroesophageal reflux in patients with hiatus hernia is caused by mechanisms other than transient LES relaxations. Gastroenterology 2000;119:1439–46.
39. Vantrappen G, Janssens J. Gastro-oesophageal reflux disease, an important cause of angina-like chest pain. Scand J Gastroenterol 1989;24: 73–9.
40. Venables TL, Newland RD, Patel AC, Hole J, Wilcock C, Turbitt ML. Omeprazole 10 milligrams once daily, omeprazole 20 milligrams once daily, or ranitidine 150 milligrams twice daily, evaluated as initial therapy for relief of symptoms of gastro-oesophageal reflux disease in general practice. Scand J Gastroenterol 1997; 32:965–73.
41. Voutilainen M, Sipponen P, Mecklin JP, Juhola M, Farkkila M. Gastroesophageal reflux disease: prevalence, clinical, endoscopic and histopathological findings in 1,128 consecutive patients referred for endoscopy due to dyspeptic and reflux symptoms. Digestion 2000;61:6–13.

42. Wang HH, Mangano MM, Antonioli DA. Evaluation of T-lymphocytes in esophageal mucosal biopsies. Mod Pathol 1994;7:55–8.
43. Winter HS, Madara JL, Stafford RJ, Grand RJ, Quinlan JE, Goldman H. Intraepithelial eosinophils: a new diagnostic criterion for reflux esophagitis. Gastroenterology 1982;83:818–23.

Barrett Esophagus

44. Biddlestone LR, Barham CP, Wilkinson SP, Barr H, Shepherd NA. The histopathology of treated Barrett's esophagus. Squamous reepithelialization after acid suppression and laser and photodynamic therapy. Am J Surg Pathol 1998;22:239–45.
45. Blot WJ, Devesa SS, Fraumeni JF Jr. Continuing climb in rates of esophageal adenocarcinoma: an update. JAMA 1993;270:1320.
46. Blot WJ, Devesa SS, Kneller RW, Fraumeni JF Jr. Rising incidence of adenocarcinoma of the esophagus and gastric cardia. JAMA 1991:265; 1287–9.
47. Brand DL, Ylvisaker JT, Gelfand M, Pope CE 2nd. Regression of columnar esophageal (Barrett's) epithelium after anti-reflux surgery. N Eng J Med 1980;302:844–8.
48. Cameron AJ, Lagergren J, Henriksson C, Nyren O, Locke GR 3rd, Pedersen NL. Gastroesophageal reflux disease in monozygotic and dizygotic twins. Gastroenterology 2002;122:55–9.
49. Cameron AJ, Lomboy CT. Barrett's esophagus. Age, prevalence and extent of columnar epithelium. Gastroenterology 1992;103:1241–5.
50. Cameron AJ, Ott BJ, Payne WS. The incidence of adenocarcinoma in columnar-lined (Barrett's) esophagus. N Engl J Med 1985;313:857–9.
51. Clark GW, Smyrk TC, Burdiles P, et al. Is Barrett's metaplasia the source of adenocarcinomas of the cardia? 1994;129:609–14.
52. Crabb DW, Berk MA, Hall TR, Conneally PM, Biegel AA, Lehman GA. Familial gastroesophageal reflux and development of Barrett's esophagus. Ann Int Med 1985;103:52–4.
53. Dahms BB, Rothstein FC. Barrett's esophagus in children: a consequence of chronic gastroesophageal reflux. Gastroenterology 1984;86:318–23.
54. Deviere J, Buset M, Dumonceau JM, Rickaert F, Cremer M. Regression of Barrett's esophagus with omeprazole. N Engl J Med 1989;320:1497–8.
55. Dietz J, Meurer L, Maffazzoni R, Furtado AD, Prolla JC. Intestinal metaplasia in the distal esophagus and correlation with symptoms of gastroesophageal reflux disease. Dis Esophagus 2003;16:29–32.
56. Falk JW. Barrett's esophagus. Gastroenterology 2002;122:1569–91.
57. Hassall E. Columnar-lined esophagus in children. Gastroenterol Clin N Am 1997;26:533–48.
58. Jass JR. Mucin histochemistry of the columnar epithelium of the oesophagus: a retrospective study. J Clin Pathol 1981;34:866–70.
59. Jochem VJ, Fuerst PA, Fromkes JJ. Familial Barrett's esophagus associated with adenocarcinoma. Gastroenterology 1992;102:1400–2.
60. Lapertosa G, Baracchini P, Fulcheri E. Mucin histochemical analysis in the interpretation of Barrett's esophagus—results of a multicenter study. Am J Clin Pathol 1992;98:61–6.
61. Lee JI, Park H, Jung HY, Rhee PL, Song CW, Choi MG. Prevalence of Barrett's esophagus in an urban Korean population: a multicenter study. J Gastroenterol 2003;38:23–7.
62. McClave SA, Boyce HW, Gottfried MR. Early diagnosis of columnar-lined esophagus: a new endoscopic diagnostic criterion. Gastrointest Endosc 1987:33;413–6.
63. Nishimaki T, Holscher AH, Schuler M, Bollschweiler E, Becker K, Siewert JR. Histopathologic characteristics of early adenocarcinoma in Barrett's esophagus. Cancer 1991;68:1731–6.
64. Ormsby AH, Goldblum JR, Rice TW, et al. Cytokeratin subsets can reliably distinguish Barrett's esophagus from intestinal metaplasia of the stomach. Hum Pathol 1999;30:288–94.
65. Ormsby AH, Vaezi MF, Richter JE, et al. Cytokeratin immunoreactivity patterns in the diagnosis of short-segment Barrett's esophagus. Gastroenterology 2000;119:683–90.
66. Philips RW, Wong RK. Barrett's esophagus: natural history, incidence, etiology and complications. Gastrointest Clin N Am 1991;20:791–6.
67. Rex DK, Cummings OW, Shaw M, et al. Screening for Barrett's esophagus in colonoscopy patients with and without heartburn. Gastroenterology 2003;125:1670–7.
68. Sampliner RE. Practice guidelines on the diagnosis, surveillance, and therapy of Barrett's esophagus. The Practice Parameters Committee of the American College of Gastroenterology. Am J Gastroenterol 1998;93:1028–32.
69. Spechler SJ. The columnar-lined esophagus. History, terminology, and clinical issues. Gastroenterol Clin North Am 1997;26:455–6.
70. Spechler SJ, Goyal RK. Barrett's esophagus. N Engl J Med 1986;315:362–71.
71. Spechler SJ, Schimmel EM, Dalton JW, Doos W, Trier JS. Barrett's epithelium complicating lye ingestion with sparing of the distal esophagus. Gastroenterology 1981;81:580–3.
72. Talley NJ, Cameron AJ, Shorter RG, Zinsmeister AR, Phillips SF. *Campylobacter pylori* and Barrett's esophagus. Mayo Clin Proc 1988;63:1176–80.

73. Tytgat GN. Endoscopic diagnosis of columnar-lined esophagus. Motility 1989;7:14–5.
74. Tytgat GN. What are the endoscopic criteria for diagnosing columnar metaplasia? In: Guili R, Tygat GN, DeMeester TR, Galmiche JP, eds. The esophageal mucosa. Amsterdam: Elsevier; 1994: 795–8.
75. Watson DI, Jamieson GG. Antireflux surgery in the laparoscopic era. Brit J Surg 1998;85:1173–84.
76. Wesdorp IC, Bartelsman J, Schipper ME, Tytgat GN. Effect of long-term treatment with cimetidine and antacids in Barrett's oesophagus. Gut 1981;22:724–7.
77. Winters C Jr, Spurling TJ, Chobanian SJ. Barrett's esophagus. A prevalent occult complication of gastroesophageal reflux disease. Gastroenterology 1987;92:118–24.
78. Womack C, Harvey L. Columnar epithelial lined oesophagus (CELO) or Barrett's oesophagus: mucin histochemistry, dysplasia and invasive adenocarcinoma. J Clin Pathol 1985;38:477–8.

Eosinophilic Esophagitis

79. Faubion WA Jr., Perraulat J, Burgart LJ, Zein NN, Clawson M, Freese DK. Treatment of eosinophilic esophagitis with inhaled corticosteroids. J Pediatr Gastroenterol Nutr 1998;27:90–3.
80. Fox VL, Nurko S, Furuta GT. Eosinophilic esophagitis: it's not just kid's stuff. Gastrointest Endosc 2002;56:260–70.
81. Kelly KJ, Lazenby AJ, Rowe PC, Yardley JH, Perman JA, Sampson HA. Eosinophilic esophagitis attributed to gastroesophageal reflux: improvement with an amino acid-based formula. Gastroenterology 1995;109:1503–12.
82. Liacouras CA, Wenner WJ, Brown K, Ruchelli E. Primary eosinophilic esophagitis in children: successful treatment with oral corticosteroids. J Pediatr Gastroenterol Nutr 1998;26:380–5.
83. Orenstein SR, Shalaby TM, Di Lorenzo C, et al. The spectrum of pediatric eosinophilic esophagitis beyond infancy: a clinical series of 30 children. Am J Gastroenterol 2000;95:1422–30.
85. Rothenberg ME. Eosinophilic gastrointestinal disorders (EGID). J Allergy Clin Immunol 2004;113:11–28.
84. Rothenberg ME, Mishra A, Collins MH, Putnam PE. Pathogenesis and clinical features of eosinophilic esophagitis. J Allergy Clin Immunol 2001;108:891–4.
86. Ruchelli E, Wenner W, Voytek T, Brown K, Liacouras C. Severity of esophageal eosinophilia predicts response to conventional gastroesophageal reflux therapy. Pediatr Dev Pathol 1999;2:15–8.
87. Walsh SV, Antonioli DA, Goldman H, et al. Allergic esophagitis in children: a clinicopathologic entity. Am J Surg Pathol 1999;23:390–6.

Bacterial Infections

88. Damtew B, Frengley D, Wolinsky E, Spagnuolo PJ. Esophageal tuberculosis: mimicry of gastrointestinal malignancy. Rev Infect Dis 1987;9: 140–6.
89. Walsh TJ, Belitsos NJ, Hamilton SR. Bacterial esophagitis in immunocompromised patients. Arch Intern Med 1986;146:1345–8.

Viral Esophagitis

90. McDonald GB, Sharma P, Hackman RC, Meyers JD, Thomas ED. Esophageal infections in immunosuppressed patients after marrow transplantation. Gastroenterology 1985;88:1111–7.
91. Rattner HM, Cooper DJ, Zaman MB. Severe bleeding from herpes esophagitis. Am J Gastroenterol 1985;80:523–5.
92. Weber JN, Thom S, Barrison I, et al. Cytomegalovirus colitis and oesophageal ulceration in the context of AIDS: clinical manifestations and preliminary report of treatment with foscarnet (phosphonoformate). Gut 1987;28:482–7.
93. Whitley RJ. Neonatal herpes simplex virus infections. J Med Virol 1993;1:13–21.

Fungal Esophagitis

94. Forsmark CE, Wilcox CM, Darragh TM, Cello JP. Disseminated histoplasmosis in AIDS: an unusual case of esophageal involvement and gastrointestinal bleeding. Gastroint Endosc 1990;36:604–5.
95. Kodsi BE, Wickremesinghe C, Kozinn PJ, Iswara K, Goldberg PK. *Candida* esophagitis: a prospective study of 27 cases. Gastroenterology 1976;71: 715–9.

Corrosive Esophagitis

96. Cello JP, Fogel RP, Boland R. Liquid caustic ingestion spectrum of injury. Arch Intern Med 1980;140:501–4.
97. Zargar SA, Kochhar R, Nagi B, Mehta S, Mehta SK. Ingestion of corrosive acids. Spectrum of injury to upper gastrointestinal tract and natural history. Gastroenterology 1989;97:702–7.

Drug-Associated Esophagitis

98. Bonavina L, Demeester TR, McChesney L, Schwizer W, Albertucci M, Bailey RT. Drug-induced esophageal strictures. Ann Surg 1987; 206:173–83.
99. Brewer AR, Smyrk TC, Bailey RT Jr, Bonavina L, Eypasch EP, Demeester TR. Drug-induced esophageal injury. Histopathological study in a rabbit model. Dig Dis Sci 1990;35:1205–10.
100. Kikendall JW. Pill esophagitis. J Clin Gastroenterol 1999;28:298–305.

101. Seidner DL, Roberts IM, Smith MS. Esophageal obstruction after ingestion of a fiber-containing diet pill. Gastroenterology 1990;99:1820–2.

Boerhaave's Syndrome

102. Salo JA. Spontaneous rupture and functional state of the esophagus. Surgery 1992;112:897–900.

Melanosis

103. Kawamura O, Sekiguchi T, Kusano M, et al. Endoscopic ultrasonographic abnormalities and lower esophageal sphincter function in reflux esophagitis. Dig Dis Sci 1995;40:598–605.
104. Piccone VA, Klopstock R, Leveen HH, Sika J. Primary malignant melanoma of the esophagus associated with melanosis of the entire esophagus. J Cardiovasc Surg 1970;59:864–70.

Nevus

105. Krajewska IA, Moore L, Howard-Brown J. White sponge nevus presenting in the esophagus—case report and literature review. Pathology 1992;24:112–5.
106. Lam KY, Law S, Chan GS. Esophageal blue nevus: an isolated endoscopic finding. Head Neck 1001;23:506–9.
107. Timmer R, Seldenrijk CA, v Gorp LH, Dingemans KP, Bartelsman JF, Smout AJ. Esophageal white sponge nevus associated with severe dysphagia and ondynophagia. Dig Dis Sci 1997;42: 1914–8.

Glycogen Acanthosis

108. Bender MD, Allison J, Cuartas F, Montgomery C. Glycogenic acanthosis of the esophagus: a form of benign epithelial hyperplasia. Gastroenterology 1973;65:373–80.
109. Glick SN, Teplick SK, Goldstein J, Stead JA, Zitomer N. Glycogenic acanthosis of the esophagus. AJR Am J Roentgenol 1982;139: 683–8.
110. Kay PS, Soetikno RM, Mindelzun R, Young HS. Diffuse esophageal glycogenic acanthosis: an endoscopic marker of Cowden's disease. Am J Gastroenterol 1997;92:1038–40.
111. McGarrity TJ, Wagner Baker MJ, Ruggiero FM, et al. GI polyposis and glycogenic acanthosis of the esophagus associated with PTEN mutation positive Cowden syndrome in the absence of cutaneous manifestations. Am J Gastroenterol 2003;98:1429–34.

Amyloidosis

112. Bjerle P, Ek B, Linderholm H, Steen L. Oesophageal dysfunction in familial amyloidosis with polyneuropathy. Clin Physiol 1993;13:57–69.
113. Cekin AH, Boyacioglu S, Gursoy M, et al. Gastroesophageal reflux disease in chronic renal failure patients with upper GI symptoms: multivariate analysis of pathogenetic factors. Am J Gastroenterol 2002;97:1352–6.
114. Costigan DJ, Clouse RE. Achalasia-like esophagus from amyloidosis. Successful treatment with pneumatic bag dilatation. Dig Dis Sci 1983;28:763–5.
115. Estrada CA, Lewandowski C, Schubert TT, Dorman PJ. Esophageal involvement in secondary amyloidosis mimicking achalasia. J Clin Gastroenterol 1990;12:447–50.
116. Kanai H, Kashiwagi M, Hirakata H, et al. Chronic intestinal pseudo-obstruction due to dialysis-related amyloid deposition in the propria muscularis in a hemodialysis patient. Clin Nephrol 2002;53:394–9.
117. Khan GA, Lewis FI, Dasgupta M. Beta 2-microglobulin amyloidosis presenting as esophageal perforation in a hemodialysis patient. Am J Nephrol 1997;17:524–7.
118. Rubinow A, Burakoff R, Cohen AS, Harris LD. Esophageal manometry in systemic amyloidosis. A study of 30 patients. Am J Med 1983;75:951–6.
119. Suris X, Moya F, Panes J, del Olmo JA, Sole M, Munoz-Gomez J. Achalasia of the esophagus in secondary amyloidosis. Am J Gastroenterol 1993;88:1959–60.

Diabetes

120. Annese V, Bassotti G, Caruso N, et al. Gastrointestinal motor dysfunction, symptoms, and neuropathy in noninsulin-dependent (type 2) diabetes mellitus. J Clin Gastroenterol 1999;29:171–7.
121. Kinekawa F, Kubo F, Matsuda K, et al. Relationship between esophageal dysfunction and neuropathy in diabetic patients. Am J Gastroenterol 2001;96:2026–32.

Cystic Fibrosis

122. Dab I, Malfroot A. Gastroesophageal reflux: a primary defect in cystic fibrosis? Scand J Gastroenterol 1988;23:125–31.
123. Gregory PC. Gastrointestinal pH, motility/transit and permeability in cystic fibrosis. J Pediatr Gastroenterol Nutr 1996;23:513–23.
124. Heine RG, Button BM, Olinsky A, Phelan PD, Catto-Smith AG. Gastro-oesophageal reflux in infants under 6 months with cystic fibrosis. Arch Dis Child 1998;78:44–8.
125. Ledson MJ, Tran J, Walshaw MJ. Prevalence and mechanisms of gastro-oesophageal reflux in adult cystic fibrosis patients. J R Soc Med 1998;91:7–9.

Autoimmune Diseases

126. Anselmino M, Zaninotto G, Costantini M, et al. Esophageal motor function in primary Sjogren's syndrome: correlation with dysphagia and xerostomia. Dig Dis Sci 1997;42:113–8.
127. Belafsky PC, Postma GN. The laryngeal and esophageal manifestations of Sjogren's syndrome. Curr Rheumatol Rep 2003;5:297–303.
128. Grande L, Lacima G, Ros E, Font J, Pera C. Esophageal motor function in primary Sjogren's syndrome. Am J Gastroenterol 1993;88: 378–81.
129. Kjellen G, Fransson SG, Lindstrom F, Sokjer H, Tibbling L. Esophageal function, radiography, and dysphagia in Sjogren's syndrome. Dig Dis Sci 1986;31:225–9.
130. Palma R, Freire A, Freitas J, et al. Esophageal motility disorders in patients with Sjogren's syndrome. Dig Dis Sci 1994;39:758–61.
131. Tsianos EB, Chiras CD, Drosos AA, Moutsopoulos HM. Oesophageal dysfunction in patients with primary Sjogren's syndrome. Ann Rheum Dis 1985;44:610–3.

Dermatologic Diseases

132. Ahmed AR, Newcomer VD. Bullous pemphigoid: clinical features. Clin Dermatol 1987;5:6–12.
133. Hanson RD, Olson KD, Rogers RS. Upper aerodigestive tract manifestations of cicatricial pemphigoid. Ann Otol Rhinol Laryngol 1988;97:493–9.
134. Kern IB, Eisenberg M, Willis S. Management of oesophageal stenosis in epidermolysis bullosa dystrophia. Arch Dis Child 1989;64:551–6.
135. Kuechle MK, Hutton KP, Muller SA. Angiotensin-converting enzyme inhibitor-induced pemphigus: three case reports and literature review. Mayo Clin Proc 1994;69:1166–71.
136. Rogers DL. Acanthosis nigricans. Semin Dermatol 1991;10:160–3.

Graft Versus Host Disease

137. McDonald GB, Sullivan KM, Schuffler MD, Shulman HM, Thomas ED. Esophageal abnormalities in chronic graft-vs-host disease in humans. Gastroenterology 1981;80:914–21.
138. Minocha A, Mandanas RA, Kida M, Jazzar A. Bullous esophagitis due to chronic graft-versus-host disease. Am J Gastroenterol 1997;92:529–30.

4 DISEASES OF THE STOMACH

CLINICAL PRESENTATION OF GASTRIC DISEASES AND WHAT THE CLINICIAN WANTS TO KNOW

Dyspepsia, among the most common gastrointestinal symptoms (2,5,10), is treated with empiric therapies. Treatment generally reflects the physician's interpretation that the symptoms are arising from the upper luminal gastrointestinal tract. Unfortunately, one third of the patients with this symptom either fail to respond (13), or relapse, necessitating investigations to establish a more definitive diagnosis to guide additional therapy. It is in this setting that the multidisciplinary efforts of the gastroenterologist, pathologist, and radiologist are required to determine the etiology of clinically pertinent pathologic processes. While the relevance of diagnosing fungating masses or large ulcerations is obvious, the pathologic diagnosis of clinically and endoscopically "overt erythema," "patchy gastritis," or "erosive disease" constitutes a major challenge to the clinician who must decide whether to treat the patient and if so, with what.

MUCOSAL BARRIER: STRUCTURE AND FUNCTION

The mucosal barrier consists of preepithelial, epithelial, and postepithelial defenses (fig. 4-1); these defenses act against the diffusion of gastric acid and pepsin from the gastric lumen. Adherent mucus provides a stable, unstirred layer that allows surface neutralization of acid by mucosal bicarbonate secretion (1). Mucous cells also secrete lipid into the mucus, which coats the epithelium lining the gastric lumen with a nonwettable surface, thereby protecting the mucosa against the action of water-soluble hydrogen ions and pepsin. Tight junctions (3,6) and mucosal blood flow, as well as mucosal cytoprotectants (15), are other components of the gastric mucosal barrier.

The gastric cytoprotectants include immunoglobulins (9), prostaglandins (14), heat shock proteins (12), growth factors (7), sulfhydryl donors such as glutathione (11), and neuropeptides (4). Growth factors stimulate gastric mucosal growth and accelerate healing of mucosal damage. Mucosal blood flow brings bicarbonate, oxygen, and nutrients to the luminal surface and removes hydrogen ions from the same region (10).

All of these defenses protect the mucosa from injury. When they fail, back diffusion of luminal acid, tissue acidosis, vascular compromise, mucosal congestion, and tissue necrosis develop.

MUCOSAL REPAIR

When the gastric mucosa is damaged, it regenerates from a stem cell zone located in the mucous neck region (fig. 4-2). Various factors

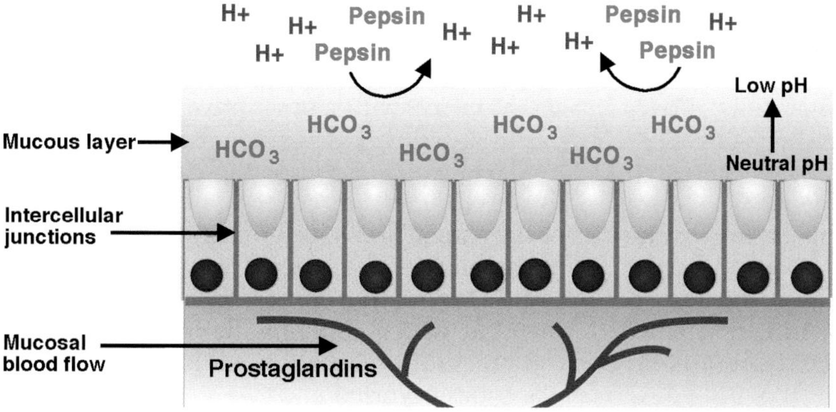

Figure 4-1

STRUCTURE OF THE GASTRIC MUCOSAL BARRIER

See text for details.

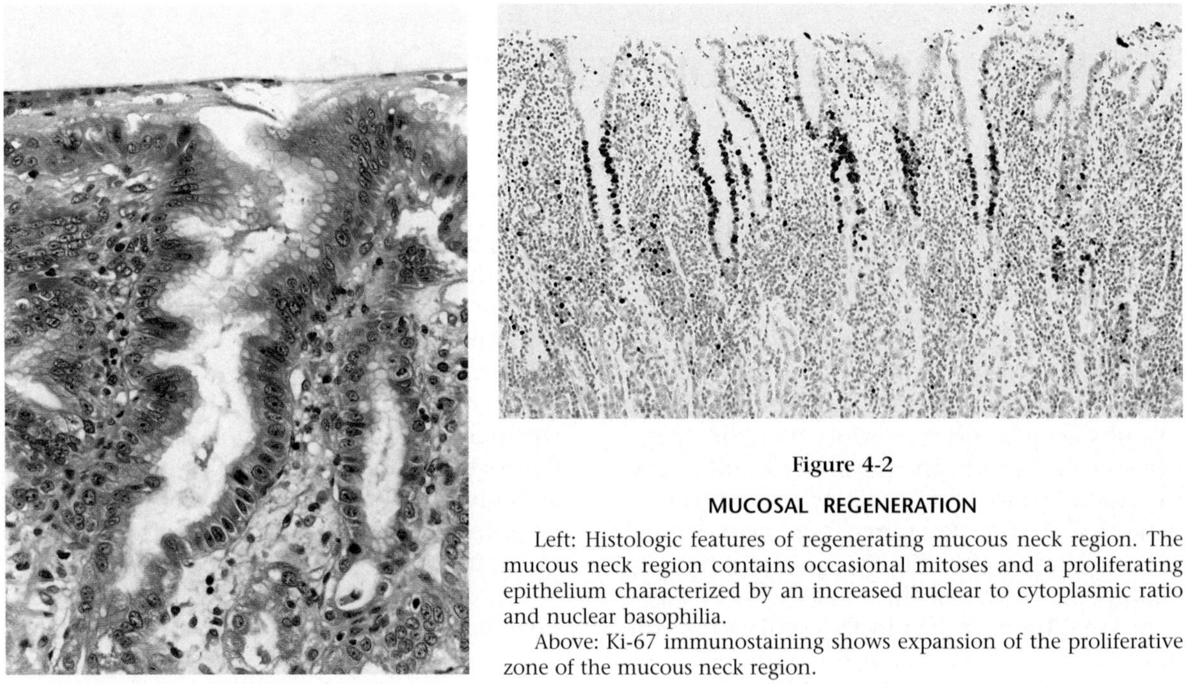

Figure 4-2

MUCOSAL REGENERATION

Left: Histologic features of regenerating mucous neck region. The mucous neck region contains occasional mitoses and a proliferating epithelium characterized by an increased nuclear to cytoplasmic ratio and nuclear basophilia.

Above: Ki-67 immunostaining shows expansion of the proliferative zone of the mucous neck region.

contribute to gastric mucosal repair. Prostaglandins limit the initial injury to the surface epithelium and lamina propria. A cap of mucus, cellular debris, and plasma proteins forms within seconds of the epithelial injury and traps plasma shed from the underlying microcirculation. This cap protects the lamina propria from luminal acid and limits the extent of the injury. Mucosal reepithelialization, a process that requires epithelial migration across an intact basal lamina, occurs rapidly, ensuring quick restoration of surface epithelial continuity.

Proliferative responses of the pluripotential stem cells in the mucous neck region also contribute to epithelial reepithelialization. Stem cells differentiate into foveolar cells above, and specialized glandular epithelial cells below the mucous neck region, reconstituting the normal architecture within a few days. Proliferating mucous neck cells appear mucin-depleted and contain abundant basophilic cytoplasm resulting in an increased nuclear to cytoplasmic ratio, increased mitoses, nuclei with vesicular chromatin, and a prominent, solitary, eosinophilic nucleolus (fig 4-2).

PATHOLOGIC EVALUATION OF GASTRIC BIOPSIES

A systematic approach to the histologic examination of gastric biopsies facilitates their evaluation, and provides the discipline for establishing a differential diagnosis that includes specific diagnostic entities. Sometimes, more than a single abnormality is present, as in coexisting *Helicobacter* and cytomegalovirus infections. It is important to recognize that many agents cause gastric injury without generating much inflammation, as typified by the chemical gastropathies; the absence of significant inflammation does not exclude the presence of mucosal injury. From time to time, a biopsy will simply defy a diagnostic category; in this situation, one might be left with a descriptive "diagnosis."

Initial biopsy evaluation should begin with a careful examination of the requisition information to ascertain the relevant clinical features of the patient and to determine the site of origin of the biopsy. The latter is very important because a biopsy that appears to be relatively normal, but which contains the wrong epithelial cell types for the location, indicates that metaplasia has occurred.

Table 4-1

FEATURES TO BE EVALUATED IN GASTRIC BIOPSIES

Are all parts of the biopsy the same, or are there focal differences? If focal differences exist, do they affect:
- the surface?
- the epithelium? If yes, then which part of epithelium (foveolar, glandular, or endocrine cells)
- the stroma?
- or all of these sites?
- the antrum?
- the fundus?
- the cardia?

Is there gastritis? If inflammation is present, is it:
- acute, chronic, mixed, granulomatous, eosinophilic, plasmacytic, lymphocytic?
- in the surface, pits, mucous neck region, glands, stroma?
- does it destroy the epithelium?

Is there an obvious etiology for the changes? Are there microorganisms or erosions?

Is there evidence of cellular differentiation? If not, is the lack of differentiation due to regeneration or neoplasia?

Is there obvious cancer or dysplasia elsewhere?

Is there architectural distortion? Can you line the glands up in your mind's eye in a more or less parallel fashion?

Is the ratio of the glands to stroma normal?
- if not, is the alteration due to too much stroma?
- is the alteration due to the loss of normal mucosal components?
- is there an increased cellularity of either component?

Is there atrophy? If so, where is it?

Is there metaplasia? If so, is it:
- intestinal?
- pyloric?
- pancreatic?
- ciliated?

Is the mucosa expanded? If so, is it by:
- inflammation?
- pit expansion?
- glandular expansion?
- an abnormal cellular infiltrate?

Are the vessels normal? If not, are they:
- dilated?
- thrombosed?
- thickened?
- dysplastic?
- neoplastic?

The first determination that should be made is whether the biopsy is normal or abnormal. It should be examined for the presence of gastritis, gastropathy, vasculopathy, mucosal expansion, or other abnormalities. The biopsy should also be examined to assess its overall histologic architecture. Answers to the questions listed in Table 4-1 allow recognition of the salient features of gastrointestinal injury and initial categorization into a specific pathologic entity. Jumbo biopsies may be used to generate biopsy material in individuals in whom the gastroenterologist suspects either the presence of a submucosal mass or gastric mucosal fold disease. This suspicion must be present before the endoscopy is started, since a larger diameter endoscope must be used to accommodate the jumbo biopsy forceps. Additionally, this large endoscope is not well tolerated by patients, who are awake during the procedure.

EXAMINATION OF SURGICAL GASTRECTOMY SPECIMENS

It is rare to receive a resection specimen today for a benign gastric disease, unless some catastrophic event, such as a perforation, has occurred. If such a specimen is received, the extent of the resection specimen should be assessed. The external surface of the stomach should be evaluated for any alterations and it should then be opened along the greater curvature, unless a gross lesion is present in this site. It is easiest to appreciate the extent of the gastric resection in the opened specimen, since the tan-white mucosa of the esophagus is readily differentiated from the pinkish red, granular gastric mucosa. When there is coexisting Barrett esophagus, pinkish granular mucosa may extend into the esophagus. In this situation, the proximal extension of the stomach can be determined by locating the proximal termination of the gastric folds. Distally, the duodenum is recognizable beyond the thickened pyloric sphincter. The mucosa usually is pinkish tan. If the patient has peptic disease, the duodenum may appear finely granular due to the presence of peptic duodenitis and Brunner gland hyperplasia.

In resections performed for peptic ulcer disease, it is important to identify the duodenum and document its presence, since it indicates the adequacy of an antral resection. Similarly, the proximal margin should be confirmed as oxyntic to ensure that complete antrectomy is performed. The entire mucosa must be examined, and the presence of erosions, ulcers, or other focal lesions noted. The nature of the mucosal folds should be evaluated to determine if they are flattened or increased in thickness. When ulcers are identified, their number, depth, and diameter should be noted. It is important to note whether an ulcer cavity is filled with blood or whether a visible vessel is present. In some patients with multiple peptic ulcerations, a small duodenal gastrin-producing tumor may be present. Careful examination of cross-sectional mucosal slices may be required to identify it. Suspicion that a gastrin-producing tumor may be present should be aroused if both multiple ulcers and gastric fold thickening are present. In this setting, the entire duodenal segment may be submitted for histologic examination. Individual lesions should be diagrammatically recorded and/or photographed. Prior endoscopic or radiologic intervention, such as injection with hypertonic saline or epinephrine, electric cautery, or embolization, may influence the pathologic findings.

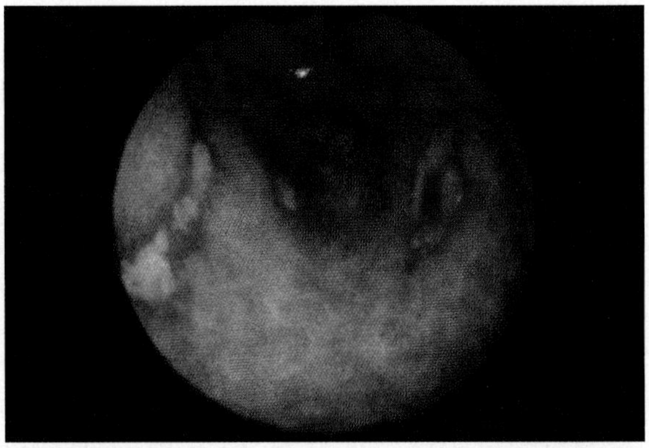

Figure 4-3

EROSIVE GASTRITIS

There are small punctate areas of mucosal erosion and hyperemia.

If it is necessary to take sections of the entire mucosa, strips can be rolled up, pinned, and placed in 10 percent formalin to be embedded in paraffin to create an "anchovy-like" roll. The resection specimen should be fixed quickly due to its propensity to undergo autolysis. We find it useful to pin resection specimens out on a cork board and suspend them upside down in 10 percent neutral buffered formalin, placing paper towels or other wicking substances between the cork board and the specimen itself. Once the stomach is completely fixed, sections can be taken carefully. Visible lesions should be sampled.

GASTRITIS

Histologically, *gastritis* is defined as gastric inflammation. Clinically, gastritis presents as abdominal discomfort, pain, heartburn, or nausea and vomiting. Endoscopically, gastritis is defined by the presence of visible mucosal alterations (fig. 4-3). Terms used to describe the endoscopic features are listed in Table 4-2. Gastritis is usually divided into acute and chronic forms. It is also classified by etiology or by its dominant histologic features. Clinical symptoms, endoscopic findings, and histologic features often fail to correlate with one another. Occasionally, when the endoscopist sees what may

Table 4-2

ENDOSCOPIC FEATURES OF GASTRITIS

Edema (swelling): This is readily diagnosed when severe. The mucosa appears glistening and may be paler than normal.

Erythema (redness): Unequivocal increase in the redness of the mucosa. A beefy red mucosa correlates with severe erythema. The process may appear focal or diffuse.

Friability: Minor trauma, such as probing with a closed biopsy forceps, causes punctate hemorrhage or frank oozing.

Exudate: Gray-yellow (sometimes brownish or greenish) material adherent to the mucosal surface. Exudate may tenaciously adhere to the mucosa. It may be punctate or form patches, streaks, or plaques. An underlying process (e.g., ulceration) may be present.

Erosion: Break in the mucosa. Flat erosions correspond to necrotic foci that do not extend beyond the muscularis mucosae. Their number and location may vary.

Raised erosion (varioliform erosion): Discrete lesions of elevated mucosa capped by a central defect. They are often superimposed on the gastric folds.

Rugal hyperplasia or hyperrugosity (fold enlargement): The folds do not flatten (or only partially flatten) when the stomach is insufflated with air.

Rugal atrophy: Thinning of mild or moderate degree or ultimate disappearance of the gastric rugae.

Vascular pattern: A vascular pattern is not visible endoscopically in the normal gastric mucosa. When it is present, it results from mucosal thinning accompanied by the appearance of ramifying vessels.

Intramucosal bleeding spots: Loss of the vascular integrity leads to intramucosal or intraluminal extravasation of blood. It appears as petechiae or as larger reddish brown or dark black ecchymotic spots, streaks, or flecks.

Nodularity (granularity): Lack of evenness of the mucosa. Elevated areas may be visible.

appear to be severe gastritis, the pathologist may find nothing remarkable, and vice versa.

Acute Gastritis

Definition. *Acute gastritis* has an acute onset and short duration. Inflammation, if present, consists of polymorphonuclear leukocytes. *Cushing ulcers* are associated with serious brain injury, intracranial neurosurgical procedures, or increased intracranial pressure. *Curling ulcers* affect burn patients. Other synonyms for acute gastritis are *active gastritis, acute hemorrhagic gastritis, erosive gastritis, stress gastritis,* and *ulcerative gastritis*. The term *chronic erosive gastritis* is also synonymous with *lymphocytic* or *varioliform gastritis*.

Demography. Acute gastritis accounts for up to 25 percent of hospital admissions of patients with acute upper gastrointestinal bleeding (26).

Etiology. Acute gastritis complicates toxic injury and major physiologic disturbances (Table 4-3). To determine the exact etiology, correlation with the clinical features is required.

The major physiologic factors implicated in the development of acute gastritis are increased gastric acid secretion and failure of any component of the mucosal barrier system. Mucosal ischemia is the common denominator of stress-associated lesions, but reperfusion also

Table 4-3

MAJOR CAUSES OF ACUTE GASTRITIS

Physiologic Stresses
- Uremia
- Severe burns
- Congestive heart failure
- Infections and sepsis
- Major surgery
- Trauma
- Respiratory failure
- Major central nervous system injury

Toxic Stresses
- Alkaline and bile reflux
- Ingestion of
  - Certain foods
  - Alcohol
  - Drugs, especially nonsteroidal antiinflammatory drugs (NSAIDs)
- Corrosive agents

Circulatory Stresses
- Shock and hypovolemia
- Ischemia
- Portal hypertension
- Hypotension

significantly contributes to gastric mucosal injury (22). Systemic acidosis, a common finding in shock, contributes to the development of mucosal erosions by lowering cellular pH levels. Cardiac dysfunction, hemorrhage, shock, and sepsis also redistribute blood flow away from subepithelial capillaries, causing mucosal hypoxia. The hypoxia may persist after recovery from the initial injury, especially since mucosal arterioles contract, further reducing tissue oxygenation (72).

Pathophysiology. Hypoxia directly damages the mucosa via oxygen metabolic deprivation, tissue acidosis, vascular compromise, and mucosal congestion, thereby destroying mucosal defenses and rendering the mucosa vulnerable to acid and peptic attack. Neutrophils play a major role in generating both ischemic and reperfusion injury (38). They release vasoactive mediators that modify vascular tone, reduce mucosal blood flow, and increase vascular permeability. This leads to loss of normal mucosal cytoprotection, allowing mucosal injury to progress beyond what would otherwise have resulted from the initial injurious event. Neutrophil-derived oxygen-free radicals also cause cellular damage.

Clinical Features. Patients with acute gastritis typically present with gastrointestinal pain and bleeding. Bleeding begins 3 to 7 days following a physiologically stressful event or following the ingestion of injurious substances. The bleeding ranges from occult blood loss to massive hemorrhage originating from innumerable foci of mucosal damage. When erosive gastritis evolves into acute or chronic ulcers, the bleeding becomes more severe and hematemesis may result.

Gross Findings. Acute gastritis is hemorrhagic or nonhemorrhagic, erosive or nonerosive. Erosive gastritis and stress ulcers typically appear as multiple lesions located anywhere in the stomach, although they tend to predominate proximally. Erosions are discrete, superficial, oval or circular areas of mucosal necrosis and tissue loss measuring less than 5 mm in diameter (usually less than 2 mm). They typically have sharply defined edges (fig. 4-3). Ulcers, if present, usually measure less than 1 cm in diameter. The ulcer base appears grayish yellow and hemorrhagic, with slightly raised, congested, regenerative margins. The intervening gastric mucosa often appears diffusely congested and contains numerous, small petechial hemorrhages (fig. 4-4). Alternatively, the mucosa appears diffusely hemorrhagic without a discrete lesion. In severe diffuse hemorrhagic gastritis, the stomach may be filled with blood.

Radiographic studies reflect disease severity. Findings range from nonspecific thickening of the gastric folds and spasm, which are difficult to distinguish reliably from normal, to frank ulceration (fig. 4-5). Classic air-contrast fluoroscopy shows multiple, tiny contrast collections in shallow erosions.

Microscopic Findings. Mucosal changes range from focal hyperemia, edema, surface erosions, and acute inflammation to massive mucosal necrosis, sloughing, ulceration, and eventual scarring (figs. 4-6, 4-7). The number and types of inflammatory cells present depend on the etiology.

Early acute gastritis exhibits superficial mucosal inflammation, edema, and hyperemia with subepithelial hemorrhage but without actual erosion formation. Such a lesion may be difficult to distinguish from biopsy trauma. More severe disease shows extreme vascular congestion and dilatation with lamina propria hemorrhage (figs. 4-6, 4-7). The mucosa contains superficial fibrin deposits (fig. 4-7).

Erosions result in tissue loss that does not extend into the submucosa. Sloughed necrotic tissue lies above a relatively normal mucosa (fig. 4-7). The eroded cavity may contain an exudate of proteinaceous fluid, cellular debris, neutrophils, and red blood cells.

During its acute phase, acute gastritis shows vascular engorgement, interstitial hemorrhage, superficial necrosis, neutrophils in the pits and glands, and variable epithelial damage. During the healing phase, there is epithelial regeneration (fig. 4-8), pit elongation, nuclear enlargement, mucus depletion, and numerous mitoses. The superficial epithelium acquires a pseudostratified or syncytial appearance. Regenerating epithelium may exhibit alarming cytologic features that should not be mistaken for carcinoma. Table 4-4 compares the features of regenerative and neoplastic mucosae.

Differential Diagnosis. The differential diagnosis of acute gastritis includes chemical gastropathy, drug-induced gastritis, infectious gastritis, and a number of other entities (Table 4-3).

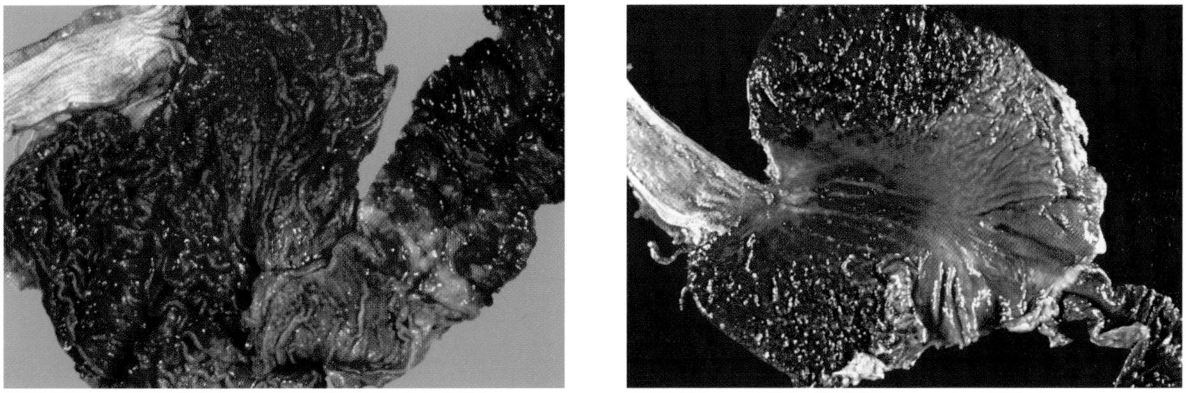

Figure 4-4

EROSIVE GASTRITIS

Gross appearance of the stomach opened along the greater curvature.

Left: Diffuse involvement of the gastric and duodenal mucosa by erosive changes. Both sites show marked mucosal erythema without specific punctate hemorrhages.

Right: Erosive changes are confined to the proximal stomach and duodenum. Both diffuse and punctate lesions are identified.

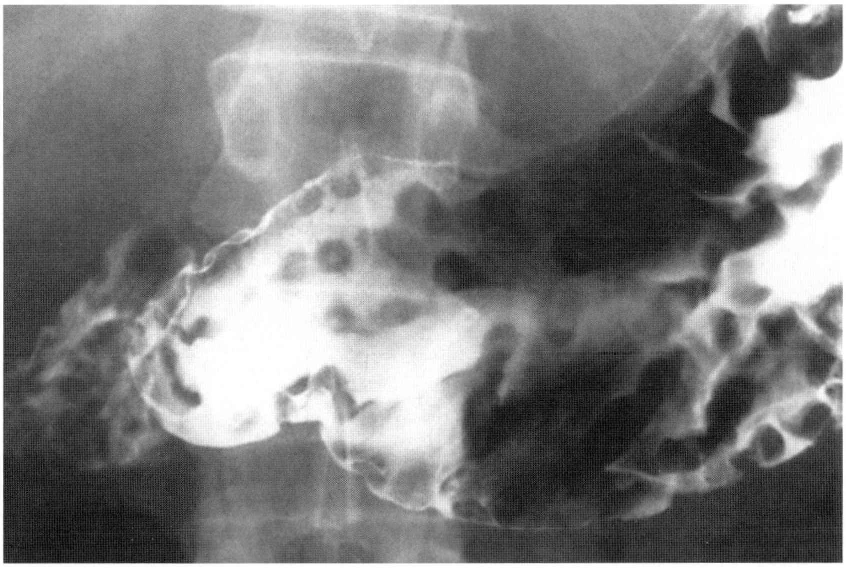

Figure 4-5

EROSIVE GASTRITIS

A spot radiograph of the gastric fundus from a double-contrast upper gastrointestinal study shows multiple, complete, varioliform, shallow erosions surrounded by halos of edema. The pattern is thought to be more typical of chronic erosive gastritis than acute hemorrhagic gastritis in which the erosions are often less complete and less obvious radiographically. (Fig. 2 from Poplack W, Paul RE, Goldsmith M, et al. Demonstration of erosive gastritis by the double-contrast technique. Radiology 1975:117;519–21.)

Treatment and Prognosis. Treatment consists of removal of the inciting factor, acid reduction with antisecretory agents, and administration of mucosal protectants, such as sucralfate. The acute gastritis usually heals days to weeks following removal of the causative factor(s). In patients with deeper lesions, complete regeneration of the gastric glands rarely occurs and mild mucosal scarring results.

Animal Models. Numerous animal models exist for producing acute gastritis. Animal studies involve the production of vasoconstriction, diversion of gastric mucosal blood flow, and the administration of specific etiologic agents in various types of animals.

Helicobacter Pylori Gastritis

Definition. *Helicobacter pylori* (HP) *gastritis* includes the entire spectrum of gastric mucosal changes induced by HP infections.

Demography. HP infections occur worldwide, and the age at which a patient becomes

Figure 4-6

EROSIVE GASTRITIS

A: Fibrin thrombi and an eosinophilic coagulum are often present at the surface. The surface epithelium becomes denuded and the upper portions of the pits lack their epithelial lining. This pattern mimics that seen in early intestinal ischemia (see chapter 7).

B: The superficial mucosa appears congested and shows interstitial and subepithelial hemorrhage.

C: Higher magnification view of B.

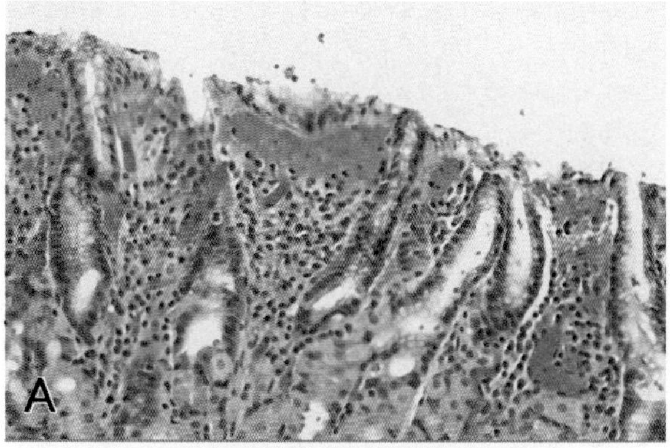

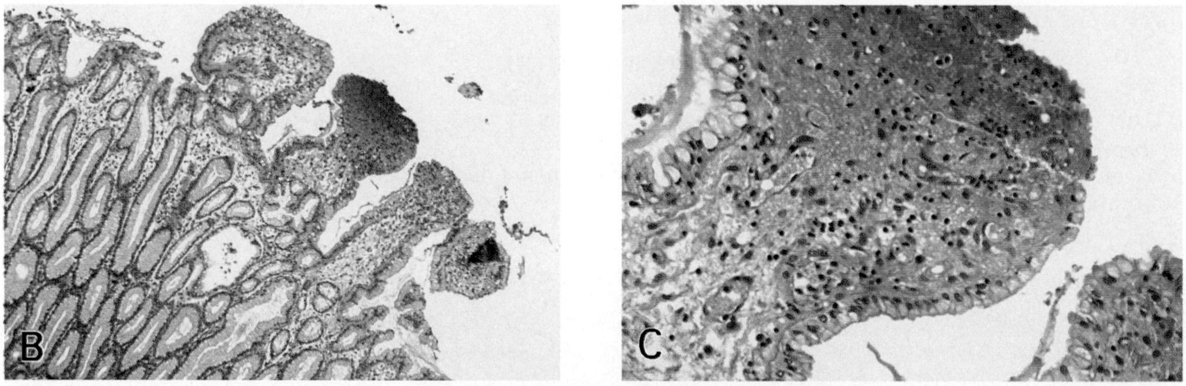

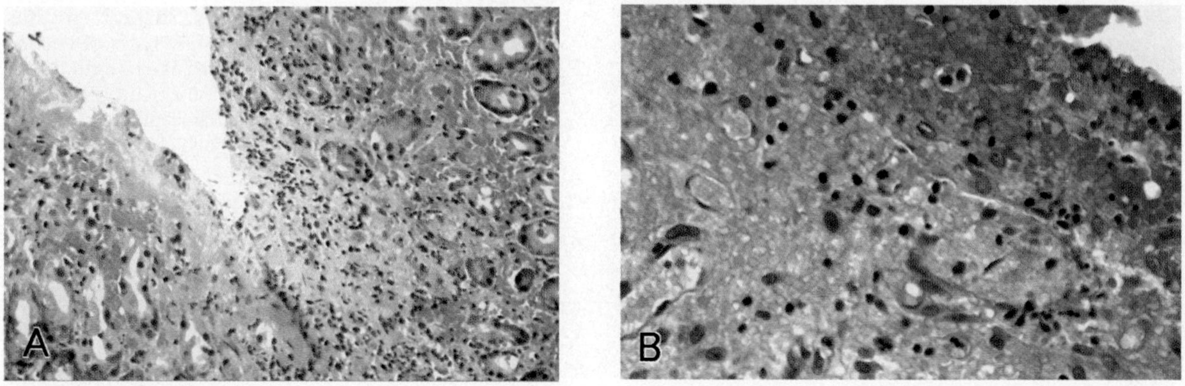

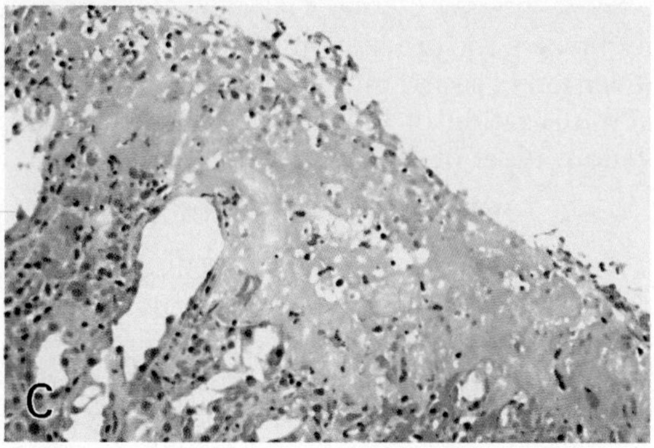

Figure 4-7

EROSIVE GASTRITIS

A: Extravasated red blood cells and edema replace the normal architecture of the lamina propria.

B: A coagulum of extravasated red blood cells, dying epithelial cells, and inflammatory cells is present. No epithelium is identifiable on the surface.

C: Often, superficial portions of the lesion consist of areas of coagulation necrosis and dying cells.

infected reflects local hygiene. High-density living facilitates disease transmission and correlates with a lower socioeconomic status, a family history of peptic ulcer disease, and pediatric HP-related gastrointestinal illnesses. Infants and children are most susceptible to HP infections. HP infection is transmitted person-to-person (77), from drinking infected water (47), and by the fecal-oral route (67).

The prevalence of HP infections increases rapidly with age. Infection prevalence in developing countries can be as high as 75 percent by age 25. In industrialized countries, 60 percent or more of patients over age 60 have evidence of HP infection. In the United States, blacks (70 percent) and Hispanics have higher rates of infection than whites (34 percent) (58). Obesity or type II diabetes predisposes to HP colonization secondary to decreased gastric motility.

Pathophysiology. Bacterial motility and the production of various enzymes, cytotoxins, and hemolysins are important in the pathogenesis of HP-associated gastritis and gastric ulcers. HP normally resides in the unstirred layer overlying the gastric mucosa. The organisms move down through this viscous environment to attach to the apical cell membranes of foveolar cells (fig. 4-9), preferentially attaching at or near intercellular junctions. Bacterial adhesins recognize specific cell surface proteins, facilitating

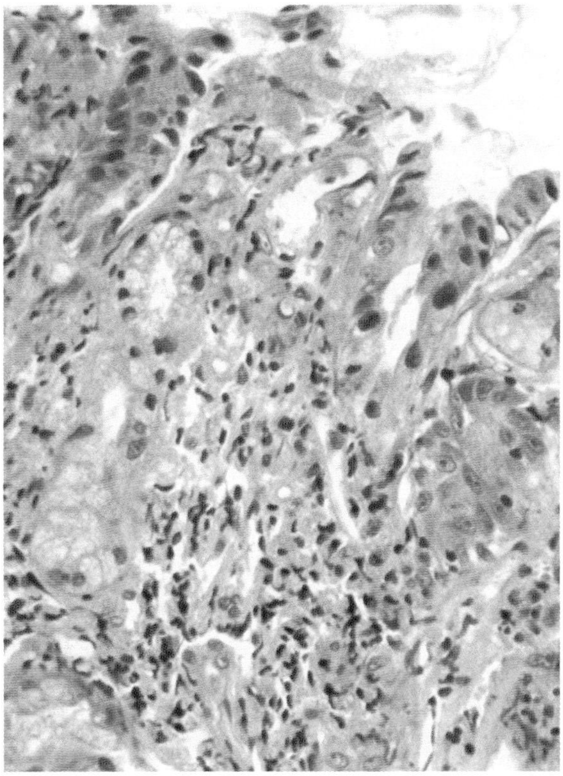

Figure 4-8

MUCOSAL REGENERATION FOLLOWING EROSIVE GASTRITIS

The epithelial cells appear mucin depleted, with prominent nuclei increasing the nuclear to cytoplasmic ratio.

Table 4-4

COMPARISON OF REGENERATIVE VERSUS NEOPLASTIC MUCOSA

Change	Regeneration	Neoplasia
Cellular immaturity	Present	Present
Mucin loss	Present	Present
Increased N/C ratio[a]	Usually absent, but may be present	Present
Nuclear atypia	If present typically minimal	Usually present
Basal location of nuclei	Usually retained	Often lost
Atypical mitoses	Usually absent	Often present
Nucleoli	Prominent and single	Multiple and irregular in size and shape
Glandular architecture	Usually retained, with glands lying in parallel with one another	Often distorted; individual glands may appear very irregular
Relationship to intestinal metaplasia	May involve metaplastic epithelium	Often involves metaplastic epithelium, especially in intestinal type gastric cancers
Acute inflammatory background	Usually present	Usually absent unless ulcerated
Chronic inflammatory background	May be present	Always present unless atrophy has occurred

[a]N/C ratio = nuclear to cytoplasmic ratio.

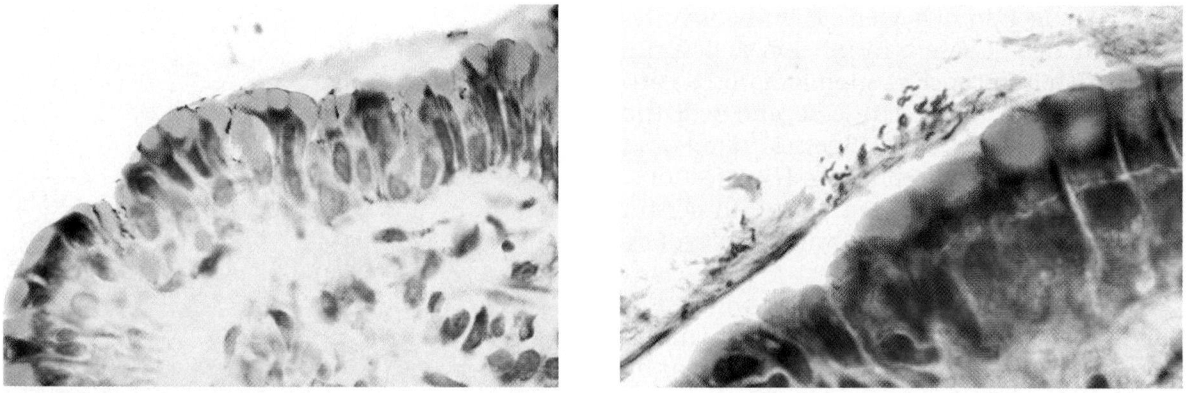

Figure 4-9

HELICOBACTER PYLORI

Left: Organisms are adherent to the foveolar epithelium.

Right: Numerous organisms lie in the mucinous layer overlying the epithelium. (Left and right figures are stained with Alcian yellow. Mucin stains yellow; organisms stain blue.)

epithelial colonization (31,37). Bacteria unable to adhere to the epithelium are eliminated from the mucosa.

Differences in the availability of specific receptors have been suggested as a means to explain genetic differences in susceptibility to infection with HP (21). HP weakens the intercellular junctions, allowing the organisms to penetrate junctional complexes and move down along lateral cell membranes (fig. 4-9). As a result, intercellular spaces widen and fill with neutrophils. The latter phagocytize the HP. HP also alters mucin release into the gastric lumen and causes mucous granule depletion, which, together with bacterial enzymes, results in loss of mucosal barrier integrity, allowing mucosal acid and pepsin diffusion to further contribute to mucosal damage. HP also promotes neutrophil adhesion to endothelial cells and vascular emigration, activities mediated by adhesion molecules on both the endothelium and neutrophils.

HP infections generate significant cellular and humoral responses via antigenic stimulation of mucosal monocytes and T cells. These inflammatory cells produce numerous cytokines, prostaglandins, proteases, and reactive oxygen metabolites which further damage the mucosa. Some of the cytokines promote adhesion of leukocytes to endothelial cells; others recruit additional leukocytes to the infected site. Stimulated B cells differentiate into immunoglobulin (Ig)M, IgA, and IgG antibody-producing cells. IgA promotes complement-dependent phagocytosis and the killing of HP by neutrophils. Secretory IgA synergizes with IgG to promote antibody-dependent cell-mediated cytotoxicity by human neutrophils, monocytes, and lymphocytes. High levels of HP-specific IgG antibodies correlate with severe antral gastritis and dense HP antral colonization. Some antibodies cross react with the gastric mucosa, contributing to the development of chronic gastritis (53).

Bacterial products mediating tissue injury include lipopolysaccharides (61), chemotactic factors (32), vacuolating cytotoxin (VacA) (56), cytotoxin-associated antigen (CagA) (19), heat shock proteins (50), and outer membrane inflammatory protein (81). The presence of CagA is associated with a more prominent inflammatory tissue response and an increased risk of symptomatic outcome (20,71).

Relationship of HP to Gastric Diseases. HP plays a significant role in the genesis of several gastric diseases (Table 4-5). The development of gastritis, ulcers, gastric carcinoma, and gastric lymphoma all involve interactions between environmental (i.e., infection with HP) and genetic factors (Table 4-6). The risk for developing gastric ulcers is highest in the nonatrophic forms of gastritis, whereas cancer is associated with severe atrophic gastritis.

Identification of HP Infection. Diagnostic tests for HP include bacterial culture, histologic or cytologic examination, rapid urease-based

Table 4-5

DISEASES SHOWING A STRONG RELATIONSHIP WITH *HELICOBACTER PYLORI* INFECTION

Chronic gastritis
Chronic active gastritis
Multifocal atrophic gastritis
Follicular gastritis
Gastric and duodenal ulcers
Gastric adenocarcinoma
Gastric lymphoma

Table 4-6

HELICOBACTER PYLORI–ASSOCIATED DISEASE COMPARISON

High Acid Secretors	Low Acid Secretors
Antral gastritis	Antral and corpus gastritis
Healthy corpus	Impaired antral and corpus function
Increased antral gastrin due to lost D-cell function	Increased antral gastrin
Increased acid	Decreased acid
Increased risk of duodenal ulcer	Increased gastric cancer

tests, carbon 13 and carbon 14 breath tests, and serologic studies. Histologic examination equals or even surpasses culture, especially when positive. The patchy nature of the infection, however, requires examination of a minimum of two biopsies: one from the gastric antrum and one from the body. The greater the number of biopsies, the greater the diagnostic yield, especially in individuals with low bacterial densities. Recommendations to maximize diagnostic yield include the use of large-cup biopsy forceps, obtaining at least three samples (from the lesser curve angularis, the greater curve prepyloric antrum, and greater curve body), proper mounting and preparation of specimens, and use of an appropriate stain (35).

The occasional need for an immediate diagnosis prompted the development of the more rapid *Campylobacter*-like organism (CLO) test, which is based on bacterial urease production. Gastric brushings or tissues are placed in a urea solution. The HP, if present, produce urease, resulting in ammonia production. The ammonia alkalinizes a solution that contains a pH-sensitive indicator causing a color change (fig. 4-10).

Since culture, cytologic or histologic examination, and rapid urease-based examinations all require endoscopy, noninvasive diagnostic tests that do not require an endoscopic procedure were developed. The most popular of these are the carbon13 and carbon14 breath tests. Patients with possible HP infection receive orally administered carbon-labeled urea. Bacterial urease, if present, releases the labeled carbon that is absorbed into the blood, converted to bicarbonate, and expired as radiolabeled CO_2. The presence of radiolabeled CO_2 in expired air confirms the presence of HP. Such tests are rapid and reasonably easy to perform. The test is often used to confirm eradication of the infection. Another new noninvasive diagnostic test is a stool antigen test (HpSA test). Sensitivity and specificity of this test vary compared to histologic examination and urea breath tests (58,74).

Various HP strains can be differentiated using restriction fragment length polymorphism (RFLP) analysis of polymerase chain reaction (PCR)-amplified DNA. Antibiotic-resistant forms of the organism may be detectable by ribotyping. Ribotyping also creates genetic fingerprints and allows epidemiologic studies to be performed on HP organisms.

Clinical Features. The clinical features of HP-associated gastritis include the presence of upper abdominal pain, dyspepsia, and emesis. Many patients remain asymptomatic.

Gross Findings. Endoscopic changes include several antral changes, including erosions, mucosal nodularity, spotty erythema, and altered mucosal markings. Alteration in the endoscopic appearance of collecting venules is helpful in differentiating normal from HP gastritis (63).

Microscopic Findings. HP, a Gram-negative, motile, flagellated bacterium, measuring approximately 0.3 µm in width and 5 µm in length, generally assumes a curved, sinuous, or gently spiraled shape (fig. 4-9). HP is readily identified in hematoxylin and eosin (H&E)-stained sections as thin, wavy, blue rods lying in the mucus overlying or attached to foveolar epithelium (fig. 4-11), in the crevices between the foveolar cells, or within the

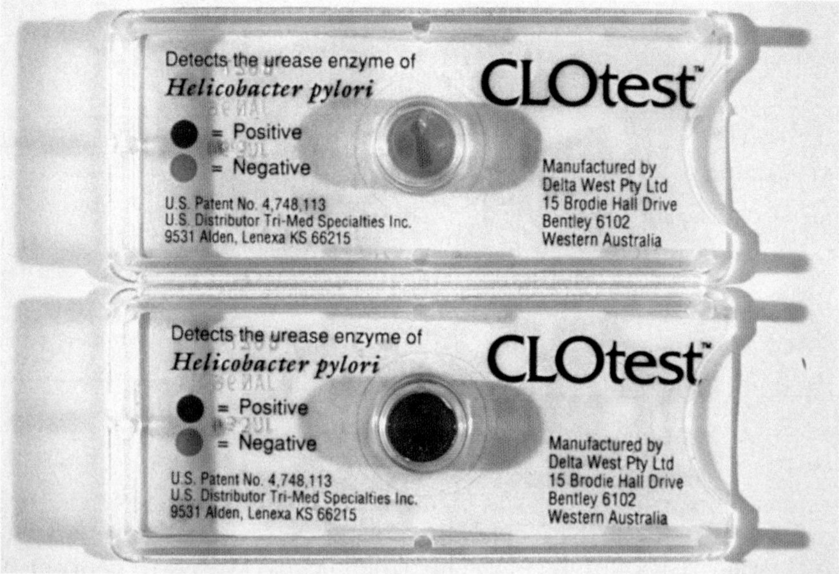

Figure 4-10

CLO TEST FOR *H. PYLORI*

The upper slide is negative; the lower slide, positive. The color change in the well of the lower slide is a result of urease reaction.

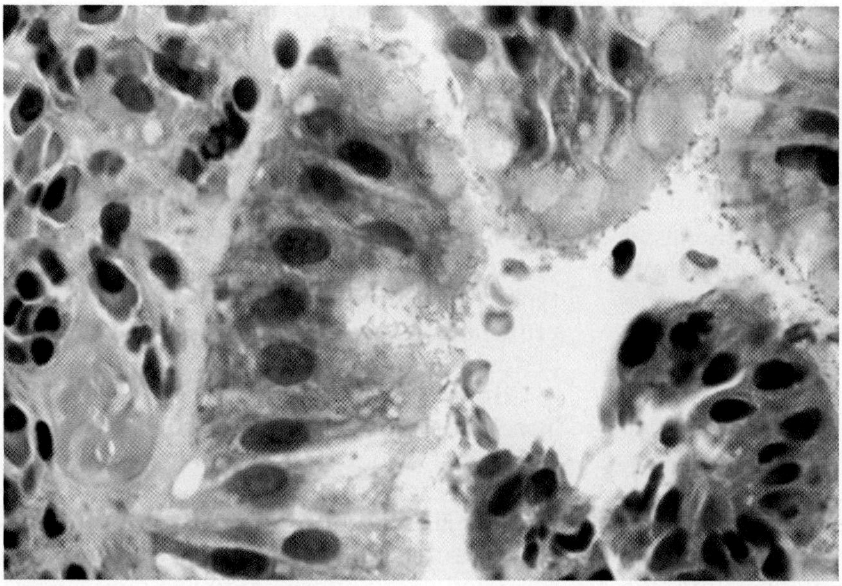

Figure 4-11

***H. PYLORI* GASTRITIS**

Several fragments of gastric epithelium are present. Those with residual mucin in the foveolar cells are covered by numerous *H. pylori* organisms.

pit lumens. HP sometimes become coccoid in shape when patients receive antibiotics, but helicobacillary forms invariably coexist with the coccoid forms.

Various special stains enhance bacterial detection (Table 4-7). A combination of Steiner, hematoxylin, and Alcian blue stains (the Genta stain) has the advantage of combining a silver-based stain for the organism and a stain that identifies areas of intestinal metaplasia on one slide (36). It also allows a more accurate distinction of the bacteria from mucinous debris. The use of monoclonal antibodies may be especially helpful in identifying coccoid forms. We use an H&E-stained section to examine the biopsy, and if organisms are easily seen in such a preparation, additional special stains are not used unless specifically requested by the clinician. If we see chronic active gastritis and do not see obvious HP, then we will perform special stains. We formerly used the Diff-Quik stain, but have recently replaced it with an immunohistochemical/immunostain because the latter is easier to interpret.

Table 4-7

STAINS USED TO DETECT *HELICOBACTER PYLORI* INFECTION

Acridine orange	Gram
Alcian yellow	Immunohistochemical staining
Brown-Hopps	Loeffler methylene blue
Cresyl violet	Steiner
Dieterle silver	Toluidine blue
Diff-Quik	Warthin-Starry
Genta	Wright-Giemsa
Giemsa	

HP-Associated Acute Gastritis. HP gastritis always involves the antrum, but it may diffusely affect the remaining stomach. HP infections begin as an acute gastritis with a marked neutrophilic infiltrate in the mucous neck region. Neutrophils do not usually infiltrate the superficial epithelium where the organisms are located. Both the neutrophils and the HP destroy the epithelium, causing mucous neck cell hyperplasia. The toxin produced by the organism induces cytoplasmic swelling and vacuolization, micropapillary change, mucin loss, desquamation of surface foveolar cells, and erosions, resulting in loss of epithelial mucosal barrier function. Pure acute gastritis is almost never seen; by the time patients are biopsied, they usually have chronic active gastritis.

Chronic Active (Nonatrophic) Gastritis. In chronic active gastritis, the changes seen with acute gastritis are superimposed on a background of chronic inflammation (fig. 4-12). Neutrophils, eosinophils, basophils, macrophages, monocytes, plasma cells, and mast cells infiltrate the mucosa. Neutrophils infiltrate the lamina propria and mucous neck region of the gastric glands. In severe infections, neutrophilic aggregates in the pit lumens form abscesses. The superficial epithelium degenerates and the epithelial loss leads to mucous neck cell hyperplasia. This results in elongated, distorted, tubular, and pseudopapillary structures. Regenerating cells form a multicellular layer with indistinct intercellular borders, creating syncytial polypoid excrescences. The regenerating mucous neck cells are characterized by mucin loss, cytoplasmic basophilia, increased mitotic activity, and hyperchromatic stratified nuclei, changes sometimes mimicking epithelial dysplasia. The enlarged nuclei retain smooth, regular nuclear membranes. Within a few days of HP eradication, the surface changes rapidly reverse, and the epithelial cells acquire their normal shape and spatial organization. When active superficial gastritis becomes quiescent, the acute inflammation, edema, and vascular congestion disappear, and the epithelium returns to normal. The lamina propria still contains increased numbers of mononuclear cells.

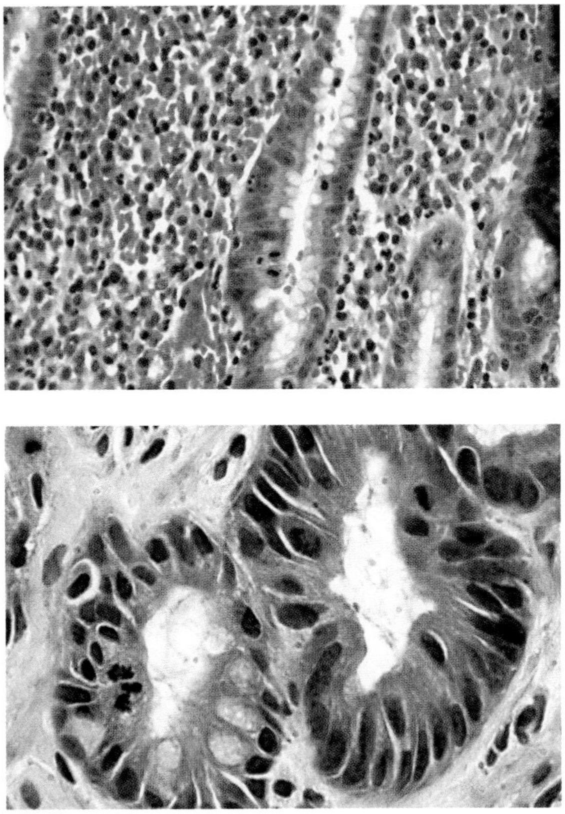

Figure 4-12

CHRONIC ACTIVE GASTRITIS

Top: This area of the mucous neck region contains mitotic figures and is infiltrated by neutrophils. The surrounding lamina propria contains a mononuclear cell infiltrate consisting of lymphocytes and plasma cells; occasional neutrophils are present.

Bottom: Area of the mucous neck demonstrates mitoses and nuclear enlargement.

Early, the chronic inflammation, which consists of dense lymphocytic and plasma cell infiltrates, remains confined to the superficial gastric mucosa, often along the lesser curvature in the antrum. The lymphoplasmacytosis of the superficial lamina propria then extends into the glandular compartment. With time, the inflammation becomes confluent and transmucosal. Lymphoid aggregates develop in over 80 percent of HP-infected patients, creating a lesion termed *follicular gastritis* (fig. 4-13). Follicular gastritis, an immune response to the bacteria, is most prominent in the antrum and is significantly less prevalent proximally. Its presence serves as a useful histologic marker of HP infection.

Eventually, most patients with chronic HP infections develop chronic pangastritis, followed by multifocal atrophy. These changes result from both the infection and the inflammatory infiltrate. Additionally, HP-associated antibodies that cross react with the gastric mucosa and other factors, such as bile reflux and dietary irritants, induce further mucosal damage. As atrophy develops, areas of intestinal metaplasia replace the native gastric mucosa.

Chronic Atrophic Gastritis. In some individuals, chronic active superficial gastritis progresses to atrophic gastritis (55). Such progression leads to three patterns of atrophic gastritis: body predominant (diffuse corporal) atrophic gastritis, antral predominant atrophic gastritis, and both antral and body (multifocal) atrophic gastritis. Antral predominant atrophic gastritis is the most common and multifocal atrophic gastritis is the least common of the three (51).

The antral mucosa shows loss of antral glands, which can be identified by a decrease in the mucosal thickness. The atrophic antral glands are replaced by metaplastic glands, most commonly of the intestinal type. In the early stages, prominent lymphocytic infiltration is present in the mucosa; this is replaced by fibrosis in the later stage. Atrophic gastritis in the body has similar histologic findings as autoimmune gastritis.

Differential Diagnosis. The differential diagnosis of HP gastritis depends in part on which features predominate histologically. The presence of chronic active gastritis with neutrophils in the mucous neck region is virtually pathognomonic for HP. Lesser degrees of active chronic gastritis may also be seen in patients with *Helicobacter heilmannii* infections. Once the active inflammation subsides, the entities in the differential diagnosis of chronic gastritis are autoimmune gastritis and lymphocytic gastritis. Fundic gastritis and antral gastritis are compared in Table 4-8. Lymphocytic gastritis differs from the chronic gastritis associated with HP infection in that an intraepithelial lymphocytosis dominates the histologic findings (see figs. 4-30, 4-31). If there is a proliferation of lymphoid tissues in HP gastritis, the intense mucosal lymphocytic and plasmacytic infiltrate may be severe enough to require distinction from a mucosa-associated lymphoid tissue (MALT) lymphoma.

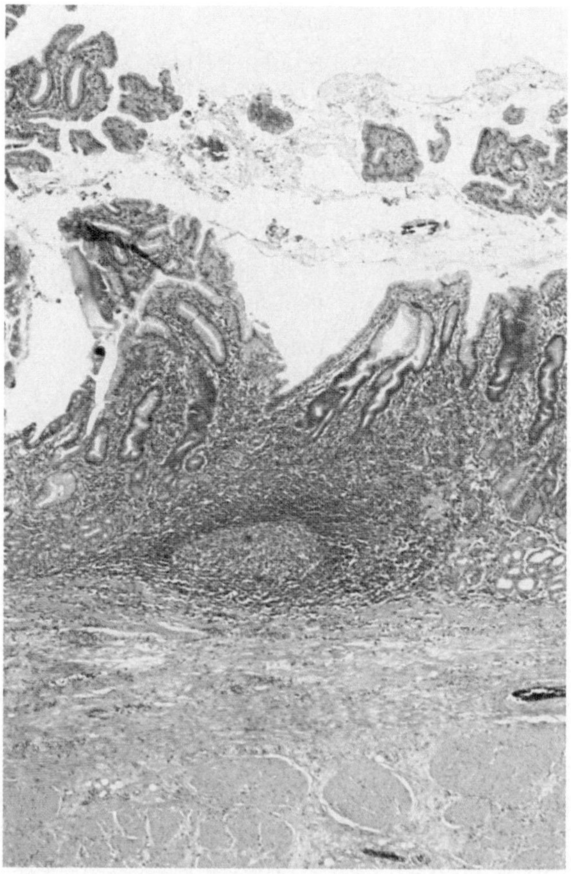

Figure 4-13

FOLLICULAR GASTRITIS

Prominent lymphoid aggregates form in the basal portion of the mucosa. They often contain germinal centers, as in this case.

Treatment and Prognosis. Eradication of the infection is achieved in more than 90 percent of patients with a 14-day regimen of proton pump inhibitors together with two antimicrobial drugs. Treatment of dyspeptic symptoms with proton pump inhibitors may alter the pattern of HP infection as HP migrates from the

Table 4-8

COMPARISON OF ANTRAL AND FUNDIC GASTRITIS

Features	Antral Gastritis	Fundic Gastritis
Distribution	Antral and then spreads proximally	Fundus and body, spares the antrum
Etiology	*H. pylori* infection combined with dietary factors	Antibody against H^+,K^+-ATPase proton pump in parietal cells
Acid levels	Variable	Hypochlorhydria or achlorhydria
Gastrin levels	Low or normal	Elevated
Antibodies to parietal cells	Absent	Present
Antibodies to intrinsic factor	Absent	Present
Pernicious anemia	Absent	Present
Peptic ulcers	Present	Absent
Metaplasia	Intestinal, ciliated, pancreatic	Intestinal, pyloric, ciliated, pancreatic
Endocrine cell hyperplasia	Not usually present	ECL[a] hyperplasia, antral G-cell hyperplasia, carcinoid tumors
Chronic active gastritis	Present	Absent
Pepsinogen levels	May be low, depending on disease extent	Low
Foveolar hyperplasia	May be present	May be present
Complications	Peptic ulcer disease, gastric carcinoma, MALT[b] lymphomas	Gastric carcinoma, gastric carcinoid tumors

[a]ECL = enterochromaffin-like.
[b]MALT = mucosa-associated lymphoid tissue.

antrum to the fundus and activity of the antral gastritis is decreased. A test to confirm eradication should not be performed within 4 weeks of the end of the treatment course.

The prognosis of patients with HP infections depends on the extent of the damage by the time the infection is detected and treated. In patients with early lesions, treatment of the infection may stop gastric damage. In individuals with atrophic gastritis, peptic ulcer disease, or some form of malignancy, the prognosis is determined by the more severe consequences of the infection.

Animal Models. Numerous animal models exist for evaluating the pathophysiology of HP infections and their ability to generate the gastritis as well as ulcer disease, lymphomas, and carcinomas.

Helicobacter Heilmannii Gastritis

Definition. *Helicobacter heilmannii gastritis* consists of those mucosal changes that result from infection with *Helicobacter heilmannii*.

Demography. *H. heilmannii* (formerly called *Gastrospirillum hominis*) infects both humans (children and adults) and small animals.

Etiology. *H. heilmannii* is closely related to HP. Like HP, *H. heilmannii* is a Gram-negative, urease-producing bacterium, but is larger (size, 3.5 to 7.5 µm) and more tightly coiled (more than three coils) than HP (17,44).

Clinical Features. Patients with *H. heilmannii* infections either remain asymptomatic or present with a gastritis that is generally milder than that produced by HP organisms.

Microscopic Findings. *H. heilmannii* more commonly infects the gastric antrum than the gastric body. Unlike HP, which closely adheres to the gastric epithelium, *H. heilmannii* organisms usually lie free in the gastric lumen or deep in the gastric pits and necks of the pyloric glands, with little or no epithelial attachment. The organisms are easier to see than HP because of their larger size (fig. 4-14). The resulting chronic active gastritis is milder than that produced by HP (45).

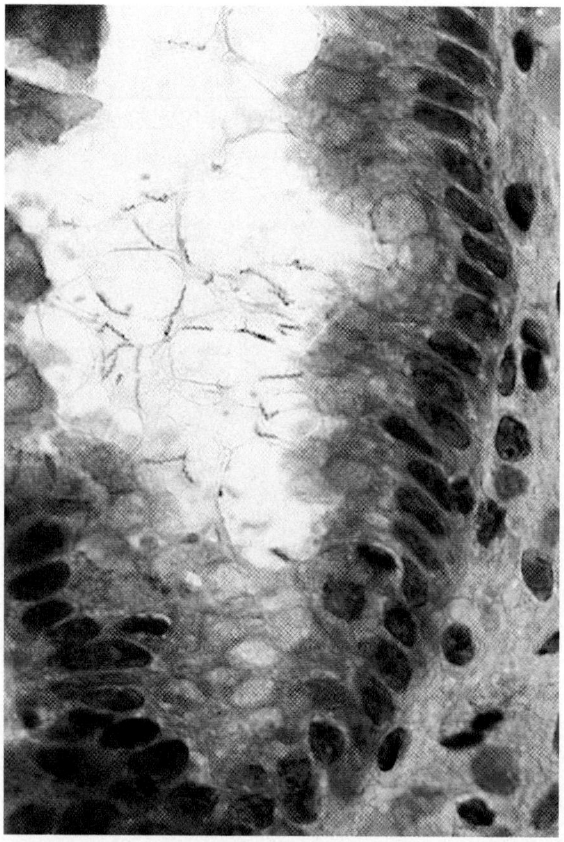

Figure 4-14

H. HEILMANNII INFECTION

Long, tightly coiled bacteria are in the mucus. The length (10 to 15 µm) and coiled appearance differentiate *H. heilmannii* from *H. pylori*. (Fig. 2-30 from Emory TS, Carpenter HA, Gostout CJ, Sobin LH. Atlas of gastrointestinal endoscopy & endoscopic biopsies. Washington DC: Armed Forces Institute of Pathology; 2000:91.)

Treatment. Treatment is the same as for HP gastritis.

Suppurative Gastritis

Definition. *Suppurative gastritis* is a severe form of gastritis resulting from bacterial infection in patients with poor host defenses. It consists of a marked acute inflammatory reaction and abscess formation in the gastric wall. When air-filled spaces are also present, the entity may be termed *emphysematous gastritis*.

Demography. Most examples of suppurative gastritis antedate the antibiotic era and usually affect severely debilitated individuals with chronic illnesses.

Etiology. Infections with pyogenic bacteria cause suppurative gastritis. The most common organisms that cause emphysematous gastritis are *Clostridium* sp, *Escherichia coli*, *Streptococcus*, *Enterobacter* sp, and *Pseudomonas aeruginosa*. Microbial culture identifies the specific organism.

Clinical Features. Patients present with dramatic episodes of nausea, vomiting, fever, and severe, acute, noncolicky epigastric pain, which are associated with leukocytosis. Commonly, peritonitis or pleural effusions develop. Some patients develop localized abscesses. The clinical course resembles that of patients with a perforated viscus; shock and death often ensue.

Gross Findings. The dilated stomach appears extensively necrotic, with marked mural thickening due to the presence of intense submucosal edema. Gas-filled spaces are present and fibrinous serous adhesions may be seen.

Microscopic Features. There is marked acute inflammation, with or without microabscesses; prominent edema; and hemorrhage. In some cases, the mucosa appears focally necrotic; in others, the mucosa is completely destroyed and covered by a mucopurulent exudate. Widespread intravascular thrombosis involving mural vessels causes secondary ischemic gangrenous necrosis. Transmural inflammation develops in severe cases. The muscularis propria appears variably inflamed and necrotic. Air spaces, similar to those in pneumatosis intestinalis, are present. A Gram stain demonstrates bacteria in the tissues.

Treatment and Prognosis. The mortality rate approaches 100 percent unless the affected part of the stomach is resected.

CHEMICAL GASTROPATHY

Definition. *Chemical gastropathy* is the presence of foveolar hyperplasia, muscle fibers in the lamina propria, edema, and vasodilatation in the absence of an increase in acute or chronic inflammatory cell infiltrates. *Reactive gastropathy* is an alternative term for this condition; however, the morphologic changes of chemical gastropathy indicate a number of specific etiologies and that is why we prefer to use more specific terminology than reactive gastropathy.

Etiology. Chemical gastropathy results from the presence of surface damaging agents in the gastric lumen, including alkaline reflux, alcohol, nonsteroidal antiinflammatory drugs (NSAIDs), and probably a host of less well-defined etiologies. Similar changes also occur in uremic patients. The histologic features of all of the chemical gastropathies resemble one another, making it impossible to determine the exact etiology, in the absence of identifiable bile in the biopsy or a pertinent clinical history.

Alkaline reflux gastritis develops in patients with abnormal pyloric sphincter function from previous surgical intervention, chronic alcohol ingestion, or aging. Reflux can occur any time after the initial operation, and its onset may be delayed for decades. The surgical interventions that can cause secondary alkaline reflux include partial gastrectomy with anastomosis, truncal vagotomy with pyloroplasty, and cholecystectomy.

In reflux gastritis, alkaline secretions, pancreatic enzymes, and bile salts that are present in the duodenal contents damage the gastric mucosa. Bile salts increase mucosal permeability to hydrogen ions by binding to the apical end of the foveolar cells. Bile inhibits mucosal bicarbonate secretion and therefore decreases the pH gradient between the epithelium and the luminal acid (46). The acid then either causes vasoconstriction or directly damages the mucosal epithelium. The amount of reflux often correlates with symptom severity, but endoscopic and histologic features rarely correlate with one another. The most severe changes occur in the antrum, where often there is clear-cut evidence of gastritis at the time of endoscopy, namely, hyperemia, edema, friability, and bile staining of the gastric mucosa. The pathophysiologic effects of NSAIDs are discussed in the section on drug-induced gastritis.

Uremia damages mucosal barrier function and stimulates gastrin production (75). The latter results in cell proliferation in the mucous neck region and preferential differentiation of stem cells into parietal and enterochromaffin-like (ECL) cells. The surface epithelial cells show increased acidification from the acid produced by the expanded parietal cell mass. Mucus production decreases, resulting in a thinned mucus gel layer, which in the face of the increased acid levels, leads to further mucosal damage. Abnormal bile salt formation and increased bile acid production also cause uremic gastropathy and ulcer formation.

Gross Findings. The most common endoscopic abnormality in chemical gastropathy is the presence of intramucosal hemorrhage; this can vary in size from petechiae to large ecchymoses. There may be slow oozing rather than rapid blood loss.

Microscopic Findings. Chemical gastropathy is suspected when pit expansion, mucus depletion, and superficial edema are present in the absence of an active inflammatory infiltrate, bacteria, atrophy, metaplasia, ulcers, polyps, or enlarged fold disease. The histologic features are subtle and often overlooked unless suspected. Gastropathy may not even seem to be present. The principal histologic features are listed in Table 4-9. All of the listed features may be present, but are not needed to make the diagnosis (fig. 4-15).

The foveolar cells appear mildly mucin depleted and vacuolated, especially in patients who have undergone previous gastric surgery. The lack of an inflammatory response contrasts with the degree of the hyperplasia.

Differential Diagnosis. The histologic changes overlap with those seen in alcoholic gastropathy, stress gastropathy, or NSAID-induced gastropathy. Therefore, it is impossible to determine the etiology of the gastritis (unless bile is found in the biopsy) in the absence of the appropriate history, and even then it may be impossible. Hyperplastic polyps may have some overlapping features with chemical gastropathy and they are frequently associated with prior gastrectomy. A clinical history of polyp is helpful in establishing the diagnosis. Often, however, the endoscopist describes biopsies from areas of chemical gastropathy as "nodular." Other features seen in hyperplastic polyps include cystically dilated glands, distorted glands with an irregular branching and serrated appearance, and expansion of the lamina propria by the glands.

Treatment and Prognosis. Treatment consists of administering prokinetic agents. In reflux gastropathy, cholestyramine may bind bile salts and reduce the mucosal injury. Occasionally, surgical diversion is necessary.

Animal Models. Numerous animal models exist for the production of alkaline reflux gastropathy, as well as other forms of chemical gastropathy.

CHRONIC GASTRITIS

Chronic gastritis is any gastritis in which the histologic features are dominated by the presence of a chronic inflammatory cell infiltrate. Chronic gastritis can be classified as active when neutrophils are present.

Table 4-9

HISTOLOGIC FEATURES OF CHEMICAL GASTROPATHY

Mucosal edema
Hypercellularity and expansion of the gastric pits (with increased mitotic activity) resulting in glandular elongation and tortuosity
Capillary congestion and vasodilation within the superficial lamina propria
Mucin depletion
Foveolar hyperplasia and villiform transformation of the mucosa
Increased numbers of smooth muscle fibers in the lamina propria
Absence of acute inflammation except in the presence of an erosion
Bile in the glands (helpful if present, but not always seen)

A concise, widely accepted classification scheme for chronic gastritis has not emerged. The classification scheme commonly utilized is the modified Sydney system (fig. 4-16) (27,29). Its goal is to relate the gastritis to its etiology. The Sydney classification system requires that biopsies be examined from both the antrum and the body, since each area is assessed separately. Five histologic variables are independently graded (fig. 4-16). Table 4-10 lists the definition and grading guidelines for each of the histologic features used in the Sydney system.

Nonspecific chronic gastritis has many etiologies, which produce similar or overlapping histologic features. This results in a poor correlation among clinical symptoms, endoscopic features, and histology. There are three distinct forms of chronic gastritis based on the topographic distribution of the damage: *diffuse antral, fundic,* and *multifocal gastritis*. Diffuse antral gastritis (DAG) and multifocal antral gastritis (MAG) are sometimes referred to as type B, or environmental, gastritis, and they share HP infection as an etiologic factor. The major difference between the two is that DAG is not atrophic, and acid and pepsin secretion probably also play an etiologic role.

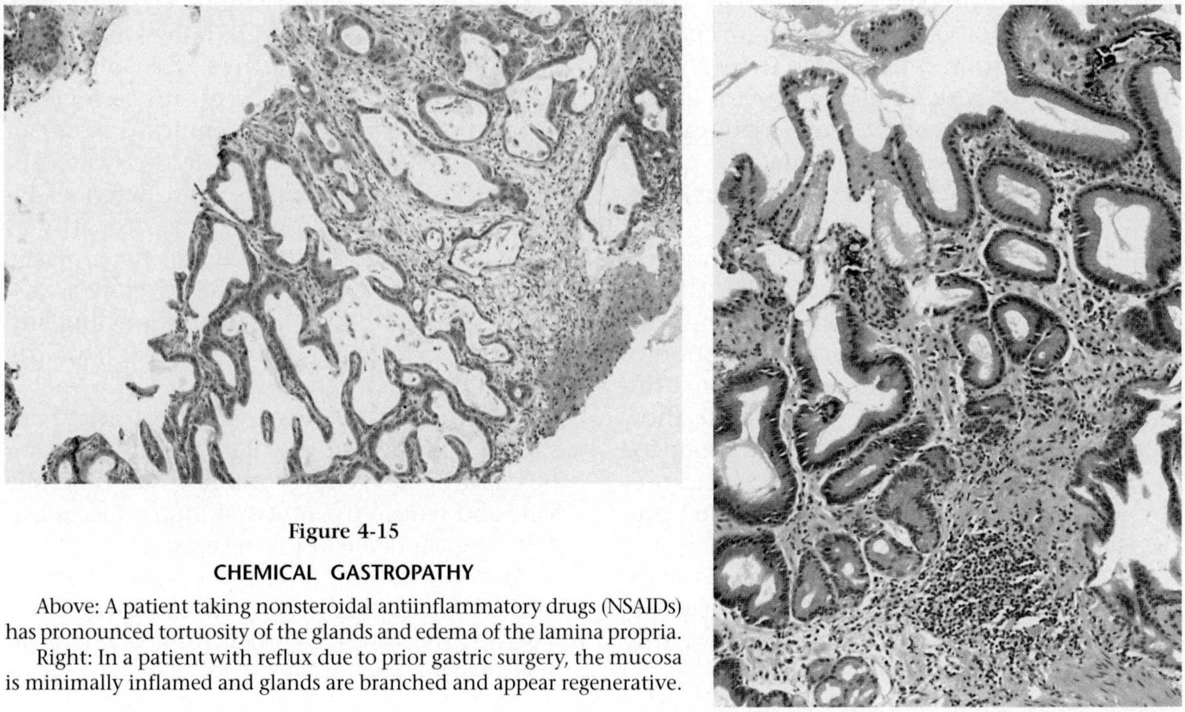

Figure 4-15

CHEMICAL GASTROPATHY

Above: A patient taking nonsteroidal antiinflammatory drugs (NSAIDs) has pronounced tortuosity of the glands and edema of the lamina propria.

Right: In a patient with reflux due to prior gastric surgery, the mucosa is minimally inflamed and glands are branched and appear regenerative.

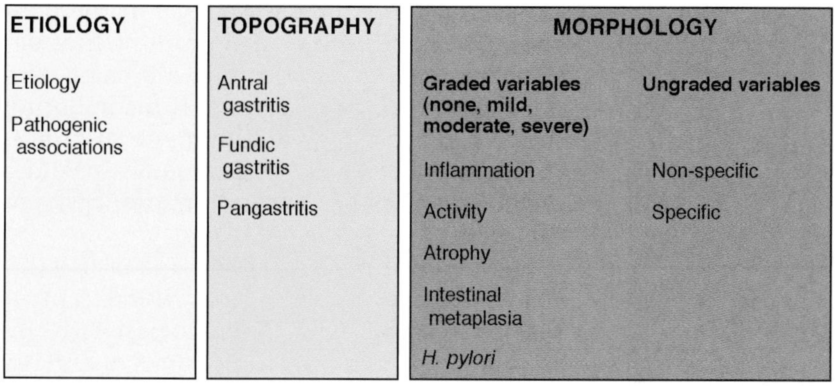

ETIOLOGY
Etiology
Pathogenic associations
TOPOGRAPHY
Antral gastritis
Fundic gastritis
Pangastritis
MORPHOLOGY
Graded variables (none, mild, moderate, severe)
Inflammation
Activity
Atrophy
Intestinal metaplasia
H. pylori
Ungraded variables
Non-specific
Specific

Figure 4-16

SYDNEY SYSTEM OF CLASSIFICATION FOR CHRONIC GASTRITIS

Pathologic features are evaluated in several topographic areas. Five features are graded and other features that may be present are ungraded.

Table 4-10

DEFINITIONS AND GRADING GUIDELINES FOR THE SYDNEY SYSTEM

Feature	Definition	Grading Guidelines
Chronic inflammation	Increase in lymphocytes and plasma cells in the lamina propria	Mild, moderate, or severe increase in density
Activity	Neutrophilic infiltration of the lamina propria, pits, or surface epithelium	<1/3 of pits and surface infiltrated = mild; 1/3–2/3 = moderate; >2/3 = severe
Atrophy	Loss of specialized glands from either antrum or corpus	Mild, moderate, or severe loss
Intestinal metaplasia	Intestinal metaplasia (all subtypes) of the epithelium	<1/3 of mucosa involved = mild; 1/3-2/3 = moderate; >2/3 = severe
H. pylori	Density of *Helicobacter*-like organisms overlying epithelium	Scattered organisms covering <1/3 of the surface = mild colonization; large clusters or a continuous layer >2/3 of surface = severe; intermediate numbers = moderate

The mucosa of patients with chronic gastritis is often sampled in order to establish the presence of the gastritis, to delineate its geographic extent, to judge the degree of activity, to detect the presence of HP organisms that may be treated, and to rule out the presence of complications such as peptic ulcer disease or various tumors.

Autoimmune Gastritis

Definition. *Autoimmune gastritis* preferentially localizes to the fundus and body and results from the presence of antibodies directed against parietal cells. Affected patients also often have antibodies against intrinsic factor and the gastrin receptor. Synonyms include *fundic gastritis* and *type A gastritis*.

Demography. In most countries, only a minority of patients (less than 5 percent) with chronic gastritis have autoimmune gastritis (70). The disease tends to affect people of Scandinavian or northern European origin and is rare among other ethnic groups. Not only do patients have demonstrable antibodies against parietal cells, but so do their first-degree relatives, suggesting that genetic influences play a role in the pathogenesis of the disease (52).

Etiology. The antibodies are directed against the catalytic subunit of the H^+K^+-ATPase proton pump and pepsinogen (59), and may develop spontaneously. Patients receiving methyldopa treatment also develop antibodies against parietal cells and subsequent chronic autoimmune gastritis (52). The gastritis disappears upon cessation of the drug. Atrophic autoimmune gastritis affects approximately 25 percent of patients with dermatitis herpetiformis (69).

Pathophysiology. The acid-secreting mucosa is progressively destroyed by immunologic injury directed primarily at the parietal cells; chief cells, however, are also destroyed in the

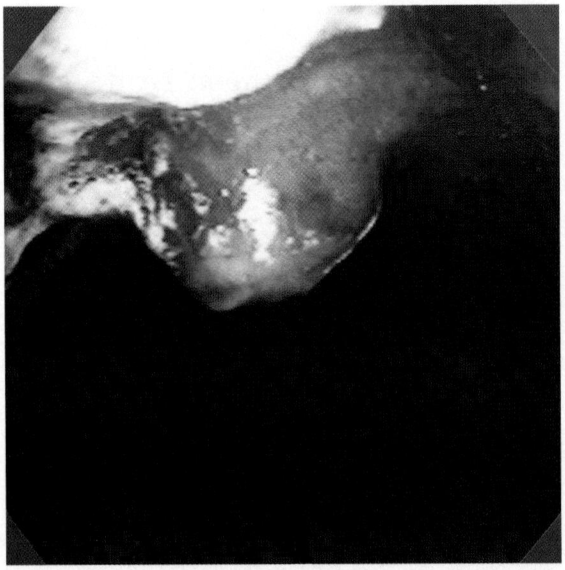

Figure 4-17

GASTRIC CARCINOID

Gastric carcinoid is seen in the fundus of a patient with hypergastrinemia due to autoimmune atrophic gastritis.

process. Eventually, this results in the complete loss of the specialized oxyntic mucosa and oxyntic glandular atrophy. Hypochlorhydria or achlorhydria develops and serum pepsinogen group 1 levels fall. The hypochlorhydria stimulates antral G-cell hyperplasia. Increased serum gastrin levels lead to enterochromaffin-like (ECL)-cell hyperplasia in the oxyntic mucosa and foveolar hyperplasia.

Patients with autoimmune gastritis often have pernicious anemia due to the presence of an autoantibody to intrinsic factor that inhibits distal ileal vitamin B12 absorption. The development of pernicious anemia, particularly in the elderly, is insidious, typically occurring 6 to 18 years following the initial diagnosis of gastritis. The patients often have autoantibodies directed against other organs as well. As a result, they may have coexisting Hashimoto's thyroiditis, idiopathic hypoadrenalism, idiopathic hypoparathyroidism, or insulin-dependent diabetes. The postpartum state aggravates autoimmune gastritis in some patients (16).

Clinical Features. In individuals with pernicious anemia, the diagnosis usually becomes obvious because the patient presents with chronic megaloblastic anemia. Alternatively, the presence of an elevated serum gastrin level in the presence of achlorhydria is diagnostic. Other patients present with the complications of atrophic gastritis or the diagnosis is made during the workup for other autoimmune disorders. Symptoms referable to the gastrointestinal tract include diarrhea, malabsorption, dyspepsia, or symptoms related to a malignancy.

Gross Findings. The antrum is usually spared with autoimmune gastritis except in severe cases. The changes may coexist with HP-associated gastritis. Gastric atrophy manifests as mucosal thinning and loss of the rugal folds. The submucosal vessels become increasingly more visible. Endoscopically, the presence of easily discernible gastric vasculature should alert the physician to the probability of atrophic gastritis. It is useful for the endoscopist to determine the pH of the resting gastric juice and biopsy all nodules and visible lesions to exclude an associated gastric carcinoid or other neoplasm (fig. 4-17).

Microscopic Findings. There are three histologic stages of autoimmune gastritis: superficial gastritis, atrophic gastritis, and gastric atrophy. The distinction between these three stages relates to the location of the inflammation in the mucosa and the extent of the glandular atrophy. In *superficial gastritis*, the inflammatory infiltrate remains localized to the superficial mucosa lying between the gastric pits, and glandular atrophy is minimal or absent. The lamina propria infiltrate contains lymphocytes and plasma cells. In *atrophic gastritis*, the inflammatory infiltrate involves the entire thickness of the mucosa, and there is marked glandular atrophy with a severe reduction in the number of parietal and chief cells (fig. 4-18). In *gastric atrophy*, there is complete loss of the glands and minimal inflammation. Eventually, the fundic mucosa is completely replaced by metaplastic pyloric or intestinal type glands. Sequential biopsy studies show that autoimmune gastritis progresses from superficial gastritis to atrophic gastritis over a period of 15 to 20 years (23).

Patients with long-standing autoimmune gastritis develop antral G-cell hyperplasia as a result of achlorhydria. G cells can be present in large numbers in the antropyloric mucosa, usually exhibiting an irregular and random spatial distribution that ranges between one and four

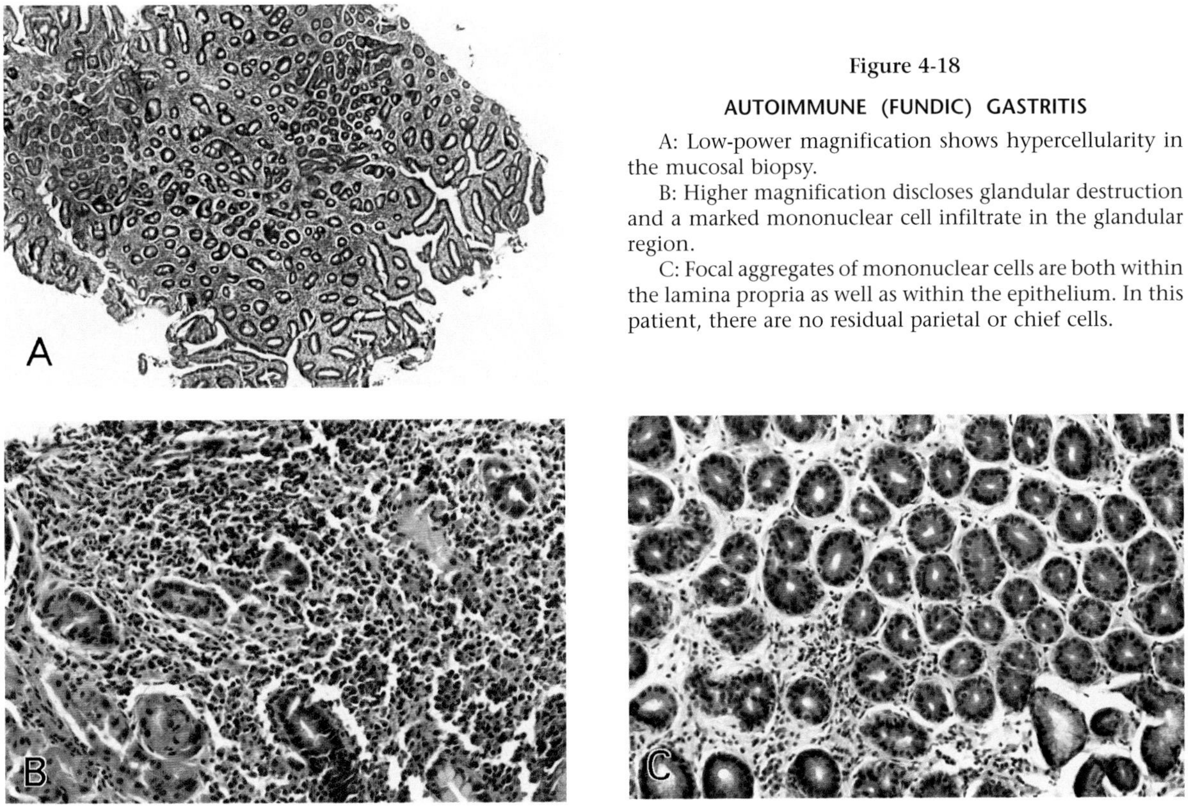

Figure 4-18

AUTOIMMUNE (FUNDIC) GASTRITIS

A: Low-power magnification shows hypercellularity in the mucosal biopsy.

B: Higher magnification discloses glandular destruction and a marked mononuclear cell infiltrate in the glandular region.

C: Focal aggregates of mononuclear cells are both within the lamina propria as well as within the epithelium. In this patient, there are no residual parietal or chief cells.

cells/gland. The foveolar mucosa may become hyperplastic once G-cell hyperplasia develops. Multifocal gastric ECL hyperplasia, micronests, and multifocal carcinoid tumors also develop in the atrophic and metaplastic gastric body secondary to the G-cell hyperplasia in the antral mucosa (fig. 4-19).

ECL-cell hyperplasia passes through a series of stages, ranging from a diffuse increase in argyrophilic cells, through linear and nodular aggregates, to intramucosal and frankly invasive carcinoid tumors. *Simple hyperplasia*, the earliest stage, consists of a diffuse increase in ECL cells, scattered singly or in clusters of up to three cells/gland. The cells appear somewhat enlarged and although they are diffusely distributed throughout the upper, middle, and lower third of the mucosal thickness, they appear more prominent in the lower third. The hyperplastic cells are present in the atrophic fundic glands and pyloric metaplastic glands but not in the intestinal metaplastic glands. *Linear hyperplasia* is diagnosed when a linear, semilinear, or daisy chain-like configuration of ECL cells is present along the glandular basement membrane. The next stage, designated as *micronodular hyperplasia*, consists of solid micronodular ECL cell nests measuring 100 to 150 mm in size (the average diameter of a gastric gland). These can be seen using H&E-stained sections and are variously described as argyrophil cell clusters, microcarcinoids, or endocrine cell micronests. The micronests may be bounded by an intact basement membrane contiguous with that of the rest of the gland or lie in the basoglandular portion of the mucosa disassociated from the glands lying freely in the lamina propria abutting the muscularis mucosae. Still others may appear trapped within a widened and somewhat ragged muscularis mucosae.

Adenomatous hyperplasia consists of interglandular micronodular lesions, each with an intact basement membrane. As each micronodule enlarges, the basement membrane breaks down, and the nuclear to cytoplasmic ratio increases. This dysplastic stage marks the borderline between the clearly hyperplastic stages preceding it and the neoplastic stage of a fully developed carcinoid tumor. These lesions range

Figure 4-19

ENTEROCHROMAFFIN-LIKE CELL HYPERPLASIA

A: Hematoxylin and eosin (H&E) stain of a gastric biopsy in a patient with fundic gastritis. At low magnification, numerous small, dark, cellular nests are seen in the lamina propria.

B: When stained with an antibody to synaptophysin, both the intraglandular proliferations as well as proliferations in the lamina propria are highlighted in a specimen from the same biopsy.

C: Endocrine cell hyperplasia and endocrine micronests are in the lamina propria in another patient.

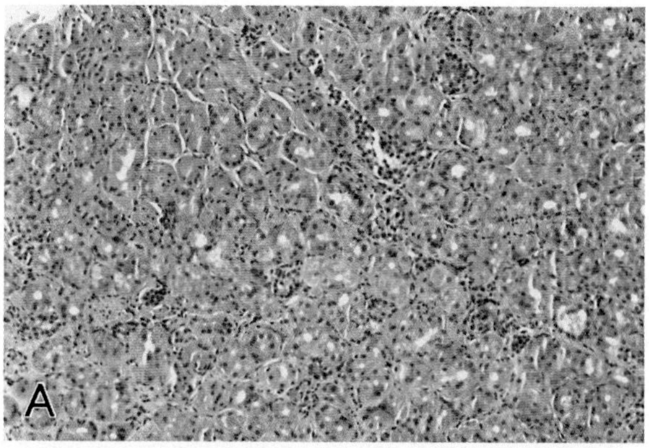

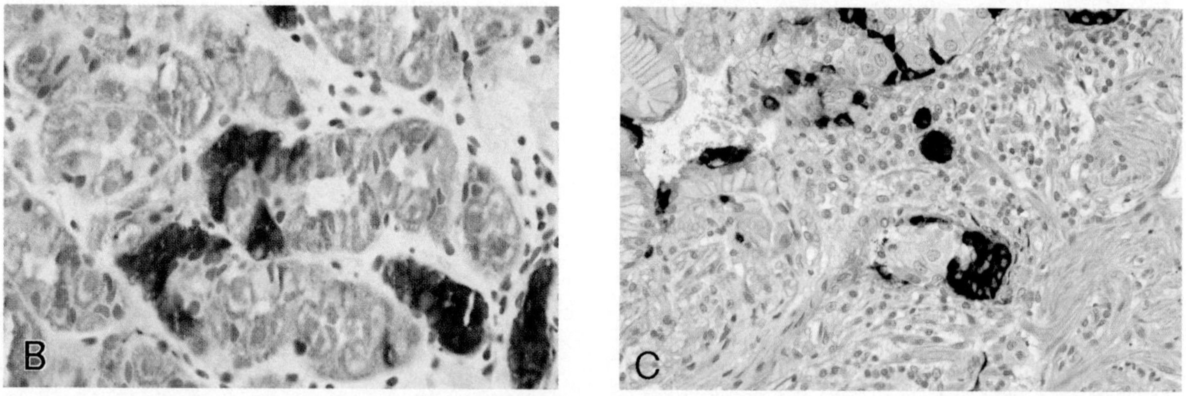

in size from 150 μm to 0.5 mm and progress from enlarging micronodules to microinvasive lesions and nodules with newly formed stroma. The carcinoid stage is characterized by nodular infiltrating growths measuring over 0.5 mm.

Differential Diagnosis. The differential diagnosis of autoimmune gastritis has several aspects. The first is determining whether the chronic gastritis is autoimmune or a form of environmental gastritis, or possibly both diseases. The diagnosis rests on examination of biopsies from the oxyntic mucosa that show evidence of gastritis, parietal and chief cell destruction, or atrophy. The next consideration concerns the presence of glandular atypia and determining whether the glands are reactive, dysplastic, or malignant. The presence of antral G-cell hyperplasia raises another set of diagnostic possibilities (Table 4-11). If ECL hyperplasia is present, gastric carcinoid tumor is a diagnostic possibility.

Treatment and Prognosis. Autoimmune gastritis predisposes to the development of gastric adenocarcinoma through an intervening step of intestinal metaplasia. The metaplastic mucosa becomes dysplastic (fig. 4-20) and then frankly malignant. The dysplasia always arises in the intestinalized mucosa. Some patients have adenocarcinomas and coexisting multiple carcinoid tumors in a setting of diffuse endocrine cell hyperplasia and autoimmune gastritis. Antrectomy reverses the oxyntic endocrine cell hyperplasia, but it is not used in the absence of endocrine neoplasia. Multiple small carcinoids arising in the setting of chronic atrophic gastritis are usually indolent, and do not warrant gastrectomy. Patients deficient in vitamin B12 require lifelong B12 administration. In the United States, endoscopic surveillance is not considered to be cost-effective; however, endoscopy must be performed should symptoms referable to the upper gastrointestinal tract develop.

Animal Models. A murine model of autoimmune gastritis results from neonatal thymectomy (63).

Chronic Antral Gastritis

Definition. *Chronic antral gastritis* begins in the antrum and then extends proximally.

Demography. Antral gastritis accounts for most cases of chronic gastritis. The incidence of

Table 4-11

DIFFERENTIAL DIAGNOSIS OF HYPERGASTRINEMIA

Primary	
	Zollinger-Ellison syndrome
	Primary G-cell hyperplasia
	G-cell hyperresponsiveness
Secondary	
	Chronic atrophic gastritis
	Retained excluded antrum
	Acromegaly
	Gastric outlet obstruction
	Long-term therapy with H_2-receptor blockers or proton pump inhibitors
	Chronic renal failure
	Post vagotomy
	Hypercalcemia
	Systemic mastocytosis

antral gastritis varies from country to country and parallels that of gastric cancer. In countries with a high incidence of gastric cancer, such as Japan or Colombia, antral gastritis appears early in life and increases to affect approximately 90 percent of the population by age 60 (16).

Etiology. Major contributors to the development of antral gastritis are HP infection and a high salt and nitrite intake.

Clinical Features. Patients with antral gastritis frequently become symptomatic because of associated peptic ulcer disease rather than the gastritis per se. Some patients with antral gastritis have excessive excretion of acid, pepsin, and gastrin.

Gross Findings. The distribution of gross and endoscopic abnormalities varies, depending on whether the patient has the diffuse or multifocal form of chronic antral gastritis. Grossly and endoscopically, the stomach may appear normal or it may show evidence of mild gastritis as evidenced by the presence of mucosal erythema. When atrophic gastritis develops, the stomach becomes lined by a thin, smooth mucosa with loss of the rugal folds (fig. 4-21). In severe atrophy, the mucosa appears translucent with prominent submucosal veins showing through it.

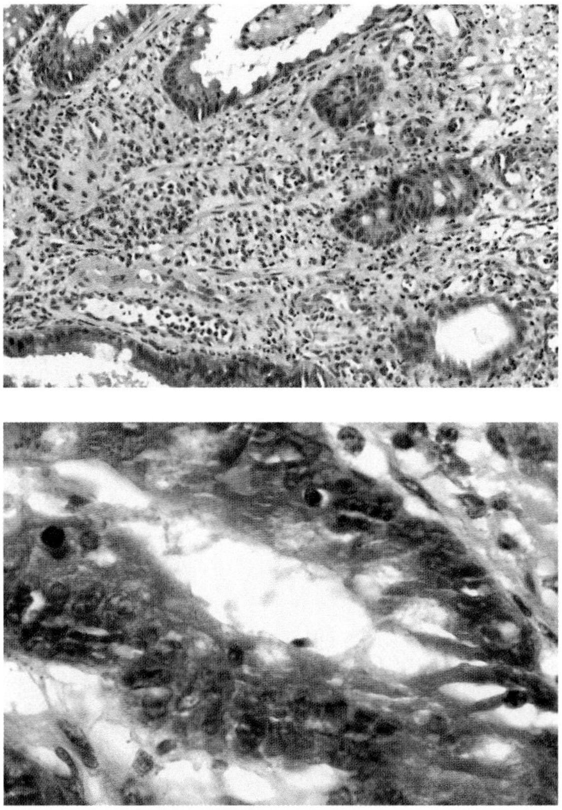

Figure 4-20

INTESTINAL METAPLASIA IN AUTOIMMUNE GASTRITIS

Areas of intestinal metaplasia (top) sometimes become dysplastic (bottom).

Microscopic Findings. Early, the inflammation is confined to the superficial gastric mucosa (superficial gastritis). Chronic superficial gastritis usually progresses to the next stage, chronic atrophic gastritis (figs. 4-22–4-24), over a period of 15 to 20 years (25). Inflammation extends deep into the mucosa, damaging the glands and causing chronic atrophic gastritis. Intestinal metaplasia develops. The inflammation is characterized by an intense, interstitial, mononuclear infiltrate that consists of mature lymphocytes and plasma cells (fig. 4-22). Follicular gastritis occurs frequently. The epithelium may appear mucin depleted and there may be elongation of the pits. All stages in the evolution of chronic gastritis often coexist within a single stomach.

The lesions first appear on the lesser curvature (25) and then on both sides of the antral-

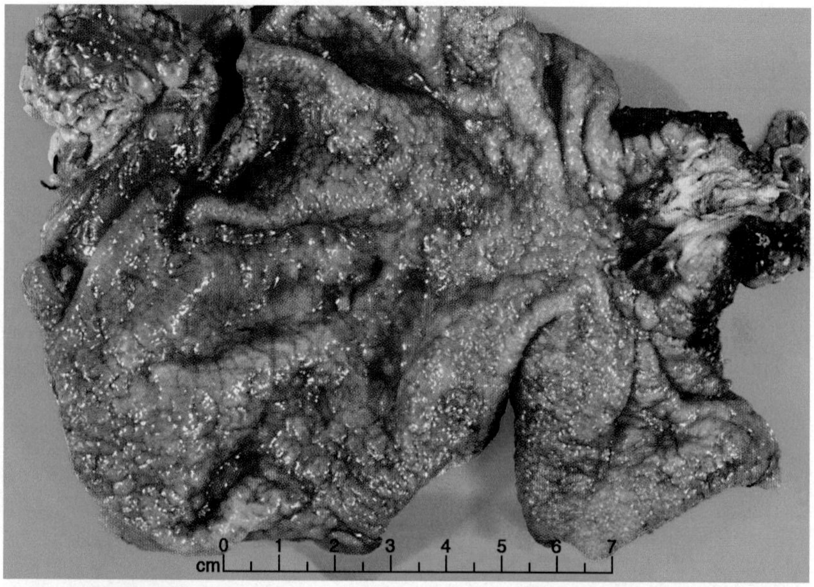

Figure 4-21

GROSS APPEARANCE OF CHRONIC GASTRITIS

Often, the rugal folds are lost and the mucosa appears thinned and diffusely hemorrhagic.

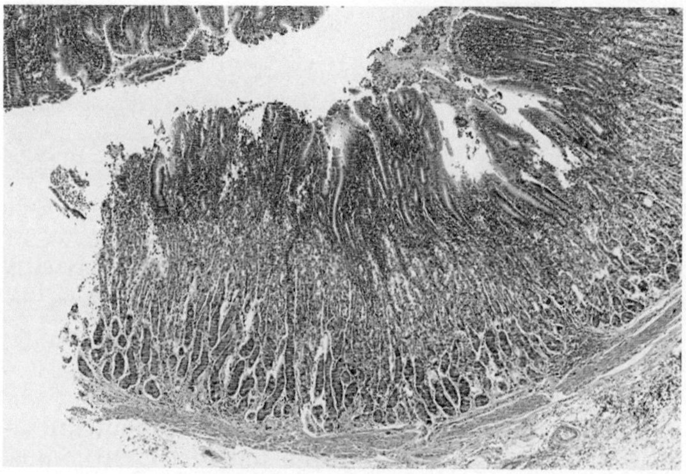

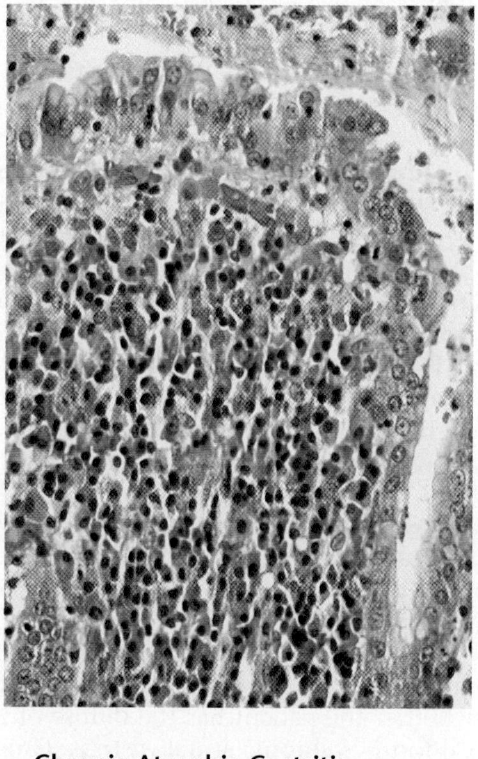

Figure 4-22

CHRONIC SUPERFICIAL GASTRITIS

Above: Early chronic gastritis shows restriction of the mononuclear cell infiltrate to the upper mucosa. The infiltrate appears as a dense basophilic band.

Right: Higher magnification of superficial epithelium and upper lamina propria shows a dense mononuclear cell infiltrate.

corporal junction in the shape of an inverted V. The inflammation spreads proximally along the lesser curvature. These atrophic foci coalesce and, in advanced cases, cover extensive mucosal areas. Eventually, the entire stomach may be replaced by metaplastic mucosa. Fundic glands never completely disappear, however, and pernicious anemia rarely develops.

Chronic Atrophic Gastritis

Definition. *Chronic atrophic gastritis* is characterized by a marked or complete loss of the specialized glands of either the antrum or the fundus, depending on the etiology of the underlying chronic gastritis.

Etiology. Chronic atrophic gastritis can affect patients with any form of chronic gastritis.

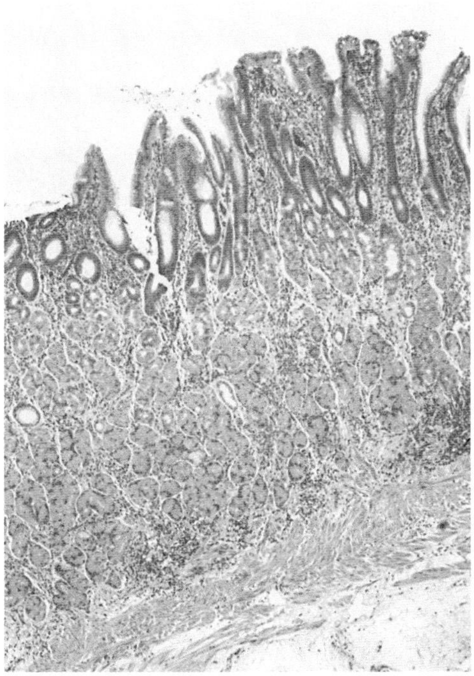

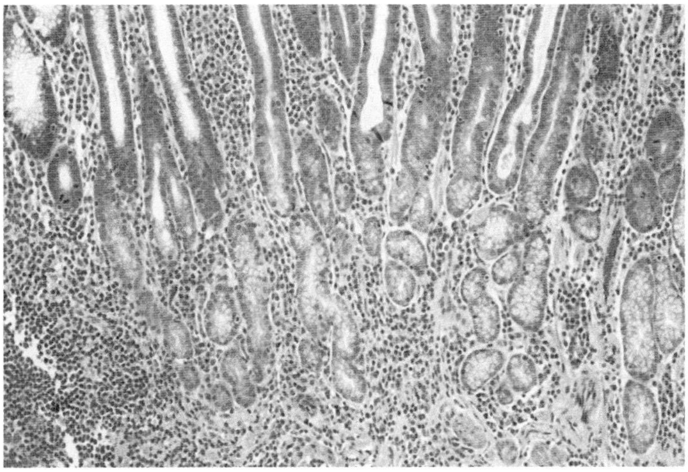

Figure 4-23

CHRONIC ATROPHIC GASTRITIS

Left: Inflammation is present throughout the full thickness of the mucosa.

Above: Higher magnification shows the inflammation in the lower portion of the mucosa and some evidence of glandular atrophy.

Microscopic Findings. The pathologic features of chronic atrophic gastritis depend on the etiology of the gastritis. Both chronic antral and autoimmune gastritis show a marked inflammatory infiltrate consisting of plasma cells, lymphocytes, and variable numbers of eosinophils in all levels of the lamina propria (fig. 4-22). The inflammation leads to cell dropout from both the pits and glands. The distance between individual glands increases and the reticulin fibers of the lamina propria collapse upon one another. Chronic progressive atrophy of the specialized epithelium results in an almost total loss of acid- and pepsinogen-secreting cells in chronic fundic gastritis and antral glands in chronic antral gastritis. As the mucosa thins, and as glands disappear, the bases of the pits come to rest on the muscularis mucosae. The muscularis mucosae becomes hypertrophic and sometimes splits, sending smooth muscle strands into the overlying lamina propria. In advanced atrophic gastritis, the glands disappear, the inflammation recedes, and the cellularity of the lamina propria returns to normal. Increasing degrees of atrophy are associated with cystic glandular dilatation, epithelial atypia, and metaplasia.

Metaplasia in Chronic Gastritis

Definition. Metaplasia is the replacement of one mature cell type for another. Five major types of metaplasia affect the gastric mucosa: intestinal, pyloric, pancreatic, ciliated, and squamous. These metaplasias are defined by the type of epithelium that replaces the gastric epithelium indigenous to a particular region. Thus, *pancreatic metaplasia* consists of pancreatic acini replacing part of the mucosa; *intestinal metaplasia* is the replacement of the gastric glands or pits by either small or large intestinal epithelium; pyloric metaplasia is the replacement of the oxyntic mucosa by antropyloric glands; *ciliated metaplasia* is the replacement of the gastric glands anywhere in the stomach by ciliated epithelium. This epithelium often lines cystically dilated glands. In the rarest form of metaplasia, *squamous metaplasia*, the gastric mucosa is replaced by squamous epithelium.

Demography. Metaplasias are very common in the stomach affected by chronic gastritis. The two most common forms of metaplasia are intestinal and pyloric metaplasia. The risk factors for developing intestinal metaplasia resemble those of gastric cancer in high-risk populations. Diets deficient in fresh fruits and vegetables

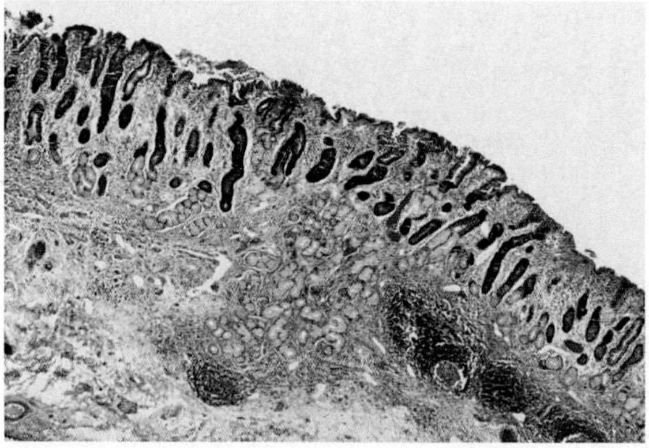

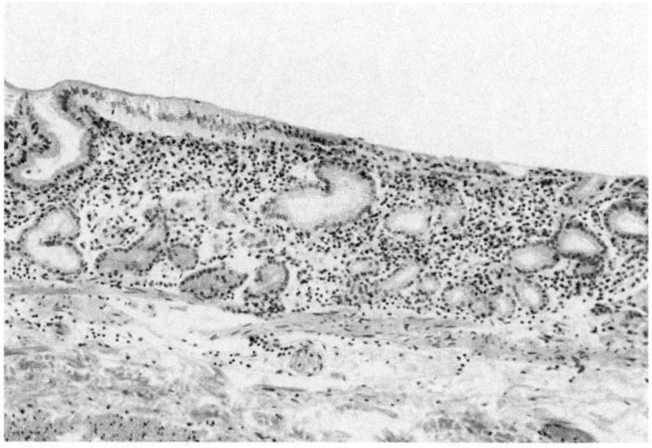

Figure 4-24

CHRONIC ATROPHIC GASTRITIS

Left: This patient has severe atrophic gastritis. Almost all of the glands have disappeared and the mucosa has become thinned.

Right: The end stage of chronic atrophic gastritis is gastric atrophy, as seen here. There are virtually no glands remaining and the mucosa is extremely thin. The normal architecture of the pits is also distorted.

combined with a high salt and nitrite intake are common to both conditions (25,73). Chronic gastritis precedes the metaplasia.

Etiology. The usual etiology of all the metaplasias is chronic gastritis.

Clinical Features. There are no specific clinical features associated with intestinal metaplasia. The clinical features are those of the underlying chronic gastritis.

Gross Findings. No specific gross findings are associated with the various forms of metaplasia. The gross features reflect the underlying disorder. Intestinal metaplasia usually occurs in an atrophic stomach.

Microscopic Findings. *Pyloric Metaplasia.* The earliest stage of pyloric metaplasia is the loss of the specialized cells in the oxyntic mucosa (fig. 4-25). Instead of giving rise to specialized peptic or parietal cells, the mucous neck cells give rise to a simpler, mucin-secreting glandular epithelium. Ultimately, the metaplastic glands become indistinguishable from the antral glands. Pyloric metaplasia first affects body glands closest to the antral junction, producing antral expansion at the expense of the body mucosa. It may be very difficult to determine whether pyloric metaplasia is present if the location of the biopsy is not known, especially if the patient has had a previous gastrectomy with removal of the distal stomach.

Ciliated Cell Metaplasia. Ciliated cells develop deep to areas of intestinal metaplasia. They develop in the mucosa of patients with gastric ulcers, dysplasia, or adenocarcinoma. The affected cells resemble antral rather than metaplastic intestinal cells since they make pepsinogen. As the atrophic, cystically dilated glands enlarge, the intrinsic pressure of the retained mucus results in cellular atrophy and ciliary disappearance.

Intestinal Metaplasia. Intestinal metaplasia is a common form of gastric metaplasia. It begins at the antral-corpus junction in a patchy, multifocal fashion, and then spreads both distally and proximally to involve the antrum and fundus. It occurs most frequently, and with the most intensity, along the lesser curvature, at the junction of the pylorus and corpus. This area of intestinal metaplasia frequently coexists with a band of metaplasia on both the anterior and posterior gastric walls at the junction of the pylorus and corpus. Gastric resections stained for alkaline phosphatase highlight the extent of the intestinal metaplasia (73).

Intestinal metaplasia originates from the mucous neck region. Intestinal goblet and absorptive cells replace the superficial epithelium. Initially, only the type of epithelium changes, but later the mucosal architecture acquires a small intestinal villiform shape, often exhibiting Paneth cells at the base of the glands.

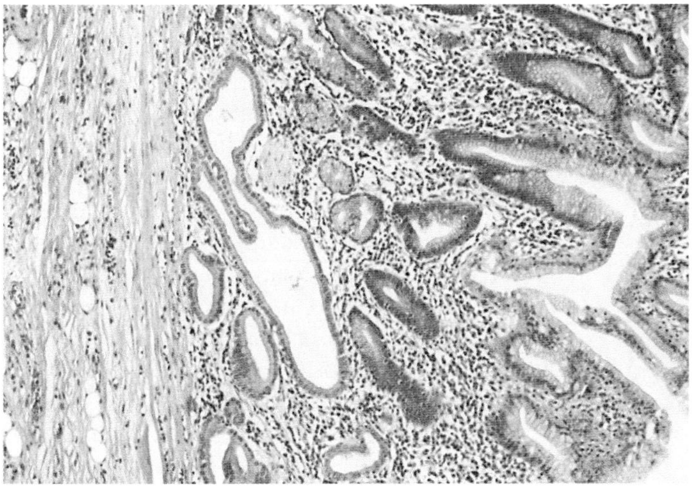

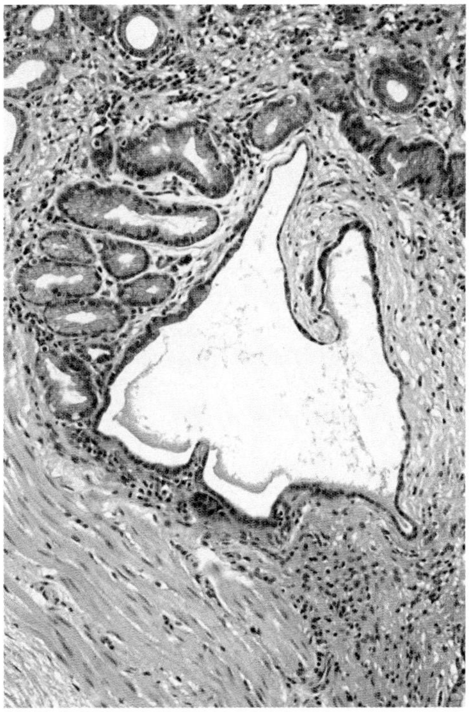

Figure 4-25

PYLORIC METAPLASIA

Above: This patient with chronic fundic gastritis had three types of metaplasia, two of which are shown here: pyloric and pancreatic.

Right: Higher magnification shows the cytologic features of both the pyloric and pancreatic metaplasias.

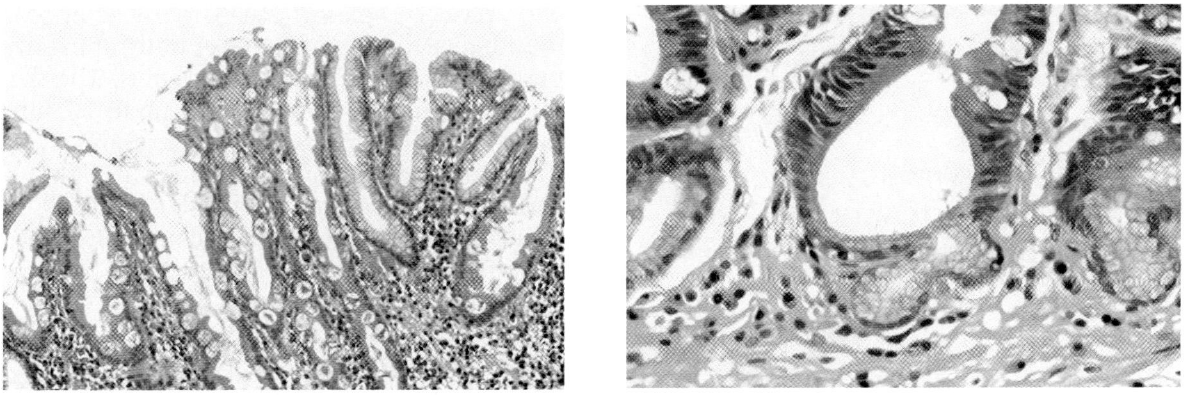

Figure 4-26

COMPLETE INTESTINAL METAPLASIA

Left: The superficial portion of the mucosa has glands with a normal pit lining as well as others lined by metaplastic cells. These cells resemble those seen in the small intestine.

Right: Higher magnification of the lower portion of an antral gland partially replaced by complete intestinal metaplasia.

Intestinal metaplasia is divided into two types that are often delineated by the use of special stains. The earliest metaplastic change, small intestinal metaplasia, consists of enterocytes with well-developed brush borders alternating with sialomucin-secreting goblet cells. Paneth cells may be present. This type of metaplasia is also referred to as type I, or complete, metaplasia (fig. 4-26) (49). The epithelium resembles normal small bowel with mucin-negative absorptive cells and Alcian blue–positive goblet cells.

In colonic metaplasia, both neutral and acidic mucin-producing goblet cells are present, but well-developed absorptive cells are absent. This type of metaplasia is also called type II, or incomplete, metaplasia (fig. 4-27). The absorptive cells lack a well-developed brush border

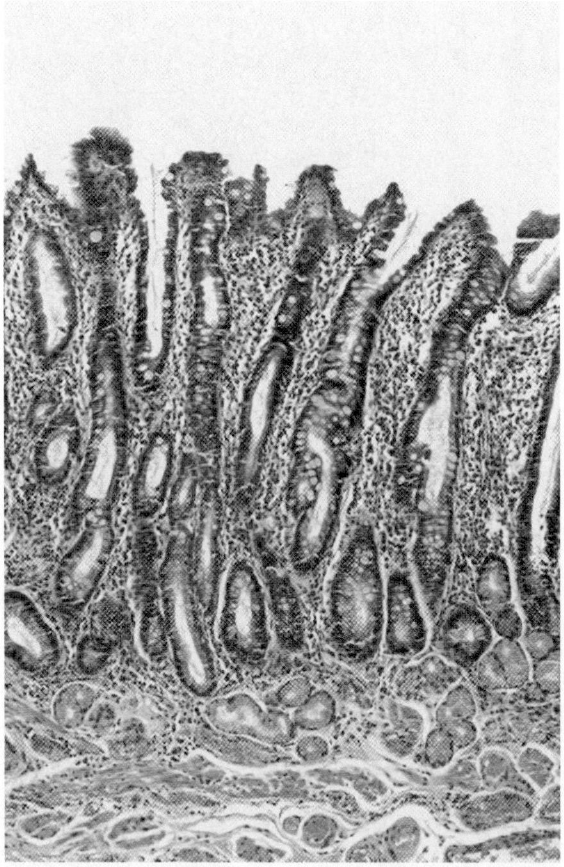

Figure 4-27

INCOMPLETE METAPLASIA

Incomplete metaplasia more closely resembles colon.

and the goblet cells contain sulfomucins (49). Paneth cells are absent.

The nature of the mucin present is best appreciated using special stains. Normal gastric surface epithelial cells contain periodic acid–Schiff (PAS)-positive, Alcian blue–negative neutral mucin. The sialomucin of complete intestinal metaplasia is PAS positive, Alcian blue positive at pH 2.5, but Alcian blue negative at pH 0.5 (fig. 4-28). It also stains with high iron diamine stains. Sulfomucin is weakly PAS positive but is Alcian blue positive at pH 2.5 and pH 0.5, and contains a high iron diamine content. Both types of metaplasia contain endocrine cells indigenous to either the small or large intestine.

Pancreatic Metaplasia. Metaplastic pancreatic acinar cells usually lie among, or at the bottom of, the gastric glands, where they form single or multiple nests and lobules (fig. 4-29). The metaplastic cells have a truncated pyramidal shape, a rim of deeply basophilic basal cytoplasm, and numerous small, acidophilic, weakly PAS-positive, refractile granules in the middle and apical cytoplasm (29). The nuclei appear round, relatively small, and centrally or basally located, with a prominent nucleolus. The size of each lobule varies, measuring up to 1.7 mm in diameter. The mucous cells intermingle with the acinar cells within the lobules (fig. 4-29). Larger lobules contain tubules or small cystic spaces reminiscent of dilated ductules. The metaplastic tissue continues into the gastric

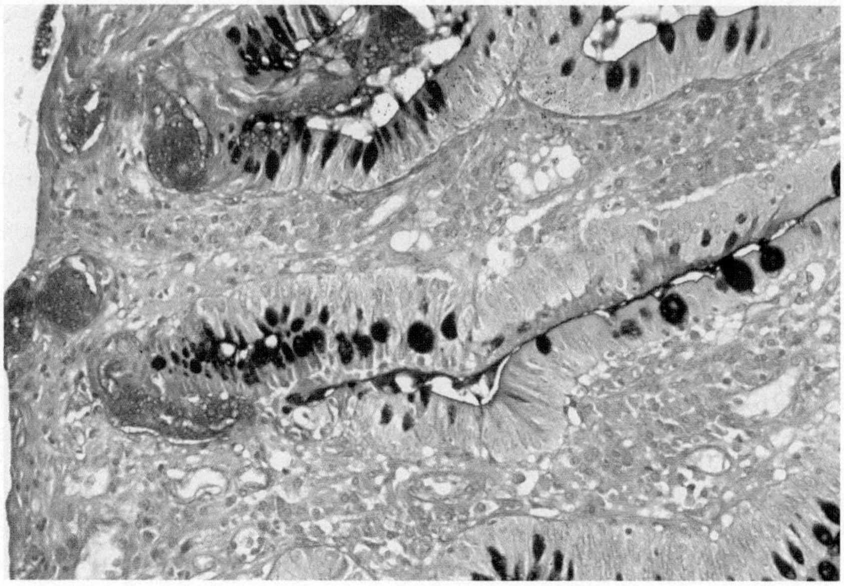

Figure 4-28

INTESTINAL METAPLASIA

Alcian blue–periodic acid–Schiff (PAS) stains both acidic (blue) and neutral (red) mucins.

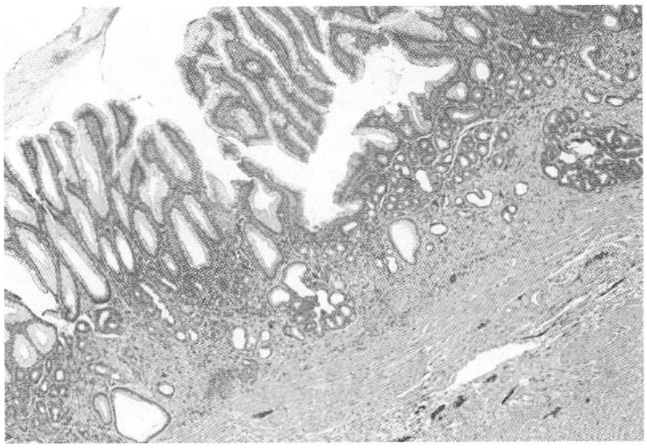

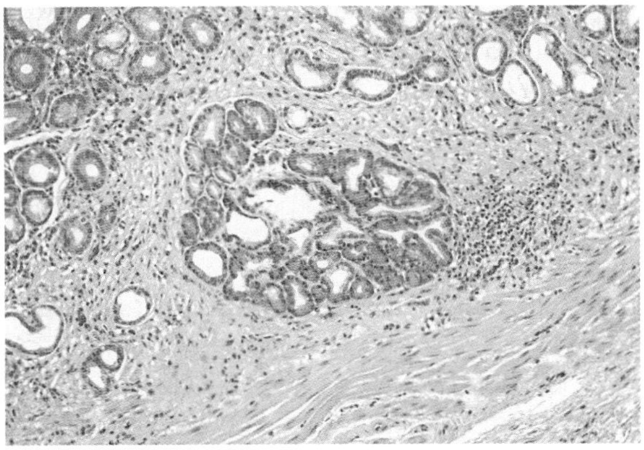

Figure 4-29

PANCREATIC METAPLASIA

Left: Low-power microscopy shows lobules of pancreatic cells among islands of pyloric metaplasia in a patient with chronic autoimmune gastritis.

Right: Medium-power view shows both pancreatic lobules and antral glands. This section is from the cardia.

glands. Less commonly, acinar cells lie scattered individually or in small foci among the gastric glands, sometimes with neuroendocrine cells. The presence of pancreatic metaplasia significantly correlates with the presence of chronic gastritis or intestinal and pyloric metaplasia in the adjacent mucosa (29).

Gastric pancreatic cells occur in 3.4 percent of pediatric patients. They occur in the antrum on a background of either normal or minimally inflamed mucosa, without coexisting atrophy or metaplasia (54). Pediatric lesions differ from those seen in adults due to the absence of the small duct-like structures present in adult cases. Additionally, pediatric cases contain amphicrine cells with a hybrid cell phenotype consisting of acinar and endocrine differentiation.

Differential Diagnosis. The main entity in the differential diagnosis is pancreatic heterotopia. Metaplastic pancreatic tissue differs from pancreatic heterotopia in that well-delineated nodules of pancreatic parenchyma, which often include ducts and their surrounding muscle fibers and islets, are absent. Heterotopic pancreas usually lies in the submucosa and muscularis propria, whereas pancreatic metaplasia lies in the basal mucosa and superficial submucosa.

Prognosis. The presence of intestinal metaplasia serves as a useful marker for the presence of chronic gastritis. The risk of gastric cancer increases in proportion to the extent of gastric intestinal metaplasia. The risk of dysplasia and carcinoma is higher in patients with type II (colonic) metaplasia than type I (small intestinal) metaplasia (70).

LYMPHOCYTIC GASTRITIS

Definition. *Lymphocytic gastritis,* also termed *chronic erosive gastritis,* is an intense, intraepithelial, T-cell infiltrate involving the gastric pits and surface epithelium. In its most severe form, lymphocytic gastritis is diagnosed as *varioliform gastritis*.

Demography. Lymphocytic gastritis affects 0.83 to 4.50 percent of individuals, mainly middle-aged and elderly men (40,41,78).

Etiology. The etiology is unknown. Recent findings provide compelling evidence that lymphocytic gastritis can occur as a manifestation of celiac sprue or sprue-like disease (26). It may occur as a part of the intraepithelial lymphocytosis seen in celiac sprue along with lymphocytic enteritis and lymphocytic colitis (80). Lymphocytic gastritis is also seen in patients with HP infection (64). Patients with gastric lymphoma have an increased prevalence of lymphocytic gastritis (60), as do patients with gastric adenocarcinoma (43). Associations with Menetrier's disease (39,71), human immunodeficiency virus (HIV) infection (80), Crohn's disease (77), and ticlopidine administration (18) have also been suggested. The entity may result from some form of autoimmune injury or hypersensitivity to some unknown antigen. It may also reflect the presence of some dietary substance, reflux of duodenal contents, or another as yet unidentified factor.

Clinical Features. Most patients with lymphocytic gastritis present with epigastric pain resembling peptic ulcer disease, dyspepsia, anorexia, and weight loss. It is possible that some symptoms result from the presence of concurrent disorders, such as celiac disease or lymphocytic colitis. Other patients remain asymptomatic.

Gross Findings. The characteristic endoscopic change is the presence of enlarged, bumpy, hyperemic, rugal folds, which result from alternating areas of mucosal hyperplasia and erosion. The enlarged folds bear variably sized and shaped nodules showing surface erosions, or aphthous ulcers surrounded by mucosal hyperemia (41). Thick mucus covers the irregularly thickened folds. The mucosal elevations persist after the erosions heal, and they may resemble sessile hyperplastic polyps. Lymphocytic gastritis in patients with celiac disease is more likely to involve the antrum whereas corpus-dominant lymphocytic gastritis is more likely to represent HP infection (42,80).

Radiographically, the enlarged gastric rugal folds exhibit distinctive 0.3- to 1.0-cm discrete nodules that appear as radiolucent halos; central barium flecks are distributed along their surfaces. These folds are most prominent in the gastric body and fundus and occasionally they extend into the antrum (78).

Microscopic Findings. Biopsies demonstrate areas of mucosal degeneration and regeneration coexisting with marked intraepithelial lymphocytosis (fig. 4-30). The epithelium shows loss of apical mucin and appears flattened. Mature intraepithelial T lymphocytes crowd the surface and the superficial pit epithelium (41,78). The process spares the deeper glands. Normally, there are 4 to 6 lymphocytes/100 epithelial cells, but in lymphocytic gastritis they are increased, with an average of 46 lymphocytes/100 epithelial cells. Usually, the number of epithelial lymphocytes is obviously increased and formal counting is not required. If counting is necessary, 25 lymphocytes/100 epithelial cells is considered the minimum for diagnosis (66). They display the CD8-positive cytotoxic suppressor T-lymphocyte phenotype. A clear halo often surrounds the lymphocytes. The gastric pits acquire a corrugated and dilated appearance and their lumens may contain abundant mucus admixed with polymorphonuclear leukocytes, forming pit abscesses. The lamina propria also contains increased numbers of lymphocytes. Lymphocytic gastritis may involve both the antrum and the body, and patients may develop glandular atrophy. In the severe form of the disease, extensive surface erosion occurs (fig. 4-31).

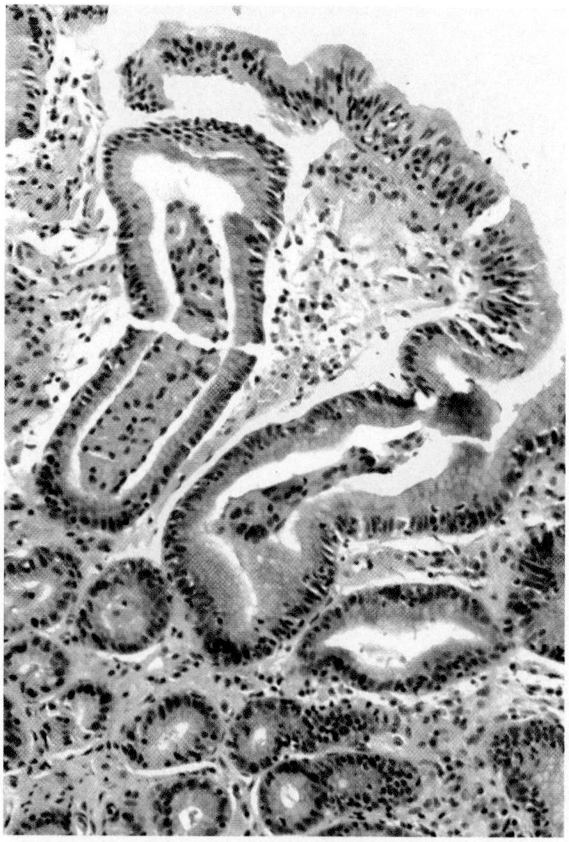

Figure 4-30

LYMPHOCYTIC GASTRITIS

The foveolar epithelium lining the surface and pits in the superficial portion of the mucosa is infiltrated by an increased number of lymphocytes. The epithelium appears mucin depleted.

Differential Diagnosis. The differential diagnosis of lymphocytic gastritis has two aspects. The first concerns the identity of the cells with the prominent halos. A number of entities mimic this pattern, including ECL hyperplasia, the presence of dystrophic goblet cells, or the presence of a

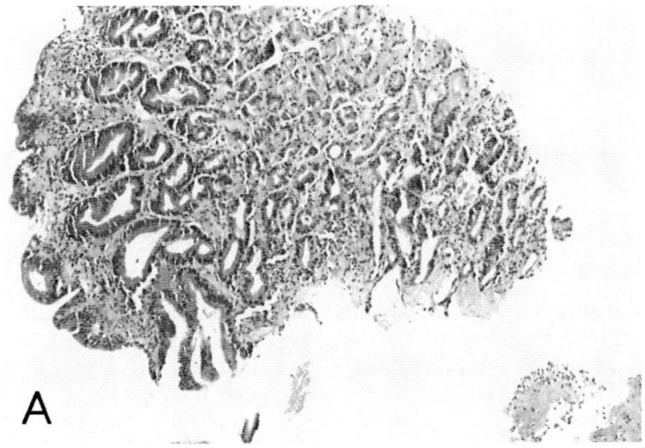

Figure 4-31

LYMPHOCYTIC GASTRITIS

A: Low-power magnification of a biopsy with regenerating glands and surface erosions.

B: The erosions are shown at higher magnification.

C: At high power, intraepithelial lymphocytosis with edema is seen in the lamina propria. The usual features of chronic gastritis are not present.

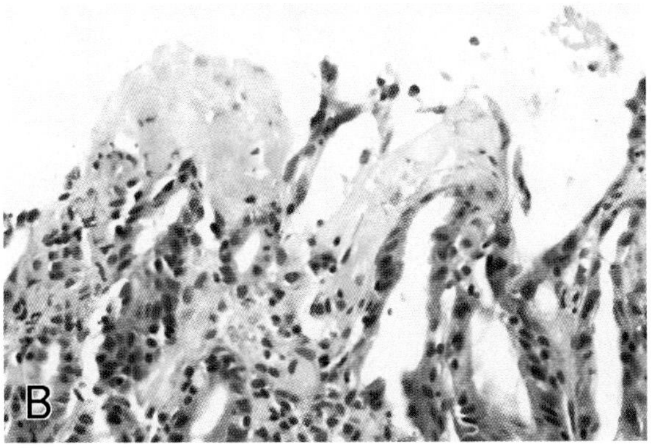

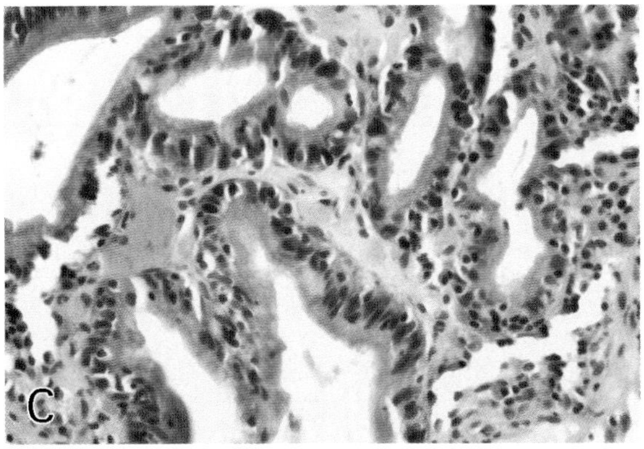

fixation artifact. Immunohistochemical stains for lymphocytic, endocrine, and epithelial cell lineages allow identification of the cell type.

Once the cells are identified as lymphocytes, then the differential diagnosis lies between a neoplastic and a benign lymphoid infiltrate. In the stomach, most neoplastic lymphoid lesions are MALT proliferations consisting of B cells. In contrast, lymphocytic gastritis results from an infiltration of T cells (Table 4-12). Unlike lymphocytic gastritis, MALT lymphoma shows glandular destruction and lymphoepithelial lesions, which are defined as a group of three or more lymphocytes clustered together in the epithelium. In addition, lymphoma cells infiltrate the muscularis mucosae and have a monocytoid morphology with Dutcher bodies.

Treatment and Prognosis. Associated celiac disease should be excluded. If present, it should be treated with dietary modification. If present, HP infection should be treated with antibiotics.

GRANULOMATOUS GASTRITIS

Granulomatous gastritis is any gastric disorder associated with the presence of granulomas. As used here, the term granuloma refers to a compact collection of mature mononuclear cells consisting of either macrophages or epithelioid cells that exist alone or are accompanied by necrosis or other inflammatory cells. Multinucleated giant cells may or may not be present.

Gastric granulomas complicate numerous conditions (Table 4-13). The specific diagnosis depends on the clinical history, histologic appearance, evaluation of other gastrointestinal and visceral lesions, and the use of special stains or other ancillary diagnostic techniques. The identification of granulomas within gastric biopsies often prompts the use of specialized stains for mycobacteria and fungi to rule out a treatable infection. Interpretation of the biopsy is facilitated by obtaining clinical Information with regard to: 1) travel history (to exclude certain infections); 2) the presence of associated disorders including Crohn's disease, immunosuppression, vasculitis, sarcoidosis, tuberculosis, or histoplasmosis; 3) the presence of an associated gastric carcinoma; 4) the use of illicit drugs; and 5) the presence of a sexually transmitted disease.

Table 4-12

DISTINCTIONS BETWEEN LYMPHOCYTIC GASTRITIS AND MUCOSA-ASSOCIATED LYMPHOID TISSUE (MALT) LYMPHOMA

Feature	Lymphocytic Gastritis	MALT Lymphoma
Lymphocyte number	Significantly increased	Significantly increased
Lymphocyte distribution	Single cells or linear arrangement in the epithelium	Clusters of three or more lymphocytes in the epithelium
Lymphocyte type and distribution	Mature T cells; similar intensity of distribution of lymphocytes in superficial and deep lamina propria	Monocytoid B cells; denser infiltrate in the deep lamina propria with predominant monocytoid B cells
Perilymphocytic halo	Common	Uncommon
Significant epithelial destruction	No	Yes
Cytologic atypia of the lymphocytes	No	Yes
Diffuse lamina propria infiltration and gland destruction by atypical lymphocytes	No	Yes

Table 4-13

GRANULOMATOUS DISEASES OF THE STOMACH

Infectious		
	Bacterial	Syphilis Mycobacterial infections Whipple's disease (rare) *Helicobacter pylori* (not typical)
	Fungal	Histoplasmosis South American blastomycosis Phycomycosis (rare) *Cryptococcus* Coccidioidomycosis
	Parasitic	Anisakidosis Schistosomiasis Strongyloidiasis
Idiopathic		Crohn's disease Sarcoidosis Isolated granulomatous gastritis
Miscellaneous		Chronic granulomatous disease of childhood Allergic granulomatosis and vasculitis Plasma cell granulomas Tumoral amyloidosis Rheumatoid nodules Gastric perforation Complications of peptic ulcer disease Malakoplakia Granulomas seen in drug addicts
Neoplastic		Associated with gastric carcinoma Associated with gastric lymphoma Langerhans cell histiocytosis
Foreign body granulomas		Food Suture Barium Retained surgical sponges or lap pads Talc Beryllium

The most common cause of granulomatous gastritis is Crohn's disease (30,68), followed by idiopathic isolated granulomatous gastritis in one study (30) or sarcoidosis in another (68). Most granulomas occur in the antrum.

Infections Associated with Granuloma Formation

Granulomatous gastritis develops in response to several types of infection, including tuberculosis, syphilis, and fungal and HP infections (Table 4-13). Granulomatous gastritis develops in 1.1 percent of HP cases (68). The granulomas form late in the disease course, after the host has become sensitized to the organism. Small sarcoid-like granulomas lie in the gastric lamina propria and sometimes HP organisms can be found within them. Macrophages may ingest antibody-coated bacteria, stimulating the histiocytic response. Granulomas are also seen in patients with parasitic infections, especially in anisakidosis and schistosomiasis. Additional features of each of these infections are more extensively discussed in chapter 10.

Gastric Crohn's Disease

Definition. *Crohn's disease* (CD) is an idiopathic inflammatory disease that affects the gastrointestinal tract from the mouth to the anus. It is extensively discussed in chapter 15.

Demography. The stomach is the principal location of CD in less than 4 percent of patients, but abnormalities may be appreciated endoscopically in up to 15 percent (48). Microscopic inflammation is more common and may be detected in 8 to 75 percent of patients (65,79). In 50 percent of the patients, the inflammation is considered to be direct involvement by CD. Gastric mucosal granulomas can be detected in approximately 10 percent of cases (79). Patients with gastric involvement often have duodenal involvement as well.

Clinical Features. Upper gastrointestinal pain, nausea, and vomiting result from gastric outlet obstruction. The lesions may simulate a gastric malignancy clinically. Rare patients present with giant gastric ulcers.

Gross Findings. Endoscopic, radiographic, and gross abnormalities include mucosal granularity and nodularity with cobblestoning; multiple aphthous, linear, or serpiginous ulcers; thickened antral folds; and antral narrowing. Hypoperistalsis and duodenal strictures are present in patients with severe gastric CD. Extensive gastric involvement may resemble linitis plastica due to the prominent intramural thickening and rigidity, and luminal narrowing (33). Radiographically, the changes localize to the antrum, progressing to a "ram's horn" or "shofar" configuration.

Microscopic Findings. Patients with CD gastritis have a pattern of patchy and focally active gastritis with acute inflammation in the pits (pit abscesses) or glands, producing a pattern similar to the focal active colitis pattern characteristic of CD colitis (68). Granulomas affect 14 to 33 percent of patients. The focality of the process should alert one to the possibility of CD, since focal inflammation is uncommon in antral biopsies from patients with HP infections. There are often focal, subepithelial, dense accumulations of macrophages throughout the mucosa. A diffuse mononuclear cell infiltrate in the lamina propria is associated with acute gastric pit inflammation and gastric gland atrophy. This contrasts with a bland, noninflammatory background observed in patients with sarcoidosis (68). Normal mucosa separates the areas of patchy, chronic, active gastritis, unless the patient has HP infection. Lymphoid aggregates are also common; they are found in all layers of the bowel wall, contrasting with follicular gastritis, which remains restricted to the area of the mucosal-muscularis mucosae junction. A prominent lymphoplasmacytic infiltrate often surrounds the granulomas. Neural hyperplasia may also be present. Severe cases exhibit transmural inflammation, fissures, and typical undermining ulcers as well as prominent lymphoid follicles, serosal and submucosal fibrosis, and possibly, sarcoid-like granulomas (fig. 4-32).

The diagnosis of gastric CD is easily made in the presence of florid disease and in the setting of disease elsewhere in the gut. The diagnosis is more difficult, however, when gastric involvement is the first manifestation of the disease. The diagnosis should be considered in patients without known CD in whom irregularly distributed inflammatory foci are seen in the gastric mucosa with the presence of glandular abscesses, focal fibrosis, and lymphoid proliferation in the lamina propria, particularly in the absence of HP infection. An ulcer that does not respond to antisecretory therapy should suggest the possibility of gastric CD.

Differential Diagnosis. The differential diagnosis includes any of the entities listed in Table 4-13. The three main diagnostic entities are shown in Table 4-14. The other major differential diagnosis is with HP infection, since both disorders may present with predominantly antral disease, and both may exhibit granulomas, acute inflammation, and chronic inflammation. The focality of the lesions in CD, however, contrasts with the diffuse nature of HP gastritis.

Treatment and Prognosis. Protein pump inhibitors may provide some symptomatic improvement; otherwise, medical therapy is as for intestinal disease. Occasionally, resection is required for gastric outlet obstruction or intractable symptomatic fistulas.

Foreign Body Granuloma

Definition. *Foreign body granulomas* are collections of histiocytes and giant cells that surround foreign material.

Demography. Foreign body granulomas usually affect postsurgical patients, patients with parasitic infections, or those with ulcerating diseases.

Etiology. In patients with parasitic infections, histiocytes and giant cells surround either the

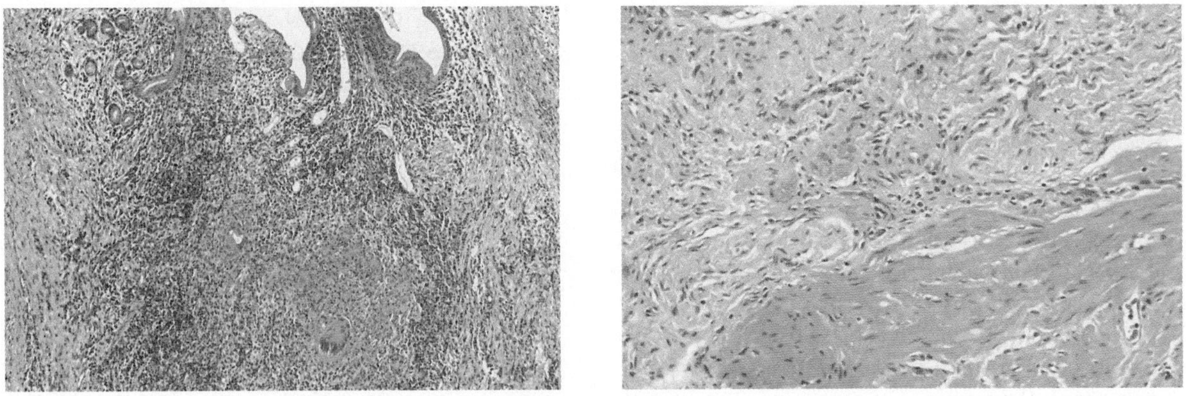

Figure 4-32

GASTRIC CROHN'S DISEASE

Left: Low-power magnification shows focal inflammation and a granuloma surrounded by a dense lymphoplasmacytic infiltrate.

Right: Sometimes there is marked neural hyperplasia in the submucosa or the myenteric plexus.

Table 4-14

COMPARISON OF GASTRIC CROHN'S DISEASE, SARCOIDOSIS, AND ISOLATED GRANULOMATOUS GASTRITIS

Features	Crohn's Disease	Sarcoidosis	Isolated Granulomatous Gastritis
Major location of changes	Antrum	Antrum	Antrum
Focal active gastritis	Present	Absent	Absent
Isolated lymphoid aggregates	Present	Absent	Absent
Fissures and undermining ulcers	Present	Absent	Absent
Evidence of other gastrointestinal involvement	Usually present	May be present	Absent
Compact granulomas	Present	Present	Present
Associated nonspecific inflammation	Present	Present	Usually absent

larvae (as in anisakidosis) or ova (as in schistosomiasis) and form *foreign body granulomas*. *Suture granulomas* occur in the anastomotic sites in postsurgical patients. *Food granulomas* occur in individuals with current or past mucosal ulcerating diseases. The small mucosal defects allow gastric juice and small food particles access to deeper layers of the gastric wall. The gastric acid produces partial necrosis, increasing the size of the mucosal defect, thereby allowing more food to enter. *Barium granulomas* also affect the stomach.

Microscopic Findings. Food granulomas (fig. 4-33) appear as amorphous, eosinophilic, granulomatous masses, sometimes containing vegetable cells recognizable by their thick, bricklike cell walls. Palisading epithelioid histiocytes and foreign body giant cells surround the food particles. Food granulomas can undergo secondary fibrosis or calcification. Severe mucosal fibrosis may result in pyloric stenosis.

Suture granulomas are discovered incidentally or present as masses consisting of variable fibrosis, abscess formation, and granulomatous responses (fig. 4-34). When nonresorbable sutures are used, residual suture material is evident.

In barium granulomas, collections of macrophages containing refractile, greenish gray, foamy cytoplasm are typically seen. Nodules may measure up to 2 cm in diameter.

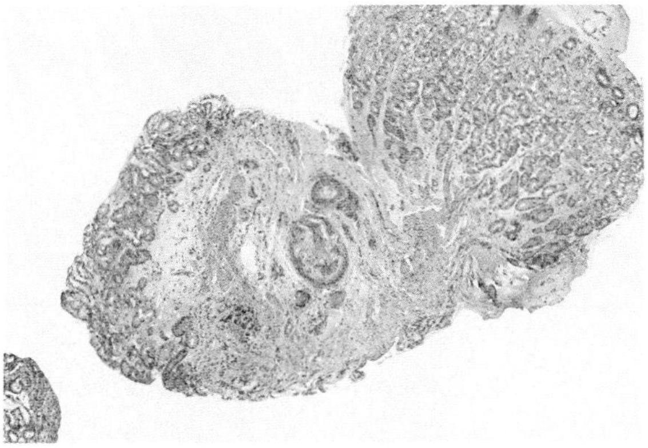

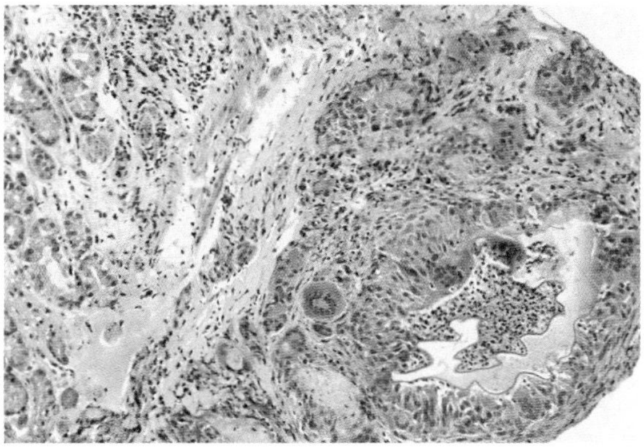

Figure 4-33

FOOD GRANULOMA

Left: Low-power magnification shows a mass-like lesion in the submucosa. The overlying mucosa is inflamed.

Right: Higher magnification of the granuloma with a central eosinophilic coagulum surrounded by palisading epithelioid cells.

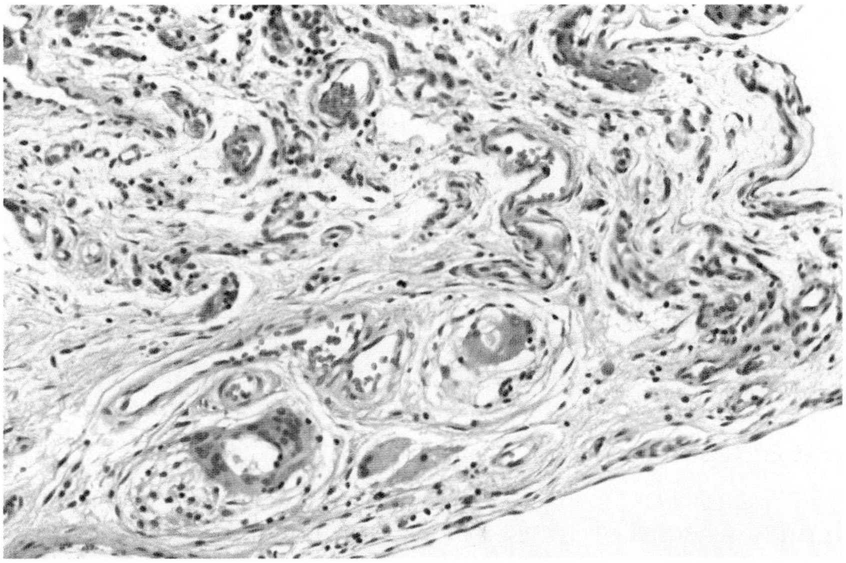

Figure 4-34

SUTURE GRANULOMA

Giant cells surround suture remnants in this biopsy taken from an anastomotic line.

Differential Diagnosis. The differential diagnosis includes all the entities listed in Table 4-13.

Granulomatous Gastritis Associated with Malignancy

Definition. *Granulomatous gastritis associated with malignancy* is a granulomatous response that forms in the gastric mucosa and the draining gastric lymph nodes of individuals with gastric malignancies (epithelial and hematologic).

Etiology. The granulomas presumably result from an immune response to the tumor.

Gross Findings. This form of granulomatous gastritis has no specific gross features. The gross findings reflect those of the malignancy, not the granuloma.

Microscopic Findings. The granulomas typically lie in the basal part of the non-neoplastic mucosa (fig. 4-35). They also surround, or intermingle with, infiltrating tumor. The granulomas resemble those of sarcoid and may affect all levels of the gastric wall.

Prognosis and Treatment. The treatment is for the cancer. The impact of the presence of the granulomas on the cancer is uncertain.

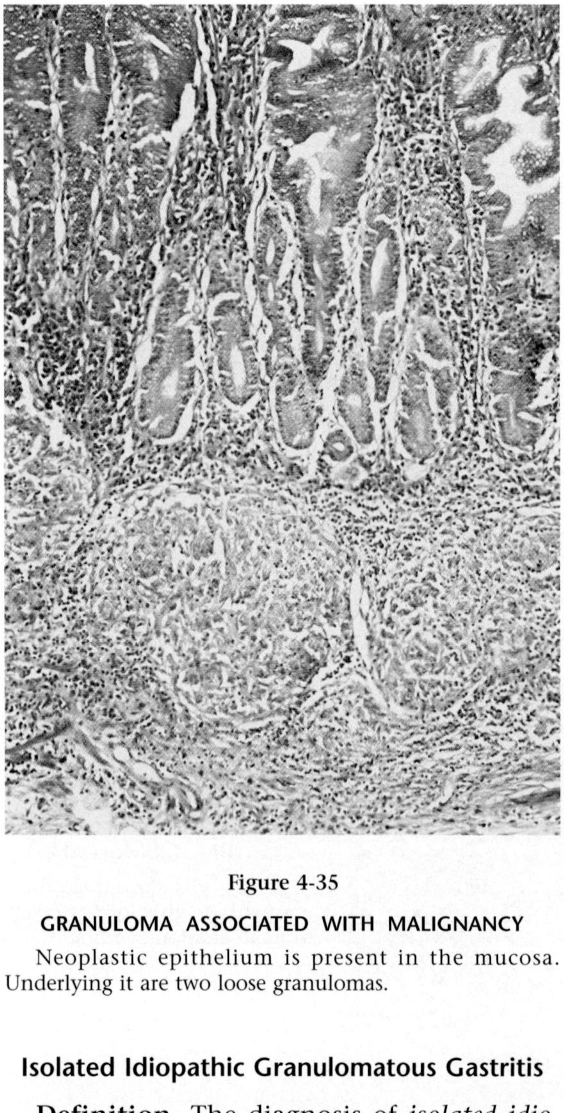

Figure 4-35

GRANULOMA ASSOCIATED WITH MALIGNANCY

Neoplastic epithelium is present in the mucosa. Underlying it are two loose granulomas.

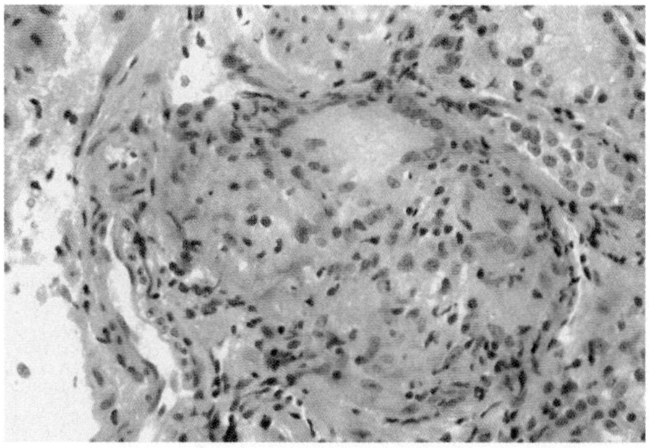

Figure 4-36

ISOLATED GRANULOMATOUS DISEASE

This patient had no evidence of sarcoidosis, Crohn's disease, or other explanation for granulomas.

Isolated Idiopathic Granulomatous Gastritis

Definition. The diagnosis of *isolated idiopathic granulomatous gastritis* is made when other entities associated with granuloma formation have been excluded. Excluding other entities that cause granulomas is increasingly difficult, since HP infections are associated with granuloma formation. It is assumed that the granulomatous inflammation that coexists with chronic active gastritis results from HP.

Demography. The incidence depends on how frequently other diseases can be excluded, most notably gastric CD, sarcoidosis, or HP infection.

Etiology. This is unknown. Controversy exists as to whether isolated idiopathic granulomatous gastritis represents a distinctive entity or whether it represents an isolated or limited form of gastric sarcoidosis or CD (33,68).

Clinical Features. Symptomatic patients usually present over age 40 years with epigastric pain, weight loss, and vomiting secondary to pyloric obstruction. Approximately 25 percent of patients develop hematemesis.

Gross Findings. The predominant findings consist of antral narrowing and rigidity.

Microscopic Findings. The pathologic changes of idiopathic granulomatous gastritis parallel those seen in sarcoidosis and CD (fig. 4-36). Transmural, noncaseating granulomatous inflammation is present predominantly in the antrum. The inflammation and fibrosis rarely extend beyond the mucosa. Ulcers similar to peptic ulcers develop, but the slit-shaped ulcers and fissures typical of CD are absent. In a third of cases, regional lymph nodes become involved.

Differential Diagnosis. In a review, Shapiro et al. (68) analyzed all cases of granulomatous gastritis occurring at the Cleveland Clinic between 1975 and 1994, and concluded the following: 1) in most cases of granulomatous gastritis a diagnosis of CD or sarcoidosis could be established; 2) the background inflammatory pattern is helpful in suggesting a diagnostic category for granulomatous gastritis; 3) granulomatous gastritis is not associated with HP per se; however, if known cases of CD and sarcoid are excluded, an association with HP infection and granulomatous gastritis cannot be ruled out; and 4) isolated idiopathic granulomatous gastritis, if it exists, is extremely rare.

Table 4-15

MORPHOLOGIC AND CLINICAL MANIFESTATIONS OF GIANT GASTRIC FOLDS

	Surface Mucous Cells	Body Glandular Component	Gastrin Level	Ulcers	Protein Loss	ECL[a] Hyperplasia
Zollinger-Ellison syndrome	Normal	Hyperplastic	Elevated	Present	Absent	Present
Hypertrophic hypersecretory gastropathy	Hyperplastic	Hyperplastic	Normal	Present	Absent	Absent
Menetrier's disease	Hyperplastic	Atrophy	Normal	Absent	Present	Absent
Hypertrophic hypersecretory protein-losing gastropathy	Hyperplastic	Hyperplastic	Normal	Absent	Present	Absent

[a]ECL = enterochromaffin-like.

COLLAGENOUS GASTRITIS

Definition. *Collagenous gastritis* is a characteristic thickening of the subepithelial collagen table lying beneath the surface foveolar cells, coexisting with gastritis. It resembles the subepithelial fibrosis that develops in the small intestine (collagenous sprue) and in the colon (collagenous colitis).

Demography. Collagenous gastritis is a rare form of gastritis. It develops in the gastric corpus, in the setting of chronic gastritis.

Etiology. The etiology of collagenous gastritis is unknown and its relationship to collagenous sprue and collagenous colitis remains to be defined.

Gross Findings. Grossly, the gastric corpus may appear nodular and erythematous.

Microscopic Findings. Biopsies reveal patchy, chronic, active gastritis with a striking focal thick band of subepithelial collagen, which measures 20 to 75 mm in thickness.

HYPERTROPHIC GASTROPATHIES

Four well-defined hypertrophic gastropathies exist (Table 4-15). Distinct clinical features define each syndrome, although several entities show some overlap (83,91). Individual patients may lack classic clinical, laboratory, or histologic features. Additionally, some patients with hypertrophic gastric folds are not easily classified and the diagnosis requires knowledge of the histologic, clinical, endoscopic, and radiologic findings.

Menetrier's Disease

Definition. *Menetrier's disease* is characterized by the four following criteria: 1) a pure foveolar cell hyperplasia that creates giant mucosal folds predominantly affecting the fundus and sometimes affecting the antrum; 2) low acid levels; 3) mucosal protein loss; and 4) histology that consists of gastric pit hyperplasia and oxyntic glandular atrophy.

Demography. Menetrier's disease is the most common hypertrophic gastropathy, accounting for two thirds of cases. It usually affects men (three times more frequently than women) in the 4th to 6th decades of life (83). Menetrier's disease sometimes affects children and, very rarely, young infants.

Etiology. The etiology is generally unknown. In children, allergies, autoimmune reactions, and infections may play an etiologic role, with proteins, such as those in cow's milk, often precipitating the disease. In pediatric cases and in some adult cases, cytomegalovirus infection is suspected as the etiologic agent (87). There may also be a relationship to lymphocytic gastritis (92). Although not generally considered to be a genetic disorder, familial cases do exist, leading some to suggest that the disease is inherited in both an autosomal dominant and an autosomal recessive fashion. Patients with Menetrier's disease may have a marked increase in the expression of transforming growth factor-alpha (TGFα) (84) or epidermal growth factor (EGF). Data from animal models suggest that growth factors may play an etiologic role.

Clinical Features. *Adults.* Menetrier's disease begins insidiously, and gradually becomes increasingly symptomatic. Signs and symptoms characteristically wax and wane, so that different features come and go. Symptoms include epigastric pain, bloating, anorexia, vomiting,

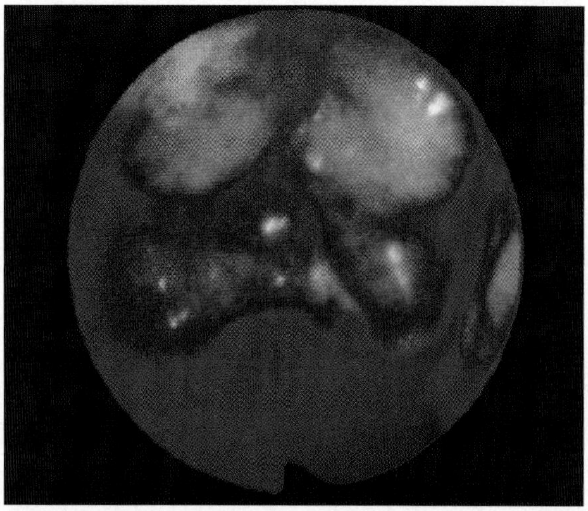

Figure 4-37

MENETRIER'S DISEASE

Endoscopic appearance of enlarged gastric folds.

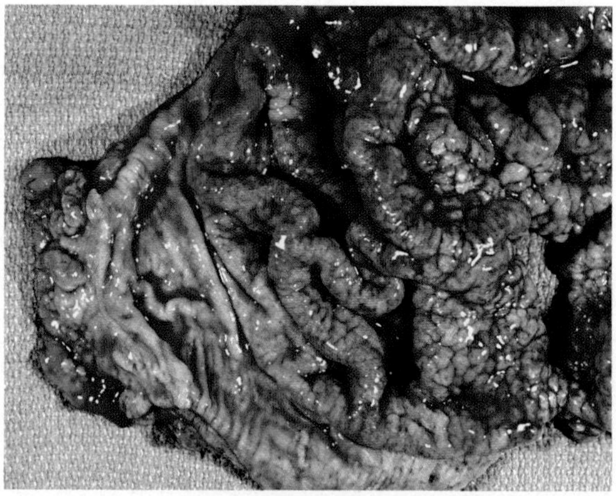

Figure 4-38

MENETRIER'S DISEASE

Opened resection specimen shows thickening of the gastric folds, especially proximally.

weight loss, diarrhea, peripheral edema, and bleeding. Some patients describe a rash and food hypersensitivity. There is diffuse enlargement of the gastric folds, especially proximally, with marked mucus hypersecretion. The latter leads to severe hypoproteinemia, especially hypoalbuminemia and hypochlorhydria, and a tendency to develop peripheral edema. Eosinophilia affects up to 61 percent of adults. Laboratory findings include anemia, low IgG levels, and low total protein levels.

Extraintestinal phenomena include severe or recurrent pulmonary infections and pulmonary edema. Some patients show an unusually frequent association with coexisting thrombotic cardiovascular disease, predisposing them to myocardial infarcts, pulmonary emboli, small bowel infarcts, and venous thromboses occurring at a young age. Other associations include coexisting esophageal or gastric cancer, and anorexia nervosa. Not all manifestations of the disease are present at the same time.

Children. In young children, the disease is usually self-limited, with spontaneous reversal of protein loss (85,90). This contrasts with the adult form of the disease that may be so prolonged and severe that it may require gastrectomy. Marked periorbital or facial edema affects 88 percent of children. Emesis, abdominal pain, and anorexia are other common symptoms. Frank upper gastrointestinal bleeding develops in only 12 percent of children contrasting with 20 to 40 percent of adults. The antrum can be markedly involved (87), contrasting with the adult form of the disease. Affected children develop atypical lymphocytosis and transient hepatosplenomegaly, and have cytomegalovirus demonstrable in the blood, urine, and gastric tissues (87). Coexisting HP and cytomegalovirus infections occur.

Gross Findings. Grossly, the stomach exhibits a bulky, thickened wall characterized by marked enlargement of the mucosal folds. Mucosal folds vary from 4 mm to 4 cm in height and resemble cerebral convolutions. The disease predominantly affects the body and fundus, generally sparing the antrum (figs. 4-37, 4-38), except in children where the reverse is true. Thick mucin may cover the mucosa. In severe disease, the lesions may extend into the antrum.

Radiographic criteria for diagnosing Menetrier's disease include: 1) thick, nonuniform, tortuous, angular gastric folds; 2) ragged, nodular, crinkled and spiculated appearance of the greater curvature; 3) a thickened gastric wall; and 4) a fine reticulated barium pattern produced by irregular mucus mixing (fig. 4-39). Motility disturbances include delayed gastric emptying, pylorospasm with antral narrowing, and sluggish peristalsis.

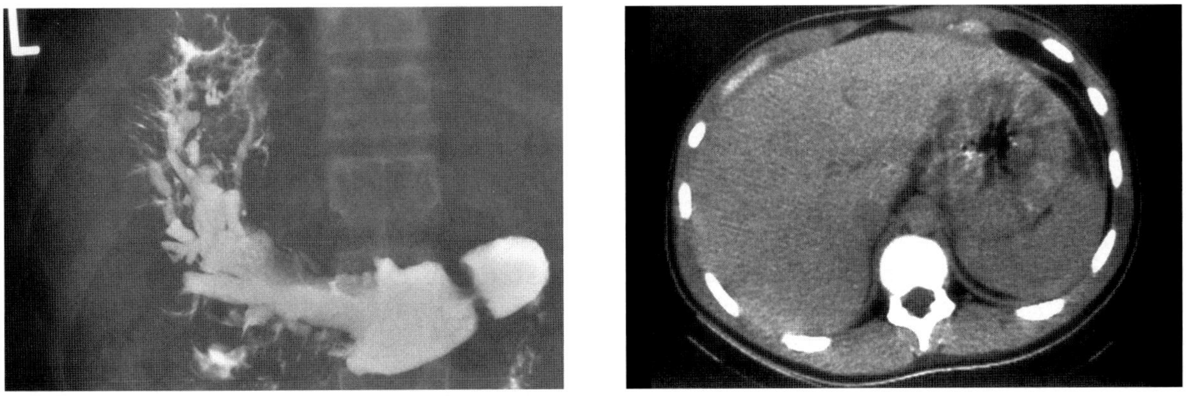

Figure 4-39

MENETRIER'S DISEASE

Left: An image from a single-contrast upper gastrointestinal radiograph shows marked thickening and irregularity of the folds in the proximal portion of the stomach relatively sparing the antrum. The finding is classic for Menetrier's disease but not completely specific. Zollinger-Ellison syndrome, in particular, may show similar findings.

Right: Computerized tomography (CT) scan demonstrates the proximal fold thickening.

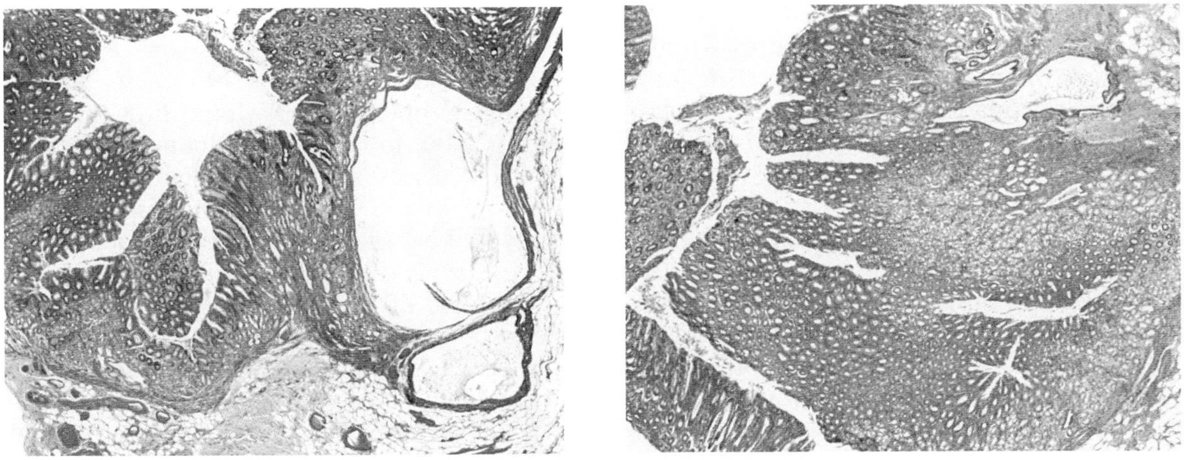

Figure 4-40

MENETRIER'S DISEASE

Left: The mucosal folds appear thickened due to an expansion of the gastric pits. Often, there are prominent cysts that extend into the submucosa, as in this case.

Right: Mucosal expansion.

Microscopic Findings. The most striking histologic features of Menetrier's disease are foveolar hyperplasia and glandular atrophy. Foveolar cells that maintain their normal polarity line the elongated, tortuous, corkscrew-shaped and dilated, mucin-filled gastric pits. The mucus-secreting cells in the elongated pits extend to the base of the mucosa. The glands become variably cystic (fig. 4-40) and may extend into the superficial submucosa, producing gastritis cystica profunda. Superficial edema and variable, but usually minimal, degrees of inflammation are present in the lamina propria. The inflammatory infiltrate consists of neutrophils, eosinophils, lymphocytes, and occasional plasma cells. Lymphangiectasia may develop. The muscularis mucosae becomes hypertrophic, hyperplastic, distorted, and fragmented, sending smooth muscle extensions into the lamina propria. The degree of protein loss correlates with the pit hyperplasia, edema, and superficial inflammation.

As the disease runs its course, an atrophic mucosa with intestinal metaplasia develops, with the loss of the superficial inflammation and edema. Granulomas develop in some patients with spontaneous disease resolution. Progressive hypochlorhydria results from gradual replacement of the oxyntic glandular compartment by expanding pit compartments, thereby compromising the parietal cell mass and resulting in decreased acid secretion.

Differential Diagnosis. Mucosal biopsies document the presence or absence of classic forms of the hypertrophic hyperplastic gastropathies and rule out the presence of tumors that expand the gastric wall. Gastric biopsies, however, are inadequate for complete diagnosis since all giant fold disorders share an expanded mucosa and it is difficult to obtain a full thickness mucosal biopsy unless giant forceps are used. In Menetrier's disease, a biopsy usually contains either pure foveolae, suggesting focal foveolar hyperplasia or the top of a hyperplastic polyp, or else the mucosa appears normal. The presence of the hyperplastic foveolar cells in a biopsy alone is insufficient to establish a diagnosis of Menetrier's disease since foveolar cell hyperplasia occurs in other settings. The differential diagnosis usually includes localized mucosal expansions, including those seen at the margins of a peptic ulcer, the prolapsed expansile mucosa of a gastroenterostomy stoma, reflux gastropathy, and some gastric polyps, particularly hyperplastic polyps and polyps found with the Canada-Cronkhite syndrome (see chapter 16). Biopsies of all of these lesions may look identical, particularly when they are superficial in nature. For this reason, it is important to correlate the histologic findings with the typical clinical syndrome.

In adults, Menetrier's disease may also resemble lymphoma, acid hypersecretory states, or lymphocytic gastritis, especially since about one third of patients with lymphocytic gastritis present with weight loss, anorexia, protein loss, and peripheral edema. Patients with Menetrier's disease, however, lack marked intraepithelial lymphocytosis.

Treatment and Prognosis. Menetrier's disease may undergo spontaneous remission, especially in children, and may also improve following antisecretory therapy. The associated protein-losing gastropathy may require specific nutritional support. Surgery may be necessary in intractable cases. Five percent of patients develop carcinoma; some concurrently, others after the diagnosis of Menetrier's disease. It is likely that the patients who develop cancer do so from the associated chronic gastritis rather than the underlying Menetrier's disease, although the associated elevated growth factor levels may play a role in cancer development.

Animal Models. A gastropathy resembling Menetrier's disease occurs in transgenic mice overexpressing TGFα (88).

Zollinger-Ellison Syndrome

Definition. *Zollinger-Ellison syndrome* (ZES) combines peptic ulceration and hypergastrinemia. It is also known as *hypersecretory hypergastrinemia with protein loss*.

Demography. ZES affects 0.1 percent of all patients with duodenal ulcer disease. Studies among European populations show an incidence of 0.2 to 0.4 cases/million population/year. The disease occurs in patients ranging in age from 7 to 90 years (89), with most patients diagnosed between the 3rd and 5th decades of life. There is no sex predominance.

Etiology. ZES results from gastrin hypersecretion by gastrinomas, endocrine cell tumors located in the pancreas or in the bowel wall, particularly in the first portion of the duodenum. Less commonly, gastrin is hypersecreted from severe G-cell hyperplasia (85,93). In approximately 20 percent of cases, the pancreatic neoplasm is part of multiple endocrine neoplasia syndrome type 1.

Pathophysiology. Excessive gastrin production serves as the stimulus for increased gastric acid secretion and it is the excessive acid production that produces many of the clinical features of the syndrome. Gastrin is a trophic hormone with multiple cellular targets, the major one of which is the parietal cell. These cells become hyperplastic, secreting acid and completing a negative feedback loop by inhibiting G-cell secretion. Gastrin also increases the growth of chief cells, ECL cells, and foveolar epithelium. A marked parietal and chief cell hyperplasia (83, 91) expands the gastric glands, causing rugal

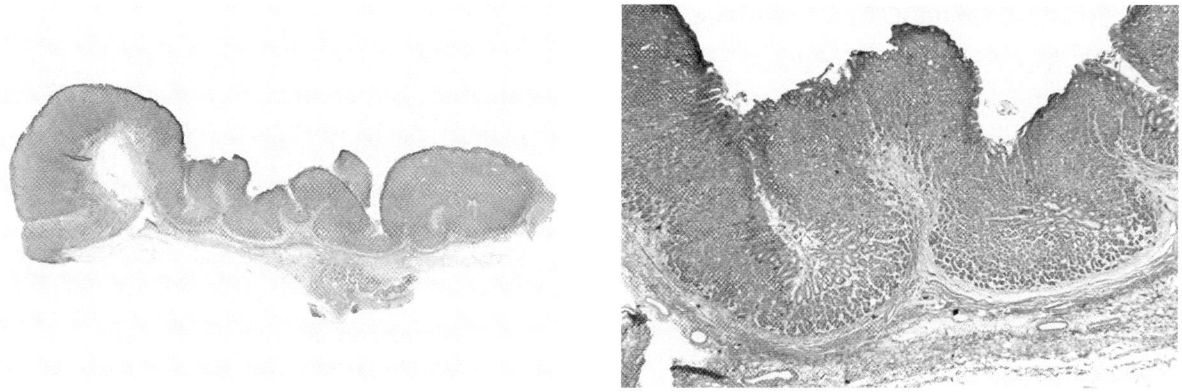

Figure 4-41

ZOLLINGER-ELLISON SYNDROME

Left: Whole mount section of the diffuse mucosal thickening.
Right: Higher magnification shows that this is the result of a marked expansion of the glandular mucosa. The pits are extremely shortened.

hypertrophy, acid hypersecretion, and subsequent peptic ulceration. ECL hyperplasia results in increased histamine production, further stimulating acid production by parietal cells.

Clinical Features. The usual presenting symptoms are recurrent abdominal pain and diarrhea. Abdominal pain affects 70 to 95 percent of patients; diarrhea affects 33 to 75 percent of patients. Both symptoms result from excessive acid secretion. The acid hypersecretion may be mild and indistinguishable from that seen with ordinary duodenal ulcer. Some patients lack all the features of ZES. Peptic ulcer may be absent, and diarrhea with steatorrhea may be the only clinical manifestation.

Gross Findings. Giant rugal folds cover the body and fundus but spare the antrum. The surfaces of the folds appear uniformly exaggerated, coarsely granular, or finely cobblestoned. These expanded folds thicken the gastric mucosa 1½ to 2 times normal. Endoscopically, ulcers, often multiple, are seen. There may be copious amounts of resting gastric juice, coexistent duodenal ulcers, and reflux esophagitis.

Microscopic Findings. The oxyntic glands become lengthened and contain hypertrophic and hyperplastic parietal cells. The increased parietal cell mass comprises a progressively larger percentage of the glands, filling their entire length down to their bases and crowding out other cell populations. Parietal cells also extend into the neck regions or higher, coming closer to the luminal surface than usual. In some cases, parietal cells completely populate the mucosal glands. Large numbers of parietal cells may be present in the antrum, an area that usually lacks parietal cells. Foveolae appear normal in length or shortened (fig. 4-41). Antral glands and pits are of normal size (85,93). Hyperplastic ECL cells may be seen among the fundic glands. Cystic changes are absent, contrasting with Menetrier's disease.

Differential Diagnosis. The differential diagnosis includes the entities listed in Table 4-15 and pseudo-ZES (see below). In ZES, endoscopic biopsies may appear normal since the pits are likely to be normal and the expanded glandular component is not easy to appreciate. The only hint of ZES is the finding of hyperplastic parietal cells high in the mucosa in the mucous neck regions, a phenomenon not usually found in other conditions.

Treatment and Prognosis. The prognosis of patients with ZES relates more to the type of tumor causing the disease than to the gastric changes. The main predictor of survival is the presence of liver metastasis. Resection offers the only hope for cure. Up to 50 percent of primary lesions are extrapancreatic. Proton pump inhibitors are necessary to block the acid hypersecretion and have been effective in reducing the morbidity and mortality from exsanguinating upper gastrointestinal hemorrhage.

Pseudo-Zollinger-Ellison Syndrome

Definition. *Pseudo-Zollinger-Ellison syndrome* (pseudo-ZES) results from primary antral G-cell hyperplasia and hyperfunction.

Demography. Pseudo-ZES is a rare pediatric disorder in which G-cell hyperplasia, hyperfunction, or both occur without a clearly identifiable or predisposing cause.

Etiology. The syndrome likely has a multifactorial etiology. Most familial cases result from a genetic defect in normal regulation of G-cell function and/or proliferation. Patients with nonfamilial forms of the disease have increased antral G-cell sensitivity to intragastric food stimulation.

Clinical Features. Pseudo-ZES causes clinical and biochemical features that resemble peptic ulcer disease and ZES. Children sometimes present with nonspecific symptoms of abdominal pain or upper gastrointestinal bleeding (84). The gastrin hyperfunction results in hypergastrinemic hyperchlorhydria, but it does not always present clinically as ulcer disease. Rather, it may only cause nonspecific gastrointestinal symptoms. The diagnosis requires a high degree of clinical suspicion and demonstration of basal hypergastrinemia and acid hypersecretion; differentiation from duodenal ulcer disease and classic ZES is critical for clinical management. Diagnosis is achieved using provocative tests. Patients exhibit basal acid hypersecretion, elevated fasting plasma gastrin levels, enhanced gastric response to meals, high basal serum pepsinogen levels, and severe duodenal ulcer disease.

Microscopic Findings. The microscopic findings resemble those of ZES.

Treatment and Prognosis. Since patients with primary antral G-cell hyperplasia do not have a gastrin-producing tumor, the hypergastrinemia (which is of antral origin) reverts to normal following antrectomy.

Hypertrophic, Hypersecretory Gastropathy

Definition. *Hypertrophic, hypersecretory gastropathy* combines body glandular hyperplasia, normal surface components, and peptic ulcer disease, but it differs clinically from ZES by the absence of hypergastrinemia. The patients lack pancreatic tumors or G-cell hyperplasia. Some authors consider this a form of ZES (83).

Etiology. This syndrome may result from hypersensitivity of the parietal cells to gastrin stimulation rather than to hypergastrinemia and may overlap with pseudo-ZES.

Gross Findings. Endoscopically, there is a diffusely nodular mucosa with prominent rugal folds, resembling ZES.

Microscopic Findings. The histologic features resemble those found in patients with ZES.

Hypertrophic, Hypersecretory Gastropathy with Protein Loss

Definition. *Hypertrophic, hypersecretory gastropathy with protein loss* consists of giant gastric folds, hypersecretion, protein loss, and a clinical presentation that represents a cross between Menetrier's disease and ZES. It is also known as *mixed type of hyperplastic gastropathy*.

Demography. This is the rarest form of giant fold disease.

Clinical Features. Most patients complain of epigastric pain, asthenia, anorexia, weight loss, edema, and vomiting. There may be no symptoms, hypersecretion, or protein loss, or there may be hypersecretion without protein loss, depending on the degree of hyperplasia of the various components and the relative proportion of the cell types. Enteric protein loss and hypoalbuminemia exist in most cases. Occasionally, a concomitant gastric ulcer is found. Some patients, however, remain asymptomatic.

Microscopic Findings. There is foveolar hyperplasia with deep cysts and mild glandular hyperplasia with increased numbers of lymphocytes and plasma cells.

Helicobacter Pylori–Associated Hypertrophic Gastropathy

Helicobacter pylori–associated hypertrophic gastropathy is the hypertrophic gastropathy that results from HP infection. This hypertrophic gastropathy may represent a special form of HP gastritis (88).

Some patients with HP infection exhibit hypertrophic gastric folds and a protein-losing enteropathy. Biopsies demonstrate the presence of a chronic or mixed acute and chronic gastritis, with or without ulceration. The pit-to-gland ratio is normal and the increased mucosal thickness results from edema and inflammation.

Eradicating the HP infection restores the normal architecture.

LOCALIZED HYPERTROPHIC DISORDERS

Focal Hyperplasia

Definition. *Focal hyperplasia* is localized mucosal expansion.

Etiology. A number of entities cause localized mucosal hyperplasia. The lesions lie adjacent to healed peptic ulcers, neoplasms, and surgical stomas. Polyps, which are believed to represent an exuberant regenerative response of gastric foveolar cells, develop in anastomotic sites 1 to 18 years following gastrectomy. Numerous factors contribute to the genesis of the lesions seen in the postsurgical stomach, including chronic bile reflux, stomal ischemia secondary to mucosal prolapse, and mucosal deformities resulting from the anastomosis. Patients who undergo Billroth II procedures may develop G-cell proliferation after the procedure. Patients with tumors may produce growth factors that stimulate localized mucosal growth. There is a direct correlation between the degree of mucosal thickening and EGF expression by some tumors.

Gross Findings. Focal hyperplasia creates lesions that measure up to 5 mm in diameter. They are frequently multiple and arise in the antrum. Lesions surrounding stomas may present as a solitary sessile polyp or as a linear arrangement of polyps encircling the gastric side of the stoma.

Microscopic Findings. The gastric pits have an increased depth or diameter, with saccular dilatations. The stroma increases and appears edematous and/or inflamed, widely separating the gastric glands. The base of the lesion contains fibrous connective tissue replacing or extending through the muscularis mucosae. Histologically, these proliferative lesions resemble hyperplastic polyps in that they contain proliferating nondysplastic foveolar cells (fig. 4-42). The epithelium appears regenerative and surface erosions with cellular loss may be found. The adjacent mucosa is often atrophic. The hypertrophic muscularis mucosae appears irregularly frayed, and cystic glands penetrate into the submucosa, producing gastritis cystica profunda. Each of the mucosal protrusions closely relates to the rugal folds without distinct borders between the lesions and the folds.

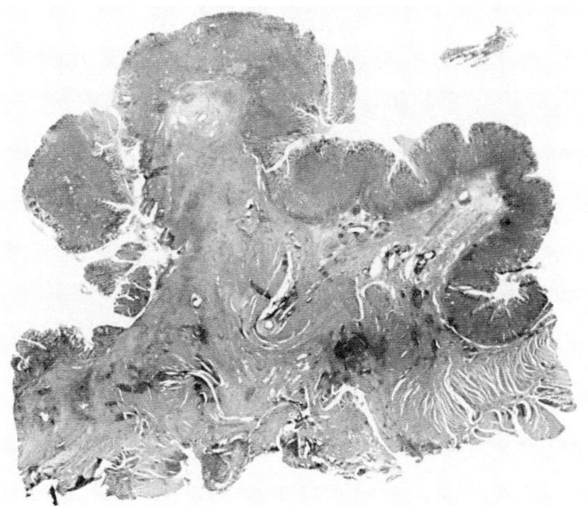

Figure 4-42

LOCALIZED POLYPOID HYPERPLASIA

Localized polypoid hyperplasia overlying an anastomotic site.

Treatment and Prognosis. The natural history of these lesions is controversial, and it remains unclear whether they represent an intermediate stage between chronic stomal gastritis and stomal cancer.

GASTRIC POLYPS

Gastric polyps are found in 2.0 to 8.7 percent of gastric examinations, usually as incidental findings (97,100). The polyps may be neoplastic or non-neoplastic, with most (80 to 90 percent) being non-neoplastic. They may be multiple or solitary (50 to 87 percent of cases [100]), and some complicate polyposis syndromes (Table 4-16). Gastric polyps affect all age groups, but they peak in the 5th to 7th decades, except in individuals with a polyposis syndrome, in which case they occur earlier.

The two main types of non-neoplastic polyps are hyperplastic polyps and fundic gland polyps (96); less commonly, neoplastic (adenomatous) polyps develop. Lesions that may present as gastric polyps include Brunner gland heterotopia, inflammatory fibroid polyps, pancreatic heterotopia, carcinoid tumors, and hamartomatous polyps (96,105).

Table 4-16

DIFFERENTIAL DIAGNOSIS OF GASTRIC POLYPS

Hyperplastic polyps
Fundic gland polyps
Inflammatory polyps
Inflammatory fibroid polyps
Hamartomatous polyps
Adenomas
Polyps in polyposis syndromes
Familial adenomatous polyposis
Peutz-Jeghers syndrome
Juvenile polyposis
Cowden's syndrome
Cronkhite-Canada syndrome
Carcinoid tumors
Heterotopic tissue
Pancreas
Brunner glands
Stromal tumors
Lipomas

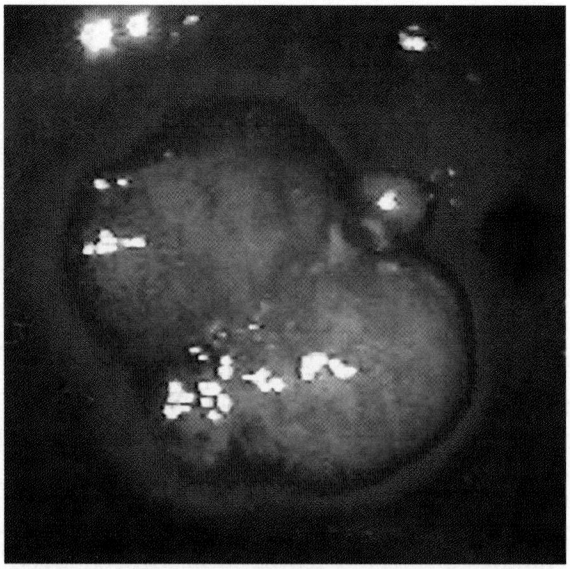

Figure 4-43

HYPERPLASTIC POLYP

Endoscopically, these lesions appear polypoid and bosselated.

Symptoms, when present, are usually vague and nonspecific. Some patients present with mild bleeding. Pedunculated lesions may prolapse through the pylorus causing obstruction. Clinical and endoscopic features are rarely able to distinguish the various types of polyps prior to histologic examination.

Hyperplastic Polyp

Definition. *Hyperplastic polyps* are localized, non-neoplastic mucosal expansions consisting of elongated, tortuous, sometimes cystically dilated foveolae supported by an edematous lamina propria and distended vessels. Synonyms include *gastritis polyposa, retention polyps,* and *hyperplasiogenic polyps*.

Demography. Forty-five to 90 percent of gastric polyps are hyperplastic (104,105). They develop in men and women with equal frequency, with a median age of 69 years; these lesions also arise in children. Some arise with concomitant chronic atrophic gastritis, hypochlorhydria, low levels of pepsinogen 1, and hypergastrinemia, a setting consistent with autoimmune gastritis (93,99). A possible relationship exists with HP infections (102).

Clinical Features. Larger polyps twist on their stalks, leading to superficial ulceration, hemorrhage, or pyloric prolapse. The latter results in intermittent gastric outlet obstruction.

Gross Findings. Hyperplastic polyps are usually small, smooth, lobulated, sessile or pedunculated (figs. 4-43, 4-44), sometimes umbilicated lesions measuring less than 2 cm in diameter. Rare polyps are larger and simulate carcinoma. Multiple polyps that may appear confluent occur in 20 to 33 percent of patients. Hyperplastic polyps develop throughout the stomach, in both the body and antrum, and occasionally at the gastroesophageal junction (95).

Microscopic Findings. Most hyperplastic polyps arise on a background of chronic gastritis. Histologically, they consist of a proliferation of surface foveolar cells lining exaggerated, elongated, branched, sometimes cystically dilated pits (fig. 4-45). Mucosal cysts can be quite prominent. Hypertrophic foveolar cells, resembling goblet cells, may be present. The pits extend from the surface deep into the stroma. The glands in hyperplastic polyps are usually of the antral type, even when the polyps arise in the body or fundus (sometimes referred to as *mixed fundic-antral hyperplastic polyps*), although occasionally, oxyntic glandular mucosa is seen. A prominent stroma separates the glands. This stroma often becomes edematous and infiltrated

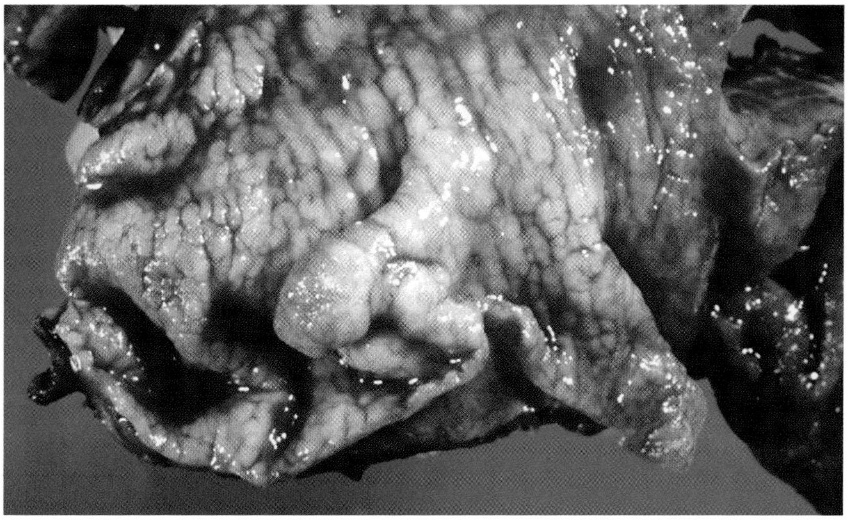

Figure 4-44

HYPERPLASTIC POLYP

Several hyperplastic polyps with typical lobulated structure are in a partial resection specimen.

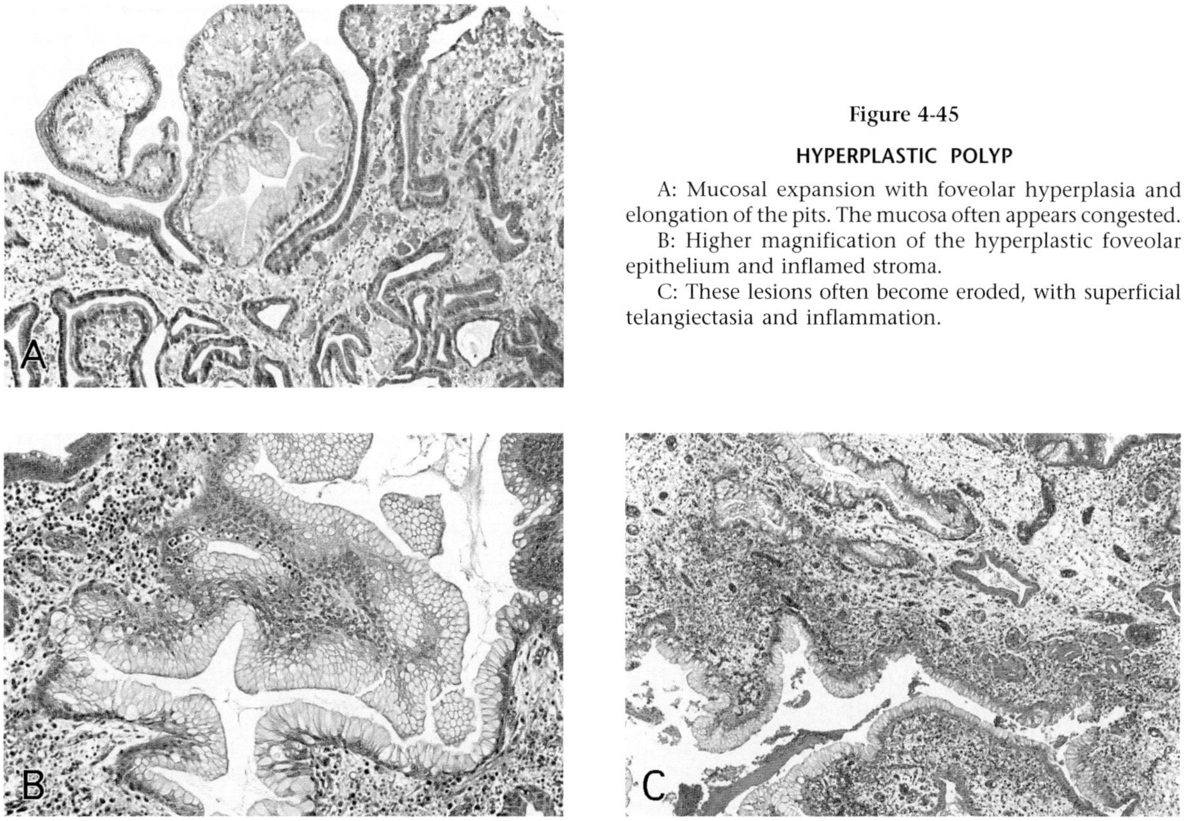

Figure 4-45

HYPERPLASTIC POLYP

A: Mucosal expansion with foveolar hyperplasia and elongation of the pits. The mucosa often appears congested.

B: Higher magnification of the hyperplastic foveolar epithelium and inflamed stroma.

C: These lesions often become eroded, with superficial telangiectasia and inflammation.

by inflammatory cells, particularly by plasma cells, lymphocytes, and eosinophils. Smooth muscle fibers extend upward from the splayed muscularis mucosae. Patchy fibrosis may develop.

Erosion of the surface, with subsequent regeneration, produces reactive atypia in the lining epithelium, which is characterized by cytoplasmic eosinophilia, an enlarged nucleus, and a cuboidal cell shape. In some cases, it may be difficult to distinguish the regenerating foveolar epithelium from adenomatous epithelium. In order to separate the two, one should the suspicious cells within their context. The presence of clear-cut regeneration in adjacent areas or inflammation should indicate a reparative and not an adenomatous lesion. Atypia is either absent or minimal and often regenerative in nature, especially in areas of surface erosion (fig. 4-45). Neutrophils are especially prominent in ulcerated areas. Eroded hyperplastic polyps may also contain atypical mesenchymal cells with marked nuclear pleomorphism and atypical mitotic figures. These cells blend in with the typical granulation tissue. Vascular proliferations resembling granulation tissue develop superficially near areas of inflammation.

Differential Diagnosis. Superficial biopsies of small polyps disclose mixtures of hyperplastic and inflammatory tissue similar to that seen in areas of chronic gastritis. In such biopsies, the polypoid nature of the lesion may not be readily appreciated if the appropriate clinical information is not provided. The most important feature to be assessed is the presence or absence of adenomatous, dysplastic, or malignant epithelium. The latter is extremely unlikely in the absence of intestinal metaplasia.

Treatment and Prognosis. The treatment of hyperplastic polyps is endoscopic removal in order to determine their nature and to prove that the lesions are benign. Because hyperplastic polyps represent a reactive change of the normal mucosa, they are not genuine neoplasms; however, neoplastic changes can develop within them, especially in individuals with multiple polyps. Of interest is the report that hyperplastic polyps exhibit clonality and contain *ras* gene mutations (100). When dysplasia develops within hyperplastic polyps, it generally resembles the adenomatous epithelium found in the colon. Areas of adenomatous change are generally more extensive than the areas of atypia seen in focally eroded polyps.

Fundic Gland Polyp

Definition. *Fundic gland polyps*, also known as *cystic hamartomatous epithelial polyps*, consist of localized expansions of oxyntic mucosa.

Demography. Fundic gland polyps were initially described in patients with familial adenomatous polyposis coli (FAP). The frequency of fundic polyps in FAP patients ranges from 30 to 56 percent, affecting patients in the 2nd and 3rd decades of life. Fundic gland polyposis also occurs in the absence of FAP, affecting up to 1.4 percent of the general population. Compared with non-FAP cases, FAP patients with fundic gland polyps have a lower male to female ratio, a younger mean age at diagnosis, and a higher proportion of multiple polyps. The youngest patient in one study was 8 years old. In contrast, non-FAP patients develop their polyps in middle age.

Etiology. The etiology of these lesions is unclear. Some believe that they represent hamartomas. They are frequently found in patients undergoing treatment with proton pump inhibitors. As a result, it has been hypothesized, but not yet proven, that these lesions result from the increased gastrin levels that follow inhibition of gastric acid secretion.

The role of the germline mutation in the *APC* gene found in FAP patients in predisposing to fundic gland polyps is unclear. A recent study found β-catenin gene mutations in 29 of 35 sporadic fundic gland polyps (103). *APC* mutations appear to occur in sporadic fundic gland polyps with dysplasia (94).

Clinical Features. The number of polyps may decrease or increase over time. Circulatory disturbances of the pedicles, torsion, or mechanical traction resulting in autoamputation may cause polyps to disappear.

Gross Findings. Fundic gland polyps developing in the setting of FAP may result in a carpet of several hundred polyps, each usually measuring less than 5 mm in diameter. These polyps have a sessile base and a smooth-domed surface. In sporadic cases, polyps usually number less than 50; often they are solitary. They appear as minute mucosal bumps measuring 1 to 5 mm in diameter. Fundic gland polyps are the same color as the surrounding mucosa. Most lesions arise in the fundic mucosa but rare lesions arise in the antrum.

Microscopic Findings. No histologic differences exist between FAP-associated fundic gland polyps and non-FAP–associated lesions (101). Histologically, they represent localized hyperplastic expansions of the deep epithelial compartment of the oxyntic mucosa (fig. 4-46). Masses of distorted oxyntic glands lie close to the luminal surface, and they contain scattered, cystically dilated pits and glands. The overlying pits appear shortened or absent. The

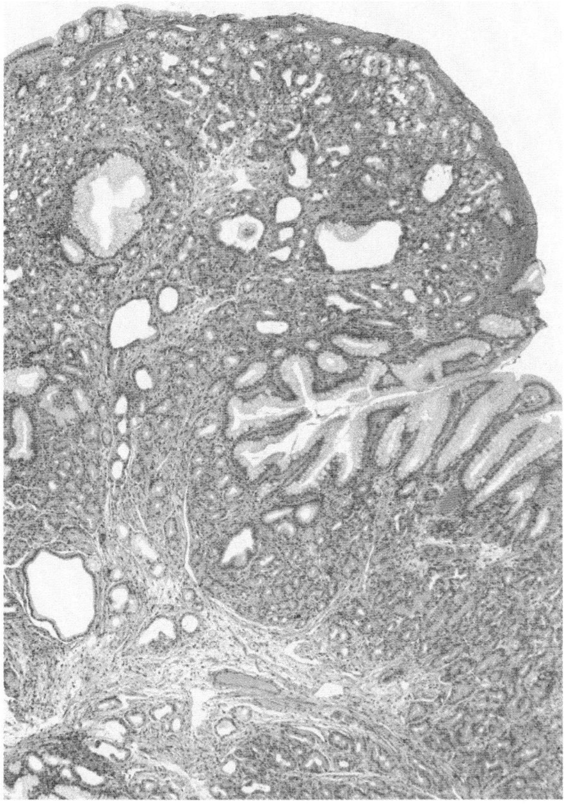

Figure 4-46

FUNDIC GLAND POLYP

The polyps result from expansion of the oxyntic glands and the pits become shortened. Here, the junction of a fundic gland polyp is seen, with more or less normal mucosa on the right. The polyp itself often develops cystic dilatations.

branched tubular glands are lined by chief cells, parietal cells, and mucous neck cells, and they open into the pits. The mucin in the surface foveolar cells stains intensely with the PAS stain, but is negative with Alcian blue stains for acidic mucin. Most fundic gland polyps show an increase in smooth muscle content, often in a pericystic distribution.

Fundic gland polyps probably develop from the progressive dilatation and infolding of glandular buds to produce irregular tortuous glands and microcysts. Proliferating cells are found in the mucous neck region as well as in the epithelium lining the microcysts and in the glands directly adjacent to microcysts. The presence of these aberrantly located proliferative cells may explain the histogenesis of the polyp (101).

Treatment and Prognosis. Treatment consists of endoscopic removal to confirm their identity and to exclude other lesions. Fundic gland polyps have little malignant potential, but they serve as a marker for FAP, especially in patients with multiple lesions who are not taking proton pump inhibitors.

Isolated Hamartomatous Polyp

Definition. *Isolated hamartomatous polyps* consist of a submucosal mass of oxyntic glands in a framework of smooth muscle. They are also termed *submucosal heterotopia of gastric glands.*

Microscopic Findings. Isolated hamartomatous polyps consist of a mixture of haphazardly arranged fundic type glands, smooth muscle tissue, and focal accumulations of mature lymphoid tissue, supported by normal lamina propria. The glands may appear cystically dilated or may be compact, as in the normal stomach. There are mucous cells resembling those of the gastric foveolar epithelium as well as rare antral or cardiac type glands containing the endocrine cells indigenous to the mucosal site.

Differential Diagnosis. The major entity in the differential diagnosis is the Peutz-Jeghers polyp. Clinically, patients with hamartomatous polyps lack the classic features of Peutz-Jeghers polyps, which are usually mucosally based lesions with possible submucosal extensions that contain characteristic arborizing muscle bundles. In contrast, isolated hamartomatous polyps are predominantly submucosal in location and lack arborizing smooth muscle bundles.

Gastric Polyps in Polyposis Syndromes

Many generalized polyposis syndromes affect the stomach. Patients with juvenile polyposis, familial adenomatous polyposis, Peutz-Jeghers syndrome, Cronkhite-Canada syndrome, and Cowden's disease all may develop gastric lesions. The polyposis syndromes are discussed in chapter 16.

GASTRIC XANTHOMA

Definition. *Xanthomas* are bland collections of foamy, lipid-containing histiocytes (xanthoma cells) arranged in pavement-like patterns in the upper lamina propria immediately beneath the surface epithelium. *Xanthelasma* and *lipid islands* are synonymous terms for this entity.

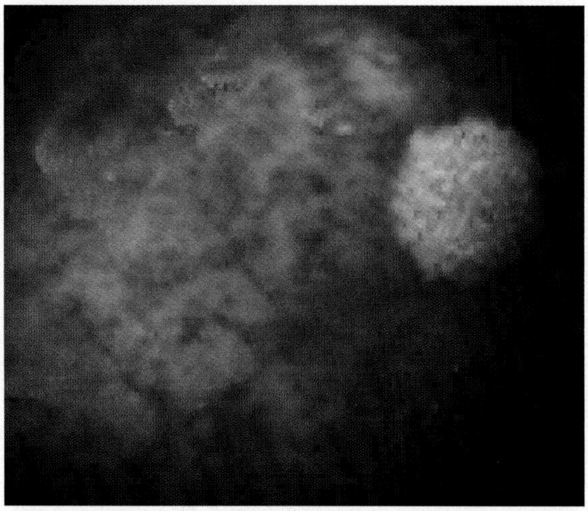

Figure 4-47

GASTRIC XANTHOMA

Endoscopic examination reveals a typical yellow island.

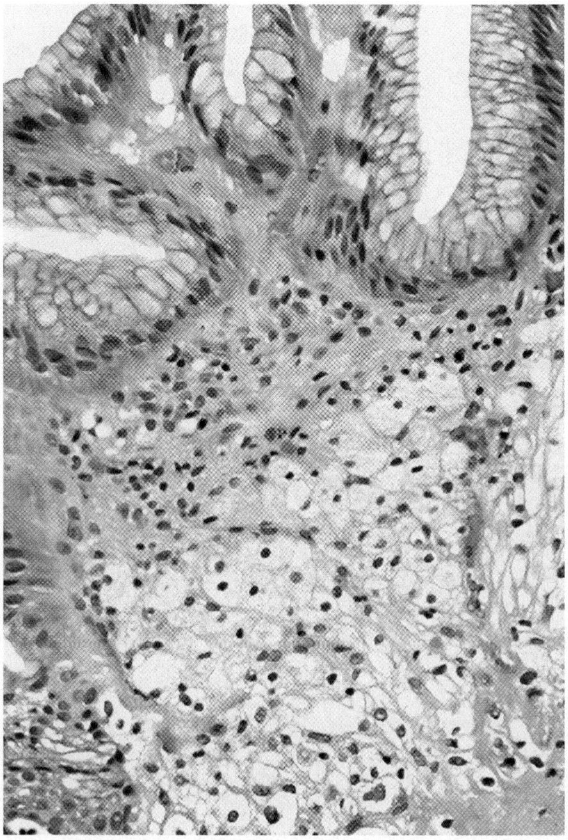

Figure 4-48

GASTRIC XANTHOMA

Clusters of pale-staining, foamy histiocytes are in the lamina propria.

Demography. The frequency of gastric xanthoma is said to be 18 percent in gastrectomy specimens and as high as 53 percent among autopsies (106–108).

Etiology. The etiology of xanthomas is unknown but they never occur in the normal gastric mucosa. Patients often have evidence of bile reflux, varying degrees of gastritis, gastric surgery, or even associated cancer. Some patients have associated cholesterolosis of the gallbladder. They sometimes develop in patients with cholestasis and then regress once the cholestasis disappears.

Gross Findings. Xanthomas appear to the endoscopist as single or multiple, well-demarcated, circular-oval, whitish yellow plaques measuring 1 to 10 mm but rarely exceeding 5 mm (fig. 4-47). They are often multiple and occur frequently along the lesser curvature of the fundus and prepyloric region (106).

Microscopic Findings. These lamina propria–based histiocytic collections displace gastric glands and foveolae and occasionally extend into the submucosa. The cytologically bland cells contain abundant, foamy, finely vacuolated cytoplasm (fig. 4-48). The cells are PAS negative, and lymphocytes, plasma cells, and macrophages are associated with the foam cells (106). These lipid islands stain with the macrophage marker KP1 and the foam cells contain low-density lipoproteins (LDL) and oxidized LDL (107).

Differential Diagnosis. The differential diagnosis includes Whipple's disease and certain fungal infections, such as histoplasmosis. These entities may be ruled out with the use of special stains. The differential diagnosis also includes the diffuse form of gastric carcinoma. Signet ring cell carcinomas tend to be composed of cells with eccentric nuclei. In contrast, xanthoma cells usually have central nuclei. In cases where there is doubt, a negative cytokeratin immunostain rules out diffuse gastric carcinoma.

Brunner Gland Heterotopia

Heterotopic Brunner glands may accompany heterotopic pancreas or may be seen alone. The prepyloric antrum is the most frequently affected site. Histologically, the lesion resembles duodenal Brunner gland hyperplasia.

REFERENCES

Clinical Presentation of Gastric Diseases

1. Allen A, Leonard AJ, Sellers LA. The mucus barrier: its role in gastroduodenal mucosal protection. J Clin Gastroenterol 1988;10:S93–8.
2. Frank L, Kleinman L, Ganoczy D, et al. Upper gastrointestinal symptoms in North America: prevalence and relationship to healthcare utilization and quality of life. Dig Dis Sci 2000;45: 809–18.
3. Gasbarrini G, Montalto M. Structure and function of tight junctions. Role in intestinal barrier. Ital J Gastroenterol Hepatol 1999;31:481–8.
4. Gyires K. Neuropeptides and gastric mucosal homeostasis. Curr Top Med Chem 2004;4(1): 63–73.
5. Heading RC. Prevalence of upper gastrointestinal symptoms in the general population: a systematic review. Scand J Gastroenterol Suppl 1999;231:3–8.
6. Hollander D. Clinician's guide through the tight junctions. Ital J Gastroenterol Hepatol 1999;31: 435–9.
7. Konturek PC, Konturek SJ, Brzozowski T, Ernst H. Epidermal growth factor and transforming growth factor-alpha: role in protection and healing of gastric mucosal lesions. Eur J Gastroenterol Hepatol 1995;7:933–7.
8. Locke GR 3rd. Prevalence, incidence and natural history of dyspepsia and functional dyspepsia. Baillieres Clin Gastroenterol 1998;12:435–42.
9. Mestecky J, McGhee JR, Eslon CO. Intestinal IgA system. Immunol Allergy Clin North Am 1988; 8:349.
10. Sorbye H, Svanes K. The role of blood flow in gastric mucosal defense, damage and healing. Dig Dis 1994;12:305–17.
11. Szabo S, Nagy L, Plebani M. Glutathione, protein sulfhydryls and cysteine proteases in gastric mucosal injury and protection. Clin Chim Acta 1992;206:95–105.
12. Tsukimi Y, Okabe S. Recent advances in gastrointestinal pathophysiology: role of heat shock proteins in mucosal defense and ulcer healing. Biol Pharm Bull 2001;24:1–9.
13. Veldhuyzen van Zanten SJ, Flook N, Chiba N, et al. An evidence-based approach to the management of uninvestigated dyspepsia in the era of *Helicobacter pylori*. Canadian Dyspepsia Working Group. CMAJ 2000;162:S3–23.
14. Wallace JL. Nonsteroidal anti-inflammatory drugs and the gastrointestinal tract. Mechanisms of protection and healing: current knowledge and future research. Am J Med 2001; 110(1A):19S–23S.
15. Wright NA. Interaction of trefoil family factors with mucins: clues to their mechanism of action? Gut 2001;48:293–4.

Gastritis

16. Allen A, Flemstrom G, Garner A, Kivilaakso E. Gastroduodenal mucosal protection. Physiol Rev 1993;73:823–57.
17. Andersen LP, Boye K, Blom J, Holck S, Norgard A, Elsborg L. Characterization of a culturable "*Gastrospirillum hominis*" (*Helicobacter heilmannii*) strain isolated from human gastric mucosa. J Clin Microbiol 1999;37:1069–76.
18. Arnold R, Koop H. Omeprazole: long-term safety. Digestion 1989;44:77–86.
19. Atherton JC. CagA: a role at last. Gut 2000;47:330–1.
20. Atherton JC, Cao P, Peek RM Jr, Tummuru MK, Blaser MJ, Cover TL. Mosaicism in vacuolating cytotoxin alleles of Helicobacter pylori. Association of specific vacA types with cytotoxin production and peptic ulceration. J Biol Chem 1995;270:17771–7.
21. Boren T, Falk P, Roth KA, Larson G, Normark S. Attachment of *Helicobacter pylori* to human gastric epithelium mediated by blood group antigens. Science 1993;262:1892–5.
22. Brzozowski T, Konturek PC, Pajdo R, et al. Brain-gut axis in gastroprotection and cholecystokinin against ischemia-reperfusion induced gastric lesions. Physiol Pharmacol 2001;52:583–602.
23. Burman P, Kampe O, Kraaz W, et al. A study of autoimmune gastritis in the postpartum period and a 5-year follow-up. Gastroenterology 1992;103:934–42.
24. Chamberlain CE. Acute hemorrhagic gastritis. Gastroenterol Clin North Am 1993;22:843–73.
25. Correa P. The epidemiology and pathogenesis of chronic gastritis: three etiologic entities. Front Gastrointest Res 1980;6:98–108.
26. Diamanti A, Maino C, Niveloni S, et al. Characterization of gastric mucosal lesions in patients with celiac disease: a prospective controlled study. Am J Gastroenterol 1999;94:1313–9.
27. Dixon MF, Genta RM, Yardley JH, Correa P. Histological classification of gastritis and Helicobacter pylori infection: an agreement at last? The International Workshop on the Histopathology of Gastritis. Helicobacter 1997; 2(suppl 1):S17–24.

28. Dixon M, Genta R, Yardley J, Correa P. Classification and grading of gastritis: the updated Sydney System. Am J Surg Pathol 1996;20:1161–81.
29. Doglioni C, Laurino L, Dei Tos AP, et al. Pancreatic (acinar) metaplasia of the gastric mucosa. Histology, ultrastructure, immunocytochemistry, and clinicopathologic correlations of 101 cases. Am J Surg Pathol 1993;17:1134–43.
30. Ectors NL, Dixon MF, Geboes KJ, et al. Granulomatous gastritis: a morphological and diagnostic approach. Histopathology 1993;23:55–61.
31. Evans DG, Evans DJ Jr, Moulds JJ, Graham DY. N-acetylneuraminyllactose-binding fibrillar hemagglutinin of *Campylobacter pylori*: a putative colonization factor antigen. Infect Immun 1988;56:2896–906.
32. Evans DJ Jr, Evans DG, Takemura T, et al. Characterization of a *Helicobacter pylori* neutrophil-activating protein. Infect Immun 1995;63:2213–20.
33. Fahimi HD, Deren JJ, Gottlieb LS, Zamcheck N. Isolated granulomatous gastritis: its relationship to disseminated sarcoidosis and regional enteritis. Gastroenterology 1963;45:161–75.
34. Feldman M, Friedman LS, Sleisenger MH, eds. Sleisenger & Fordtran's gastrointestinal and liver disease: pathophysiology/diagnosis/management, vol. 2, 7th ed. Philadelphia: Saunders; 2002:812–3.
35. Genta RM, Graham DY. Comparison of biopsy sites for the histopathologic diagnosis of *Helicobacter pylori*: a topographic study of *H. pylori* density and distribution. Gastrointest Endosc 1994;40:342–5.
36. Genta RM, Robason GE, Graham DY. Simultaneous visualization of *Helicobacter pylori* and gastric morphology: a new stain. Hum Pathol 1994;25:221–6.
37. Gold BD, Dytoc M, Huesca M, et al. Comparison of *Helicobacter mustelae* and *Helicobacter pylori* adhesion to eukaryotic cells in vitro. Gastroenterology 1995;109:692–700.
38. Granger DN. Role of xanthine oxidase and granulocytes in ischemia-reperfusion injury. Am J Physiol 1988;255:H1269–75.
39. Haot J, Bogomoletz QV, Jouret A, Mainguet P. Menetrier's disease with lymphocytic gastritis. Hum Pathol 1991;22:379–6.
40. Haot J, Hamichi L, Wallez L, Mainguet P. Lymphocytic gastritis: a newly described entity: a retrospective endoscopic and histological study. Gut 1988;29:1258–64.
41. Haot J, Jouret A, Willette M, Goussin A, Mainguet P. Lymphocytic gastritis—prospective study of its relationship with varioliform gastritis. Gut 1990;31:282–5.
42. Hayat M, Arora DS, Wyatt JI, O'Mahony S, Dixin MF. The pattern of involvement of the gastric mucosa in lymphocytic gastritis is predictive of the presence of duodenal pathology. J Clin Pathol 1999;52:815–9.
43. Hayat M, Everett S. Lymphocytic gastritis, *Helicobacter pylori*, and gastric cancer: is vitamin C the common link? Nutrition 1999;15:402–3.
44. Heilmann KL, Borchard F. Gastritis due to spiral shaped bacteria other than *Helicobacter pylori*: clinical, histological, and ultrastructural findings. Gut 1991;32:137–40.
45. Hilzenrat N, Lamoureux E, Weintrub I, Alpert E, Lichter M, Alpert L. *Helicobacter heilmannii*-like spiral bacteria in gastric mucosal biopsies. Prevalence and clinical significance. Arch Pathol Lab Med 1995;119:1149–53.
46. Hojgaard L, Mertz Nielsen A, Rune SJ. Peptic ulcer pathophysiology: acid, bicarbonate, and mucosal function. Scand J Gastroenterol Suppl 1996;216:10–5.
47. Hulten K, Han SW, Enroth H, et al. *Helicobacter pylori* in the drinking water in Peru. Gastroenterology 1996;110:1031–5.
48. Isaacs KL. Upper gastrointestinal tract endoscopy in inflammatory bowel disease. Gastrointest Endosc Clin N Am 2002;12:451–62.
49. Jass JB. The role of intestinal metaplasia in the histogenesis of gastric carcinoma. J Clin Pathol 1980;33:801–10.
50. Kansau I, Labigne A. Heat shock proteins of *Helicobacter pylori*. Aliment Pharmacol Ther 1996;10:51–6.
51. Karnes WE Jr, Samloff IM, Siurala M, et al. Positive serum antibody and negative tissue staining for *Helicobacter pylori* in subjects with atrophic body gastritis. Gastroenterology 1991;101:167–74.
52. Konturek PK, Brzozowski T, Konturek SJ, Dembinski A. Role of epidermal growth factor, prostaglandin, and sulfhydryls in stress-induced gastric lesions. Gastroenterology 1990;99:1607–15.
53. Kreuning J, Lindeman J, Biemond I, Lamers CB. Relation between IgG and IgA antibody titres against *Helicobacter pylori* in serum and severity of gastritis in asymptomatic subjects. J Clin Pathol 1994;47:227–31.
54. Krishnamurthy S, Integlia MJ, Grand RJ, Dayal Y. Pancreatic acinar cell clusters in pediatric gastric mucosa. Am J Surg Pathol 1998;22:100–5.
55. Kuipers EJ, Uyterlinde AM, Pena AS, et al. Long-term sequelae of *Helicobacter pylori* gastritis. Lancet 1995;345:1525–8.
56. Leunk RD, Johnson PT, David BC, Kraft WG, Morgan DR. Cytotoxic activity in broth-culture filtrates of *Campylobacter pylori*. J Med Microbiol 1988;26:93–9.

57. Makristathis A, Pasching E, Schutze K, et al. Detection of *H. pylori* in stool specimens by PCR and antigen enzyme immunoassay. J Clin Microbiol 1998;36:2772–4.
58. Malaty HM, Evans DG, Evans DJ, Graham DY. *Helicobacter pylori* in Hispanics: comparison with blacks and whites of similar age and socioeconomic class. Gastroenterology 1992;103:813–6.
59. Mardh S, Song YH. Characterization of antigenic structures in auto-immune atrophic gastritis with pernicious anaemia. The parietal cell H,K-ATPase and the chief cell pepsinogen are the two major antigens. Acta Physiol Scand 1989;136:581–7.
60. Miettinen A, Karttunen TJ, Alavaikko M. Lymphocytic gastritis and *Helicobacter pylori* infection in gastric lymphoma. Gut 1995;37:471–6.
61. Moran AP. The role of lipopolysaccharide in *Helicobacter pylori* pathogenesis. Aliment Pharmacol Ther 1996;10:39–50.
62. Mori Y, Fukuma K, Adachi Y, et al. Parietal cell autoantigens involved in neonatal thymectomy-induced murine autoimmune gastritis. Studies using monoclonal autoantibodies. Gastroenterology 1989;97:364–75.
63. Nakayama Y, Horiuchi A, Kumagai T, et al. Discrimination of normal gastric mucosa from *Helicobacter pylori* gastritis using standard endoscopes and a single observation site: studies in children and young adults. Helicobacter 2004;9:95–9.
64. Niemela S, Karttunen T, Kerola T, Karttunen R. Ten year follow up study of lymphocytic gastritis: further evidence on *Helicobacter pylori* as a cause of lymphocytic gastritis and corpus gastritis. J Clin Pathol 1995;48:1111–6.
65. Oberhuber G, Puspok A, Oesterroicher C, et al. Focally enhanced gastritis—a frequent type of gastritis in patients with Crohn's disease. Gastroenterology 1997;112:698–706.
66. Owen DA. Gastritis and carditis. Modern Pathology 2003;16:325–41.
67. Parsonnet J, Shmuely H, Haggerty T. Fecal and oral shedding of *Helicobacter pylori* from healthy infected adults. JAMA 1999;282:2240–5.
68. Shapiro JL, Goldblum JR, Petras RE. A clinicopathologic study of 42 patients with granulomatous gastritis. Is there really an "idiopathic" granulomatous gastritis? Am J Surg Pathol 1996;20:462–70.
69. Silen W, Ito S. Mechanisms for rapid re-epithelialization of the gastric mucosal surface. Ann Rev Physiol 1985;47:217–29.
70. Silva R, Dinis-Ribeiro M, Lopes C, et al. A follow up model for patients with atrophic chronic gastritis and intestinal metaplasia. J Clin Pathol 2004;57:177–82.
71. Spechler SJ, Fischbach L, Feldman M. Clinical aspects of genetic variability in *Helicobacter pylori*. JAMA 2000;283:1264–6.
72. Stark ME, Szurszewski JH. Role of nitric oxide in gastrointestinal and hepatic function and disease. Gastroenterology 1992;103:1928–49.
73. Stemmermann GN. Intestinal metaplasia of the stomach. Cancer 1994;74:556–64.
74. Vaira D, Malfertheiner P, Megraud F, et al. Diagnosis of *Helicobacter pylori* infection with a new non-invasive antigen-based assay. HpSA European study group. Lancet 1999;354:30–3.
75. Var C, Gultekin F, Candan F, et al. The effects of hemodialysis on duodenal and gastric mucosal changes in uremic patients. Clin Nephrol 1996;45:310–4.
76. Vincent P, Gottrand F, Pernes P, et al. High prevalence of *Helicobacter pylori* infection in cohabiting children. Epidemiology of a cluster, with special emphasis on molecular typing. Gut 1994;35:313–6.
77. Weinstein WM. Emerging gastritides. Curr Gastroenterol Rep 2001;3:523–7.
78. Wolber R, Owen D, DelBuono L, Appleman H, Freeman H. Lymphocytic gastritis in patients with celiac sprue or sprue-like intestinal disease. Gastroenterology 1990;98:310–5.
79. Wright CL, Riddell RH. Histology of stomach and duodenum in Crohn's disease. Am J Surg Pathol 1998;22:383–90.
80. Wu TT, Hamilton SR. Lymphocytic gastritis: association with etiology and topology. Am J Surg Pathol 1999;23:153–8.
81. Yamaoka Y, Kwon DH, Graham DY. A M(r) 34,000 pro-inflammatory outer membrane protein (oipA) of *Helicobacter pylori*. Proc Natl Acad Sci USA 2000;97:7533-8. Erratum in: Proc Natl Acad Sci USA 2000;97:11133.

Hypertrophic Gastropathies

82. Annibale B, Bonamico M, Rindi G, et al. Antral gastrin cell hyperfunction in children: a functional and immunocytochemical report. Gastroenterology 1991;101:1547–51.
83. Appelman HD. Localized and extensive expansions of the gastric mucosa: mucosal polyps and giant folds. In: Appelman HD, ed. Pathology of the esophagus, stomach, and duodenum. New York: Churchill Livingstone; 1984:79–120.
84. Bluth RF, Carpenter HA, Pittelkow MR, Page DL, Coffey RJ. Immunolocalization of transforming growth factor-alpha in normal and diseased human gastric mucosa. Hum Pathol 1995;26:1333–40.

85. Coad NA, Shah KJ. Menetrier's disease in childhood associated with cytomegalovirus infection: a case report and review of the literature. Br J Radiol 1986;59:615–20.
86. Dempsey PJ, Goldenring JR, Soroka CJ, et al. Possible role of transforming growth factor alpha in the pathogenesis of Menetrier's disease: supportive evidence from humans and transgenic mice. Gastroenterology 1992;103:1950–63.
87. Eisenstat D, Griffiths A, Cutz E, et al. Acute cytomegalovirus infection in a child with Menetrier's disease. Gastroenterology 1995;109: 592–5.
88. Hill ID, Sinclair-Smith C, Lastovica AJ, Bowie MD, Emms M. Transient protein losing enteropathy associated with acute gastritis and *Campylobacter pylori*. Arch Dis Child 1987;62:1215–9.
89. Isenberg JI, Walsh JH, Grossman MI. Zollinger-Ellison syndrome. Gastroenterology 1973;65: 140–65.
90. Knight J, Ma'tlak M, Condon V. Menetrier's disease in children: report of a case and review of the pediatric literature. Pediatr Pathol 1983;1: 179–84.
91. Komorowski RA, Caya JG. Hyperplastic gastropathy. Clinicopathologic correlation. Am J Surg Pathol 1991;15:577–85.
92. Wolfsen HC, Carpenter HA, Talley NJ. Menetrier's disease: a form of hypertrophic gastropathy or gastritis? Gastroenterology 1993; 104:1310–19.

Gastric Polyps

93. Abraham S, Singh V, Yardley J, Wu TT. Hyperplastic polyps of the stomach: associations with histologic pattern of gastritis and gastric atrophy. Am J Surg Pathol 2001;25:500–7.
94. Abraham SC, Park SJ, Mugartegui L, Hamilton SR, Wu TT. Sporadic fundic gland polyps with epithelial dysplasia. Am J Pathol 2002;161: 1735–42.
95. Abraham SC, Singh V, Yardley J, Wu T. Hyperplastic polyps of the esophagus and esophagogastric junction: histologic and clinicopathologic findings. Am J Surg Pathol 2001;25:1180–7.
96. Borch K, Skarsgard J, Franzen L, Mardh S, Rehfeld JF. Benign gastric polyps: morphological and functional origin. Dig Dis Sci 2003;48: 1292–7.
97. Dekker W. Clinical relevance of gastric and duodenal polyps. Scand J Gastroenterol 1990;25:7–12.
98. Dijkhuizen SM, Entius MM, Clement MJ, et al. Multiple hyperplastic polyps in the stomach: evidence for clonality and neoplastic potential. Gastroenterology 1997;112:561–6.
99. Haruma K, Yoshihara M, Sumii K, et al. Gastric acid secretion, serum pepsinogen I, and serum gastrin in Japanese with gastric hyperplastic polyps or polypoid-type early gastric carcinoma. Scand J Gastroenterol 1993;28:633–7.
100. Ming SC, Goldman H. Gastric polyps. A histogenetic classification and its relation to carcinoma. Cancer 1965;18:721–36.
101. Odze RD, Marcial MA, Antonioli D. Gastric fundic gland polyps: a morphological study including mucin histochemistry, stereometry, and MIB-1 immunohistochemistry. Hum Pathol 1996;27:896–903.
102. Ohkusa T, Takashimizu I, Fujiki K et al. Disappearance of hyperplastic polyps in the stomach after eradication of *Helicobacter pylori*: a randomized, clinical trial. Ann Intern Med 1998; 129:712–5.
103. Sekine S, Shibata T, Yamauchi Y, et al. Beta-catenin mutations in sporadic fundic gland polyps. Virchows Arch 2002;440:381–6.
104. Snover DC. Benign epithelial polyps of the stomach. Pathol Annu 1985;20:302–29.
105. Stolte M, Sticht T, Eidt S, Ebert D, Finkenzeller G. Frequency, location, and age and sex distribution of various types of gastric polyp. Endoscopy 1994;26:659–65.

Gastric Xanthoma

106. Domeloff L, Eriksson S, Helander HF, Janunger KG. Lipid islands in the gastric mucosa after resection for benign ulcer disease. Gastroenterology 1977;72:14–8.
107. Kaiserling E, Heinle H, Itabe H, Takano T, Remmele W. Lipid islands in human gastric mucosa: morphological and immunohistochemical findings. Gastroenterology 1996;110: 369–74.
108. Terruzzi V, Minoli G, Butti G, Rossini A. Gastric lipid islands in the gastric stump and in non-operated stomach. Endoscopy 1980;12:58–62.

5 PEPTIC ULCER DISEASES

A major insight of the last 10 to 20 years is that gastric peptic ulcers primarily result from altered gastric mucosal defenses whereas duodenal ulcers develop in association with increased acid production. It has also become clear that *Helicobacter pylori* infection plays a vital role in peptic ulcer development in both sites. Other factors that play a role in peptic ulcer disease include the use of nonsteroidal antiinflammatory drugs (NSAIDs), cigarette smoking, the presence of chronic renal disease, and excessive alcohol consumption. Disturbed motility predisposes to active ulceration in the duodenum due to prolonged mucosal contact with acid containing material from the stomach.

NORMAL GASTRIC DEFENSE MECHANISMS

The stomach has evolved a complex mucosal cytoprotection system in order to withstand the hostile environment present within it (see chapter 4). Adherent mucus provides a stable unstirred layer that neutralizes acids at the luminal surface. In addition, this unstirred layer acts as a permeability barrier to luminal pepsin. Acid reaching the mucosal surface is neutralized by bicarbonate secreted into the mucus layer covering the epithelium (1,12). The net result is that the pH in the gastric lumen is approximately 2.0, while that at the mucosal surface is increased to approximately 7.0 (3,11). Mucus also lubricates the stomach and facilitates the movement of food, thereby avoiding mucosal abrasions from coarse foods. In addition, the mucous cells secrete lipid, which coats the epithelial membranes lining the gastric lumen with a nonwettable surface, thereby protecting them against the action of water-soluble hydrogen ions and pepsin (2,5). Tight junctions also constitute a major structural component of the gastric mucosal barrier. Breaking the mucosal barrier leads to mucosal damage because it allows hydrogen ions, pepsin, and bile acids to back-diffuse into the mucosa.

Mucosal blood flow brings bicarbonate, oxygen, and nutrients to the luminal surface and removes hydrogen ions from the same region (4). The autonomic nervous system controls mucosal gastric blood flow. Nitric oxide, prostaglandins, epidermal growth factor, and transforming growth factor-alpha also regulate mucosal blood flow.

Some cytoprotectants are naturally present in the gastric mucosa. These include prostaglandins and sulfhydryl donors such as glutathione and neuropeptides (6,7,9,10). Prostaglandins play a major role in mucosal protection (8) by mediating mucus and bicarbonate secretion, inhibiting acid secretion at the level of the parietal cell, and regulating mucosal blood flow.

Normal mucosal defenses become altered in patients with gastric ulcers because of several factors. One factor is an increased proportion of low molecular weight dextrans in the gastric mucous layer, which results in weaker mucus (13), reduced mucosal hydrophobicity, and impaired prostaglandin production in patients taking NSAIDs. The association between NSAID ingestion and peptic ulcer formation is dramatic (see below).

PATHOGENESIS OF PEPTIC ULCERS

Role of *Helicobacter Pylori*

It is now recognized that infection with the bacterium *Helicobacter pylori* (HP) is a major etiologic factor in many forms of gastric disease, including peptic ulcer. Approximately 95 percent of patients with duodenal ulcers and 70 to 93 percent of patients with gastric ulcers have an associated HP infection (44). The mucosa, weakened by HP infection, becomes susceptible to acid attack, especially in the presence of increased gastric acid secretion, leading to peptic ulceration (20,23,44,45)

The corkscrew-like movement of the organisms and their production of various enzymes play important roles in the pathogenesis of

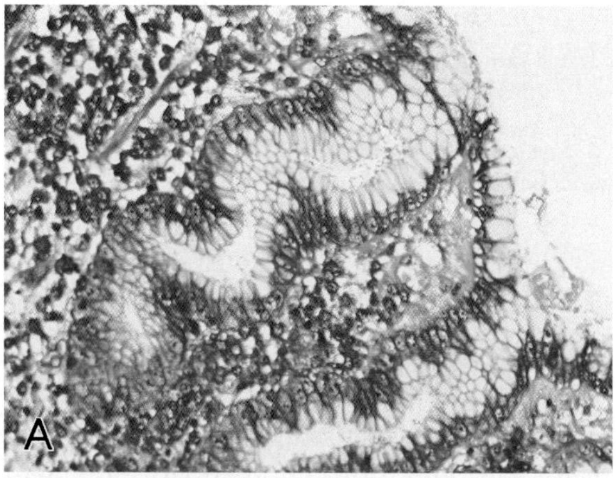

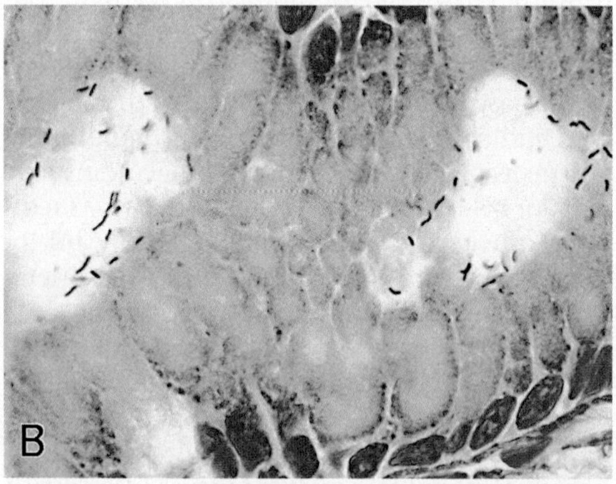

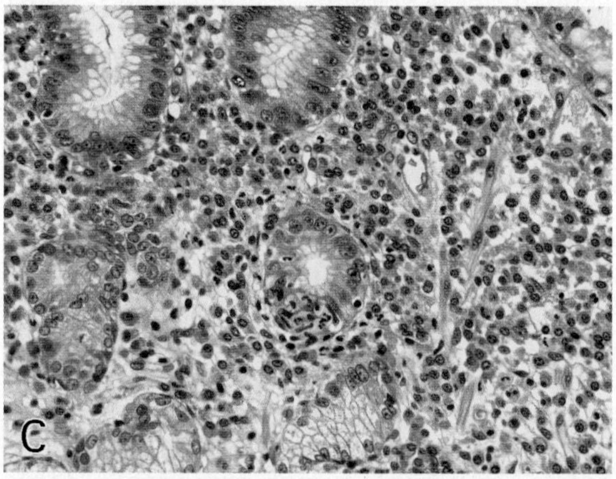

Figure 5-1

***HELICOBACTER PYLORI* GASTRITIS**

A: A Diff-Quik–stained preparation shows numerous curved bacteria in the mucus overlying the mucosal surface. Other organisms adhere to the apical and lateral aspects of the gastric foveolar cells.

B: Wenger-Angritt stain shows abundant organisms. (Fig. 2-29 from Emory TS, Carpenter HA, Gostout CJ, Sobin LH. Atlas of gastrointestinal endoscopy & endoscopic biopsies. Washington DC: Armed Forces Institute of Pathology; 2000:91.)

C: The inflammatory infiltrate associated with *H. pylori* includes a dense population of lymphocytes and plasma cells within the lamina propria, as well as neutrophils infiltrating the necks of the gastric glands.

gastritis and gastric ulcer (18,25,50,52–54). The majority of HP organisms reside in the unstirred layer of the gastric mucus, but some organisms bind to the luminal aspect of gastric foveolar cells (fig. 5-1). The organisms are motile, possessing one to five polar flagella (17). These flagella allow them to move freely within the mucous layer, and to reach the epithelial surface to which they attach (19,28).

HP organisms preferentially attach at or near intercellular junctions, perhaps reflecting the availability of nutrients or preferred metabolites diffusing through the junctional spaces. Once the intracellular junctions become weakened, the organisms penetrate the junctional complexes and move down along the lateral cell membranes of the surface foveolar cells. Generally, they do not invade the underlying lamina propria (33,35).

HP alters the release of intracellular mucins into the gastric lumen (41). The proteases produced by the organism further damage the epithelial protective layer by digesting gastric mucin (50,52,53). Organisms lying free in the mucus cause less epithelial damage than organisms located between, and even within, cells (33).

The powerful enzyme, urease, is produced by HP and has many functions. It protects the organisms against the acid environment of the stomach by creating an alkaline microenvironment (54). It also acts as an epithelial cytotoxin (51,54) and disrupts the intercellular tight junctions in a manner that allows cells to remain viable but also allows luminal contents, including acid, to flow between them (51). Organisms that fail to produce urease are incapable of gastric colonization and die in the acidic environment of the stomach (26,39,48).

HP organisms induce gastric inflammatory infiltrates composed of lymphocytes, plasma cells, macrophages, and neutrophils (fig. 5-1). This inflammation invariably disappears following eradication of the organisms. The inflammation is probably induced by bacterial products such as urease, porins, hemolysin, paf-acether, and cytotoxins (24,29,36,38,58,61). HP water extracts can promote neutrophil endothelial interactions (63).

Additionally, the organisms induce inflammation through direct contact with the gastric epithelium and induction of subsequent cytokine release (16).

HP infections result initially in acid hyposecretion, followed by normal gastric acid secretion, and finally, hypersecretion (27,40,42). Gastric acid secretion increases due to several mechanisms, and the acid hypersecretion reverses with eradication of the infection (31,34). Parietal cells gradually become atrophic as the HP-induced gastritis extends proximally to involve the oxyntic mucosa, thereby decreasing gastric acid secretory capacity. Patients with an increased parietal cell mass and hyperchlorhydria who become infected with HP organisms exhibit antral restriction of the gastritis because the high acid levels protect the corpus from bacterial adhesion and inflammation. Such patients develop acid-induced duodenal foveolar metaplasia, which becomes colonized by HP, eventually leading to active chronic duodenitis and, potentially, duodenal ulcer formation.

Not all individuals colonized with HP develop symptomatic gastric disease. This fact suggests that different strains of the bacteria vary in their pathogenicity. Approximately 50 percent of HP stains possess a *vacA* gene that encodes a vacuolating cytotoxin (22,29,36). The vacA cytotoxin produces vacuolation in many types of epithelial cells (29,36). Essentially all HP strains possess some form of the *vacA* gene, but it is a specific allelotype (s1-m1) that is associated with greater pathogenicity of the organisms (14,15). Some studies have found that HP strains expressing the vacA cytotoxin are more commonly found in patients with peptic ulcer disease than among HP-infected individuals with superficial gastritis alone (22,29,30,43,49,55).

Another potential virulence factor produced by approximately 60 percent of HP strains is cagA. A strong correlation is observed between the presence of the *cagA* gene and the production of vacuolating cytotoxin (21,59). Recent evidence suggests that the *cagA* gene is part of the so-called cag pathogenicity island, a cluster of approximately 15 genes that is absent in HP strains that do not produce the cagA protein. The presence of the cag pathogenicity island is associated with greater activity of gastritis and an increased degree of surface epithelial degeneration in the stomachs of infected individuals. CagA positivity has been strongly associated with the development of peptic ulcers in many studies (32,43,46,55,56). In some populations, however, cagA-positive HP strains do not appear to be associated with increased disease risk (37,47).

The type and grade of gastritis strongly predict the risk of a coexisting peptic ulcer. The risk of coexisting duodenal or gastric ulcers increases with the increasing grade of atrophic antral gastritis and decreases with an increasing grade of atrophic gastritis in the gastric body. These observations correlate with the fact that cagA-producing strains of HP are more likely to produce intense gastric inflammation, and therefore, are more frequently associated with the development of peptic ulcers. Ulcer recurrence is less frequent in patients whose HP infections have been eradicated than in those with continuing evidence of infection (57).

A third potential virulence factor, iceA, has recently been identified. The iceA1 allelic variant of the HP *iceA* gene has been linked to the development of peptic ulcer disease in one study (60). Other studies have failed to confirm this association (62).

Role of Acid Secretion

The increased acid secretion seen in duodenal and distal antral ulcer patients underscores the importance of acid/peptic activity in the development of peptic ulcer disease. In most patients, the excess acid results from an increased mass of acid-secreting gastric mucosa. An extreme example of this occurs in patients with gastrinomas and Zollinger-Ellison syndrome.

Role of Nonsteroidal Antiinflammatory Drugs

NSAID use is the most common cause of macroscopic gastric injury. Gastrointestinal injury secondary to NSAID use is among the most prevalent drug side effects seen in the United States: as many as 107,000 patients are hospitalized every year for NSAID-related ulcer complications (71). NSAID use is now the most common predisposing factor contributing to hospital admissions for peptic ulcer disease in the elderly. The incidence of gastroduodenal lesions in patients on chronic therapy varies from 31 to 68 percent (66,67,69); approximately 50 percent of patients on long-term NSAID therapy have gastric erosions, and up to 25 percent have gastric ulcers. Severe and sometimes fatal upper gastrointestinal hemorrhage occurs, especially in individuals over the age of 75 (72). This may relate to the fact that gastric mucosal prostaglandin levels decrease with age (68), making the mucosa more vulnerable to NSAID-induced injury. NSAIDs cause several types of injury, including acute mucosal hemorrhages, erosions, and chronic ulceration.

NSAIDs exert their effects on the gastric mucosa through several mechanisms. They cause defects in the normal gastric mucosal barrier, in part through their inhibition of prostaglandin synthesis. This effect occurs because NSAIDs act through inhibition of cyclooxygenase, a molecule essential for the production of eicosanoids such as prostaglandins E2 and I2. Cyclooxygenase inhibition also results in the production of metabolites such as leukotrienes, as arachidonic acid metabolism is shunted from the cyclooxygenase to the lipoxygenase pathway (64). The analgesic effects of NSAIDs occur mainly through inhibition of cyclooxygenase-2 (COX-2), while inhibition of cyclooxygenase-1 (COX-1) results in the deleterious effects on the gastric mucosal barrier. It is hoped that with the recent development of NSAIDs that specifically inhibit COX-2, the negative effects of these drugs on the gastroduodenal mucosa will be minimized. While recent studies suggest that this may be the case (65), potential benefits can be negated by co-therapy with salicylates. Unfortunately, the cost of COX-2 inhibitors is two to three times that of conventional NSAIDs.

NSAIDs also inhibit gastric mucosal secretion and alter cell membrane permeability, leading to acid back-diffusion into the lamina propria. In addition, they inhibit active bicarbonate secretion, alter surface phospholipids, and change mucosal blood flow.

NSAIDs usually produce acute mucosal lesions within 7 to 14 days of administration. True ulcers develop despite the fact that mucosal adaptation occurs (70,72). HP infection makes the mucosa more susceptible to NSAID-mediated damage. Conversely, NSAIDs intensify HP-induced injury.

Endoscopically, the lesions vary from erythematous patches or streaks to erosions and overt ulcerations, particularly of the gastric antrum, prepyloric area, and duodenal bulb. Histologically, the erosions or ulcers resemble stress-related changes or features of chemical gastropathy, although NSAIDs induce deeper pit inflammation than is commonly seen in other chemical gastropathies (fig. 5-2). There may be small superficial mucosal defects and extravasated red blood cells in the underlying lamina propria. The mucosa often appears edematous and regenerative. The degree of inflammation associated with these lesions tends to be minimal. Occasionally, neutrophilic infiltrates are seen at the junction of necrotic and viable tissues. Prominent eosinophilia may also be present. The diagnosis of these lesions is often problematic when based on biopsy evaluation, particularly in the absence of a history of NSAID ingestion.

Role of Steroids

Steroids do not cause as much gastric damage as NSAIDs, but they increase luminal acid loss in the presence of aspirin or bile salts. Additionally, the concomitant use of steroids and NSAIDs is associated with an up to 10-fold increased risk of upper gastrointestinal hemorrhage (74). In addition, the severity of the ulceration may be increased with concomitant steroid and NSAID use, particularly when COX-1 inhibitors are employed (75). Furthermore, steroids stimulate G-cell hyperplasia (73), indirectly increasing acid production by parietal cells. They also decrease the rate of epithelial turnover and mucin secretion, thereby impairing the healing process. For all of these reasons, steroid administration may exacerbate underlying gastric mucosal damage.

Role of Cigarette Smoking

Cigarette smoking has been linked to both the initiation and the delayed healing of gastric ulcers. Cigarette smoking has also been associated with relapse of duodenal ulcers, with nicotine exhibiting a dose-dependent effect on ulcer recurrence (76,79,80). Smoking increases the likelihood that surgery will be required for the treatment of peptic ulcer disease, and increases the risks of surgery (76).

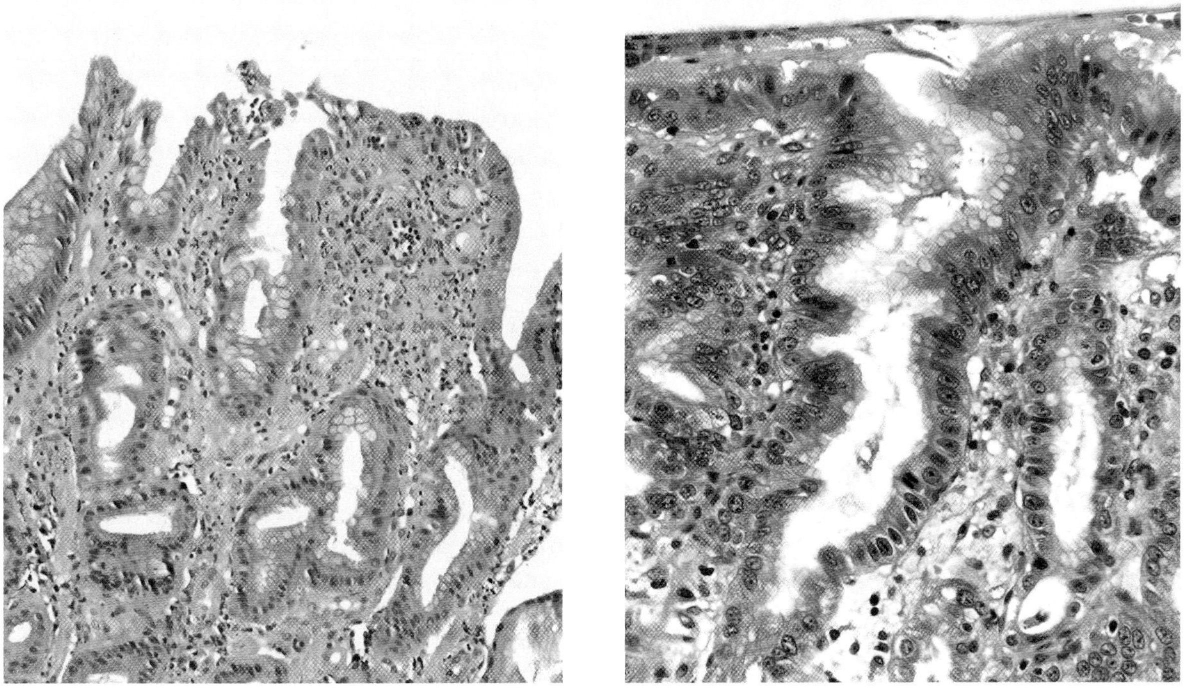

Figure 5-2

NONSTEROIDAL ANTIINFLAMMATORY DRUG (NSAID) INJURY

Left: Erosive gastritis secondary to NSAID injury. The lamina propria contains numerous acute inflammatory cells.
Right: A typical example of chemical gastropathy shows essentially no inflammation of the lamina propria, but reactive-appearing epithelial cells. The glands have a corkscrew-like appearance.

Numerous mechanisms have been proposed to explain the effect of smoking on peptic ulcer development (Table 5-1) (77,78). Traditionally, a close relationship has existed between peptic ulcers and chronic lung disease, but this association may reflect the role of smoking in both conditions.

Other Factors in Ulcer Development

Pepsins are another factor in peptic ulceration. These become irreversibly activated at an alkaline pH. An elevated level of pepsinogen 1 (PG1) is a marker of gastric peptic ulcer disease (82); the treatment of gastritis associated with peptic ulcer disease results in reduced serum PG1 levels (83). A specific pepsinogen C gene polymorphism may predict gastric ulcer risk (81).

Demography

The incidence of peptic ulcers depends on the geographic region, the age and sex of the patient, and the method used to make the diagnosis. Overall, gastric ulcers occur more frequently in individuals of increased age, a finding that is in part explained by increased NSAID use for the treatment of degenerative joint disorders in the elderly. The cumulative probability of developing a peptic ulcer, however, is

Table 5-1

EFFECTS OF SMOKING ON THE GASTRIC MUCOSA

Increased acid and pepsin secretion
Increased gastric motility and emptying
Reduced efficacy of H_2-blocker therapy
Decreased prostaglandin synthesis
Decreased mucosal blood flow
Decreased epidermal growth factor secretion
Increased risk of *Helicobacter pylori*–associated damage
Increased free radical production
Increased synthesis of cytokines
Increased bile reflux

Table 5-2

GENETIC SYNDROMES ASSOCIATED WITH PEPTIC ULCERS

Multiple endocrine neoplasia type 1
Essential tremor, congenital nystagmus, and narcolepsy
Familial forms of systemic mastocytosis
Van Allen form of amyloidosis with neuropathy, nephropathy, and peptic ulcer
Pachydermoperiostosis and hypertrophic gastropathy

Table 5-3

SITES OF PEPTIC ULCERS

Stomach
Duodenum
Barrett esophagus
Meckel diverticulum
Surgical anastomotic sites and stomas
Sites of ectopic gastric mucosa

highest in middle-aged men (aged 41 to 60 years) in whom chronic antral gastritis or chronic pangastritis is present (89). In populations at high risk for developing gastric cancer (e.g., Japanese), gastric ulcers are more common than duodenal ulcers.

A marked change has occurred in the incidence of peptic ulcer disease over the last century: current figures suggest that the overall incidence of peptic ulcer disease is declining (85). Hypotheses to explain this decline include changes in smoking habits (90), improved living conditions that decrease the likelihood of HP infection, decreased physical workload, and decreased salt intake. In contrast, the incidence of ulcers in women is increasing.

Estimates of ulcer frequency in children have also increased in recent times. Twenty to 50 percent of adults and 25 to 62 percent of children with ulcers (86,87) have a family history of peptic ulcer disease. Peptic ulcers in children, like adults, may be associated with NSAID use (88). Primary peptic ulcers in children under the age of 6 are usually gastric and affect boys and girls equally (84). Most are located in the antrum.

GASTRIC PEPTIC ULCER DISEASE

Definition. *Gastric peptic ulcer disease* is a defect occurring in the mucosal surface of the stomach, usually as a result of the action of acid and pepsin on a mucosa with impaired defense mechanisms.

Etiology. Peptic ulcers fall into three etiologic groups: those resulting from acid hypersecretion, as in Zollinger-Ellison syndrome; those due to NSAID use; and those associated with HP infection. HP-associated ulcers form the largest subset. Gastric and duodenal ulcers share overlapping epidemiologic and pathophysiologic features but also show significant differences. Prepyloric and duodenal ulcers arise in the setting of increased acid secretion and antral gastritis, whereas gastric ulcers are associated with decreased gastric acid secretion and diminished mucosal defense mechanisms. Some genetic syndromes are associated with an increased risk of developing peptic ulcers (Table 5-2)

Clinical Features. Episodic epigastric pain constitutes the most prominent clinical feature of gastric peptic ulcer disease. The pain, aggravated by meals or alcohol, often occurs at night, awakening the patient. Bleeding develops in about 20 percent of patients and is massive in 5 percent. Endoscopic visualization of a bleeding vessel or other signs of recent hemorrhage predict further bleeding and increased mortality (94,95). Juxtapyloric ulcers may cause obstruction early due to the presence of coexisting edema and pyloric stenosis as the ulcer heals and fibrosis develops.

Occasionally, a large gastric ulcer high on the lesser curvature heals to produce a scarred, constricted, hourglass-shaped stomach. Giant gastric ulcers are more likely to result in severe hemorrhage or penetrate into contiguous organs. The risk of microscopic malignancy is significantly greater in giant ulcers than in the nongiant type (91). Rarely, peptic ulcers penetrate into the pericardium and heart (96), especially in patients with previous surgery involving the esophagogastric region.

Gross Findings. The term "peptic ulcer" refers to any deep mucosal break resulting from exposure to gastric acid or pepsin. Such ulcers develop adjacent to any site containing oxyntic mucosa, including those listed in Table 5-3. Rarely, they arise in the acid-secreting mucosa itself. Acute peptic ulcers are often deep, are

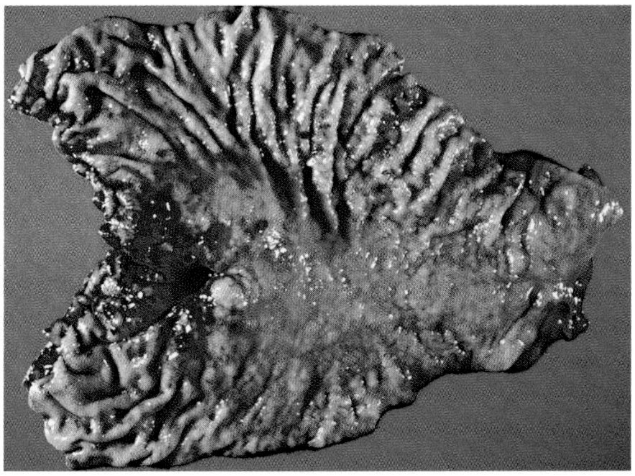

Figure 5-3

GASTRIC ULCER

Antrectomy specimen shows a punched-out, deep peptic ulcer near the antral-corpus junction.

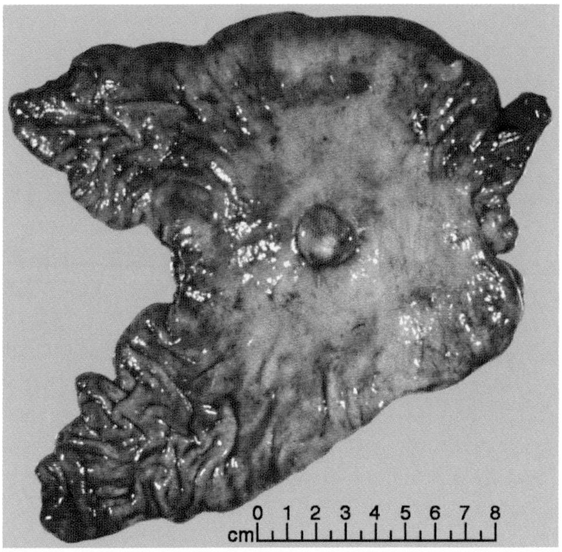

Figure 5-4

BENIGN GASTRIC ULCER

The ulcer appears punched out and has a clean-appearing base. The surrounding mucosa is flattened and atrophic.

more than 0.5 cm in diameter, penetrate the muscularis mucosae, and have little fibrous tissue at their base. Those that measure greater than 3 cm in diameter are sometimes referred to as *giant gastric ulcers*.

Gastric ulcers are usually solitary, although about 30 percent of patients have associated duodenal ulcers. Gastric peptic ulcers arise in any part of the stomach, but they typically develop on its lesser curvature, usually at the antral-corpus junction (fig. 5-3).

Benign ulcers typically appear as round to oval, sharply punched-out lesions with perpendicular walls (fig. 5-4). The surrounding mucosa appears congested and edematous, and often overhangs the margin, forming a lip and sometimes imparting a flask-shaped appearance to the ulcer. The lip of a benign peptic ulcer should not appear rolled or heaped up. The mucosa away from the ulcer also often appears atrophic with flattened mucosal folds (fig. 5-4). Scarring at the ulcer base often causes puckering of the surrounding mucosal folds, causing them to radiate away from the ulcer in a spoke-like fashion. The ulcer base should appear smooth and cream colored or pearly gray unless hemorrhage has occurred. In contrast, ulcerated carcinomas tend to be shallow, irregular, bowl-shaped lesions with rolled or heaped up, sloping borders. Their bases appear necrotic and flattened out. The ulcer often distorts the rugal folds in such a way that they do not converge toward it or, if they do, they terminate short of it.

Ulcer depth varies; deeper ulcers may perforate through the stomach wall, extending into adjacent structures. Giant gastric ulcers are more likely to penetrate than nongiant ulcers (91).

Microscopic Findings. A gastric biopsy differentiates benign gastric ulcers from ulcerated invasive carcinomas. Multiple biopsies taken from the ulcer edge increase the chance of making a correct diagnosis. The likelihood of obtaining a positive cancer diagnosis increases from 45 percent when four biopsies are taken to 99 percent when eight or more are taken (92). It may be technically impossible, however, to perform this many biopsies under some circumstances.

Histologically, four zones characterize chronic ulcers: 1) a superficial layer of polymorphonuclear leukocytes and fibrin debris; 2) an underlying layer of coagulation necrosis; 3) a deeper layer of granulation tissue; and 4) a deepest layer of fibrosis at the ulcer base (fig. 5-5). The latter often disrupts the muscularis mucosae and the submucosa, and can be highlighted using a trichrome stain. The vessels at the ulcer base usually show an obliterative endarteritis. The extent of this change governs the magnitude of hemorrhage that occurs should the vessels become eroded.

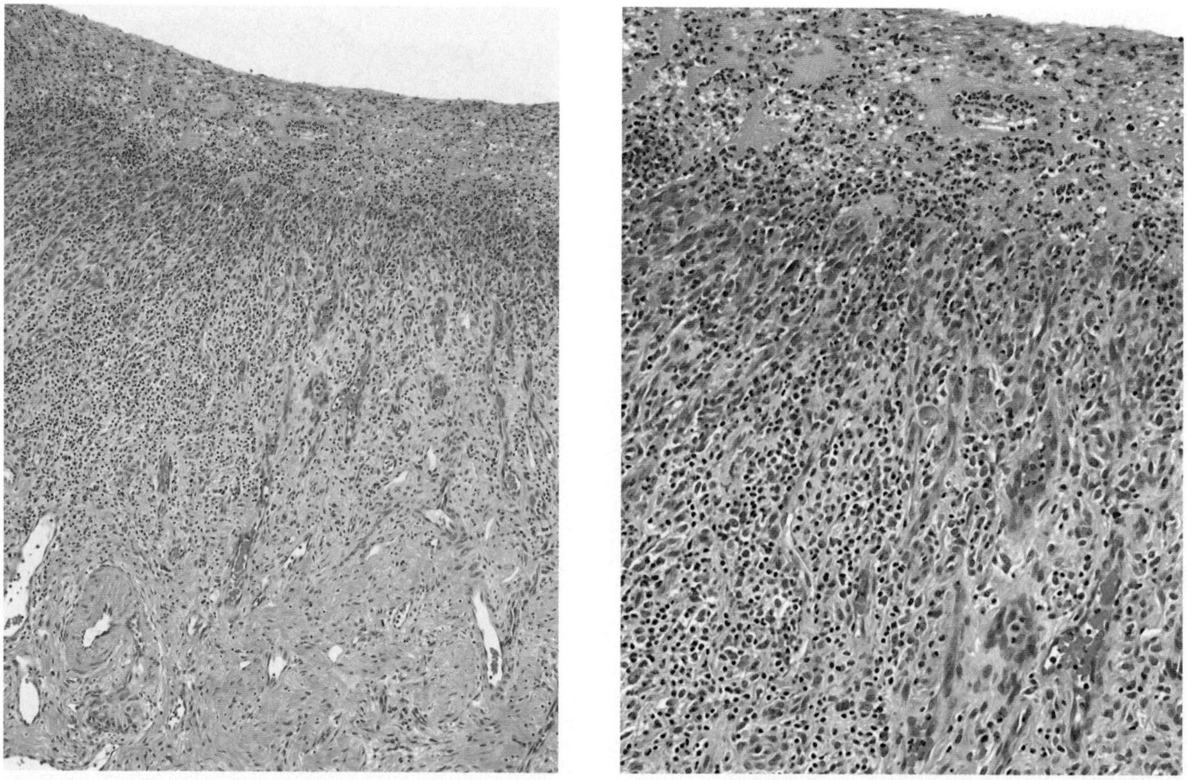

Figure 5-5

ULCER HISTOLOGY

Left: Low-power microscopy shows the layers that comprise a typical peptic ulcer. A superficial layer of fibrin and an acute inflammatory exudate are over a layer of granulation tissue. Under the granulation tissue is a layer of fibrosis.

Right: Higher-power view shows the inflamed granulation tissue in the ulcer base.

Candida may also colonize the ulcer base. If the organism does not invade the underlying tissues, it has no clinical significance, nor does it necessarily prolong the healing process.

Acute peptic ulcers do not contain the four zones described above. A polymorphonuclear exudate replaces the epithelium and moderate amounts of granulation tissue fill the ulcer center. The remaining mucosa appears regenerative, with immature cells and occasional mitotic figures. Scarring is absent.

Histologic examination of bleeding gastric ulcers usually reveals a small, eroded artery in the ulcer crater (fig. 5-6). The larger the eroded artery, the more likely that death will result. Arterial diameter ranges from 1.5 to 3.4 mm in 25 percent of patients with fatal bleeding ulcers (94). Histologically, the blood vessel may show evidence of aneurysmal dilatation, intense arteritis, and endarteritis obliterans.

Peptic ulcers begin to heal by the inward migration of a single epithelial layer at the ulcer edge (fig. 5-7). The proliferating mucosa grows downward and extends over the ulcer surface. This single cell layer may entirely cover the surface of small ulcers (less than 2 cm). Simple mucous glands also develop. Mucosal islands may become entrapped in the fibrous or granulation tissue, and may be mistaken for invasive carcinoma. Away from the ulcer, the mucosa appears normal or exhibits chronic gastritis. Prominent collections of chronic inflammatory cells that are associated with neural hyperplasia may be seen in the gastric wall adjacent to the ulcer. This finding could suggest a diagnosis of Crohn's disease if one were unaware of the presence of a nearby healing ulcer. The neuromuscular changes that occur in association with peptic ulcers may result in disordered gastric motility.

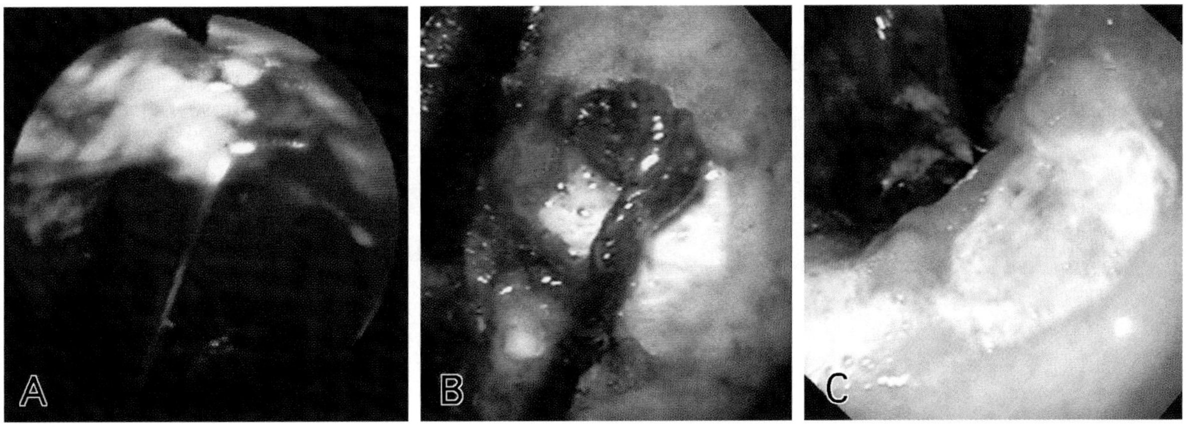

Figure 5-6

BLEEDING ULCER

A: Endoscopic view of an actively bleeding gastric ulcer.

B: Another ulcer that is not actively bleeding, but shows an overlying blood clot, suggesting a previous episode of hemorrhage.

C: Endoscopic appearance of the ulcer following removal of the blood clot.

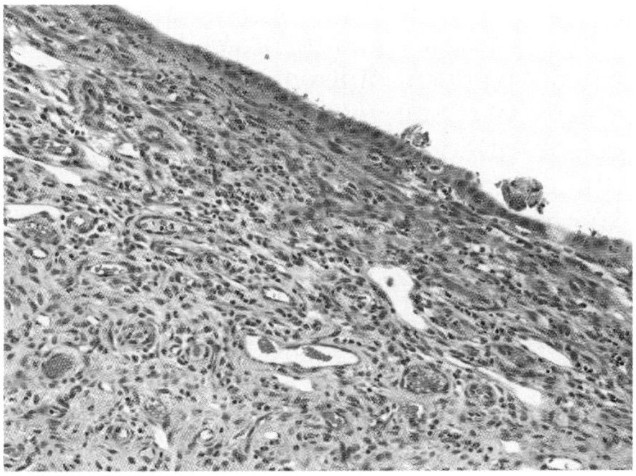

Figure 5-7

HEALING ULCER

A single layer of cuboidal epithelial cells is seen migrating inward to reepithelialize this gastric ulcer. Organizing granulation tissue underlies the new epithelial layer.

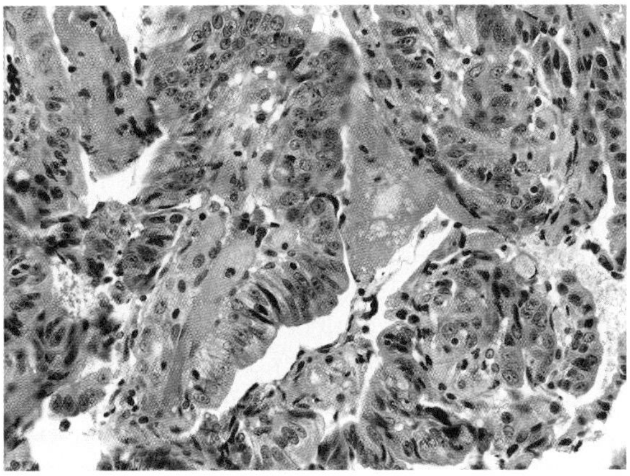

Figure 5-8

EPITHELIAL CHANGES ADJACENT TO A GASTRIC ULCER

The epithelium shows marked atypia with increased nuclear to cytoplasmic ratios, large hyperchromatic nuclei, and prominent nucleoli. Scattered acute inflammatory cells are present, suggesting that the histologic changes are likely reactive.

The serosa underlying a peptic ulcer often appears fibrotic, demonstrates fat necrosis, or shows areas of mesothelial hyperplasia. The fibrosis and fat necrosis thicken the gastric wall. Adhesions develop and extensive areas of mesothelial hyperplasia may be trapped within the inflammatory process. Regional lymph nodes become enlarged and reactive in appearance.

Differential Diagnosis. One of the most difficult tasks facing the pathologist is to distinguish malignant cells from the regenerative atypia invariably present in areas of gastritis adjacent to ulcers (fig. 5-8) (93). Reactive fibrosis at the base or sides of a chronic ulcer crater can distort the regenerating glands and suggest the possibility of tissue invasion, particularly in the presence of a partially healed ulcer where epithelial regeneration is still occurring. Under

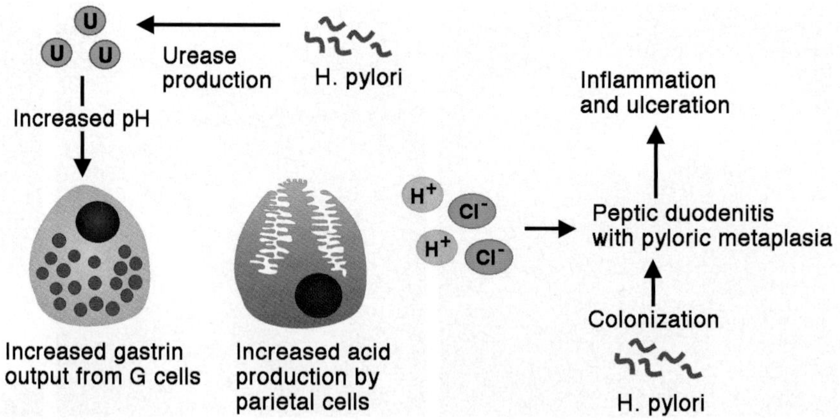

Figure 5-9

DUODENAL ULCER DEVELOPMENT

The diagram depicts the pathophysiology of duodenal ulcer development.

such circumstances, it is imperative to recognize the classic cytologic hallmarks of malignancy before making a diagnosis of cancer.

When the pathologist cannot unequivocally distinguish regenerative epithelium from carcinoma, a subsequent rebiopsy, once the inflammation subsides, may be warranted if a strong clinical suspicion for cancer exists. If, on the other hand, the clinical features suggest that the lesion is benign and reactive, the patient can be treated medically for 4 to 6 weeks, then reevaluated and additional biopsies taken at that time. A useful rule of thumb is that any chronic gastric ulcer that has been histologically diagnosed as benign should be followed by the gastroenterologist until ulcer healing is complete. Larger ulcers take longer to heal. Ongoing NSAID intake may retard healing.

The use of immunostains for cytokeratin may help to determine whether or not single cells have extended into the lamina propria. Such preparations should be carefully interpreted because isolated non-neoplastic cells can remain entrapped in the granulation or fibrous tissue at the base of gastric ulcers. Alternatively, residual epithelial remnants from the associated gastritis may be present. Cytokeratin positivity occasionally can be found in nonepithelial cells, especially near the peritoneal surface. Such cytokeratin-positive, spindled submesothelial cells do not communicate with the gastric mucosa and usually fail to show other epithelial features, such as epithelial membrane antigen immunoreactivity. The cytokeratin-positive cells are also vimentin immunoreactive.

The distinction between chronic ulcers and ulcerating cancers is further facilitated by examination of the muscularis propria. Deep ulcers and their scars result in fibrous replacement of the muscle layer, whereas the muscularis propria deep to a cancer usually remains intact and nonfibrotic, and may even become accentuated.

DUODENAL PEPTIC DISEASES

Peptic duodenitis and *peptic duodenal ulcers* essentially represent different phases of the same process. As a result, many patients who initially present with duodenitis later develop a duodenal ulcer. Peptic duodenitis results from chronic overexposure to hydrochloric acid from the stomach and is usually confined to the duodenal bulb.

Peptic duodenitis progresses to erosive peptic duodenitis with superficial loss of the duodenal mucosa and then to frank peptic ulceration. Factors leading to duodenal ulcer formation include mucosal inflammation, weakening of the mucus bicarbonate barrier, superficial epithelial cell damage, increased serum gastrin levels with defective feedback control, an increase in parietal cell mass in some patients, and the development of gastric metaplasia. Colonization by HP organisms further weakens mucosal defenses.

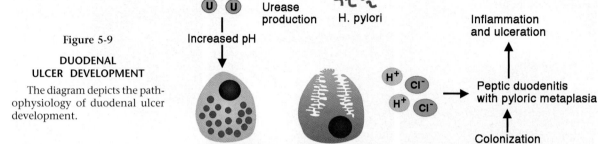

HP colonize areas of foveolar metaplasia in peptic duodenitis and play a major role in the genesis of peptic ulcer disease (fig. 5-9) (99–103). Patients with duodenal HP infection generally have coexisting gastric infection. Once colonized, the organisms propagate and increase areas of the foveolar metaplasia (103). The metaplastic epithelium becomes inflamed by the same mechanisms that exist in the stomach. The urease produced by HP in the stomach increases the gastric pH, which in turn stimulates antral G cells, resulting in increased gastrin release and increased gastric acid secretion. This then leads to an increased duodenal acid load. Treatment of the infection enhances ulcer healing and reduces ulcer recurrence, further confirming the etiologic relationship of HP with duodenal ulcer.

Role of Genetic Factors

The increased incidence of duodenal ulcers among first-degree relatives and patients with blood type group O (98) and an elevated concentration of serum pepsinogen 1 suggests that genetic factors play some role in duodenal ulcer pathogenesis. This hypothesis is supported by the discovery of familial clusters of ulcer patients with elevation of the same pepsinogen group 1 fractions. The hyperpepsinogenemia reflects an increased gastric pepsin-secreting and acid-secreting cell mass (97).

Peptic Duodenitis

Gross Findings. The gross appearance of peptic duodenitis varies from simple mucosal erythema to mucosal friability and nodularity. The erythema results from the shunting of blood to the villous tips induced by increased hydrochloric acid. Severe cases exhibit erosions and ulcers. With long-standing disease, mucosal atrophy, thickening, or irregularity may be present. Areas of nodularity usually correspond to areas of Brunner gland hyperplasia.

Microscopic Findings. The principal histologic features of peptic duodenitis are: 1) inflammatory cells in the epithelium or lamina propria; 2) altered epithelial cell morphology due to degeneration, regeneration, or metaplastic changes; 3) mucosal hemorrhage and edema; and 4) Brunner gland hyperplasia. In the most severe forms of duodenitis, villous atrophy can be seen.

The presence of foveolar cell metaplasia (gastric surface epithelial metaplasia) provides a helpful clue to the diagnosis of peptic duodenitis (fig. 5-10). Foveolar metaplasia probably represents an adaptive response to duodenal hyperacidity and may protect against ulceration because, like the surface epithelium of the stomach, this epithelium has a number of defense mechanisms that protect it from acid. Histologically, the metaplastic cells appear as fully developed gastric mucous cells or they may demonstrate features intermediate between gastric and intestinal cells.

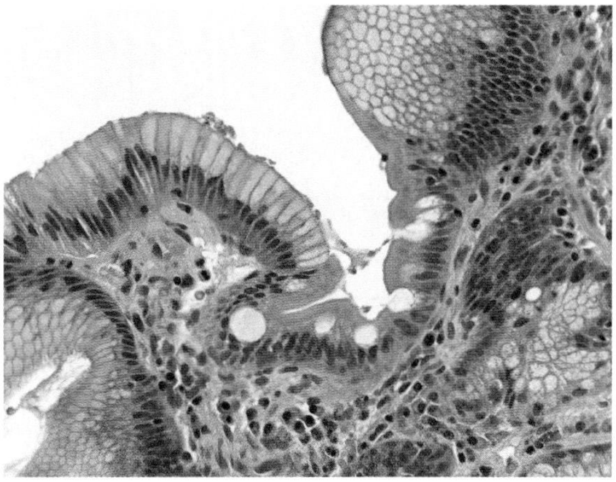

Figure 5-10

PEPTIC DUODENITIS WITH GASTRIC FOVEOLAR METAPLASIA

On the left, the epithelial lining is composed of cells with an appearance similar to the gastric surface epithelium. In the center, residual enterocytes and goblet cells that normally make up the small intestinal epithelium are seen. Eosinophils are prominent.

HP organisms may colonize areas of foveolar cell metaplasia using the same mechanisms as in the stomach. The bacteria are much more likely to be seen when the metaplasia is extensive. The organisms inhibit the secretion of proximal duodenal mucosal bicarbonate. The result is decreased acid neutralization in the duodenal lumen and further exacerbation of peptic injury to the duodenal mucosa. The gastric metaplasia may disappear after treatment of the HP infection.

Endoscopically identified nodular duodenitis usually occurs secondary to hyperplasia of the Brunner glands in the submucosa and mucosa of the duodenum. Histologically, the glands appear identical to normal Brunner glands except that they are increased in number and size (fig. 5-11). The glands retain their lobular architecture, but the lobules vary in size, and fibromuscular strands stretch between them. No capsule surrounds the glands. Larger polypoid lesions may become superficially eroded.

Brunner gland hyperplasia is an adaptive response to the increased luminal acid that accompanies peptic duodenitis. Brunner glands normally produce alkaline secretions that neutralize duodenal luminal acid. Hypergastrinemia also plays an etiologic role in the hyperplasia,

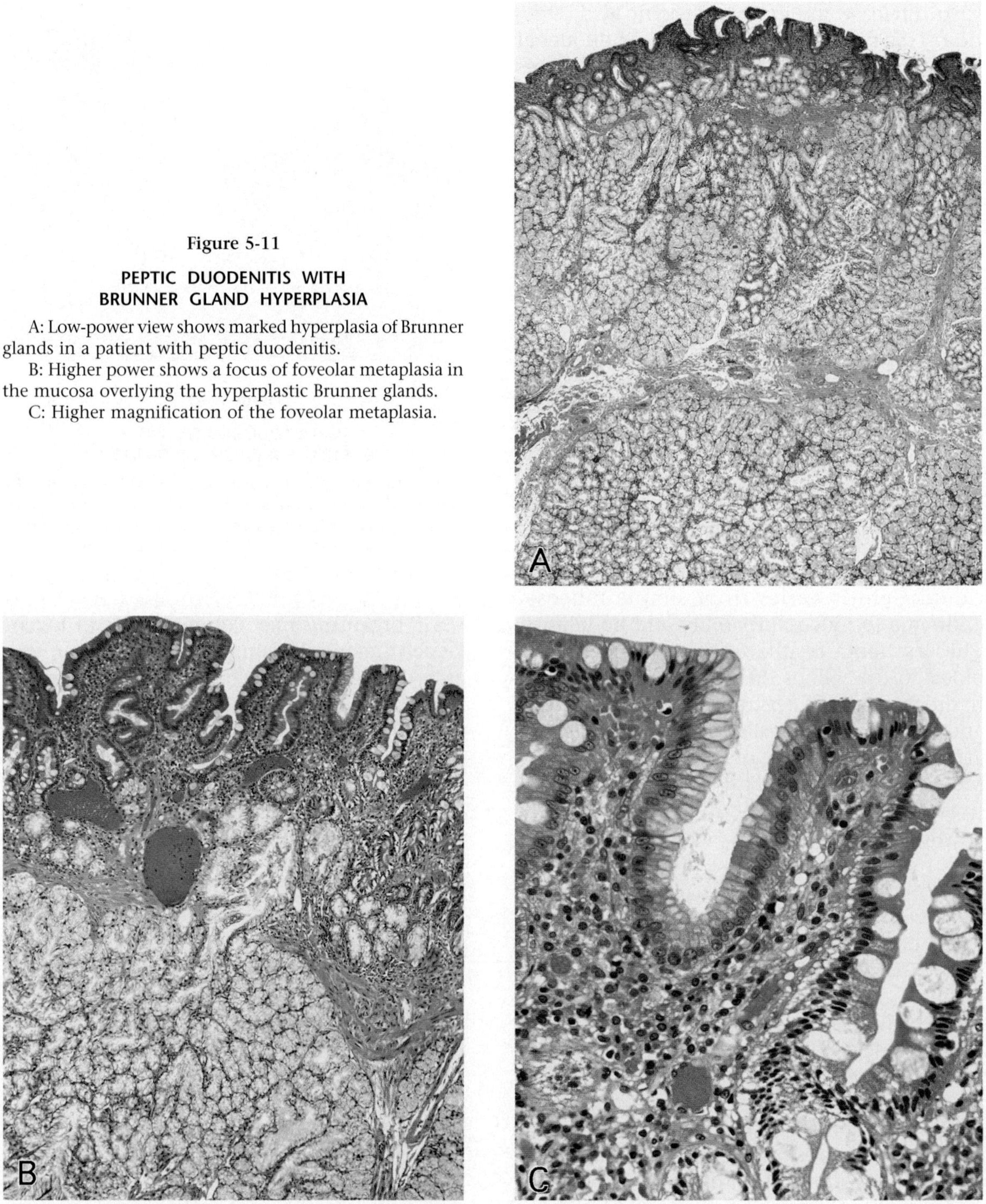

Figure 5-11

PEPTIC DUODENITIS WITH BRUNNER GLAND HYPERPLASIA

A: Low-power view shows marked hyperplasia of Brunner glands in a patient with peptic duodenitis.

B: Higher power shows a focus of foveolar metaplasia in the mucosa overlying the hyperplastic Brunner glands.

C: Higher magnification of the foveolar metaplasia.

presumably through its trophic effects on the cells of Brunner glands. Occasionally, the hyperplastic area may assume the characteristics of a polypoid mass that may ulcerate and bleed, and if particularly large, may lead to mechanical problems including gastric outlet obstruction.

Most of the histologic features of peptic duodenitis are nonspecific. Similar findings

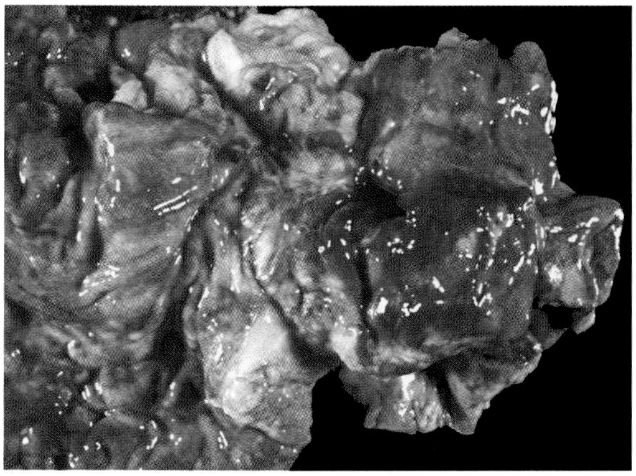

Figure 5-12

DUODENAL ULCER

A deep ulcer in the proximal portion of the duodenum.

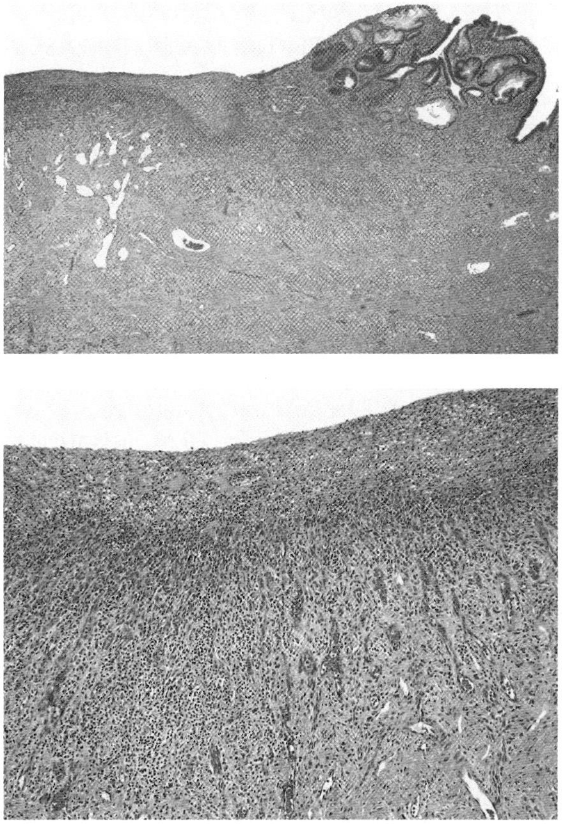

Figure 5-13

DUODENAL ULCER

Top: Low-power view of a duodenal ulcer with adjacent peptic duodenitis. Even at low power, foveolar epithelium can be appreciated at the ulcer edge.

Bottom: The ulcer is similar to those seen in the stomach.

occur in patients with Crohn's disease, drug-induced injury, stress-induced duodenitis, and certain infectious diseases.

Duodenal Ulcer

Clinical Features. Patients with duodenal ulcers experience general symptoms of dyspepsia and intermittent abdominal pain. Duodenal ulcers are more likely to perforate, bleed, or cause obstruction than are gastric ulcers. In some cases, the bleeding may be massive. Recurrent bleeding affects 13.6 to 32.0 percent of patients, especially those older than 60 years of age (104,108). Duodenal ulcers also occur in children. In young patients, the clinical presentation is often atypical. Children with cystic fibrosis are particularly prone to develop duodenal ulcers due to decreased duodenal bicarbonate secretion.

Duodenal ulcers may be multiple. Patients with multiple ulcers have lower healing rates and higher mean fasting and meal-stimulated serum gastrin levels than those with single ulcers. The presence of multiple ulcers should arouse the suspicion of NSAID use or Zollinger-Ellison syndrome. Patients with Zollinger-Ellison syndrome also have ulcers in the second and third portions of the duodenum or jejunum and/or repeated penetrating or perforating ulcers in the third portion of the duodenum or first portion of the jejunum.

Gross Findings. Usually, duodenal ulcers appear circular or oval, and measure less than 3 cm in maximum diameter (fig. 5-12). Ulcers measuring greater than 3 cm in diameter are unusual. Ulcers located in the posterior portion of the duodenal bulb are more likely to bleed than those situated elsewhere (107) because two sizable vessels, the pancreaticoduodenal and the gastroduodenal arteries, lie in the vicinity. Penetration of the duodenal wall by an ulcer may result in erosion of one or both of these vessels, producing massive hemorrhage. Ulcer scarring may lead to the formation of a prestenotic diverticulum.

Microscopic Findings. Histologically, duodenal ulcers resemble their counterparts in the stomach. Features of peptic duodenitis are often seen in the adjacent nonulcerated mucosa (fig. 5-13).

TREATMENT AND PROGNOSIS FOR PATIENTS WITH PEPTIC ULCER DISEASE

The treatment of peptic ulcers depends on several factors, the most important of which are whether the patient is infected with HP and whether the patient is taking NSAIDs. In general, all patients with peptic ulcer disease should be advised to stop smoking. Prophylaxis with maintenance antisecretory agents may need to be considered in those patients who present with an ulcer complication, those who have numerous co-morbidities, or those who cannot discontinue anti-inflammatory agents.

HP-Infected Patients. In 1994, a National Institutes of Health consensus conference recommended that all patients with peptic ulcer and HP infection should be given antimicrobial therapy (109). Optimal therapy for HP-associated peptic ulcer disease includes treatment with combinations of antibiotics and antisecretory agents. The antibiotics that appear to be most effective in eradicating HP organisms are clarithromycin and metronidazole. These drugs may be used in combination with other antibiotics such as tetracycline or amoxicillin. The selection of an antibiotic regimen should depend on local prevalence rates of antibiotic-resistant HP strains (112). The addition of bismuth-containing compounds to the treatment regimen may enhance ulcer healing through stimulation of prostaglandin synthesis and bicarbonate secretion.

First-line therapies are generally effective in eradicating HP infection 90 to 95 percent of the time. In some patients, second-line therapy, consisting of a proton pump inhibitor, bismuth, tetracycline, and either metronidazole or clarithromycin, is necessary. The choice of whether to use metronidazole or clarithromycin depends on which drug was initially given as a first-line therapy: if metronidazole-containing first-line therapy was unsuccessful, then the second-line treatment should contain clarithromycin, and vice versa.

Patients Taking NSAIDs. Optimally, patients with peptic ulcers who are taking an NSAID should stop the drug, if possible. In many cases, however, NSAID cessation is not an option. In such patients, administration of the prostaglandin E1 analogue, misoprostol, may facilitate ulcer healing when used in combination with antisecretory agents (110). In addition, misoprostol may be effective in preventing the development of gastritis and peptic ulcers in patients receiving NSAIDs (111). Some studies suggest that proton pump inhibitors may be as or more effective than misoprostol in promoting ulcer healing in patients on NSAIDs (106). Proton pump inhibitors have fewer side effects and are better tolerated by most patients than misoprostol.

Another effective method of treating patients with NSAID-induced ulcers is substituting a nonspecific COX inhibitor for a specific COX-2 inhibitor. A recent study suggests that celecoxib (a COX-2 inhibitor) was as effective as diclofenac plus omeprazole in preventing recurrent bleeding from peptic ulcers (105). Major drawbacks to this therapy are renal toxicity, fluid retention, hypertension, possible associations with cardiac events, and cost.

Patients Without HP Infection or NSAID Use. Peptic ulcer patients who are negative for HP and are not taking NSAIDs can usually be successfully treated with antisecretory therapy alone. Either H_2-blockers or proton pump inhibitors may be used.

ZOLLINGER-ELLISON SYNDROME

Etiology. The gastroduodenal changes in *Zollinger-Ellison syndrome* (ZES) consist of two major alterations: peptic ulcer disease and hypertrophic gastropathy. ZES represents the prototypic hypersecretory gastropathy. It is characterized by gastric mucosal hypertrophy and acid hypersecretion. The acid hypersecretion results in the development of multiple peptic ulcers, usually in the duodenum. Excessive gastrin production serves as the stimulus for increased gastric acid production, often as a result of a gastrin-secreting tumor (gastrinoma) located either in the pancreas or in the intestinal wall. A minority of patients with ZES show evidence of gastric G-cell hyperplasia rather than a gastrin-producing tumor.

Gastrin has multiple targets, the major one of which is the parietal cell, which secretes hydrochloric acid in the stomach. Gastrin also increases the growth of parietal cells, chief cells, enterochromaffin-like (ECL) cells, and foveolar epithelium, a factor that accounts for the hypertrophy that occurs in the gastric mucosa in patients with this disorder.

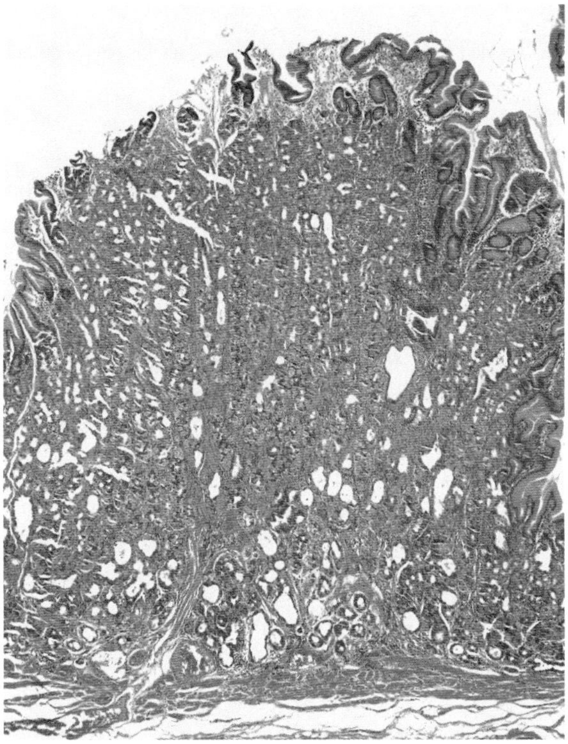

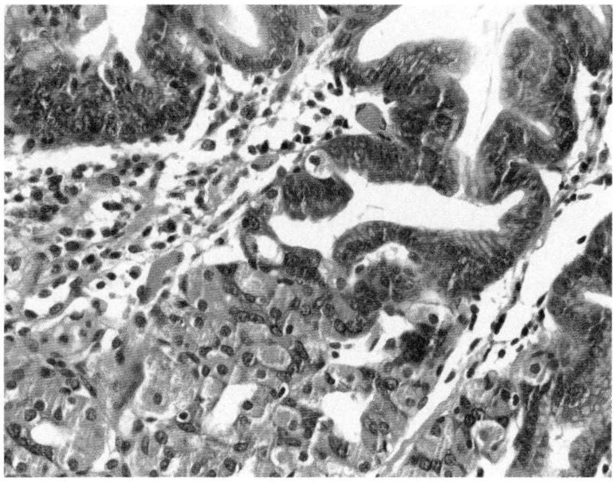

Figure 5-14

ZOLLINGER-ELLISON SYNDROME

Left: Low-power microscopy demonstrates a marked increase in the glandular component of the gastric oxyntic mucosa.

Above: On higher power, parietal cells lie in the upper portions of the gastric pits, where they are normally not present.

Clinical Features. ZES affects 0.1 percent of all patients with duodenal ulcer disease; studies among European populations have documented an incidence of between 0.2 and 0.4 case/million population/year. The disease occurs in patients ranging in age from 7 to 90 years (113), with most patients diagnosed between the 3rd and 5th decades of life. There is no major sex predominance. The usual presenting symptom is abdominal pain, which affects 70 to 95 percent of patients; diarrhea affects 33 to 75 percent of patients.

Some patients lack all features of ZES. Peptic ulcers may be absent, and diarrhea with steatorrhea may be the only clinical manifestation. The acid hypersecretion may be mild and indistinguishable from that seen with ordinary duodenal ulcer. The marked parietal and peptic cell hyperplasia (115) expands the gastric glands and causes rugal hypertrophy and acid hypersecretion with subsequent peptic ulceration.

Gross Findings. Giant rugal folds spare the antrum but cover the body and fundus. The surfaces of the folds appear uniformly exaggerated, coarsely granular, or finely cobblestoned.

Microscopic Findings. Histologic examination of the hypertrophic gastric folds reveals substantial glandular lengthening due to increased numbers of parietal cells (fig. 5-14). The increased parietal cell mass comprises a progressively larger share of the glands, filling their entire length down to the base. Parietal cells also extend into the neck regions or higher, coming closer to the surface than usual (fig. 5-14). In some cases, parietal cells completely populate the mucosal glands. Large numbers of parietal cells can also be present in the antrum, an area that usually lacks these cells. The foveolae appear normal in length or shortened.

Treatment and Prognosis. The acid hypersecretion in patients with ZES can be controlled with the use of inhibitors of H^+/K^+-ATPase, which is present on the gastric parietal cell membrane (114). As a result, the acid-mediated manifestations (ulceration, bleeding, perforation, diarrhea, and reflux) are seldom fatal. These medications do not influence tumor growth and spread. Consequently, for many patients, the tissue bulk and invasive effects of the gastrin-secreting tumor are more problematic. While localization of small lesions may be challenging, surgery, particularly for localized, nonmetastatic tumors, affords the best chance of cure (116).

REFERENCES

Normal Gastric Defense Mechanisms

1. Allen A, Cunliffe WJ, Pearson JP, Venables CW. The adherent gastric mucus gel barrier in man and changes in peptic ulceration. J Intern Med suppl 1990;732:83–90.
2. Allen A, Flemstrom G, Garner A, Kivilaakso E. Gastroduodenal mucosal protection. Physiol Rev 1993;73:823–57.
3. Engel E, Peskoff A, Kauffman GL Jr, Grossman MI. Analysis of hydrogen ion concentration in the gastric gel mucus layer. Am J Physiol 1984;247:G321–38.
4. Holzer P, Livingston EH, Guth PH. Sensory neurons signal of an increase in rat gastric mucosal blood flow in the face of pending acid injury. Gastroenterology 1991;101:416–23.
5. Kao YC, Lichtenberger LM. Phospholipid- and neutral lipid-containing organelles of rat gastroduodenal mucous cells. Possible origin of the hydrophobic mucosal lining. Gastroenterology 1991;101:7–21.
6. Konturek PK, Brzozowski T, Konturek SJ, Dembinski A. Role of epidermal growth factor, prostaglandin, and sulfhydryls in stress-induced gastric lesions. Gastroenterology 1990;99:1607–15.
7. Redfern JS, Feldman M. Role of endogenous prostaglandins in preventing gastrointestinal ulceration: induction of ulcers by antibodies to prostaglandins. Gastroenterology 1989;96:596–605.
8. Robert A. Role of endogenous and exogenous prostaglandins in mucosal protection. In: Allen A, Flemstrom G, Garner A, et al, eds. Mechanisms of mucosal protection in the upper gastrointestinal tract. New York: Raven Press; 1984:377.
9. Robert A, Eberle D, Kaplowitz N. Role of glutathione in gastric mucosal cytoprotection. Am J Physiol 1984;247:G296–304.
10. Scheiman JM, Kraus ER, Bonnville LA, Weinhold PA, Boland CR. Synthesis and prostaglandin E2-induced secretion of surfactant phospholipid by isolated gastric mucous cells. Gastroenterology 1991;100:1232–40.
11. Williams SE, Turnberg LA. Demonstration of a pH gradient across mucous adherent to rabbit gastric mucosa; evidence for a "mucous-bicarbonate" barrier. Gut 1981;22:94–6
12. Williams SE, Turnberg LA. Retardation of acid diffusion by gastric mucosa: a potential role in mucosal protection. Gastroenterology 1980;79:299–304.
13. Younan F, Pearson J, Allen A, Venables C. Changes in the structure of the mucous gel on the mucosal surface of the stomach in association with peptic ulcer disease. Gastroenterology 1982;82:827–31.

Role of *Helicobacter pylori*

14. Atherton JC, Cao P, Peek RM, Tummuru MK, Blaser MJ, Cover TL. Mosaicism in vacuolating cytotoxin alleles of *Helicobacter pylori*. J Biol Chem 1995;270:17771–7.
15. Atherton JC, Peek RM, Tham KT, Cover TL, Blaser MJ. Clinical and pathological importance of heterogeneity in vacA, the vacuolating cytotoxin gene of *Helicobacter pylori*. Gastroenterology 1997;112:92–9.
16. Blaser MJ. Ecology of *Helicobacter pylori* in the human stomach. J Clin Invest 1997;100:759–62.
17. Blaser MJ. *Helicobacter pylori*: its role in disease. Clin Infect Dis 1992;15:386–91.
18. Bode G, Malfertheiner P, Ditschuneit H. Pathogenic implications of ultrastructural findings of *Campylobacter pylori* related gastroduodenal disease. Scand J Gastroenterol Suppl 1988;142:25–39.
19. Boren T, Falk P, Roth KA, Larson G, Normark S. Attachment of *Helicobacter pylori* to human gastric epithelium mediated by blood group antigens. Science 1993;262:1892–5.
20. Chan WY, Hui PK, Chan JK, et al. Epithelial damage by *Helicobacter pylori* in gastric ulcers. Histopathology 1991;19:47–53.
21. Covacci A, Censini S, Bugnoli M, et al. Molecular characterization of the 128-kDa immunodominant antigen of *Helicobacter pylori* associated with cytotoxicity and duodenal ulcer. Proc Natl Acad Sci USA 1993;90:5791–5.
22. Cover TL, Blaser MJ. Purification and characterization of the vacuolating cytotoxin from *Helicobacter pylori*. J Biol Chem 1992;267:10570–5.
23. Crabtree JE, Covacci A, Farmery SA, et al. *Helicobacter pylori* induced interleukin-8 expression in gastric epithelial cells is associated with CagA positive phenotype. J Clin Pathol 1995;48:41–5.
24. Denizot Y, Sobhani I, Rambaud JC, Lewin M, Thomas Y, Benveniste J. Paf-acether synthesis by *Helicobacter pylori*. Gut 1990;31:1242–5.
25. Dick JD. *Helicobacter (Campylobacter) pylori*: a new twist to an old disease. Annu Rev Microbiol 1990;44:249–69.

26. Eaton KA, Brooks CL, Morgan DR, Krakowka S. Essential role of urease in pathogenesis of gastritis induced by *Helicobacter pylori* in gnotobiotic piglets. Infect Immun 1991;59:2470–5.
27. El-Omar E, Penman I, Ardill JE, Chittajallu RS, Howie C, McColl KE. *Helicobacter pylori* infection and abnormalities of acid secretion in patients with duodenal ulcer disease. Gastroenterology 1995;109:681–91.
28. Evans DG, Karjalainen TK, Evans DJ Jr, Graham DY, Lee CH. Cloning, nucleotide sequence, and expression of a gene encoding adhesion subunit protein of *Helicobacter pylori*. J Bacteriol 1993;175:674–83.
29. Figura N, Guglielmetti P, Rossolini A, et al. Cytotoxin production by *Campylobacter pylori* strains isolated from patients with peptic ulcers and from patients with chronic gastritis only. J Clin Microbiol 1989;27:225–6.
30. Goosens H, Glupczynski Y, Burette A, et al. Role of the vacuolating cytotoxin from *Helicobacter pylori* in the pathogenesis of duodenal and gastric ulcer. Med Microbiol Lett 1992;1:153–9.
31. Graham DY, Lew GM, Lechago J. Antral G-cell and D-cell numbers in *Helicobacter pylori* infection: effect of *H. pylori* eradication. Gastroenterology 1993;104:1655–60.
32. Gunn MC, Stephens JC, Stewart JA, Rathbone BJ, West KP. The significance of cagA and vacA subtypes of *Helicobacter pylori* in the pathogenesis of inflammation and peptic ulceration. J Clin Pathol 1998;51:761–4.
33. Hazell SL, Lee A, Brady L, Hennessy W. *Campylobacter pyloridis* and gastritis: association with intercellular spaces and adaptation to an environment of mucus as important factors in colonization of the gastric epithelium. J Infect Dis 1986;153:658–63.
34. Hunt RH. Hp and pH: implications for the eradication of *Helicobacter pylori*. Scand J Gastroenterol Suppl 1993;196:12–6.
35. Langenberg W, Rauws EA, Houthoff HJ, et al. Follow-up study of individuals with untreated *Campylobacter pylori*-associated gastritis and of noninfected persons with non-ulcer dyspepsia. J Infect Dis 1988;157:1245–9.
36. Leunk RD, Johnson PT, David BC, Kraft WG, Morgan DR. Cytotoxic activity in broth-culture filtrates of *Campylobacter pylori*. J Med Microbiol 1988;26:93–9.
37. Maeda S, Kanai F, Ogura K, et al. High seropositivity of anti-cagA antibody in *Helicobacter pylori*-infected patients irrelevant to peptic ulcers and normal mucosa in Japan. Dig Dis Sci 1997;42:1841–7.
38. Mai UE, Perez-Perez GI, Allen JB, et al. Surface proteins from *Helicobacter pylori* exhibit chemotactic activity for human leukocytes and are present in gastric mucosa. J Exp Med 1992;175:517–25.
39. Marshall BJ, Barrett LJ, Prakash C, McCallum RW, Guerrant RL. Urea protects *Helicobacter pylori* from the bactericidal effect of acid. Gastroenterology 1990;99:697–702.
40. McGowan CC, Cover TL, Blaser MJ. *Helicobacter pylori* and gastric acid: biological and therapeutic implications. Gastroenterology 1996;110: 926–38.
41. Micots I, Augeron C, Laboisse CL, Muzeau F, Megraud F. Mucin exocytosis: a major target for *Helicobacter pylori*. J Clin Pathol 1993;46:241–5.
42. Morris A, Nicholson G. Experimental and accidental C. pylori infection of humans. In: Blaser MJ, ed. *Campylobacter pylori* in gastritis and peptic ulcer disease. New York: Igaku-Shoin; 1989:61–72.
43. Navaglia F, Basso D, Piva MG, et al. *Helicobacter pylori* cytotoxic genotype is associated with peptic ulcer and influences serology. Am J Gastroenterol 1998;93:227–30.
44. Nomura A, Stemmermann GN, Chyou PH, Perez-Perez GI, Blaser MJ. *Helicobacter pylori* infection and the risk for duodenal and gastric ulceration. Ann Intern Med 1994;120:977–81.
45. O'Connor HJ. The role of *Helicobacter pylori* in peptic ulcer disease. Scand J Gastroenterol Suppl 1994;29:11–5.
46. Orsini B, Ciancio G, Surrenti E, et al. Serologic detection of cagA positive *Helicobacter pylori* infection in a northern Italian population: its association with peptic ulcer disease. Helicobacter 1998;3:15–20.
47. Park SM, Park J, Kim JG, et al. Infection with *Helicobacter pylori* expressing the cagA gene is not associated with an increased risk of developing peptic ulcer diseases in Korean patients. Scand J Gastroenterol 1998;33:923–7.
48. Perez-Perez GI, Olivares AZ, Cover TL, Blaser MJ. Characteristics of *Helicobacter pylori* variants selected for urease deficiency. Infect Immun 1992;60:3658–63.
49. Rautelin H, Blomberg B, Jarnerot G, Danielsson D. Nonopsonic activation of neutrophils and cytotoxin production by *Helicobacter pylori*: ulcerogenic markers. Scand J Gastroenterol 1994;29:128–32.
50. Sarosiek J, Slomiany A, Slomiany BL. Evidence for weakening of gastric mucus integrity by *Campylobacter pylori*. Scand J Gastroenterol 1988;23:585–90.
51. Segal ED, Shon J, Tompkins LS. Characterization of *Helicobacter pylori* urease mutants. Am Soc Microbiol 1992;60:1883–9.

52. Sidebotham RL, Batten JJ, Karim QN, Spencer J, Baron JH. Breakdown of gastric mucus in presence of *Helicobacter pylori.* J Clin Pathol 1991;44:52–7.
53. Slomiany BL, Bilski J, Sarosiek J, et al. *Campylobacter pyloridis* degrades mucin and undermines gastric mucosal integrity. Biochem Biophys Res Commun 1987;144:307–14.
54. Smoot DT, Mobley HL, Chippendale GR, Lewison JF, Resau JH. *Helicobacter pylori* urease activity is toxic to human gastric epithelial cells. Infect Immun 1990;58:1992–4.
55. Stephens JC, Stewart JA, Folwell AM, Rathbone BJ. *Helicobacter pylori* cagA status, vacA genotypes and ulcer disease. Eur J Gastroenterol Hepatol 1998;10:381–4.
56. Takata T, Fujimoto S, Anzai K, et al. Analysis of the expression of CagA and VacA and the vacuolating activity in 167 isolates from patients with either peptic ulcers or non-ulcer dyspepsia. Am J Gastroenterol 1998;93:30–4.
57. Treiber G, Lambert JR. The impact of *Helicobacter pylori* eradication on peptic ulcer healing. Am J Gastroenterol 1998;93:1080–4.
58. Tufano MA, Rossano F, Catalanotti P, et al. Immunobiological activities of *Helicobacter pylori* porins. Infect Immun 1994;62:1392–9.
59. Tummuru MK, Cover TL, Blaser MJ. Mutation of the cytotoxin-associated cagA gene does not affect the vacuolating cytotoxin activity of *Helicobacter pylori.* Infect Immun 1994;62:2609–13.
60. van Doorn LJ, Figueriedo C, Sanna R, et al. Clinical relevance of the cagA, vacA and iceA status of *Helicobacter pylori.* Gastroenterology 1998;115:58–66.
61. Wetherall BL, Johnson AM. Haemolytic activity of *Campylobacter pylori.* Eur J Clin Mircobiol Infect Dis 1989;8:706–10.
62. Yamaoka Y, Kodama T, Gutierrez O, et al. Relationship between *Helicobacter pylori* iceA, cagA, and vacA status and clinical outcome: studies in four different countries. J Clin Microbiol 1999;37:2274–9.
63. Yoshida N, Granger DN, Evans DJ, et al. Mechanisms involved in *Helicobacter pylori*-induced inflammation. Gastroenterology 1993;105:1431–40.

Role of Nonsteroidal Antiinflammatory Drugs

64. Brown LF, Wilson DE. Gastroduodenal ulcers: causes, diagnosis, prevention and treatment. Comp Ther 1999;25:30–8.
65. Geis GS. Update on clinical developments with celecoxib, a new specific COX-2 inhibitor: what can we expect? Scand J Rheumatol Suppl 1999;109:31–7.
66. Langman MJ. Epidemiologic evidence on the association between peptic ulceration and antiinflammatory drug use. Gastroenterology 1989;96:640–6.
67. Larkai EN, Smith JL, Lidsky MD, Graham DY. Gastroduodenal mucosa and dyspeptic symptoms in arthritic patients during chronic nonsteroidal antiinflammatory drug use. Am J Gastroenterol 1987;82:1153–8.
68. Lee M, Feldman M. Age-related reductions in gastric mucosal prostaglandin levels increase susceptibility to aspirin-induced injury in rats. Gastroenterology 1994;107:1746–50.
69. Levy M, Miller DR, Kaufman DW, et al. Major upper gastrointestinal tract bleeding: relation to the use of aspirin and other nonnarcotic analgesics. Arch Intern Med 1988;148:281–5.
70. Quinn CM, Bjarnason I, Price AB. Gastritis in patients on non-steroidal anti-inflammatory drugs. Histopathology 1993;23:341–8.
71. Singh G, Triadafilopoulos G. Epidemiology of NSAID-induced gastrointestinal complications. J Rheumatol 1999;26(Suppl 26):18–24.
72. Wilcox CM, Shalek KA, Cotsonis G. Striking prevalence of over-the-counter nonsteroidal anti-inflammatory drug use in patients with upper gastrointestinal hemorrhage. Arch Intern Med 1994;154:42–6.

Role of Steroids

73. Delaney JP, Michel HM, Bonsack ME, Eisenberg MM, Dunn DH. Adrenal corticosteroids cause gastrin cell hyperplasia. Gastroenterology 1979;76:913–6.
74. Gabriel SE, Jaakkimainen L, Bombardier C. Risk for serious gastrointestinal complications related to use of nonsteroidal anti-inflammatory drugs. A meta-analysis. Ann Intern Med 1991;115:787–96.
75. Kataoka H, Horie Y, Koyama R, Nakatsugi S, Furukawa M. Interaction between NSAIDs and steroid in rat stomach: safety of nimesulide as a preferential COX-2 inhibitor in the stomach. Dig Dis Sci 2000;45:1366–75.

Role of Cigarette Smoking

76. Korman MG, Hansky J, Eaves ER, Schmidt GT. Influence of cigarette smoking on healing and relapse in duodenal ulcer disease. Gastroenterology 1983;85:871–4.
77. Massarrat S, Enschai F, Pittner PM. Increased gastric secretory capacity in smokers without gastrointestinal lesions. Gut 1986;27:433–9.
78. Muller-Lissner SA. Bile reflux is increased in cigarette smokers. Gastroenterology 1986;90:1205–9.

79. Raiha I, Kemppainen H, Kaprio J, Koskenvuo M, Sourander L. Lifestyle, stress and genes in peptic ulcer disease: a nationwide twin cohort study. Arch Intern Med 1998;158:698–704.
80. Suadicani P, Hein HO, Gyntelberg F. Genetic and life-style determinants of peptic ulcer. A study of 3387 men aged 54 to 74 years: the Copenhagen male study. Scand J Gastroenterol 1999;34:12–7.

Other Factors in Ulcer Development

81. Azuma T, Teramae N, Hayakumo T, et al. Pepsinogen C gene polymorphisms associated with gastric body ulcer. Gut 1993;34:450–5.
82. Samloff IM, Varis K, Ihamaki T, Siurala M, Rotter JI. Relationships among serum pepsinogen I, serum pepsinogen II and gastric mucosal histology. A study in relatives of patients with pernicious anemia. Gastroenterology 1982;83:204–9.
83. Soll AH. Pathogenesis of peptic ulcer disease and implications for treatment. N Engl J Med 1990; 322:909–16.

Demography of Peptic Ulcer Disease

84. Deckelbaum RJ, Roy CC, Lussier-Lazaroff J, Morin CL. Peptic ulcer disease: a clinical study in 73 children. Can Med Assoc J 1974;111:225–8.
85. Gustavsson S, Nyren O. Time trends in peptic ulcer surgery, 1956 to 1986. A nation-wide survey in Sweden. Ann Surg 1989;210:704–9.
86. Hyman PE, Hassall E. Marked basal gastric acid hypersecretion and peptic ulcer disease: medical management with a combination H2-histamine receptor antagonist and anticholinergic. J Pediatr Gastroenterol Nutr 1988;7:57–63.
87. Kekki M, Sipponen P, Siurala, Laszewicz W. Peptic ulcer and chronic gastritis: their relation to age and sex, and to location of ulcer and gastritis. Gastroenterol Clin Biol 1990;14:217–23.
88. Len C, Hilario MO, Kawakami E, et al. Gastroduodenal lesions in children with juvenile rheumatoid arthritis. Hepatogastroenterology 1999;46:991–6.
89. Sipponen P, Seppala K, Aarynen M, Helske T, Kettunen P. Chronic gastritis and gastroduodenal ulcer: a case control study on risk on coexisting duodenal or gastric ulcer in patients with gastritis. Gut 1989;30:922–9.
90. Stemmermann GN, Marcus EB, Buist AS, MacLean CJ. Relative impact of smoking and reduced pulmonary function on peptic ulcer risk. A prospective study of Japanese men in Hawaii. Gastroenterology 1989;96:1419–24.

Gastric Ulcers

91. Chua C, Jeyaraj P, Low C. Relative risks of complications in giant and nongiant gastric ulcers. Am J Surg 1992;164:94–7.
92. Graham DY, Schwartz JT, Cain GD, Gyorkey F. Prospective evaluation of biopsy number in the diagnosis of esophageal and gastric carcinoma. Gastroenterology 1982;82:228–31.
93. Isaacson P. Biopsy appearances easily mistaken for malignancy in gastrointestinal endoscopy. Histopathology 1982;6:377–89.
94. Swain CP, Lai KC, Kalabakas AA, et al. A comparison of size and pathology of vessel and ulcer in patient dying from bleeding gastric and duodenal ulcers. Gastroenterology 1993;104: A202.
95. Swain CP, Storey DW, Bown SG, et al. Nature of the bleeding vessel in recurrently bleeding gastric ulcers. Gastroenterology 1990;98:A31.
96. West AB, Nolan N, O'Briain DS. Benign peptic ulcers penetrating pericardium and heart: clinicopathological features and factors favoring survival. Gastroenterology 1988;94:1478–87.

Duodenal Peptic Ulcer Diseases

97. Chuong JJ, Fisher RL, Chuong RL, Spiro HM. Duodenal ulcer: incidence, risk factors, and predictive value of plasma pepsinogen. Dig Dis Sci 1986;31:1178–84.
98. Edwards JH. The meaning of the associations between blood groups and disease. Ann Hum Genet 1965;29:77–81.
99. Hamlet A, Olbe L. The influence of *Helicobacter pylori* infection on postprandial duodenal acid load and duodenal bulb pH in humans. Gastroenterology 1996;111:391–400.
100. Hogan DL, Rapier RC, Dreilinger A, et al. Duodenal bicarbonate secretion: eradication of *Helicobacter pylori* and duodenal structure and function in humans. Gastroenterology 1996; 110:705–16.
101. Khulusi S, Badve S, Patel P, et al. Pathogenesis of gastric metaplasia of the human duodenum: role of *Helicobacter pylori*, gastric acid, and ulceration. Gastroenterology 1996;110:452–8.
102. Madsen JE, Vetvik K, Aase S. *Helicobacter*-associated duodenitis and gastric metaplasia in duodenal ulcer patients. APMIS 1991;99:997–1000.
103. Wyatt JI, Rathbone BJ, Sobala GM, et al. Gastric epithelium in the duodenum: its association with *Helicobacter pylori* and inflammation. J Clin Pathol 1990;43:981–6.

Duodenal Ulcer

104. Branicki FJ, Boey J, Fok PJ, et al. Bleeding duodenal ulcer. A prospective evaluation of risk factors for rebleeding and death. Ann Surg 1990;211:411–8.
105. Chan FK, Hung LC, Suen BY, et al. Celecoxib versus diclofenac and omeprazole in reducing the risk of recurrent ulcer bleeding in patients with arthritis. N Eng J Med 2002;347:2104–10.
106. Hawkey CJ, Jeffrey DM, Karrasch JA, et al. Omeprazole compared with misoprostol for ulcers associated with nonsteroidal anti-inflammatory drugs. N Eng J Med 1998;338:727–34.
107. Kang JY, Nasiry R, Guan R, et al. Influence of the site of a duodenal ulcer on its mode of presentation. Gastroenterology 1986;90:1874–6.
108. Morgan AG, Clamp SE. OMGE International upper gastrointestinal bleeding survey 1978–1986. Scand J Gastroenterol Suppl 1988;144:51–8.
109. NIH Consensus Development Panel: Helicobacter pylori in peptic ulcer disease. JAMA 1994; 272:65–9.
110. Roth S, Agrawal N, Mahowald M, et al. Misoprostol heals gastroduodenal injury in patients with rheumatoid arthritis receiving aspirin. Arch Intern Med 1989;149:775–9.
111. Silverstein FE, Graham DY, Senior JR, et al. Misoprostol reduces serious gastrointestinal complications in patients with rheumatoid arthritis receiving nonsteroidal anti-inflammatory drugs. Ann Intern Med 1995;123:241–9.
112. Tytgat GN. Treatment of peptic ulcer. Digestion 1998;59:446–52.

Zollinger-Ellison Syndrome

113. Isenberg JI, Walsh JH, Grossman MI. Zollinger-Ellison syndrome. Gastroenterology 1973;65: 140–65.
114. Metz DC, Soffer E, Forsmark CE, et al. Maintenance oral pantoprazole therapy is effective for patients with Zollinger-Ellison syndrome and idiopathic hypersecretion. Am J Gastroenterol 2003;98:301–7.
115. Neuburger P, Lewin M, de Recherche C, Bonfils S. Parietal and chief cell populations in four cases of the Zollinger-Ellison syndrome. Gastroenterology 1972;63:937–42.
116. Norton JA, Fraker DL, Alexander R, et al. Surgery to cure the Zollinger-Ellison syndrome. N Engl J Med 1999;341:635–44.

6 ACQUIRED STRUCTURAL ALTERATIONS

DIVERTICULA

A diverticulum is a circumscribed pouch or sac that originates from a hollow viscus. *Gastrointestinal diverticula* are mucosal outpouchings into or through the submucosa, or beyond. They are either congenital or acquired. Congenital diverticula are discussed in chapter 2; acquired diverticula are discussed here. Diverticula can be divided into *true diverticula* (with a wall containing all of the mural structures) or *false* or *pseudodiverticula* in which the wall lacks some mural component, such as the muscularis propria. The presence of multiple diverticula is called *diverticulosis*.

Esophageal Diverticula

Definition. *Esophageal diverticula* can be divided into pulsion or traction types. The action of intraluminal pressure forces the mucosal outpouchings in *pulsion diverticula*. An extrinsic inflammatory process retracts or pulls the gut wall outward in *traction diverticula*. Esophageal diverticula can also be classified by their location into *pharyngoesophageal, thoracic* or *epiphrenic diverticula*.

Demography. Overall, esophageal diverticula are identified in 0.15 percent of upper barium examinations (56). Zenker's (hypopharyngeal) is the most common (up to 70 percent) esophageal diverticulum. It tends to affect middle-aged or elderly individuals. Approximately 21 percent of the remaining diverticula originate in the mid-esophagus; 8.5 percent originate in the supradiaphragmatic region. Epiphrenic diverticula tend to affect men beyond middle age, supporting an acquired etiology. Patients with diffuse esophageal intramural pseudodiverticulosis range in age from 11 to 83 years (28); mostly older individuals and males are affected. These lesions are rare, affecting less than 1 percent of patients undergoing radiologic esophageal examinations (28).

Etiology and Pathophysiology. Diverticula in the proximal and distal esophagus are pulsion diverticula, whereas mid-esophageal diverticula are traction diverticula. Pulsion diverticula result from motility disturbances and associated achalasia, diffuse esophageal spasm, or other motility diseases (11,24,38). Zenker diverticula arise from defective upper esophageal sphincter function caused either by a failure to completely inhibit cricopharyngeal muscle tone or from muscular fibrosis that causes loss of sphincter compliance (9). As a result, intrabolus pressure increases to maintain normal bolus flow. This eventually leads to the development of a pulsion diverticulum at points of muscular weakness. The presence of a Zenker diverticulum may sometimes result in difficulty in intubating the esophagus at upper endoscopy, and as a result, may lead to inadvertent trauma.

Mid-esophageal traction diverticula are associated with mediastinal inflammation, which causes traction on the esophageal wall, pulling it outward as the mediastinal inflammation begins to heal. Traction diverticula have decreased in frequency with a decline in the incidence of mediastinal tuberculosis.

Epiphrenic diverticula are almost always pulsion diverticula. They arise because increased intraesophageal pressure pushes the mucosa outward in areas of muscular weakness. For this reason, epiphrenic diverticula frequently coexist with inflammatory disorders, including hiatal hernia, achalasia, diaphragmatic eventration, carcinoma, Ehlers-Danlos syndrome, and primary motility disturbances (11,16,18,49,54).

Esophageal pseudodiverticulosis has several known associations, including *Candida* infection, diabetes, gastroesophageal reflux disease (GERD), and chronic alcoholism, but it is unclear which of these associated disorders plays a role in its pathogenesis, since many are so common that the relationships may be fortuitous rather than etiologic. The cysts of esophageal pseudodiverticulosis form as a result of ductal obstruction caused by inflammation, excess mucin, or squamous debris blocking the ductal orifices.

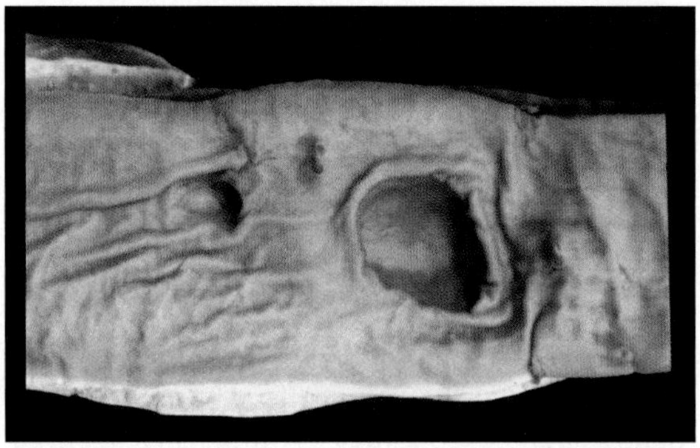

Figure 6-1

TRACTION DIVERTICULUM OF THE ESOPHAGUS

A large, wide-mouthed diverticular opening is in the mid-esophagus. (Courtesy of the Division of Gastrointestinal Pathology, Armed Forces Institute of Pathology, Washington DC.)

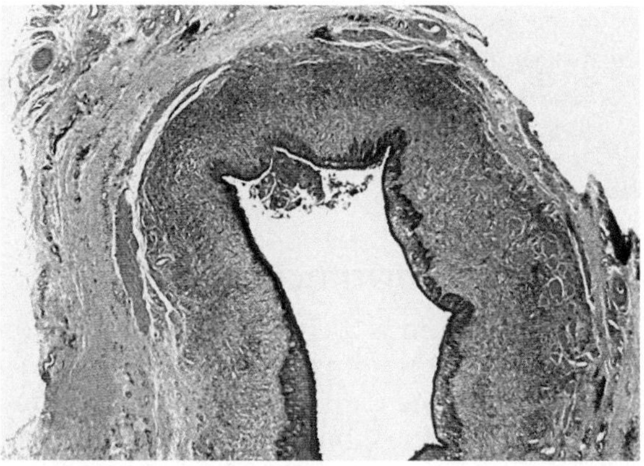

Figure 6-2

ZENKER DIVERTICULUM

The diverticulum is lined by normal-appearing squamous epithelium. The wall of the diverticulum is composed of muscularis mucosae, submucosal tissue, and strands of muscle derived from the muscularis propria. (Courtesy of the Division of Gastrointestinal Pathology, Armed Forces Institute of Pathology, Washington, DC.)

Clinical Features. Patients with Zenker diverticula complain of dysphagia, halitosis, regurgitation, and heartburn. When the diverticulum fills with food and secretions, it enlarges and compresses the esophagus, causing dysphagia, obstruction, and aspiration. Secondary bacterial colonization results in diverticulitis. Mid-esophageal diverticula are almost always discovered incidentally. Patients with diffuse esophageal intramural pseudodiverticulosis present with dysphagia and acute bolus obstruction, probably because of the association between intramural diverticulosis, dysmotility, and stricture formation (3,28,42).

Gross Findings. Esophageal diverticula develop in the pharyngoesophageal junction, just above the diaphragm, and in the mid-thorax in a frequency of 7 to 1 to 2, respectively (56). The proximally located Zenker diverticulum develops posteriorly or posterolaterally between the pharyngeal inferior constrictor muscle and fibers of the cricopharyngeus muscle, in a triangular zone of sparse musculature termed Killian dehiscence or Killian triangle (10).

Mid-esophageal diverticula develop as single or multiple saccular outpouchings of the esophageal lumen, usually near the tracheal bifurcation (24). Most are wide-mouthed. The diverticular walls consist of a variably inflamed mucosa and submucosa with an attenuated muscularis propria (fig. 6-1). The globular and wide-mouthed epiphrenic diverticula arise in the distal third of the esophagus, usually projecting from the terminal 4 cm of the right posterior esophageal wall. Esophageal diverticula can become quite large (up to 10 cm), although they usually measure less than 2 cm in diameter.

In esophageal pseudodiverticulosis, the multiple, cystically dilated, submucosal glandular ducts produce a dramatic radiographic picture (3). "Flask" or "collar button"-like outpouchings varying from 1 mm to 1 cm in diameter, lie evenly distributed along the esophageal wall and correspond to the distribution of normal esophageal glands. The cysts remain intramural, extending 3 mm or less beyond the esophageal lumen (23); each cyst connects with the lumen via a small ostium. Fifty percent of cases are diffuse and 50 percent are segmental (35). Segmental disease affects the proximal third of the esophagus. Most patients have associated strictures in the same location as the intramural diverticulosis (28,35).

Microscopic Findings. The walls of esophageal diverticula consist of mucosa, submucosa, and an attenuated muscularis propria (fig. 6-2). A true muscular coat is usually absent. Squamous epithelium lines all esophageal diverticula unless they develop in an area of Barrett esophagus. Variable inflammation and prominent lymphoid follicles may be present.

In esophageal pseudodiverticulosis, dilated submucosal ducts and glands are present, often associated with acute and/or chronic inflammation and desquamated epithelium (fig. 6-3). Bacteria and fungi may secondarily colonize the cysts. Occasionally the cysts undergo squamous metaplasia. Associated submucosal fibrosis causes marked thickening of the esophageal wall and results in stricture formation.

Treatment and Prognosis. Complications of Zenker diverticulum include dysphagia, inflammation, mucosal ulcerations, and perhaps even cancer (31). The incidence of carcinoma ranges from 0.3 to 0.7 percent, affecting individuals over age 60 years who have long-standing symptomatic diverticula. Diverticulectomy and/or myotomy is the treatment of choice in those cases in which surgery becomes unavoidable. Complications of epiphrenic diverticula include obstruction, diverticulitis, perforation, mediastinitis, hemorrhage, and cancer.

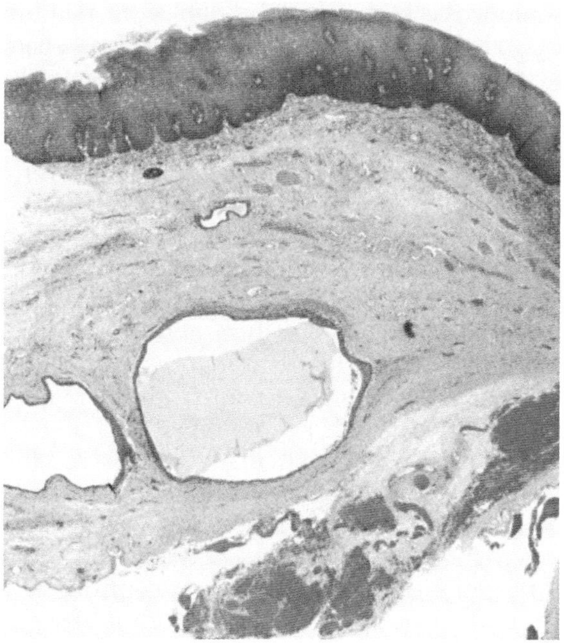

Figure 6-3

ESOPHAGEAL PSEUDODIVERTICULOSIS

Several markedly dilated submucosal glands underlie the squamous epithelium.

Gastric Diverticula

Demography. *Gastric diverticula* are not as common as other gastrointestinal diverticula. They are found in 0.1 percent of upper gastrointestinal barium studies (56).

Etiology and Pathophysiology. Gastric diverticula usually result from underlying antral disease. Predisposing conditions include ulcers, neoplasms, previous surgery, and radiation.

Gross Findings. *Pulsion diverticula* typically arise on the posterior wall of the proximal stomach near the cardia, in areas where the gastric wall is congenitally weak. The lesion may be mildly inflamed. *Traction diverticula* arise in the antrum in areas of previous damage from inflammatory processes. They are invariably inflamed (13).

Microscopic Findings. Gastric diverticula consist of all the gastric layers but with an attenuated muscularis propria. If the diverticulum develops adjacent to an ulcer, then regenerative epithelium, granulation tissue, or scar tissue may be present.

Small Intestinal Diverticula

Demography. Most *small intestinal diverticula* occur in the duodenum. Duodenal diverticula are found in 1 to 6 percent of radiologically examined small intestines and in an average of 8.6 percent of autopsies (31). They complicate peptic ulcer disease, choledocholithiasis (21), duodenal obstruction, and genetic or systemic disorders. *Small intestinal diverticulosis*, a heterogenous disorder, affects 1.3 to 4.6 percent of the population (26). It consists of single or multiple diverticula predominantly involving the jejunum. Jejunal diverticula develop seven times more commonly than ileal diverticula (51); men are affected twice as frequently as women and most patients are over age 40 (26). Underlying neuromuscular disorders predispose to small intestinal diverticulosis (26). The pathologic features of the underlying motility disorders are described in chapter 17.

Etiology and Pathophysiology. Most duodenal diverticula develop as a result of chronic peptic ulcer disease (12). The ulcerating process causes fibrosis of the muscularis propria and abnormal contractility. Jejunal diverticula also result from areas of transmural fibrosis and atrophy, or underlying neural or other abnormalities. Uncoordinated muscular contractions lead to focal areas of increased intraluminal pressure, which cause mucosal and submucosal herniation through weakened areas in the bowel wall. Diverticula begin as a pair of small outpouchings along the mesenteric border where the intestinal wall is weakest, where the penetrating arteries pierce the muscular and serosal coats. These outpouchings enlarge until they meet and eventually fuse, forming a single thin-walled diverticulum.

Clinical Features. Most patients with duodenal diverticula remain asymptomatic but sphincter of Oddi dysfunction, obstructive jaundice, hemorrhage, perforation, or acute pancreatitis may develop (22,43,56). The vast majority of patients with jejunal diverticula are asymptomatic; the diverticula are discovered incidentally at the time of surgery, autopsy, or radiographic examination. When small intestinal diverticula cause symptoms, it is usually due to inflammation, torsion, intussusception, obstruction, bleeding, perforation, or malabsorption. The last is particularly likely when patients develop large diverticula that act like blind loops and accumulate microorganisms. Vitamin B12 deficiency leading to macrocytic anemia may develop because of bacterial overgrowth within the diverticulum (34).

Gross Findings. Acquired duodenal diverticula usually develop in the first portion of the duodenum when complicating peptic ulcer disease, and in a juxtapapillary location when they result from ampullary inflammation. They are usually solitary (fig. 6-4). In patients with diffuse small intestinal diverticulosis, diverticula tend to be larger in the proximal jejunum and become smaller and fewer distally. As many as 400 diverticula, ranging in size from 1 to 22 cm in diameter, can be present (26).

Microscopic Findings. The diverticula are lined by mucosa, muscularis mucosae, submucosa, and an attenuated muscularis propria (fig. 6-5). The mucosa usually demonstrates crypt hyperplasia, villous atrophy, and chronic inflammation. These changes probably result from intestinal stasis and bacterial overgrowth. Lipid-containing histiocytes often lie in the mucosa, submucosa, and lymphatic vessels, close to the collar of muscularis propria surrounding the diverticular neck (27). Pneumatosis intestinalis complicates jejunal diverticular disease in some instances (57). If diverticulitis develops, the inflammation localizes to the diverticulum.

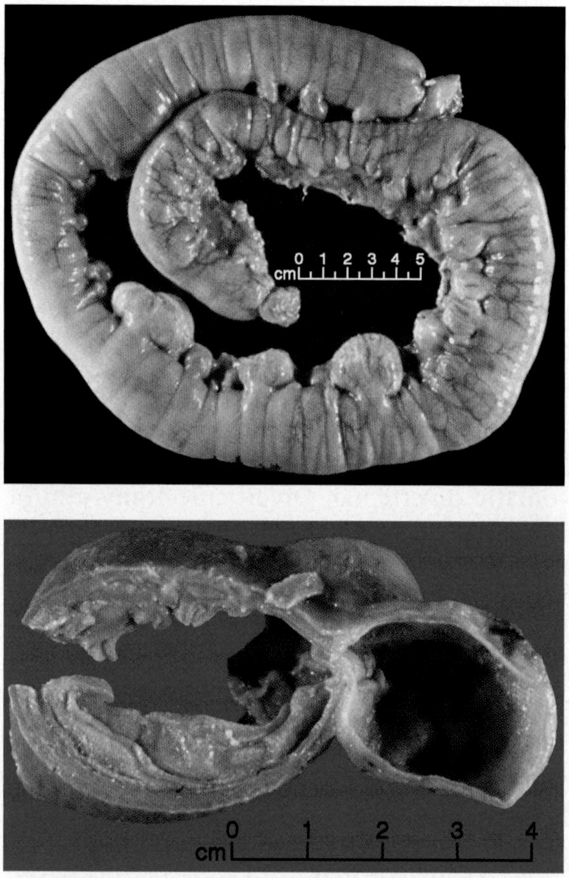

Figure 6-4

SMALL INTESTINAL DIVERTICULOSIS

Top: Jejunal resection specimen has multiple diverticular outpouchings along its length.

Bottom: A large diverticulum (right) projects from the wall of the small intestine.

Treatment and Prognosis. Small intestinal diverticula perforate, bleed, become inflamed, and undergo the complications listed in Table 6-1. These complications lead to morbidity and mortality rates as high as 40 percent. Resection is the treatment of choice.

Appendiceal Diverticula

Demography. Most *appendiceal diverticula* are acquired (14). Both sexes are equally affected. Incidence estimates range from 0.004 percent to 2.8 percent (6,7,30). Acute appendicitis with focal destruction of the muscularis propria accounts for most appendiceal diverticula. Patients with cystic fibrosis or tumors tend to

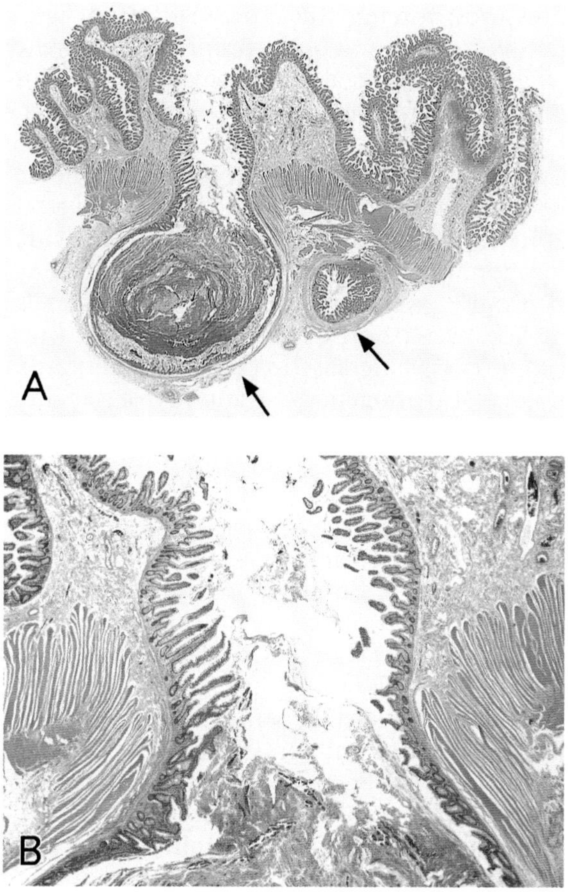

Figure 6-5

SMALL INTESTINAL DIVERTICULUM

A: Prominent small intestinal diverticula are seen. The muscularis propria appears thicker than usual.

B: Low-power view shows the neck of the larger diverticulum lined by normal-appearing small intestinal mucosa. The muscularis propria is thickened and shows the typical separation of muscle bundles seen in diverticular disease in the colon.

C: The diverticulum is filled with inspissated fecal material.

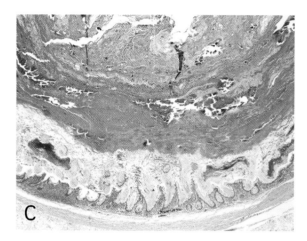

develop appendiceal diverticula secondary to chronic luminal obstruction.

Gross Findings. Appendiceal diverticula are usually small and multiple, measuring 0.2 to 0.5 mm. They occur along the mesenteric and antimesenteric borders of the appendix, at the site of penetrating arteries (19), giving the appendix a beaded appearance (7). They typically arise in the distal appendix.

Microscopic Findings. Appendiceal diverticula resemble colonic diverticula. When they become inflamed, the inflammation localizes to the diverticulum but may also extend into the remainder of the appendix producing appendicitis, periappendicitis, or periappendiceal abscesses. Extensive inflammation may distort, obliterate, or disrupt the diverticulum.

Colonic Diverticula

Definition. In the colon, the term *diverticulosis* refers to the presence of multiple diverticula, with or without the accompanying

Table 6-1

COMPLICATIONS ASSOCIATED WITH SMALL INTESTINAL DIVERTICULOSIS

Acute mechanical intestinal obstruction
From enteroliths, diverticulitis, or volvulus
From pressure on the intestine by filled diverticula
Chronic intestinal obstruction
Without apparent mechanical obstruction (pseudo-obstruction)
From stricture or adhesions secondary to chronic diverticulitis
Inflammatory disturbances varying from mild inflammation to gangrene
Intestinal hemorrhage
Intestinal stasis
Bacterial stasis in diverticulum creating "blind loop syndrome" resulting in malabsorption, B12 deficiency
Steatorrhea, anemia, weight loss, and hypoproteinemia
Rupture
Foreign bodies
Neoplasia

muscle abnormality found in classic diverticular disease. The term *diverticular disease* is used to describe a specific clinical disorder with a defined radiologic and pathologic appearance in which there is a characteristic muscle abnormality, usually but not invariably accompanied by the presence of diverticula. When a muscular abnormality occurs in the absence of established diverticula, the term *prediverticular disease* is sometimes used (40).

Demography. The incidence of large intestinal diverticular disease varies with national origin, cultural background, and diet (50,52). Colonic diverticular disease is prevalent in the United States and other Westernized countries (8,52), and affects both sexes equally (53). The frequency correlates with advancing age. Diverticula are found in up to 66 percent of colons examined with barium enema in Western countries (46). The increasing incidence of diverticular disease seen in Japan (41,44), South Africa (50), and Israel (29) results from the introduction of a Western-type diet in these countries. Asians often have right-sided diverticulosis, although diverticulosis involving the right and left side of the colon (bilateral diverticular disease) has increased in incidence in recent years (37). Some patients with a solitary rectal diverticulum have scleroderma (48). Children with colonic diverticulosis often have underlying Marfan's or Ehlers-Danlos syndrome or associated polycystic kidney disease (1).

Etiology and Pathophysiology. Three major factors are required for the development of colonic diverticula: 1) a higher pressure within the colonic lumen than the ambient peritoneal pressure; 2) a weak point within the intestinal wall through which the mucosa can herniate; and 3) biophysical changes in the colonic wall as a result of aging. Age-related changes in the tensile strength of the colonic wall cause contraction and shortening of the taeniae coli, and redundant mucosal folds that narrow the colonic lumen. Aging; decreased dietary fiber intake; consumption of beef, beef fat, and salt; lack of physical activity; and the presence of constipation all correlate with the development of diverticular disease. Decreased luminal fiber and lower stool volume requires more colonic segmentation to propel fecal material forward (46). The increased segmentation generates greater intraluminal pressures; forcing the mucosa through weak points in the muscularis propria (45), usually where penetrating arteries pierce the muscularis propria. Diverticula arising between the mesenteric and antimesenteric taeniae are usually more advanced than those located on the antimesenteric border, probably because the blood vessels entering the colonic wall are smaller in the latter location. The pronounced muscularis propria hypertrophy present in patients with diverticular disease, even before the formation of diverticula, supports the increased colonic segmentation theory of pathogenesis. The rarity of rectal diverticula may be related to the lower luminal pressure and greater retroperitoneal support in this region compared to the sigmoid colon.

Genetic factors seem to play a role in the evolution of diverticular disease, because diverticula preferentially arise in the right colon among Asians (53) and young patients, contrasting with a location in the sigmoid and left colon in Caucasians and older individuals (4,47).

Because diverticula often lack a muscular layer, secretions and fecal material easily enter them. The feces are not easily expelled and they harden into fecaliths that block the diverticular orifice, leading to diverticulitis.

Clinical Features. Most people with large intestinal diverticulosis remain asymptomatic; 10 to 25 percent of patients become symptomatic, usually due to the development of diverticulitis (4). Most symptomatic individuals are between the ages of 50 and 70. The symptoms of diverticulosis may be accentuated by the increasing constipation seen in older patients.

Acute diverticulitis varies in severity. Clinical features of left-sided diverticulitis include lower abdominal pain, made worse by defecation, and signs of peritoneal irritation, including muscle spasm, guarding, rebound tenderness, fever, and leukocytosis. Some patients develop recurrent, left lower quadrant, colicky pain without clinical or pathologic evidence of acute diverticulitis. Patients have alternating bouts of constipation and diarrhea. Acute diverticulitis of the right colon ranges in frequency from 0.7 to 1.5 percent. Patients present with right lower quadrant abdominal pain and periumbilical pain radiating to the right lower quadrant. Most patients have elevated levels of white blood cells, erythrocyte sedimentation rates, and C-reactive protein. Symptom duration may be short and rectal examination may reveal the presence of a tender mass.

Once diverticulitis develops, the subsequent clinical course depends on bacterial virulence and host defenses. Complications are more common in individuals using nonsteroidal anti-inflammatory drugs (NSAIDs) (2), perhaps because the drugs mask the symptoms of earlier disease or because NSAIDs interfere with natural mucosal defenses (see chapter 8). Life-threatening complications occur more commonly among patients with chronic renal failure or on high-dose steroid therapy (17).

If acute inflammation involves all layers of the bowel wall, the diverticulum may perforate, leading to peritonitis. Perforated diverticula can also remain confined, especially when they occur in the mesentery, by local fibrosis or abscess formation. Abscesses may track into the bladder or adjacent bowel, forming fistulas. Fistulas that extend below the peritoneal reflection can reach the skin, urinary bladder, or adjacent loops of bowel.

Bleeding affects 10 to 30 percent of patients with diverticular disease. It is usually overt and clinically obvious, but may vary from occult bleeding to massive hemorrhage. It often results from erosion of the penetrating artery in the wall of the diverticulum by a fecalith. The bleeding typically occurs suddenly, without signs or symptoms of diverticulitis, and stops spontaneously in 70 to 80 percent of patients (33). The blood appears bright red or maroon but can appear melanotic, especially if it comes from the right colon. Colonoscopy is the investigation of choice for suspected lower gastrointestinal bleeds. Endoscopic intervention can be performed if a bleeding diverticulum is identified; however, usually the bleeding is self-limited, and the actual involved diverticulum cannot be identified.

Gross Findings. Barium enema often establishes the diagnosis of diverticulosis. An early change is the presence of fine mural serrations known as the prediverticular state or myochosis. "Sawtooth" luminal irregularities reflect associated muscle spasm. A contracted haustral pattern may also be seen. The sigmoid colon becomes shortened and distorted, causing it to acquire a concertina-like appearance, with bunched, redundant mucosal folds. These can significantly narrow the colonic lumen and may cause obstruction, with dilatation proximal to the area of obstruction.

Diverticula, mucosal flask-shaped outpouchings, can develop throughout the entire length of the colon, although most commonly they occur in the distal colon. In the Western world, 90 percent of patients have sigmoid involvement and 20 percent have pancolonic involvement. In contrast, Asians, particularly individuals from Japan, Singapore, and China, develop multiple right colon diverticula (5,52). When the diverticula are fully developed, they remain permanently distended and extracolonic in location. Since symptomatic diverticulitis remains a relative contraindication to contrast studies, computerized tomography (CT) best demonstrates acute left-sided colonic diverticulitis (15) and its complications, particularly abscesses (18).

Since the muscular abnormalities are the most striking and consistent part of diverticular disease, pronounced muscular hypertrophy provides a clue to its presence (39). The taeniae coli are much thicker than normal, developing an almost cartilaginous consistency. The circular layer also thickens, gaining a corrugated appearance, which corresponds to the interdigitating muscle processes. These changes are most prominent in the sigmoid colon and may extend for variable distances proximally.

Diverticula commonly appear as two parallel rows of beaded outpouchings between the longitudinal muscle or taeniae coli at sites corresponding to the location of penetrating arteries (fig. 6-6). The diverticula project through and beyond the circular muscle layer of the bowel wall so that they come to lie in the pericolonic fat and are covered by a thin layer of longitudinal muscle. Diverticula usually measure less than 1 cm in diameter; rarely, they reach diameters up to 25 cm (fig. 6-7). The diverticula associated with scleroderma differ from the usual diverticula in that they are often square-mouthed. This results from almost complete replacement of the muscularis propria by fibrous tissue. There are usually associated broad bands of scarring.

When bleeding occurs, the exact bleeding point can be difficult to identify. If a bleeding point is seen, a histologic section through a

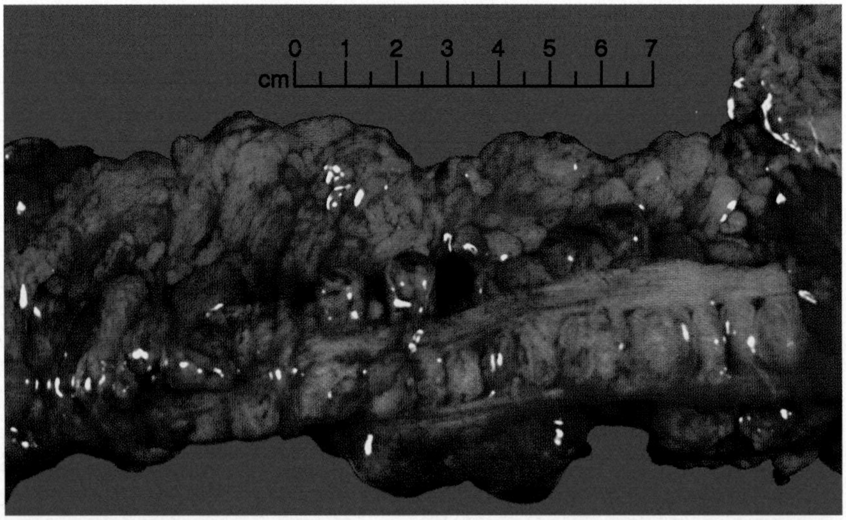

Figure 6-6

COLONIC DIVERTICULOSIS

Numerous smooth, round outpouchings project from the colonic wall. They are aligned in a row along the length of the taeniae coli.

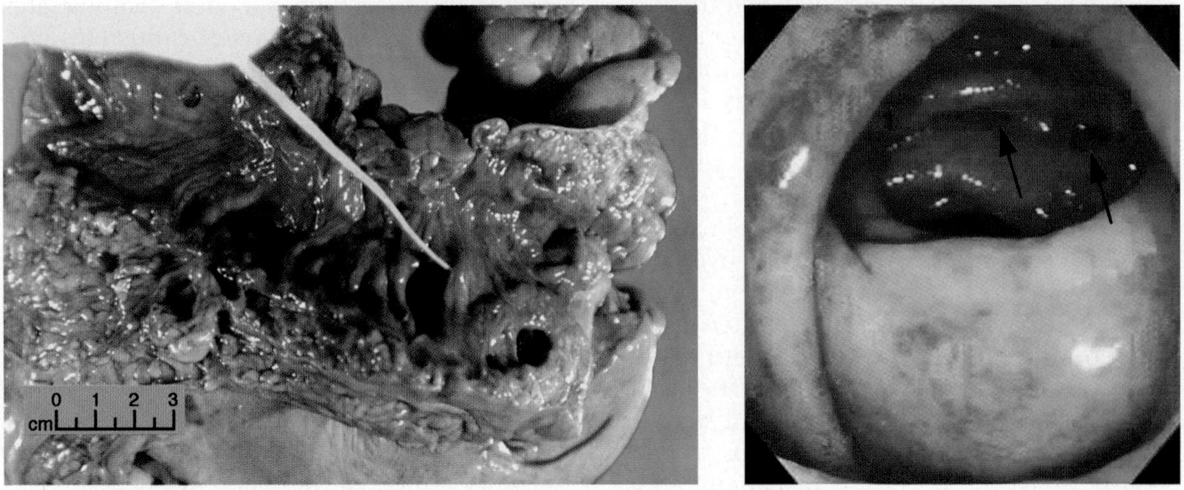

Figure 6-7

COLONIC DIVERTICULA

Left: Several large diverticula extend through the colonic wall.
Right: Endoscopic view in a patient with diverticulitis. The openings to several diverticula are visible (arrows).

diverticulum can identify the bleeding source. The chance of detecting the bleeding site increases by probing each diverticular opening with a cotton-tipped probe. Arteriolar rupture always occurs on the side of the vessel facing the bowel lumen.

The mucosa surrounding diverticular orifices may become slightly elevated, simulating mucosal polyps. Tonic muscular contractions produce redundant, accordion-like mucosal folds. Grossly, these appear as localized swellings or exaggerations of the mucosal folds or as larger, leaf-like, smooth-surfaced "polyps" with broad bases (25). The lesions may be single or multiple.

Colonoscopic examination in patients with diverticulosis-associated colitis shows confluent granularity and friability affecting the area of the sigmoid colon surrounding the diverticular ostia (fig. 6-8). The colonic mucosa proximal and distal to the area of diverticulosis appears endoscopically normal (39). Not uncommonly, a diagnosis of Crohn's disease is entertained due to the segmental nature of the colonoscopic findings. The biopsy can often differentiate

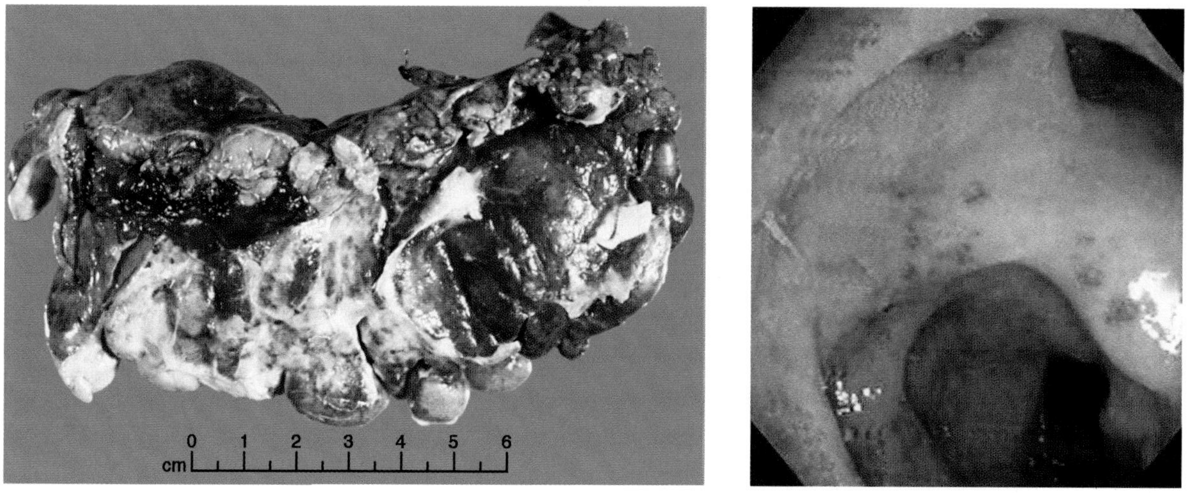

Figure 6-8

DIVERTICULITIS-ASSOCIATED COLITIS

Left: Opened colon in a patient with diverticulitis. The mucosal surface is markedly erythematous and granular. Adherent inflammatory exudates have the appearance of pseudomembranes. There is marked thickening of the colonic wall.

Right: Endoscopically, the mucosal surface demonstrates foci of erythema and erosion. A diverticular opening is identifiable in the upper right.

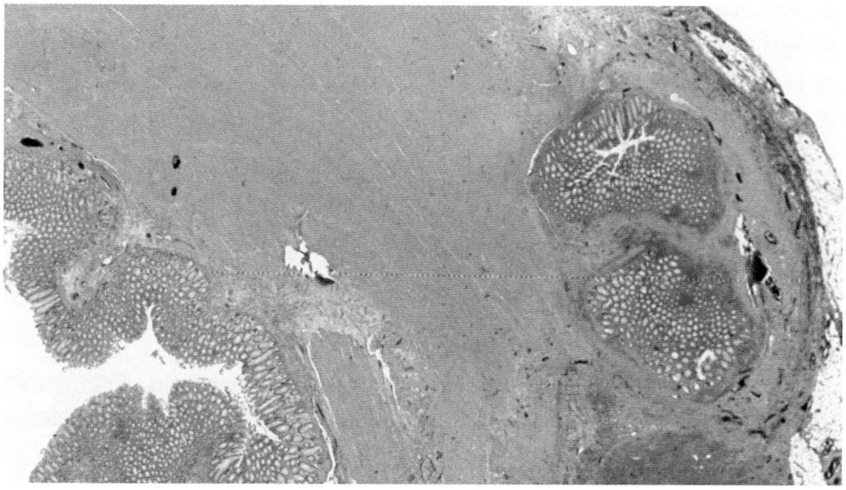

Figure 6-9

COLONIC DIVERTICULOSIS

Several diverticula of the colonic wall are cut in cross section on the outer aspect of the specimen.

between the two entities if the pathologist is made aware of the presence of diverticulosis in the segment of interest.

Microscopic Findings. The histologic features of the bowel wall depend on whether there is simple diverticulosis or complications. The major pathologic abnormalities of uncomplicated diverticulosis include a thickened muscularis propria and diverticular outpouchings (figs. 6-9, 6-10). The latter are usually lined by the mucosa, muscularis mucosae, submucosa, and variable amounts of muscularis propria. Later, the muscularis propria disappears as the diverticula extend beyond the colonic wall. The resulting thin-walled diverticula are unsupported by other tissues. Many eventually become inflamed.

The mucosa surrounding diverticula may be thrown up into redundant mucosal folds (25). Redundant mucosal folds appear polypoid, with increased mucosal height, crypt elongation, mucosal distortion, edema, vascular congestion, and hemorrhage, and possibly associated with thrombi, hemosiderin deposition, erosions,

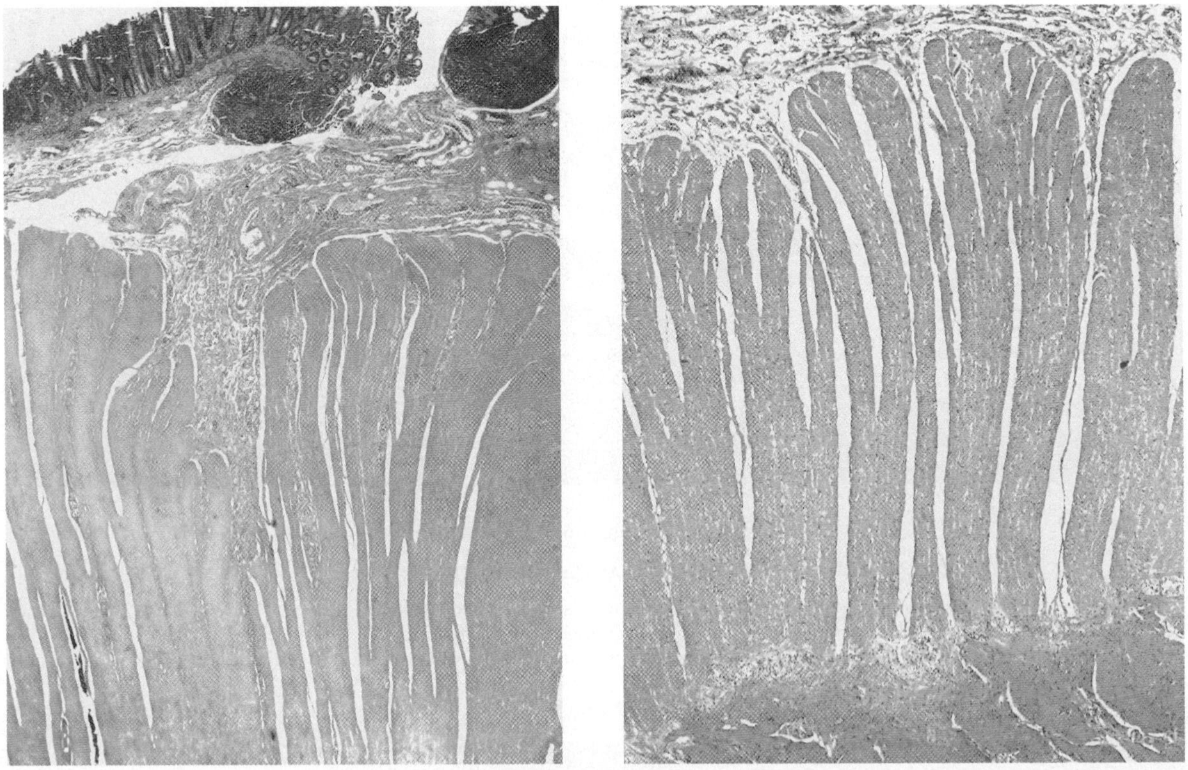

Figure 6-10

MUSCULAR CHANGES IN COLONIC DIVERTICULOSIS

Left: The muscularis propria is markedly thickened.
Right: The muscle fibers separate from one another creating a characteristic clefted pattern.

granulation tissue, and fibrosis. The fibers of the muscularis mucosae extend high into the lamina propria, producing changes resembling those seen in mucosal prolapse. The mucosa may also appear hyperplastic or it may have a thickened collagen table, mimicking collagenous colitis. This resemblance is further accentuated if there is mild colitis associated with the thickened collagen table.

In *diverticular disease–associated colitis* (also termed *crescentic colitis* or *isolated sigmoiditis*), the histologic changes may exactly mimic those found in inflammatory bowel disease (IBD) (fig. 6-11). Changes include a lymphoplasmacytic and eosinophilic expansion of the lamina propria with cryptitis, crypt abscesses, basal lymphoid aggregates, distorted crypt architecture, basal plasmacytosis, surface epithelial sloughing, focal Paneth cell metaplasia, and granulomatous cryptitis (32). The only way to distinguish isolated sigmoiditis from IBD is to interpret the findings in the context of the entire clinical, gross, and endoscopic picture (20,32). All of these changes lie near the diverticula and are not present away from the diverticula, distinguishing this lesion from ulcerative colitis or Crohn's disease. In some cases, it may be impossible to distinguish between these entities.

Trauma within a diverticulum may induce asymmetric intimal vascular proliferations and vessel injury, predisposing it to rupture and bleeding (36). The arterial walls duplicate the internal elastic lamina and exhibit eccentric medial thinning, which is most marked on the luminal side. The myenteric plexus may appear abnormal and disorganized.

When diverticulitis develops, the diverticula become infiltrated by acute inflammatory cells, followed by chronic inflammation (fig. 6-12). As the inflammation extends, the mucosa ulcerates and abscesses, or fistulas may form. There may be broad areas of mucosal ulceration,

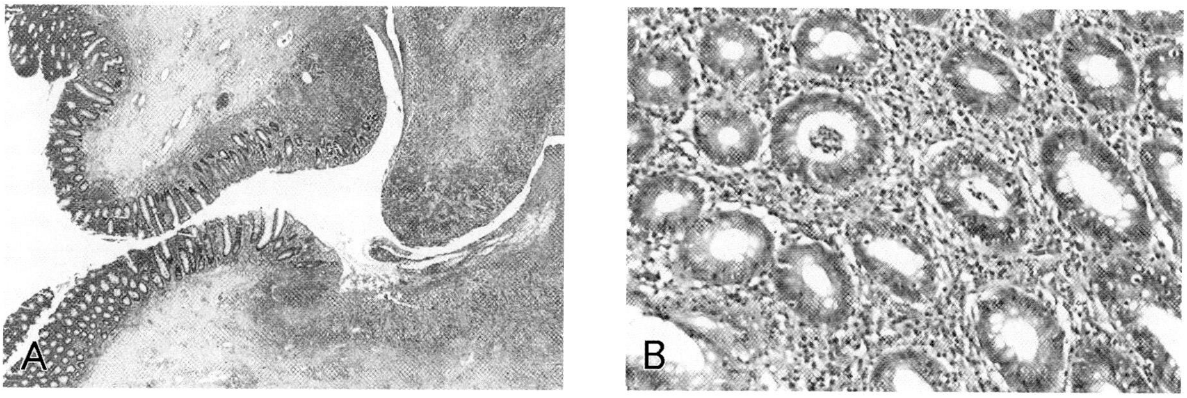

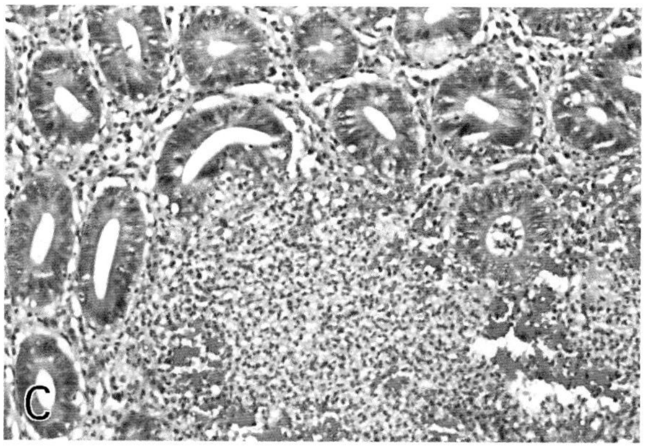

Figure 6-11

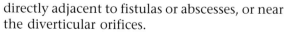

DIVERTICULAR DISEASE–ASSOCIATED COLITIS

A: A large area of ulceration is seen in the colon. The adjacent intact mucosa shows mild architectural changes.

B: High-power view of the mucosa demonstrates the presence of cryptitis and a crypt abscess. The surrounding lamina propria contains a dense inflammatory infiltrate composed mainly of lymphocytes and plasma cells.

C: Crypt rupture is also present.

D. The inflammation is transmural. Lymphoid aggregates similar to those seen in Crohn's disease lie in the subserosal soft tissue.

E: Rarely, granulomas are seen, a feature that may also simulate the histologic appearance of Crohn's disease.

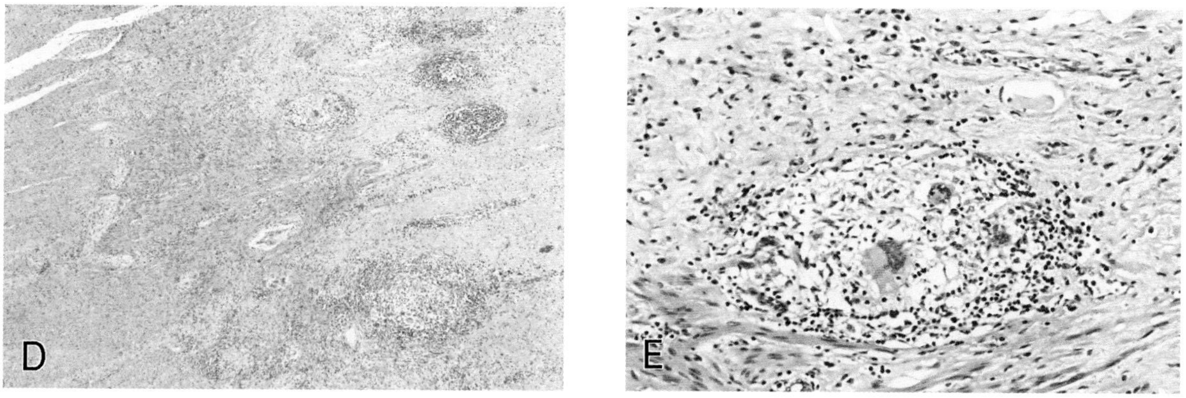

directly adjacent to fistulas or abscesses, or near the diverticular orifices.

Because diverticulosis occurs commonly in the Western world, it often coexists with other diseases, including adenomas and carcinomas, idiopathic IBD, and other forms of colitis. Only rarely do carcinomas arise within a diverticulum.

Differential Diagnosis. It is important to distinguish between congenital and acquired diverticula, since the latter often result from underlying pathology either in the bowel itself or in a structure outside the bowel. The most important feature distinguishing the two is the absence of an intact muscularis propria in acquired diverticula.

Another major diagnostic problem is differentiating IBD from diverticulosis-associated colitis. Diverticulosis-associated colitis is clearly diagnosed in a resection specimen from a patient with obvious diverticulosis or diverticulitis and the inflammatory changes can be related to the distribution of the diverticula.

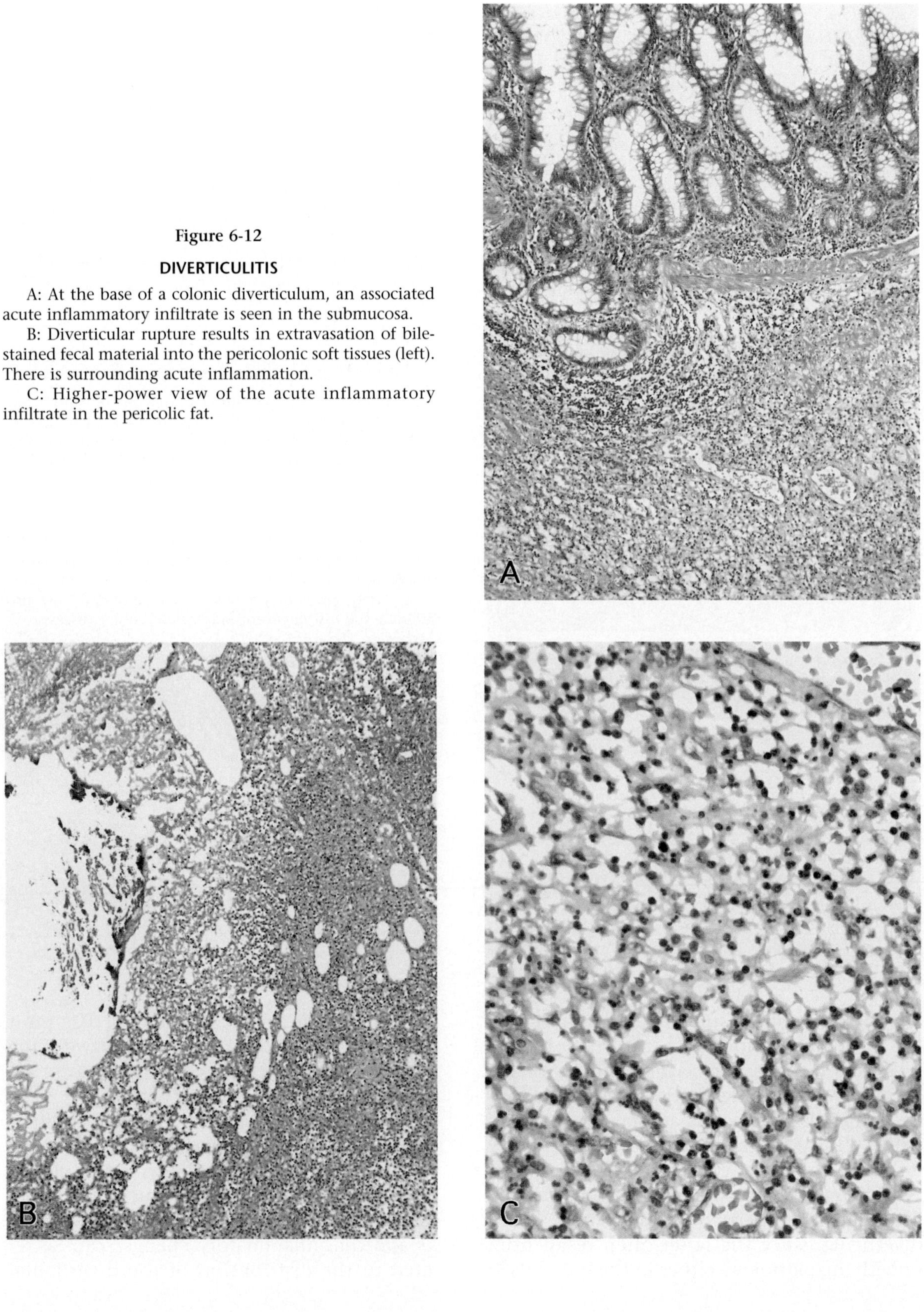

Figure 6-12

DIVERTICULITIS

A: At the base of a colonic diverticulum, an associated acute inflammatory infiltrate is seen in the submucosa.

B: Diverticular rupture results in extravasation of bile-stained fecal material into the pericolonic soft tissues (left). There is surrounding acute inflammation.

C: Higher-power view of the acute inflammatory infiltrate in the pericolic fat.

Given the frequency with which diverticulosis is encountered in the population and the frequency of colonic biopsies, however, diverticulosis-associated colitis may cause unrecognized diagnostic difficulties when interpreting biopsy specimens, and may be falsely interpreted as representing either IBD or collagenous colitis. This is particularly problematic because the chronic colitis of diverticular disease shows a similar distribution as IBD. If the endoscopist biopsies both the area around the diverticula and areas remote from them, the biopsies will show a patchy distribution of the inflammation, distinguishing the changes of sigmoiditis from ulcerative colitis. Additionally, since diverticula rarely occur in the rectum, the "rectal sparing" that occurs in colitis associated with diverticular disease should help distinguish it from ulcerative colitis. If it is not known whether the patient has diverticulosis, then a diagnosis of Crohn's disease may be considered, especially since lymphoid aggregates are commonly dispersed throughout the colonic wall in diverticulosis.

When diverticula rupture, forming abscesses and peridiverticulitis, the features overlap with those seen in Crohn's disease. Features that suggest the presence of Crohn's disease complicating diverticular disease include the presence of ulcers away from the diverticula, fissures, and internal fistulas other than colovesical or colovaginal fistulas. If acute inflammatory masses are present in diverticular disease, they may grossly resemble a carcinoma. Additionally, the colonic wall may become thickened by pericolonic, postinflammatory fibrosis, also grossly simulating a neoplasm or IBD. To further complicate the matter, patients may have both IBD and diverticular disease. Patients with ulcerative colitis who also have diverticulosis may have extension of their mucosal disease into a diverticulum, perhaps obliterating the underlying architecture, resulting in an appearance of a primary fistula and creating changes that mimic those of Crohn's disease.

Treatment and Prognosis. Surgical resection is performed in patients with complications of diverticulitis, such as perforation, obstruction, or hemorrhage. The complication rates are highest in those patients in whom the surgery is performed as an emergency. Patients may die from recurrent pericolic abscesses, peritonitis, fecal peritonitis, bleeding, or bowel obstruction.

INTUSSUSCEPTION

Definition. An *intussusception* results from the invagination or telescoping of an intestinal segment (the intussusceptum) into the next part of the intestine, which forms a sheath around it (the intussuscipiens). Intussusceptions are classified as primary (without an identifiable cause) or secondary (due to a preexisting lesion). Appendiceal intussusception is sometimes referred to as inside-out appendix, inverted appendix, appendiceal invagination, or appendiceal prolapse.

Demography. Intussusception is one of the most common abdominal emergencies of early childhood. Two thirds of cases occur in infancy, with a peak incidence between 3 and 5 months of age (58,65,80). It is also the most common cause of intestinal obstruction in children (69,78). The incidence varies considerably in different parts of the world (77). Some patients have a strong family history of intussusception (70). Interestingly, there appears to be a high incidence of intussusception in doctors' families (81). In the United States there is a male predominance of 2 to 1 and a seasonal prevalence with two peaks, one in the winter and one in the summer (65). Patients are typically well nourished, without a history of gastrointestinal disease.

Etiology. There are numerous causes of intussusception (Table 6-2) (68). Some infantile intussusceptions are primary without an identifiable cause. Most, however, result from an adenovirus infection causing hyperplasia of Peyer patches. Children over age 6 and adults have a demonstrable lead point in 80 to 90 percent of cases (77); some are tumor related (66).

Pathophysiology. During an intussusception, the intussusceptum is drawn into the intussuscipiens by peristalsis until it can go no further because of mesenteric traction. The intussusceptum forms the lead point that becomes ensheathed by the bowel distal to the point of the intussusception. The intussusception constricts the lumen and compresses the mesentery between the inner intussusceptum and the ensheathing intussuscipiens, blocking both venous outflow and the arterial supply, and leading to secondary ischemia. As a result, the

Table 6-2

CAUSES OF INTUSSUSCEPTION

Congenital Abnormalities
Congenital diverticula
Duplications
Enterogenous cysts
Heterotopic tissues
Malrotations
Infections
Adenovirus
Epstein-Barr virus
Herpesvirus
Mycobacteria
Yersinia
Clostridium difficile
Parasites
Tumor-Like Conditions
Endometriosis
Hamartomatous or inflammatory polyps
Lipomatous hypertrophy of the ileocecal valve
Localized lymphoid hyperplasia
Pneumatosis intestinalis
Neoplasms
Other
Complications of surgery
Cystic fibrosis
Fecaliths
Foreign bodies, including bezoars
Gastrojejunostomy tubes
Hematomas
Motility disorders
Redundant sigmoid colon

intussusception continues to swell, causing bowel obstruction and possibly gangrene.

Clinical Features. The diagnosis of an intestinal intussusception is based on clinical symptoms, physical examination, and imaging techniques that include plain films, ultrasound, and barium or air enemas. The classic triad of symptoms is intermittent crampy abdominal pain, vomiting, and passage of stool mixed with blood and mucus. Significant positive predictors of intussusception include the presence of a sausage-shaped right upper quadrant mass (positive predictive value [PPV], 94 percent); gross blood in the stool (PPV, 80 percent); blood on rectal examination (PPV, 78 percent); the triad of intermittent abdominal pain, vomiting, and right upper quadrant mass (PPV, 93 percent); and the triad with occult or gross blood per rectum (PPV, 100 percent) (67). Abdominal spasm and tenderness may make the mass difficult to detect.

In infants, the pain manifests as episodic screaming attacks that persist for 4 to 5 minutes. The infant pulls up its knees in distress. The acute episode is followed by a 10- to 20-minute interval of complete relief (59). Infants with prenatal intussusception present with intestinal atresia and develop signs of intestinal obstruction immediately after birth. Babies usually have a pathologic lead point and the colon is almost always involved (82).

Appendiceal intussusceptions tend to affect males, particularly in their adolescence, but patients range in age from 8 months to 75 years (71,72,84). They present with features of acute appendicitis. The lesion may also remain asymptomatic, only to be discovered incidentally, e.g., when presenting as a cecal polyp. Duodenal intussusception may produce symptoms of biliary obstruction, and hematemesis may rarely occur (60). Internal rectal intussusception can develop into total rectal prolapse (73). Intussusceptions may be chronic or recurrent. Children exhibit a high recurrence rate (20 percent) (78).

Radiologic Findings. Intussusceptions are confirmed by the presence of the donut, target, coiled-spring, crescentic, or pseudokidney sign during ultrasonography; such a sign is present in over 95 percent of cases (61,64,67). Intussusceptions tend to have a curved, sausage-like form with a concavity toward the root of the mesentery. The sensitivity and specificity of ultrasonographic examination are 98.5 and 100 percent, respectively (79). Intussusception may also be detected by CT scans. When contrast is used, a characteristic "target" appearance of concentric rings can be seen. Fluoroscopic images obtained during air enemas can depict or exclude lead points, although this technique is not very sensitive and many patients require surgical exploration (74).

Gross Findings. Ileocolic intussusceptions account for more than 80 percent of cases. In children, lymphoid hyperplasia associated with an adenovirus infection often acts as the lead point and the ileum invaginates into the colon (59,62,63). Intussusceptions develop anywhere in the colon, but are most common at the hepatic flexure (75). They also affect the appendix and much of the small intestine. Duodenal and gastric intussusceptions are rare (62).

Appendiceal intussusceptions take several forms. In one form, the distal appendix intussuscepts into the proximal appendix. In other forms, the proximal appendix intussuscepts into the cecal appendicular valvular opening or the whole appendix intussuscepts into the cecum, presenting as a cecal "polyp."

No matter where the intussusception occurs, the gross findings show the invaginated gastrointestinal segment if the intussusception has not spontaneously reduced (fig. 6-13). Variable external and internal signs of ischemia may be visible, ranging from mild petechial hemorrhages to frank gangrenous necrosis. If the patient has had recurrent bouts of intussusception, the serosal surface may show adhesions.

Microscopic Findings. The intussuscepted bowel may show the features of the intussusception, the pathology of the predisposing cause, and secondary ischemia. The histologic changes differ depending on whether it is an acute, chronic, or acute superimposed on chronic intussusception. In patients with chronic or recurrent intussusceptions, the muscularis mucosae sometimes buckles upward, indicating the lead point of the intussusception, and the subserosal or even intramural vessels may show evidence of a "pulling artifact," with tethering in the same direction as the muscularis mucosae. Similar traction forces probably act on the mucosa, muscularis propria, and subserosal vessels. Recurrent intussusceptions can produce florid submucosal vascular proliferations that may be so pronounced as to raise the possibility of a primary vascular neoplasm (76). Characteristically, there are also prominent muscular hypertrophy and neural hyperplasia.

In children with adenovirus infections, the lymphoid tissue is markedly hyperplastic and the epithelium overlying the lymphoid hyperplasia at the lead point is damaged or even necrotic. Intranuclear viral inclusions appear as reddish globules surrounded by halos or as poorly demarcated purple nuclear smudges.

Most intussusceptions show variable degrees of ischemia (fig. 6-14). The histologic features of the ischemia resemble gastrointestinal ischemia due to other causes. They reflect the length of time that the injury lasted and the degree of vascular compromise that occurred (see chapter 7).

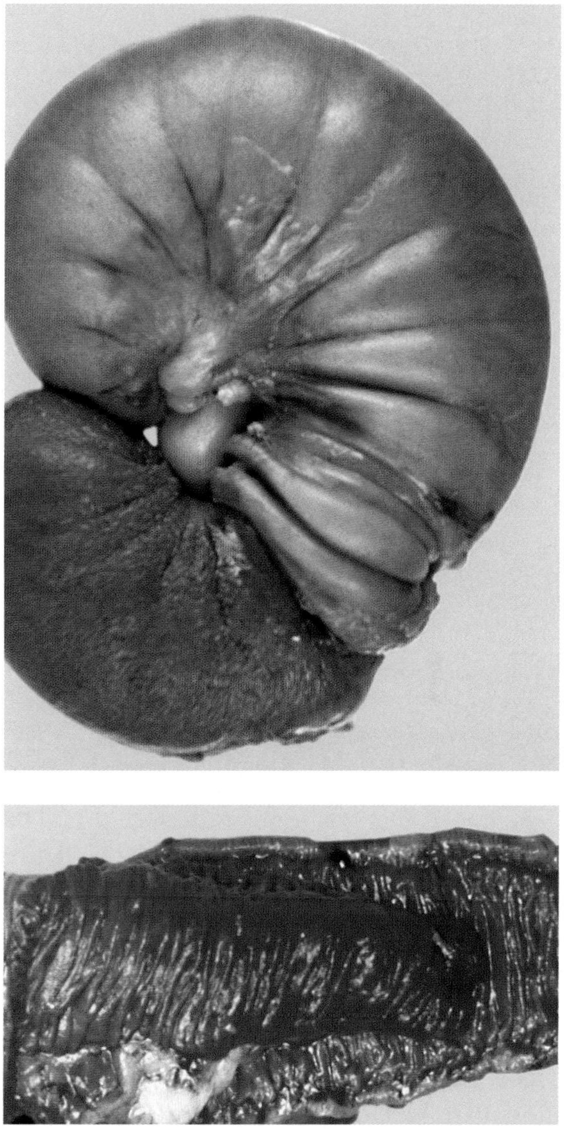

Figure 6-13

INTUSSUSCEPTION

Top: The external aspect of a segment of intussuscepted small bowel. The serosal surface of the intussusceptum is granular and somewhat dusky.

Bottom: Opened specimen shows the invaginated portion of intussuscepting intestine. The lead point appears hemorrhagic.

In appendiceal intussusceptions, the histology appears "inside-out," with the epithelium lying on the external surface of the tissue and the submucosa and muscularis propria lying inside the mucosa (see chapter 13). The epithelium appears hyperplastic, inflamed, or eroded,

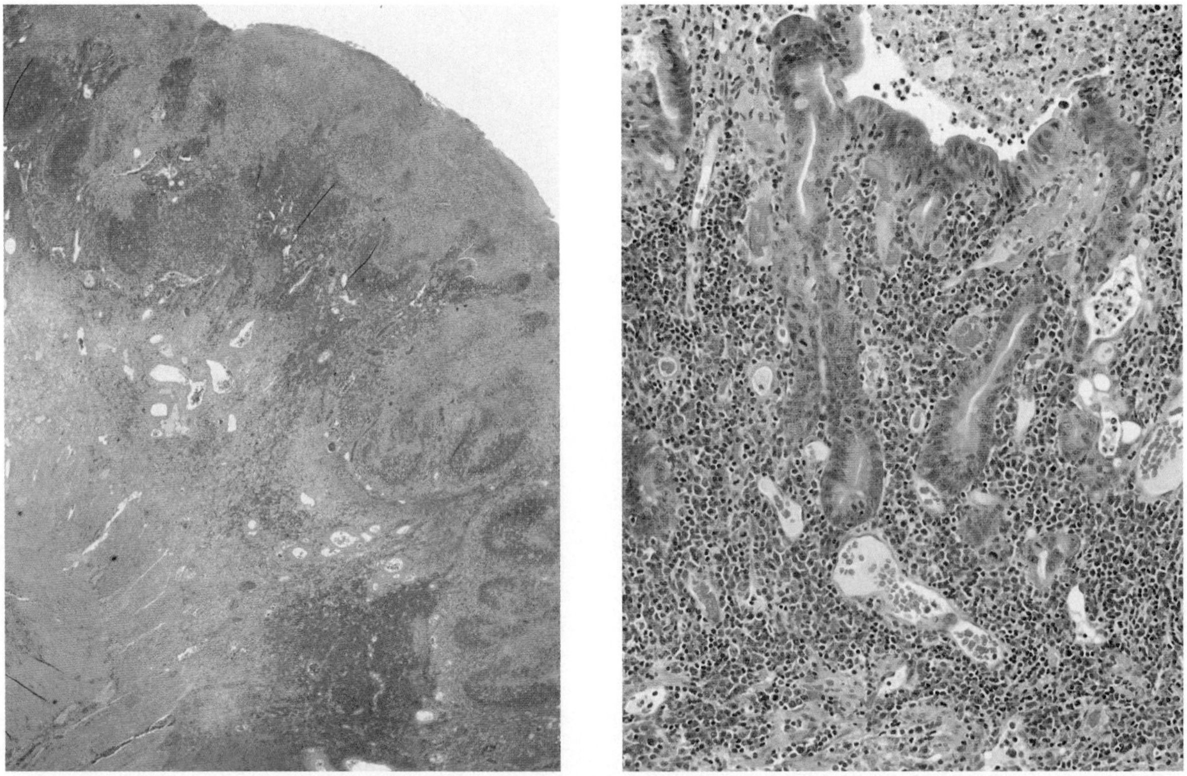

Figure 6-14

INTUSSUSCEPTION

Left: An intussuscepted segment of small intestine shows diffuse ischemic injury to the mucosa with ulceration and hemorrhage.

Right: Higher-power view shows glands with evidence of ischemic injury. The lamina propria contains dilated, congested capillaries and a dense chronic inflammatory infiltrate.

especially if secondary ischemia has occurred. The submucosa becomes edematous and the muscularis propria may appear hyperplastic, fibrotic, or as though it has been subjected to traction. A helpful clue to the diagnosis is the presence of both the circular and longitudinal layers of the muscularis propria with its myenteric plexus in the submucosa of a polypoid lesion. The muscular layers maintain a normal relationship with one another and with the submucosa and mucosa. Sometimes the bowel wall appears to have two muscularis propriae. The amount of tissue inversion seen depends on the extent of the intussusception.

Diagnosing a resected, unreduced intussusception is not difficult. Recurrent or past intussusceptions that spontaneously reduce may be more difficult to recognize. Histologic clues pointing to recurrent intussusception at any site include the following: 1) marked disorganization of the muscularis propria, sometimes showing features of peristaltic drag; 2) fusion of the muscularis mucosae with the underlying muscularis propria; 3) focal submucosal fibrosis; 4) marked telangiectasia; 5) evidence of healed serosal disease, including adhesions; and 6) localized mucosal hyperplasia. Sometimes the bowel wall is kinked on itself with only the muscularis propria demonstrating the twisted appearance of the previous intussusception. In patients with neoplasms, special care must be taken to ensure that the neoplasm is evaluated appropriately for its stage as well as to ensure that it has been completely resected.

Treatment and Prognosis. Some intussusceptions reduce spontaneously. In those that do not, radiologic reduction is often the first line of treatment. Successful reduction with barium, saline, or gas enemas occurs in 50 to 90 percent of patients (59,83). A complication of the treatment may be perforation and pneumoperitoneum. Intussusceptions may also be reduced manually during surgery without a need to resect the gut. Between 15 and 20 percent of cases must be resected. Indications for a surgical resection include perforation, infarction, or irreducibility. Disease duration influences the necessity for intestinal resection. Those with symptoms of more than 24 hours' duration are more likely to require intestinal resection than those with symptoms of less than 24 hours (59).

VOLVULUS

Volvulus, or *torsion*, is an axial twist of a part of the gastrointestinal tract around itself or its mesentery.

Gastric Volvulus

Pathophysiology. *Gastric volvulus* usually occurs secondary to hiatal hernias (103). The most common type of gastric volvulus, organoaxial volvulus, accounts for approximately 60 percent of cases. The stomach twists around the longitudinal axis of the lesser curvature, a position that remains relatively fixed, causing it to turn upside down. The greater curvature rotates upward, forward, and to the right, producing both proximal and distal obstruction. Anterior rotation occurs more commonly than posterior rotation. Mesenteroaxial volvulus represents 30 percent of cases and occurs around a line that runs from the center of the greater curvature to the porta hepatis. Mesenteroaxial and organoaxial volvulus can coexist. As gastric volvulus develops, the stomach progressively distends due to the accumulation of food and secretions that cannot pass forward or be regurgitated due to the presence of both distal and proximal obstruction.

Clinical Features. Gastric volvulus presents either acutely or chronically. Acute gastric volvulus results in gastric hemorrhage, ischemia, and infarction, and is easily diagnosed. Patients with subacute volvulus frequently go undiagnosed because of the presence of vague, nonspecific symptoms (99). Chronic gastric volvulus presents with intermittent dysphagia, epigastric pain, vomiting, abdominal masses, occasional hematemesis, and gastroesophageal reflux disease (98). Death can result from the sequence of obstruction, strangulation, and ischemic necrosis due to compression of the gastric vasculature.

Gross Findings. Radiologic abdominal films show gastric distension with two separate fluid levels.

Table 6-3

VOLVULUS: ETIOLOGY

Gastric Volvulus
Congenital diaphragmatic abnormalities
Lax esophageal hiatus
Periesophageal hernia
Congenital absence of intraperitoneal visceral attachments
Intestinal Volvulus
Intestinal bands
Intestinal malrotation
Intestinal diverticula
Infections and other inflammatory diseases
Motility disorders
Redundant sigmoid colon
Endometriosis
Cystic fibrosis
Pneumatosis intestinalis
Tumors
Treatment with psychotropic drugs
Previous surgery

Small Intestinal Volvulus

Definition. *Intestinal volvulus* is divided into primary and secondary forms. Primary volvulus develops in patients lacking a predisposing anatomic abnormality. Secondary volvulus affects patients with an acquired or congenital abnormality that predisposes the bowel to rotate.

Demography. Volvulus affects people of all ages, most often adults (90,92,97,104). Small bowel volvulus constitutes 8 percent of all cases of mechanical intestinal obstruction and up to 30 percent of small bowel obstructions in some countries, especially in Asia, Africa, and the Middle East, where high fiber diets are consumed. Volvulus is a rare cause of small bowel obstruction in Western Europe, Australasia, and North America. Half of the cases are primary and half are secondary. Most patients are male.

Etiology. In Africa and Asia, the etiology of intestinal volvulus is usually primary, while in Western countries predisposing conditions usually initiate volvulus formation (Table 6-3).

Clinical Features. Small bowel volvulus is a rare, but life-threatening, surgical emergency. Volvulus occurs acutely, causing complete obstruction, or intermittently, producing partial or complete obstruction with compromise of the blood supply, ischemia, gangrene, perforation, and peritonitis. Patients with intestinal obstruction have severe abdominal pain, nausea, bilious vomiting, abdominal distension, and rectal bleeding. Often the patient collapses due to occlusion of the venous return by the mesenteric twist while arterial perfusion continues. As much as 50 percent of the blood volume may accumulate within the area of the volvulus. Obstipation, tachycardia, and fever occur less commonly (90). A history of recurrent similar minor attacks is present in approximately 50 percent of patients.

Gross Findings. X rays show a closed-loop obstruction. The whirlpool sign (wrapping of the superior mesenteric vein and mesentery around the superior mesenteric artery) is used to diagnose midgut volvulus. The sensitivity, specificity, and positive predictive values of a clockwise whirlpool sign for midgut volvulus are 92 percent, 100 percent, and 100 percent, respectively (101). In developing countries, the resected small bowel is usually filled with undigested food. In ileosigmoid knotting, the ileum twists around the base of the sigmoid and both loops are often gangrenous.

Colonic Volvulus

Demography. In Western countries, volvulus is the third most frequent cause of large bowel obstruction, following cancer and diverticular disease. It accounts for 1 to 7 percent of large bowel obstructions in the United States and Britain. In developing countries, such as Africa, Iran, Pakistan, and South America, where an unrefined diet is consumed, volvulus accounts for up to 50 percent of large bowel obstructions (95). Consumption of large, high fiber meals after prolonged fasts leads to more forceful peristalsis than usual, predisposing to the development of a volvulus (97). In one county in Minnesota, its incidence is 1.47/100,000 people (87), compared to an incidence in Ghana of 12/100,000 (100). Cecal and sigmoid volvulus have a similar incidence in patients under 60 years of age; over the age of 60 the incidence of sigmoid volvulus increases. Sigmoid volvulus accounts for 40 to 80 percent of colonic volvuli (87,89), whereas volvulus of the transverse colon accounts for only 4 to 9 percent of cases (87,95,105). There is also an association with mental abnormalities (85).

Pathophysiology. The proximal colon is affected by 15 to 20 percent of colonic volvuli, usually due to a failure of the cecum and ascending colon to develop normal attachments. The sigmoid colon is also a common site of involvement. A high fiber diet and chronic constipation result in bulky stools with a volume that leads to a persistently loaded colon. In time, the persistently loaded sigmoid distends and elongates. Its two ends approximate one another, producing a narrower mesenteric attachment. The base of the sigmoid loop is narrow, providing a pinnacle for the 180° to 720° rotation. Fibrosis at the base of the mesosigmoid accentuates the narrow base. The actual precipitating cause is often a minor event, such as straining at stool or coughing.

In its early stages, a volvulus produces a check-valve effect, allowing flatus and fecal material to enter the loop but preventing them from leaving. As a result, the bowel rapidly distends. As the volvulus tightens, a complete closed loop obstruction develops leading to vascular compression and ischemic necrosis.

A variant of cecal volvulus, known as *cecal bascule*, consists of a mobile cecum but the ascending colon is fixed, allowing the cecum to fold transversely and superiorly over the ascending colon. Because it is not a true axial twist, vascular occlusion and ischemia are uncommon.

Clinical Features. Large intestinal volvulus causes intestinal obstruction and ischemia anywhere from the cecum to the sigmoid (87). It presents with asymmetric intestinal distension or palpable tympanic swelling. Partial volvulus with spontaneous twisting gives rise to recurrent bouts of lower abdominal pain (87). The diagnosis can be made from a good history and careful interpretation of plain abdominal X rays, and is usually confirmed by barium enema findings. Once a sigmoid volvulus has developed, it tends to recur, with patients developing subacute, slowly progressive attacks. Patients often provide a history of previous episodes of abdominal pain. Cecal rotations tend to occur during pregnancy

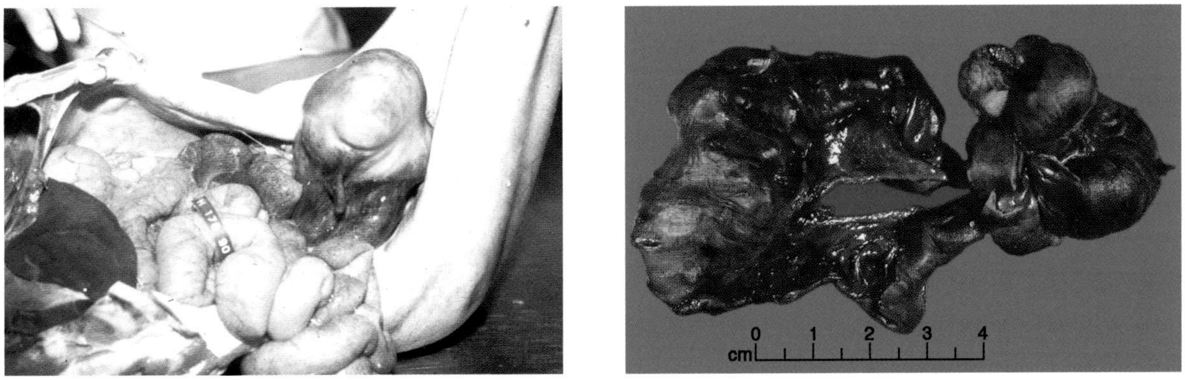

Figure 6-15

VOLVULUS

Left: Autopsy photograph of a torsed segment of intestine. The segment that has undergone volvulus is dusky in appearance, a reflection of ischemic injury.

Right: Gross photograph of a resecttion of a torsed segment of colon. The ischemic portion of the resected colon appears dark blue-brown.

or in patients with obstructing lesions in the left colon. When the rotation occurs, the cecum relocates to the left hypochondrium and becomes tensely distended and often infarcted.

Gross Findings. Cecal volvulus produces a characteristic appearance of small bowel obstruction: enormous distension of the cecum and proximal colon and displacement of the cecum into the upper abdomen (fig. 6-15). The cecum can measure up to 35 cm in circumference (88). The distension causes thinning of the intestinal wall. Radiographically, the tip of the "coffee-bean" deformity in a cecal volvulus points toward the left upper quadrant, contrasting with the "bent inner tube" or "ace of spades" deformity of sigmoid volvulus, which is usually directed toward the right (87). A barium enema may reveal a typical "bird's beak" deformity at the point of the twist. A dilated sigmoid colon that ascends cephalad to the transverse colon is a newly described and accurate finding of sigmoid volvulus. This finding has a sensitivity of 86 percent and a specificity of 100 percent (93).

In resection specimens, the gut appears twisted and may show signs of ischemia or infarction. The ischemia results from either obstruction of the arterial flow or interference with venous return. Pneumatosis intestinalis may be present. The mesentery often appears thickened with large vessels, suggesting that recurrent episodes of rotation have occurred. The thickening may help prevent ischemic necrosis.

Microscopic Findings. When the bowel becomes massively dilated, the muscularis mucosae and muscularis propria often appear markedly attenuated (88). Some cases may show a reduction in the number of ganglion cells, perhaps a manifestation of an underlying motility disorder or the massive dilatation. Histologically, the tissues show variable degrees of ischemia and necrosis.

Treatment and Prognosis. Early preoperative investigation and expedient surgery prevent bowel infarction. The initial treatment can be nonoperative decompression by proctoscopy, sigmoidoscopy, or colonoscopy, a procedure successfully carried out in many patients. The role of colonoscopic reduction in children is limited to diagnosis, immediate relief, and helping with bowel preparation before surgery (102). In patients who undergo surgery, the treatment is often simple untwisting of the bowel if the bowel is viable. Patients with gangrene require resection of the gangrenous segments and primary bowel anastomosis. The overall mortality rate of patients with sigmoid volvulus is 19.7 percent, rising to 52.8 percent if gangrenous colon is present and decreasing to 12.4 percent when the intestines are viable (86).

RECTAL MUCOSAL PROLAPSE

Definition. *Rectal prolapse* is the protrusion of some or all of the rectal layers through the anus. Rectal prolapse is either complete or

Table 6-4

CLASSIFICATION OF COMPLETE RECTAL PROLAPSE

1st degree	Protrusion of full thickness of the rectum, including the mucocutaneous junction
2nd degree	Complete prolapse without involvement of the mucocutaneous junction
3rd degree	Concealed or internal prolapse in which the rectum intussuscepts but does not pass through the anus

Table 6-5

SPECTRUM OF RECTAL PROLAPSE

Solitary rectal ulcer syndrome
Proctitis cystica profunda
Inflammatory cloacogenic polyps
Inflammatory cap polyps
Rectal intussusception

Table 6-6

CAUSES OF ANORECTAL PROLAPSE

Cystic fibrosis
Acute diarrheal diseases
Infections (bacterial, parasitic)
Inflammatory bowel disease
Lymphoid hyperplasia
Chronic constipation
Connective tissue diseases
Radiation
Previous surgery
Hemorrhoids
Bulimia nervosa
Redundant sigmoid colon
Rectal polyps
Neoplasms

incomplete, and categorized by degree as shown in Table 6-4. Complete rectal prolapse is either concealed (not externally visible at rest), externally visible with straining, or externally visible without straining. When the prolapse remains in the upper anal canal, it is called a hidden prolapse. Complete rectal prolapse is also known as *procidentia*.

Demography. A number of entities fall within the spectrum of rectal prolapse (Table 6-5). The frequency of rectal prolapse is unknown. Rectal prolapse occurs in infants; it is uncommon in childhood and early adulthood; then it increases in frequency after age 40 (122). Although 85 percent of affected adults are women, solitary rectal ulcer usually affects men (122), and is more commonly seen in young adults (113). Inflammatory cap polyp occurs more commonly in females and is usually solitary. Inflammatory cloacogenic polyps may be seen in adults as well as children.

Etiology. Rectal prolapse complicates a number of disorders (Table 6-6) (106,111,112,118–121, 123–127). Patients with mass lesions, such as polyps or tumors, often have recurrent prolapse.

Pathophysiology. Approximately 6 percent of patients with severe diarrhea develop rectal mucosal prolapse (107). Rectal prolapse also occurs in patients who strain during defecation. In older individuals, it occurs as the musculature loses its normal tone.

Several anatomic abnormalities are present in patients with rectal prolapse, including an abnormally deep rectovaginal or retrovesicle pouch, lax and atonic musculature of the pelvic floor, lack of normal rectal fixation with an elongated mesorectum, redundant rectosigmoid and sigmoid colon, and lax and atonic sphincters. These defects are probably consequences of long-standing prolapse. Hemorrhoids may also prolapse through the anus.

Repeated straining during defecation, possibly associated with muscular spasm, may create a shear on the rectal mucosa, causing traumatic ulceration. Excessive straining also facilitates mild mucosal redundancy in the anterior rectal wall. The term "solitary rectal ulcer syndrome" is a misnomer, since frank ulceration is a late feature of the disease and the ulcers may be multiple.

The ulceration that develops in mucosal prolapse syndrome is thought to result from one of the following: 1) pressure necrosis caused by mucosal impaction in the anal canal; 2) ischemia secondary to stretching and rupture of submucosal vessels; 3) trauma during digital replacement of the prolapsing mucosa; and 4) ischemia secondary to obliteration of mucosal capillaries by fibromuscular sclerosis of the lamina propria (122).

Clinical Features. Patients often become symptomatic in their 3rd or 4th decades. Symptoms include rectal bleeding, diarrhea, anorectal pain, pruritus, altered bowel habits, abdominal cramps, and difficulty defecating. The last presents as constipation, straining, increased laxative use, or incomplete rectal evacuation necessitating digital manipulation. Patients complain of perineal or intervaginal weakness, profuse mucus discharge, and the presence of something protruding from the anus following defecation, straining, or when the patient stands. Difficulty in initiating a bowel movement and a feeling of incomplete evacuation are common. Prolapse often starts with straining and as the straining continues, the rectal wall progressively infolds, filling up the rectal lumen. The tissues may remain within the rectal ampulla or prolapse through the anus. Fifty percent of patients become incontinent due to overstretching and weakness of the anal sphincter. The pudendal or perineal nerve may become entrapped by the prolapsing rectal contents, resulting in subsequent neuromuscular dysfunction.

Most patients appear physically fit without abnormalities until rectal examination is performed. Ulcerated and indurated areas are often present on the anterior or anterolateral wall. Patients may have a palpable mass on digital examination. Ulcers often straddle a rectal fold and vary in size from a few millimeters to several centimeters in diameter. The rectum remains freely mobile. Not all patients have ulcers, and in some, the only abnormality is an erythematous area, sometimes associated with polypoid mucosal projections (119). The most extreme form of rectal prolapse is one that incarcerates and cannot be reduced. Pressure on it may cause perforation (115).

The diagnosis is easy to make if the prolapse comes through the anus. The diagnosis of hidden prolapse can be difficult. Redness of the rectal mucosa, especially anteriorly at about the 6- to 7-cm level, provides a clue to the diagnosis. Inflammatory cloacogenic polyps present as small sessile polyps at the anorectal junction.

Gross Findings. The various lesions listed in Table 6-5 show overlapping features, and the relationship among the four entities is confusing. Rectal prolapse involves all of the layers of the rectum, essentially creating a rectal wall intussusception (116). The mucosa may appear erythematous or ulcerated. Polypoid lesions may be present. In solitary rectal ulcer syndrome, solitary or multiple lesions are found within 15 cm of the anal margin, usually lying on the anterior rectal wall. Inflammatory cap polyps develop on top of mucosal folds, mainly in the rectosigmoid. They appear as multiple, often umbilicated, dark red areas of granulation tissue. Patients who develop proctitis cystica profunda show mucosal edema, erythema, and a lumpy-bumpy mucosa, with increased folds; polyps or pseudopolyps; mucosal friability; oval, linear, stellate, or serpiginous ulcers; or a cauliflower-shaped mass measuring up to 5 cm in size. Cross-sections of the bowel wall show the cysts. Surface ulceration is uncommon, but loss of superficial lining cells occurs frequently. Tracts sometimes extend from the mucosa toward the mucinous cysts. The cysts may contain gelatinous or mucinous secretions.

Radiographic features include the nonspecific findings of rectal stricture, mucosal granularity, and rectal thickening (112). Mucosal prolapse syndromes may be investigated by endoscopic ultrasound examination. Ultrasonography demonstrates the normal layers and plays a role in distinguishing prolapse syndromes from malignancy or Crohn's disease (114). Endoscopically, mucosal reddening, ulceration, and edema are seen (117).

Microscopic Findings. The earliest histologic manifestation of rectal prolapse may be nothing more than mucosal erosions or ulcers, or even just nonspecific inflammation with thickening of the collagen table producing changes mimicking collagenous colitis. Ulceration is heralded by capillary dilation and congestion beneath the surface epithelium. Ulcers covered by a fibrous exudate erupt from the mucosal surface in a volcano-like fashion, producing a lesion reminiscent of pseudomembranous colitis. The ulcers never penetrate deeply into the submucosa. Later, the lamina propria becomes replaced by smooth muscle cells and fibroblasts that are arranged at right angles to the muscularis mucosae (fig. 6-16) (110). The glands appear regenerative, with mucin depletion, branching, and hyperplasia (fig. 6-16). The anal mucosa appears

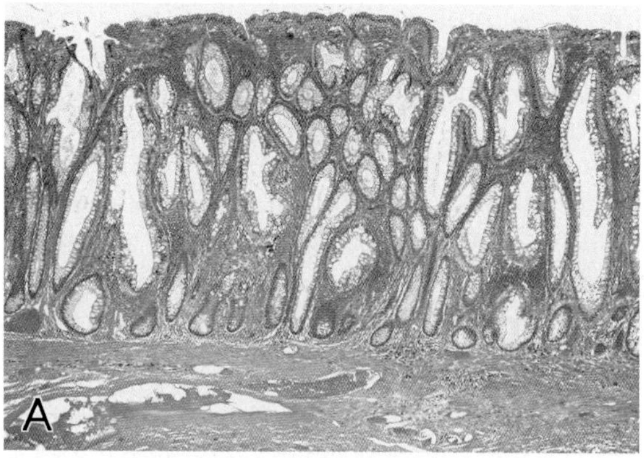

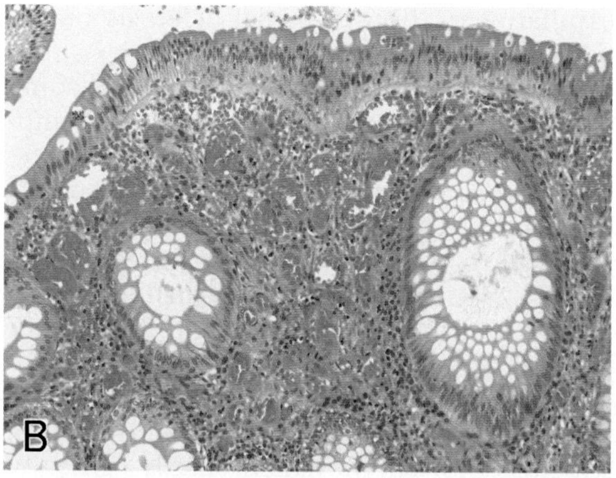

Figure 6-16

MUCOSAL PROLAPSE

A: Low-power view of congested mucosa and submucosa. The crypts are architecturally distorted.

B: The mucosal surface is congested, and proliferating vessels appear granulation tissue-like. The features suggest the possibility of past erosion of the mucosal surface in this area.

C: Hemosiderin pigment is in the deep mucosa, an indication of previous bleeding.

D: Strands of smooth muscle extend upward between the colonic crypts in a direction perpendicular to the fibers of the muscularis mucosae.

E: Fibromuscular changes are seen in the lamina propria between the colonic glands.

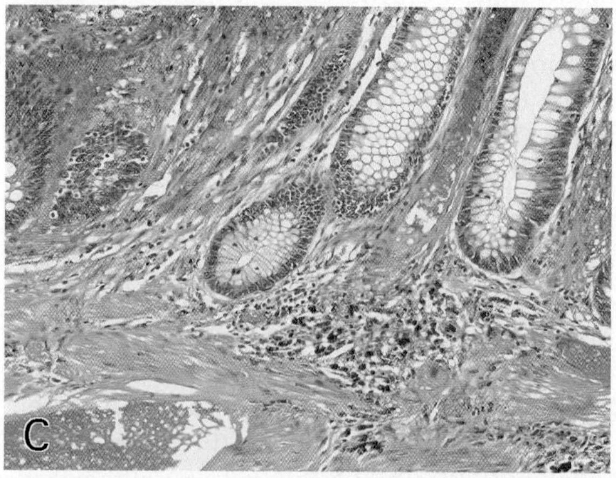

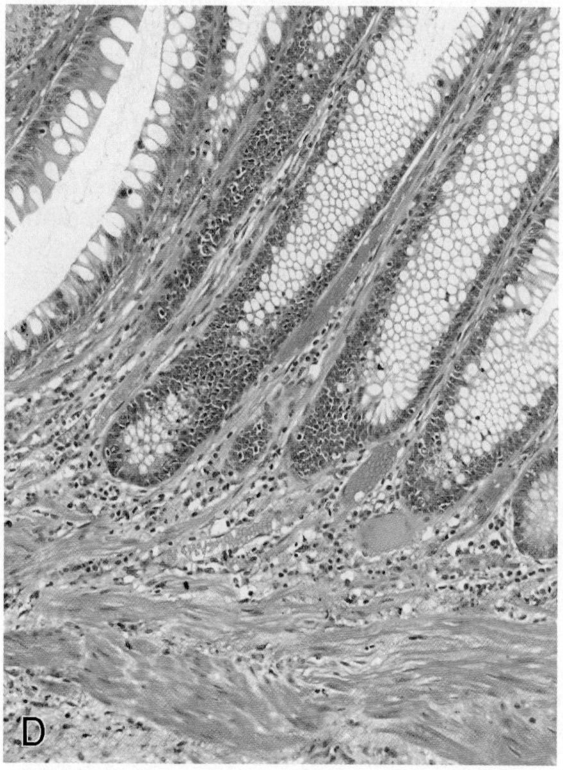

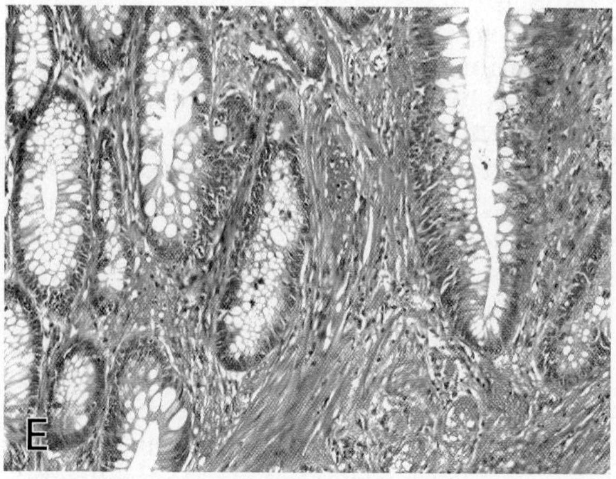

acanthotic, hyperkeratotic, congested, and chronically inflamed.

Microscopic Variants. *Inflammatory (Fibrin) Cap Polyps.* Prolapse induces colorectal and anorectal inflammatory cap polyps. Histologically, inflammatory cap polyps contain tortuous, hyperplastic crypts; fibromuscular hypertrophy, with obliteration of the lamina propria; and goblet cell hypertrophy. The tortuous glands have a serrated tubular architecture, resembling a hyperplastic polyp. Abundant mucin secretion is often present. Fibromuscular tissue frequently extends into the lamina propria in a radial fashion (109,126). The lesions get their name from the cap of granulation tissue and fibrin that covers their surface.

Inflammatory Cloacogenic Polyps. The inflammatory cloacogenic polyp (ICP) is a non-neoplastic polyp that results from transitional zone prolapse. It presents as a small sessile polyp at the anorectal junction. Histologically, ICPs contain epithelium similar to that found in the mucosa of the anal transitional zone. They may exhibit a complex tubulovillous growth pattern, often with a squamous "collar." Long, slender, delicate bundles of proliferating fibrovascular stroma, with smooth muscle fibers from the muscularis mucosae, extend into a normal or inflamed lamina propria. Simple columnar, colonic epithelium containing goblet cells and compressed absorptive cells line the villous projections (fig. 6-17). In cases with moderate to marked submucosal smooth muscle hyperplasia, bundles of smooth muscle–associated proliferating fibrous stroma extend from the submucosa into the lamina propria, usually in a plane perpendicular to the surface. ICPs display a spectrum of mucosal erosion, fibromuscular effacement of the lamina propria, thickened villiform surface mucosa, and displaced epithelium and cysts in the submucosa. The cysts contain variable amounts of mucin and inflammatory cells. Often, the epithelium at the surface appears hyperplastic. Regenerative changes may be pronounced, and may simulate dysplasia; this, coupled with displaced glands, can mimic carcinoma.

Solitary Rectal Ulcer Syndrome. Some of the histologic changes of solitary rectal ulcer syndrome result from an impaired mucosal blood supply during the prolapse. In the acute phase of the disease, the crypts appear elongated and lined by immature basophilic epithelium. Fibrovascular components proliferate in the lamina propria and the epithelium becomes hyperplastic and cystically dilated. Telangiectasia is a common finding. The mucosa may become extremely hyperplastic and polypoid, and may even resemble adenoma because of the villiform architecture that may develop. The features of solitary rectal ulcers include fibrous obliteration of muscle fibers and mucosal reactive hyperplasia with villous configuration or mild pseudoinvasion. Fibrosis may be present, but is usually a late event. This change may be accentuated using trichrome stains. Biopsies of these lesions often show the nonspecific changes of mucosal inflammation, necrosis, and regeneration.

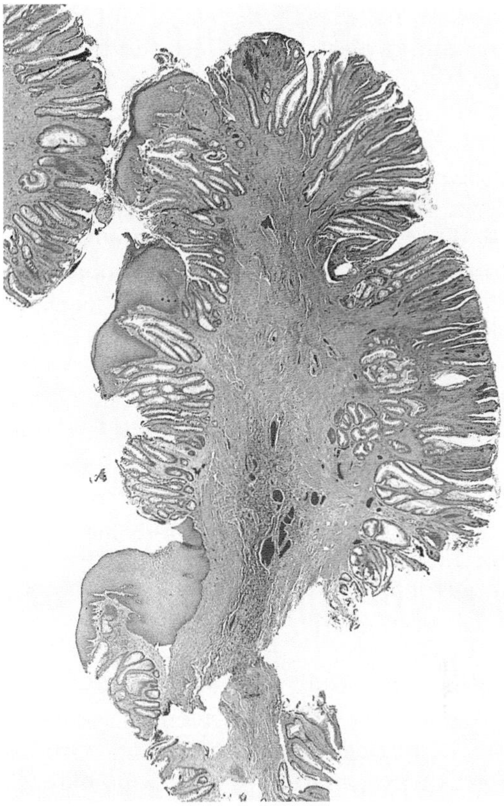

Figure 6-17

INFLAMMATORY CLOACOGENIC POLYP

Alternating villoglandular epithelium and squamous epithelium cover the polyp. (Fig. 2-62 from Atlas of Tumor Pathology, Fascicle 32, Third Series.)

Colitis/Proctitis Cystica Profunda. Mucosal ulceration and healing can also lead to the presence of cysts lined by colonic epithelium deep in the submucosa. The histologic features of proctitis cystica profunda resemble those of colitis cystica profunda (see next section). Other histologic findings reflect ischemia secondary to vascular compression, especially when the prolapse becomes impacted in the upper end of the anal canal. Localized trauma, especially if the prolapse is digitally replaced, also causes some of the histologic features.

Special Techniques. The pathophysiology of defecatory disorders is complex and multifactorial, and requires multiple tests to provide the comprehensive information required to arrive at an appropriate diagnosis and therapeutic planning. Among these, anorectal manometry is extremely useful since it provides objective evidence of poor rectoanal coordination, weak anal sphincters, or changes that support a diagnosis of obstructive defecation. Other tests, such as the balloon expulsion test, may serve as screening tools for patients with constipation. In patients with fecal incontinence, anal endosonography may localize the sphincter defect and aid surgical reconstruction. The pudendal nerve latency test provides a pathophysiologic basis for a weak anal sphincter. Imaging techniques, such as defecography, may provide useful information regarding levator ani dysfunction (121). Defecography shows failed relaxation of the puborectis muscle preventing bolus passage and resulting in abnormal perineal descent (112).

Differential Diagnosis. Rectal prolapse does not usually pose a diagnostic problem. We have seen instances, however, in which unrecognized prolapse in children has led to a misdiagnosis of IBD due to the presence of inflammation, fibrosis, ulcers, or fistulas complicating the prolapse. When the mucosal prolapse results in thickening of the subluminal collagen table, the changes may mimic those found in collagenous colitis.

ICPs may resemble neoplastic lesions since the disordered tubulovillous growth pattern and regenerative atypia of many suggest a neoplastic process. The overall benign reactive appearance of the glandular epithelium, the lack of desmoplasia, and the fibromuscular hyperplasia of the muscularis mucosae and lamina propria in ICPs should make their diagnosis possible. The lesion is also distinct from Peutz-Jeghers polyps that only rarely involve the anal canal. The nature of proliferating fibroblastic stroma along with perpendicular organization of the muscle fibers in ICP contrast with arborizing muscle fibers in Peutz-Jeghers polyps and serve to distinguish the two lesions. Furthermore, ICP is usually an isolated lesion, whereas Peutz-Jeghers polyps usually form part of a more generalized syndrome.

Endometriosis may mimic colitis cystica profunda and the distinction between the two lesions can be difficult. The major difference is the nature of the epithelium, particularly in the absence of the typical endometrial stroma accompanying the endometrial lining epithelium in the latter. Immunostains for estrogen receptor, progesterone receptor, and CD10 may be helpful when the stroma is sparse. Proctitis cystica profunda can also mimic a mucinous carcinoma. The bland appearance of the glandular epithelium, the presence of surrounding lamina propria, the absence of an associated desmoplastic stroma, and the absence of a dysplastic surface lesion distinguish proctitis cystica profunda.

Treatment and Prognosis. Rectal prolapse in children usually corrects itself (113); otherwise injection sclerotherapy may be used to treat rectal prolapse in children (108). Persistent rectal prolapse, especially in adults, is usually managed by surgery, with the most common technique being rectopexy, with or without sigmoid resection. The surgical management can be expected to alleviate the prolapse but not necessarily fecal incontinence. The surgical procedure should not only correct the prolapse, but also help improve bowel and sphincter function. Despite these surgical techniques, there is an overall recurrence rate of greater than 15 percent. In the future, the development of new biocompatible materials may offer alternative therapies.

GASTRITIS, ENTERITIS, AND COLITIS CYSTICA PROFUNDA

Definition. In *gastritis, enteritis,* and *colitis cystica profunda*, glandular epithelium is displaced into the submucosa, typically following ulceration due to mucosal inflammation. Characteristically, the displaced glands form submucosal cysts. These lesions are all similar and are named differently based on their location.

Demography. Enteritis cystica profunda occurs less commonly than its colonic counterpart, colitis cystica profunda (128); gastritis cystica profunda is even rarer. Patients with diffuse colitis cystica profunda (122) range in age from 4 to 68 years, with a mean of 33 years. Males outnumber females by a ratio of 7 to 1. Gastritis cystica profunda primarily affects men in the 7th decade of life (134).

Etiology. Mucus submucosal retention cysts develop following episodes of inflammation and ulceration, such as occur in patients with severe infection, ischemic enterocolitis, or IBD. Associated diseases include Crohn's disease (128,129), Peutz-Jeghers syndrome (133), congenital anomalies, and ulcerative colitis (140). Areas near lymphoid follicles represent points of weakness in the muscularis mucosae, facilitating mucosal herniation (140). Colitis cystica profunda may also follow pelvic radiation (138), neoadjuvant radio/chemotherapy for rectal or esophageal carcinoma, or previous surgery. In the last situation, the cystic lesions are often in anastomoses. Displaced epithelium results from epithelial implantation into the submucosa, muscularis propria, or serosa following mucosal ulceration, herniation (as occurs in adenomas or Peutz-Jeghers polyps), or formation of mucosal microdiverticula (132). Mucosal repair following regeneration of an ulcer leaves the detached epithelium buried in the submucosa. It eventually is covered by an intact mucosa. Displaced epithelium also results from epithelialization of fissures or fistulous tracts.

Clinical Features. Patients may remain asymptomatic or present with the signs and symptoms of the underlying cause of the lesion, i.e., infection, IBD, etc. Symptomatic patients may present with rectal bleeding or passage of mucus and blood. Some patients have diarrhea, tenesmus, and crampy abdominal pain. Endoscopy may show the presence of a nodular mucosa. Intestinal lesions can cause intestinal obstruction (131) or intussusception (135) as they enlarge and form a mass.

Gross Findings. Colitis cystica profunda presents either as a localized lesion or diffusely as multiple lesions. When multiple lesions are present, they are scattered throughout the large intestine. Localized colitis cystica profunda involves any portion of the colon, but usually affects the rectum in the setting of prolapse. Grossly, the bowel wall appears thickened. The cut surface discloses numerous cystic submucosal spaces. These are often quite prominent and glisten because of their mucinous content. They are variable in size, but may measure up to 2 cm in diameter. The mucosa overlying such lesions usually demonstrates histologic evidence of active or healed inflammation.

Microscopic Findings. Cysts in gastritis cystica profunda develop in the submucosa or in the muscularis mucosae of the gastric body and antrum (fig. 6-18). They arise from displaced mucin-producing heterotopic gastric glands. Sometimes chief and parietal cells lie scattered among the mucin-secreting epithelial cells. A normal-appearing lamina propria usually surrounds the displaced gastric glands. Coexisting areas of hemosiderin deposition and fibrosis attest to episodes of previous injury, and suggest that the displaced epithelium does not represent a neoplastic process. Sometimes the cyst lining disappears due to pressure atrophy from large intracystic mucinous accumulations. The muscularis mucosae may appear hypertrophic and frayed.

In enteritis and colitis cystica profunda, flattened epithelium completely or partially lines submucosal mucin-filled cysts. Cuboidal or columnar epithelium resembling normal small intestinal or colonic mucosa usually lines newly formed cysts (fig. 6-19). Since the submucosal cyst lining appears benign, confusion with a malignant process is generally not a problem. Serial sections may demonstrate a communication between the cysts and the mucosal surface. Older cysts often lack an epithelial lining and are surrounded by fibrous tissue and/or a polymorphic inflammatory infiltrate, hemosiderin, or foreign body giant cells (136). The material in the cysts may calcify or ossify. Fibrosis is usually moderate but can be significant, extending into the muscularis propria or even into the serosa (128, 130,133,136,137). As with gastric cysts, lamina propria often surrounds the displaced glands (fig. 6-19), distinguishing the lesion from invasive carcinoma. If the patient has had a barium examination, the barium may extend into the lumen of the displaced glands, further confirming the presence of epithelial displacement.

Differential Diagnosis. Sometimes it is difficult to determine whether the displaced

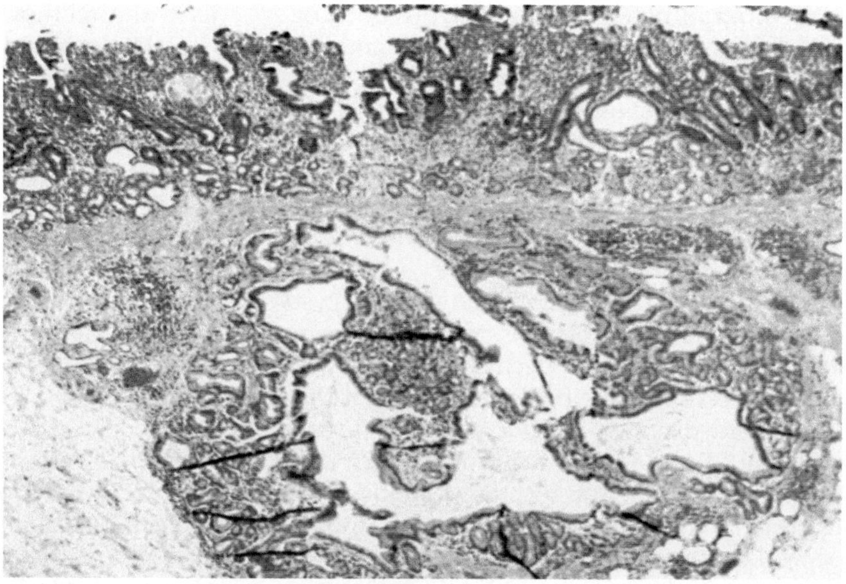

Figure 6-18

GASTRITIS CYSTICA PROFUNDA

Dilated glands are within the submucosa of the stomach. These are surrounded by normal-appearing lamina propria.

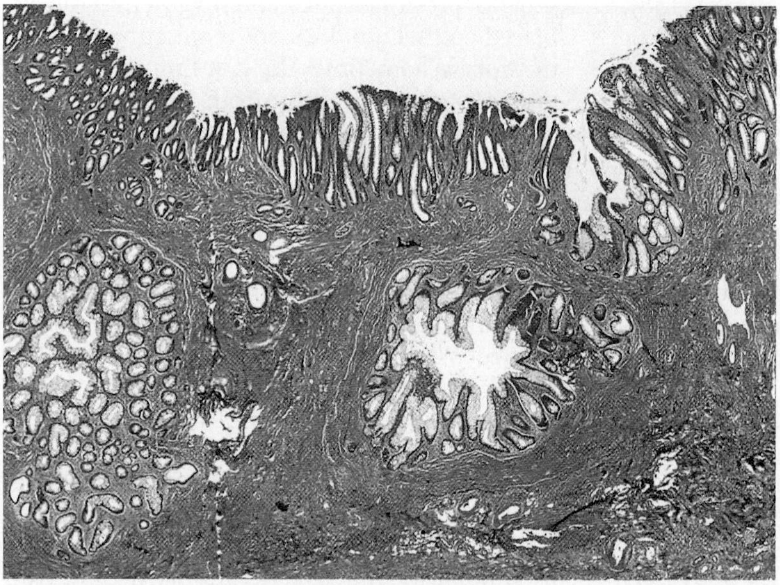

Figure 6-19

COLITIS CYSTIC PROFUNDA

Two nests of rectal mucosa with lamina propria are embedded in the fibromuscular stroma beneath the distorted and altered mucosa. (Fig. 2-69 from Atlas of Tumor Pathology, Fascicle 32, Third Series.)

epithelium represents an invasive mucinous carcinoma or merely displaced epithelium, especially when lamina propria does not surround the glands or when the benign epithelium produces excessive amounts of mucin, resulting in large mucinous cysts containing scant epithelial elements. The traditional histologic and cytologic features distinguish invasive from noninvasive epithelium. Features that help to rule out malignancy include the absence of cytologic atypia, lack of desmoplasia, and the presence of surrounding lamina propria. In some cases, it may be impossible to determine whether one is dealing with displaced epithelium or an invasive cancer. Sometimes, careful sampling and examination of the surface epithelium helps resolve the diagnostic dilemma. If the surface epithelium appears dysplastic, the possibility of an invasive lesion increases.

Another lesion that may superficially resemble colitis cystica profunda causing localized cystic masses with variable degrees of inflammation is endometriosis. The endometrial epithelial lining should not contain mucin and the stroma surrounding the glands should be denser endometrial stroma rather than the looser lamina propria typical of intestinal mucosa.

Treatment and Prognosis. No treatment is necessary for this lesion. The underlying cause of the inflammation and ulceration may require therapy, however. The preferred treatment is local excision to avoid a local mass lesion (139).

ANAL FISSURES

Definition. An *anal fissure* is a painful tear or split in the distal anal canal. Most acute fissures heal spontaneously, but some become chronic. Chronic anal fissures are defined in terms of chronology and morphology. Most surgeons regard the persistence of a fissure for longer than 6 weeks to be an indication of chronicity. Morphologically, the presence of visible transverse internal anal sphincter muscle fibers characterizes a chronic anal fissure (151).

Demography. Anal fissures affect individuals of all ages, including infants (145). They occur with greater frequency in individuals with anal carcinoma, acquired immunodeficiency syndrome (AIDS), tuberculosis, and sexually transmitted diseases (144). Anal fissures are also extremely common in patients with Crohn's disease (141,146,154).

Etiology. Chronic anal fissures develop secondary to persistent contraction of the internal anal sphincter. Localized ischemia may also play a role in their etiology (153). Patients with anal fissures typically have high anal resting pressures and infrequent relaxation of the internal anal sphincter (143). The posterior commissure of the anal canal is less well perfused than the remainder of the anoderm, and increased activity of the internal anal sphincter further decreases the blood supply to this region (149,153).

Clinical Features. Anal fissures are both easy to diagnose and easy for an inexperienced examiner to miss. Anal fissures typically cause severe pain after defecation and bright red rectal bleeding. They are diagnosed by everting the anal canal using the opposing traction of the patient's buttocks. A sentinel skin tag may be present that alerts the examiner to the presence of a fissure. Anal and rectal ulcers commonly are associated with anal fissures.

Gross and Microscopic Findings. Anal fissures occur in the midline, particularly posteriorly. Fissures off the midline suggest the presence of an underlying disorder, such as Crohn's disease, carcinoma, or human immunodeficiency virus (HIV) infection (152). Histologically, anal fissures have granulation tissue, acute inflammatory infiltrates, and often a foreign body type giant cell reaction.

Treatment and Prognosis. Most patients with a newly diagnosed anal fissure should have an initial trial of conservative therapy, since most acute fissures will heal with this approach. In patients with less severe disease, topical glycerol trinitrate is the first line of treatment, since it relieves the pain and causes the fissure to heal (143). An alternative treatment is local injection with botulinum toxin, which leads to symptom relief and scarring of the fissure (147,148). Botulinum toxin decreases resting anal pressure by preventing the release of acetylcholine from presynaptic nerve terminals (142).

Since internal anal sphincter tone is mediated by nitric oxide (NO), efforts have been made to provide exogenous sources of NO (153). Thus, another treatment is the topical application of the nitrogen donor, isosorbide dinitrate. It reduces the anal pressure and increases anorectal blood flow, allowing fissures to heal (153).

Patients unresponsive to medical therapy may undergo surgical treatment. Surgical procedures for treating chronic anal fissures include anal stretch, open or closed lateral sphincterotomy, posterior midline sphincterotomy, and less commonly, dermal flap coverage of the fissure (150).

FISTULAS AND SINUSES

Definitions. The term *fistula* ordinarily implies the presence of an inflammatory tract between two epithelial-lined surfaces. The term *sinus* refers to a tract with only one open end. *Enteroenteric fistulas* are communications between two portions of the gastrointestinal tract. *Bouveret's syndrome* is a cholecystoduodenal or choledochoduodenal fistula resulting from the passage of a gallstone into the duodenal bulb with subsequent gastric outlet obstruction (161). *Aortoenteric fistulas* are communications between the gastrointestinal tract and the aorta. *Gastrocutaneous* and *enterocutaneous fistulas* are a communication between the stomach and intestine, respectively, and the skin.

Demography. Cholecystoduodenal or choledochoduodenal fistula with gallstone ileus

Table 6-7
ETIOLOGY OF GASTROINTESTINAL FISTULAS
Cancer
Trauma
Inflammatory conditions
Appendicitis
Behcet's syndrome
Chronic diarrhea
Crohn's disease
Diverticulitis
Pancreatitis
Peptic ulcers
Vasculitis
Chemical injury
Foreign bodies
Previous surgery
Radiotherapy
Drugs

is a rare disease that affects primarily the elderly, and demonstrates a female to male ratio of approximately 4 to 1 (157). Aortoenteric fistulas also usually affect the elderly. Children with *perianal abscesses,* or fistula-in-ano, present from ages 22 days to 18 years (145). The vast majority of affected children are boys.

Etiology. Fistulas result from three major etiologies: inflammation, trauma, and malignancy (Table 6-7). Esophageal fistulas often result from primary mucosal esophageal disease (reflux or cancer), disease extension in the lungs or mediastinum (infection or cancer), or trauma (esophageal intubation).

Aortoenteric fistulas usually result from disorders involving either the aorta (usually atherosclerosis or following the insertion of an aortic bypass graft), or intrinsic gastrointestinal disease. The blood vessel most commonly perforated by an esophageal foreign body (such as a nasogastric tube) is the aorta, 1 to 5 cm from the origin of the subclavian artery, where the esophagus lies closest to it.

Most anal fistulas represent a complication of infection of the anal glands. Fistulas may also develop secondary to other disorders, most commonly Crohn's disease. Anal fistulas are often complex lesions involving different tissue planes and causing varying degrees of sphincter involvement and destruction. Anal fistula may also result from the presence of heterotopic gastric mucosa and duplications due to the presence of oxyntic mucosa and secondary peptic ulceration.

For several reasons, most anal fistulas develop in the posterior midline of the anorectal ring. First, there is less muscular support for the skin and subcutaneous tissues in this region and as a result, the skin in the area shows a greater tendency to split during descent and eversion of the anal canal during defecation. Second, the anterior rectal wall forms an almost straight line with the anus. This differs from the posterior wall where the rectal ampulla bulges posteriorly toward the hollow of the sacrum so that it forms almost a right angle with the anus. When defecation occurs, the posterior area, which has the least muscular support, almost entirely bears the weight of the fecal contents, and is, therefore, subject to injury.

Clinical Features. *Esophagus.* The symptoms of esophageal fistulas often reflect the underlying pathology. Esophageal-pulmonary fistulas allow food to enter the lung, leading to pneumonitis and pneumonia. Esophageal-aortic fistulas result in rapid death from exsanguination. Initial symptoms include acute epigastric or retrosternal pain.

Small Intestine. Small intestinal fistulas most often result as a complication of Crohn's disease. This entity is discussed in greater detail in chapter 15. They may also develop when a patient with large intestinal neoplasia has a tumor that grows into an adjacent loop of small bowel. Clinical symptoms result either from the inflammation or from the presence of an associated mass lesion. Enteric-aortic graft fistulas cause hematochezia or melena with hematemesis.

Anus. Anal fistulas produce a persistent or intermittent discharge from the fistula opening, leading to the development of perianal dermatitis. Patients tend to develop multiple fistulas. Circumferential spread of a septic process results in horseshoe fistula, which demonstrates one or several openings connected to each other. The classification of anal fistulas is shown in Table 6-8. Anal fistulas are intersphincteric, trans-sphincteric, suprasphincteric, and extrasphincteric, in decreasing order of frequency (158).

Gross Findings. In Bouveret's syndrome, the usual route of fistulization is from the gallbladder to the duodenum (164). A series of upper gastrointestinal endoscopy studies is the best way to visualize the lesion (157,160).

Aortoenteric fistulas involve the duodenum, the esophagus, and other gastrointestinal sites. They develop in the abdominal aorta in 71 percent of cases and the descending thoracic aorta in 29 percent.

In resection specimens, uncomplicated chronic fistulas are often identified by the presence of a cord-like thickening, which may be better appreciated by palpation than by visual inspection of the specimen. A fistulous tract may also be probed in order to identify it (fig. 6-20). Injection of methylene blue or some other dye helps delineate the course of the fistula.

The external opening of anal fistulas is usually within 5 cm of the anus. Magnetic resonance imaging (MRI) can be used to image the anorectal area in patients with fistula-in-ano, but it only correctly identifies the fistula in approximately 50 percent of patients. Fistula-in-ano may have internal openings or external openings, or it may empty into an abscess cavity (163). Some patients have bilateral fistula-in-ano. A relationship exists between the presence of perianal abscess and the development of fistula-in-ano (155).

Microscopic Findings. The lining of fistulas usually consists of granulation or fibrous tissue and variable amounts of inflammation, depending on the age of the process. When the

Table 6-8

CLASSIFICATION OF ANAL FISTULAS

Intersphincteric: The tract runs between the internal and external sphincteric muscle. It is low if it runs low into the skin and high if it runs under the rectum.
Simple low tract
High blind tract
High tract with rectal opening
Rectal opening without a perineal opening
Ectorectal extension
Secondary to pelvic disease
Trans-sphincteric: The tract runs through the external sphincter and through the ischiorectal fossa to the perianal gland.
Uncomplicated
High blind tract
Suprasphincteric: The tract runs between and above the intersphincter space, above the external sphincter and back into the ischiorectal fossa to the perianal gland.
Uncomplicated
Blind tract
Extrasphincteric: This is secondary to pelvic sepsis rather than anal gland infarction and discharges through the ischiorectal fossa to the skin.
Secondary to anal fistula
Secondary to trauma
Secondary to anal rectal disease

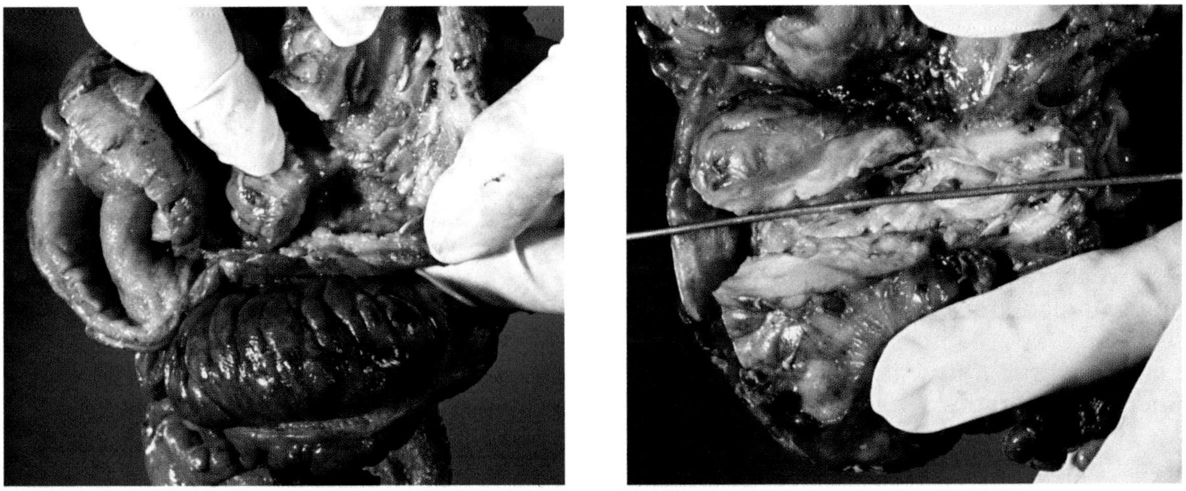

Figure 6-20

FISTULA

Left: A fistulous tract exists between the colon and small intestine.
Right: The tract is more easily seen when a probe is inserted into it.

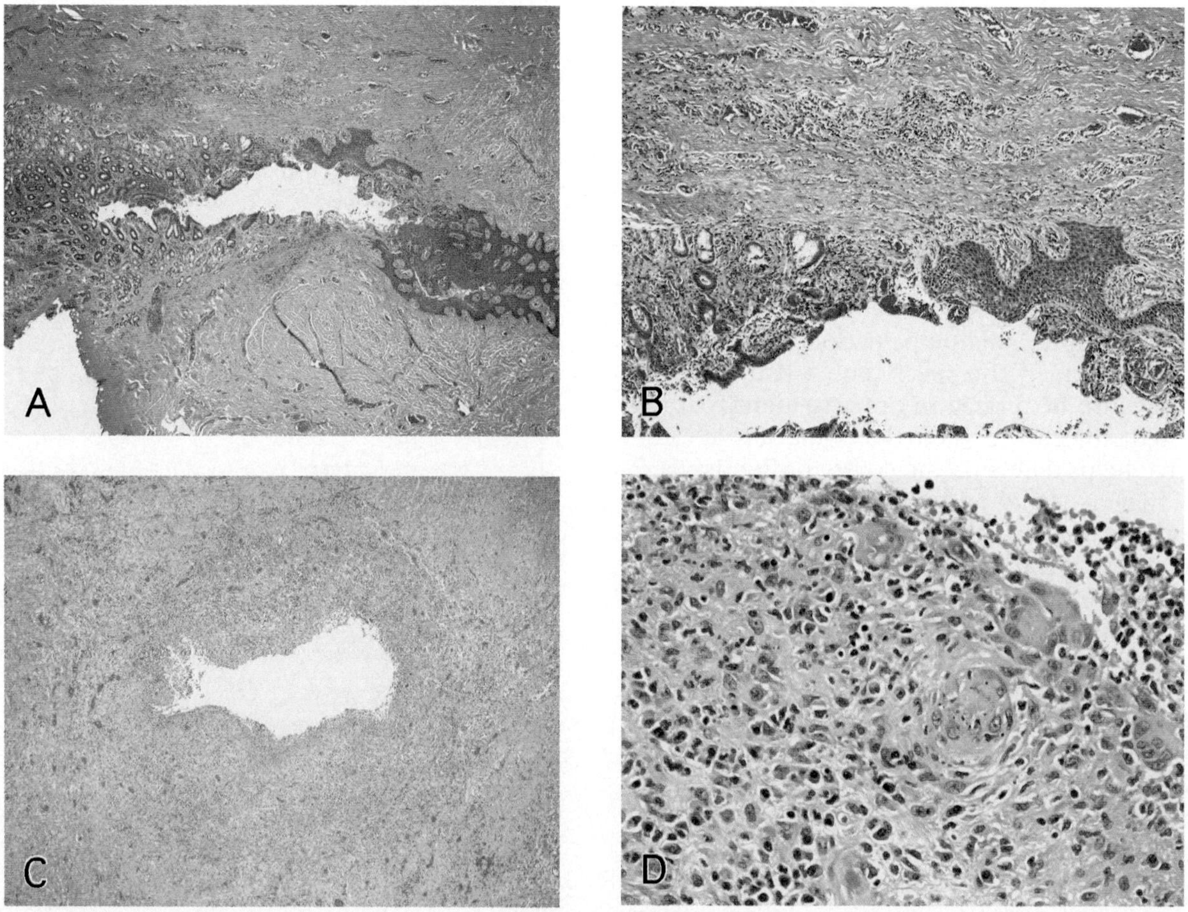

Figure 6-21

FISTULAS

A: Gastrocutaneous fistula. The tract is partially lined by gastric type and squamous epithelium.

B: The surrounding stroma shows chronic inflammation and fibrosis.

C: Fistula tract in a patient with Crohn's disease. No epithelial lining is present in this case. The tract is lined by granulation tissue infiltrated with inflammatory cells.

D: Higher-power view shows granulation tissue, inflammation, and foreign body giant cell reaction.

intestinal contents gain access to a fistula, a granulomatous response may develop. Acute lesions contain numerous inflammatory cells and granulation tissue along the length of the fistula (fig. 6-21). Epithelial ingrowth can occur, especially in anal fistulas, at either end of the tract, leading to the development of a secondary epidermoid cyst (fig. 6-21). Giant cell reactions frequently complicate fistula-in-ano, especially if oil-based medications were used to treat the disease.

Differential Diagnosis. *Anorectum.* Several disorders must be considered in the differential diagnosis of fistula-in-ano (Table 6-7). Crohn's disease is the most likely lesion to be confused with a simple fistula. This is particularly true since only about 50 percent of the fistulas developing in the setting of anal Crohn's disease contain sarcoid-like granulomas suggesting the diagnosis. Hidradenitis suppurativa is differentiated by the presence of multiple perianal skin openings and the fact that the opening in the anal canal lies distal to the dentate line. A pilonidal sinus with perianal extension and infected perianal sebaceous cyst may also be considered. Additionally, carcinomas (mostly low grade) may develop in long-standing fistulas after many decades. Anal canal carcinomas, particularly anal duct carcinomas, may present clinically as chronic fistulous tracts.

Treatment and Prognosis. Exsanguination is the major cause of death when gastrointestinal fistulas involve blood vessels (159).

The majority of anal fistulas are anatomically simple and easy to treat, but others are high or anatomically complex and have the potential to become major management problems. Transsphincteric fistulas are more complex than intersphincteric fistulas. Trans-sphincteric and high fistulas are more likely to occur in females and in patients with previous perianal sepsis or surgery for fistulas. Simple fistulas have external openings close to the posterior midline whereas posterolateral external openings are predictive of complex fistulas (156).

More advanced anal fistulas are treated with sphincterotomy, fistulotomy, marsupialization, and endorectal advancement (158). Lateral internal sphincterotomy is the mainstay of treatment for chronic anal fissures. Endorectal sonography allows identification of patients who might be at increased risk for postoperative incontinence; an anal advancement flap can be used for these patients. Sphincterotomy permanently weakens the internal sphincter and may lead to anal deformity and incontinence. Some fistulas recur. Factors associated with fistula recurrence include a complex form of fistula, horseshoe extension, failure to delineate the lateral location of a fistulous opening, previously fistula surgery, and the experience of the surgeon (158).

The complications of untreated anorectal infections include perirectal abscesses and anal, rectovaginal, rectovesical, and ischiorectal fistulas. Anorectal strictures are a late complication, usually occurring 2 to 6 cm from the anal orifice. Perianal abscesses are drained.

LACERATIONS, PERFORATIONS, HEMATOMAS

Definition. *Lacerations* are mucosal tears that extend into but not through the gastrointestinal wall. *Perforations* are transmural gaps in the integrity of the gastrointestinal wall that allow air and luminal contents to exit the bowel into the surrounding structures. The term *Mallory-Weiss syndrome* refers to painless gastrointestinal bleeding resulting from esophageal or gastroesophageal mucosal lacerations, usually following severe vomiting. *Boerhaave's syndrome* is a spontaneous rupture that occurs at the gastroesophageal junction. *Stercoral perforations* are due to pressure necrosis from fecal masses. *Hematomas* are localized collections of blood within the wall of the gastrointestinal tract.

Demography. Mallory-Weiss tears occur as a result of sudden, often violent increases in intraabdominal pressure compared to intrathoracic pressure. This can occur during vomiting, childbirth, weight lifting, defecation, or trauma (167,176,185,209). They also complicate upper endoscopy with an incidence of 0.07 to 0.49 percent (179,195,199). In some patients, vomiting precipitates tears of preexisting ulcers or thermal burns (173). Less traumatic events, even snoring, can produce partial esophageal tears, usually above the cardia (193). Most patients with Mallory-Weiss tears are in their 3rd to 5th decades and there is a slight male predominance (209).

Boerhaave's syndrome typically affects alcoholic males between the ages of 40 and 60 years, although the disease affects children (182,213) and neonates on rare occasion (171,191,201). The average age of patients with these lesions is 63. Ninety-five percent of spontaneous complete tears (Boerhaave's syndrome) are associated with vomiting (171). Patients may also have a history of NSAID use, hiatal hernia, or gastroduodenal ulcer disease (169).

The median age of patients with stercoral perforations is 60 years, with an age range of 16 to 89. Forty-five percent are men and 55 percent women. Twenty-three percent of patients are in chronic nursing homes or similar environments (206). Ingestion of the following materials may predispose patients to constipation: aluminum hydroxide, codeine or other narcotics, clay mixtures, constipating sedatives, and paper (pica) (206). Many patients with stercoral perforations have renal failure and severe constipation which is due to nonabsorbable antacids, particularly magnesium and aluminum hydroxide gels, and cation exchange resins used to treat their hyperkalemia (196,197,212).

Etiology. Perforations result from many pathologic conditions (Table 6-9). In countries with poor hygiene, infections often cause the perforation (166,178,181,198). In Western countries, foreign bodies, ischemia, Crohn's disease,

Table 6-9

PERFORATIONS: ETIOLOGY

Appendicitis
Behcet's syndrome
Boerhaave's syndrome
Corrosive injury
Crohn's disease
Drug injury (numerous drugs)
Ehlers-Danlos syndrome
Gastrointestinal obstruction
Infections
Ischemia
Meconium ileus
Motility disorders
Peptic ulcer disease
Radiation injury
Structural defects
Trauma
Tumors
Ulcers due to any cause

tumors, trauma resulting from blunt or penetrating injuries, instrumentation, foreign body impaction, diverticula, and radiation therapy are the most common causes (184,200). Eating, falling, the use of anticoagulants, or the Heimlich maneuver may all precipitate esophageal perforations (168,204). Other antecedent events include abdominal blows, straining at stool, parturition, epileptic seizures, asthma, prolonged hiccups, and neurologic diseases (171), as well as accidental introduction of compressed air into the esophagus (165). Therapeutic intervention, such as dilatation, hemostasis, stent placement, foreign body removal, cancer palliation, and endoscopic ablation techniques increase the risk of perforation from the insertion of flexible fiberoptic endoscopes (170, 186,187,207,210). Esophageal perforations also result from surgical instrumentation or surgical procedures, most commonly fundoplication and esophageal myotomy (205). Esophageal hematomas can be spontaneous or secondary to trauma, toxic ingestion, or interventions.

Pathophysiology. Nausea is associated with closure of the pylorus, distension of the stomach, and retrograde pulsion of the gastric contents from the antrum toward the cardia. If retching or forceful vomiting follows, there is abrupt movement of the diaphragm upward. This coincides with a rapid increase in intra-abdominal pressure leading to the propulsion of the gastric cardia into the thoracic cavity through the hiatus (190). If this is forceful enough, a longitudinal laceration follows. Hiatal hernia is found in over 75 percent of patients with Mallory-Weiss tears (194). With large hiatal hernias, the injury appears more distal because of the greater amount of herniated stomach, whereas with absent or small hiatal hernias, the injury occurs at or just below the gastroesophageal junction (211). In the Mallory-Weiss syndrome, vomiting increases the pressure gradient between the abdomen and the thorax, resulting in distal esophageal ballooning or herniation of the stomach. Once the pressure gradient reaches a certain critical level, the areas of least distensibility, such as the submucosa and mucosa, rupture while the muscular layer remains intact (188).

In Boerhaave's syndrome, the sudden development of a pressure gradient between the internal portion of the viscus and its external supporting tissues usually is the cause of gastrointestinal rupture (203). The antecedent events vary. The viscus may become overdistended by food, drink, gas, or any combination thereof.

Stercoral perforation most commonly occurs in the rectosigmoid (177). Reasons for this are: 1) local pressure from structures surrounding the rectosigmoid that keep it from distending; 2) the presence of hard feces in this area; and 3) the presence of a relatively narrow intestinal lumen. Perforation often occurs during difficult bowel movements. Local pressure from the stool causes the ischemia and subsequent necrosis and perforation (175,178). The situation is made worse by loss of normal mucosal barrier function, often due to coexisting uremia as well as immunosuppression in renal transplant patients.

Clinical Features. The clinical and pathologic features of disruption of mucosal integrity depend on the depth of the tissue disruption and the site of the damage. The deeper the disruption, the more severe the clinical findings. The presentation of esophageal perforations may vary with the site of injury. The classic triad is pain, fever, and the presence of subcutaneous or mediastinal air. Respiratory complications are also common.

Most patients with Mallory-Weiss tears present with gastrointestinal bleeding following retching or emesis. In a minority of patients, melena or hematochezia is the sole presentation.

Severe vomiting followed by excruciating, constant chest pain are the classic clinical signs of Boerhaave's syndrome. Hematemesis occurs at times, and the clinical features and radiologic findings often point to an intrathoracic catastrophe. The clinical features of Boerhaave's syndrome mimic those of instrument perforation, with pain being the presenting symptom in the majority of patients; 25 percent of patients are in shock (165). Atypical chest pain may mimic an acute thoracic aortic dissection (183). The nonspecific symptomatology delays the correct diagnosis, often resulting in significant complications.

Patients with esophageal hematomas have severe chest pain; they may also have dysphagia, odynophagia, and hematemesis. Patients are commonly thought to have an acute cardiac event or dissecting aneurysm. Distinction from a cardiac ischemic event is critical because this condition is worsened by anticoagulation. Precipitating factors such as retching, vomiting, coughing, or foreign body impaction occur in 50 percent of patients (192).

Many patients with stercoral perforations complain of a long history of chronic constipation. Stercoral ulceration with perforation is uncommon but it can be fatal, since patients often develop peritonitis. Such patients typically present with symptoms and signs suggestive of an acute abdomen. An abdominal mass is sometimes palpable.

Gross Findings. Radiologic studies are the key to establishing the diagnosis of esophageal perforation. A standard chest radiograph and an upper abdominal X ray can establish the diagnosis by showing subcutaneous emphysema, pneumomediastinum, and mediastinal air fluid levels, or they may suggest the diagnosis by the presence of mediastinal widening, pneumothorax, hydrothorax, pleural effusion, or pulmonary infiltrates (214). Contrast studies confirm the site of perforation.

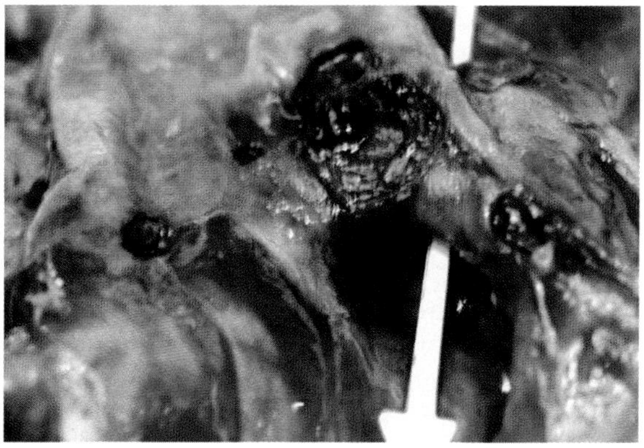

Figure 6-22

MALLORY-WEISS TEAR

A large, hemorrhagic defect is seen in the distal esophagus.

In Mallory-Weiss syndrome, single or multiple lacerations lie along the long axis of the distal esophagus in the right lateral area, crossing the esophageal-gastric junction or lying in the gastric fundus (fig. 6-22). Over 75 percent of lacerations are limited to the stomach. They average 1.5 cm in length but may extend up to 4.0 cm or more. Grossly, these lesions have a linear or cleft-like appearance, and, if examined acutely, are covered by clotted blood.

Boerhaave's syndrome may be diagnosed on CT scan by the presence of a collapsed esophagus and air dissecting through the fascial planes, in a circular fashion around the great vessels, and outlining the aorta and the esophagus. If radiographic contrast material is inserted into the esophagus, a large amount will enter the mediastinum. Characteristically, in Boerhaave's syndrome the rent is linear and longitudinal, and occurs most commonly in the left lateral posterior position, 1 to 3 cm above the cardioesophageal junction (189). This is the weakest part of the esophagus. The tears measure 1 to 20 cm in length, with an average of 2 cm; the mucosal part of the tear is usually longer than the muscular part.

Most small intestine perforations occur in the duodenum, especially in Western countries, perhaps due to the presence of an underlying duodenal diverticulum, gallstones, or peptic ulcer disease.

The most common site of colonic perforation is the sigmoid colon. The next site is the rectosigmoid followed by the cecum, transverse colon, descending colon, and splenic flexure (206). Perforation is single in the majority of cases, although multiple perforations may occur (208). Almost all perforations occur on the antimesenteric border of the colon (208). Most resection specimens show features of colonic loading with scybala and fibrinous exudates, and external evidence of inflammation, necrosis, and friability. The mucosa is ulcerated in a geographic pattern, with round or ovoid perforations occurring centrally in the ulcerated area. Fecal material is often present within or through the bowel wall.

Microscopic Findings. Histologically, esophageal lacerations usually involve only the mucosa and submucosa; they rarely extend into the muscularis propria. At the base of the tear, acute inflammation and numerous ruptured arterioles and small veins are seen. Submucosal hematomas may form and dissect for a distance beyond the tear. In rare situations, Mallory-Weiss lesions present as a submucosal mass (202). In these cases, collections of blood or inflammatory debris gain submucosal access to form a pseudotumor.

The lesion in Boerhaave's syndrome is seldom examined microscopically (except at the time of autopsy in fatal cases). When it is, acute inflammation, fibrinous exudates, and necrosis are seen.

Stercoral ulceration features ulceration of the colonic wall with acute and chronic inflammation.

Differential Diagnosis. Stercoral perforations usually result from a localized hard fecal mass, commonly of a diameter equal to or greater than the colon, with characteristics similar to those of a tumor. These fecal masses are often referred to as fecal or stercoraceous masses, fecalomas, stercoromas, and scybala.

Treatment and Prognosis. The optimal management of esophageal perforation is controversial. Because the nature and sites of perforation vary, the therapy chosen needs to be tailored to the clinical setting. This includes consideration of the patient's esophageal pathology, the hemodynamic consequences of the perforation, and whether the perforation is confined. Despite the type of therapy chosen, delays in diagnosis and treatment are associated with increased morbidity and mortality. Some consider nonoperative management since there is a high morbidity associated with emergency esophagectomy (172). Up to 50 percent of patients treated with primary repair of a perforation require additional surgery (180). Patients with minimal symptoms of fever, absence of shock and sepsis, and with a nontransmural or well-contained tear may be considered for nonoperative management. Nonoperative therapy consists of broad-spectrum antibiotics, parenteral alimentation, and diversion through oral and nasoesophageal suction. Surgery is the intervention of choice in patients with large, noncontained esophageal perforations or clinical signs of sepsis or shock. A gastrostomy or jejunostomy may be necessary to provide nutritional support until the patient is able to resume oral intake.

Most patients with Mallory-Weiss tears have a benign clinical course with evidence of healing in the first 36 hours to 3 days. More than 90 percent of lesions stop bleeding spontaneously. Patients with persistent active bleeding may require additional therapy. Endoscopic therapy with either multipolar electrocoagulation or injection therapy is usually effective in stopping the bleeding. Selective infusion of vasopressin in the celiac or left gastric artery is successful in some cases (174). Gastric embolization may be needed. Surgical intervention with oversewing is rarely necessary. Surgical resection is only used if bleeding is massive; mortality is rare.

The tears in Boerhaave's syndrome must be immediately repaired surgically if the patient is to survive. Unfortunately, the syndrome is frequently misdiagnosed as an acute abdomen, pancreatitis, or cardiac arrest. The current mortality rate is approximately 31 percent (169). Persistent reflux often follows repair of the rupture (203).

The mortality rate associated with stercoral perforation is high, even following surgery. Patients treated conservatively have a much higher mortality rate. Death usually results from uncontrolled sepsis.

STRICTURES

Definition. *Strictures* are areas of narrowing, usually due to scarring following an inflammatory condition.

Etiology. A number of conditions cause strictures (Table 6-10).

Pathophysiology. Repetitive, prolonged exposure to any inflammatory agent can cause transmural inflammation which leads to fibrosis, loss of gastrointestinal wall compliance, and stricture development.

Clinical Features. The clinical presentation of strictures reflects their location. Strictures often develop over a period of time so that symptom onset is insidious. In the esophagus, strictures cause dysphagia. In the stomach, they cause gastric outlet obstruction. In the intestines, they cause partial or complete obstruction. Two of the most common conditions associated with stricture formation are gastroesophageal reflux disease and Crohn's disease. Strictures also complicate radiation therapy. Clinically, strictures, especially focal ones, must be distinguished from carcinomas, which can develop at inflammatory sites. One of the most effective ways of evaluating a stricture is to perform endoscopic brushings of the surface of the lesion, since the densely fibrotic scar tissue may be exceedingly difficult to biopsy.

Table 6-10

CAUSES OF STRICTURES

Acute pancreatitis	Ischemia
Behcet's syndrome	Peptic ulcer disease
Corrosive injury	Radiation
Crohn's disease	Reflux
Diverticulitis	Sarcoidosis
Drug-induced injury	Scleroderma
Graft versus host disease	Tumors
Infections (tuberculosis, herpes simplex virus, cytomegalovirus)	

Gross Findings. Most strictures present as areas of thickening and/or narrowing (figs. 6-23–6-25). The cut surface typically shows varying degrees of fibrosis.

Microscopic Findings. Histologically, strictures consist of variably inflamed fibrous tissues. The mucosal surface may appear eroded, or it may be covered by epithelium that appears normal, atrophic, or regenerative, depending on the underlying cause of the stricture formation.

CHANGES ASSOCIATED WITH PREVIOUS SURGERY

Definition. The functional definition of *short bowel syndrome* is the malabsorptive state that often follows massive resection of the small intestine. Anatomically, short bowel syndrome is defined as a residual jejunoileum measuring less than 75 cm in length (215,233,235). *Anastomotic ulcers* develop at or near anastomotic sites. Many terms have been used to describe anastomotic ulcers following gastrectomy, including *stomal ulcer, gastrojejunal ulcer*, and *jejunal ulcer*.

Demography. Short bowel syndrome follows small intestinal resection for many reasons including malignancy, radiation injury, and vascular insufficiency. Intestinal transplantation is used to treat children with irreversible intestinal failure who are dependent on total parenteral nutrition. Pediatric candidates for intestinal transplantation are those who undergo extensive intestinal resections for necrotizing enterocolitis and intestinal congenital anomalies, including total aganglionosis, volvulus, gastroschisis, and atresia (215) as well as those with functional disorders such as intestinal pseudo-obstruction, microvillous inclusion disease, juvenile polyposis, and trauma (229). The incidence of extreme short bowel syndrome in

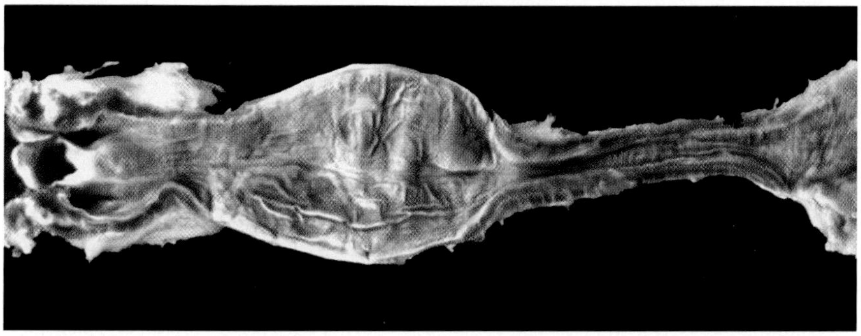

Figure 6-23

STRICTURE OF THE ESOPHAGUS

The lumen is narrowed distally and dilated proximally. (Courtesy of the Division of Gastrointestinal Pathology, Armed Forces Institute of Pathology, Washington, DC.)

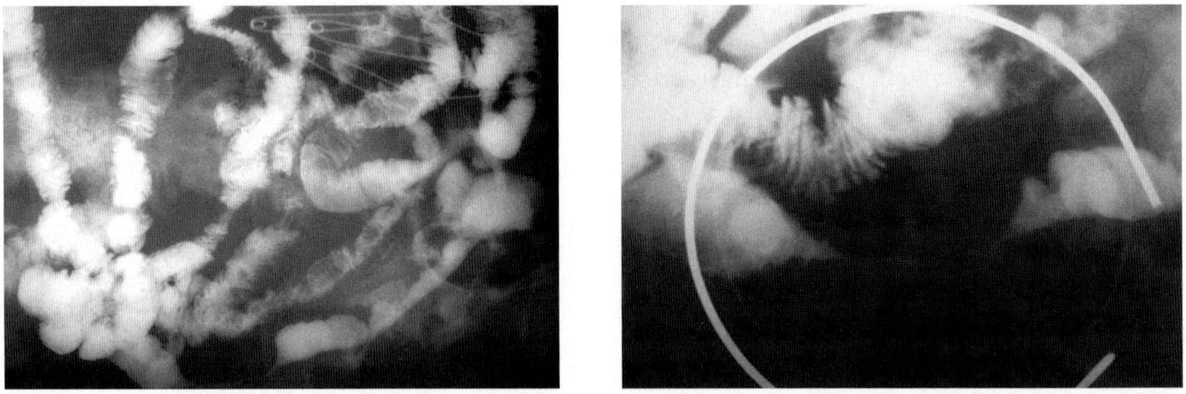

Figure 6-24

SMALL INTESTINAL STRICTURE IN A PATIENT PREVIOUSLY TREATED WITH RADIATION

Left: Small bowel series shows a long segment of strictured small intestine. Only a thin line of barium is seen in the narrowed segment of bowel.

Right: Spot film showing the strictured area.

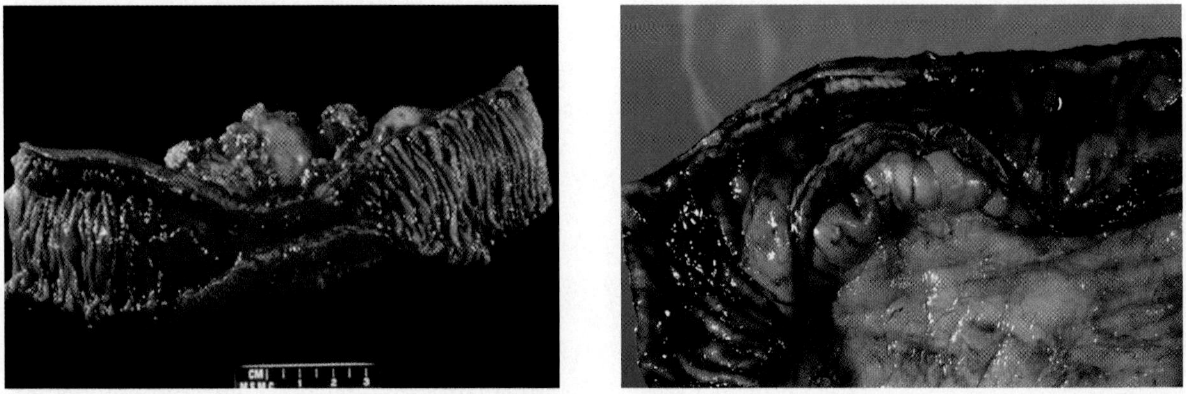

Figure 6-25

SMALL INTESTINAL ISCHEMIC STRICTURE

Left: An unfixed specimen with scarring resembles a carcinoma-like apple core lesion. (Courtesy of the Division of Gastrointestinal Pathology, Armed Forces Institute of Pathology, Washington, DC.)

Right: A fixed specimen with marked narrowing of the small bowel lumen.

newborn infants is difficult to assess but it is estimated to be between 0.3 and 0.5/10,000 births a year (215). Volvulus and Crohn's disease may require massive small intestinal resection in both adults and children.

Pathophysiology. The impact of small intestinal resection depends on the site and extent of the resection and the degree of morphologic and functional adaptation that occurs in the residual bowel (221,227,228,234). Adaptive responses also affect the large intestine, increasing both its growth and mucosal permeability (232). Intestinal digestive and absorptive functions do not parallel the degree of compensatory mucosal hyperplasia (224). Because the small intestine differs in its functions along its length, resections of different segments result in different consequences. Ileal resections are less well tolerated than jejunal ones.

No reliable data exist regarding the length of small intestinal mucosa that can be resected before malabsorption occurs. Studies suggest that one third of the jejunum can be resected without severe effects and that resection of 40 to 50 percent of the total length of the small intestine is usually well tolerated, but more massive resection frequently results in short bowel syndrome (225). In the case of distal ileal resection, especially if the ileocecal valve is removed, lesser degrees of resection may result in malabsorption. The loss of the ileocecal valve and proximal colon predisposes the residual small bowel mucosa to exposure to colonic microorganisms.

Clinical Features. *Changes Following Gastric Surgery.* Patients often exhibit malabsorption following gastric surgery. The afferent loop of a Billroth II gastrectomy is at risk for the development of bacterial overgrowth. Vagotomy and pyloroplasty contribute to reduced gastric acid secretion, predisposing to bacterial or fungal colonization of the blind loop.

Short Bowel Syndrome. Malabsorption of both macronutrients and micronutrients is common. In some patients, caloric and protein needs can be adequately met enterally but vitamin and mineral deficiencies result. In the case of massive small bowel resection, the patient may be committed to lifelong dependence on parenteral nutrition or may require intestinal transplantation.

Gross Findings. *Anastomotic Ulcers.* The normal mucosal pattern disappears and the mucosal folds become reddened, friable, irregular, blunted, cobblestoned, and edematous, with areas of ulceration intermingled with punctate hemorrhages. In patients with a history of antrectomy, anastomotic ulcers develop at or near the anastomosis between the stomach and small bowel, most frequently on the jejunal side, either opposite the stoma or in the efferent loop approximately 1 cm from the anastomotic line. Such ulcers tend to penetrate deeply, often into adjacent organs such as the liver, pancreas, or transverse colon. Radiologically, only about half of such ulcers are correctly diagnosed since a surgical deformity at the anastomotic site may mimic or conceal the ulcer.

Microscopic Findings. *Changes Associated with Previous Gastric Surgery.* Small intestinal mucosal changes in patients who have undergone previous gastric surgery range from a completely normal appearance to mild, patchy, villous atrophy and crypt hypoplasia. Some patients exhibit dense chronic inflammation.

Short Bowel Syndrome. The histologic features of short bowel syndrome differ, depending on the etiology. If it results from healed necrotizing enterocolitis, the intestinal wall will show segmental fibrosis (often transmural in nature) and chronic inflammation. If the patient had a previous resection, the bowel may appear normal or there may be histologic features of the disease for which the resection was undertaken. Villous height increases following intestinal resection. The degree of villous enlargement is proportional to the amount of intestine resected. Villous enlargement is greatest immediately distal to the resection and tapers off. There is an increase in the number of cells per unit length of villus. The number of intestinal stem cells also increases.

Anastomotic Ulcers. Nonspecific mucosal and submucosal inflammation complicates surgical anastomoses. Villous atrophy and intense mucosal and submucosal inflammation may be present. These chronic inflammatory infiltrates consist of lymphocytes, eosinophils, monocytes, and histiocytes. The bowel wall becomes fibrotic and scarred, with destruction of the muscularis propria and the neural plexuses.

Ileostomies. Biopsies of the ileostomy site may show the effects of the surgery with suture granulomas, nonspecific inflammatory changes, dysplasia, or even carcinoma.

Treatment and Prognosis. *Short Bowel Syndrome.* Management of short bowel syndrome is a gradually changing, multistep process (230). During the early postoperative phase, parenteral nutrition is administered and the complications of fluid and electrolyte imbalance rectified. Gradual transition to continuous enteral nutrition and subsequent dietary therapy constitutes the next phase of management. Complications such as nutrient deficiency states, liver disease, and bacterial overgrowth may occur

Potential long-term survival in infants with short bowel syndrome depends on the length of intestine remaining, and whether or not the ileocecal valve is present. Overall, the mortality rate among infants with short bowel syndrome is 15 to 25 percent (215,217,219,220,222,226). In adults, a remnant small bowel length of less than 50 cm correlates with increased mortality (223).

Chronic complications of short bowel syndrome include cholelithiasis, parenteral nutrition-induced liver disease, nutrient deficiency states, and small bowel bacterial overgrowth (231). Fluid and sodium losses in patients with short bowel syndrome can be treated with antidiarrheals, octreotide, omeprazole, or H2 blockers (to reduce rebound acid hypersecretion), but intravenous supplementation is still required.

Animal Models. In experimental animals, 24 to 48 hours after bowel resection the remaining small intestine undergoes an adaptive response characterized by epithelial hyperplasia. The villi lengthen and the intestinal absorptive surface increases so that digestive and absorptive functions gradually improve (216,218). The ileum has a greater capacity to adapt than the jejunum.

CHANGES ASSOCIATED WITH EATING DISORDERS

Definition. *Anorexia nervosa* is defined by four criteria: 1) failure to maintain minimal weight for height and age; 2) fear of fatness; 3) distorted body image; and 4) amenorrhea. *Bulimia nervosa* is an eating disorder characterized by periodic food binges that are followed by purging. The purging usually takes the form of self-induced vomiting, laxative abuse, and/or diuretic abuse. Bulimia is defined by: 1) binge eating; 2) feeling of lack of control; 3) compensatory action to negate binge effects; 4) two binges/week for 3 months; and 5) overconcern with body weight and shape (239). *Binge eating disorder* is a newly recognized entity in which patients eat large amounts of food while feeling a loss of control over their eating. This disorder differs from bulimia nervosa in that the patients do not purge afterward.

Demography. Eating disorders affect an estimated 5 million Americans each year. These illnesses include anorexia nervosa, bulimia nervosa, binge eating disorder, and their variants. Eating disorders typically affect adolescent girls or young women, although 5 to 15 percent of cases of anorexia nervosa and bulimia nervosa, and 40 percent cases of binge eating disorder, occur in boys and men (236). An estimated 3 percent of young women have these disorders (237). The mortality rate associated with anorexia nervosa (0.56 percent/year) is more than 12 times the mortality rate among young women in the general population (243).

Etiology. The disorders appear to be caused by a combination of genetic, neurochemical, psychodevelopmental, and sociocultural factors (237).

Clinical Features. Clinically, patients are often hypotensive, with bradycardia and hypothermia, and have an extremely low weight. Other findings associated with anorexia nervosa include dry skin, hypercarotenemia, and atrophy of the breasts. Laboratory findings are often normal in these patients. Amenorrhea is a cardinal manifestation of anorexia nervosa but oligomenorrhea or amenorrhea may also occur in patients of normal weight who have bulimia nervosa (242). Gastric perforation or Boerhaave's syndrome can complicate bulimic attacks (240,241). Esophageal complications include esophagitis, erosions, and ulcers that result from self-induced vomiting and frequent exposure of the esophageal mucosa to gastric acid (238). Patients with anorexia nervosa lose weight by self-induced starvation. Bulimic forms of the disease combine dietary restrictions with episodes of binging, vomiting, and other forms of purging. The patients may develop rectal prolapse due to constipation, laxative use, overzealous exercise, and increased intra-abdominal pressure from forced vomiting.

Gross Findings. The esophagus may show erythema, erosion, or ulceration as a result of induced vomiting. In patients who develop gastric perforation, the stomach appears dilated and necrotic.

Microscopic Findings. Histologically, the changes of severe reflux esophagitis are seen in bulimic patients.

ARTERIOVENOUS MALFORMATION

Definition. Gastrointestinal vascular anomalies occur in both inherited and genetic disorders; in the setting of previous injury or radiation to the bowel; and with coexisting aortic valvular stenosis, cardiac, pulmonary, or hepatic disease, and hemodialysis. Camilleri et al. (251) suggest separation of vascular anomalies into type 1, arteriovenous malformations with angiodysplasia and vascular ectasia; type 2, multiple phlebectasias; type 3, telangiectasias including those with hereditary or genetic backgrounds; type 4, hemangiomas sometimes including hereditary forms; and type 5, disorders of connective tissue affecting blood vessels.

The terms *angiodysplasia* and *arteriovenous* (AV) *malformation* are often used interchangeably. At time of surgery, an AV malformation may be detectable as a pulsating mass. The lesion consists of a localized increase in the number and size of blood vessels without the features of hemangioma.

Demography. The most common type of vascular malformation is angiodysplasia, which usually involves the right colon (252,256,259), although it also affects other sites. The true incidence of angiodysplasia is unknown since the lesion is difficult to demonstrate surgically and pathologically. Angiodysplastic lesions are incidental findings in 3 to 6 percent of individuals undergoing colonoscopy and in up to 25 percent of the elderly (245). Angiodysplasia usually affects persons over 50 years of age, although it can affect individuals of any age; average patient age is 70 years.

Etiology. Controversy surrounds the etiology of angiodysplasia. Arguments favoring an acquired origin include its association with aortic stenosis, underlying inflammatory gastrointestinal conditions, and hereditary von Willebrand's disease (252,260,282). Mechanical factors may play a role in some cases, with vigorous peristalsis or increased intraluminal pressure causing shunting of blood into the submucosal AV system. Boley (246,247) has proposed that the lesions result from chronic low-grade obstruction of submucosal veins. Normal intermittent distention of the cecum and right colon causes recurrent obstruction to venous outflow, especially where veins penetrate the muscularis propria. This increases the back pressure, resulting in the formation of AV shunts. The pattern of involvement points to the dilatation of submucosal veins as the initial morphologic change, lending credibility to the notion that recurrent obstruction plays a role in its etiology. This obstruction, repeated over many years during the muscular contraction and distention of the colon, results in dilatation and tortuosity of the submucosal veins and then retrograde involvement of the venules of the arteriolar-capillary venular units. Ultimately, the capillary rings surrounding the crypts dilate and the competency of the precapillary sphincters is lost, thus producing a small AV communication.

Pathophysiology. Local factors may be important in the pathogenesis of angiodysplasia. These include intermittent venous obstruction, increased intraluminal pressure, intermittent abnormal arterial flow, and local vascular degeneration.

Clinical Features. Patients with angiodysplasia present either with overt gastrointestinal bleeding or anemia. Bleeding from these lesions can be massive and recurrent. Coagulation abnormalities contribute to episodic bleeding (260). Numerous studies show an association between bleeding from angiodysplasia and the presence of aortic stenosis (244,247,282). Valve replacement causes cessation of the recurrent bleeding (252). This suggests that the aortic stenosis does not cause the lesion but contributes to the bleeding from it (247).

Gross Findings. Angiodysplasias are frequently multiple, measure less than 5 mm in diameter, and primarily involve the cecum and right colon. The lesions are often flat. They usually consist of small (1 to 2 mm or less) or larger (over 5 mm) cherry red, fan-shaped mucosal lesions with a tense central vessel and radiating foot processes (fig. 6-26). Mucosal erosions may be present. If the lesion is examined under the dissecting microscope, multiple, often coalescent vascular channels with adjacent arteries and veins stand out as "coral reefs" against the normal capillary "honeycomb" pattern of the colonic mucosa. Sometimes a gross specimen is received in which the angiodysplasia has been cauterized, in which case the lesion may appear as a heaped-up ulcer.

Microscopic Findings. Histologically, angiodysplasia consists of abnormal numbers of dilated, distorted arteries and veins lined by endothelium (fig. 6-27). The vessels have an abnormal distribution and aberrant morphology, and probably represent true AV malformations. The earliest abnormality is the presence of dilated (twice normal diameter), thin-walled, submucosal veins that may occur in the absence of mucosal involvement. The dilated, thin-walled vessels do not demonstrate sclerosis. The architecture of the overlying gastrointestinal glands is not altered and the lamina propria is not significantly inflamed.

As the disease progresses, mucosal abnormalities become more pronounced. Increased numbers of dilated and deformed vessels are seen in the mucosa and submucosa, eventually leading to distortion of the mucosal architecture and mucosal erosion. The walls of the vessels in the submucosa appear irregularly thickened and often massively dilated (fig.

Figure 6-26

ANGIODYSPLASIA

A: Small, flat, stellate hemorrhagic lesions on the colonic mucosal surface.

B: Endoscopic view with similar-appearing, flat, hemorrhagic foci on the mucosal surface.

C: Endoscopic view of a larger area of angiodysplasia.

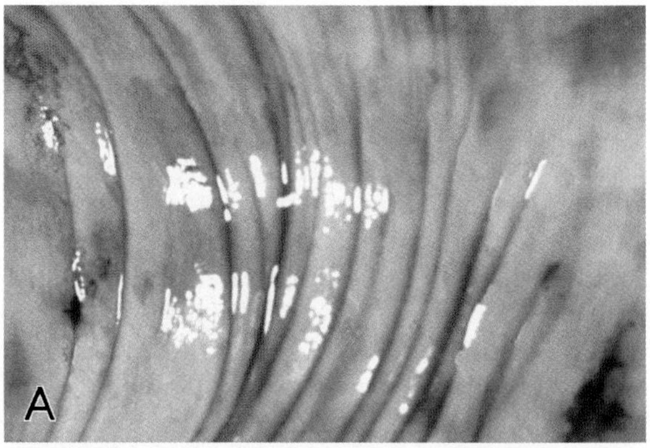

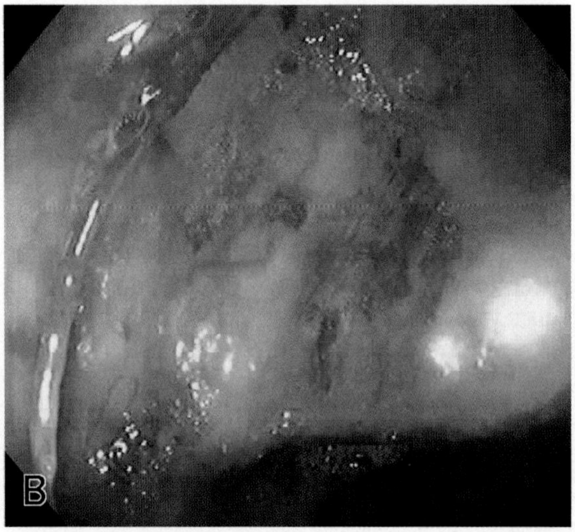

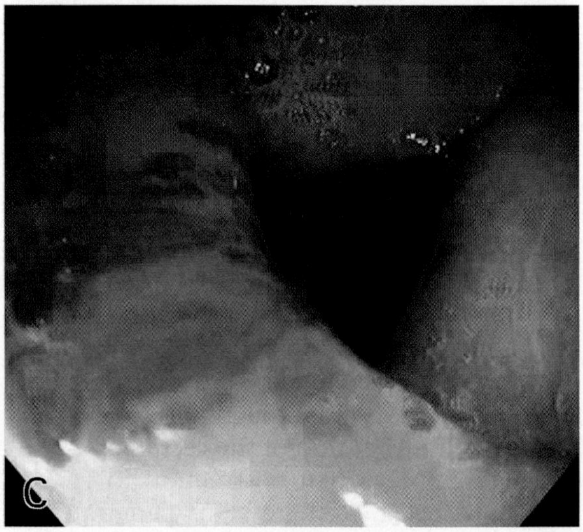

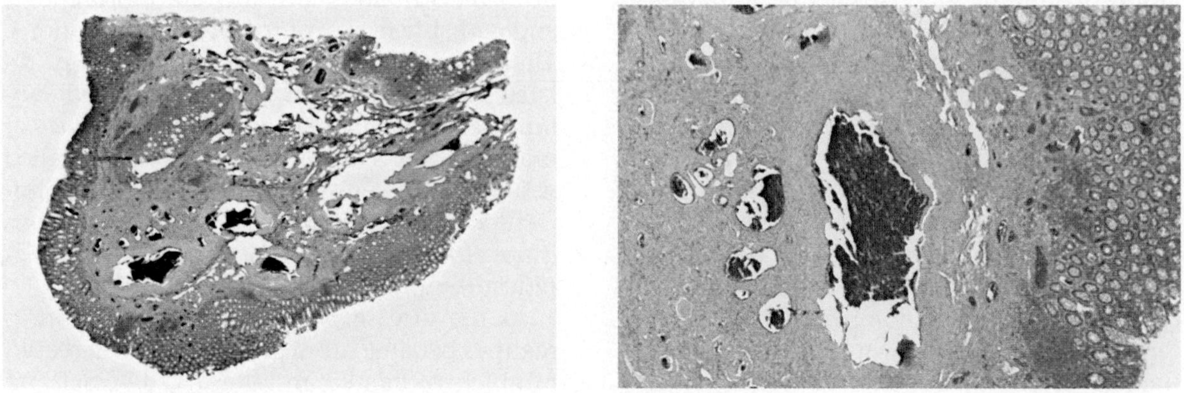

Figure 6-27

ANGIODYSPLASIA

Left: Several thickened, ectatic vessels lie within the colonic submucosa.

Right: Higher-power view shows the irregular, thickened, abnormal submucosal vessels making up the lesion.

6-28). As the lesions advance, the mucosal glands become displaced by the proliferating blood vessels. Only a layer of endothelial cells may separate the vascular channels from the intestinal lumen. Mucosal lesions are always associated with submucosal vascular abnormalities. Occasionally, the submucosal vessels show mild to moderate sclerotic changes, sometimes with atheromatous emboli. Organized and recanalized thrombi may be present in larger veins. The walls of the vessels in the submucosa appear irregularly thickened and often massively dilated. Some vascular ectasias extend the full thickness, from the serosa through the muscularis propria to the submucosa and mucosa.

Special Techniques. Most angiodysplasias are mucosal and submucosal lesions that are not always visible externally to the surgeon or the pathologist, although transillumination occasionally leads to their recognition. A helpful way to identify the vascular abnormality in resection specimens is to have the surgeon cannulate the major vessels at the time of the resection, leaving the cannulas in place. When the specimen is received in the laboratory, the pathologist can inject a combination of India ink and a radiopaque dye into the specimen and then X ray it. The specimen can then be fixed and sections taken. The India ink will remain visible within the abnormal vessels.

Differential Diagnosis. The presence of distorted and malformed vessels distinguishes this lesion from hemangioma or telangiectasia.

Treatment and Prognosis. Some patients need resection because of massive blood loss. Removal of the involved segment cures the disorder.

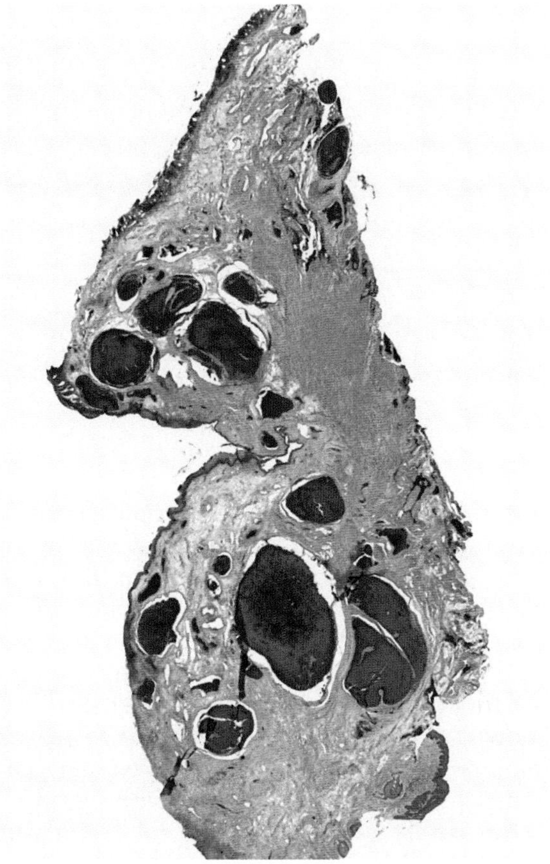

Figure 6-28

HEMORRHOID

Dilated vascular spaces are underlying the anal mucosa and perianal skin. (Courtesy of the Division of Gastrointestinal Pathology, Armed Forces Institute of Pathology, Washington, DC.)

CALIBER-PERSISTENT ARTERY

Definition. *Caliber-persistent artery* is the presence of an abnormally large artery lying horizontally in the submucosa. This entity is also termed *cirsoid aneurysm* and *Dieulafoy lesion*.

Demography. Caliber-persistent artery tends to affect middle-aged and elderly men. The median age of patients is 52 to 54 years, but patients range in age from 16 to 91 (274). The lesions most commonly involve the stomach, but they can occur anywhere in the gastrointestinal tract.

Etiology. The lesion was previously thought to reflect aneurysmal dilatation of a submucosal vessel. Today, however, it is considered to represent a congenital anomaly.

HEMORRHOIDS

Definition. Definitions of hemorrhoid-associated lesions are shown in Table 6-11.

Demography. The prevalence of hemorrhoids is not increased in patients with portal hypertension but the prevalence of anorectal varices and colopathy is higher in these patients. Hemorrhoids rarely develop in individuals under the age of 30, except in pregnant women.

Pathophysiology. Hemorrhoids represent the distal displacement of the anal cushions, tissue that is normally present in the anal mucosa and that becomes more prominent with age. These

Table 6-11

DEFINITION OF LESIONS ASSOCIATED WITH HEMORRHOIDS

External hemorrhoids: dilated venules at the inferior hemorrhoidal plexus located below the dentate line.
Internal hemorrhoids: the anal cushions located above the dentate line prolapse.
First degree hemorrhoid: anal cushions slide down beyond the dentate line upon straining.
Second degree hemorrhoids: the anal cushions prolapse through the anus on straining but reduce spontaneously.
Third degree hemorrhoids: the anal cushions prolapse through the anus upon straining or exertion and require manual replacement into the anal canal.
Fourth degree hemorrhoids: the prolapsed hemorrhoid stays out all the time and cannot be reduced.
Strangulated hemorrhoids: when a sphincter spasm occurs in the presence of irreducible prolapsed hemorrhoids, both the external and internal hemorrhoids become engorged, the blood supply is compromised, and the hemorrhoids become strangulated.

cushions consist of arterioles, venules, and AV communications. Hemorrhoids develop when the supporting tissues of the anal cushion lose their strength and the mucosa becomes more susceptible to the effects of straining at stool, resulting in bleeding and protrusion. The precise function of the anal cushions remains unknown, although they are believed to play a role in anal continence. During the act of defecation, they become engorged with blood.

Hereditary and environmental factors, as well as individual habits, may account for variations in hemorrhoid size, presentation, or symptoms. Factors that predispose to hemorrhoid formation include chronic straining, pregnancy, low fiber diet, anal sphincter spasm, hereditary factors, and tumors (267). As the veins dilate, the overlying mucosa stretches until it eventually protrudes into and down the anal canal. If further dilation of the hemorrhoidal plexus occurs, then secondary hemorrhoids form between the primary ones. When internal hemorrhoids protrude through the anal sphincter, they become strangulated due to sphincter contraction.

Clinical Features. Patients complain of bright red blood on toilet tissue or coating the stool and a vague feeling of rectal discomfort. The discomfort increases when the hemorrhoids enlarge or prolapse through the anus, an event often accompanied by edema and sphincteric spasm. Prolapse, if untreated, becomes chronic as the muscularis stays stretched and the patients complain of constant soiling of underclothing with very little pain. Complications of hemorrhoids include superficial ulceration, thrombosis, necrosis, inflammation, fissure formation, and hemorrhagic infarction with strangulation. Hemorrhoidal thrombosis causes pain, inducing many patients to seek medical help. Later, organization of thrombotic areas results in the formation of fibrous polyps or anal skin tags.

Microscopic Findings. Histologically, hemorrhoids consist of anorectal mucosa covering a plexus of thin-walled, dilated vascular spaces (fig 6-28). These sometimes contain a large amount of smooth muscle in their walls. Variable degrees of hemorrhage, thrombosis, ulceration, and fibrosis are present. Recanalized thrombi are frequently present.

Differential Diagnosis. A number of neoplasms may present clinically as hemorrhoids. These include squamous cell carcinomas, melanoma, and carcinoid tumors. For this reason, it is critical that hemorrhoids be examined histologically.

Treatment and Prognosis. Hemorrhoidal thrombosis may resolve spontaneously with eventual fibrosis or may require surgical removal. Sometimes phenol is injected into the anorectal area in order to sclerose the vasculature. Under these circumstances, there may be an interstitial inflammatory response that may acquire granulomatous features.

VARICES

Definition. *Varices* are dilatations of venous channels. The veins become thickened and sclerotic.

Demography. Varices develop throughout the gastrointestinal tract, although they are most common in the esophagus. Lower esophageal varices develop in up to 90 percent of patients with cirrhosis, particularly in those with alcoholic cirrhosis. Mean patient age is 50 years, and there is a slight male predominance. Feldman et al. (261) found a frequency of large intestinal varices of 0.07 percent in an autopsied population.

Etiology. Sites where varices form reflect the embryonic juxtaposition of visceral and systemic vascular plexuses. Portal hypertension not only causes dilatation of the preexisting natural shunts and creation of collateral vessels, but also reopens embryonic vessels, particularly the periumbilical veins, producing caput medusae.

In patients with portal hypertension varices develop at sites of portosystemic anastomoses. The coronary-azygous system is the primary portal-systemic channel in 50 percent of cases; in 25 percent, the inferior mesenteric and internal iliac systems represent the primary portal-systemic channel. Portal-systemic communications also exist in the rectum.

A common vascular bypass (the coronary-azygous system) that becomes dilated in portal hypertension lies in the area below the esophagus. Here portal blood flow is diverted through the gastric coronary veins, into the esophageal submucosal plexus veins, to the azygous veins, and eventually back to the systemic circulation. This submucosal venous plexus dilates to form esophageal varices. The most common causes of lower esophageal varices are cirrhosis, schistosomiasis, and extrahepatic portal venous obstruction. Upper esophageal varices result from compression of the superior vena cava. Right-sided cardiac insufficiency produces esophageal venous distention as part of the syndrome of congestive heart failure. Bleeding results from rupture, because of increased pressure, or from thinning of the overlying supporting structures, rather than from mucosal erosions caused by acid pepsin digestion (286). Venous stasis and subsequent anoxia produce necrosis and epithelial ulceration, thereby increasing the risk of bleeding. Epithelial destruction occurs over extremely dilated superficial submucosal varices. Thrombosis is rare but perivenous edema and necrosis of the adjacent epithelium are often present, as are hemorrhage and submucosal inflammation. In long-standing stasis, fibrosis becomes prominent.

Most patients with gastric varices have portal hypertension and esophageal varices. Gastric varices also complicate portocaval shunts. The patients develop high systemic venous pressure in the presence of normal portal venous pressure, causing the formation of collateral vessels from the systemic to the portal veins. Varices can also develop as isolated lesions secondary to splenic vein thrombosis or complicate gastric torsion.

Small intestinal varices develop in the same settings as esophageal varices, but they are less common and less well known. Varices result from liver disease in approximately 90 percent of cases. The presence of adhesions, enterostomies, or previous injury (248,253,283) favors their formation, especially if portal hypertension is present. Patients with pancreatitis and splenic vein thrombosis also develop colonic varices (249). Colonic varices may also occur on a familial basis in the absence of portal hypertension (267,276).

Clinical Features. Varices usually do not cause symptoms until they rupture, at which time they produce massive hematemesis or hematochezia. Rupture may occur without an apparent triggering event. Many patients with esophageal varices have an antecedent history of vomiting. In some patients, the bleeding arises from concomitant portal hypertensive gastropathy, Mallory-Weiss tears, or peptic ulcer disease. Bleeding is usually substantial and dramatic. Many patients have concomitant coagulopathy as a result of impaired hepatic synthetic function, and thrombocytopenia due to associated hypersplenism.

Gross Findings. Grossly, varices appear as discrete, large veins protruding into the lumen, or as multiple smaller venules occupying the lamina propria. Endoscopically, esophageal varices appear as bluish, sinuous, linear mucosal elevations that are most prominent below the aortic arch, especially as one approaches the distal esophagus (fig. 6-29). Submucosal varices grossly appear as tortuous dilated veins distributed in the long axis of the distal esophagus, protruding directly beneath the mucosa (fig. 6-30). Varices may be difficult to detect at the time of pathologic examination (usually at autopsy) because they collapse unless special efforts are made to keep them blood-filled. In some cases, transillumination highlights their presence.

Gastric varices usually surround the cardioesophageal junction. They appear as localized,

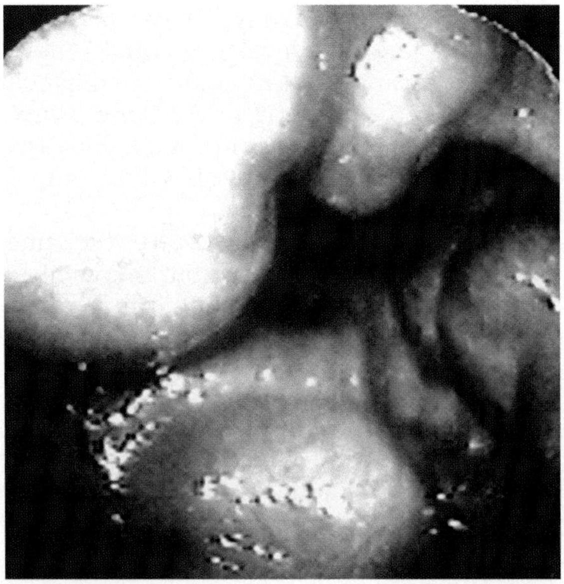

Figure 6-29

ENDOSCOPIC APPEARANCE OF ESOPHAGEAL VARICES

Large, blue-black, dilated and congested veins bulge into the esophageal lumen.

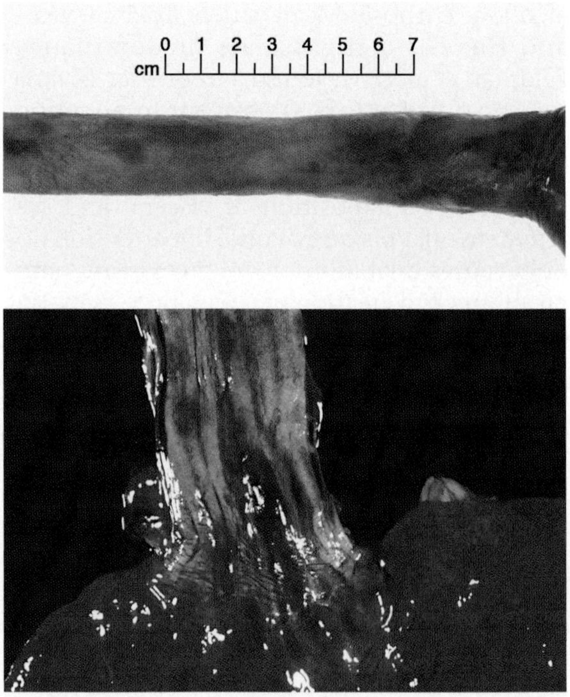

Figure 6-30

ESOPHAGEAL VARICES

Top: The veins appear enlarged and blue-purple.

Bottom: Another specimen shows prominent dilated veins in the distal esophagus. Grossly, esophageal varices may be difficult to visualize in resected or autopsy specimens because the congested veins collapse. A prominent vascular pattern, however, may be observed in the distal esophagus.

polypoid, or multiple rounded submucosal projections. These vessels do not have the bluish cast seen in the esophagus due to increased mucosal thickness. Their varicose features are usually obvious. Classically, gastric varices present radiographically as a cluster of submucosal, polypoid nodules near the gastroesophageal junction. They may appear soft and pliable. It is important that the endoscopist not biopsy "blue polyps," since they may bleed.

Microscopic Findings. Histologically, varices appear as dilated, intraepithelial or subepithelial blood-filled channels (fig. 6-31). Evidence of old thrombosis, hemorrhage, superimposed inflammation, or fibrosis suggests previous rupture. Vessels deeper in the esophageal wall may be massively thickened and sclerotic. Thrombosis is rare but perivenous edema and necrosis of the adjacent epithelium are often present, as are hemorrhage and submucosal inflammation. In long-standing stasis, fibrosis becomes prominent. The histologic features of varices throughout the gastrointestinal tract are similar.

Differential Diagnosis. The differential diagnosis of gastric varices includes portal hypertensive gastropathy and gastric antral vascular ectasia. These lesions may coexist.

Treatment and Prognosis. Patients with varices and an alcoholic history have a poorer prognosis than those with varices from other etiologies. The longer the duration of cirrhosis and low-grade vascular lesions, the greater the risk of developing large varices. Patients with cirrhosis and ruptured esophageal varices stand a 40 percent chance of dying from the initial bleed. If they survive the initial episode, their probability of remaining alive for 1 year is about 30 percent.

Beta-blockers are the treatment of choice to prevent variceal bleeding. During the acute bleed, all patients should receive vasoconstrictors and endoscopic treatment. Injection sclerotherapy controls acute variceal bleeding in many patients by either thrombosing veins or fibrosing the overlying mucosa. Fibrosis occurs late and it is often transmural. Sclerotherapy results in complications in over 20 percent of individuals, including bleeding, reflux esophagitis, necrosis,

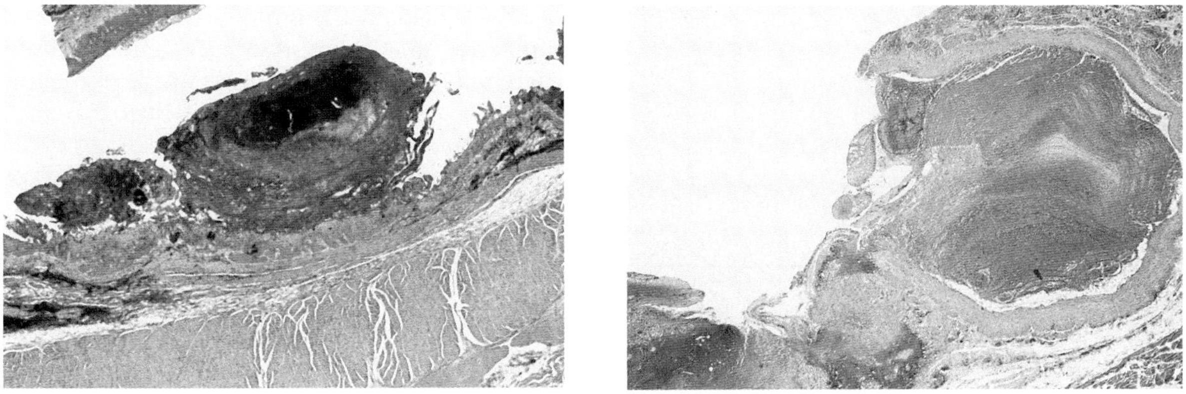

Figure 6-31

ESOPHAGEAL VARICES

Left: A large, dilated, submucosal vein appears partially thrombosed.
Right: Ruptured esophageal varix. The overlying mucosa is eroded, and the vessel wall is no longer intact.

ulcers, tears, abscess formation, perforations, strictures, mediastinal stenosis, esophageal dysmotility, and bacteremia (246,250,289). Some of these complications are transient, whereas others are more chronic.

Tracheoesophageal fistulas may result from the treatment of esophageal varices and the placement of Sengstaken-Blakemore tubes. Prolonged placement of a tube weakens the esophageal wall, precipitating ulcer formation and eventually leading to fistula development. Because of the high complication rate associated with sclerotherapy, endoscopic ligation with an elastic "O" ring offers an alternate therapy and has become the procedure of first choice for the treatment of esophageal varices. The varices are ligated endoscopically and strangled with small elastic O rings, which drop off after a few days, following thrombosis of the underlying varices. The incidence of clinically significant complications is far less than with endoscopic sclerotherapy. Multiple sessions may be required to achieve variceal eradication. Treatment failure should lead to consideration of a transjugular intrahepatic portosystemic shunt (257,272).

PORTAL HYPERTENSIVE VASCULOPATHY

Portal Hypertensive Colopathy

Definition. *Portal hypertensive vasculopathy* is a general term for the widespread gastrointestinal mucosal venous and capillary ectasia seen in association with portal hypertension. The changes may affect any region of the gastrointestinal tract, but are most commonly seen in the stomach. Other terms for this entity are *portal colopathy, portal hypertensive colopathy, portal hypertensive intestinal vasculopathy,* and *portal hypertensive enteropathy*. Colonic portal hypertensive disease is discussed here; portal hypertensive gastropathy is discussed separately below.

Demography. In patients with portal hypertension, both portal hypertensive enteropathy and portal hypertensive colopathy have been reported. Most investigators report a frequency of vascular ectasias of between 48 to 52 percent (254,262,275), with a risk of bleeding from portal hypertensive colopathy estimated at between 0 and 8 percent (254,262). Although hemorrhoids and rectal varices are reported to be the most common causes of lower gastrointestinal bleeding in patients with portal hypertension (264,269), another cause of both acute and chronic lower gastrointestinal hemorrhage in these patients is an increased incidence of changes of the intestinal microvasculature in the mucosa (262,277,287).

Etiology and Pathophysiology. The underlying mechanism for the formation of portal hypertensive colopathy is unclear but both portal hypertension and the associated hyperkinetic circulatory state may play a role in its genesis. A hepatic venous pressure gradient of greater than 12 mm Hg is necessary for the

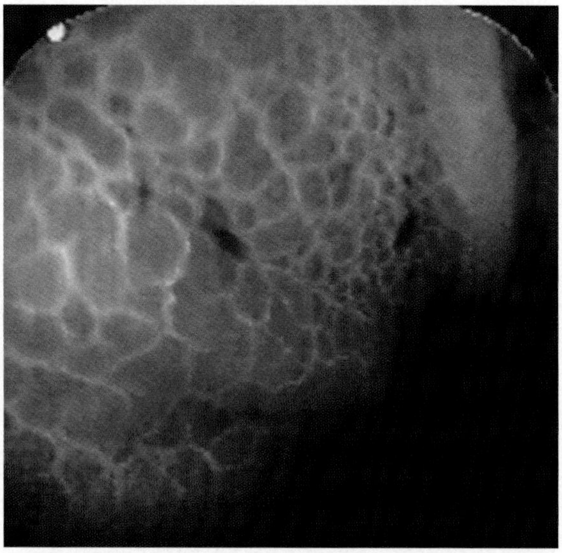

Figure 6-32

PORTAL HYPERTENSIVE GASTROPATHY

The endoscopic features are characteristic, with a reticular network imparting a "snakeskin" appearance to the mucosa.

development of gastroesophageal varices and upper gastrointestinal bleeding (263).

Clinical Features. Patients with portal hypertension may bleed from variceal portosystemic collaterals or specific nonvariceal lesions. Little information is available on portal hypertensive intestinal vasculopathy involving the small bowel or colon (258,273,277–280).

Gross Findings. Endoscopically, the colonic mucosal changes in patients with portal hypertension include telangiectasias or angiodysplasia-like lesions, erythematous patches, and varices (262,264,285). Mucosal vascular changes occur throughout the entire colon in the setting of portal hypertension (273). Endoscopic findings that suggest vascular lesions in cirrhotic patients with dilated vessels on histologic examination include patchy erythema, punctate red macules, telangiectasia, and occasionally visible vessels that are bleeding.

Microscopic Findings. Mucosal vascular dilatation is present in over 70 percent of cases. The spectrum of colonic lesions in portal hypertension includes anorectal/colorectal varices, angiodysplasia-like lesions, telangiectasias, and cherry-red spots (254,255,262,271,273,275,288). Mucosal edema with erythema caused by dilated capillaries can also be present (287). In addition, there may be reactive changes in the crypt epithelium as well as focal infiltration of the lamina propria by neutrophils in some cases.

Treatment and Prognosis. Small intestinal or colonic lesions may be treated with transjugular intrahepatic portosystemic shunt placement.

Portal Hypertensive Gastropathy

Definition. *Portal hypertensive gastropathy* consists of gastric mucosal damage and gastric vasculopathy in the setting of portal hypertension.

Demography. Up to 95 percent of patients with cirrhosis and portal hypertension develop portal hypertensive gastropathy.

Etiology and Pathophysiology. Passive congestion of the portal system and its associated hemodynamic disturbances play a role in the genesis of the gastropathy (265). The patients exhibit increased mucosal blood flow contrasting with the significant reduction seen in patients with chronic gastritis (266).

Clinical Features. Patients present with gastric mucosal abnormalities, anemia, and gastrointestinal hemorrhage.

Gross Findings. The mucosa appears "beefy" red, with multiple petechial hemorrhages, red spots, acute ulcers, and erosions. Often, a characteristic mosaic pattern of a white reticular network outlines central erythematous areas (fig. 6-32) (278). This imparts a "snakeskin" appearance to the mucosa.

Microscopic Findings. The hallmark of portal hypertensive gastropathy is venular ectasia affecting mucosal capillaries and veins (fig. 6-33). This is accompanied by submucosal venous dilatation. The vascular congestion damages the mucosa, probably in a manner that resembles the mechanisms seen in stress gastritis. The congested, dilated vasculature predisposes the mucosa to localized areas of hypoxia, thereby leading to localized erosions and inflammation. Occasional cases demonstrate prominent arterial intimal hyperplasia, diffuse duplication, and focal fragmentation of the internal elastica. Gastric varices are usually present.

Differential Diagnosis. The endoscopic diagnosis is usually characteristic and is not easily confused with gastric antral vascular ectasia (GAVE), varices, or angiodysplasia. Pathologically,

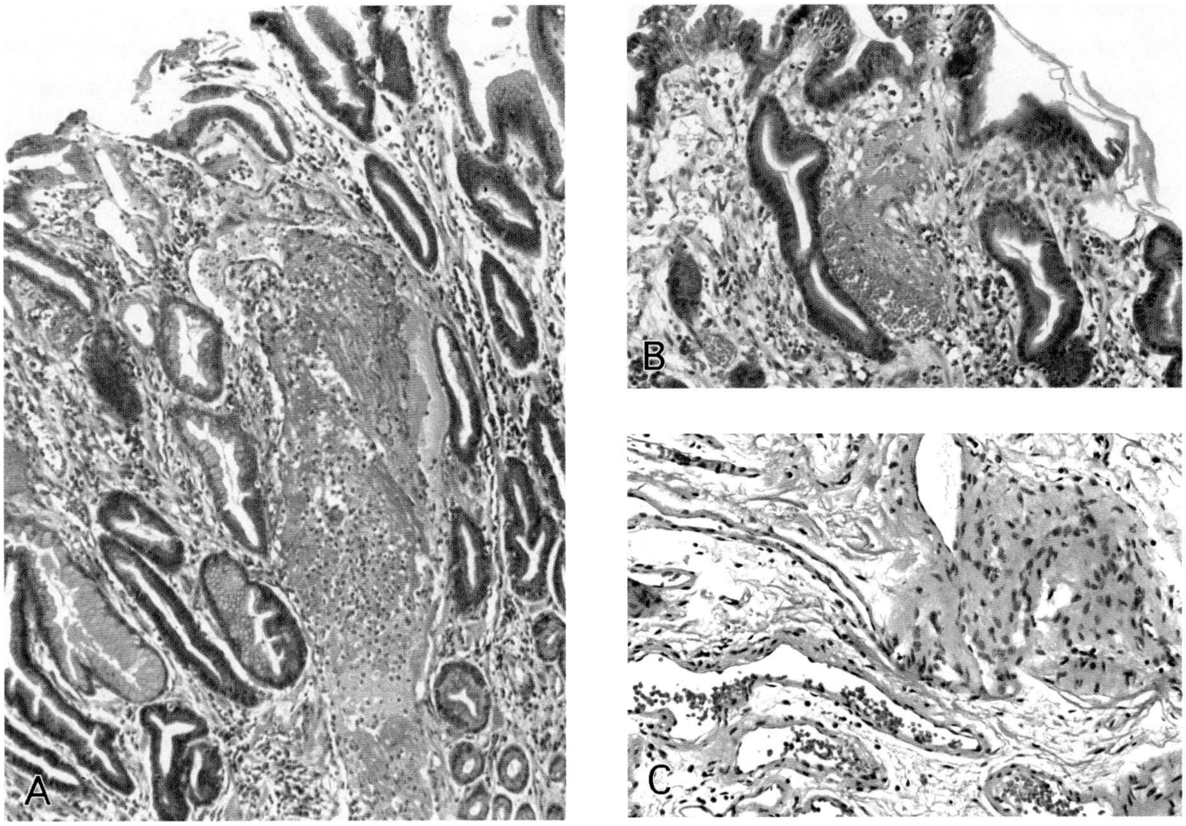

Figure 6-33

PORTAL HYPERTENSIVE GASTROPATHY

A: The mucosal venules are markedly dilated. The surrounding mucosa appears regenerative and the lamina propria is infiltrated with chronic inflammatory cells.

B: Regenerative glands and a surface lined by foveolar cells that are mucin depleted. The capillaries are dilated.

C: Similar vascular changes may be found in the submucosa.

however, portal hypertensive gastropathy may show features that overlap with those of GAVE and varices. Portal hypertensive gastropathy usually affects the body of stomach, while GAVE affects the antrum.

Treatment and Prognosis. Strategies that reduce the portal venous pressure (propranolol, portosystemic shunting) may be necessary to reverse the gastropathy should bleeding become problematic.

GASTRIC ANTRAL VASCULAR ECTASIA

Definition. *Gastric antral vascular ectasia* (GAVE) affects the vessels of the antrum (hence the name) and produces characteristic endoscopic and histologic changes (270,284). *Watermelon stomach* is another name for this disease.

Demography. GAVE predominantly affects women, with a female to male ratio of 17 to 4. Patients range in age from 35 to 80 years, with an average age of 66.5 years (270).

Etiology. The etiology of GAVE is unclear. Many patients have cirrhosis; some have associated autoimmune connective tissue disorders or have undergone bone marrow transplantation. Other factors that are possibly associated with GAVE include vascular disease of the liver, oral busulfan as part of a conditioning regimen, and growth factor use after a transplant. Motility disturbances may also play a role. Some patients have hypergastrinemia.

Clinical Features. GAVE is an unusual, but important, cause of severe gastrointestinal bleeding and iron deficiency anemia.

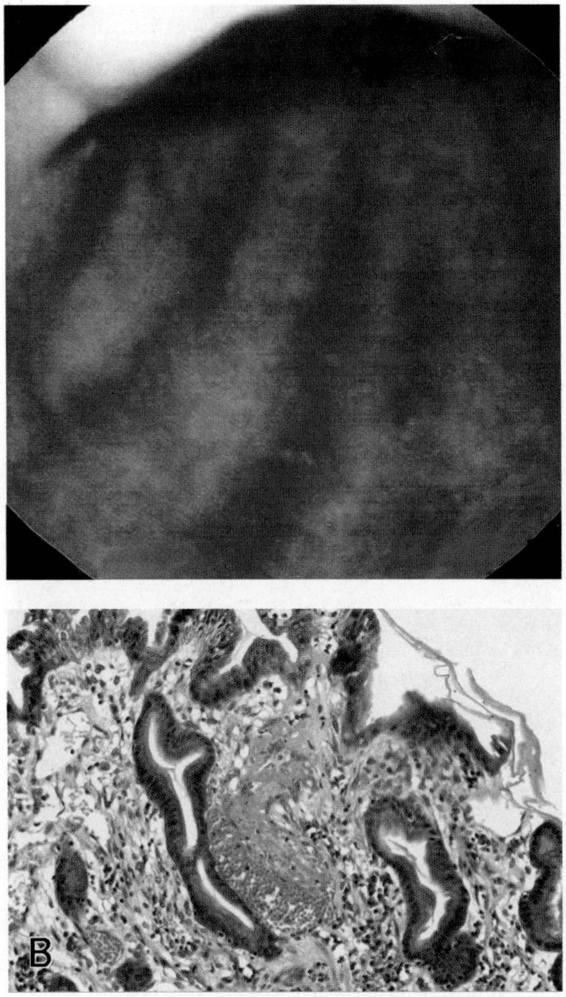

Figure 6-34

WATERMELON STOMACH

Top: Endoscopic appearance shows linear mucosal stripes. (Fig. 2-99 from Emory TS, Carpenter HA, Gostout CJ, Sobin LH. Atlas of gastrointestinal endoscopy & endoscopic biopsies. Washington DC: Armed Forces Institute of Pathology; 2009:117.)

Bottom: At autopsy, linear stripes are seen in the mucosa.

Gross Findings. The distinctive endoscopic appearance of nearly parallel, intensely red, longitudinal stripes situated at the crests of hyperplastic mucosal folds and traversing the gastric antrum prompted Jabbari et al. (270) to coin the phrase "watermelon stomach." These stripes correspond to markedly dilated, tortuous mucosal capillaries (fig. 6-34). Ultrasonography may show hyperechoic focal thickening of the inner layers of the gastric wall.

Microscopic Findings. The characteristic findings of GAVE consist of markedly dilated mucosal capillaries that often contain fibrin thrombi, with variable edema and interstitial hemorrhage in the surrounding tissue. These dilated capillaries are surrounded by fibrohyalinosis and coexist with fibromuscular hyperplasia of the lamina propria (figs. 6-35, 6-36). The fibrohyalinosis that appears as a homogeneous light pink substance in H&E-stained sections helps differentiate GAVE from severe portal hypertensive gastropathy (270,284). The mucosa also usually shows a coexisting patchy, mild, chronic inflammatory infiltrate in the superficial lamina propria of the gastric antrum. Atrophic gastritis with intestinal metaplasia may be present. The muscularis mucosae may appear thickened and hyperplastic. Submucosal vessels appear dilated and congested but vascular malformations are absent. The lesions may be associated with hyperplasia of vasoactive intestinal polypeptide- and serotonin-containing endocrine cells. The serotonin may cause the vascular dilatation and sclerosis.

Differential Diagnosis. The endoscopic findings are characteristic. The histologic differential diagnosis includes gastric varices and portal hypertensive gastropathy. These lesions are compared in Table 6-12.

Treatment and Prognosis. The lesion may be treated with laser therapy. Antrectomy may be necessary in nonresponsive cases.

MUCOSAL TELANGIECTASIAS

Definition. *Telangiectasia* generally refers to dilation of preexisting vessels, whereas *angiomatosis* refers to new vessel growth.

Demography and Etiology. Gastrointestinal telangiectasias occur as isolated lesions within the gastrointestinal tract where they occur concomitantly with telangiectasias elsewhere, especially in the skin. They may be spontaneously acquired or hereditary. The cause of telangiectasia is unknown, however, there is an association with hemodialysis. Telangiectasias may also be the result of systemic or cutaneous diseases, including scleroderma, systemic lupus erythematosus, syphilis, or cirrhosis. Essential or idiopathic telangiectasias result from progressive dilatation of blood vessels independent of preceding or coexistent skin lesions in systemic disease.

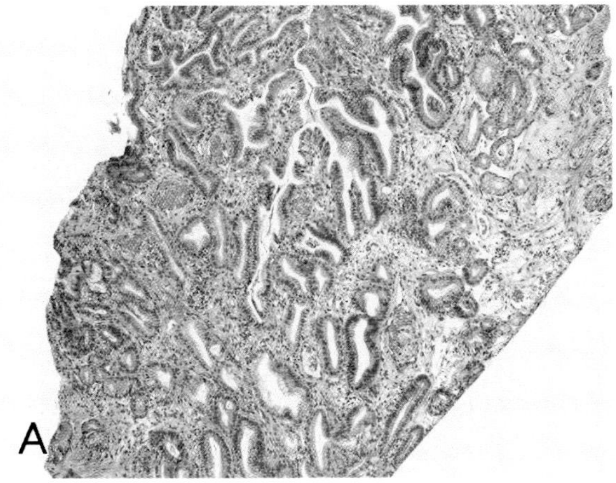

Figure 6-35

GASTRIC ANTRAL VASCULAR ECTASIA

A: Antral mucosa with numerous dilated mucosal vessels.
B: Fibrin thrombi are in many of these vessels.
C: A partially thrombosed mucosal venule.

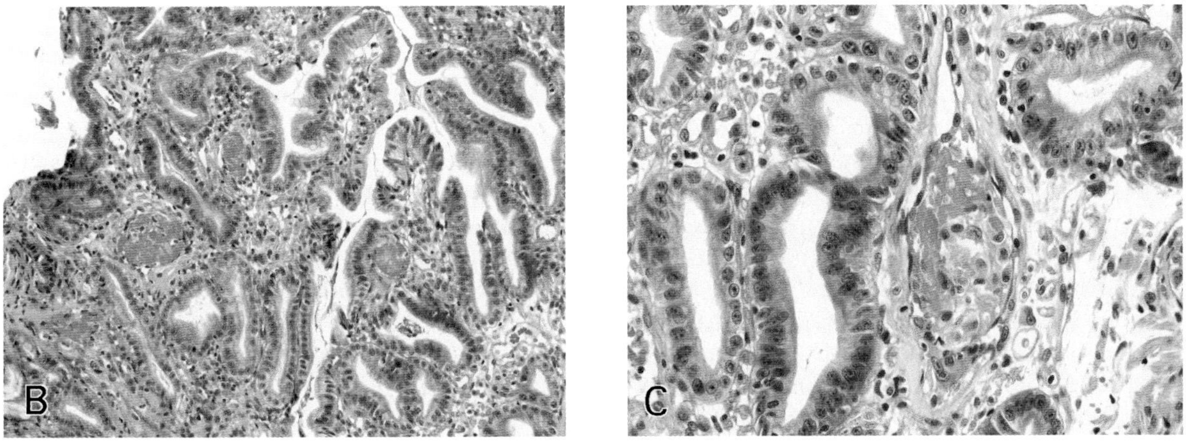

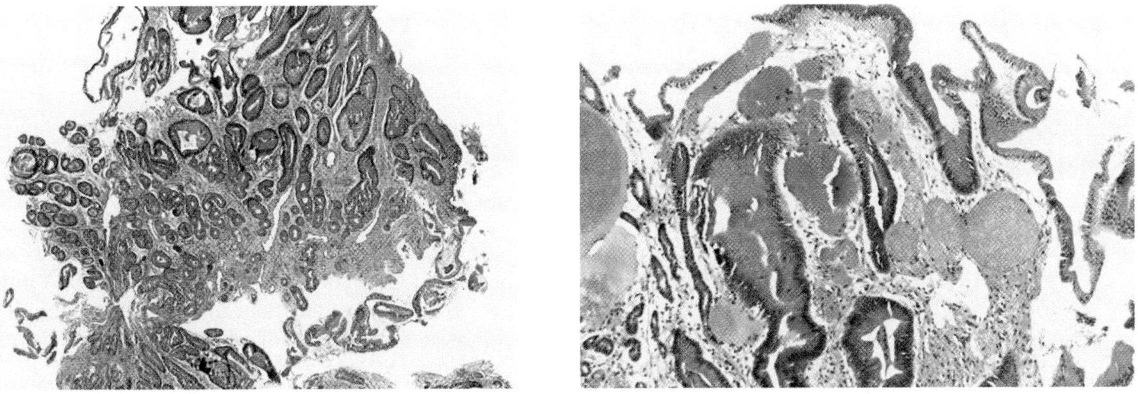

Figure 6-36

GASTRIC ANTRAL VASCULAR ECTASIA

Left: Dilated vessels without thrombi and little surrounding gastritis.
Right: The vessels are more dilated. (Specimens in these two figures came from two different patients with characteristic endoscopic features.)

Table 6-12

COMPARISON OF PORTAL GASTROPATHY AND GASTRIC ANTRAL VASCULAR ECTASIA (GAVE)

Feature	Portal Gastropathy	GAVE
Location	Fundus and corpus	Antrum
Degree of ectasia	Mild ectasia	Marked ectasia
Presence of cirrhosis	Always	30% of patients
Presence of fibrohyalinosis	No	Yes
Presence of thrombosis	No	Yes
Vascular spindle cell proliferation	No	Yes
Anemia and hemorrhage	Low incidence	High incidence
Endoscopic lesions	Diffuse erythema	Appear as microvessels with antral stripes
Liver disease severity	More severe	Less severe
Sex	More common in men	Predominantly in women

Clinical Features. Generalized telangiectasias are characterized by widespread cutaneous distribution; progression or permanence of the lesions; accentuation by dependent positioning; absence of coexisting epidermal or dermal changes such as atrophy, purpura, and depigmentation; and follicular involvement. Spontaneous bleeding does not occur but disease progression is common. Gastrointestinal mucosal aspects of hereditary hemorrhagic telangiectasia include millet seed- to pinhead-sized bright red spots in the mucosa that are circular and slightly raised (281). Patients with hereditary syndromes have telangiectasias involving many organs, including the skin and gastrointestinal tract.

Gross Findings. The telangiectatic areas appear as small, flattened and reddish lesions with fern-like margins. The lesions can be detected endoscopically or angiographically.

Microscopic Findings. Histologically, telangiectasias consist of dilated, thin-walled, distended vascular channels in the mucosa and submucosa.

Treatment and Prognosis. Endoscopic ablation of symptomatic lesions remains the treatment of choice.

REFERENCES

Diverticula

1. Almy TP, Howell DA. Diverticular disease of the colon. N Engl J Med 1980;302:324–31.
2. Campbell K, Steele RJ. Non-steroidal anti-inflammatory drugs and complicated diverticular disease: a case-control study. Br J Surg 1991; 78:190–1.
3. Castillo S, Aburashed A, Kimmelman J, Alexander LC. Diffuse intramural esophageal pseudodiverticulosis. New cases and review. Gastroenterology 1977;72:541–5.
4. Chappuis CW, Cohn I Jr. Acute colonic diverticulitis. Surg Clin North Am 1988;68:302–13.
5. Chia JG, Wilde CC, Ngoi SS, Goh PM, Ong CL. Trends of diverticular disease of the large bowel in a newly developed country. Dis Colon Rectum 1991;34:498–501.
6. Collins DC. A study of 50,000 specimens of the human vermiform appendix. Surg Gynecol Obstet 1955;101:437–45.
7. Collins DC. 71,000 human appendix specimens, a final report summarizing forty years' study. Am J Proctol 1963;14:265–81.
8. Connell AM. Pathogenesis of diverticular disease of the colon. Adv Intern Med 1977;22:377–95.

9. Cook IJ, Gabb M, Panagopoulos V, et al. Pharyngeal (Zenker's) diverticulum is a disorder of upper esophageal sphincter opening. Gastroenterology 1992;103:1229–35.
10. Costantini M, Zaninotto G, Rizzetto C, Narne S, Ancona E. Oesophageal diverticula. Best Pract Res Clin Gastroenterol 2004;18:3–17.
11. Debas HT, Payne S, Cameron AJ, Carlson HC. Physiopathology of lower esophageal diverticulum and its implications for treatment. Surg Gynecol Obstet 1980;151:593–600.
12. Eggert A, Teichmann G, Wiltman DH. The pathological implications of duodenal diverticula. Surg Gynecol Obstet 1982;154:62–4.
13. Eras P, Beranbaum S. Gastric diverticula: congenital and acquired. Am J Gastroenterol 1972; 57:120.
14. Esparza AR, Pan CM. Diverticulosis of the appendix. Surgery 1970;67:922–8.
15. Feldberg MA, Hendriks MJ, van Waes PF. Role of CT in diagnosis and management of complications of diverticular disease. Gastrointest Radiol 1985;10:370–7.
16. Gage-Whote L. Incidence of Zenker's diverticulum with hiatus hernia. Laryngoscope 1988;98: 526–30.
17. Galbraith P, Bagg MN, Schabel SI, Rajagopalan PR. Diverticular complications of renal disease. Gastrointest Radiol 1990;15:259–62.
18. Garcia JB, Bengochea JB, Wooler GH. Epiphrenic diverticula of the esophagus. J Thorac Cardiovasc Surg 1972;63:114–7.
19. George DH. Diverticulosis of the vermiform appendix in patients with cystic fibrosis. Hum Pathol 1987;18:75–9.
20. Gore S, Shepherd NA, Wilkinson SP. Endoscopic crescenteric fold disease of the sigmoid colon: the clinical and histopathological spectrum of a distinctive endoscopic appearance. Int J Colorectal Dis 1992;7:76–81.
21. Hagege H, Berson A, Pelletier G, et al. Association of juxtapapillary diverticula with choledocholithiasis but not with cholecystolithiasis. Endoscopy 1992;24:248–51.
22. Juler JL, List JW, Stemmer EA, Connolly JE. Duodenal diverticulitis. Arch Surg 1969;99:572–78.
23. Kataoka H, Higa T, Koono M. An autopsy case report of diffuse esophageal intramural pseudodiverticulosis. Acta Pathologica 1992;42:837–40.
24. Kaye MD. Oesophageal motor dysfunction in patients with diverticula in the mid-thoracic oesophagus. Thorax 1974;29:666–72.
25. Kelly, JK. Polypoid prolapsing mucosal folds in diverticular disease. Am J Surg Pathol 1991;15: 871–8.
26. Krishnamurthy S, Kelly MM, Rohrmann CA, Schuffler MD. Jejunal diverticulosis: a heterogeneous disorder caused by a variety of abnormalities of smooth muscle or myenteric plexus. Gastroenterology 1983;85:538–47.
27. Lee FD. Submucosal lipophages in diverticula of the small intestine. J Pathol Bacteriol 1966; 92:29–34.
28. Levine MS, Moolten DN, Herlinger H, Laufer I. Esophageal intramural pseudodiverticulosis. A reevaluation. Am J Radiol 1986;147:1165–70.
29. Levy N, Stermer E, Simon J. The changing epidemiology of diverticular disease in Israel. Dis Colon Rectum 1985;28:416–8.
30. Lipton S, Estrin J, Glasser I. Diverticular disease of the appendix. Surg Gynecol Obstet 1989;168: 13–6.
31. Localio A, Stahl WM. Diverticular disease of the alimentary tract. Part II: The esophagus, stomach, duodenum and small intestine. Curr Prob Surg 1968;5:1–47.
32. Makapugay LM, Dean PJ. Diverticular disease-associated chronic colitis. Am J Surg Pathol 1996;20:94–102.
33. McGuire HH Jr. Bleeding colonic diverticula: a reappraisal of natural history and management. Ann Surg 1994;220:653–6.
34. Meagher AP, Porter AJ, Rowland R, et al. Jejunal diverticulosis. Aust N Z J Surg 1993;63:360–6.
35. Medeiros LJ, Doos WG, Balogh K. Esophageal intramural pseudodiverticulosis: a report of two cases with analysis of similar, less extensive changes in 'normal' autopsy esophagi. Hum Pathol 1988;19:928–31.
36. Meyers MA, Alonso DR, Gray GF, Baer JW. Pathogenesis of bleeding colonic diverticulosis. Gastroenterology 1976;71:577–83.
37. Miura S, Kodaira S, Aoki H, Hosoda Y. Bilateral type diverticular disease of the colon. Int J Colorectal Dis 1996;11:71–5.
38. Morgenstern L, Weiner R, Michel SL. 'Malignant' diverticulitis. A clinical entity. Arch Surg 1979;114:1112–6.
39. Morson BC. The muscle abnormality in diverticular disease of the colon. Proc R Soc Med 1963;56:798–800.
40. Morson BC, Dawson EM, Day DW, Jass JR, Price AB, Williams GT. Morson and Dawson's gastrointestinal pathology. Oxford: Blackwell; 1990.
41. Munakata A, Nakaji S, Takami H, Nakahima H, Iwane S, Tuchida S. Epidemiologic evaluation of colonic diverticulosis and dietary fiber in Japan. Tohoku J Exp Med 1993;171:145–51.
42. Murney RG Jr, Linne JH, Curtis J. High-amplitude peristaltic contractions in a patient with esophageal intramural pseudodiverticulosis. Dig Dis Sci 1983;28:843–7.

43. Nagakawa T, Kanno M, Ueno K, et al. Intrabiliary pressure measurement by duodenal pressure loading for the evaluation of duodenal parapapillary diverticulum. Hepatogastroenterology 1996;43:1129–34.
44. Nakada T, Ubukata H, Goto Y, et al. Diverticular disease of the colon at a regional general hospital in Japan. Dis Colon Rectum 1995;38:755–9.
45. Painter NS. Diverticular disease of the colon. Br Med J 1968;3:475–9.
46. Painter NS, Burkitt DP. Diverticular disease of the colon: a deficiency disease of Western civilization. Br Med J 1971;2:450–4.
47. Parks TG. Natural history of diverticular disease of the colon. A review of 521 cases. Br Med J 1969;4:639–42.
48. Plasvic BM, Raider L, Drnobsek VH, Kogutt MS. Association of rectal diverticula and scleroderma. Acta Radiol 1995;36:96–9.
49. Rasmussen PC, Jensen BS, Winther A. Oesophageal achalasia combined with epiphrenic diverticulum. A case report. Scand J Thorac Cardiovas Surg 1988;22:81–2.
50. Segal I, Solomon A, Hunt JA. Emergence of diverticular disease in the urban South African black. Gastroenterology 1977;72:215–9.
51. Steiner A, Geist A, Scheinfeld A. Non-Meckelian diverticula of the small intestine. Int Surg 1967;47:597–601.
52. Stemmermann GN, Yatani R. Diverticulosis and polyps of the large intestine: a necropsy study of Hawaii Japanese. Cancer 1973;31:1260–70.
53. Sugihara K, Muto T, Morioka Y, Asano A, Yamamoto Y. Diverticular disease of the colon in Japan. A review of 615 cases. Dis Colon Rectum 1984;27:531–7.
54. Toyohara T, Kaneko T, Araki H, Takahashi K, Nakamura T. Giant epiphrenic diverticulum in a boy with Ehlers-Danlos syndrome. Pediatr Radiol 1989;19:437.
55. Uomo G, Manes G, Ragozzino A, Cavallera A, Rabitti PG. Periampullary extraluminal duodenal diverticula and acute pancreatitis: an underestimated etiological association. Am J Gastroenterol 1996;91:1186–8.
56. Wheeler D. Diverticula of foregut. Radiology 1947;49:476–82.
57. Zakhour HD, Clark RG. Intramural gas cysts in a case of diverticular disease of the jejunum. Histopathology 1982;6:363–9.

Intussusception

58. Bissett GS 3rd, Kirks DR. Intussusception in infants and children: diagnosis and therapy. Radiology 1988;163:141–5.
59. Bruce J, Huh YS, Cooney DR, Karp MP, Allen JE, Jewett TC Jr. Intussusception: evolution of current management. J Pediatr Gastroenterol 1987;6:663–74.
60. Brynitz S, Rubinstein E. Hematemesis caused by jejunogastric intussusception. Endoscopy 1986; 18:162–4.
61. del Posso B, Albillos JC, Tejedor D. Intussusception: ultrasound findings with pathologic correlation—the crescent-in-doughnut sign. Radiology 1996;199:688–92.
62. Dennison WM, Shaker M. Intussusception in infancy and childhood. Br J Surg 1970;57:679–84.
63. Ein SH, Stephens CA. Intussusception: 354 cases in 10 years. J Pediatr Surg 1971;6:16–27.
64. Eklof OA, Johanson L, Lohr G. Childhood intussusception: hydrostatic reducibility and incidence of leading points in different age groups. Pediatr Radiol 1980;40:136–43.
65. Fanconi S, Berger D, Rickham PP. Acute intussusception: a classic clinical picture. Helv Paediatr Acta 1982;37:345–52.
66. Felix EL, Cohen MH, Bernstein AD, Schwartz JH. Adult intussusception: case report of recurrent intussusception and a review of the literature. Am J Surg 1976;131:758–61.
67. Harrington L, Connolly B, Hu X, Wesson DE, Babyn P, Schuh S. Ultrasonographic and clinical predictors of intussusception. J Pediatr 1998;132:836–9.
68. Hsu HY, Kao CL, Huang LM, et al. Viral etiology of intussusception in Taiwanese childhood. Pediatr Infect Dis J 1998;17:893–8.
69. Kuruvilla TT, Naraynsingh V, Raju GC, Manmohansingh LU. Intussusception in infancy and childhood. Trop Geogr Med 1988;40:342–6.
70. Kurzbart E, Cohen Z, Yerushalmi B, Yulevich A, Newman-Heiman N, Mares AJ. Familial idiopathic intussusception: a report of two families. J Pediatr Surg 1999;34:493–4.
71. Mann WJ, Fromowitz F, Saychek T, Madariaga JR, Chalas E. Endometriosis associated with appendiceal intussusception. J Reprod Med 1984;29:625–9.
72. Martin LF, Tidman MK, Jamieson MA. Appendiceal intussusception and endometriosis. J Can Assoc Radiol 1980;31:276–7.
73. Mellgren A, Schultz I, Johansson C, Dolk A. Internal rectal intussusception seldom develops into total rectal prolapse. Dis Colon Rectum 1997;40:817–20.
74. Miller SF, Landes AB, Dautenhahn LW, et al. Intussusception: ability of fluoroscopic images obtained during air enemas to depict lead points and other abnormalities. Radiology 1995;197: 493–6.

75. Ravitch MM. Intussusception. In: Welch KJ, Randolph JG, Ravitch MM, O'Neill JA, Rowe M, eds. Pediatric surgery, 4th ed. Chicago: Yearbook Medical Publishers; 1986:868–82.
76. Ramsden KL, Newman J, Moran A. Florid vascular proliferation in repeated intussusception mimicking primary angiomatous lesion. J Clin Pathol 1993;46:91–2.
77. Reijnen JA, Festen C, Joosten HJ, Van Wieringen PM. Atypical characteristics of a group of children with intussusception. Acta Paediatr Scand 1990;79:675–9.
78. Schuh S, Wesson DE. Intussusception in children 2 years of age or older. Can Med Assoc J 1987;136:269–72.
79. Shanbhogue RL, Hussain SM, Meradji M, Robben SG, Vernooij JE, Molenaar JC. Ultrasonography is accurate enough for the diagnosis of intussusception. J Pediatr Surg 1994;29: 324–7.
80. Stringer MD, Pablot SM, Brereton RJ. Paediatric intussusception. Br J Surg 1992;79:867–76.
81. Tangi VT, Bear JW, Reid IS, Wright JE. Intussusception in Newcastle in a 25 year period. Aust NZJ Surg 1991;61:608–13.
82. Wang NL, Yeh ML, Chang PY, et al. Prenatal and neonatal intussusception. Pediatr Surg Int 1998;13:232–6.
83. Wright VM. Intussusception. In: Spitz L, Coran AG, eds. Rob & Smith's operative surgery, pediatric surgery, 5th ed. London: Chapman & Hall Medical; 1995:396–401.
84. Yates LN. Intussusception of the appendix. Int Surg 1983;68:231–3.

Volvulus

85. Anderson JR, Lee D. The management of acute sigmoid volvulus. Br J Surg 1981;68:117–20.
86. Ballantyne GH. Review of sigmoid volvulus. History and results of treatment. Dis Colon Rectum 1982;25:494–501.
87. Ballantyne GH, Brandner MD, Beart RW Jr, Ilstrup DM. Volvulus of the colon. Incidence and mortality. Ann Surg 1985;202:83–92.
88. Collure DW, Hameer HR. Loss of ganglion cells and marked attenuation of bowel wall in cecal dilatation. J Surg Res 1996;60:385–8.
89. Echenique Elizondo M, Amondarain Arratibel JA. Colonic volvulus. Rev Esp Enferm Dig 2002; 94:201–10.
90. Frazee RC, Mucha P Jr, Farnell MB, Van Heerden JA. Volvulus of the small intestine. Ann Sur 1988;208:565–8.
91. Gibney EJ. Volvulus of the sigmoid colon. Surg Gynecol Obstet 1991;173:243–55.
92. Gurleyik E, Gurleyik G. Small bowel volvulus: a common cause of mechanical intestinal obstruction in our region. Eur J Surg 1998;164:51–5.
93. Javors BR, Baker SR, Miller JA. The northern exposure sign: a newly described finding in sigmoid volvulus. AJR 1999;173:571–4.
94. McIntyre RC, Bensard DD, Karrer FM, Hall RJ, Lilly JR. The pediatric diaphragm in acute gastric volvulus. J Am Col Surg 1994;178:234–8.
95. Mellor MF, Drake DG. Colonic volvulus in children: value of barium enema for diagnosis and treatment in 14 children. AJR 1994;162:1157–9.
96. Miller D, Pasquale M, Seneca R, Hodin E. Gastric volvulus in the pediatric population. Arch Surg 1991;126:1146–9.
97. Perry EG. Intestinal volvulus: a new concept. Aust NZ J Surg 1983;53:483–6.
98. Samuel M, Burge DM, Griffiths DM. Gastric volvulus and associated gastro-oesophageal reflux. Arch Dis Childhood 1995;73:462–4.
99. Schaefer DC, Nikoomenesh P, Moore C. Gastric volvulus: an old disease process with some new twists. Gastroenterologist 1997;5:41–5.
100. Schagen van Leeumeen JH. Sigmoid volvulus in a West African population. Dis Colon Rectum 1985;28:712–6.
101. Shimanuki Y, Aihara T, Takano H, et al. Clockwise whirlpool sign at color Doppler US: an objective and definite sign of midgut volvulus. Radiology 1996;199:261–4.
102. Starling JR. Initial treatment of sigmoid volvulus by colonoscopy. Ann Surg 1979;190:36–9.
103. Teague WJ, Ackroyd R, Watson DI, Devitt PG. Changing patterns in the management of gastric volvulus over 14 years. Br J Surg 2000;87: 358–61.
104. Vaez-Zadeh K, Dutz W, Nowrooz-Zadeh M. Volvulus of the small intestine in adults: a study of predisposing factors. Ann Surg 1969;169:265–71.
105. Zinkin LD, Katz LD, Rosin JD. Volvulus of the transverse colon: report of case and review of the literature. Dis Colon Rectum 1979;22:492–6.

Rectal Mucosal Prolapse

106. Beighten PH, Murdoch JL, Votteler T. Gastrointestinal complication of the Ehlers-Danlos syndrome. Gut 1969;10:1004–8.
107. Bhimma R, Rollins NC, Coovadia HM, Adhikari M. Post-dysenteric hemolytic uremia syndrome in children during an epidemic of *Shigella* dysentery in Kwazulu/Natal. Pediatr Nephrol 1997;11:560–4.
108. Chan WK, Kay SM, Laberge JM, Gallucci JG, Bensoussan AL, Yazbeck S. Injection sclerotherapy in the treatment of rectal prolapse in infants and children. J Pediatr Surg 1998;33:255–8.
109. Chetty R, Bhathal PS, Slavin JL. Prolapse-induced inflammatory polyps of the colorectum and anal transitional zone. Histopathology 1993;23:63–7.

110. Corman ML. Rectal prolapse in children. Dis Colon Rectum 1985;28:535–9.
111. Freeman NV. Rectal prolapse in children. J R Soc Med 1984;77:9–12.
112. Goei R, Baeten C, Arends JW. Solitary rectal ulcer syndrome: findings at barium enema study and defecography. Radiology 1988;168:303–6.
113. Groff DB, Nagaraj HS. Rectal prolapse in infants and children. Am J Surg 1990;160:531–2.
114. Hizawa K, Iida M, Suekane H, et al. Mucosal prolapse syndrome: diagnosis with endoscopic US. Radiology 1994;191:527–30.
115. Hovey MA, Metcalf AM. Incarcerated rectal prolapse—rupture and ileal evisceration after failed reduction: report of a case. Dis Colon Rectum 1997;40:1254–7.
116. Ihre T. Internal procidentia of the rectum—treatment and results. Scand J Gastroenterol 1972;7:643–6.
117. Ihre T. Intussusception of the rectum and the solitary ulcer syndrome. Ann Med 1990;22: 419–23.
118. Lock G, Holstege A, Lang B, Scholmerich J. Gastrointestinal manifestations of progressive systemic sclerosis. Am J Gastroenterol 1997;92: 763–71.
119. Madigan MR, Morson BC. Solitary ulcer of the rectum. Gut 1969;10:871–81.
120. Malik M, Stratton J, Sweeney WB. Rectal prolapse associated with bulimia nervosa: report of seven cases. Dis Colon Rectum 1997;40: 1382–5.
121. Rao SS, Sun WM. Current techniques of assessing defecation dynamics. Dig Dis 1997;1:64–77.
122. Rutter KR, Riddell RH. The solitary ulcer syndrome of the rectum. Clin Gastroenterol 1975; 4:505–30.
123. Stern RC, Izant RJ Jr, Boat TF, Wood RE, Matthews LW, Doershuk CF. Treatment and prognosis of rectal prolapse in cystic fibrosis. Gastroenterology 1982;82:707–10.
124. Traisman E, Conlon D, Sherman JO, Hageman JR. Rectal prolapse in two neonates with Hirschsprung's disease. Am J Dis Child 1983;137:1126–7.
125. Traynor LA, Michner WM. Rectal procidentia: a rare complication of ulcerative colitis: report of two cases in children. Cleve Clin J Med 1966;33:115–7.
126. Williams GT, Bussey HJ, Morson BC. Inflammatory cap polyps of the large intestine. Br J Surg 1985:72;133–40.
127. Zempsky WT, Rosenstein BJ. The cause of rectal prolapse in children. Am J Dis Child 1988; 142:338–9.

Gastritis, Enteritis, and Colitis Cystica Profunda

128. Aftalion B, Lipper S. Enteritis cystica profunda associated with Crohn's disease. Arch Pathol Lab Med 1984;108:532–3.
129. Alexis J, Lubin J, Wallack M. Enteritis cystica profunda in a patient with Crohn's disease. Arch Pathol Lab Med 1989;113:947–9.
130. Baillie EE, Abell MR. Enteritis cystica polyposa. Am J Clin Pathol 1970;54:643–9.
131. Bentley E, Chandrasoma P, Cohen H, Radin R, Ray M. Colitis cystica profunda: presenting with complete intestine obstruction and recurrence. Gastroenterology 1985;89:1157–61.
132. Clark RM. Microdiverticula and submucosal epithelial elements in ulcerative and granulomatous disease of the ileum and colon. Can Med Assoc J 1970;103:24–8.
133. Dippolito AD, Aburano A, Bezouska CA, Happ RA. Enteritis cystica profunda in Peutz-Jeghers syndrome: report of a case and review of the literature. Dis Colon Rectum 1987;30:192–8.
134. Franzin G, Novelli P. Gastritis cystica profunda. Histopathology 1981;5:535–47.
135. Karnak I, Gogus S, Senocak ME, Akcoren Z, Hicsonmez A. Enteritis cystica profunda causing ileoileal intussusception in a child. J Pediatr Surg 1997;32:1356–9.
136. Kyriakos M, Condon SC. Enteritis cystica profunda. Am J Clin Pathol 1978;69:77–85.
137. O'Donnell N. Enteritis cystica profunda revisited. Hum Pathol 1987;18:1300–1.
138. Valiulis AP, Gardiner GW, Mahoney LJ. Adenocarcinoma and colitis cystica profunda in a radiation-induced colonic stricture. Dis Colon Rectum 1985;28:128–31.
139. Yamagiwa H. Protruded variants in solitary ulcer syndrome of the rectum. Acta Pathol Jpn 1988;38:471–8.
140. Zidi SH, Marteau P, Piard F, Coffin B, Favre JP, Rambaud JC. Enterocolitis cystica profunda lesions in a patient with unclassified ulcerative enterocolitis. Dig Dis Sci 1994;39:426–32.

Anal Fissures

141. Bernard D, Morgan S, Tasse D. Selective surgical management of Crohn's disease of the anus. Can J Surg 1986;29:318–21.
142. Blasi J, Chapman ER, Link E, et al. Botulinum neurotoxin A selectively cleaves the synaptic protein SNAP-25. Nature 1993;365:160–3.
143. Farouk R, Gunn J, Duthie GS. Changing patterns of treatment for chronic anal fissure. Ann R Coll Surg Engl 1998;80:194–6.
144. Fellous K. Anal fissures and fissurations. Rev Prat 2001;51:32–5.

145. Festen C, van Harten H. Perianal abscess and fistula-in-ano in infants. J Ped Surg 1998; 33:711–3.
146. Hobbiss JH, Schoffield PF. Management of perianal Crohn's disease. J R Soc Med 1982;75: 414–7.
147. Jost WH. One hundred cases of anal fissure treated with botulinum toxin: early and long-term results. Dis Colon Rectum 1997;40:1029–32.
148. Jost WH, Schrank B. Chronic anal fissures treated with botulinum toxin injections: a dose-finding study with Dysport. Colorectal Dis 1999;1:26–8.
149. Klosterhalfen B, Vogel P, Rixen H, Mittermayer C. Topography of the inferior rectal artery: a possible cause of chronic, primary anal fissure. Dis Colon Rectum 1989;32:43–52.
150. Lindsey I, Jones OM, Cunningham C, Mortensen NJ. Chronic anal fissure. Br J Surg 2004;91: 270–9.
151. Nelson R. A systematic review of medical therapy for anal fissure. Dis Colon Rectum 2004;47:422–31.
152. Nelson RL. A review of operative procedures for anal fissure. J Gastrointest Surg 2002;6:284–9.
153. Schouten WR, Briel JW, Auwerda JJ, De Graaf EJ. Ischaemic nature of anal fissure. Br J Surg 1996;83:63–5.
154. Sweeney JL, Ritchie JK, Nicholls RJ. Anal fissure in Crohn's disease. Br J Surg 1988;75:56–7.

Fistulas and Sinuses

155. al-Salem AH, Qaisaruddin S, Qureshi SS. Perianal abscess and fistula in ano in infancy and childhood: a clinicopathological study. Pediatr Pathol Lab Med 1996;16:755–64.
156. Barwood N, Clarke G, Levitt S, Levitt M. Fistula-in-ano: a prospective study of 107 patients. Aust N Z J Surg 1997;67:98–102.
157. Frattaroli FM, Reggio D, Gaudalaxara A, Illomei G, Lomanto D, Pappalardo G. Bouveret's syndrome: case report and review of the literature. Hepatogastroenterology 1997;44:1019–22.
158. Garcia–Aguilar J, Belmonte C, Wong WD, Goldberg SM, Madoff RD. Anal fistula surgery. Factors associated with recurrence and incontinence. Dis Colon Rectum 1996;39:723–9.
159. Grande J, Ackermann DM, Edwards WD. Aortoenteric fistulas. A study of 28 autopsied cases spanning 25 years. Arch Pathol Lab Med 1989;113:1271–5.
160. Heinrich D, Meier J, Wehrli H, Buhler H. Upper gastrointestinal hemorrhage preceding development of Bouveret's syndrome. Am J Gastroenterol 1993;85:777–80.
161. Patel NM, Lo A, Bobowski SL. Gastric outlet obstruction secondary to a gallstone (Bouveret's syndrome). J Clin Gastroenterol 1985;7:277–8.
162. Rodriguez-Moreno D, Moreno-Gonzalez E, Jimenez-Romero C, et al. Duodenal obstruction by gallstones (Bouveret's syndrome). Presentation of a new case and literature review. Hepatogastroenterology 1997;44:1351–5.
163. Scholefield JH, Berry DP, Armitage NC, Wastie ML. Magnetic resonance imaging in the management of fistula in ano. Int J Colorectal Dis 1997;12:276–9.
164. Scott CA, Davis WB. Cholecystoduodenal fistula with duodenal bulb obstruction. Case reports (Bouveret's syndrome). Mo Med 1984; 81:69–72.

Lacerations and Perforations

165. Abbott OA, Mansour KA, Logan WD Jr, Hatcher CR Jr, Symbas PN. Atraumatic so-called "spontaneous" rupture of the esophagus. A review of 47 personal cases with comments on a new method of surgical therapy. J Thorac Cardiovasc Surg 1970;59:67–83.
166. Badejo OA, Arigbabu AO. Operative treatment of typhoid perforation with peritoneal irrigation: a comparative study. Gut 1980;21:141–5.
167. Baker RW, Spiro AH, Trnka YM. Mallory-Weiss tear complicating upper endoscopy: case reports and review of the literature. Gastroenterology 1982;82:140–2.
168. Barone JE, Robilotti JG, Comer JV. Conservative treatment of spontaneous intramural perforation of the esophagus. Gastroenterology 1980;74:165–7.
169. Brauer RB, Liebermann-Meffert D, Stein HJ, Bartels H, Siewert JR. Boerhaave's syndrome: analysis of the literature and report of 18 new cases. Dis Esophagus 1997;10:64–8.
170. Byrne JP, Armstrong GR, Attwood SE. Restoration of the normal squamous lining in Barrett's esophagus by argon plasma coagulation. Am J Gastroenterol 1998;93:1810–5.
171. Callaghan J. The Boerhaave syndrome (spontaneous rupture of the oesophagus). Br J Surg 1972;59:41–4.
172. Cameron JL, Kieffer RF, Hendrix TR, Mehigan DG, Baker RR. Selective non-operative management of contained intra-thoracic esophageal perforation: it is safe? J Thorac Cardiovasc Surg 1996;111:114–21.
173. Derrick JR, Wilkinson AH, Howard JM. Perforation of stress ulcers of the esophagus following thermal burns. Arch Surg 1957;75:17–20.
174. Fisher RG, Schwartz JT, Graham DY. Angiotherapy with Mallory-Weiss tear. AJR 1980;134: 679–84.
175. Gekas P, Schuster MM. Stercoral perforation of the colon. A case report and review of the literature. Gastroenterology 1981;80:1054–8.
176. Graham DY, Schwartz JT. The spectrum of the Mallory-Weiss tear. Medicine 1977;57:307–18.

177. Grinvalsky HT, Bowerman CI. Stercoraceous ulcers of the colon: relatively neglected medical and surgical problem. JAMA 1959;171:1941–6.
178. Guyton DP, Evans D, Schrieber H. Stercoral perforation of the colon: concept of operative management. Am Surg 1985;51:520–2.
179. Haddad N, Al-Kawas F, Benjamin S, Fleischer D, Nguyen C. Incidence and natural history of iatrogenic Mallory-Weiss tears during upper endoscopy. Am J Gastroenterol 1993;88:1592–7.
180. Iannettoni MD, Vlessis AA, Whyte RI, Orringer MB. Functional outcome after surgical treatment of esophageal perforation. Ann Thorac Surg 1997;64:1606–10.
181. Ihekwaba FN. Ascaris lumbricoides and perforation of the ileum: a critical review. Br J Surg 1979;66:132–4.
182. Inculet R, Clark C, Girvan D. Boerhaave's syndrome and children: a rare and unexpected combination. J Pediatr Surg 1996;31:1300–1.
183. Jaworski A, Fischer R, Lippmann M. Boerhaave's syndrome. Computed tomographic findings and diagnostic considerations. Arch Intern Med 1988;148:223–4.
184. Kinuya S, Hwang EH, Ikeda E, Yokoyama K, Michigishi T, Tonami N. Mallory-Weiss syndrome caused by iodine-131 therapy for metastatic thyroid carcinoma. J Nucl Med 1997;38:1831.
185. Knauer LM. Mallory-Weiss syndrome. Characterization of 75 Mallory-Weiss lacerations in 528 patients with upper gastrointestinal haemorrhage. Gastroenterology 1976;71:5–8.
186. Lee J, Lieberman D. Complications related to endoscopic hemostasis techniques. Gastrointest Endosc Clin North Am 1996;6:305–22.
187. Lightdale CJ, Heier SK, Marcon NE, et al. Photodynamic therapy with porfimer sodium versus thermal ablation therapy with Nd:YAG laser for palliation of esophageal cancer: a multicenter randomized trial. Gastrointest Endosc 1995;42:507–12.
188. Lion-Cachet J. Gastric fundal mucosal tears. Br J Surg 1963;50:985–6.
189. Mackler SA. Spontaneous rupture of the esophagus; an experimental and clinical study. Surg Gynecol Obstet 1952;95:345–56.
190. Mallory GK, Weiss SW. Hemorrhages from lacerations of the cardiac orifice of the stomach due to vomiting. Am J Med Sci 1929;178:506–12.
191. McCartney J, Dobrow J, Hendrix TR. Boerhaave syndrome. Johns Hopkins Med J 1979;144:28–33.
192. McIntyre AS, Ayres R, Atherton J, Spiller RC, Cockel R. Dissecting intramural haematoma of the oesophagus. Q J Med 1998;91:701–5.
193. Merrill JR. Snore-induced Mallory-Weiss syndrome. J Clin Gastroenterol 1987;9:88–9.
194. Michel L, Serrano A, Malt RA. Mallory-Weiss syndrome. Evaluation of diagnostic and therapeutic patterns over two decades. Ann Surg 1980;192:716–12.
195. Montalvo RD, Lee R. Retrospective analysis of iatrogenic Mallory-Weiss tears occurring during upper gastrointestinal endoscopy. Hepatogastroenterology 1996;43:174–7.
196. Nadkarni KM, Shetty SD, Kagzi RS, Pinto AC, Bhalerao RA. Small-bowel perforations. Arch Surg 1981;116:53–7.
197. Nellgard P, Cassuto J. Inflammation as a major cause of fluid losses in small-bowel obstruction. J Gastroenterol 1993;28:1035–41.
198. Noussias MP. Spontaneous rupture of the bowel. Br J Surg 1962;50:195–8.
199. Penston JG, Boyd EJ, Wormsley KG. Mallory-Weiss tears occurring during endoscopy: a report of seven cases. Endoscopy 1992;24:262–5.
200. Putzki H, Ledwoch J, Dueben W, Mlasowsky B, Heymann H. Nontraumatic perforations of the small intestine. Am J Surg 1985;149:375–7.
201. Rogers LF, Puig AW, Dooley BN, Cuello L. Diagnostic considerations in mediastinal emphysema: a pathophysiologic-roentgenologic approach to Boerhaave's syndrome and spontaneous pneumomediastinum. Am J Roentgenol Radium Ther Nucl Med 1972;115:495–511.
202. Romeu J. Pseudotumor in the Mallory-Weiss syndrome. Am J Gastroenterol 1978;70:83–4.
203. Salo JA, Sepalla KM, Pitkaranta PP, Kivilaakso EO. Spontaneous rupture and functional state of the esophagus. Surgery 1992;112:897–900.
204. Sams JS. Dangers of the Heimlich maneuver for esophageal obstruction. N Eng J Med 1989;321:980–1.
205. Schauer PR, Meyers WC, Eubanks S, Norem RF, Franklin M, Pappas TN. Mechanisms of gastric and esophageal perforations during laparoscopic Nissen fundoplication. Ann Surg 1996;223:43–52.
206. Serpell JW, Nicholls RJ. Stercoral perforation of the colon. Br J Surg 1990;77:1325–9.
207. Silvis SE, Nebel O, Rogers G, Sugawa C, Mandelstam P. Endoscopic complications—results of the American Society for Gastrointestinal Endoscopy survey. JAMA 1976;235:928–30.
208. Strutynsky N, Orbon D. Stercoral perforation of the descending colon appearing radiographically as pneumomediastinum. Mt Sinai J Med 1987;54:436–8.
209. Sugawa C, Masuyama H, Walt AJ. Mallory-Weiss syndrome. Contemp Surg 1985;27:51–8.
210. Tytgat GN, den Hartog Jager C, Bartelsmen JF. Endoscopic prosthesis for advanced esophageal cancer. Endoscopy 1987;18:32–9.
211. Watts HD. Lesions brought on by vomiting: the effect of hiatus hernia on the site of injury. Gastroenterology 1976;71:683–8.

212. Waxman I, Firas HA, Bass B, Glouderman M. PEG ileus: a new cause of small bowel obstruction. Dig Dis Sci 1991;36:251–4.
213. Woolford TJ, Birzgalis AR, Lundell C, Farrington WT. Vomiting in pregnancy resulting in oesophageal perforation in a 15-year-old. J Laryngol Otol 1993;107:1059–60.
214. Younes Z, Johnson DA. The spectrum of spontaneous and iatrogenic esophageal injury. J Clin Gastroenterol 1999;29:306–17.

Changes Associated with Previous Surgery

215. Caniano DA, Starr J, Ginn-Pease ME. Extensive short-bowel syndrome in neonates: outcome in the 1980s. Surgery 1989;105:119–24.
216. Cooper A, Floyd TX, Roos AJ, Bishop HC, Templeton JM, Ziegler MM. Morbidity and mortality of short bowel syndrome acquired in infancy: an update. J Pediatr Surg 1984:10;711–8.
217. Coran AG, Spivak D, Teitelbaum DH. An analysis of the morbidity and mortality of short-bowel syndrome in the pediatric age group. Eur J Pediatr Surg 1999;9:228–30.
218. Dorney SF, Ament ME, Berquist WE, Vargas H, Hassall E. Improved survival in very short small bowel of infancy with use of long-term parenteral nutrition. J Pediatr 1985:106;521–5.
219. Galea MH, Holliday H, Carachi R, Kapila L. Short-bowel syndrome: a collective review. J Pediatr Surg 1992;27:592–6.
220. Goulet OJ, Revillon Y, Jan D, et al. Neonatal short bowel syndrome. J Pediatr 1991;119:18–23.
221. Hanson WR, Osborne WO. Epithelial cell kinetics in the small intestine of the rat 60 days after resection of 70 percent of the ileum and jejunum. Gastroenterology 1971;60:1087–97.
222. Mayr JM, Schober PH, Weissensteiner Y, Hollwarth ME. Morbidity and mortality of the short-bowel syndrome. Eur J Pediatr Surg 1999;9:231–5.
223. Messing B, Crenn P, Beau P, Boutron-Ruault MC, Rambaud JC, Matuchansky C. Long-term survival and parenteral nutrition dependence in adult patients with the short bowel syndrome. Gastroenterology 1999;117:1043–50.
224. O'Loughlin E, Winter M, Shun A, Hardin JA, Gall DG. Structural and functional adaptation following jejunal resection in rabbits: effect of epidermal growth factor. Gastroenterology 1994;107:87–93.
225. Rickham PP. Massive intestinal resection in newborn infants. Ann R Coll Surg Engl 1967; 41:480–5.
226. Thakur A, Chiu C, Quiros-Tejeira RE, et al. Morbidity and mortality of short-bowel syndrome in infants with abdominal wall defects. Am Surgeon 2002;68:75–9.
227. Thompson JS. Growth of neomucosa after intestinal resection. Arch Surg 1987;122:316–9.
228. Tilson MD, Wright HK. The effect of resection of the small intestine upon the fine structure of the intestinal epithelium. Surgery 1972;134: 992–4.
229. Todo S, Tzakis A, Abu-Elmagd K, et al. Clinical intestinal transplantation. Transplant Proc 1993;25:2195–7.
230. Vanderhoof JA. Short bowel syndrome in children and small intestinal transplantation. Pediatr Clin North Am 1996:43;533–50.
231. Vanderhoof JA, Langnas AN. Short–bowel syndrome in children and adults. Gastroenterology 1997:113;1767–78.
232. Vazquez CM, Molina MT, Ilundain A. Distal small bowel resection increases mucosal permeability in the large intestine. Digestion 1988;40:168–72.
233. Wallander J, Ewald U, Läckgren, Gerdin B, Tufveson G. Extreme short bowel syndrome in neonates: an indication for small bowel transplantation? Transplantation 1992;24:1230–5.
234. Weisbrodt NW, Nemeth PR, Bowers RL, Weems WA. Functional and structural changes in intestinal smooth muscle after jejunoileal bypass in rats. Gastroenterology 1985;88:958–63.
235. Wilmore DW. Factors correlating with a successful outcome following extensive intestinal resection in newborn infants. J Pediatrics 1972; 80:88–95.

Changes Associated with Eating Disorders

236. Andersen AE. Eating disorders in males. In: Brownell KD, Fairburn CG, eds. Eating disorders and obesity: a comprehensive handbook. New York: Guilford Press; 1995:177–87.
237. Becker AE, Grinspoon SK, Klibanski A, Herzog DB. Eating disorders. N Engl J Med 1999:340: 1092–7.
238. Cuellar RE, Van Thiel DH. Gastrointestinal consequences of the eating disorders: anorexia nervosa and bulimia. Am J Gastroenterol 1986;81:1113–24.
239. McClain CJ, Humphries LL, Hill KK, Nickl NJ. Gastrointestinal and nutritional aspects of eating disorders. J Am Coll Nutr 1993;12:466–74.
240. Nakao A, Isozaki H, Iwagaki H, Kanagawa T, Takakura N, Tanaka N. Gastric perforation caused by a bulimic attack in an anorexia nervosa patient: report of a case. Surg Today 2000;30:435–7.
241. Overby KJ, Litt IF. Mediastinal emphysema in an adolescent with anorexia nervosa and self-induced emesis. Pediatrics 1988;81:134–6.
242. Pirke KM, Dogs M, Fichter MM, Tuschl RJ. Gonadotrophins, oestradiol and progesterone during the menstrual cycle in bulimia nervosa. Clin Endocrinol 1988;29:265–70.

243. Sullivan PF. Mortality in anorexia nervosa. Am J Psychiatry 1995;152:1073–4.

Acquired Vascular Lesions

244. Baum S, Athanasoulis CA, Waltman AC, et al. Angiodysplasia of the right colon. AJR Am J Roentgenol 1977;129:787–94.
245. Baydur A, Korula J. Cardiorespiratory effects of endoscopic esophageal variceal sclerotherapy. Am J Med 1990;89:477–82.
246. Boley SJ, Brandt LJ. Vascular ectasias of the colon—1986. Dig Dis Sci 1986;3(suppl):26S–42S.
247. Boley SJ, Sammartano JR, Brandt LJ, Sprayregen S. Vascular ectasias of the colon. Surg Gynecol Obstet 1979;119:353–9.
248. Bruet A, Fingerhut A, Lopez Y, et al. Ileal varices revealed by recurrent hematuria in a patient with portal hypertension and Mekong schistosomiasis. Am J Gastroenterol 1983;78:346–50.
249. Burbige EJ, Tarder G, Carson S, Eugene J, Frey CF. Colonic varices, a complication of pancreatitis with splenic vein thrombosis. Am J Dig Dis 1978;23:752–5.
250. Caletti GC, Brocchi E, Labriola E, Gasbarrini G, Barbara L. Pericarditis: a probably overlooked complication of endoscopic variceal sclerotherapy. Endoscopy 1990;22:144–5.
251. Camilleri M, Chadwick VS, Hodgson HJ. Vascular anomalies of the gastrointestinal tract. Hepatogastroenterology 1984;31:149–53.
252. Cappell MS, Lebwohl O. Cessation of recurrent bleeding from gastrointestinal angiodysplasias after aortic valve replacement. Ann Intern Med 1986;105:54–7.
253. Cappell MS, Price JB. Characterization of the syndrome of small and large intestinal variceal bleeding. Dig Dis Sci 1987;32:422–7.
254. Chen LS, Lin HC, Lee FY, Hou MC, Lee SD. Portal hypertensive colopathy in patients with cirrhosis. Scand J Gastroenterol 1996;31:490–4.
255. Chawla Y, Dilawari JB. Anorectal varices: their frequency in cirrhotic and non-cirrhotic portal hypertension. Gut 1991;32:309–11.
256. Clouse RE, Costigan DJ, Mills BA, Zuckerman GR. Angiodysplasia as a cause of upper gastrointestinal bleeding. Arch Intern Med 1985;145:458–61.
257. Dagher L, Patch D, Burroughs A. Management of oesophageal varices. Hosp Med 2000;61:711–7.
258. De Weert TM, Gostout CJ, Wiesner RH. Congestive gastropathy and other upper endoscopic findings in 81 consecutive patients undergoing orthotopic liver transplantation. Am J Gastroenterol 1990;85:573–6.
259. Duray PH, Marcal JM Jr, LiVolsi VA, Fisher R, Scholhamer C, Brand MH. Small intestinal angiodysplasia in the elderly. J Clin Gastroenterol 1984;6:311–9.
260. Duray PH, Marcal JM Jr, LiVolsi VA, Fisher R, Scholhamer C, Brand MH. Gastrointestinal angiodysplasia: a possible component of von Willebrand's disease. Hum Pathol 1984;15:539–44.
261. Feldman M, Smith VM, Warner CG. Varices of the colon. Report of three cases. JAMA 1962;179:729–30.
262. Ganguly S, Shiv KS, Bathia V, Lahoti D. The prevalence and spectrum of colonic lesions in patients with cirrhotic and noncirrhotic portal hypertension. Hepatology 1995;21:1226–31.
263. Garcia–Tsao G, Groszmann RJ, Fisher RL, Conn HO, Atterbury CE, Glickman M. Portal pressure, presence of gastroesophageal varices, and variceal bleeding. Hepatology 1985;5:419–24.
264. Goenka MK, Kochar R, Nagi B, Metha SK. Rectosigmoid varices and other mucosal changes in patients with portal hypertension. Am J Gastroenterol 1991;86:1185–9.
265. Haas PA, Fox TA, Haas GP. The pathogenesis of hemorrhoids. Dis Colon Rectum 1984;27:442–50.
266. Hawkey CJ, Amar SS, Daintith HA, Toghill PJ. Familial varices of the colon occurring without evidence of portal hypertension. Br J Radiol 1985;58:677–9.
267. Hosking SW, Smart HL, Johnson AG, Triger DR. Anorectal varices, haemorrhoids, and portal hypertension. Lancet 1989;1:349–52.
268. Iwao T, Toyonaga A, Ikegami M, et al. Portal vein hemodynamics in cirrhotic patients with portal hypertensive gastropathy: An echo-Doppler study. Hepatogastroenterology 1994:41;230–4.
269. Iwao T, Toyonaga A, Sumino M, et al. Portal hypertensive gastropathy in patients with cirrhosis. Gastroenterology 1992:102;2060–5.
270. Jabbari M, Cherry R, Lough JI, Daly DS, Kinnear DG, Goresky CA. Gastric antral vascular ectasia: the watermelon stomach. Gastroenterology 1984:87;165–70.
271. Katz JA, Rubin RA, Cope C, Holland G, Brass CA. Recurrent bleeding from anorectal varices: successful treatment with a transjugular intrahepatic portosystemic shunt. Am J Gastroenterol 1993;88:1104–7.
272. Knechtle SJ, Rikkers LF. Current management of esophageal variceal bleeding. Adv Surg 1999;33:439–58.
273. Kozarek RA, Botoman VA, Bredfeldt JE, Roach JM, Patterson DJ, Ball TJ. Portal colopathy: prospective study of colonoscopy in patients with portal hypertension. Gastroenterology 1991;101:1192–7.
274. Miko TL, Thomazy VA. The caliber persistent artery of the stomach: a unifying approach to gastric aneurysms, Dieulafoy's lesion and submucosal arterial malformation. Hum Pathol 1988;19:914–21.

275. Misra SP, Dwivedi M, Misra V. Prevalence and factors influencing hemorrhoids, anorectal varices, and colopathy in patients with portal hypertension. Endoscopy 1996;28:340–5.
276. Morini S, Caruso F, De Angelis P. Familial varices of the small and large bowel. Endoscopy 1993;25:188–90.
277. Naveau S, Bedossa P, Poynard T, Mery B, Chaput JC. Portal hypertensive colopathy: a new entity. Dig Dis Sci 1991;36:1774–81.
278. Ohta M, Hashizume M, Higashi H, et al. Portal and gastric mucosal hemodynamics in cirrhotic patients with portal-hypertensive gastropathy. Hepatology 1994:20;1432–6.
279. Quintero E, Piqué JM, Bouabi JA, et al. Gastric mucosal vascular ectasias causing bleeding in cirrhosis: a distinct entity associated with hypergastrinemia and low serum levels of pepsinogen I. Gastroenterology 1987;93:1054–61.
280. Rabinovitz M, Yoo YK, Schade RR, Dindzans VJ, Van Thiel DH, Gavaler JS. Prevalence of endoscopic findings in 510 consecutive individuals with cirrhosis evaluated prospectively. Dig Dis Sci 1990;35:705–10.
281. Renshaw JF. Multiple hemorrhagic telangiectasia with special reference to gastroscopic appearance. Cleveland Clin Q 1939;6:226–30.
282. Shbeeb I, Prager E, Love J. The aortic valve. Colonic axis. Dis Colon Rectum 1984;27:38–41.
283. Stansby G, Meyrick-Thomas J, Lewis AA. Pericolostomy varices. J Royal Coll Surg Edinburgh 1990;35:109–10.
284. Suit PF, Petras RE, Bauer TW, Petrini JL Jr. Gastric antral vascular ectasia. A histologic and morphometric study of "the watermelon stomach." Am J Surg Pathol 1987:11;750–7.
285. Tam TN, Ng WW, Lee SD. Colonic mucosal changes in patients with liver cirrhosis. Gastrointest Endosc 1995:42;408–12.
286. Terblanche J, Burroughs AK, Hobbs KE. Controversies in the management of bleeding esophageal varices. N Engl J Med 1989;320: 1469–75.
287. Viggiano TR, Gostout CJ. Portal hypertensive intestinal vasculopathy: a review of the clinical, endoscopic, and histopathologic features. Am J Gastroenterol 1992;87:944–54.
288. Yamakado S, Kanazawa H, Kobayashi M. Portal hypertensive colopathy: endoscopic findings and the relation to portal pressure. Intern Med 1995:35;153–7.
289. Zeller FA, Cannan CR, Prakash UB. Thoracic manifestations after esophageal variceal sclerotherapy. Mayo Clin Proc 1991;66:727–32.

7 ISCHEMIA AND OTHER VASCULAR DISORDERS

GASTROINTESTINAL ISCHEMIA

Ischemia is a generic term encompassing a number of conditions that lead to a decrease in blood flow and oxygen supply to the intestinal wall, with or without an increase in oxygen demand. Gastrointestinal ischemia includes a broad spectrum of conditions, which differ in onset, duration, cause of injury, and type of vessels involved. In the last 20 years, our understanding of the etiology and pathogenesis of ischemic conditions has evolved significantly. Like many other gastrointestinal disorders, ischemia is a diagnosis made after appropriate correlation of clinical, radiologic, and histologic findings. The pathologist should make an attempt to identify the etiology of the ischemic injury since therapy is based on correction of its underlying cause.

Demography

The incidence of ischemic injury to the small and large intestines varies depending upon the etiology. Acute mesenteric ischemia accounted for 0.1 percent of admissions to a large tertiary care center (2); chronic ischemia accounts for 1/2,000 hospital admissions.

Intestinal ischemia may affect any part of the gastrointestinal tract of individuals of any age, including infants. The small intestine is more prone to ischemic injury than other parts of the gastrointestinal tract. In general, the elderly are more prone to ischemic injury than younger individuals. Small intestinal ischemic necrosis following an acute ischemic event predominantly affects elderly individuals with underlying cardiovascular diseases. Chronic intestinal ischemia (abdominal angina) results from chronic mesenteric vascular insufficiency and severe anoxia, without complete cessation of the blood flow. It tends to affect middle-aged or older patients with advanced vasoocclusive disease involving the celiac axis and the superior mesenteric artery, usually secondary to arteriosclerosis of the mesenteric vessels. Disorders leading to mechanical obstruction of the blood flow, such as torsion, prolapse, herniation, or intussusception, make up a large part of the ischemic lesions seen by pathologists.

Ischemia developing in a younger person who has no apparent predisposing factors, such as cardiac failure, cardiac arrhythmia, or the use of drugs known to cause ischemia, should be investigated for an underlying primary vascular disorder. Gastrointestinal complaints are seen in 25 to 79 percent of patients with polyarteritis nodosa (1,3). Gastrointestinal involvement is seen in up to 75 percent of children with Henoch-Schönlein purpura (4); abdominal symptoms precede the typical purpuric rash of this disease in 14 to 36 percent of cases.

Unusual causes of ischemia include hypercoagulable states, infection, and vascular conditions limited to the gastrointestinal tract. These make up a small, probably underestimated, component of gastrointestinal ischemia.

Etiology

Intestinal ischemia results from a wide variety of causes (Table 7-1). The most common cause of acute mesenteric ischemia is a thromboembolic event superimposed on an atherosclerotic vascular disorder (6). Atheromatous embolization, either from migration of intracardiac mural thrombi or following aortic catheterization, can result in localized or widespread acute abdominal ischemia.

Nonocclusive mesenteric ischemia is an underdiagnosed condition with a relatively poor prognosis. It is caused by hypoperfusion of the gut and is precipitated by congestive cardiac failure, cardiac arrhythmia, hypotension, dehydration, shock, and large volume shifts. Nonocclusive mesenteric ischemia is responsible for 20 to 30 percent of cases of acute intestinal ischemia (5).

Mesenteric venous thrombosis is an uncommon lesion seen in young patients with hypercoagulable states or as an idiopathic lesion in

Table 7-1

CAUSES OF INTESTINAL ISCHEMIA

Acute vascular occlusion
Thrombosis
Embolism
Nonocclusive mesenteric ischemia
Atherosclerosis
Necrotizing enterocolitis
Pig bel
Neonatal necrotizing enterocolitis
Vasculitides and vasculopathies (see Table 7-2)
Hypercoagulable states
Drug effects (see Table 7-4)
Vascular compression
Volvulus
Intussusception
Celiac axis compression
Infections (see Table 7-3).
Amyloidosis
Radiation damage
Diabetes mellitus

Table 7-3

INFECTIONS WITH AN ISCHEMIC PATTERN OF INJURY

Clostridium difficile
Enterotoxigenic *Escherichia coli* O157:H7
Staphylococcal enterocolitis
Cytomegalovirus
Aspergillus sp
Candida sp

older individuals. A number of small and large vessel vasculitides and vasculopathies cause intestinal ischemia (Table 7-2). Their diagnosis is based primarily on extraintestinal manifestations and laboratory evaluation.

A number of infections can cause ischemia or an ischemic pattern of injury (Table 7-3). The most commonly involved organisms are *Clostridium difficile* (pseudomembranous colitis), enterotoxigenic *Escherichia coli* O157:H7, and cytomegalovirus. Although, a number of drugs (Table 7-4) have been associated with intestinal ischemia, nonsteroidal antiinflammatory drugs (NSAIDs), cocaine, oral contraceptives, and certain antibiotics (antibiotic-associated pseudomembranous colitis) are the four most common causes of drug-induced ischemic injury.

Mechanical obstruction can lead to ischemia in a number of different conditions (Table 7-5). Intussusception is the most common mechanical cause of vascular occlusion in pediatric patients. Adhesions, volvulus, and strangulated hernia are frequent causes of mechanical obstruction in adults.

Table 7-2

GASTROINTESTINAL VASCULAR DISORDERS

Affecting large, medium, and small blood vessels
Takayasu's arteritis
Giant cell arteritis
Churg-Strauss syndrome
Predominantly affecting large and medium blood vessels
Crohn's disease
Predominantly affecting medium and small blood vessels
Radiation damage
Polyarteritis nodosa
Kawasaki's disease
Wegener's granulomatosis
Buerger's disease
Vasculitis associated with connective tissue diseases
Fungal vasculitis
Behcet's syndrome
Danlos-Ehlers syndrome
Predominantly affecting small blood vessels
Henoch-Schönlein syndrome
Hypersensitivity vasculitis
Hypocomplementemic vasculitis
Cytomegalovirus vasculitis
Rickettsial vasculitis
Cryoglobulinemia
Predominantly affecting veins and venules
Mesenteric inflammatory venoocclusive disease
Mesenteric phlebosclerosis

Table 7-4

DRUGS ASSOCIATED WITH INTESTINAL ISCHEMIA

Nonsteroidal antiinflammatory drugs
Oral contraceptive pills
Cocaine
Antibiotic-associated (pseudomembranous) colitis
Immunosuppressive agents
Potassium salts
Digitalis
Alpha-interferon
Interleukin-2

Table 7-5

MECHANICAL CAUSES OF ISCHEMIA

Adhesions
Intussusception
Volvulus
Strangulated hernia
Severe obstruction
Celiac axis compression
Congenital bands

Pathophysiology

All forms of ischemic damage share the underlying feature of a blood supply that fails to meet the local tissue demands required to fulfill normal functions and/or maintain normal structure. The pathogenesis of ischemic damage depends on enough blood being supplied to the ischemic segment to prevent complete death, but insufficient blood flow to meet the metabolic needs of the injured bowel. When the blood flow falls below a critical level so that oxygen uptake is limited, the tissues become hypoxic. Prolonged cessation of blood flow to any organ inevitably results in cell death because of the diminished delivery of oxygen and metabolic substrates and the accumulation of potentially cytotoxic end products of anaerobic metabolism.

When the blood supply to a tissue is interrupted, a sequence of chemical events is initiated that leads to cellular dysfunction, cellular and interstitial edema, and ultimately, cell death. Oxygen, as a basic cell fuel, is crucial to cell function. Aerobic metabolism replenishes the high-energy phosphate bonds required for normal cell function. A lack of oxygen results in anaerobic metabolism and an increased local concentration of lactic acid. The resulting acidosis alters normal enzyme kinetics. Fewer high-energy bonds are created, and the cell is deprived of the energy needed to maintain homeostasis (10). Different tissues and different areas within the same tissue withstand hypoxia for different time periods.

The small intestinal blood supply must be reduced by more than 50 percent to induce detectable tissue injury (7). Adaptive mechanisms that prevent injury with less than a 50 percent reduction in blood flow include increased oxygen extraction and oxygen redistribution within the intestinal wall to those areas with high metabolic demands. If the blood supply is cut off for more than 2 hours, it takes approximately 1 week for the mucosa to recover (9). If reflow is not established, the bowel can become totally necrotic.

Reversible ischemic damage depends on several factors: 1) the nature of the intestinal vasculature; 2) luminal bacterial virulence; and 3) the duration of the ischemic episode (9). The extent and duration of the ischemia determine the depth of the tissue injury.

The first detectable sign of ischemic bowel injury is increased capillary permeability, the cause of the associated characteristic submucosal edema. With prolonged ischemia, mucosal permeability further increases so that morphologically detectable mucosal epithelial cell injury occurs. Mucosal cells are shed at an increased rate, and damage to the plasma membrane of unshed cells results in leakage of cytoplasmic enzymes (8). Decreased cellular nucleotide metabolism, decreased mucus production, and anoxic necrobiosis associated with lysosomal rupture all damage the mucosa and make it vulnerable to the action of lysosomal and digestive enzymes. Arteriolar spasm and decreased perfusion pressure accentuate the extent of the ischemic damage. Necrosis and subsequent bacterial invasion develop when the mucosal barrier becomes defective. The initial pathologic result of ischemia is submucosal edema and mucosal coagulative necrosis. If flow is reestablished, an acute inflammatory reaction develops.

Pathophysiology of Ischemic Damage and Reperfusion Injury. When a tissue becomes ischemic, a sequence of chemical reactions is initiated that ultimately leads to cellular dysfunction and necrosis. No single process represents the critical event in ischemia-induced tissue injury. Depletion of cellular energy stores and accumulation of toxic metabolites contribute to cell death. Reestablishing blood flow (reperfusion) is required to reverse the ischemic injury, since it allows cellular regeneration and washout of toxic metabolites. Thus, reperfusion is a prerequisite for recovery from ischemic injury.

Reperfusion of ischemic tissues, however, also leads to a sequence of events that paradoxically injures the tissues (11–13,15). In fact, most of the injury that occurs in the ischemic gastrointestinal tract occurs during the period of reperfusion, in a process known as reperfusion injury. The severity of reperfusion injury depends on the duration of the preceding hypoxia. The reperfusion component of ischemic injury is more pronounced after partial than total intestinal ischemia (14). Reperfusion of the ischemic intestine results in the production of reactive oxygen metabolites and activated neutrophils.

Role of Oxygen Free Radicals. A free radical is defined as any molecule that possesses one or more unpaired electrons in its outermost shell (27). Oxygen-derived free radicals (Table 7-6) are generated within the first 2 to 3 minutes of reperfusion or reoxygenation (27,29,32,36–38, 42). Because of their ability to participate in reactions involving the transfer of single electrons, most free radicals are highly reactive molecules, capable of inducing considerable damage (28). Oxygen radicals are capable of damaging almost any molecule found in living cells, including proteins, carbohydrates, DNA, and unsaturated lipids within the cellular and mitochondrial membranes (38). The most damaging effect of free radicals is lipid peroxidation, which results in structural and functional cell damage (30).

Plasma membrane changes result from ischemic injury and lead to a loss of sodium and calcium ion balance, followed by acidosis, osmotic shock, chromatin clumping, and nuclear pyknosis (35). Sodium ions move into the cell, drawing with them a volume of water to maintain osmotic equilibrium with the surrounding interstitial space. Potassium ions escape from the cell into the interstitium (20). These changes are accompanied by activation of mitochondrial phospholipases, a precipitous loss of oxidative phosphorylation, and a drop in adenosine triphosphate (ATP) production leading to a failure of synthetic and homeostatic capabilities. Calcium overload leads to mitochondrial membrane dysfunction and irreversible damage (21). Secondary autolysis, with swelling of lysosomes, dilatation, vesiculation of the endoplasmic reticulum, leakage of enzymes and proteins, and loss of cellular compartmentalization follow. As a result of these factors, membrane integrity cannot be maintained, and the cell dies (29).

Table 7-6

OXYGEN-DERIVED FREE RADICALS

Superoxide (O_2-)
Inactivates specific enzymes
Is the precursor to hydrogen peroxide (H_2O_2)
Is a highly reactive hydroxyl radical
Hydrogen peroxide (H_2O_2)
Is a powerful oxidant
Inactivates DNA
Hydroxyl radicals (OH·)
Form via Fenton reaction
Most reactive of the free radicals
Cause lipid peroxidation
Inactivate enzymes
Inhibit cell transport
Perhydroxyl radicals
Stronger oxidant than superoxide
Are cytotoxic
Inactivate proteins
Singlet oxygen
Inactivates proteins
Initiates lipid peroxidation
Hypochlorite (HOCl)
Damages cell membranes

The end result is increased microvascular permeability and mucosal damage.

Under physiologic conditions, small amounts of free radicals are produced in almost all aerobic cells, but under normal conditions, the reactive oxidative molecules are effectively neutralized by endogenous free radical scavengers such as superoxide dismutase and glutathione peroxidase (28). After ischemia, however, the sudden reintroduction of oxygen into the tissues causes the unleashing of free radical cascades, which overwhelm endogenous defense mechanisms. Most oxygen radicals generated in the reperfused intestine are derived from the hypoxanthine-xanthine oxidase system (23,41). Xanthine oxidase is produced by enterocytes and endothelial cells (22).

Neutrophils also represent a major source of reactive oxygen metabolites (ROMs), including superoxide (O_2-), hydrogen peroxide (H_2O_2), hydroxyl (OH), hypochlorite (HOCl), and certain n-chloramines. Superoxide and hydrogen peroxide increase mucosal and vascular permeability, recruit and activate neutrophils, and act as the precursors of more damaging hydroxyl radicals via the Fenton and myeloperoxidase reactions (18,24,33,40). Transition metals, such as iron, play important roles in free radical reactions, particularly in the formation of the extremely reactive hydroxyl radical via the Fenton reaction. Hypochlorite acts as a potent oxidant that directly damages membrane-associated targets or indirectly damages them by forming less reactive chloramines that diffuse across the membrane and attack cytoplasmic components (18,24,39). Luminal aggressive factors (such as pancreatic proteases, especially trypsin) further contribute to the mucosal damage (26) and potentiate bacterial translocation and sepsis. This proteolytic activity may be especially important in the rapid conversion of xanthine dehydrogenase to xanthine oxidase (19).

Nitric oxide (NO) is as an important intracellular messenger molecule that modulates immune function, blood vessel dilatation, and neural transmission (34). NO is generated by the NO synthetase (NOS) present in macrophages, granulocytes, neurons, endothelial cells, epithelial cells, and smooth muscle cells (17). ROMs produced by activated macrophages and neutrophils react with NO to form the cytotoxic metabolitc, peroxynitrate (OONO-) (16). NOS inhibitors provide nearly complete protection against reperfusion injury (31).

The intestinal interstitium, which is continuously bathed in extracellular fluid, also provides some interstitial and epithelial protection, since it contains significant amounts of antioxidants, such as glutathione (25). The sustained production of neutrophil-derived oxidants by large numbers of extravasated cells, however, overwhelms this protective milieu and in the process alters normal intestinal structure and function.

Role of Neutrophils. Neutrophil-endothelial cell interactions are a prerequisite for the microvascular injury induced by ischemia and reperfusion (43,47). Following reperfusion, there is a significant increase in leukocytes. Far fewer leukocytes adhere to the villous microvasculature than to that of the deeper mucosa, serosa, or mesentery.

Hypoxia induces endothelial cells to produce various adhesion molecules including: 1) integrins, 2) members of the immunoglobulin superfamily, and 3) selectins (45). These powerful chemoattractants and chemoactivators act in concert to attract leukocytes and platelets to reperfused sites and to promote their adherence, transendothelial migration, and activation (51,52). As a result, a massive mucosal influx of neutrophils occurs (44). Adhesion molecules slow the motion of leukocytes in the microvasculature, causing them to roll in the vessels. This rolling behavior allows other adhesive mechanisms to operate. As a result, the slowly rolling neutrophil firmly adheres to the endothelium via the CD11/CD18 adherence glycoprotein complex (48). As the neutrophil becomes activated, CD11/CD18 expression increases and L-selectin is shed from the neutrophil membrane (49). Activated neutrophils adhere to and migrate across the endothelium and cause local destruction by releasing free radicals, proteolytic enzymes (collagenase, elastase, and cathepsins), peroxide, cytokines (46,53), platelet activating factor, and the eicosanoids, leukotriene B4 and thromboxane B2 (50). Intravascular adherence of red blood cells may plug the microvasculature, particularly capillaries and venules, further contributing to the tissue hypoxia. Neutrophils attract other neutrophils and platelets by releasing chemotactic humoral mediators, such as leukotriene B4, thromboxane A2, and platelet-activating factor (54).

Role of Platelets. Endothelial cells synthesize tissue plasminogen activator, which catalyzes the formation of plasmin, a protease that has both aggregatory and inhibitory effects on platelets. Platelets attach to damaged endothelium via specific receptors, and release a plasminogen activator inhibitor that neutralizes endothelium-associated plasminogen activator. Platelets also attach to stimulated neutrophils and monocytes, and bind to vascular walls by adhering to leukocytes already bound to the endothelium. Products released from aggregating platelets enhance the expression of adhesive proteins by the endothelium. Platelet activation enhances endothelial production of endothelin 1, an extremely potent vasoconstrictor, and causes the formation and release of platelet activating factor, a lipid inflammatory mediator.

Platelet activating factor induces platelet aggregation, adhesion to endothelial cells, and release of vasoconstrictive substances.

Role of Prostaglandins. The eicosanoids, a group of phospholipid mediators, are intimately involved in ischemic injury. They also play a major role in the pathophysiology of the shock-like states associated with sepsis and/or endotoxemia. Of particular interest is the relationship that exists between prostacyclin (PGI2), responsible for vasodilatation and platelet disaggregation from vascular endothelia, and thromboxane (TxA2), responsible for vasoconstriction and platelet aggregation. Platelets contain the enzyme thromboxane synthetase, and hence synthesize TxA2. TxA2 production increases as the platelets traverse vessels with irregular endothelial surfaces (such as in arteriolosclerosis). The increased thromboxane levels lead to vasospasm and thrombosis, thereby producing ischemia and infarction. On the other hand, normal vascular endothelium lacks thromboxane synthetase, but possesses prostacyclin synthetase, which leads to formation of PGI2 and its stable end product PGF1-alpha. PGI2 is a vasodilator and potent inhibitor of platelet aggregation, and allows platelets to flow freely through the vessels.

Another group of eicosanoids produced through the lipoxygenase pathway are the leukotrienes. Leukotrienes C4, D4, and E4 cause vasoconstriction. Leukotriene B4 stimulates aggregation and adhesion of leukocytes to the vascular endothelium.

The most recently described group of eicosanoids is the lipoxins. Lipoxins A4 and B4 are produced by the interaction between platelets and neutrophils. Lipoxins may represent negative regulators of leukotriene action. They inhibit neutrophil chemotaxis and adhesion, and cause vasodilatation.

Loss of Mucosal Barrier Function. The elements of the gastrointestinal mucosal barrier are shown in Table 7-7 (55). Mucosal epithelial cells function as a semipermeable barrier between the lumen and the intestinal wall. Typical intestinal epithelial cells have microvilli on their apical surfaces, with a filamentous brush border glycocalyx at the tip (59). These structures help prevent foreign antigen penetration into the underlying tissues. The epithelial cells also produce functional molecules such as defensins (56), trefoil factors (58), and mucin, which protect the human host. Microbes of all types are trapped in the mucus layer and are expelled from the intestine by peristalsis. In addition, proteolytic enzymes facilitate the digestion of the harmful polypeptides and diminish their immunogenic properties (60). These cells also express major histocompatability (MHC) class II receptors which facilitate antigen presentation to immune cells as needed.

Table 7-7

ELEMENTS OF THE GASTROINTESTINAL MUCOSAL BARRIER

Luminal/Epithelial	Function
Epithelium	Innate immune response Antigen presentation Block penetration of ingested antigen
Defensins	Antimicrobial peptides
Trefoil factors	Protection from bacterial toxins, chemicals, and drugs
Mucus/mucin	Entrap microbes Block penetration of ingested antigens
Proteolytic enzymes	Breakdown of ingested antigens
Secretory IgA	Block adhesion of antigen to epithelial surface
Bile acids	Breakdown of ingested antigens
Intestinal peristalsis	Expel microbes Block penetration of ingested antigens
Indigenous microflora	Competition for essential nutrients, secretion of antibiotic-like substances, chemical modification of fat and bile acids, stimulation of peristalsis
Gut-associated lymphoid tissue (GALT)	
IgA, IgG, IgM	Systemic immunity
Lymphoid follicles in lamina propria	Antigen clearance
Intraepithelial lymphocytes	Innate and acquired immune response

Ischemic damage leading to leakiness in the mucosal and microvascular barriers allows the toxic metabolites that are generated during ischemia-reperfusion injury to gain access to the systemic circulation. Mucosal damage also allows luminal contents, such as bacteria, toxins, and proteolytic enzymes, to circulate as well. These factors may contribute to both sepsis and multiple organ failure following an episode of shock (57).

Acute Mesenteric Ischemia

Definition. *Acute mesenteric ischemia* is a sudden reduction of intestinal oxygen supply due to alterations in mesenteric arterial or venous circulation. *Acute intestinal ischemia* is an alternative term.

Demography. The prevalence of mesenteric vein thrombosis ranges from 0.003 percent in general hospital populations to 0.05 percent of autopsied patients (107). Venous thrombosis accounts for 5 to 15 percent of all cases of mesenteric ischemia and infarction (109). Ischemia can affect any age group; however, acute mesenteric ischemia, particularly secondary to mesenteric arterial thrombosis and nonocclusive mesenteric ischemia, are more common in middle-aged to elderly persons.

Etiology and Pathophysiology. Acute mesenteric ischemia generally stems from the interruption of blood flow within the superior mesenteric artery or vein. Acute intestinal ischemia is a gastrointestinal emergency that may occur as a consequence of mesenteric arterial occlusion, nonocclusive low flow states, mesenteric vein thrombosis, or arteritis. Thrombosis and embolization of the mesenteric artery are the main causes (95) and occur with equal frequency; nonocclusive mesenteric ischemia is the third most common cause, the incidence of which has declined in the last two decades.

Acute colonic ischemia is often a reversible condition caused by a mismatch between blood flow and metabolic requirements in elderly individuals. Common predisposing conditions include atherosclerotic arterial diseases, hypotension, chronic renal failure, and medications. Conditions associated with acute ischemia are described in detail below.

Arterial Occlusive Disease. Arterial occlusive disease occurs secondary to thrombosis, embolism, or hemorrhage underlying an atheromatous plaque. The occlusion may involve one or all of the three intestinal arterial trees: the celiac axis, the superior mesenteric artery, and the inferior mesenteric artery. The superior mesenteric artery is most frequently affected. Atheromatous occlusion usually progresses slowly enough for a collateral circulation to develop. Therefore, intestinal infarction secondary to the atheromatous occlusion of a single vessel is rare (approximately 50 percent of patients over the age of 50 have atheromatous narrowing or occlusion of the celiac axis). Thrombi over atheromatous plaques frequently occupy the proximal few centimeters of the affected artery (66,74).

Embolic occlusion accounts for one third to half of cases of mesenteric vascular occlusion (95,104). Massive, acute, and often fatal embolism usually results from the migration of an intracardiac mural thrombus complicating heart disease. Cholesterol emboli migrate from aortic plaques, especially following catheterization, resulting in localized or widespread intraabdominal ischemia. Valvular endocarditis may shed small mycotic emboli.

Superior mesenteric artery emboli typically lodge at bifurcation points or distal to the origin of a major branch point. An embolus present in the superior mesenteric artery proximal to the origin of the ileocolic artery is called a major embolus (73). An embolus present distally in the superior mesenteric artery or one of its branches is called a minor embolus. These differences in location frequently dictate the therapeutic approach (67). Multiple emboli are present in approximately 20 percent of cases (75). The generalized mesenteric vasoconstriction that follows embolism causes additional ischemic damage.

Occlusions also result from aortic aneurysms, aortic dissections, vasculitis, and tumors that externally compress vessels.

Ischemia in Low-Flow States (Nonocclusive Ischemia). Low-flow states occur when the mesenteric arteries and veins are patent, but the blood flow through them is too slow to deliver enough oxygenated blood for the metabolic needs of the intestine. Such states usually result from decreased cardiac output following primary cardiac disease (infarction or arrhythmia), hypovolemia, shock, mesenteric arterial-to-arterial and arterial-to-venous shunting, and a combination of low mesenteric flow and mesenteric arterial sclerosis and vasoconstriction (108). Even though the blood supply to the superficial part of the mucosa is fairly well maintained during shock, hypoxic injury still develops within 1 to 2 hours. Several pathogenic mechanisms account for the ischemic necrosis: 1) vasoconstriction with increased resistance to blood flow; 2) redistribution of blood flow away from the mucosa; 3) increased capillary filtration via relaxation of the precapillary sphincter smooth muscle fibers; and 4) intestinal countercurrent mechanisms in the villi that shunt oxygen away from the villus tips (89).

During shock, blood flow velocity significantly slows (90), requiring an effective short-circuiting mechanism for oxygen at the base of the villi. Some oxygen short-circuiting also occurs in the villus countercurrent exchanger when the villus exhibits a very low resting PO_2 (78). As a result, regional hypoxia develops at the villous tips, even though the overall oxygen extraction efficiency remains high. This explains why the villous tips become anoxic first, and why early and minimal injury always occurs first at the villous tip. When sepsis complicates the shock, the splanchnic organs require increased oxygen (63,80). This further enhances the hypoxic injury, leading to increased mucosal necrosis and bacterial penetration through the intestinal mucosa, further increasing the level of sepsis.

Nonocclusive intestinal ischemia also complicates hemodialysis and abnormalities in acid-base balance. The latter reduces flow through the patent, but acutely contracted, arteries (103). Drugs such as diuretics, digoxin, anesthetics, alpha-adrenergic vasoconstrictors, and amphetamines (89) further reduce the circulating blood volume by causing splanchnic vasoconstriction. Digitalis acts at the level of arteriolar smooth muscle where it increases resistance to blood flow, resulting in hypoxia.

Mesenteric Venous Thrombosis. Mesenteric venous thrombosis is a relatively rare disease, primarily affecting persons in their 6th and 7th decades of life (61). Conditions predisposing to mesenteric venous thrombosis are listed in Table 7-8. When mesenteric venous thrombosis occurs in younger persons, an underlying predisposing condition should be sought (75,77–79, 81,83,87,88,91,93,94,98,99,101). There is no identifiable predisposing cause in 25 to 50 percent of cases.

Multiple etiologic factors may exist in any one patient. For example, a patient requiring splenectomy may have a preexisting abnormality involving the coagulation system, may

Table 7-8

FACTORS PREDISPOSING TO MESENTERIC VENOUS THROMBOSIS

Hypercoagulable states
Oral contraceptives
Liver disease
Inflammatory bowel disease
Renal disease
Factor V Leiden mutation
Protein C deficiency
Protein S deficiency
Antithrombin III deficiency
Plasminogen deficiency
Heparin cofactor II deficiency
Lupus anticoagulant
Polycythemia vera
Estrogen therapy
Cryoglobulinemia
Defective generation of plasminogen activator
Hyperviscosity syndrome
Sickle cell anemia
Thrombocytopenia
Thrombocytosis
Paraneoplastic states (especially pancreatic cancer)
Vascular injury following surgery or trauma
Inflammatory conditions
Pancreatitis
Diverticulitis
Appendicitis
Peritonitis
Cholangitis
Inflammatory bowel disease
Pelvic or intraabdominal abscess
Phlebitis
Abnormal blood flow
Postoperative dehydration
Sepsis
Cirrhosis
Blunt abdominal trauma
Prior splenectomy
Disseminated intravascular coagulation
Parasitic infestations
Schistosomiasis
Ancylostoma ceylanicum
Ascaris
Carcinoma
Pancreatic cancer
Carcinoma metastatic to the pancreas
Carcinomatosis
Vascular compression by tumors or inflammatory processes
Impaired venous drainage
Volvulus
Internal and external hernias
Portal hypertension
Postrenal transplant

experience intraoperative trauma to regional veins, and may develop a transient thrombocytosis caused by the splenectomy (98).

Approximately 95 percent of all mesenteric thromboses involve the superior mesenteric vein and lead to ischemia or infarction of the small bowel or proximal colon (83). In the remainder of cases, the inferior mesenteric vein is involved, with the principal changes affecting the distal colon. In a small number of cases, thrombosis develops over an extended time period, permitting the development of collateral venous drainage from the involved intestinal segments. Thrombosis following hypercoagulable states originates in the smaller venous branches and progresses into the major trunks (74). Thrombosis secondary to cirrhosis, neoplasia, or operative injury begins at the site of obstruction and extends peripherally.

Regardless of the cause of the mesenteric venous thrombosis, egress of blood from the intestine becomes impaired, causing the mesenteric arterial pressure to rise and arterial blood flow to slow. This leads to the development of ischemia.

Mechanical Obstruction of Venous Return. Mechanical obstruction of venous return is caused by a number of conditions (see Table 7-5). These mechanical alterations are discussed in chapter 6.

Clinical Features. The clinical features of intestinal ischemia are frequently nonspecific in the early stages and require a high degree of suspicion to allow for early intervention and a favorable prognosis (74). Abdominal pain is the usual presenting complaint (102). In later stages, patients develop features of paralytic ileus with vomiting, abdominal distension, hypotension, and septicemia.

Most of the abnormal laboratory findings are associated with late-stage disease. These include leukocytosis, metabolic acidosis, and elevation of serum amylase, serum D-lactate, and serum D-dimer (62,90,97).

Radiologic Findings. Imaging studies, particularly computerized tomography (CT) scans with contrast enhancement, duplex ultrasonography, magnetic resonance imaging (MRI), and mesenteric angiography, can pinpoint a specific etiology in some cases.

Plain X Ray. Abdominal plain films are usually normal in early ischemia (105). As the ischemia progresses, formless loops of bowel, thickening of the bowel wall, and "thumb printing" of the bowel wall develop. Any radiologic abnormality on plain X ray portends a poor outcome (74).

Duplex Ultrasonography. Duplex ultrasonography is useful to assess blood flow in the superior mesenteric artery and the portal vein. It can detect occlusion and thrombosis of these vessels (96). It can only consistently evaluate proximal portions of the major vessels (85); the peripheral branches cannot be visualized (71). Patients with nonocclusive mesenteric ischemia may have normal duplex ultrasonography results despite vasoconstriction.

Computerized Tomography. CT scan may be helpful in diagnosing acute mesenteric ischemia. Unfortunately, however, as with other radiologic methods, the early signs on CT scan are relatively nonspecific (65). Early signs of acute mesenteric ischemia include bowel wall thickening and luminal dilatation. Highly suggestive late signs include pneumatosis and mesenteric or portal venous gas, both of which indicate the presence of necrotic bowel (86,106). Contrast-enhanced CT scanning is the procedure of choice to diagnose acute mesenteric venous thrombosis (68,78,100). Lack of opacification, a central lucency in the lumen, and dilated collaterals in the mesentery are diagnostic. Magnetic resonance angiography is also being utilized as a noninvasive diagnostic test.

Mesenteric Angiography. Direct imaging of the splanchnic vasculature by mesenteric angiography is the mainstay of diagnosis in occlusive and nonocclusive forms of mesenteric ischemia (64,69,70,72). It has a high sensitivity (74 to 100 percent), and specificity (100 percent) with minimal complications (74). Aortography is the best imaging technique to detect superior mesenteric artery thrombosis. Emboli are detected by the presence of one or more filling defects, with partial or complete obstruction. Angiography is the only means available to diagnose nonocclusive ischemia. Nonocclusive mesenteric ischemia shows the following diagnostic features on angiogram: 1) narrowing and irregularity of the superior mesenteric artery branches; 2) spasm of the mesenteric arcades; and 3) impaired filling of the intramural vessels (64,103). Angiography also helps to rule out occlusive causes of ischemia. In a small number of patients with mesenteric venous thrombosis, angiography is required to delineate the thrombosed vein.

Treatment and Prognosis. Urgent laparotomy is appropriate when acute mesenteric vascular occlusion is suspected in a patient with shock. Time-consuming radiologic workup in such patients may lead to a delay in instituting therapy in an urgent situation.

In other patients with arterial or venous thrombosis, infusion of vasodilators or thrombolytic agents may be used as treatment at the time of diagnostic study. Colonic ischemia involving the watershed area in the region of the splenic flexure is invariably due to nonocclusive ischemia, and can be managed in most patients without recourse to invasive radiology or surgery.

A number of growth factors like erythropoietin, epidermal growth factor, and hepatocyte growth factor are being evaluated as potential agents that may protect the intestinal mucosal epithelium against ischemic damage (66,74,104).

Patients with acute mesenteric ischemia have a mortality rate of 60 to 100 percent (72,92). Those with colonic ischemia have a lower mortality rate than those with acute mesenteric ischemia. However, patients with gangrenous colonic ischemia who require surgical resection, incur a greater than 50 percent mortality rate (80).

Chronic Mesenteric Ischemia

Definition. *Chronic mesenteric ischemia* is a gradually developing ischemic condition that occurs most frequently in older females (112). It is also known as *abdominal angina*.

Etiology. Chronic intestinal ischemia results from chronic mesenteric vascular insufficiency and severe anoxia, without complete cessation of blood flow. It tends to affect patients with advanced vaso-occlusive disease involving the celiac axis and the superior mesenteric artery. The occlusion is usually secondary to severe occlusive arteriosclerosis of the mesenteric vessels (111), but it may also complicate aortic aneurysms. Chronic mesenteric ischemia is also caused by celiac artery compression syndrome, in which the celiac artery is compressed by the median arcuate ligament or by a neoplasm.

Pathophysiology. Slowly growing atherosclerotic obstruction is usually the source of the ischemia. Most patients develop adequate collateral circulation, which provides sufficient blood to prevent symptomatic ischemic damage (112).

Clinical Features. Since the gastrointestinal tract requires a greater blood flow during the postprandial period (from 20 percent when fasting to 35 percent postprandial) (112), patients characteristically complain of postprandial pain. They may also experience weight loss. Extensive workup to rule out gastric, pancreatic, biliary, or colonic pathology is negative. The radiographic techniques discussed below help establish the diagnosis. Early diagnosis and treatment are imperative to prevent intestinal infarction.

Endoscopic Findings. Endoscopy is helpful in evaluating colonic ischemia. Ischemia affects the colon more commonly at the splenic flexure and rectosigmoid due to poor collateral circulation in these areas. Characteristically, the ischemia gives rise to segmental abnormalities including erythema, edema, and ulceration. For most, however, an unequivocal diagnosis of ischemia cannot be made without a biopsy unless mucosal gangrene is present. The endoscopic features and distribution of the changes may be similar to those resulting from toxigenic *Escherichia coli* infection, NSAID-induced injury, tuberculosis, or Crohn's disease.

Gross Findings. Gross examination of intestinal resection specimens should not only include evaluating the features of ischemia, but determining the extent of ischemic damage, the viability of the margins, and the etiology of the ischemia. Examination of the fresh specimen helps identify the features of ischemia more easily than examination of a fixed specimen. Features of intestinal damage due to ischemia are similar, no matter what the underlying cause is.

Early on, the ischemic bowel appears edematous and pale with submucosal edema, congestion, hemorrhage, and focal mucosal sloughing. The muscularis propria usually appears normal in early lesions. As the disease progresses, the serosa becomes dusky and dark red due to the accumulation of large amounts of intraluminal blood (fig. 7-1). The serosa loses its glistening appearance and appears dull. The mucosa becomes necrotic and ulcerated. The ulcers are discrete and can be serpiginous. Pseudomembranes may be present (fig. 7-2). In the advanced stage, transmural necrosis develops (fig. 7-3). The bowel wall becomes thin and friable

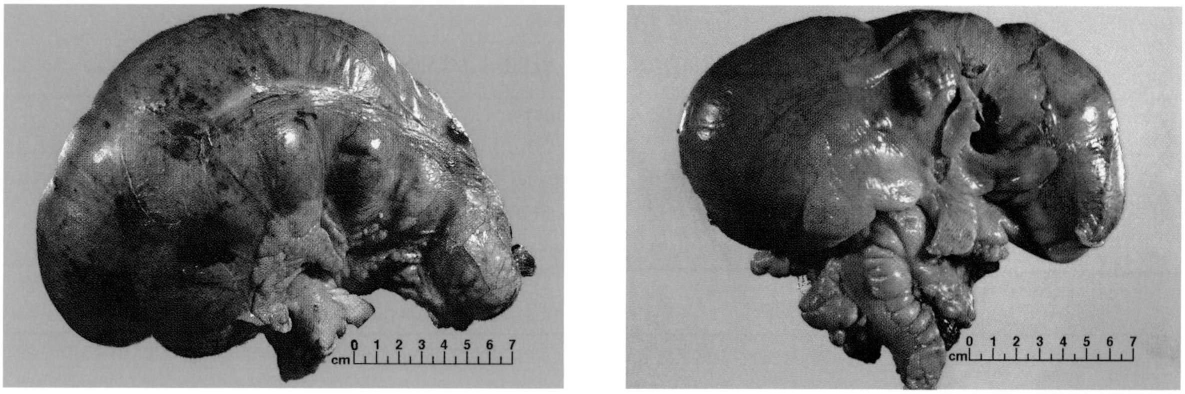

Figure 7-1

COLONIC ISCHEMIA

Left: The serosal surface of this cecectomy specimen appears dusky blue-brown.

Right: Another colon resection specimen shows patchy green-brown serosal discoloration. Green-yellow, fibrinopurulent material adheres to the serosal surface in these areas.

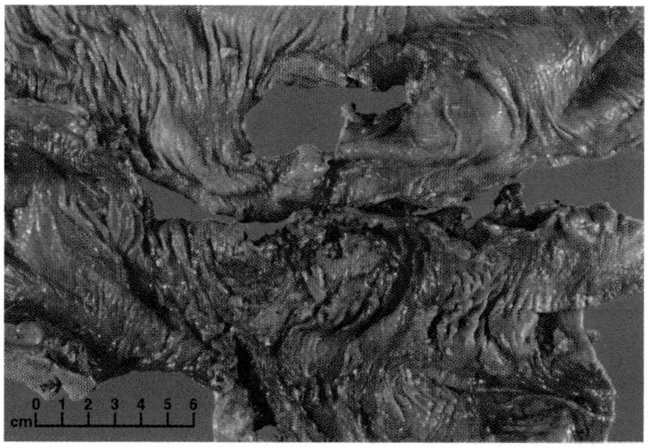

Figure 7-2

COLONIC ISCHEMIA

An opened colectomy specimen shows patchy erythema and adherent pseudomembranes.

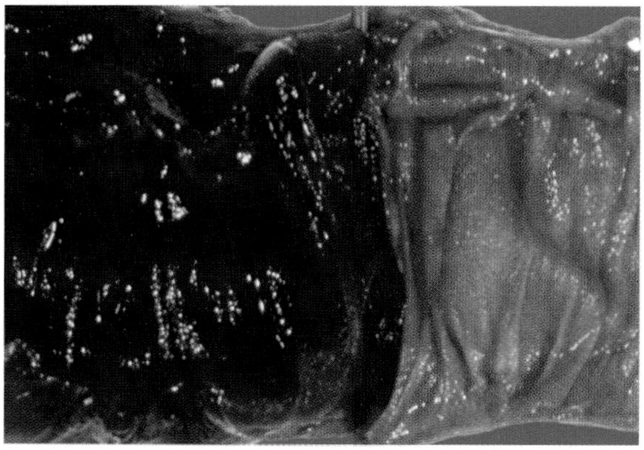

Figure 7-3

ADVANCED SMALL INTESTINAL ISCHEMIC INJURY

The ischemic intestine on the left is blue-black, while the adjacent intestine on the right appears relatively unaffected. Ischemic injury is often geographic, as depicted here, depending on which portion of the blood supply is affected.

and the serosa becomes purplish green. Pneumatosis intestinalis (gas within the bowel wall) develops and a perforation may be present at this stage. Chronic or recurrent bouts of ischemia lead to fibrosis and strictures (fig. 7-4).

The site and degree of ischemia vary depending upon the size of the vessel involved. In most cases of acute mesenteric ischemia, the superior mesenteric artery or its branches are involved. A classification (Table 7-9) based on the site of involvement of the superior mesenteric artery may be clinically useful (110).

Gross examination is as important as microscopic examination in deciding the underlying etiology of the intestinal ischemia. Volvulus, intussusception, and strangulated hernia are diagnosed either preoperatively or intraoperatively. Sometimes, an unreduced intussusception is received in surgical pathology and gross examination helps to identify not only the intussusception, but its components as well.

Mesenteric vessels should be examined for the presence of possible thrombi, emboli,

Table 7-9

FULLEN'S ANATOMIC CLASSIFICATION OF SUPERIOR MESENTERIC ARTERY INJURY

Zone	Injured Segment	Grade	Ischemia Class	Bowel Affected
I	Trunk proximal to first major branch	1	Maximal	Jejunum, ileum, right colon
II	Trunk between inferior pancreaticoduodenal and middle colic segments	2	Moderate	Major segment, small bowel, right colon
III	Trunk distal to middle colic segment	3	Minimal	Minor segment of small bowel or right colon
IV	Segmental branches	4	None	No ischemic bowel

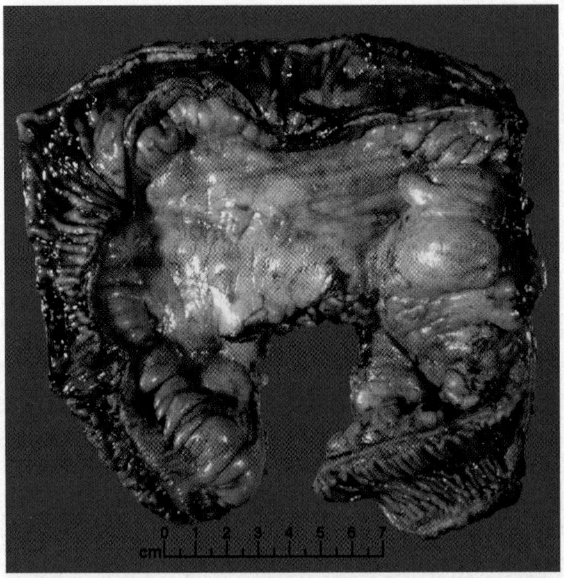

Figure 7-4

CHRONIC ISCHEMIC INJURY

Small intestinal resection specimen shows several areas of luminal narrowing secondary to previous episodes of ischemia.

atherosclerosis, and nodularity. In addition, the mesenteric vessels should always be histologically sampled to document their status. In some cases, a proximally located mesenteric artery thrombosis is not present in the surgical pathology specimen. Mesenteric venous thrombosis appears as numerous, cord-like thrombosed veins lying in a thick hemorrhagic and edematous mesentery.

In patients with polyarteritis nodosa, a nodular appearance of the artery is characteristic but uncommonly detected grossly. Mucosal ulcers seen in such patients are typically well demarcated, located on the antimesenteric border, and may be deeply penetrating. The mucosa in patients with Henoch-Schönlein purpura exhibits small, superficial petechial hemorrhages and erosions associated with edema, hemorrhage, and congestion. Patients with Behcet's syndrome preferentially develop ulcers in the terminal ileum and cecum.

Microscopic Findings. *Biopsy Specimens.* Pathologists rarely encounter a small intestinal biopsy for interpretation of ischemic changes. More commonly, a diagnosis of ischemia is made in colonic biopsies.

In the acute stage, early lesions are limited to separation and loss of the surface epithelium. The epithelial damage then progresses toward the crypt bases. The lamina propria becomes edematous and hemorrhagic, and contains dilated vessels (fig. 7-5). Crypt dropout, mucosal necrosis, and ulceration develop in the next stage (fig. 7-6). The lamina propria shows fibrin deposition in vessels or in the extravascular connective tissue. In severe cases, the crypts dilate and become lined by an attenuated epithelium (fig. 7-7). Cryptitis and acute inflammation in the lamina propria are present as reperfusion is established (fig. 7-8). The crypts fill with mucus and inflammatory debris, eventually leading to pseudomembrane formation (fig. 7-8). These changes are often patchy in distribution.

After the initial ischemic event, fibrin and granulation tissue replace areas of ulceration. Acute inflammation disappears and chronic inflammatory cells, lymphocytes, plasma cells, and macrophages infiltrate the mucosa. Macrophages enter the area to remove red blood cells from areas of hemorrhage, resulting in hemosiderin-laden macrophages (fig. 7-9). These iron-containing cells are an important diagnostic feature of ischemia.

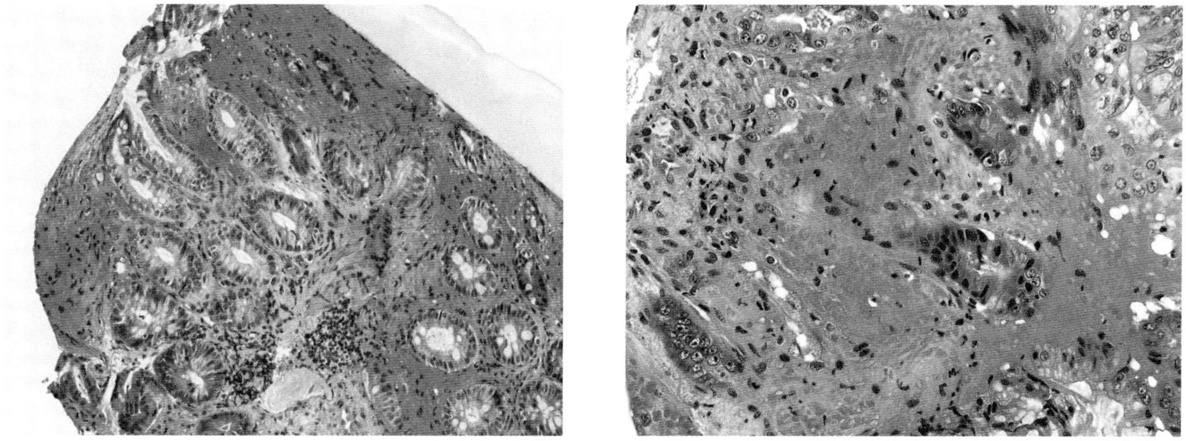

Figure 7-5

ISCHEMIA IN A COLONIC BIOPSY SPECIMEN

Left: The lamina propria appears hemorrhagic, and the crypts in the upper portion of the photograph have a mucin-depleted, regenerative appearance.

Right: Another area shows lamina propria hemorrhage and loss of the superficial portion of the crypt epithelium. Scattered neutrophils are present, an indication that some degree of reperfusion has taken place.

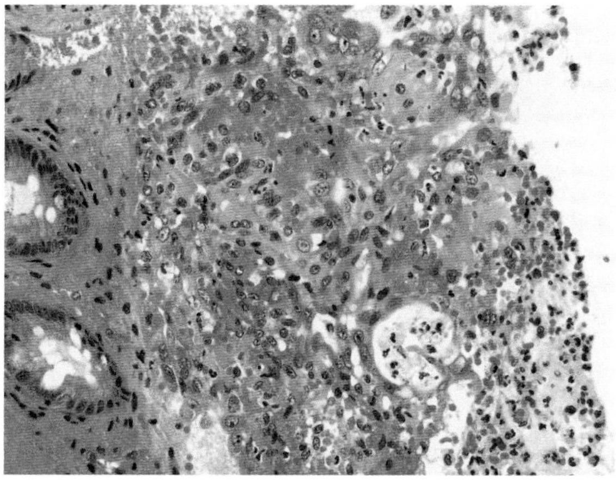

Figure 7-6

ISCHEMIC COLITIS

More advanced ischemic injury than is seen in figure 7-5. There is evidence of mucosal erosion and neutrophilic infiltration. The lamina propria is hemorrhagic.

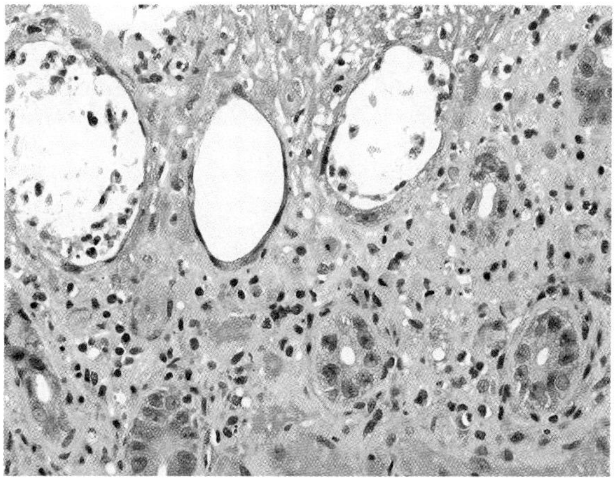

Figure 7-7

ISCHEMIC COLITIS

The crypts in this case of ischemic colitis appear withered, and are lined by flat, attenuated epithelium. Scattered neutrophils are present in the crypts. The surrounding colonic glands are smaller than usual and mucin depleted.

In chronic ischemia, the epithelium shows architectural distortion, marked regenerative activity, Paneth cell metaplasia, and endocrine cell hyperplasia (fig. 7-10). In some cases, a prominent submucosal collection of mononuclear cells is present; this may present as lymphoplasmacytosis in the deep lamina propria, simulating inflammatory bowel disease.

In addition to establishing a diagnosis of ischemia, the pathologist should attempt to determine the underlying etiology of the injury. Clues to the etiology are shown in Table 7-10.

Resection Specimens. Bowel resection is the most common type of specimen on which the diagnosis of intestinal ischemia is made. The

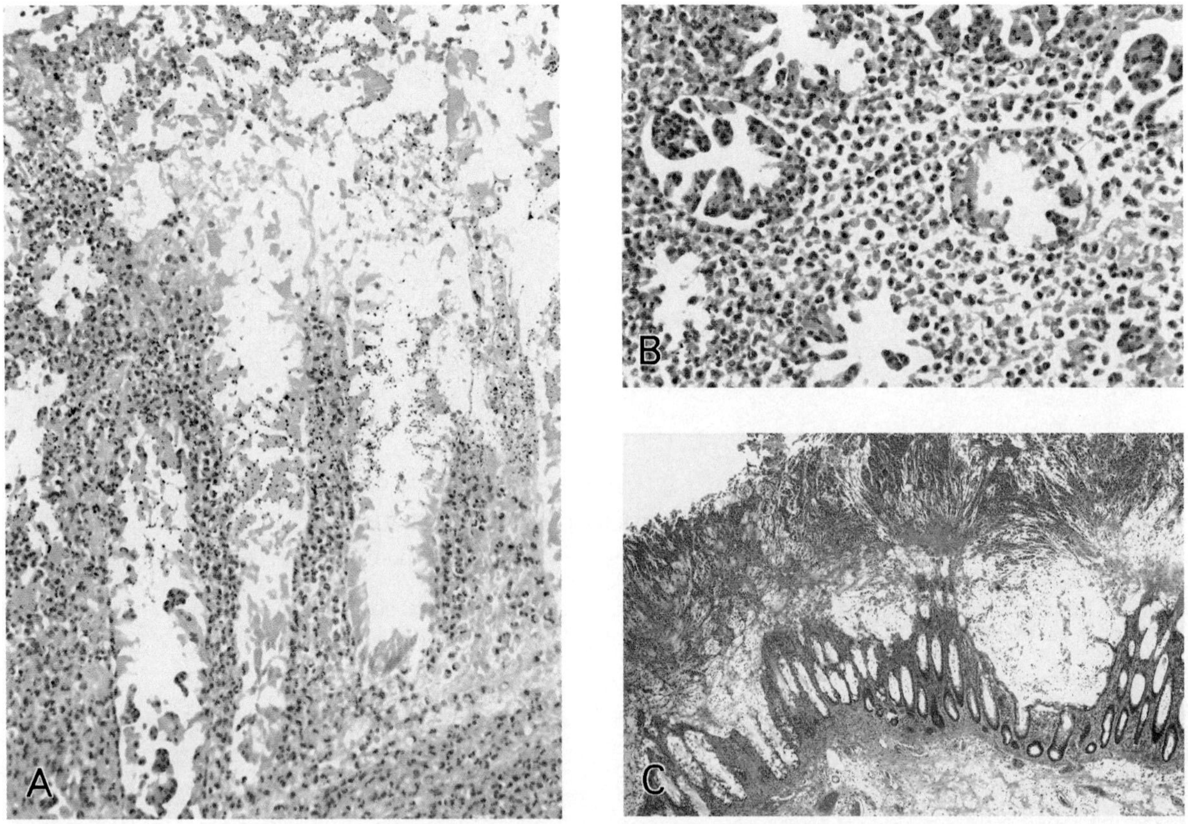

Figure 7-8

REPERFUSION INJURY

A: Typical ischemic necrosis of the colonic mucosa. The crypt architecture is still discernible, but the epithelium has been lost. The lamina propria contains a dense neutrophilic infiltrate, a sign that reperfusion of the area has occurred.

B: Higher-power view shows a dense neutrophilic infiltrate within the lamina propria and infiltrating the remaining glands.

C: Low-power view shows the presence of a pseudomembrane adherent to the mucosal surface following reperfusion. The pseudomembrane is composed of neutrophils, fibrin, extruded mucin, and necrotic cellular debris.

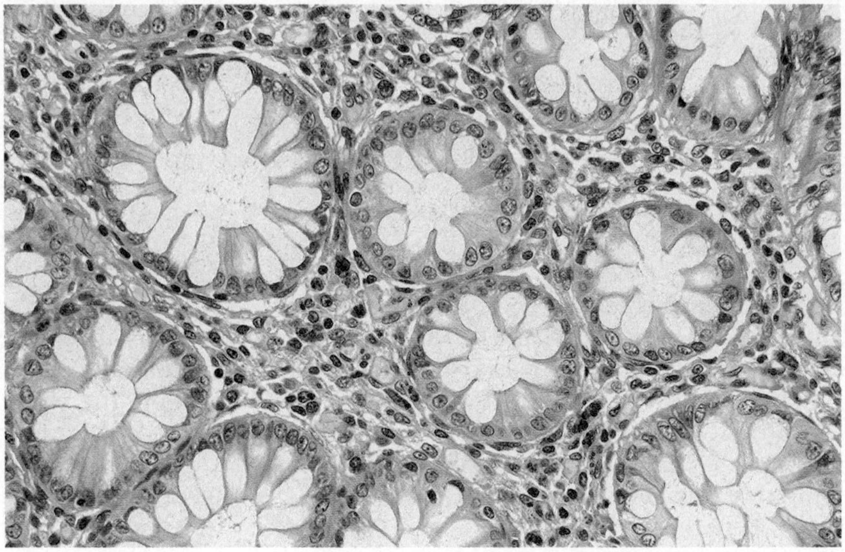

Figure 7-9

HEALING ISCHEMIC COLITIS

Yellow-brown hemosiderin is in the lamina propria in this colonic biopsy specimen. This feature is often indicative of a previous episode of ischemia.

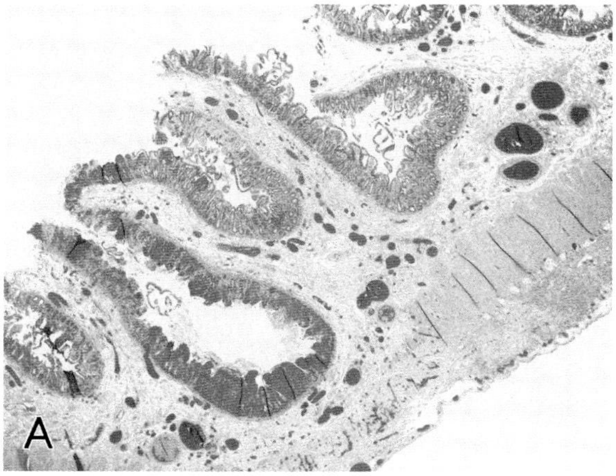

Figure 7-10

ACUTE AND CHRONIC ISCHEMIC INJURY

A: Low-power photomicrograph shows a segment of small intestine with marked vascular congestion. There is patchy ischemic necrosis. The patient had a history of previous ischemic enterocolitis and mesenteric venous thrombosis.

B: Higher-power view shows patchy acute ischemic injury superimposed on more chronic ischemic changes. The acute injury is characterized by superficial epithelial loss and surface erosion. The surrounding mucosa shows distortion of the crypt architecture and prominent regenerative epithelial changes.

C: Crypt branching is present in this section, a feature seen in chronic injury. The crypt epithelium appears mucin depleted and regenerative. Occasional neutrophils are seen in the surface epithelium and within the lamina propria. Capillaries are dilated, malformed, and sinusoidal.

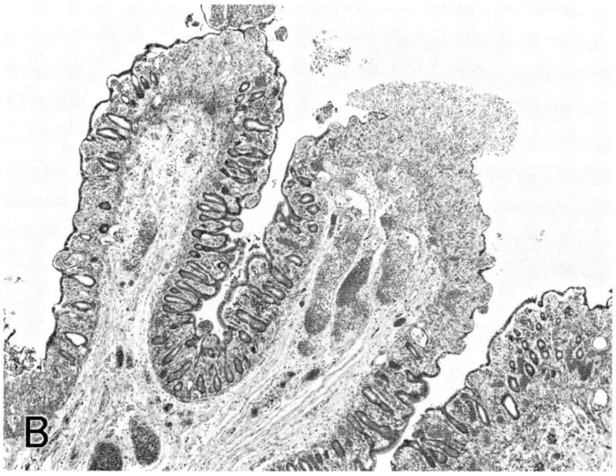

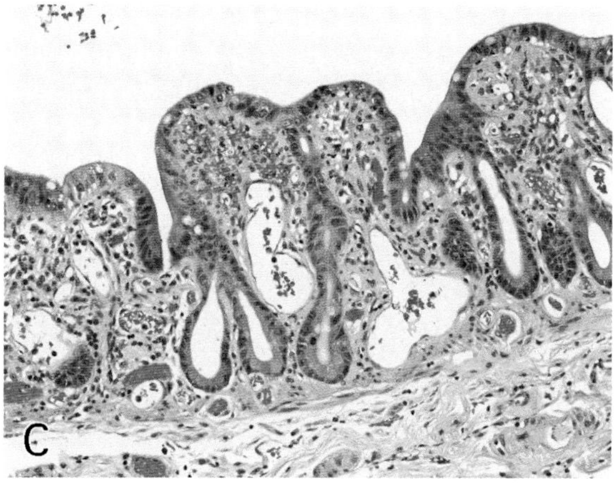

role of the pathologist in such cases is to determine the etiology of the ischemia, assess the viability of the resection margins, and rule out other pathologic abnormalities.

Early damage includes epithelial detachment and intercellular edema. Membrane-bound cytoplasmic blebs develop on the basal side of the enterocytes, leading to epithelial detachment (fig. 7-11). The process advances from the villous tips to the crypt bases (fig. 7-12). Gradually the lining epithelial cells detach and ghosts of the villi are left behind. The lamina propria becomes edematous and congested, leading to villous blunting and crypt dilatation. Submucosal edema is one of the earliest signs of ischemia. Depending on the duration and severity of the injury, mucosal and submucosal necrosis may be present (fig. 7-12). In the most severe cases, transmural necrosis occurs. Intravascular fibrin thrombi may be identified. Fibrin thrombi in necrotic areas can be either the cause of or the effect of the necrosis (fig. 7-13). If similar intravascular fibrin thrombi are found in non-necrotic

Table 7-10

COAGULATION DISORDERS LEADING TO GASTROINTESTINAL ISCHEMIA

Hemolytic uremic syndrome
Thrombotic thrombocytopenic purpura
Homocystinuria
Köhlmeier-Degos disease
Disseminated intravascular coagulation associated with sepsis
Protein C deficiency
Protein S deficiency
Paroxysmal nocturnal hemoglobinuria

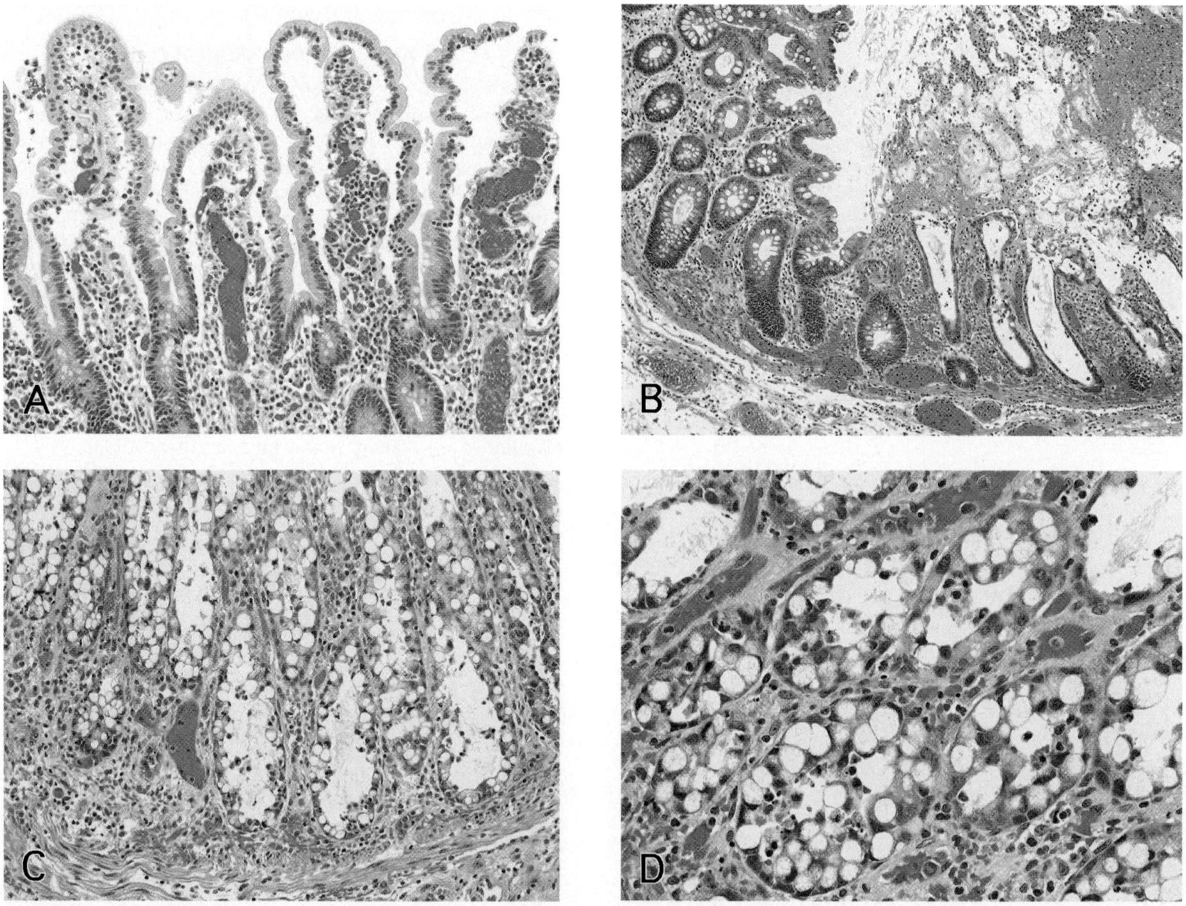

Figure 7-11

EARLY ISCHEMIC INJURY

A: The earliest visible changes of ischemia are shown here. The epithelium of this segment of small intestine has become detached from the underlying basement membrane. The mucosal capillaries are congested.

B: Low-power photomicrograph of ischemic colitis shows an essentially normal mucosa on the left, and early ischemic changes on the right. The ischemic mucosa appears congested, and the epithelium of the superficial portion of the crypts is sloughing away from the basement membrane.

C: Higher-power view of the affected colonic crypts shows discohesive, sloughing epithelial cells.

D: Goblet cells in some affected glands have a dystrophic appearance.

regions, it is likely that these are the cause of the ischemia.

If reperfusion is established, marked congestion, hemorrhage, and emigration of neutrophils in the lamina propria occur. Intraepithelial neutrophils also become prominent and pseudomembranes develop. Pseudomembranes consist of fibrin, neutrophils, other inflammatory cells, and granulation tissue. In subacute or chronic cases, fibrosis, hemosiderin-laden macrophages, and serosal adhesions are present. The remaining epithelium may show marked regenerative changes.

It is possible to identify the etiology of ischemia in some cases. Small and large vessels in the intestine and mesentery should be evaluated for emboli or other occlusive diseases, as described above (fig. 7-14). Unusual causes, including viral infection, parasitic infection, fungal vasculitis, certain connective tissue diseases like scleroderma, and hypercoagulable states, may be diagnosed by light microscopy or the use of special stains. The pathologic features of specific lesions are described below.

Differential Diagnosis. Because ischemic changes are often segmental and patchy in

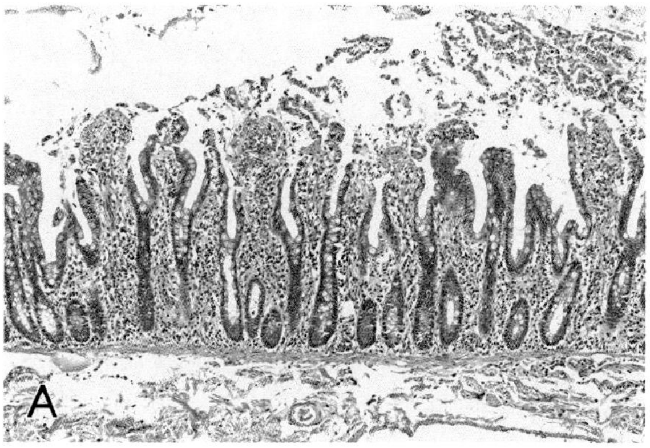

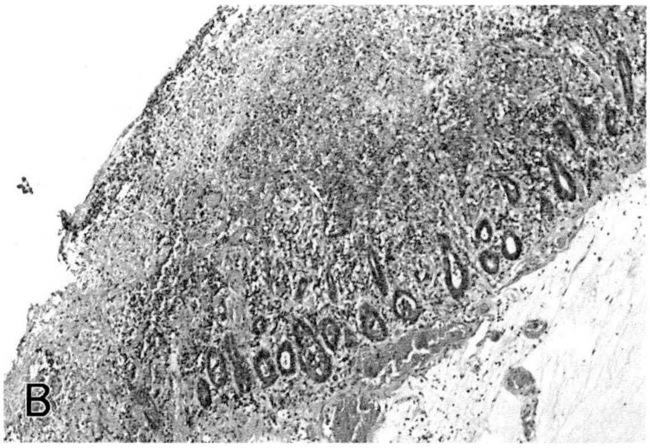

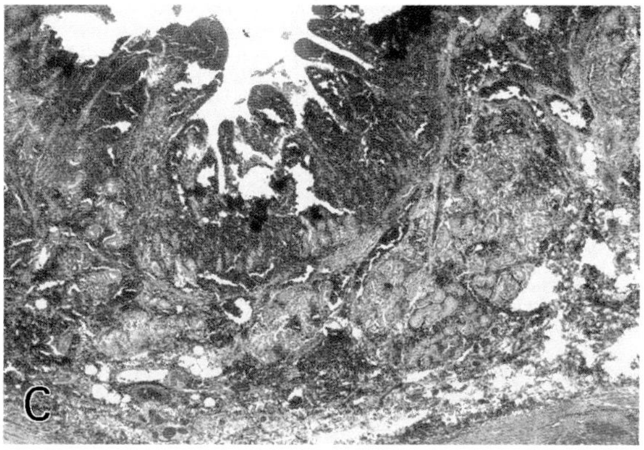

Figure 7-12

SMALL INTESTINAL ISCHEMIA

A: Early ischemic injury with loss of the epithelium overlying the villus tips. The superficial lamina propria is congested.

B: More advanced ischemia with loss of the epithelium lining almost the full length of the crypt.

C: In this case of duodenal infarction, there is full-thickness coagulative necrosis of the small intestinal wall. The tissues are congested and hemorrhagic, but inflammatory infiltrates are not present because reperfusion did not occur.

distribution, the changes may mimic Crohn's disease. Marked fibrosis and hemosiderin-laden macrophages in the lamina propria, however, are more evident in chronic ischemic colitis than in inflammatory bowel disease. In addition, the older age of the patient; the presence of coexisting systemic ischemic diseases, occlusive vascular changes in mucosal and submucosal arteries, and glandular ghosts; and the absence of rectal involvement, transmural lymphoid aggregates, and granulomas are helpful features that differentiate ischemia from other lesions.

Complications of Ischemic Injury. Untreated acute ischemia can lead to severe complications. Transmural infarction leads to metabolic acidosis, hypotension, cardiac failure, sepsis, and endotoxic shock. Reparative changes following ischemia can lead to stricture formation as early as 2 to 8 weeks after the initial injury. Loss of a large segment of intestine can lead to short bowel syndrome with malabsorption. A shortened segment of bowel with impaired motility may lead to bacterial overgrowth.

Neonatal Necrotizing Enterocolitis

Definition. *Neonatal necrotizing enterocolitis* (NEC) is a rapidly progressive, acute ischemic condition that affects premature infants at the time of the initiation of enteral feeding.

Demography. NEC affects 2 to 22 percent of all premature infants (119). It can occur at any time in the first 3 months of life, but its peak incidence is around the time when infants are started on oral foods (2 to 4 days old).

Etiology and Pathophysiology. Four factors play a critical role in the pathogenesis of NEC: 1) prematurity; 2) establishment of enteral feeding; 3) intestinal mucosal ischemia; and 4) the presence of luminal bacteria in the affected bowel loops (115,116). Premature neonates have a limited capacity to maintain oxygen uptake during periods of hypoxia and feeding (113). In addition, the immature enzymatic composition of the premature neonatal intestine does not allow complete digestion of food, thereby favoring bacterial growth. Decreased cardiac output due to fetal asphyxia also contributes to the ischemia in most cases. Umbilical vein catheterization

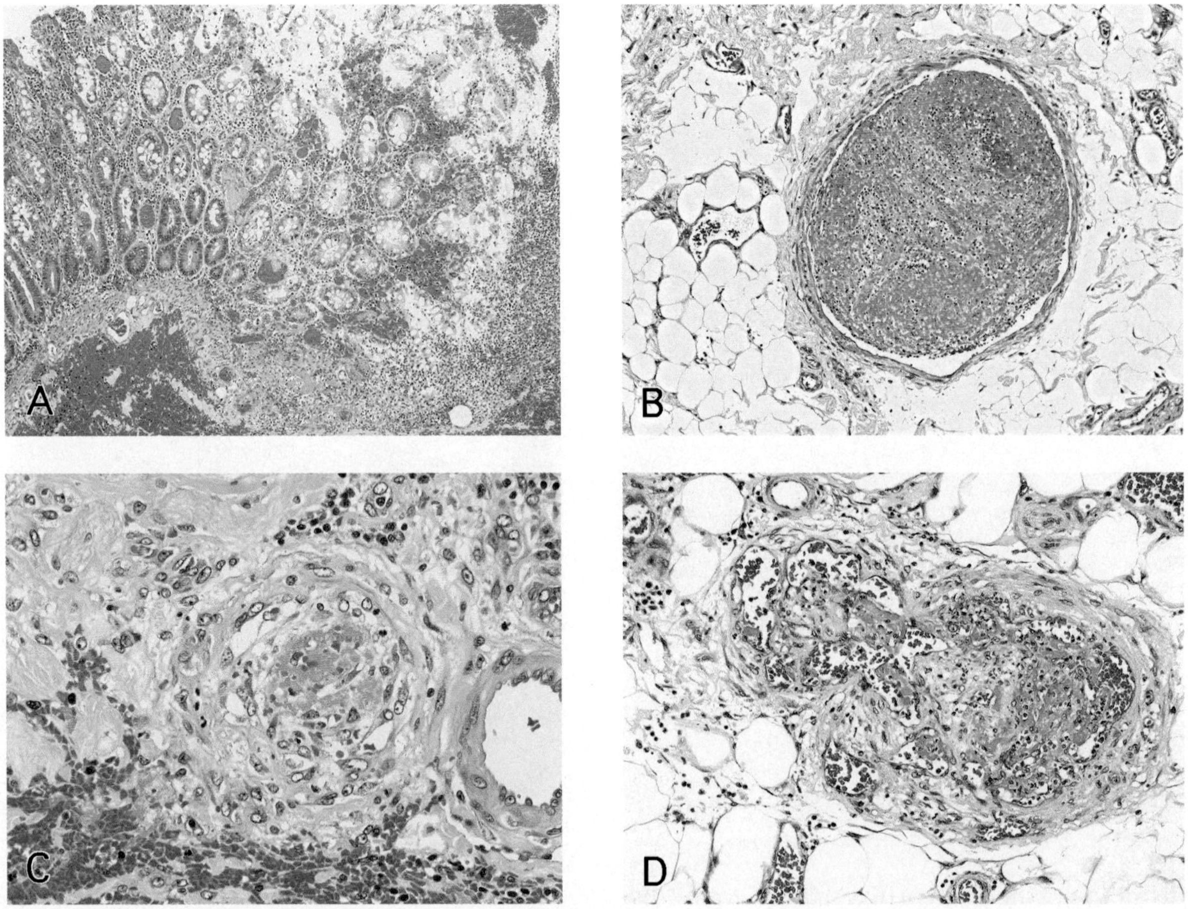

Figure 7-13

INTRAVASCULAR THROMBI IN ISCHEMIC INJURY

A: Fibrin thrombi are commonly seen in areas of ischemic necrosis. When present in an area of injury, it is not possible to determine whether the thrombi represent a primary cause of the ischemia or are a secondary change in necrotic tissues.

B: Thrombi identified in non-necrotic tissues most likely represent primary phenomena that are probably responsible for the ischemic injury seen in other regions of the bowel.

C: Sometimes thrombi of varying ages can be seen. The one depicted in this photograph appears to be organizing.

D: Later stage of organization demonstrating recanalization of a previously thrombosed vessel.

causes localized vasospasm, which can further compromise intestinal blood flow. Intestinal mucosal injury allows protein and bacterial toxins to pass into the portal circulation. These toxins reach the immature liver and then damage Kupffer cells and hepatocytes, so that the toxins are not detoxified and gain access to the systemic circulation. The endotoxemia leads to hypotension and systemic shock.

Intestinal ischemia, bacterial colonization, or formula feeding stimulates proinflammatory mediators, which activate a series of events leading to bowel necrosis (116). The proinflammatory mediators include interleukin-8, interleukin-2, and nitrous oxide (117,118).

Gross Findings. The gross findings of NEC are similar to those found in severe ischemia (fig. 7-15). Pneumatosis intestinalis is commonly present. NEC often involves the ileum and right colon; the stomach is also involved in a large number of cases (114). Affected bowel segments appear dilated, necrotic, friable, and gangrenous. The external surface is shaggy, with adhesions between the loops.

Microscopic Findings. The histologic findings in NEC resemble those seen in severe

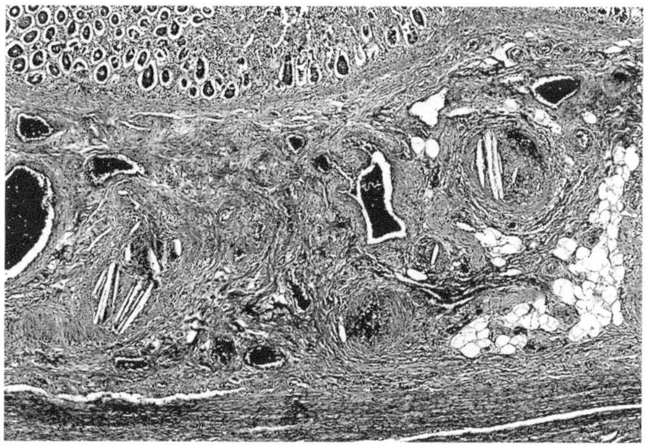

Figure 7-14

ATHEROMATOUS EMBOLI

Clear, needle-like spaces typical of cholesterol emboli lie in submucosal vessels. (Fig. 3-114 from Emory TS, Carpenter HA, Gostout CJ, Sobin LH. Atlas of gastrointestinal endoscopy & endoscopic biopsies. Washington DC: Armed Forces Institute of Pathology; 2000:229.)

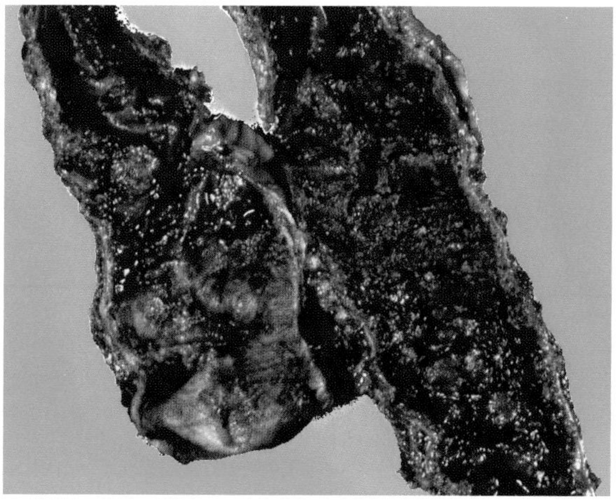

Figure 7-15

NECROTIZING ENTEROCOLITIS

The entire bowel wall appears dusky. The mucosal surface is hemorrhagic and ulcerated. The gross features resemble those of severe ischemia of any cause.

ischemia (fig. 7-16). Gas-filled cysts are present in the submucosa due to pneumatosis intestinalis. As with other resection specimens, the status of the resection margins and the extent of the ischemia should be evaluated as these factors influence long-term outcome. If possible, the unaffected bowel should be examined for other abnormalities including the absence of ganglion cells, changes of cystic fibrosis, or presence of congenital viral infections.

Treatment and Prognosis. NEC is a devastating disease with a fatal outcome in up to 40 percent of cases. Surgical resection of the affected bowel is the treatment of choice. Chronic complications include short bowel syndrome, which may require intestinal transplantation (120), and neurodevelopmental morbidity (121).

NEC in Adults. NEC can develop in adults, particularly in older individuals. Ischemia is the underlying cause. The mechanism is poorly understood and vascular occlusion is not usually demonstrable. The pathologic features are identical to those seen in severe ischemia due to other causes.

Tropical Necrotizing Enterocolitis (Enteritis Necroticans)

Tropical necrotizing enterocolitis, also known as *enteritis necroticans*, affects patients of all ages in developing countries. It is rare in developed countries, where it is generally confined to adults with chronic disease (122). Ischemia is the initial insult. Dietary factors and infections contribute to its pathogenesis. The jejunum is the most frequently involved site. Pigbel, seen in Papua New Guinea, is a classic example of this group of diseases (123). This lesion is described in more detail in chapter 10.

Acute Segmental Obstructive Enteritis

Definition. *Acute segmental obstructive enteritis* is an uncommon pediatric ischemic condition of unknown etiology which frequently involves the small intestine. Synonyms include *segmental necrotizing enteritis, nonspecific jejunitis, regional jejunitis*, and *segmental obstructing acute jejunitis*.

Demography. This is primarily a pediatric disorder (125). The disease appears to be seasonal in nature, with most cases occurring in summer and early fall (126). It was initially believed that acute segmental obstructive enteritis was limited to malnourished patients in third world countries. It has now been reported in developed countries and in well-nourished children.

Etiology. The etiopathogenesis of this condition is unclear. It may be due to toxins produced by Gram-negative bacilli or due to a localized allergic reaction (127).

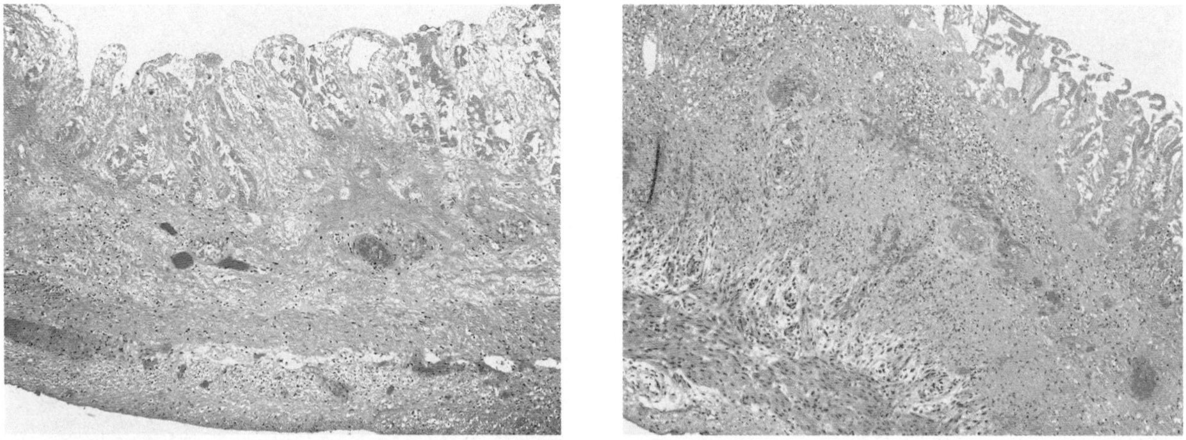

Figure 7-16

NECROTIZING ENTEROCOLITIS

Left: Low-power photomicrograph of full-thickness coagulative necrosis of the small intestine.

Right: Higher-power view shows a few viable cells remaining within mostly necrotic mucosa and submucosa. The muscularis propria in this area is still preserved.

Clinical Features. Clinically, the condition is characterized by bilious vomiting, fever, leukocytosis, severe abdominal pain, and signs of intestinal obstruction. Small bowel radiographs show segmental narrowing with proximal dilation, a feature diagnostically useful for this condition (124).

Pathologic Findings. The jejunum is most frequently affected, followed by the ileum (124). The colon is affected in only a few cases and is associated with involvement of the small intestine. Varying degrees of segmental ischemia are present on pathologic examination; the changes range from edema and minimal congestion to gangrenous necrosis with multiple perforations.

Treatment and Prognosis. The disease usually has a self-limited course and lasts 10 to 14 days (124). Surgery is usually not required, except in cases in which transmural ischemic necrosis and peritonitis develop.

Bowel Infarction in Dialysis Patients

Dialysis patients, particularly those on hemodialysis, are at risk for developing nonocclusive mesenteric ischemia (128,131). Multiple factors play a role in the development of the ischemia. Large volume shifts occurring during hemodialysis stimulate splanchnic vasoconstriction and ischemia. In addition, patients with renal disease are prone to develop hypertension and occlusive arterial disease. Hypotensive episodes, an anion gap, and metabolic acidosis can aggravate the intestinal ischemia. Many patients on dialysis have accelerated atheromatous disease, particularly if they are diabetic, and chronic constipation, resulting in increased intraluminal pressure, which can result in decreased perfusion.

The small and large intestines are equally affected by the ischemic process (130). No unique pathologic features are present in hemodialysis patients. The changes resemble ischemia due to other causes. Multiple infarctions may develop. Up to 20 percent of the mortality rate of patients on dialysis is attributable to nonocclusive mesenteric ischemia (129). Early diagnosis is critical to prevent potential life-threatening complications.

GASTROINTESTINAL ISCHEMIA SECONDARY TO SYSTEMIC VASCULITIS

Ischemia can be caused by an immune- and/or nonimmune-mediated inflammatory process involving the blood vessels of the gastrointestinal tract. Intestinal vasculitis is an unusual cause of mesenteric ischemia. It results in chronic arterial insufficiency in most of the cases, and sometimes in acute mesenteric ischemia. The diagnosis is based primarily on extraintestinal manifestations and serologic tests. Gastrointestinal vascular disorders are listed in Table 7-2.

Polyarteritis Nodosa

Definition. *Polyarteritis nodosa* (PAN) is an antineutrophil cytoplasmic antibody (ANCA)-associated vasculitis affecting medium-sized blood vessels.

Demography. Up to 30 percent of cases are associated with hepatitis B infection. An association with hepatitis C has also been described (145).

Etiology. Immune complex damage has been proposed as the etiologic mechanism for the vasculitis, particularly in patients with hepatitis B (136). Circulating immune complexes containing viral proteins have been implicated in the pathogenesis. The majority of patients have wild-type hepatitis B infection, characterized by HBe antigenemia and high hepatitis B virus replication (133).

Besides hepatitis B, other viruses, including human immunodeficiency virus (HIV) and parvovirus B19 have been proposed as etiologic factors (133). Patients often have other autoimmune diseases, with rheumatoid arthritis and systemic lupus erythematosus being the most common. Deposition of immune complexes in the blood vessels leads to fibrinoid necrosis and thrombotic, occlusive, ischemic, and hemorrhagic events in the affected tissues.

Clinical Features. Abdominal symptoms occur in 25 to 50 percent of patients with PAN (133,138), and abdominal pain is the most frequent complaint, followed by diarrhea and other gastrointestinal symptoms. Thirty-six percent of patients exhibit only gastrointestinal manifestations (135).

Mesenteric vessels are affected in 25 to 30 percent of the cases. Branching points are most frequently involved (132). Other systemic manifestations include renal artery vasculitis, central nervous system vasculitis, cutaneous vasculitis, pulmonary vasculitis, mononeuritis multiplex, fever, and musculoskeletal symptoms. Abnormal laboratory findings include a high erythrocyte sedimentation rate, anemia, leukocytosis, and thrombocytosis.

Mesenteric arteriograms are abnormal in up to 80 percent of patients (133). Multiple saccular abdominal fusiform aneurysms as well as arterial tapering and beading are seen throughout the celiac axis.

Gross Findings. The nodular appearance of the vessels is a characteristic but uncommon finding. Well-demarcated ulcers develop on the intestinal antimesenteric border. Resection specimens show varying degrees of ischemic damage. Perforation can be present and is a poor prognostic sign.

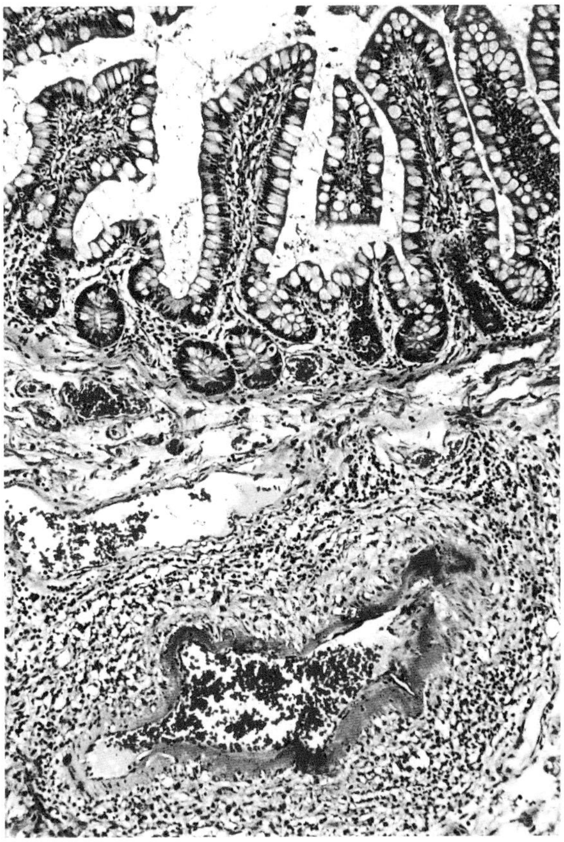

Figure 7-17

POLYARTERITIS NODOSA

Fibrinoid necrosis of the wall of a submucosal artery is associated with a perivascular lymphocytic infiltrate. The overlying mucosa appears normal. (Fig. 3-104 from Emory TS, Carpenter HA, Gostout CJ, Sobin LH. Atlas of gastrointestinal endoscopy & endoscopic biopsies. Washington DC: Armed Forces Institute of Pathology; 2000:225.)

Microscopic Findings. The findings are limited to small and medium-sized arteries. Transmural inflammation and edema of the arterial wall are characteristic (fig. 7-17). The inflammatory infiltrate predominantly consists of neutrophils and eosinophils, with a few mononuclear cells. Fibrinoid necrosis accompanies the inflammation of the arterial wall. Giant cells are absent. Destruction of the arterial wall leads to pseudoaneurysm formation. Superimposed thrombosis can be present. In the resolving and healing stages, the acute inflammation is replaced by predominantly mononuclear inflammation, granulation tissue, and fibrosis of the vessel wall. The bowel wall shows features of ischemia, as described above.

Treatment and Prognosis. Immunosuppressive agents like cyclophosphamide, methotrexate, and steroids are the mainstay of therapy. The presence of gastrointestinal symptoms is suggested to be a poor prognostic factor in patients with PAN (132). Early diagnosis and timely intervention are essential to prevent serious complications.

Henoch-Schönlein Purpura

Definition. *Henoch-Schönlein purpura* (HSP) is a small vessel vasculitis that involves the skin, gastrointestinal tract, kidney, and joints. HSP is a multisystem disorder characterized by a symmetric, nontraumatic, nonthrombotic, painless purpuric rash largely involving the skin of the legs and buttocks, along with arthritis, nephritis, hematuria, and gastrointestinal injury. HSP is also known as *anaphylactoid purpura*.

Demography. HSP is the most common vasculitis in children, although it can develop at any age (142).

Etiology. The vasculitis is caused by immunoglobulin (Ig)A-dominant immune complex deposition in small arteries, capillaries, and venules. HSP results from vascular entrapment of circulating IgA immune complexes. As a result, deposits of IgA, fibrinogen, and C3 lie in vessel walls. Immune complexes, which have a relative absence of other immunoreactants, distinguish HSP from other forms of necrotizing vasculitis because the latter typically contain deposits of IgG or IgM rather than IgA. A number of drugs have been implicated in the genesis of the immune response in HSP. Antigenic stimulation also may result from respiratory tract infections, insect stings, and immunizations.

Clinical Features. Gastrointestinal involvement is present in up to two thirds of children with HSP (143). Abdominal pain precedes the development of typical purpuric spots in 14 to 36 percent of the cases. Patients also present with gastrointestinal bleeding (139). Fifty percent of patients have melena and 15 percent develop hematemesis (140).

Endoscopic Findings. Any bowel segment may be affected, but the duodenum, jejunum, and ileum are the most frequently involved. Endoscopic findings include multiple irregular ulcers, petechiae, and mucosal redness. Hematoma-like protrusions may be seen; these are associated with the presence of leukocytoclastic vasculitis on biopsy (141).

Gross Findings. The bowel appears edematous and congested, with mottling, purulent exudates, and superficial erosions. Transmural infarction is rare. When submucosal hematomas are present, they can act as lead points for intussusception (143).

Microscopic Findings. Variable features of ischemia are present in the vessel walls. The small vessels show fibrinoid necrosis, and neutrophilic and mononuclear infiltrates in the vascular wall and in the perivascular soft tissues (fig. 7-18). Fibrin thrombi may be present. It is prudent to examine the vessels in non-necrotic areas to evaluate the features of vasculitis and determine whether the vascular inflammation is a primary or secondary event.

Treatment and Prognosis. Massive gastrointestinal bleeding, stricture formation, intussusception, and pseudomembranous colitis are complications that can occur in patients with HSP. Intestinal perforation and peritonitis may develop in a few cases.

Microscopic Polyangiitis

Definition. *Microscopic polyangiitis* is a small vessel vasculitis involving arterioles, venules, and capillaries.

Pathophysiology. Unlike HSP and PAN, microscopic polyangiitis is not associated with immune complex deposition. Rather, the disease is associated with the antineutrophil cytoplasmic antibody, p-ANCA. These antibodies are detected by their reactivity against neutrophilic myeloperoxidase. Their titers may fluctuate, sometimes decreasing with treatment or during remission. There is some evidence that ANCAs of IgM subclass are associated with pulmonary hemorrhage and severe glomerulonephritis (145).

Clinical Features. Microscopic polyangiitis is associated with pauci-immune crescentic glomerulonephritis. The kidney is the most common organ involved, followed by lung, skin, and gastrointestinal tract. Gastrointestinal

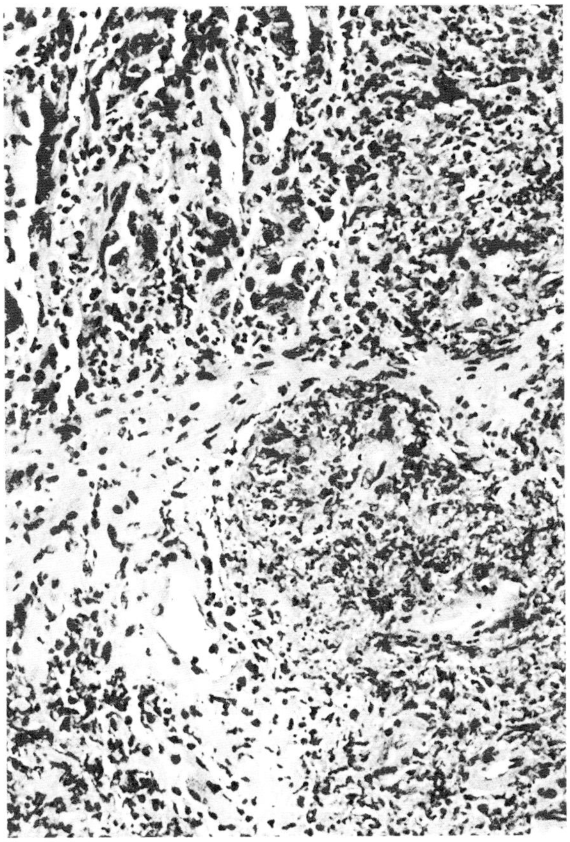

Figure 7-18

HENOCH-SCHÖNLEIN VASCULITIS

Thrombosed submucosal venule with neutrophilic destruction of the vessel wall (leukocytoclastic vasculitis). The mucosa is acutely inflamed, making the underlying vascular lesion difficult to recognize. (Fig. 3-102 from Emory TS, Carpenter HA, Gostout CJ, Sobin LH. Atlas of gastrointestinal endoscopy & endoscopic biopsies. Washington DC: Armed Forces Institute of Pathology; 2000:225.)

symptoms are reported in 29 to 58 percent of cases (144). Abdominal pain is the usual complaint followed by gastrointestinal bleeding. Although common, gastrointestinal symptoms are not usually the presenting complaint in patients with microscopic polyangiitis.

Endoscopic Findings. The endoscopic findings are similar to those described in HSP.

Microscopic Findings. Endoscopic biopsies show features of ischemia and small vessel leukocytoclastic vasculitis as described in HSP (fig. 7-19). Unlike PAN, medium-sized blood vessels are not involved. The diagnosis is primarily based on the identification of extraintestinal manifestations and a positive p-ANCA titer.

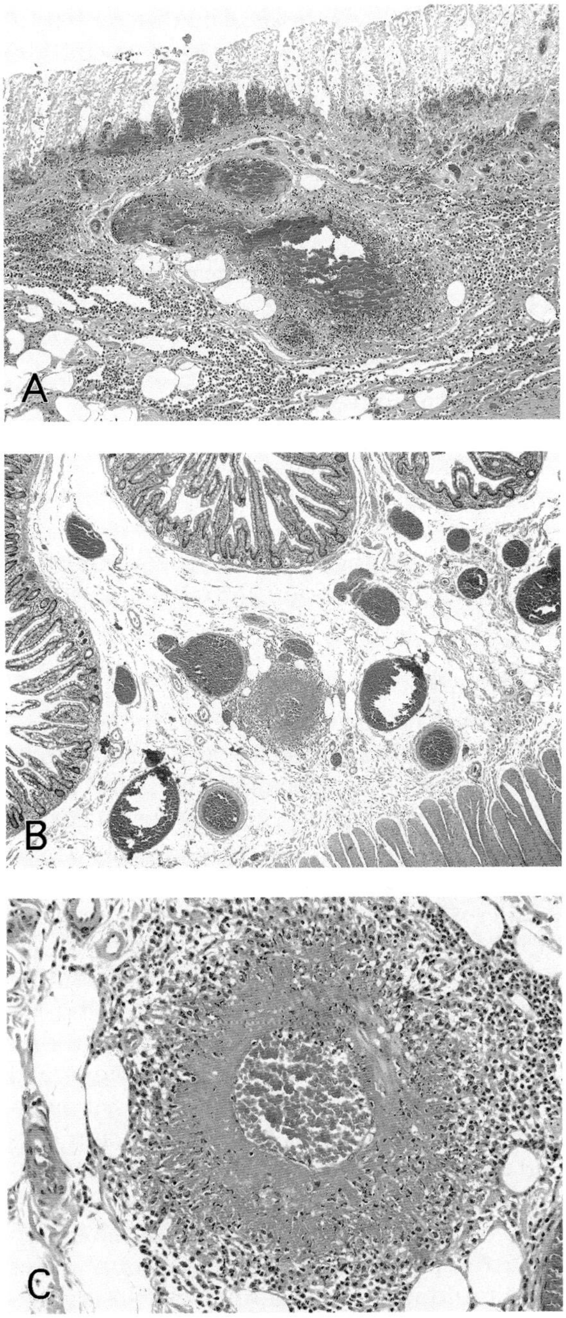

Figure 7-19

MICROSCOPIC POLYANGIITIS

A: The colon has the typical features of ischemic injury. A submucosal vessel appears to be inflamed. In areas of ischemic damage, it is often difficult to separate primary vascular injury from changes that occur secondary to ischemia.

B: Submucosal vessels in areas remote from the ischemic bowel show evidence of vasculitis, confirming a primary vasculitic process.

C: Higher-power view of a small submucosal vessel with active transmural inflammation and fibrinoid necrosis.

Differential Diagnosis. The differential diagnosis includes other small vessel vasculitides including HSP and drug-induced vasculitis. The differential diagnosis of ANCA-associated conditions is shown in Table 7-11.

Treatment and Prognosis. Immunosuppressive agents like cyclophosphamide and steroids are the mainstay of treatment. Close monitoring of renal function is required as patients may develop rapidly progressive glomerulonephritis.

Wegener's Granulomatosis

Definition. *Wegener's granulomatosis* is a granulomatous necrotizing vasculitis that involves small and medium-sized vessels of the upper respiratory tract, lungs, kidney, and gastrointestinal tract.

Pathophysiology. Like microscopic polyangiitis, Wegener's granulomatosis is not associated with immune complex damage. It is associated with the antineutrophil cytoplasmic antibody, c-ANCA (antibody against proteinase 3).

Clinical Features. Gastrointestinal involvement is unusual and the literature is limited to either case reports or small series of cases (147). When Wegener's granulomatosis does affect the gastrointestinal tract, any part may be involved from esophagus to colon (146).

Microscopic Findings. The histologic findings include nonspecific inflammation, ischemia, vasculitis, and granuloma formation. The granulomas characteristically are necrotizing, with palisading epithelioid histiocytes arranged around the necrotic foci. The vasculitis involving small and medium-sized vessels is characterized by infiltration by neutrophils and mononuclear cells and fibrinoid necrosis of the vessel wall. Multinucleated giant cells are frequently present in areas of vasculitis and/or in the granulomas.

Differential Diagnosis. Infectious causes of granulomatous inflammation should always be excluded.

Treatment and Prognosis. Immunosuppressive agents like cyclophosphamide, methotrexate, and steroids are the primary mode of therapy. Plasmapheresis has been suggested as an alternative in certain nonresponsive cases.

Churg-Strauss Syndrome

Definition. *Churg-Strauss syndrome* (CSS) is a small vessel vasculitis that is associated with granulomatous inflammation of the respiratory tract, asthma, and peripheral eosinophilia.

Pathophysiology. CSS belongs to the ANCA-associated pauciimmune vasculitides, along with microscopic polyarteritis and Wegener's granulomatosis. The ANCA-associated vasculitides are compared in Table 7-11.

Clinical Features. Gastrointestinal involvement occurs in 50 percent of patients (148). Abdominal pain, bleeding, and, less often, perforation and infarction are seen (149,150).

Gross Findings. Resection specimens show multiple ulcers of irregular size and shape. The ulcers may be deep and associated with perforation.

Microscopic Findings. Gastrointestinal involvement includes transmural eosinophilic infiltration of the stomach and duodenum resembling eosinophilic gastroenteritis, as well as multiple gastric, small intestinal, and colonic ulcers (151). Histologic examination shows small and medium-sized vessel vasculitis, necrotizing granulomas, and increased tissue eosinophils (fig. 7-20). The vasculitis involves both arteries and veins, and can be seen at all levels of the intestinal wall. Patchy areas of infarction are associated with the vasculitis.

Differential Diagnosis. The differential diagnosis includes other ANCA-associated vasculitides

Table 7-11

DISEASES ASSOCIATED WITH ANTINEUTROPHIL CYTOPLASMIC ANTIBODIES

Association with c-antineutrophil cytoplasmic antibody (ANCA)
Wegener's granulomatosis
Polyarteritis
Association with p-ANCA
Idiopathic crescentric glomerulonephritis
Churg-Strauss syndrome
Polyarteritis nodosa with visceral involvement
Ulcerative colitis
Crohn's disease with presentation resembling that of ulcerative colitis
Rheumatoid arthritis
Chronic hepatitis
Primary sclerosing cholangitis
Primary biliary cirrhosis

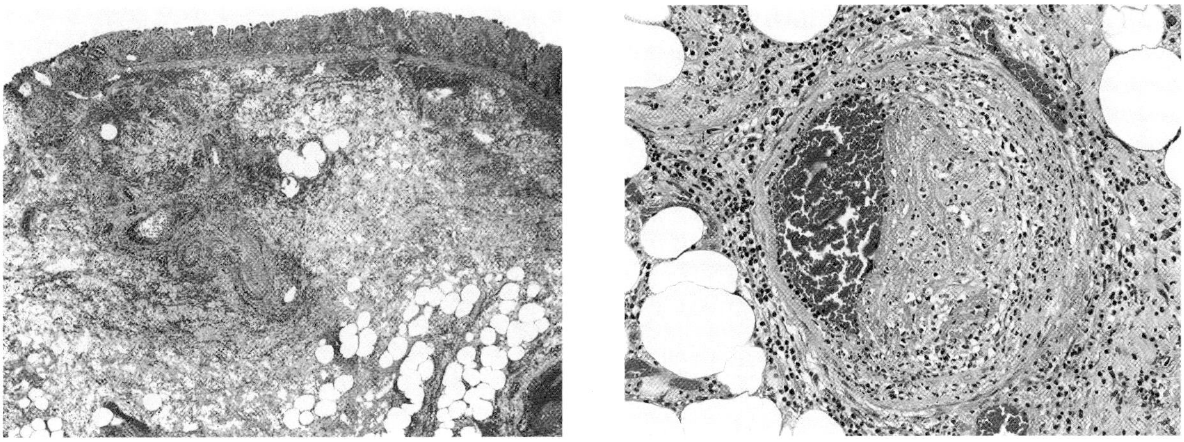

Figure 7-20

CHURG-STRAUSS SYNDROME

Left: A cluster of colonic submucosal vessels shows evidence of vasculitis. The overlying mucosa is ischemic.
Right: A submucosal vein is partially thrombosed and infiltrated by inflammatory cells, many of which are eosinophils. Numerous eosinophils are also present in the surrounding stroma. (Courtesy of Dr. John Hart, University of Chicago, Chicago, IL.)

(Table 7-11) and conditions associated with gastrointestinal mucosal eosinophilia. Correlation with systemic manifestations and laboratory results is required to exclude CSS as a possible cause of mucosal eosinophilia. If pulmonary manifestations are present, CSS should be differentiated from allergic bronchopulmonary aspergillosis. The presence of invasive fungal organisms in the lung biopsy is a diagnostic feature of the latter.

Treatment and Prognosis. Cyclophosphamide and steroids are effective in most cases. High-dose intravenous immunoglobulin is used in resistant cases.

Kawasaki's Disease

Definition. *Kawasaki's disease* is an acute febrile illness associated with vasculitis of medium-sized arteries.

Demography. Kawasaki's disease usually occurs in children, with a peak incidence in the first year of life (154).

Etiology. The pathogenesis of the disease is unknown. Several theories have been proposed, including the possibility of infection by a toxin-producing microorganism and of a superantigen-driven process (153). The vasculitis results from an immunoregulatory defect characterized by T-cell activation, secretion of cytokines, polyclonal B-cell activation, and production of autoantibodies to endothelial or smooth muscle cells.

Clinical Features. The hallmark of Kawasaki's disease is the mucocutaneous lymph node syndrome, which includes an erythematous rash, mucositis of the oropharyngeal mucosa, conjunctivitis, and nonsuppurative lymphadenitis. Kawasaki's disease often has a component of necrotizing arteritis, which affects medium-sized blood vessels. Kawasaki's disease is a leading cause of acquired heart disease in children in the United States.

Gastrointestinal involvement is rare. When it does occur, it can be of several types, including focal mucositis and focal colitis (152). Intestinal pseudoobstruction and massive gastrointestinal hemorrhage have also been described.

Microscopic Findings. Histologic findings include features of ischemia, vasculitis affecting medium-sized blood vessels, and nonspecific acute and chronic colitis. The vasculitis is similar to that seen in polyarteritis nodosa; however, the degree of necrosis is often less in the vasculitis associated with Kawasaki's disease as compared to PAN. It is necessary to differentiate Kawasaki's disease from PAN, as therapy is different. Differentiation is primarily based on extraintestinal manifestations.

Treatment and Prognosis. Intravenous immunoglobulin is often effective in controlling the progression and coronary artery involvement in Kawasaki's disease. The prognosis is worse if the coronary artery is involved.

Thromboangiitis Obliterans

Definition. *Thromboangiitis obliterans* (TAO) is a nonarteriosclerotic, segmental, progressive, inflammatory vasoocclusive disease of unknown etiology. It is also known as *Buerger's disease*.

Demography. TAO occurs almost exclusively in susceptible young men who are habitual tobacco users, usually with onset of symptoms before the age of 40 years. The condition is far more common in Japan, India, and Israel than in the United States and Europe. There is an increased prevalence of the disease in patients with human leukocyte antigen (HLA)-A9, HLA-B5, and HLA-DRB1.

Etiology. TAO affects the small and medium-sized arteries and veins of the extremities. Its etiology is unknown. The endothelial injury may be caused by tobacco, cellular toxins produced during the phagocytosis of smoking byproducts, or immune complexes.

Clinical Features. TAO is primarily a disease affecting the arteries of the distal extremities. Common symptoms are claudication, loss of skin turgor, and hair loss. In advanced stages of the disease, ischemic ulcerations with gangrenous necrosis develop.

Gastrointestinal involvement is rare; less than 100 such cases have been described in the literature. Mesenteric arteries are most frequently involved, followed by small vessels. Mesenteric TAO can present as acute or chronic ischemia (155), although chronic ischemia is more common. Patients also present with intestinal obstruction due to stricture and fibrosis. Acute mesenteric ischemia may lead to gastrointestinal bleeding, acute abdominal pain, and peritonitis.

Gross Findings. The gross intestinal findings are similar to those of other forms of ischemia. Acute ischemic injury is characterized by areas of ulceration, mucosal edema, congestion, and perforation. Chronic ischemia shows fibrosis, stricture, and atrophy of the intestinal wall. The lumens of small to medium-sized mesenteric vessels may be narrowed.

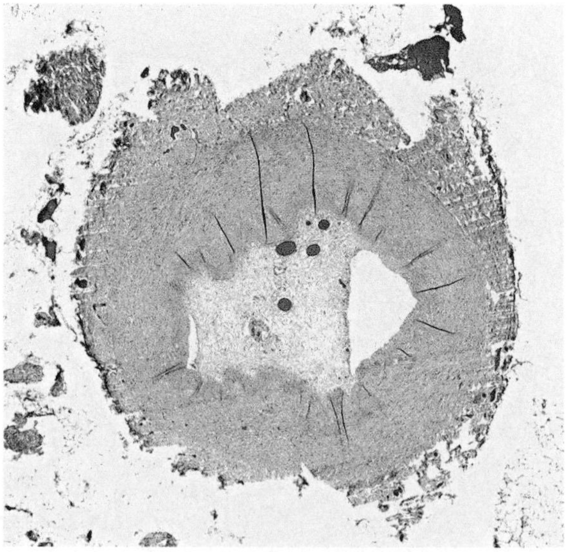

Figure 7-21

THROMBOANGIITIS OBLITERANS

A mesenteric vessel in a patient with extensive colonic ischemic necrosis secondary to thromboangiitis obliterans. The vessel lumen is almost completely obliterated by a proliferation of fibrous tissue.

Microscopic Findings. The histologic findings are those of acute and chronic ischemia. Acute and chronic inflammation permeates the arterial walls, accompanied by organized and recanalized vascular thrombosis (fig. 7-21). Characteristically, vascular thrombi contain small microabscesses, with aggregates of neutrophils surrounded by macrophages and lymphocytes.

Differential Diagnosis. An absence of medial necrosis and the nature of the associated extraintestinal manifestations distinguish TAO from PAN.

Treatment and Prognosis. Treatment depends upon whether the ischemic injury is acute or chronic. Smoking cessation is recommended for all patients. Intestinal perforation with peritonitis is the most prevalent fatal complication of the disease.

Malignant Atrophic Papulosis

Definition. *Malignant atrophic papulosis*, also termed *Kohlmeier-Degos disease*, is a rare multisystem vasculopathic disorder (158,160).

Demography. Malignant atrophic papulosis occurs most commonly in early adulthood. The disease is occasionally familial.

Etiology. The etiopathogenesis is unknown. It may be an immune complex-mediated noninflammatory vasculopathy (161).

Clinical Features. Cutaneous lesions are the initial manifestation, followed by multisystem involvement (157). Some patients with gastrointestinal involvement are asymptomatic while others present with acute abdominal symptoms, intestinal infarction, and perforation. Malabsorption due to widespread involvement of the intestines may develop (162).

Gross Findings. The characteristic gastrointestinal lesions on gross examination are conical infarcts associated with thrombi.

Microscopic Findings. The small and medium-sized vessels are affected. Early lesions consist of cellular proliferation and intimal edema. In intermediate lesions, the edema is replaced by smooth muscle proliferation. In late lesions, there is acellular intimal sclerosis with hyalinization and obliteration of the lumen. The media of the vessels remains intact in almost all cases (161). The intestine shows a variable degree of ischemic injury. The intestinal disease is recurrent and frequently fatal (158).

Differential Diagnosis. Although the vascular lesions resemble those seen in lupus erythematosus, the patients may or may not have other features of the disease (156,160).

Segmental Arterial Mediolysis

Definition. *Segmental arterial mediolysis* (SAM), formerly known as *segmental mediolytic arteritis*, is a rare condition involving abdominal splanchnic and epicardial arteries (165).

Demography. Abdominal SAM generally affects elderly individuals, whereas coronary SAM affects neonates, children, and young adults.

Etiology. The etiopathogenesis of this condition is uncertain. A proposed mechanism is an inappropriate vasospastic response in the splanchnic vascular bed in response to shock or severe hypoxemia (164). SAM may be a precursor lesion of fibromuscular dysplasia (165).

Gross Findings. This entity is most commonly encountered in resection specimens or at the time of autopsy. Aneurysms and dissecting hematomas also develop due to extensive mediolysis (165).

Microscopic Findings. Histologically, outer mediolysis expands the vascular mid and inner media. Accompanying alterations include fibrinous linear deposits at the junction of media and adventitia, and replacement of the lysed media by erythrocytes, fibrin, and granulation tissue. Inflammation is inconstant and limited to periadventitial tissues. Ultrastructural examination reveals transformation of the cytoplasmic contents of arterial medial smooth muscle into a maze of dilated edematous vacuoles.

Treatment and Prognosis. Acute abdominal hemorrhage is the most serious complication (163). Elderly patients also present with chronic intestinal ischemia.

Marfan's and Ehlers-Danlos Syndromes

Patients with *Marfan's* and *Ehlers-Danlos syndromes* develop gastrointestinal complications due to defective collagen synthesis. These include megaesophagus, intestinal hypomotility, giant jejunal diverticula, megacolon, and bacterial overgrowth (166). Aneurysmal dilatation of the mesenteric arteries is caused by the disruption of the collagen fibers in the media. Medial hemorrhage may occur. In severe cases, mesenteric artery rupture and intestinal infarction occur (167).

GASTROINTESTINAL INVOLVEMENT IN COLLAGEN VASCULAR DISEASES

Systemic Lupus Erythematosus

Definition. *Systemic lupus erythematosus* (SLE) is a multisystem autoimmune disorder that encompasses a wide range of clinical manifestations and autoantibody production.

Demography. Gastrointestinal complaints are frequent in SLE patients. Gastrointestinal vasculitis, a devastating complication of SLE, affects only 2 percent of patients (172).

Etiology. Although the exact etiology of SLE is unknown, a number of autoantibodies are associated with the disease. The most specific antibodies are anti-double stranded DNA and anti-Sm antibodies. Genetic factors have also been suggested to play a role, since family members have a high risk of developing SLE. Up to 20 percent of clinically unaffected relatives have detectable autoantibodies.

Clinical Features. Gastrointestinal symptoms are common in SLE patients. Acute abdominal pain is the usual presentation. Other symptoms include nausea, vomiting, and heartburn due to esophageal dysmotility. Malabsorption has also been described (168). There is no difference in age, sex, or autoantibody profile in patients with or without gastrointestinal vasculitis. No laboratory tests help differentiate patients with and without gastrointestinal vasculitis (170).

Gross Findings. The gross findings vary with the stage and severity of the gastrointestinal involvement. In severe acute disease, features of acute ischemia with ulceration are present. In chronic damage, the vasculitis leads to atrophy and thinning of the intestinal wall.

Microscopic Findings. The vasculitis primarily affects areas of the bowel supplied by the superior mesenteric artery, including the jejunum and ileum (170). Small vessel vasculitis involves arteries and venules. The necrotizing vasculitis is frequently associated with bowel necrosis.

Other pathologic changes seen in the gastrointestinal tract include dysmotility due to atrophy of muscle fibers, heterotopic calcification of gastric mucosa, peptic ulceration, vascular ectasia, severe mucus inspissation in intestine, serositis, hemorrhagic ileocolitis, and intussusception (169,171).

Differential Diagnosis. The differential diagnosis includes other causes of vasculitis. The final diagnosis depends on the systemic manifestations of the disease and the detection of autoantibodies.

Treatment and Prognosis. The vasculitis leads to bowel perforation, peritonitis, and fatality in some cases.

Rheumatoid Arthritis

Definition. *Rheumatoid arthritis* (RA) is an autoimmune disorder that primarily affects the musculoskeletal system but may involve multiple systems including the gastrointestinal tract.

Demography. Approximately 10 percent of patients with RA have gastrointestinal involvement (173).

Clinical Features. Patients with RA may demonstrate esophageal dysmotility due to atrophy of the muscularis propria, peptic ulcer disease, malabsorption, amyloidosis, and NSAID-induced gastrointestinal injury; the latter is the most common finding. Fewer patients develop gastrointestinal vasculitis, the most serious complication of the disease.

Rheumatoid vasculitis is seen 1 percent of patients. It appears in the setting of severe arthritis, rheumatoid nodules, and high titers of rheumatoid factor. These patients often have cutaneous vasculitis and peripheral neuritis.

Microscopic Findings. RA vasculitis involves the vessels in the intestinal wall or mesentery. Occasionally, patients develop proliferative endarteritis characterized by intimal proliferation without vascular wall inflammation or necrosis. Visceral aneurysms may develop that cause intraabdominal hemorrhage. Ischemic mucosal ulceration, bowel necrosis, perforation, pancolitis, and appendicitis have all been reported (fig. 7-22).

Treatment and Prognosis. The prognosis for patients with gastrointestinal vasculitis varies depending on whether bowel perforation has occurred or not. Patients with perforation and late-stage ischemic injury have a poor prognosis.

Behcet's Disease

Definition. *Behcet's disease* is a syndrome of oral, genital, and ocular inflammation and ulceration.

Demography. The gastrointestinal tract is infrequently involved in Behcet's disease. The disease is more common in Japan than in Western countries. Intestinal involvement is most common in men in their 4th and 5th decades.

Etiology. The underlying disease is a vasculitis involving small and large vessels.

Clinical Features. The terminal ileum and cecum are the most frequently involved gastrointestinal sites (174,175).

Gross and Endoscopic Findings. Endoscopically, the intestine shows single or multiple ulcers. Most of the ulcers are round to oval in shape. The ulcers are deep and the margins are discrete (176). They develop on the antimesenteric aspect of the intestine and exhibit a marked tendency to irregularly undermine surrounding tissues (177). Edema-like swelling with crater formation characteristically produces a "collar stud" appearance.

Microscopic Findings. Histologically, the ulcer base frequently shows either a remnant of an underlying Peyer patch or a destroyed lymphoid follicle (177). Mononuclear inflammation around the vessels, intimal thickening, thrombosis, and necrotizing lymphocytic

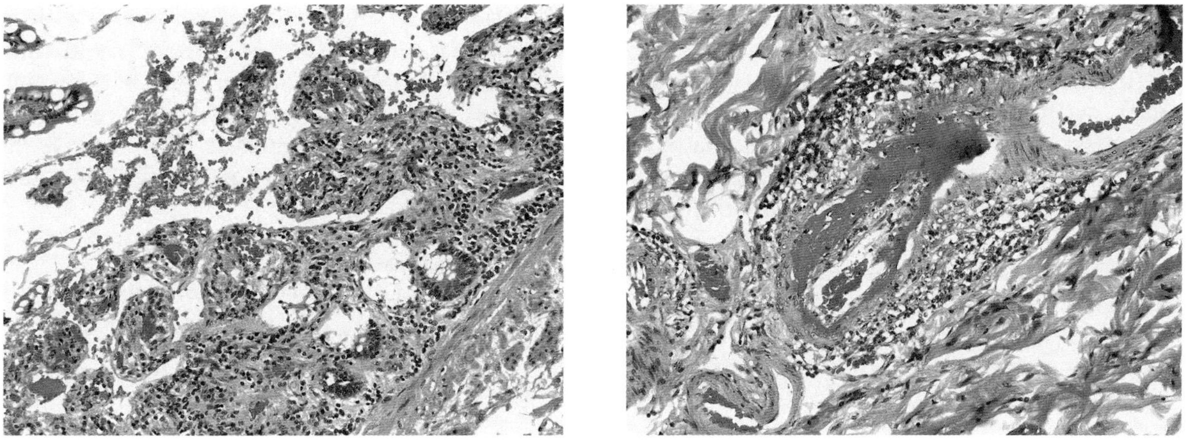

Figure 7-22

RHEUMATOID ARTHRITIS: ISCHEMIC ENTERITIS

Left: The small intestinal mucosa shows congestion and loss of the epithelium overlying the villi.
Right: Many of the submucosal vessels show prominent vasculitis associated with fibrinoid necrosis of the vessel wall.

vasculitis affecting small venules are the usual histologic features. In chronic lesions, marked submucosal fibrosis is present. Granulomas are absent. The histologic features are not specific, however, and extraintestinal manifestations are used to diagnose the disease.

Differential Diagnosis. The most common entity in the differential diagnosis is Crohn's disease. The diagnosis is primarily based on the clinical findings. The presence of granulomas, neural hyperplasia, and minimal vascular congestion favors a diagnosis of Crohn's disease.

Mesenteric Inflammatory Venoocclusive Disease

Definition. *Mesenteric inflammatory venoocclusive disease* (MIVOD) is a slowly progressive, chronic ischemic condition characterized by the inflammation of veins of the intestinal wall and pericolonic soft tissue. *Lymphocytic phlebitis* is another term for the disease.

Demography. MIVOD is a rare cause of digestive tract ischemia (180). It occurs twice as often in men as in women, and patients range in age from 24 to 78 years (181).

Clinical Features. Unexplained ischemia is the most common presentation. Patients do not have systemic disease. The diagnosis is possible only after examination of the resection specimen.

Gross Findings. Gross examination shows features of chronic ischemia as described earlier.

Microscopic Findings. The disorder selectively affects veins and venules in the submucosa, subserosa, and pericolonic soft tissue (179). Arteries and arterioles are free of inflammation. The phlebitis consists of varying degrees of lymphocytic and/or granulomatous inflammation, with or without necrosis (178). Myointimal hyperplasia is also present. There may be associated thrombosis.

Microscopic Variants. *Idiopathic myointimal hyperplasia of the mesenteric vein* is a rare cause of chronic intestinal ischemia. It is considered to be an end stage of MIVOD. Histologically, the disorder is characterized by thick-walled, bizarre, hypertrophic, arterialized veins located in the submucosa and mesentery (178).

Differential Diagnosis. It is necessary to exclude other causes of vasculitis affecting small veins, including drug-induced vasculitis, Behcet's disease, vascular changes secondary to enterocolic inflammation, and lymphoproliferative disorders.

Treatment and Prognosis. The disease appears to have an indolent course following surgery (178).

Mesenteric Phlebosclerosis

Definition. *Mesenteric phlebosclerosis* is a rare chronic ischemic condition affecting small mesenteric veins.

Demography. This rare nonthrombotic stenosis of mesenteric veins is primarily described in Asian populations. Affected patients range from 36 to 73 years of age.

Clinical Features. The disease has a gradual onset, with progression over the course of several months to years. Right lower quadrant pain and diarrhea are the usual presenting symptoms. Gastrointestinal bleeding is uncommon.

Gross Findings. Endoscopically, the bowel appears edematous, the normal vascular pattern disappears, the mucosa is bluish black, and lumens are narrowed. The disease is characterized by a continuous distribution variably extending from the terminal ileum to the colon. The right colon is the most frequently and severely affected site. The rectum is not involved and there are no skip lesions.

Gross examination of the resection specimen shows thickening of the colonic wall, disappearance of plica semilunares, and a dusky mucosa. The cut surface of the intestinal wall appears dark purple and semielastic.

Radiographic Findings. Radiographic studies are helpful in establishing the diagnosis (182-184). Plain films show multiple thread-like calcifications along the right hemicolon. Abdominal CT scans show marked thickening of and calcifications along the colonic wall. Superior mesenteric artery angiography shows tortuosity of the vasa recta and dilatation and tortuosity of veins along the vasa recta.

Microscopic Findings. Endoscopic biopsies show features of chronic ischemia. The diagnosis is based on correlating the pathologic findings with the characteristic radiographic appearance. A range of changes is present in resection specimens. The mucosa appears congested, edematous, and fibrotic. The epithelium shows features of ischemia with neutrophilic infiltrates in the superficial epithelium. Hemosiderin-laden macrophages are also present.

The distinctive features seen in the colonic wall are marked fibrous mural thickening, calcification of small mesenteric veins, deposition of collagen around the blood vessels, and the presence of foamy macrophages within the walls of blood vessels.

Treatment and Prognosis. The long-term outcome of patients with this condition is currently not known.

ISCHEMIA DUE TO COAGULATION DISORDERS

Diseases leading to microangiopathic thrombosis can involve the gastrointestinal tract (Table 7-10). These include *hemolytic uremic syndrome/thrombotic thrombocytopenic purpura (HUS/TTP), homocystinuria, factor V Leiden mutation, paroxysmal nocturnal hematuria*, and *disseminated intravascular coagulation.*

HUS/TTP is caused by toxin-producing enteric bacteria (see chapter 10). Gastrointestinal involvement is frequent in children with HUS. About 20 percent of adults with HUS/TTP have abdominal complaints. Thrombosis of small submucosal vessels and associated intramural hemorrhage are characteristic findings. In severe cases, intestinal perforation and peritonitis develop.

Patients with clotting factor abnormalities (factor V Leiden mutation, protein C and S deficiencies) have features resembling those seen in HUS/TTP. Patients with homocystinuria develop episodic thrombosis followed by fibroblastic intimal proliferation of medium-sized arteries.

ISCHEMIA CAUSED BY INFECTIONS

A number of infections involve the gastrointestinal vasculature. Fungal and cytomegalovirus infections are the most common offenders. Schistosomiasis has been shown to involve the gastrointestinal vasculature in rare case studies (185). These infections are discussed in greater detail in chapter 10.

REFERENCES

Demography of Ischemia

1. Bacon PA. Vasculitis—clinical aspects and therapy. Acta Med Scand Suppl 1987;715:157–63.
2. Feldman M, Friedman LS, Sleisenger MH, eds. Sleisenger & Fordtran's gastrointestinal and liver disease: pathophysiology, diagnosis, management, vol 2, 7th ed. Philadelphia: Saunders; 2002:2324–5.
3. Krupski W, Selzman C, Whitehall T. Unusual causes of mesenteric ischemia. Surg Clin North Am 1997;77:471–502.
4. Robson WL, Leung AK. Henoch-Schonlein purpura. Adv Pediatr 1994;41:163–94.

Etiology of Ischemia

5. Anantharaju A, Van Thiel DH. Nonocclusive mesenteric ischemia: reality. J Gastroenterol 2002;37:876.
6. Mckinsey JF, Gewertz BL. Acute mesenteric ischemia. Surg Clin North Am 1997;77:307–18.

Pathophysiology of Ischemia

7. Bulkley GB, Kvietys PR, Parks DA, et al. Relationship of blood flow and oxygen consumption to ischemic injury in the canine small intestine. Gastroenterology 1985;89:852–7.
8. Filez L, Stalmans W, Penninckx F, Kerremans R. Influences of ischemia and reperfusion on the feline small-intestinal mucosa. J Surg Res 1990;49:157–63.
9. Norris HT. Re-examination of the spectrum of ischemic bowel disease. In: Norris HT, ed. Pathology of the colon, small intestine, and anus. New York: Churchill Livingstone; 1983:109.
10. Rhodes RS, DePalma RG. Mitochondrial dysfunction of the liver and hypoglycemia in hemorrhagic shock. Surg Gynecol Obstet 1980;150: 347–52.

Pathophysiology of Ischemic Damage and Reperfusion Injury

11. Granger DN. Intestinal microcirculation and transmucosal fluid transport. Am J Physiol 1981;240:G343–9.
12. Granger DN, Hollwarth ME, Parks DA. Ischemia-reperfusion injury: role of oxygen-derived free radicals. Acta Physiol Scand (Suppl) 1986;548: 47–63.
13. Granger DN, Rutili G, McCord JM. Superoxide radicals in feline intestinal ischemia. Gastroenterology 1981;81:22–9.
14. Park PO, Haglund U, Bulkley GB, Falt K. The sequence of development of intestinal tissue injury following strangulation ischemia and reperfusion. Surgery 1990;107:574–80.
15. Schoenberg MH, Fredholm BB, Haglund U, et al. Studies on the oxygen radical mechanism involved in the small intestinal reperfusion damage. Acta Physiol Scand 1985;124:581–9.

Role of Oxygen Free Radicals

16. Beckman JS, Beckman TW, Chen J, Marshall PA, Freeman BA. Apparent hydroxyl radical production by peroxynitrite: implications for endothelial injury from nitric oxide and superoxide. Proc Natl Acad Sci USA 1990;87:1620–4.
17. Berezin I, Snyder SH, Bredt DS, Daniel EE. Ultrastructural localization of nitric oxide synthase in canine small intestine and colon. Am J Physiol 1994;266:C981–9.
18. Blake DR, Allen RE, Lunec J. Free radicals in biological systems—a review oriented to inflammatory processes. Br Med Bull 1987;43:371–85.
19. Bounous G. Acute necrosis of the intestinal mucosa. Gastroenterology 1982;82:1457–67.
20. Chaudry IH, Clemens MG, Baue AE. Alterations in cell function with ischemia and shock and their correction. Arch Surg 1981;116:1309–17.
21. Fitzpatrick DB, Karmazyn M. Comparative effects of calcium channel blocking agents and varying extracellular calcium concentrations on hypoxia-reoxygenation ischemia-reperfusion-induced cardiac injury. J Pharmacol Exp Ther 1984;228:761–8.
22. Frederiks W, Marx F, Kooij A. The effect of ischaemia on xanthine oxidase activity in rat intestine and liver. Int J Exp Pathol 1993;74:21–6.
23. Granger DN. Role of xanthine oxidase and granulocytes in ischemia-reperfusion injury. Am J Physiol 1988;255:H1269–75.
24. Grisham MB, Granger DN. Neutrophil-mediated mucosal injury. Role of reactive oxygen metabolites. Dig Dis Sci 1988;33:6S–15S.
25. Gutteridge GM, Rowley DA, Halliwell B, Westermarck T. Increased non-protein-bound iron and decreased protection against superoxide-radical damage in cerebrospinal fluid from patients with neuronal ceroid lipofuscinoses. Lancet 1982;2:459–60.
26. Haglund U. Gut ischaemia. Gut 1994;35(Suppl 1):S73–6.
27. Halliwell B. Oxidants and human disease: some new concepts. FASEB J 1987;1:358–64.
28. Halliwell B, Aruoma OI. DNA damage by oxygen-derived species. FEBS Lett 1991;281:9–19.

29. Halliwell B, Gutteridge JM. Free Radicals in biology and medicine, 2nd ed. Oxford: Clarendon Press; 1989.
30. Kellogg EW 3rd, Fridovich I. Superoxide, hydrogen peroxide and singlet oxygen in lipid peroxidation by a xanthine oxidase system. J Biol Chem 1975;250:8812–7.
31. Kubes P, Granger DN. Nitric oxide modulates microvascular permeability. Am J Physiol 1992; 262:H611–5.
32. Kukreja RC, Hess ML. The oxygen free radical system: from equations through membrane protein interactions to cardiovascular injury and protection. Cardiovasc Res 1992;26:641–55.
33. Nilsson UA, Schoenberg MH, Aneman A, et al. Free radicals and pathogenesis during ischemia and reperfusion of the cat small intestine. Gastroenterology 1994;106:629–36.
34. Salzman AL. Nitric oxide in the gut. New Horizons 1995;3:352–64.
35. Sandritter WA, Reid UN. Morphology of liver cell necrosis. In: Keppler D, ed. Pathogenesis and mechanisms of liver cell necrosis. Lancaster: MTP Press; 1975:1.
36. Svingen BA, O'Neal FO, Aust SD. The role of superoxide and singlet oxygen in lipid peroxidation. Photochem Photobiol 1978;28:803–9.
37. Tsao PS, Lefer AM. Time course and mechanism of endothelial dysfunction in isolated ischemic and hypoxic perfused rat hearts. Am J Physiol 1990;259:H1660–6.
38. Weiss SJ. Oxygen, ischaemia and inflammation. Acta Physiol Scand Suppl 1986;548:9–37.
39. Weiss SJ. Tissue destruction by neutrophils. N Engl J Med 1989;320:365–76.
40. Williams JG. Phagocytes, toxic oxygen metabolites and inflammatory bowel disease: implications of treatment. Ann R Coll Surg Engl 1990;72:253–62.
41. Zimmerman BJ, Granger DN. Oxygen free radicals and the gastrointestinal tract: role in ischemia-reperfusion injury. Hepatogastroenterology 1994;41:337–42.
42. Zweier J, Kuppusamy P, Lutty GA. Measurement of endothelial cell free radical generation: evidence for a central mechanism of free radical injury in post-ischemic tissues. Proc Natl Acad Sci USA 1988;85:4046–50.

Role of Neutrophils

43. Arfors KE, Lundberg C, Lindbom L, Lundberg K, Beatty PG, Harlan JM. A monoclonal antibody to the membrane glycoprotein complex CD 18 inhibits polymorphonuclear leukocyte accumulation and plasma leakage *in vivo*. Blood 1987;69:338–40.
44. Arndt H, Kubes P, Granger DN. Involvement of neutrophils in ischemia-reperfusion injury in the small intestine. Klin Wochenschr 1991;69:1056–60.
45. Bevilacqua M, Butcher E, Furie B, et al. Selectins: a family of adhesion receptors. Cell 1991;67: 233.
46. Caty MG, Guice KS, Oldham KT, Remick DG, Kunkel SI. Evidence for tumor necrosis factor-induced pulmonary microvascular injury after intestinal ischemia-reperfusion injury. Ann Surg 1990;212:694–700.
47. Harlan JM. Leukocyte-endothelial interactions. Blood 1985;65:513–25.
48. Harlan JM, Killen PD, Senecal FM, et al. The role of neutrophil membrane glycoprotein GP-150 in neutrophil adherence to endothelium in vitro. Blood 1985;66:167–78.
49. Kishimoto TK, Jutila MA, Berg EL, Butcher EC. Neutrophil Mac-1 and MEL-14 adhesion proteins inversely regulated by chemotactic factors. Science 1989;245:1238–41.
50. Mangino MJ, Anderson CB, Murphy MK, Brunt E, Turk J. Mucosal arachidonate metabolism and intestinal ischemia-reperfusion injury. Am J Physiol 1989;257:G299–307.
51. Milhoan K, Lane T, Bloor C. Hypoxia induces endothelial cells to increase their adherence for neutrophils: role of PAF. Am J Physiol 1992; 263:H956–62.
52. Smith CW. Transendothelial migration. In: Harlan JM, Liu DY, eds. Adhesion: its roles in inflammatory disease. New York: WH Freeman; 1992:83.
53. Welbourn CR, Goldman G, Paterson IS, et al. Pathophysiology of ischaemia-reperfusion injury: central role of the neutrophil. Br J Surg 1991;78:651–5.
54. Zimmerman GA, Prescott SM, McIntyre TM. Endothelial cell interactions with granulocytes: tethering and signal molecules. Immunol Today 1992;13:93–100.

Loss of Mucosal Barrier

55. Acheson DW, Luccioli S. Mucosal immune responses. Best Pract Res Clin Gastroenterol 2004;18:387–404.
56. Ayabe T, Satchell DP, Wilson CL, Parks WC, Selsted ME, Ouellette AJ. Secretion of microbicidal alpha-defensins by intestinal Paneth cells in response to bacteria. Nature Immunology 2000;1:113–8.
57. Haglund U. Gastro-intestinal mucosal injury in shock. In: Vincent JL, ed. Update in intensive care and emergency medicine. Berlin: Springer-Verlag; 1991:154.

58. Kindon H, Pothoulakis C, Thim L, Lynch-Devaney K, Podolsky DK. Trefoil peptide protection of intestinal epithelial barrier function cooperation interaction with mucin glycoprotein. Gastroenterology 1995;109:516–23.
59. Maury J, Nicoletti C, Guzzo-Chambraud L, Maroux S. The filamentous brush border glycocalyx. A mucin-like marker of enterocyte hyperpolarization. Eur J Biochem 1995;228:323–31.
60. Mayer L. Mucosal immunity. Pediatrics 2003; 111:1595–600.

Acute Mesenteric Ischemia

61. Abdu RA, Zakhour BJ, Dallis DJ. Mesenteric venous thrombosis—1911 to 1984. Surgery 1987;101:383–8.
62. Acosta S, Nilsson TK, Bjork M. Preliminary study of D-dimer as a possible marker of acute bowel ischemia. Br J Surg 2001;88:385–8.
63. Arvidsson D, Rasmussen I, Almqvist P, Niklasson F, Haglund U. Splanchnic oxygen consumption in septic and hemorrhagic shock. Surgery 1991;2:190–7.
64. Bakal CW, Sprayregen S, Wolf EL. Radiology in intestinal ischemia. Angiographic diagnosis and management. Surg Clin North Am 1992;72: 125–41.
65. Bartnicke BJ, Balfe DM. CT appearance of intestinal ischemia and intramural hemorrhage. Radiol Clin North Am 1994;32:845–60.
66. Boley SJ, Brandt LJ, Sammartano RJ. History of mesenteric ischemia. The evolution of a diagnosis and management. Surg Clin North Am 1997;77;275–88.
67. Boley SJ, Feinstein FR, Sammartano R, Brandt LJ, Sprayregen S. New concepts in the management of superior mesenteric artery embolus. Surg Gynecol Obstet 1981;153:561–9.
68. Boley SJ, Kaleya RN, Brandt IJ. Mesenteric venous thrombosis. Surg Clin North Am 1992; 72:183–201.
69. Boley SJ, Sprayregen S, Veith FJ, et al. An aggressive roentgenologic and surgical approach to acute mesenteric ischemia. In: Nyhus LM, ed. Surgery annual. New York: Appleton-Century-Crofits;1973:355.
70. Boos S. Angiography of the mesenteric artery 1976 to 1991: a change in the indication during mesenteric circulatory disorders. Radiologe 1992;32:154–7.
71. Bowersox JC, Zwolak RM, Walsh DB, et al. Duplex ultrasonography in the diagnosis of celiac and mesenteric artery occlusive disease. J Vasc Surg 1991;14:780–6.
72. Bradbury AW, Brittenden J, McBride K, Ruckley CV. Mesenteric ischemia: a multidisciplinary approach. Br J Surg 1995;82:1446–59.
73. Brandt LJ, Boley SJ. AGA technical review on intestinal ischemia. Gastroenterology 2000;118: 954–68.
74. Burns BJ, Brandt LJ. Intestinal ischemia. Gastroenterol Clin N Am 2003;32:1127–43.
75. Civetta JM, Kolodny M. Mesenteric venous thrombosis associated with oral contraceptives. Gastroenterology 1970;58:713–6.
76. Clavien PA, Huber O, Mirescu D, Rohner A. Contrast enhanced CT scan as a diagnostic procedure in mesenteric ischemia due to mesenteric venous thrombosis. Br J Surg 1989;76:93–4.
77. Clouse LH, Comp PC. The regulation of hemostasis: the protein C system. N Engl J Med 1986;314:1298–304.
78. Comp PC, Esmon CT. Recurrent venous thromboembolism in patients with a partial deficiency of protein S. N Engl J Med 1984;311:1525–8.
79. Cosgriff TM, Bishop DT, Hershgold EJ, et al. Familial antithrombin III deficiency: its natural history, genetics, diagnosis and treatment. Medicine 1983;62:209–20.
80. Dahn MS, Lange P, Lobdell K, Hans B, Jacobs LA, Mitchell RA. Splanchnic and total body oxygen consumption differences in septic and injured patients. Surgery 1987;101:69–80.
81. Egeberg O. Inherited antithrombin deficiency causing thrombophilia. Thromb Diath Haemorrh 1965;13:516.
82. Fitzgerald SF, Kminski DL. Ischemic colitis. Semin Colon Rectal Surg 1998;4:222–8.
83. Grendell JH, Ockner RK. Mesenteric venous thrombosis. Gastroenterology 1982;82:358–72.
84. Haglund U, Bulkley GB, Granger DN. On the pathophysiology of intestinal ischemic injury. Clinical review. Acta Chir Scand 1987;153:321–4.
85. Harward TR, Smith S, Seeger JM. Detection of celiac axis and superior mesenteric artery occlusive disease with use of abdominal duplex scanning. J Vasc Surg 1993;17:738–45.
86. Hashimoto A, Fuke H, Shimizu A, Shiraki K. Hepatic portal venous gas caused by non-obstructive mesenteric ischemia. J Hepatol 2002;37:870.
87. Hirsh J, Piovella F, Pini M. Congenital antithrombin III deficiency: laboratory diagnosis, incidence, clinical implications, and treatment with antithrombin III concentrate. Am J Med 1989;87:34S–8S.
88. Hoyle M, Kennedy A, Prior AL, Thomas GE. Small bowel ischaemia and infarction in young women taking oral contraceptives and progestational agents. Br J Surg 1977;64:533–7.
89. Johnson TD, Berenson MM. Methamphetamine-induced ischemic colitis. J Clin Gastroenterol 1991;13:687–9.

90. Kurland B, Brandt LJ, Delany HM. Diagnostic tests for intestinal ischemia. Surg Clin North Am 1992;72:85–105.
91. Lescher TJ, Brombeck CT. Mesenteric vascular occlusion associated with oral contraceptive use. Arch Surg 1977;112:1231–2.
92. Mansour MA. Management of acute mesenteric ischemia. Arch Surg 1999;134:328–30.
93. Marlar RA. Protein C in thromboembolic disease. Semin Thromb Hemost 1985;11:387–93.
94. McCullough CJ. Isolated mesenteric injury due to blunt abdominal trauma. Injury 1976;7:295–8.
95. McKinsey JF, Gewertz BL. Acute mesenteric ischemia. Surg Clin North Am 1997;77:307–18.
96. Moneta GL, Yeager RA, Dalman R, Antonovic R, Hall LD, Porter JM. Duplex ultrasound criteria for the diagnosis of splanchnic artery stenosis or occlusion. J Vasc Surg 1991;14:511–8.
97. Murray M, Gonze M, Nowak L, Cobb CF. Serum D(-) lactate levels as an aid to diagnosing acute intestinal ischemia. Am J Surg 1994;167: 575–8.
98. Nagasue N, Inokuchi K, Kobayashi M, Saku M. Mesenteric venous thrombosis occurring late after splenectomy. Br J Surg 1977;64:781–3.
99. Orozco H, Guraieb E, Takahashi T, et al. Deficiency of protein C in patients with portal vein thrombosis. Hepatology 1988;8:1110–1.
100. Rosen A, Korobkin M, Silverman PM, Dunnick NR, Kelvin FM. Mesenteric vein thrombosis. CT identification. Am J Roentgenol 1984;143:83–6.
101. Rosenberg RD. Biochemistry of heparin antithrombin interactions, and the physiologic role of this natural anticoagulant mechanism. Am J Med 1989;87:2S–9S.
102. Sack J, Aldrete JS. Primary mesenteric venous thrombosis. Surg Gynecol Obstet 1982;154: 205–8.
103. Siegelman SS, Sprayregen S, Boley SJ. Angiographic diagnosis of mesenteric arterial vasoconstriction. Radiology 1974;112:533–42.
104. Skinner DB, Zairms I, Moosa AR. Mesenteric vascular disease. Am J Surg 1974;128:835–9.
105. Smerud MJ, Johnson CD, Stephens DH. Diagnosis of bowel infarction: a comparison of plain films and CT scan in 23 cases. AJR Am J Roentgenol 1990;154:99–103.
106. van den Hauwe L, Degryse H, Coene L. Portomesenteric vein gas in mesenteric infarction. JBR-BTR 2002;85:162–3.
107. Warren S, Eberhard TP: Mesenteric venous thrombosis. Surg Gynecol Obstet 1935;61:102.
108. Wilcox MG, Howard TJ, Plaskon LA, Unthank JL, Madura JA. Current theories of pathogenesis and treatment of non-occlusive mesenteric ischemia. Dig Dis Sci 1995;40:709–16.
109. Williams LF Jr: Mesenteric ischemia. Surg Clin North Am 1988;68:331–53.

Chronic Intestinal Ischemia

110. Asensio JA, Britt LD, Borzotta A, et al. Multi-institutional experience with the management of superior mesenteric artery injuries. J Am Coll Surg 2001;193:354–65.
111. Chang JB, Stein TA. Mesenteric ischemia: acute and chronic. Ann Vasc Surg 2003;17:323–8.
112. Moawad J, McKinsey JF, Wyble CW, Bassiouny HS, Schwartz LB, Gewertz BL. Current results of surgical therapy for chronic mesenteric ischemia. Arch Surg 1997;132:613–9.

Neonatal Necrotizing Enterocolitis

113. Crissinger KD, Granger DN. Mucosal injury induced by ischemia and reperfusion in the piglet intestine: influences of age and feeding. Gastroenterology 1989;97:920–6.
114. Grosfeld JL, Molinari F, Chaet M, et al. Gastrointestinal perforation and peritonitis in infants and children: experience with 179 cases over ten years. Surgery 1996;120:650–5.
115. Kanto WP Jr, Wilson R, Breart GL, et al. Perinatal events and necrotizing enterocolitis in premature infants. Am J Dis Child 1987;141:167–9.
116. Kliegman RM. Models of pathogenesis of necrotizing enterocolitis. J Pediatr 1990;117:S2–S5.
117. Nadler EP, Dickinson E, Knisely A, et al. Expression of inducible nitric oxide synthase and interleukin-12 in experimental necrotizing enterocolitis. J Surg Res 2000;92:71–7.
118. Nanthakumar NN, Fusunyan RD, Sanderson I, Walker WA. Inflammation in developing human intestine: a possible pathophysiologic contribution to necrotizing enterocolitis. Proc Natl Acad Sci USA 2000;97:6043–8.
119. Uauy RD, Fanaroff AA, Korones SB, Phillips EA, Phillips JB, Wright LL. Necrotizing enterocolitis in very low birth weight infants: biodemographics and clinical correlates. National Institute of Child Health and Human Developmental Neonatal Research Network. J Pediatr 1991;119:630–8.
120. Vennarecci G, Kato T, Misiakos EP, et al. Intestinal transplantation for short gut syndrome attributable to necrotizing colitis. Pediatrics 2000;105:E25.
121. Vohr BR, Wright LL, Dusick AM, et al. Neurodevelopmental and functional outcomes of extremely low birth weight infants in the National Institute of Child Health and Human Development Neonatal Research Network. 1993-1994. Pediatrics 2000;105:1216–26.

Tropical Necrotizing Enterocolitis

122. Gui L, Subramony C, Fratkin J, Hughsin MD. Fatal enteritis necroticans in a diabetic adult. Mod Pathol 2002;15:66–70.
123. Petrillo TM, Beck-Sague CM, Songer JG, et al. Enteritis necroticans (pigbel) in a diabetic child. N Engl J Med 2000;342:1250–3.

Acute Segmental Obstructing Enteritis

124. Lee HC, Huang F, Hsu C, Sheu J, Shih S. Acute segmental obstructing enteritis in children. J Pediatr Gastroenterol Nutr 1994;18:82–6.
125. Narayanan R, Bhargava BN, Karba SG, Sangal BC. Segmental necrotizing jejunitis. Lancet 1987;2:1517–8.
126. Rai AN, Prasad PR, Prasad SN, Tiwari RK. Epidemic regional jejunitis: a new clinical entity? Lancet 1987;2:1020.
127. Sharma AK, Shekhawat NS, Behari S, Chandra S, Sogani KC. Non-specific jejunitis–a challenging problem in children. Am J Gastroenterol 1986;81:428–31.

Bowel Infarction in Dialysis Patients

128. Bassiouny HS. Nonocclusive mesenteric ischemia. Surg Clin North Am 1997;77:319–26.
129. Eldrup-Jorgensen J, Hawkins RE, Bredenberg CE. Abdominal vascular catastrophes. Surg Clin North Am 1997;77:1317–9.
130. John AS, Tuerff SD, Kerstein MD. Nonocclusive mesenteric ischemia in hemodialysis patients. J Am Coll Surg January 2000;190:64–88.
131. Zeier M, Wiesel M, Rambusek M, Ritz E. Nonocclusive mesenteric infarction in dialysis patients: the importance of prevention and early intervention. Nephrol Dial Transplant 1995;10:771–3.

Polyarteritis Nodosa

132. Bailey M, Chapin W, Licht H, Reynolds J. The effects of vasculitis on the gastrointestinal tract and liver. Gastroenterol Clin N Am 1998;27: 747–80.
133. Bassel K, Hartford W. Gastrointestinal manifestations of collagen-vascular disease. Semin Gastrointest Dis 1995;6:228–40.
134. Cacoub P, Maisonobe T, Thibault V, et al. Systemic vasculitis in patients with hepatitis C. J Rheumatol 2001;28:109–18.
135. Fenoglio-Preiser CM, Noffsinger AE, Stemmermann GN, Lantz PE, Listrom MB, Rilke FO. Gastrointestinal pathology: an atlas and text, 2nd ed. Philadelphia: Lippincott-Raven; 1999: 353.
136. Guillevin L, Lhote F, Cohen P, et al. Polyarteritis nodosa related to hepatitis B virus: a prospective study with long-term observation of 41 patients. Medicine 1995;74;238–53.
137. Guillevin L, Lhote F, Gayraud M, et al. Prognostic factors in polyarteritis nodosa and Churg-Strauss syndrome. A prospective study in 342 patients. Medicine 1996;75:17–28.
138. Krupski W, Selzman C, Whitehall T. Unusual causes of mesenteric ischemia. Surg Clin North Am 1997;77:471–502.

Henoch-Schönlein Purpura

139. Choong CK, Beasley SW. Intra-abdominal manifestations of Henoch-Schonlein purpura. J Paediatr Child Health 1998;34:405–9.
140. Diamond LK, Howell DA. Anaphylactoid purpura in children. Am J Dis Child 1960;99;833.
141. Esaki M, Matsumoto T, Nakamura S, et al. GI involvement in Henoch-Schonlein purpura. Gastrointest Endosc 2002;56:920–3.
142. Mills JA, Michel BA, Bloch DA, et al. The American College of Rheumatology 1990 criteria for classification of Henoch-Schonlein purpura. Arthritis Rheum 1990;33:1114–21.
143. Robson WL, Leung AK. Henoch-Schonlein purpura. Adv Pediatr 1994;41;163–94.

Microscopic Polyarteritis

144. Lhote F, Cohen P, Genereau T, Gayraud M, Guillevin L. Microscopic polyangiitis: clinical aspects and treatment. Ann Med Interne (Paris). 1996;147:165–77.
145. Ramirez G, Kamastha G, Hughes GR. The ANCA test: its clinical relevance. Ann Rheum Dis 1990; 49:741–2.

Wegener's Granulomatosis

146. Hoffman GS, Kerr S, Levitt RY, et al. Wegener's granulomatosis: an analysis of 158 patients. Ann Intern Med 1992;116;488–98.
147. Lie JT. Wegener's granulomatosis: histological documentation of common and uncommon manifestations in 216 patients. Vasa 1997;26: 261–70.

Churg-Strauss Syndrome

148. Churg J, Strauss L. Allergic granulomatosis, allergic angitis, and periarteritis nodosa. Am J Pathol 1951;27:277–94.
149. Guillevin L, Lhote F, Amouroux J, Gherardi R, Callard P, Casassus P. Antineutrophilic antibody, abnormal angiograms and pathological findings in polyarteritis nodosa and Churg-Strauss syndrome: indications for the classification of vasculitides of the polyarteritis nodosa group. Br J Rheumatol 1996;35:958–64.

150. Lhote F, Guillevin L. Polyarteritis nodosa, microscopic polyangiitis and Churg-Strauss syndrome: clinical aspects and treatment. Rheum Dis Clin North Am 1995;21:911–47.
151. Memain N, De BM, Guillevin L, Wechsler B, Meyer O. Delayed relapse of Churg-Strauss syndrome manifesting as colon ulcers with mucosal granulomas: 3 cases. J Rheumatol 2002;29:388–91.

Kawasaki's Disease

152. Chung CJ, Ryder S, Meyers W, Long J. Kawasaki's disease presenting as focal colitis. Pediatri Radiol 1996;26:455–7.
153. Meissner HC, Leung DY. Kawasaki syndrome. Curr Opin Rheumatol 1995;7:455–8.
154. Naoe S, Takahashi K, Masuda H, Tanaka N. Kawasaki's disease with particular emphasis on arterial lesions. Acta Pathol Jpn 1991;41:785–97.

Thromboangiitis Obliterans

155. Iwai T. Buerger's disease with intestinal involvement. Int J Cardiol 1998;66:S257–63.

Malignant Atrophic Papulosis

156. Black MM, Hudson PM. Atrophie blanche lesions closely resembling malignant atrophic papulosis in systemic lupus erythematosus. Br J Dermatol 1976;95:649–52.
157. Degos R. Malignant atrophic papulosis. Br J Dermatol 1979;100:21–35.
158. Feldman M, Friedman LS, Sleisenger MH, eds. Sleisenger & Fordtran's gastrointestinal and liver disease: pathophysiology, diagnosis, management, vol 2, 7th ed. Philadelphia: Saunders; 2002:347.
159. Fruhwirth J, Mischinger HJ, Werkgartner G, Beham A, Pfaffenthaller EC. Kohlmeier-Degos disease with primary intestinal manifestation. Scand J Gastroenterol 1997;32:1066–70.
160. Katz SK, Mudd LJ, Roenigk HH. Malignant atrophic papulosis involving three generations of a family. J Am Acad Dermatol 1997;37:480–4.
161. Molenaar WM, Rosman JB, Donker AJ, Houthoff HJ. The pathology and pathogenesis of malignant atrophic papulosis. A case study with reference to other vascular disorders. Pathol Res Pract 1987;182:98–106.
162. Strole WE Jr, Clark WH Jr, Isselbacher KJ. Progressive arterial occlusive disease (Kohlmeier-Degos). A frequently fatal cutaneosytemic disorder. N Eng J Med 1967;276:195–201.

Segmental Arterial Mediolysis

163. Rengstroff DS, Baker EL, Wack J, Yee LF. Intraabdominal hemorrhage caused by segmental arterial mediolysis of the inferior mesenteric artery: report of a case. Dis Colon Rectum 2004; 47:769–72.
164. Slavin RE, Cafferty L, Cartwright J Jr. Segmental mediolytic arteritis: a clinicopathologic and ultrastructural study of two cases. Am J Surg Pathol 1989;13:558–68.
165. Slavin RE, Saeki K, Bhagavan B, Maas AE. Segmental arterial mediolysis: a precursor to fibromuscular dysplasia? Mod Pathol 1995;8:287–94.

Marfan and Ehlers-Danlos Syndromes

166. Mclean AM, Paul RE Jr, Kritzman J, Farthing MJ. Malabsorption in Marfan (Ehlers-Danlos) syndrome. J Clin Gastroenterol 1985;7:304–8.
167. Stillman AE, Painter R, Hollister DW. Ehlers-Danlos syndrome type IV: diagnosis and therapy of associated bowel perforation. Am J Gastroenterology 1991;86:360–2.

GI Tract Involvement in SLE

168. Edmunds SE, Ganju V, Beveridge BR, French MA, Quinlan MF. Protein losing enteropathy in systemic lupus erythematosus. Aust N Z J Med 1988;18:868–71.
169. Hallegua DS, Wallace DJ. Gastrointestinal manifestations of systemic lupus erythematosus. Curr Opin Rheumatol 2000;12:379–85.
170. Lee CK, Ahn MS, Lee EY, et al. Acute abdominal pain in systemic lupus erythematosus: focus on lupus enteritis (gastrointestinal vasculitis). Ann Rheum Dis 2002;61:547–50.
171. Sultan SM, Ioannou Y, Isenberg DA. A review of gastrointestinal manifestations of systemic lupus erythematosus. Rheumatology 1999;38: 917–32.
172. Zizic TM, Classen JN, Stevens MB. Acute abdominal complications of systemic lupus erythematosus and polyarteritis nodosa. Am J Med 1982;73:525–31.

Rheumatoid Arthritis

173. Scott DG, Bacon PA, Tribe CR. Systemic rheumatoid vasculitis: a clinical laboratory study of 50 cases. Medicine 1981;60:288–97.

Behcet's Disease

174. Griffin JW Jr, Harrison HB, Tedesco FJ, Mills LR 4th. Behcet's disease with multiple sites of gastrointestinal involvement. South Med J 1982;75:1405–8.
175. Lee RG. The colitis of Behcet's syndrome. Am J Surg Pathol 1986;10:888–93.

176. Masugi J, Matsui T, Fujimori T, Maeda S. A case of Behcet's disease with multiple longitudinal ulcers all over the colon. Am J Gastroenterol 1994;89:778–80.
177. Takada Y, Fujita Y, Igarashi M, et al. Intestinal Behcet's disease: pathognomic changes in intramucosal lymphoid tissue and effect of a "rest cure" on intestinal lesions. J Gastroenterol 1997;32:598–604.

Mesenteric Inflammatory Venooclusive Disease

178. Flaherty M, Lie J, Haggitt R. Mesenteric inflammatory veno-occlusive disease: a seldom-recognized cause of intestinal ischemia. Am J Surg Pathol 1994;18:779–84.
179. Haber MM, Burrell M, West AB. Enterocolic lymphocytic phlebitis. J Clin Gastroenterol 1993;17:327–32.
180. Lavu K, Minocha A. Mesenteric inflammatory veno-occlusive disorder: a rare entity mimicking inflammatory bowel disease. Gastroenterology 2003;125:236–9.
181. Lie JT. Mesenteric inflammatory veno-occlusive disease (MIVOD): an emerging and unsuspected cause of digestive tract ischemia. Vasa 1997;26:91–6.

Mesenteric Phlebosclerosis

182. Ikehata A, Hiwatashi N, Kawarada H, et al. Chronic ischemic colitis associated with marked calcifications of mesenteric vessels. Report of two cases. Dig Endosc 1994;6:355–64.
183. Iwashita A, Yao T, Schlemper R, et al. Mesenteric phlebosclerosis: a new disease entity causing ischemic colitis. Dis Colon Rectum 2003;46:209–20.
184. Yao T, Iwashita A, Hoashi T, et al. Phlebosclerotic colitis: value of radiography in diagnosis—report of three cases. Radiology 2000;214:188–92.

Vasculitis Caused by Infections

185. Anayi S, Al-Nasiri N. Acute mesenteric ischaemia caused by *Schistosoma mansoni* infection. Br Med J 1987;294:1197.

8 CHEMICAL INJURY

INTRODUCTION

Demography. Chemical injury is probably far more common than is diagnosed, because pathologists rarely have sufficient clinical information to make the diagnosis. Presumably, some of the nonspecific inflammation seen throughout the gut results from chemical or drug exposure. Approximately 2 to 8 percent of patients receiving drugs experience an adverse gastrointestinal reaction, with gastrointestinal bleeding accounting for the largest burden of adverse drug-related admissions (4). Up to one third of the drug injuries affect more than a single gastrointestinal site (3,4).

Etiology. Chemical injury results from exposure to drugs, chemicals, and toxins. Some of these are exogenously derived, as in drug-induced injury; some result from the presence of gastrointestinal luminal materials in places where they ought not to be, as in gastroesophageal reflux disease or alkaline reflux gastritis (gastropathy).

Chemicals injure the gastrointestinal tract in numerous ways (Tables 8-1 and 8-2). Some drugs become entrapped, particularly in the esophagus, causing localized injury. Others are directly toxic, causing necrosis or inhibiting cell growth. In other cases, toxicity results from metabolic conversion and release of damaging endogenous mediators such as the free radical release seen in nonsteroidal antiinflammatory drug (NSAID) injury. Toxic injury generally exhibits dose-related effects. Other drugs cause ischemia via secondary events including thrombosis, decreased blood flow, vasculitis, or vasospasm (Table 8-1). Still other drugs predispose to infection, such as antibiotic-associated *Clostridium difficile* infections, or they cause motility problems.

Patients are exposed to chemical injury via 1) accidental ingestion; 2) overdose as the result of suicidal intent; 3) therapies for numerous diseases; 4) use of the drug as a preventive agent; 5) use in diagnostic tests; 6) consumption of foods that contain chemicals; 7) consumption of supplements or substances found at health food stores; or 8) via animal bites or stings. Drug injuries result from both the drugs themselves or from byproducts of food-drug (chemical) interactions. Host factors, specific meal composition and volume, and the drug or chemical type determine the nature of the interactions.

General Clinical Features of Chemical Injury. Most drugs and chemicals do not affect the gastrointestinal tract uniformly. Therefore, the clinical features depend on the location, nature, and extent of the injury, as well as on the presence or absence of complications or coexisting conditions. When patients with chemically induced injury present with symptoms related to inflammation and ulceration, the clinical presentation mimics other ulcerating diseases. Chemical injury may also manifest as malabsorption, a motility disorder, idiopathic inflammatory bowel disease (IBD), or infection. Endoscopic biopsies are usually performed to localize the lesions, to document their extent, and rule out alternative causes of the clinical manifestations.

Table 8-1

MECHANISMS OF DRUG- OR CHEMICAL-INDUCED INJURY

Act as toxins
Mediate immune reactions
Cause malabsorption
Cause bleeding
Cause ischemia
Cause allergic reactions
Affect motility
Predispose to infection
Cause damaging food-drug interactions
Cause caustic injury
Physical entrapment
Cause foreign body reactions

Table 8-2

EXAMPLES OF CHEMICAL/DRUG INJURY

Agent	Lesions
Antibiotics	Pill-associated esophagitis Pseudomembranous colitis Malabsorption (neomycin, paraaminosalicylate) Enterocolitis
Anticholinergic and antidepressant drugs	Pseudoobstruction
Anticoagulant drugs	Hemorrhages and hematomas
Cardiovascular drugs	Focal esophageal ulcers from pills (quinidine, vasopressin) Gastric and duodenal ulcers (reserpine, ethacrynic acid) Ischemic enterocolitis Malabsorption (methyldopa) Pseudoobstruction (ganglion blockers)
Caustic agents	Ulcers and strictures of the esophagus and stomach
Chemotherapeutic drugs	Ulcers and inflammation Synergism with radiation injury Malabsorption Enterocolitis
Enemas and laxatives	"Proctitis" from enemas Cathartic colon Melanosis coli
Estrogen and progesterone	Hemorrhage, thrombosis, and ischemia
Ethyl alcohol	Gastroduodenitis Mild effects on small intestine
Heavy metals	Focal esophageal ulcers from pills (ferrous sulfate) Gastric ulcers (ferrous and zinc sulfate) Enterocolitis
Nonsteroidal antiinflammatory drugs	Pill-induced esophagitis Gastroduodenitis Focal intestinal ulcers Mucosal diaphragms

The clinician often needs to differentiate chemically induced abnormalities from other disease processes that cause similar endoscopic features. For example, drug-induced esophageal ulceration may mimic gastroesophageal reflux injury, NSAID effects in the upper gastrointestinal tract may resemble peptic ulcers, and in the lower gastrointestinal tract, NSAIDs can induce endoscopic changes consistent with ischemia or idiopathic IBD. The myriad of drugs used in the transplant situation can cause an endoscopic appearance similar to that of other causes of gastritis, enteritis, and colitis. The clinician often depends on the results of the pathologic analysis to appropriately direct patient care and management.

General Pathologic Findings of Chemical Injury. The pathologic features of chemically induced injury are typically nonspecific, and the diagnosis often depends on the history and the exclusion of other conditions. Common histologic alterations include inflammation, erosions, necrosis, ulcers, ischemia, and apoptosis with epithelial loss in the proliferative zones. Microscopic clues to drug-induced injury include apoptosis, cytoplasmic vacuolation and increased intraepithelial lymphocytes (1,2), melanosis coli, and eosinophils. These features, however, are far from specific. Even with an abnormal biopsy in which eosinophils and apoptosis are prominent and a drug-induced etiology is suspected, proof positive requires resolution of the abnormalities when the drug is withdrawn and reappearance of the lesions when the drug is reinstated (1,2). Since patients are often on several drugs, these requirements are seldom fulfilled (5).

Complications include ulcers that may perforate, malabsorption from altered enterocyte morphology, pseudoobstruction from neuromuscular alterations, or stricture formation.

NONSTEROIDAL ANTIINFLAMMATORY DRUGS

Definition. *NSAID injury* is gastrointestinal damage resulting from the ingestion of nonsteroidal antiinflammatory drugs, including aspirin. Synonyms include *NSAID gastropathy* and *NSAID enteropathy*.

Demography. NSAIDs are the most commonly prescribed drugs in the Western world; the world market now exceeds $6 billion/year (29). NSAIDs are also the drugs whose complications most frequently necessitate hospitalization, especially in elderly women (12,30). Women over 75 years of age who take NSAIDs have a 5-fold increased risk of gastrointestinal hemorrhage or perforation (58). NSAIDs are primarily used to treat rheumatoid arthritis and other degenerative joint diseases, and to reduce the incidence of cancer. Aspirin is used to prevent cardiovascular and cerebrovascular thrombotic events. Its antithrombotic effects are largely mediated by its ability to acetylate and thus irreversibly inactivate platelet cyclooxygenase-1 (COX-1), the rate-limiting enzyme in thromboxane A2 synthesis. Patients on long-term NSAID therapy have a 10- to 30-fold increased risk over that of the general population for the development of a chronic refractory peptic ulcer (34). The risk of a significant gastroduodenal complication (bleeding, perforation, or gastric outlet obstruction) is 1 to 4 percent/year (9,35,53). Fortunately, there has been a decline in serious NSAID-related gastropathies due to two major factors: the use of lower doses combined with the increased use of proton pump inhibitors and the use of less toxic NSAIDs, particularly COX-2–specific inhibitors (27).

NSAIDs also damage the gastrointestinal mucosa of children, although the number of children developing significant gastrointestinal problems is low (37).

Etiology. A linear dose relationship exists between NSAID ingestion and gastrointestinal damage. This relationship is modified by host response, concomitant drug or alcohol use, route of administration, the specific drug used, and the presence of *Helicobacter pylori* infection (36). Different preparations tend to affect different portions of the gastrointestinal tract. NSAIDs that commonly induce gastrointestinal injury are listed in Table 8-3.

Table 8-3

COMMONLY USED NONSTEROIDAL ANTIINFLAMMATORY DRUGS

Acetylsalicylic acid	Misoprostol
Azapropazone	Naproxen
Diclofenac	Oxyphenbutazone
Diflunisal	Phenylbutazone
Fenoprofen	Piroxicam
Ibuprofen	Sulindac
Indomethacin	Tolmetin
Mefenamic acid	

Pathophysiology. *Esophageal Injury.* Esophagitis develops in patients on NSAIDs of all sorts. This is related, in part, to the development of reflux esophagitis due to a reduction of lower esophageal sphincter pressure and impairment of cholinergic control of lower esophageal sphincter contraction (18,29).

Gastroduodenal Injury. NSAIDs usually produce acute mucosal lesions within 7 to 14 days of administration by the mechanisms shown in figure 8-1. The normal gastroduodenal mucosa contains high concentrations of the prostaglandins PGE_2 and PGI_2, which inhibit gastric acid secretion and increase mucus production (see chapter 4). The increased vulnerability of the elderly to NSAID-induced injury may result from an age-related reduction in gastric mucosal prostaglandin levels (44,56). NSAIDs inhibit prostaglandin synthesis via their effects on COX. There are two different COX isoenzymes. COX-1 is constitutively expressed in many tissues, including the stomach. In contrast, rapidly inducible COX-2 is not expressed, or is expressed at very low levels unless the tissues are inflamed (56). Since selective COX-2 inhibitors suppress prostaglandin synthesis only at inflamed sites, they are less ulcerogenic than other NSAIDs (24,47). In addition to causing mucosal damage, NSAIDs interfere with the healing of preexisting lesions, including ulcers, by interfering with the action of mucosal growth factors, decreasing epithelial cell proliferation, decreasing angiogenesis in the ulcer bed, and slowing granulation tissue maturation (57).

Aspirin damages the gastric mucosa directly and indirectly, depending on the gastric pH. Since aspirin does not dissociate at a gastric pH of 3.5 or greater, it damages the superficial epithelium directly by acting as a physical agent (55). Insoluble aspirin preparations become embedded in the mucosa, producing circular erosions, ulcers, or mucosal cracks. Drug particles falling into these mucosal defects become "walled off" in mucus until they dissolve. In contrast, when gastric pH is 3.5 or less, aspirin indirectly damages the stomach by being absorbed. Aspirin is lipid soluble and salicylate forms following its absorption. The absorbed aspirin acts as a potent mitochondrial poison and cytotoxin, affecting mucosal barrier function, stimulating sodium transport, and increasing hydrogen ion (H+) dissipation from the mucosal surface. Salicylates also increase mucosal cellular exfoliation; ulcers develop when the rate of exfoliation

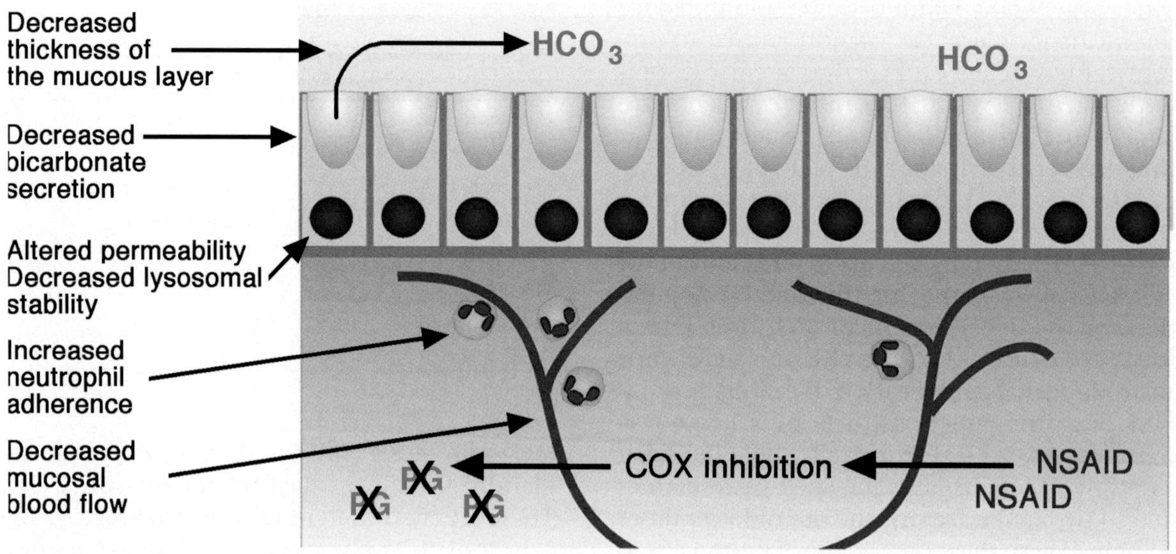

Figure 8-1

DIAGRAM OF THE EFFECTS OF NONSTEROIDAL ANTIINFLAMMATORY DRUGS (NSAIDS)

NSAIDs produce mucosal injury by inhibiting cyclooxygenase (COX) activity and reducing mucosal prostaglandin synthesis. COX is the enzyme responsible for converting arachidonic acid to prostaglandins. Reduced prostaglandin synthesis leads to an overall reduction in gastric mucosal defenses. Prostaglandins have a protective mucosal role and stimulate mucus secretion, stabilize lysosomes, and inhibit acid secretion in the stomach. NSAIDs alter mucus and bicarbonate secretion, reduce mucosal blood flow, and promote adherence of neutrophils to the vascular endothelium. NSAID-mediated cytologic damage results from a cascade of events that increases mucosal permeability and luminal hydrogen ion and pepsin leakage into the cells.

exceeds the rate of cellular regeneration. Aspirin also strongly inhibits COX-1 in the gastrointestinal mucosa, leading to its ability to induce gastrointestinal mucosal injury. This happens even at extremely low doses (21). Chronic NSAID ingestion often causes less damage than acute ingestion due to the mucosal adaptation that renders the mucosa resistant to epithelial necrosis (38,49,58).

Intestinal Injury. The pathogenesis of small intestinal NSAID-induced injury is not as well understood as gastric injury, in part, because visibly assessing the damage in the small intestine is more difficult. A key pathogenic factor is increased mucosal permeability (17), which, in conjunction with the NSAID effects on chemotaxis and neutrophil function, injures the mucosa (16) and facilitates bacterial invasion and inflammation. NSAIDs and aspirin also exacerbate underlying peptic ulcer disease and potentiate motility disorders.

Clinical Features. Clinically, over 25 percent of patients on NSAIDs experience nausea, heartburn, abdominal pain, or minor bleeding (39); approximately 60 percent of patients who take NSAIDs have clinically silent gastroduodenal damage (11). The most serious complication in long-term NSAID users is gastrointestinal bleeding (28,42), which occurs anywhere in the gut. Bleeding usually results from the presence of mucosal erosions or ulcers. Patients may also develop diarrhea and appetite loss. NSAIDs are strongly associated with an increased risk of gastrointestinal perforation (40).

Gastric erosions tend to occur acutely but they usually heal within a few days. Long-term NSAID users have an increased risk of gastric and duodenal ulcers and their complications, including bleeding, perforation, and death. Sometimes, the pill is seen lying in the ulcer (fig. 8-2). Risk factors for NSAID-related peptic ulcer complications include patient age (over 60), past history of ulcer disease, use of higher-risk NSAIDs, concurrent use of anticoagulants or corticosteroids, and the presence of serious systemic disorders. Possible other risk factors include concomitant infection with *H. pylori*, cigarette smoking, and alcohol consumption (8).

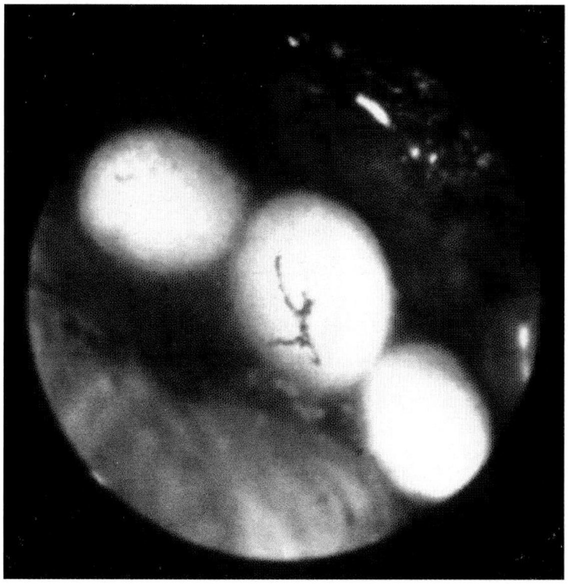

Figure 8-2

NSAID-INDUCED GASTRIC ULCER

Endoscopic appearance of gastric ulcer with three NSAID pills lying in the middle of the ulcer bed.

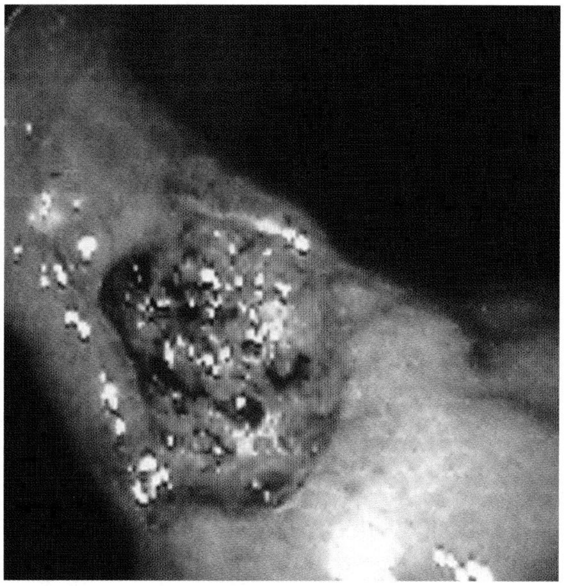

Figure 8-3

NSAID-INDUCED GASTRIC ULCER

Large gastric ulcer in a patient on NSAID therapy.

In the small intestine, NSAIDs cause bleeding, ileal dysfunction, malabsorption, diarrhea, changes in mucosal and vascular permeability (14,36,41), protein loss, ulceration, mucosal diaphragm disease, iron deficiency anemia, perforation, and death. In the colon, NSAIDs cause perforation or bleeding of preexisting colonic diverticula, relapse of IBD, microscopic colitis, and strictures, and they may exacerbate bleeding from angiodysplasias. Patients taking NSAID-containing suppositories may develop localized anorectal erosions, ulcers, and stenosis (31) that may mimic anorectal Crohn's disease or other causes of ulcerative proctitis.

Gross Findings. In patients on NSAIDs, the gastrointestinal tract may appear grossly and endoscopically normal. Additionally, erosions, ulcers, and mucosal diaphragms may develop anywhere in the gut. Because visibly assessing small intestinal damage is difficult, it has only been relatively recently that the major small intestinal effects of NSAIDs have become evident, largely through the use of radiolabeled isotopes and subsequent radiologic investigation via exclusion and permeability studies (15,22).

Esophagus. Esophagitis, esophageal ulcers, and esophageal strictures all complicate NSAID therapy (51). NSAID-induced ulcers are characteristically large, shallow, discrete, mid-esophageal ulcers surrounded by a normal mucosa.

Stomach. The stomach may appear perfectly normal or there may be changes that resemble those seen with stress ulcers. Endoscopic findings include mild erythema, petechiae, subepithelial or intramural hemorrhages, superficial necrosis, focal punctate erosions, and acute or chronic ulcers (fig. 8-3). The erosions often lie along the lesser curvature and tend to involve all of the stomach, in contrast to stress ulcers which typically occur proximally and then spread distally. Erosions may extend into the duodenum. Antral flattening in the greater curvature is a useful radiologic sign of NSAID-related gastropathy, particularly in individuals with associated erosive gastritis. NSAIDs occasionally cause gastrocolic fistulas or pyloric channel strictures.

Intestines. Intestinal lesions differ in the proximal and distal small intestine. Patients who are chronic NSAID users may develop peptic duodenal ulcers. Hemorrhage and perforation occur more commonly in NSAID-associated duodenal peptic ulcers than in those without NSAID use. Intestinal lesions may affect the entire intestine, and include villous atrophy, ulcers, strictures, areas of bleeding, mucosal diaphragms (fig. 8-4), and perforation. Duodenal lesions resemble gastric lesions, with patchy hemorrhages and erosions and acute inflammation that rapidly resolve following drug cessation. Occasionally, deep ulcers form. Smaller ulcers often surround larger ones (7). The ileum is a common site of intestinal injury.

Long-term NSAID treatment-related small intestinal ulcers are single or multiple, and vary from small, sharply demarcated, punched-out lesions on the tips of mucosal folds (fig. 8-4) to extensive deep ulcerations. The ulcers may resemble peptic ulcer disease with necrotic debris and leukocytes admixed with fibrinous exudate, often overlying granulation tissue. Fibrosis may be present. Extensive erosions can involve almost the entire small intestine (48).

Intestinal mucosal diaphragms are thought to be pathognomonic for NSAID-induced injury (41,50). The features vary depending on the stage of diaphragm development. The small intestine or colon is typically divided into variable numbers of compartments by thin circumferential membranes, creating a picture resembling that of a ring or a perforated diaphragm. Sometimes the luminal diameter narrows to less than 1 mm. The serosal aspect of the intestine usually appears normal; therefore, it is difficult to detect the intraluminal lesions by external examination. Occasionally, however, the diaphragms cause small serosal constrictions that are visible externally. The mucosa between the diaphragms usually appears normal, but it may be ulcerated or regenerative. There are three patterns of mucosal diaphragm disease: 1) an extreme exaggeration of the normal plica circularis; 2) broad-based rigid strictures consisting of dome-shaped lesions that cause a rounded hump projecting into the gastrointestinal lumen, often with a focal ulcer in the center of the hump (fig. 8-4); and 3) a conventional flat stricture. Circumferential linear ulcers may be the precursors of the mucosal diaphragm (32).

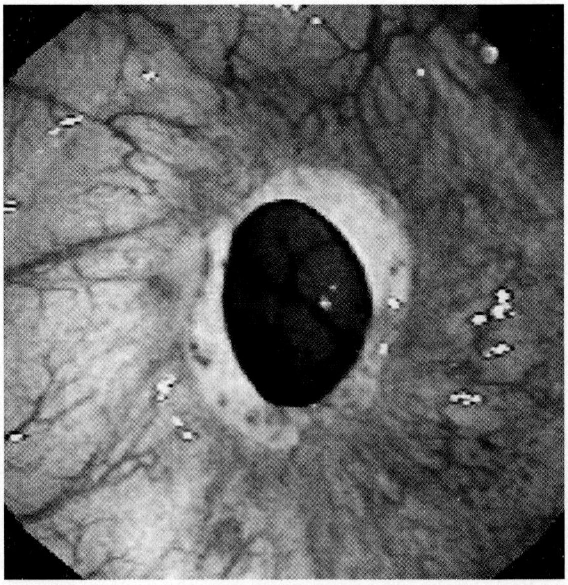

Figure 8-4

NSAID-INDUCED STRICTURE AND ULCER

Endoscopic view showing a distinctive diaphragm-like stricture with an ulcerated rim. (Fig. 4-129 from Emory TS, Carpenter HA, Gostout CJ, Sobin LH. Atlas of gastrointestinal endoscopy & endoscopic biopsies. Washington DC: Armed Forces Institute of Pathology; 2009:335.) (Figs. 8-4, 8-8–8-10, and 8-12 are from the same patient.)

Microscopic Findings. *Esophagus.* Patients on long-term NSAID therapy may have an endoscopically normal-appearing esophagus or there may be nonspecific changes, including basal cell hyperplasia. Alternatively, the esophageal mucosa may appear inflamed, eroded, or ulcerated. The histologic features of the ulcers are nonspecific. Patients may also develop reflux esophagitis. Basal cell hyperplasia may not be present, since proliferation is inhibited by the prostaglandin inhibitors (46).

Stomach. Histologically, NSAIDs cause three major types of gastric injury: 1) acute mucosal hemorrhages and erosions that produce a pattern resembling acute erosive gastritis (fig. 8-5); 2) ulcers; and 3) chemical gastropathy (fig. 8-6). Erosions and ulcers, when present, are usually small and sharply demarcated, and gastritis may or may not be present in the surrounding mucosa. These lesions heal in a manner similar to that seen with stress ulcers. The ulcer surface reepithelializes with minimal fibrosis. When ulcers are present, there is surprisingly little inflammation in the surrounding mucosa, even if the ulcers are chronic.

Patients on NSAIDs also develop changes that resemble those seen in bile (alkaline) reflux gastritis (also known as chemical gastropathy), although the changes may be more subtle. These changes include pit elongation and foveolar

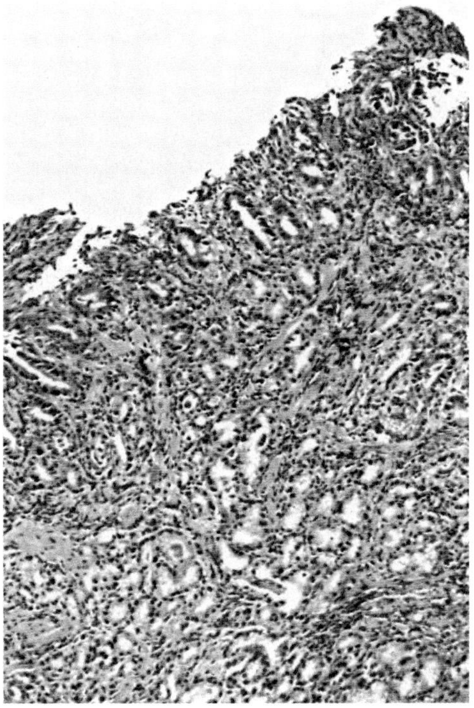

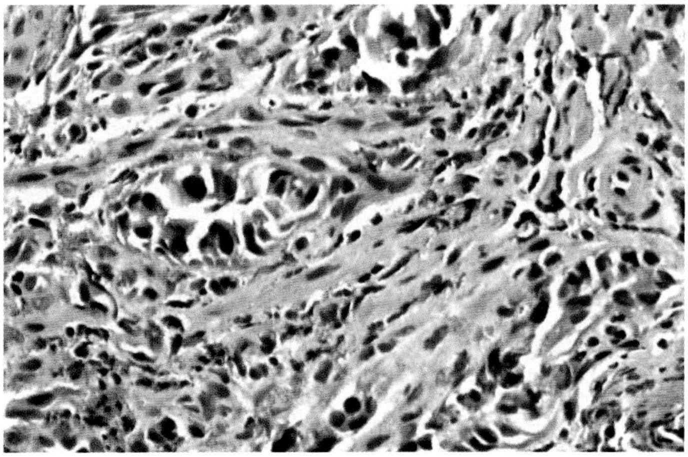

Figure 8-5

EROSIVE CHANGES WITH MARKED REACTIVE ATYPIA IN A PATIENT ON NSAIDS

Left: Low-magnification view shows eroded gastric mucosa with loss of the surface epithelium. There is severe mucin depletion of the mucous neck glands and gastric pits.

Above: Higher magnification shows significant cytologic atypia in the regenerating glands.

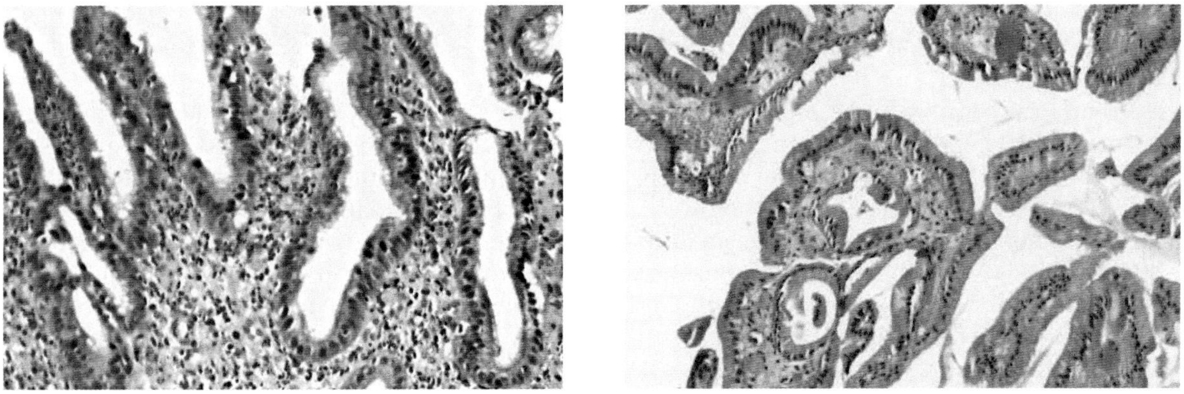

Figure 8-6

CHEMICAL GASTROPATHY IN A PATIENT ON NSAIDS

The mucosa shows villiform transformation and irregularly shaped glands.
Left: Immaturity of the epithelium with mucin depletion.
Right: More mature foveolar lining epithelium.

tortuosity, vascular congestion, mucosal villiform transformation, and muscular stranding up into the mucosa (fig. 8-7). There is a relative paucity of inflammatory cells. The sensitivity of these latter histologic changes for NSAID injury is low. Foveolar hyperplasia, one of the characteristic features of chemical gastropathy, is absent in up to 66 percent of NSAID users and prominent muscle fibers are only present in 47 percent of patients (25). Concurrent *H. pylori* gastritis may obscure the pathologic features. Acute and chronic inflammation usually surrounds NSAID-associated ulcers in *H. pylori*-infected individuals.

No single histologic parameter reliably distinguishes NSAID-associated gastric ulcers from ulcers due to other causes. Moderate to severe foveolar hyperplasia, edema, and vascular ectasia are significantly more common in NSAID

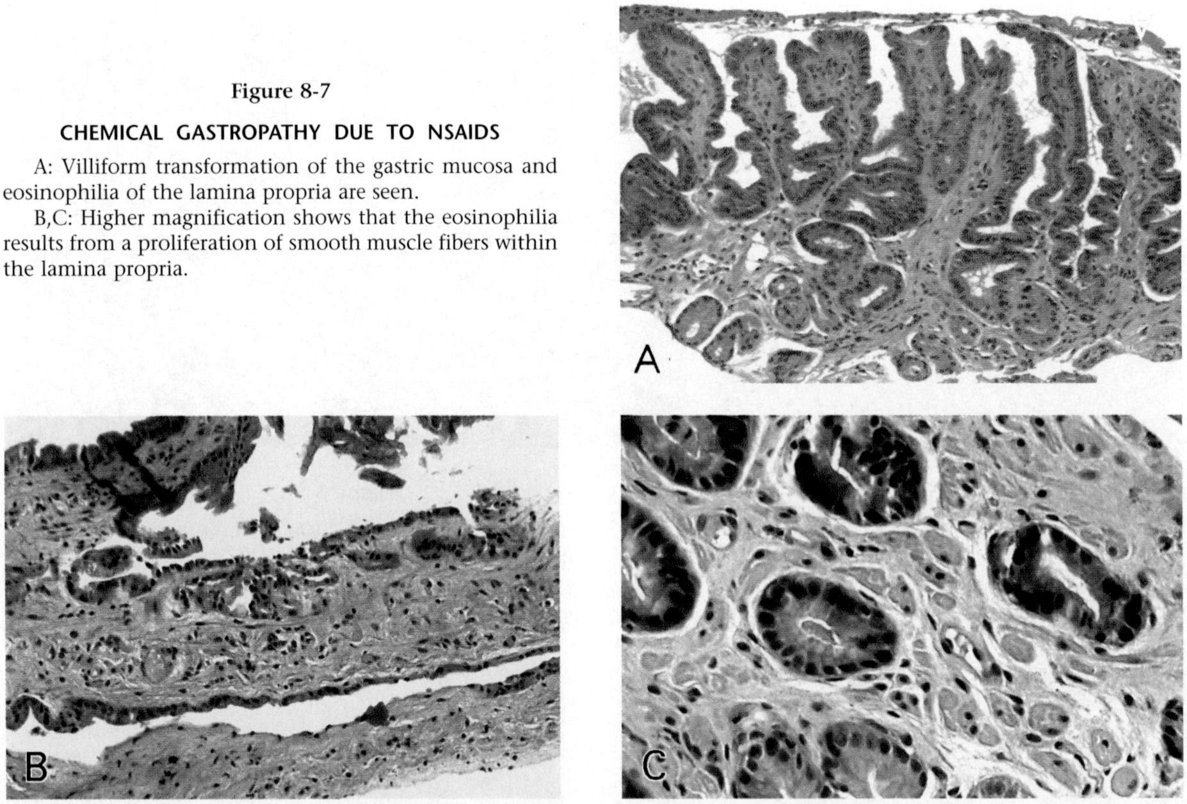

Figure 8-7

CHEMICAL GASTROPATHY DUE TO NSAIDS

A: Villiform transformation of the gastric mucosa and eosinophilia of the lamina propria are seen.

B,C: Higher magnification shows that the eosinophilia results from a proliferation of smooth muscle fibers within the lamina propria.

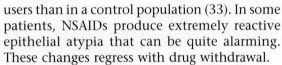

users than in a control population (33). In some patients, NSAIDs produce extremely reactive epithelial atypia that can be quite alarming. These changes regress with drug withdrawal.

Small Intestine. Early lesions in the small intestine include patchy villous tip vacuolization followed by marked focal villous blunting and lamina propria inflammation. Eventually, villous atrophy develops. In severe cases, mucosal erosions or ulcers develop on the tips of the mucosal folds (fig. 8-8). Indeed, mucosal ulceration is among the most common side effects of NSAIDs and is generally histologically nonspecific. A paucity of inflammatory cells within the ulcer bed favors NSAID damage.

Mucosal diaphragms consist of mucosa and submucosal fibrosis (figs. 8-8, 8-9) (16), often oriented perpendicularly to the luminal surface. The mucosa overlying the submucosal fibrosis and along the luminal rim of the diaphragm is usually mildly inflamed, with or without ulceration, and it may show mild architectural distortion due to repeated episodes of injury (fig. 8-10). The mucosa closer to the perimeter of the diaphragm exhibits varying degrees of villous atrophy (fig. 8-10). There may also be broader-based diaphragms composed of more densely hyalinized submucosal collagen interdigitating with the muscularis mucosae (fig. 8-11). There is often prominent mucosal eosinophilia. Significant regeneration may be present (fig. 8-12).

Large Intestine. NSAIDs exacerbate preexisting colonic diseases (Table 8-4). Mucosal ulceration is among the most common side effects of NSAID use and is generally histologically nonspecific in nature.

Several forms of colitis are associated with NSAID use. The most common is nonspecific in nature and difficult to distinguish from ulcerative colitis early in its natural history. The likelihood of a drug association increases if there is prominent apoptosis (43) and increased intraepithelial lymphocyte counts (microscopic colitis). Collagenous colitis, eosinophilic colitis, and pseudomembranous colitis are also seen.

The diagnosis of NSAID-induced colitis may be problematic since the histologic features overlap with those present in other forms of colitis. The tissues often exhibit unexpected eosinophilia. Damage may be extensive,

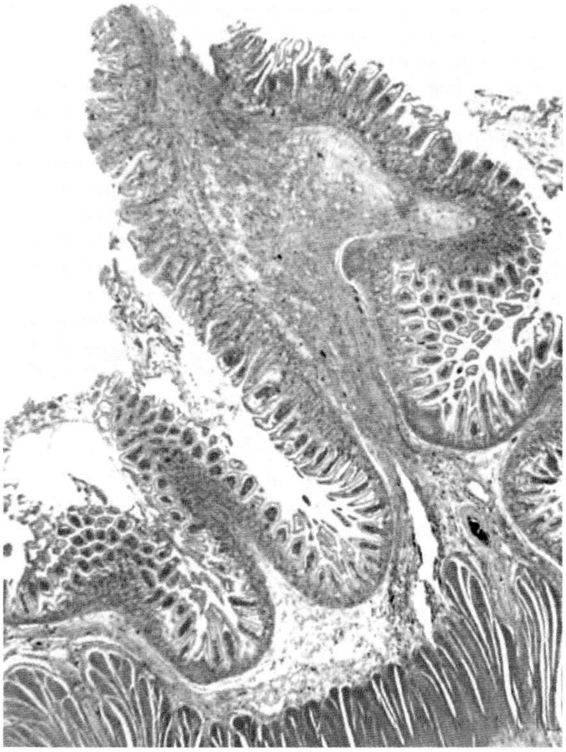

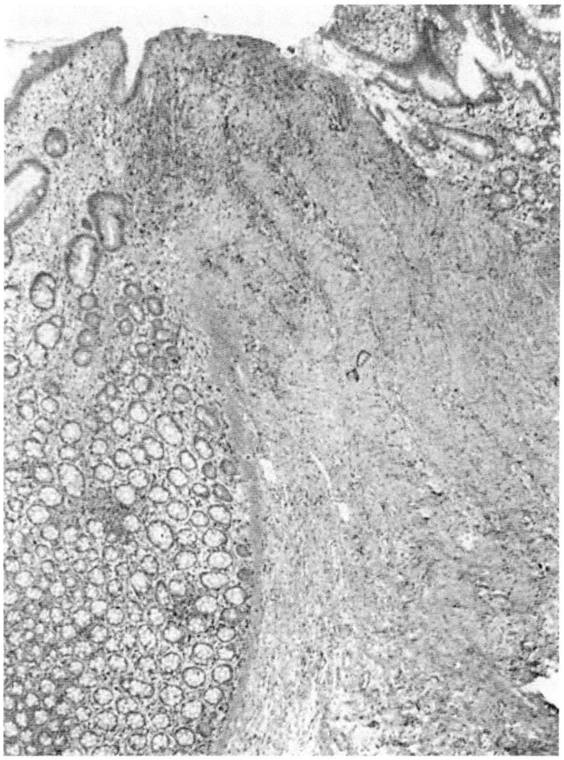

Figure 8-8

SMALL INTESTINE: MUCOSAL DIAPHRAGM DISEASE

Left: Exaggeration of the plica circularis and proliferation of connective tissue within the core of the plica. The tip of this exaggerated fold is eroded.

Right: Another area of ulceration from the same patient shows dense fibrosis and ulceration of the surface.

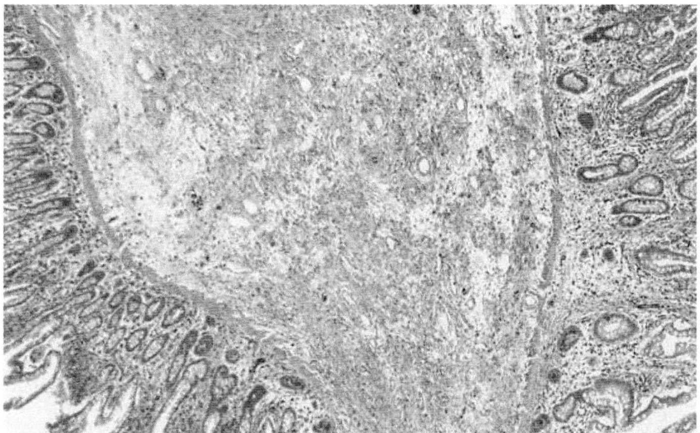

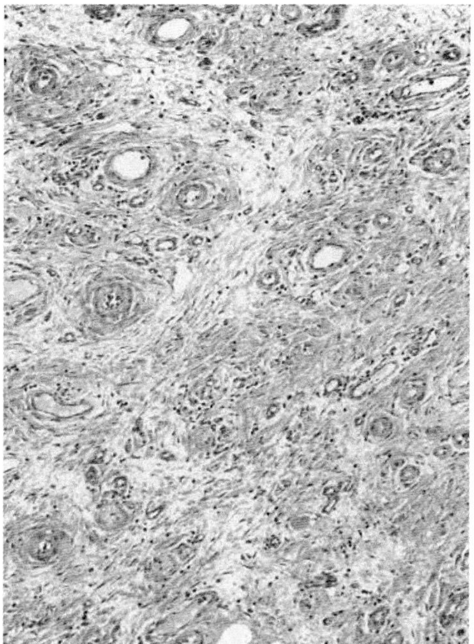

Figure 8-9

SMALL INTESTINE: MUCOSAL DIAPHRAGM DISEASE

Above: Medium magnification of the thickened plica circularis shows the damaged overlying mucosa and the proliferation of vessels and connective tissue within the submucosal tissue.

Right: Higher magnification.

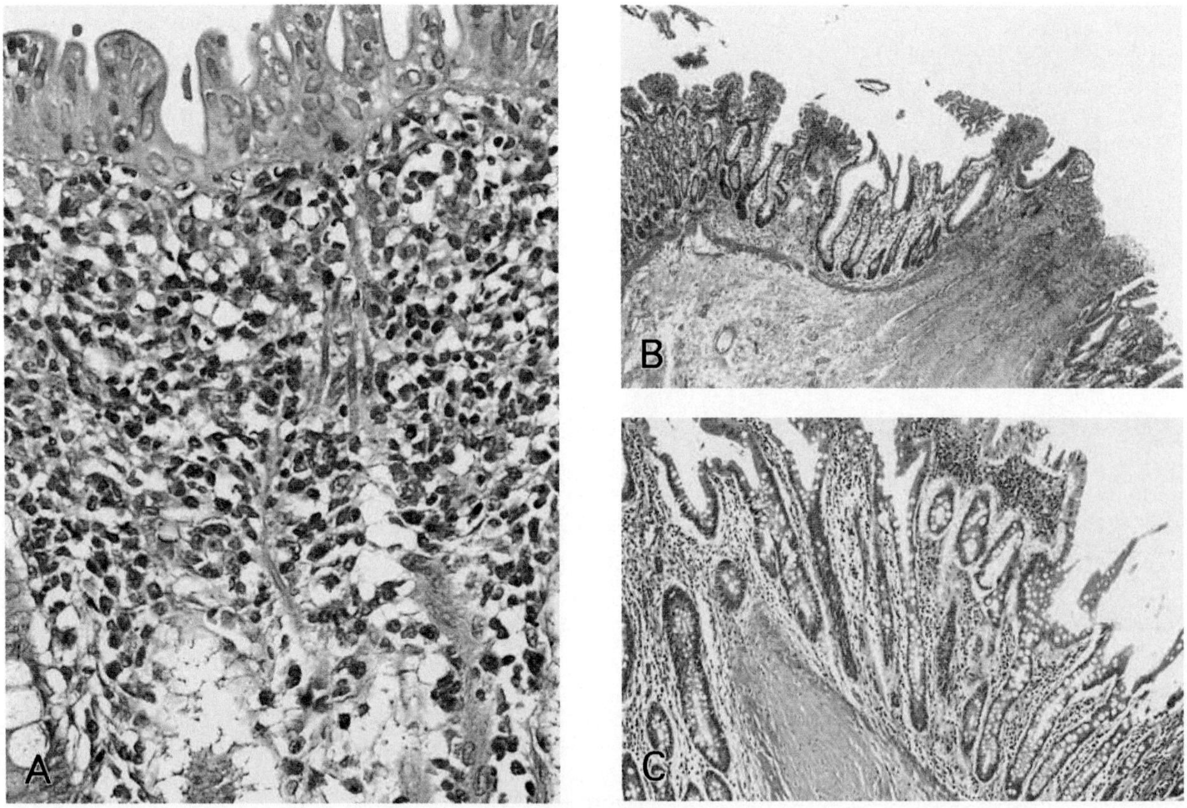

Figure 8-10

SMALL INTESTINE: MUCOSAL DIAPHRAGM DISEASE

A: A portion of the small bowel mucosa adjacent to that shown in figures 8-8 and 8-9 demonstrates regeneration and prominent mucosal eosinophilia.

B: Marked distortion of the surrounding architecture.

C: Higher magnification of the architectural distortion.

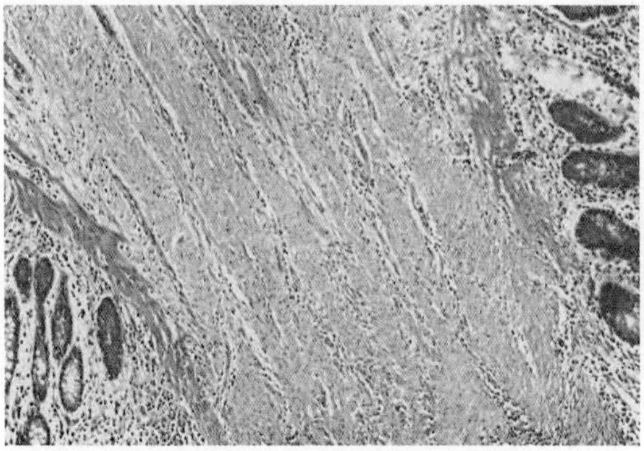

Figure 8-11

SMALL INTESTINE: MUCOSAL DIAPHRAGM DISEASE

An area of dense fibrosis is seen in the submucosa.

Table 8-4

COLONIC EFFECTS OF NONSTEROIDAL ANTIINFLAMMATORY DRUGS

Colonic ulcers
Nonspecific inflammation
Acute eosinophilic colitis
Pseudomembranous colitis
Eosinophilic colitis
Collagenous colitis
Lymphocytic colitis
Ischemic colitis
Chronic bleeding and perforation
Relapse of inflammatory bowel disease
Strictures
Complicated diverticular disease
Mucosal diaphragms

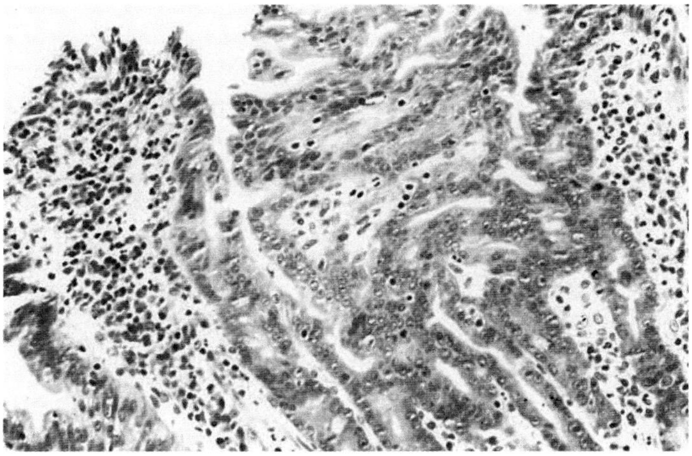

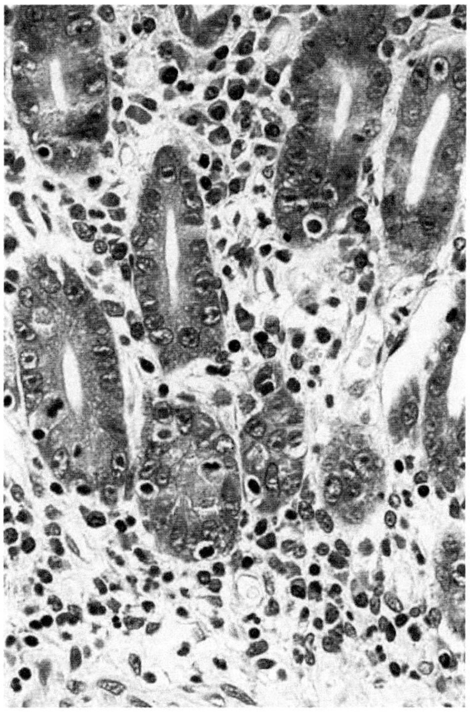

Figure 8-12

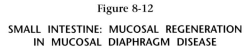

SMALL INTESTINE: MUCOSAL REGENERATION IN MUCOSAL DIAPHRAGM DISEASE

Above: The surfaces of the villi are significantly mucin depleted and have a somewhat hyperplastic appearance. Many syncytial-like cells are apparent.

Right: There is a marked increase in the number of mitotic figures in the crypts.

particularly in the proximal colon (26). Chronic damage may result in significant pyloric metaplasia (fig. 8-13). Diclofenac can cause granulomatous colonic injury (10). Large intestinal mucosal diaphragm disease resembles small intestinal diaphragm disease.

Differential Diagnosis. The gastrointestinal changes seen in NSAID injury are not specific for it. They can also be seen in stress gastritis, duodenitis, and many other forms of chemical injury, including alcohol ingestion and bile reflux. Changes shared with other causes of chemical gastropathy include foveolar hyperplasia, mucosal edema, lamina propria telangiectasia, a paucity of inflammation, and prominent muscularis mucosae fibers extending into the mucosa. Acute inflammation tends to be minimal, although occasionally it is seen at the interface of necrotic and viable tissues. The histologic features may also overlap with those of ischemia.

Focal colonic crypt injury, with neutrophilic infiltrates producing cryptitis and crypt abscesses, occurs commonly in several diseases, including ischemia, infections, IBD, obstructive colitis, and NSAID use. Intestinal strictures also occur in patients taking slow-release potassium preparations or in cystic fibrosis patients taking high-strength pancreatic supplements. The concentric luminal diaphragmatic strictures, however, are very characteristic of NSAID injury. The findings in diaphragm disease overlap with those of neuromuscular and vascular hamartoma of the small bowel (20), and the latter may in fact be the same entity as mucosal diaphragm disease. Mucosal eosinophilia can also be seen in patients with parasites, allergies, IBD, eosinophilic gastroenteritis, connective tissue disorders, and neoplasia.

Treatment and Prognosis. The most effective method for preventing NSAID-induced injury is discontinuation of the NSAID or reduction in NSAID dosage. The use of COX-2–selective drugs also offers an effective way of reducing gastrointestinal complications (18,23,52). These drugs have the benefit of selectively targeting inflamed sites and leaving uninflamed sites unaffected by the medication (34,54,59,60).

Healing of NSAID-induced upper gastrointestinal ulcers occurs if drug-induced injury is recognized early. Early treatment with antacids, H2 antagonists, prostaglandins, and other gastric cytoprotective drugs such as sucralfate may facilitate mucosal healing. Sucralfate may also

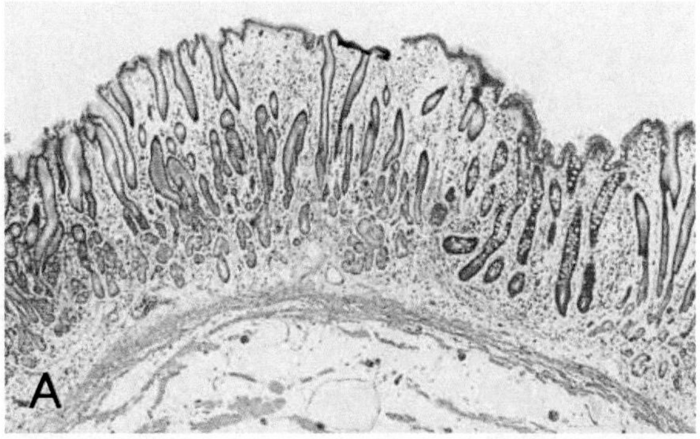

Figure 8-13

CHRONIC NSAID-INDUCED INJURY IN THE COLON

A: Low magnification shows marked architectural distortion, with pyloric metaplasia in the basal portion of the mucosa.

B: Higher magnification of the pyloric metaplasia.

C: The mucosa is very edematous with prominent crypt branching.

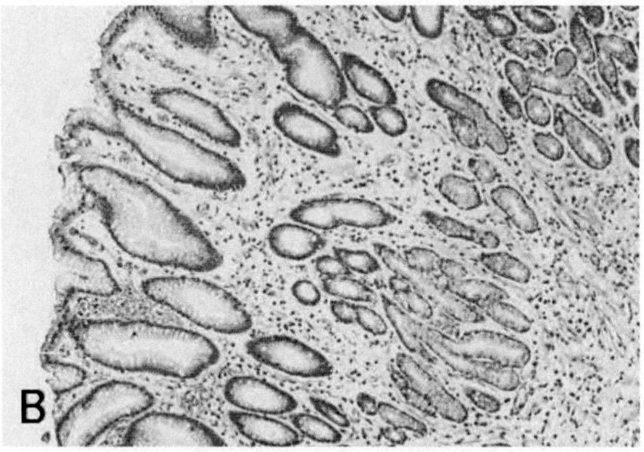

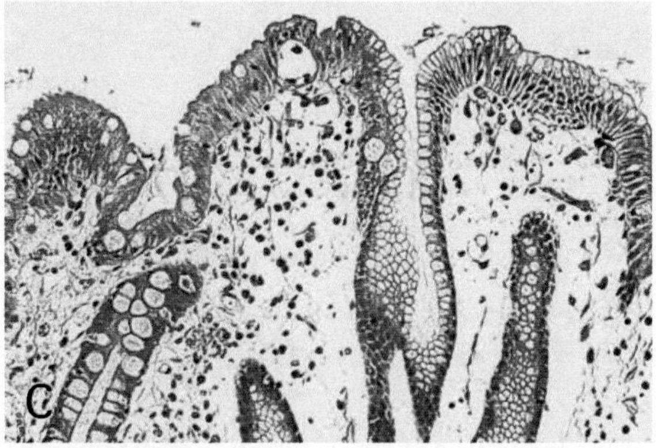

help prevent NSAID-induced erosions (6,45). Omeprazole may be used to treat or prevent NSAID-related gastroduodenal ulcers and to treat the dyspeptic symptoms (35). Symptomatic NSAID-induced strictures or stenoses need to be dilated or excised. Recently, treatment recommendations have been put forward based on risk assessment (Table 8-5) (19).

The mortality rate attributable to NSAID-related gastrointestinal toxicity is 0.22 percent/year, with an annual relative risk of 4.21 as compared with the risk for persons not using NSAIDs. Gastrointestinal complications of NSAID use may be responsible for more than10,000 deaths/year in the United States (8,13).

ALCOHOL

Definition. *Alcoholic gastritis/duodenitis* develops following excessive consumption of alcohol.

Pathophysiology. Alcohol-induced gastric damage correlates with the amount of alcohol consumed (63). Gastric alcohol-mediated injury usually requires gastric alcohol concentrations of over 10 percent (66). Since alcohol is lipid soluble (62), it directly damages the epithelium by altering cell membranes, intercellular junctions, mitochondria, endoplasmic reticulum, and the Golgi apparatus (64). There is focal separation of the cell junctions accompanied by capillary disruption and hemorrhage, with an outpouring of mucus and fibrin into the damaged mucosa. This results in epithelial sloughing that then facilitates acid back-diffusion into the mucosa. Alcohol stimulates gastric acid secretion, further augmenting the damage (fig. 8-14). Alcohol also damages the mucosal vasculature, leading to the subsequent development of mucosal hemorrhages and erosions. Mucosal vasoconstriction further contributes to the mucosal injury. Patients with *H. pylori* infection are more vulnerable to alcohol-mediated gastric mucosal damage due to the presence of an already damaged mucosal barrier. In the duodenum, alcohol-induced injury exposes the underlying tissue to the effects of luminal digestive enzymes. Neutrophil-mediated cell injury further contributes to the alcohol-induced injury (66). The effects of alcohol and NSAIDs are synergistic.

Table 8-5

STRATEGIES FOR PREVENTION OF NONSTEROIDAL ANTIINFLAMMATORY DRUG INJURY BASED ON RISK[a]

Patient Group	Strategies
Low risk (no risk factors)	Least ulcerogenic NSAIDs at lowest effective doses
Moderate risk (1-2 risk factors)[b]	Least ulcerogenic NSAID + an antisecretory agent or misoprostol COX-2[c] inhibitor
High risk (≥3 risk factors or concomitant aspirin, steroids, or warfarin)	COX-2 inhibitor + PPI or misoprostol for concomitant aspirin COX-2 inhibitor + misoprostol for concomitant warfarin COX-2 inhibitor for concomitant steroids
Very high risk (history of recent ulcer complication)	Avoid NSAIDs altogether COX-2 inhibitor + PPI and/or misoprostol

[a]Modified from Chan FK. Prevention of NSAID gastrointestinal complications—review and recommendations based on risk assessment. Aliment Pharmacol Ther 2004;19:1051–61.

[b]Old age, presence of cardiovascular diseases, use of high-dose or multiple NSAIDs, concomitant use of low-dose aspirin and other antiplatelet drugs, steroids, or warfarin.

[c]COX-2 = cyclooxygenase-2; PPI = proton pump inhibitors.

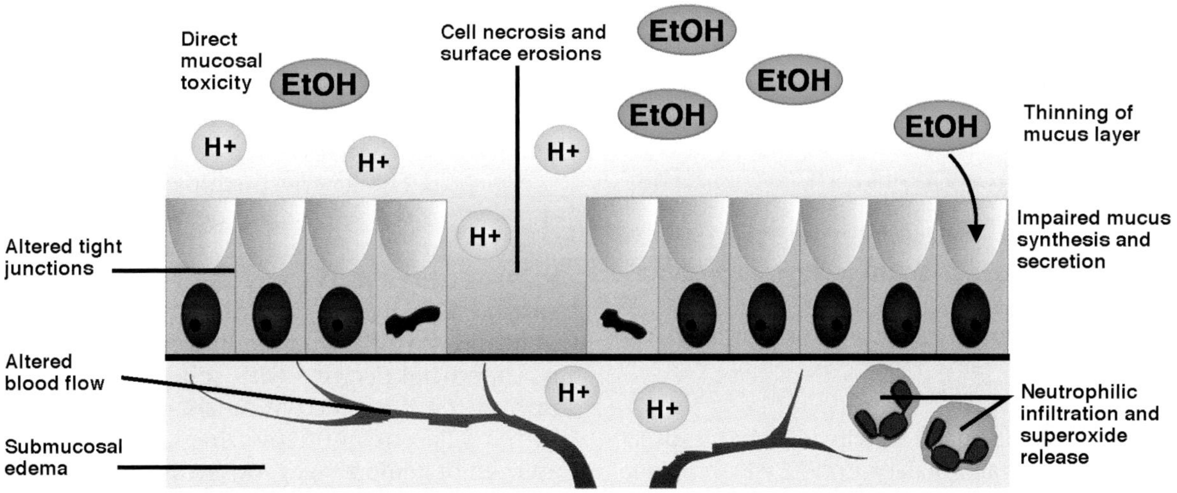

Figure 8-14

DIAGRAM OF THE PATHOPHYSIOLOGY OF ALCOHOL-INDUCED INJURY

Clinical Features. The clinical features differ depending on whether alcohol intake is acute or chronic. In alcoholics, the clinical features may be dominated by the effects of coexisting portal hypertension. Many chronic alcohol abusers develop abdominal discomfort, vomiting, diarrhea, and anorexia due either to gastritis or to hepatic disease.

Esophagus. Both acute and chronic alcohol ingestion cause esophageal dysmotility. Acute alcohol intake also decreases lower esophageal sphincter pressure (65) predisposing to reflux esophagitis.

Stomach. Alcohol ingestion results in both acute erosive and nonerosive gastritis. Many alcoholics present with gastrointestinal hemorrhage from coexisting disease, e.g., varices, portal gastropathy, peptic ulcer disease, or Mallory-Weiss tears. The magnitude of the bleed varies, depending on whether there is an associated coagulopathy. Alcohol may also cause acute "morning after" discomfort. Concomitant pancreatitis may need to be excluded in patients with severe abdominal pain.

Intestines. Chronic alcohol ingestion can cause intestinal epithelial immaturity with

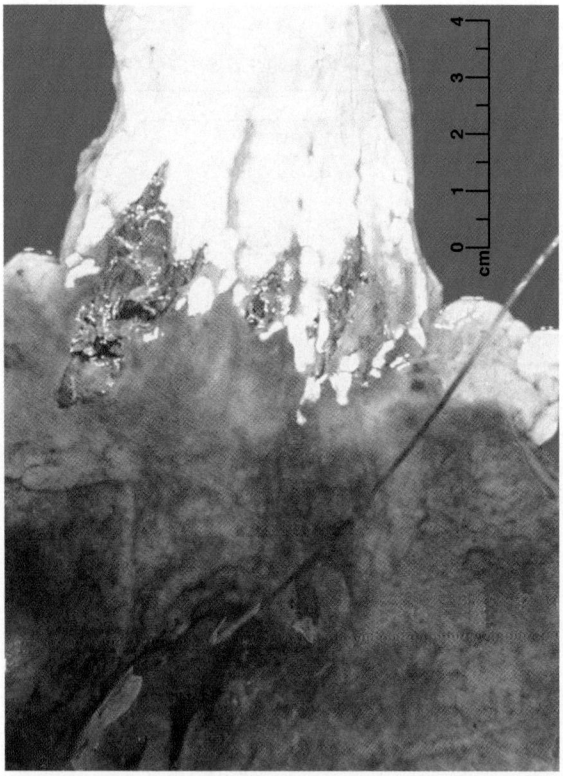

Figure 8-15

ALCOHOL-INDUCED GASTRITIS: GROSS APPEARANCE

The entire gastric mucosa is reddened. There are significant erosions at the gastroesophageal junction and there is a tear across the junction.

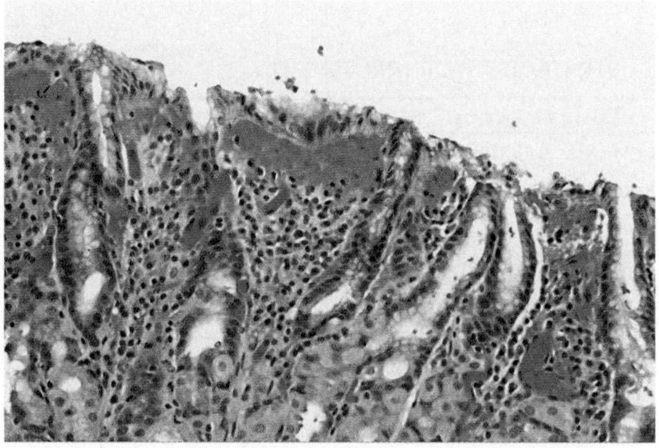

Figure 8-16

ALCOHOL-INDUCED EROSIVE GASTRITIS

The mucosa is markedly congested. (Figs. 8-16 and 8-17 are from the same patient.)

diminished enzymatic activity (61) that leads to chronic diarrhea or malabsorption. Alcohol consumption may also alter the bowel flora, further contributing to malabsorption. Discontinuing alcohol consumption corrects the diarrhea, as long as the malabsorption does not result from coexisting pancreatic insufficiency.

Gross Findings. Alcohol routinely damages the gastrointestinal mucosa, causing erosive and nonerosive esophagitis, gastritis (fig. 8-15), and duodenitis (67). The gross and endoscopic findings in the stomach and duodenum depend on the severity of the damage. The mucosa may appear congested, hemorrhagic, eroded, or ulcerated. Most damage occurs in the antrum (due to stasis), but the fundus can also be involved, as well as the mid and proximal stomach. Small intestinal mucosal damage primarily affects the proximal duodenum (68). Small intestinal changes are usually less severe than gastric changes, presumably due to lower alcohol concentrations.

Microscopic Findings. *Esophagus.* Alcohol causes esophagitis and non-neoplastic proliferative mucosal changes (69).

Stomach. The gastric histology ranges from no obvious damage to the presence of significant disease. Most histologic changes resemble those seen in either chemical gastropathy or stress gastritis. Usually, the gastric epithelial damage is mild and the inflammation minimal. There may be superficial necrosis with subepithelial hemorrhage (fig. 8-16) and prominent mucosal edema in the adjacent nonhemorrhagic mucosa. The amount of hemorrhage tends to be slightly more than that seen in patients on NSAIDs. In some patients, the edema extends deeper into the interglandular area (67). Superficial necrosis, erosions, and ulcers often coexist with these changes. The mucous neck region may appear reactive. Although controversial, it is possible that chronic alcohol ingestion produces chronic antral gastritis. Peptic ulcer disease, gastric vascular ectasia (fig. 8-17), portal gastropathy, and gastric varices may coexist with erosive gastritis or chemical gastropathy.

Intestines. Alcohol can induce acute erosive duodenitis as well as erosive gastritis. The changes mimic those induced by NSAIDs (fig. 8-18). Increased numbers of goblet cells and foveolar metaplasia are seen in the duodenum, and mild villous atrophy (68) may lead to secondary malabsorption. Patients with portal

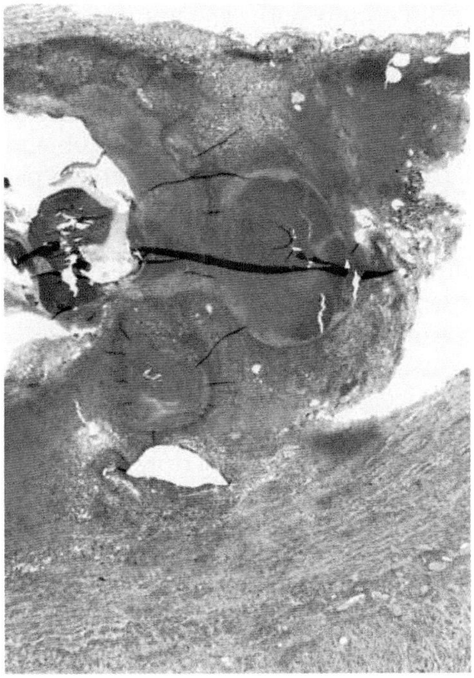

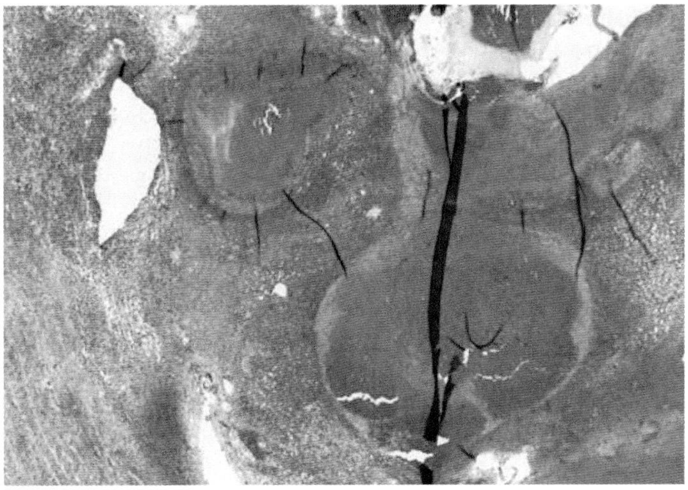

Figure 8-17

ALCOHOL-INDUCED GASTRIC INJURY

Left: Dilated and congested vessels with areas of acute and chronic inflammation.

Above: Higher magnification.

hypertension may also develop small or large intestinal varices.

Differential Diagnosis. The histologic features of alcohol-induced gastritis overlap with acute stress gastritis and chemical gastropathy due to other causes. It may be impossible to distinguish among these entities without an adequate history. The changes of portal hypertensive gastropathy may mimic those of gastric antral vascular ectasia. Many of these patients may also be consuming aspirin- or ibuprofen-containing products for their abdominal complaints so that the endoscopic and histologic picture may therefore demonstrate overlapping features.

Treatment and Prognosis. Cessation of alcohol ingestion usually results in mucosal recovery within a few days.

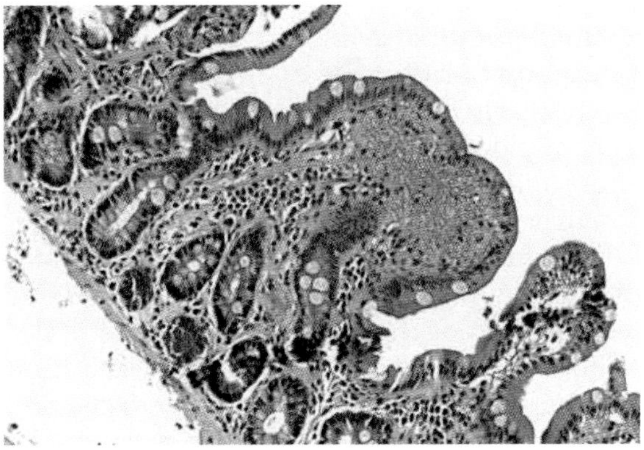

Figure 8-18

EROSIVE DUODENITIS SECONDARY TO ALCOHOL EXPOSURE

The mucosa is congested and appears chronically damaged.

CHEMOTHERAPEUTIC AGENTS

Definition. *Chemotherapy-induced gastrointestinal damage* results from the toxic effects of chemotherapeutic agents on actively replicating gastrointestinal epithelia.

Demography. The gastrointestinal tract is commonly injured by the chemotherapy used to treat cancer patients.

Etiology. Many chemotherapeutic agents damage the gastrointestinal tract. The most common are the antimetabolites, including fluoroxidin, 5-fluorouracil (5-FU) alone or in combination with leucovorin, mitomycin, cisplatin, or methotrexate. 5-FU is commonly used as an adjuvant in gastrointestinal cancer therapy. It interferes with DNA synthesis and with RNA function (76). Cyclophosphamide damages jejunal crypt cells (77a). Vinca alkaloids, such as vincristine, cause intestinal ulceration, adynamic ileus, and pseudoobstruction syndromes.

Pathophysiology. Gastrointestinal damage results from both systemic therapy and selective hepatic artery infusion chemotherapy (HAIC) used to treat hepatic tumors. Systemic chemotherapeutic agents primarily target mitotically active cells (those in the replication zones), inducing massive cell death (70); causing crypt epithelial apoptosis, cuboidalization (72), mucosal ulceration, and inflammation; and producing a lesion known as mucositis (mucosal inflammation). The degree of mucosal toxicity varies depending on the number of drugs used, their dosage, the complicating effects of surgery, the extent of tumor involvement, and the presence of concomitant radiotherapy or secondary infections. In HAIC, high drug concentrations may reach the stomach via an aberrant or collateral circulation or catheter displacement. Inadvertent infusion of 5-FU into the gastroduodenal or right gastric arteries causes necrosis and ulceration of the gastric wall. Some chemotherapeutic agents also damage the myenteric plexus, leading to motility problems.

Small intestinal cytotoxicity may result from vasospasm or a decrease in fibrinolytic activity; this results in decreased mucosal blood flow and ischemic necrosis (73). 5-FU also causes direct endothelial-independent vasoconstriction of vascular smooth muscle probably as a result of activation of protein kinase C. 5-FU may also play a role in venous thrombosis, perhaps due to activation of the coagulation cascade (73).

Both actinomycin D and adriamycin inhibit DNA repair and enhance radiation effects (83). They induce a recall phenomenon in which the drugs evoke further radiation damage after prior radiation at relatively low doses. Other drugs that increase the effects of radiotherapy include 5-FU, bleomycin, hydroxyurea procarbazine, and vinblastine. Patients on paclitaxel and carboplatin develop submucosal hemorrhages in the stomach and patchy duodenal erythema. There is a prominent arrest of cell division in the intestinal epithelium. Paclitaxel interacts with microtubule polymers and inhibits depolymerization of the microtubule, thereby blocking the cell cycle (89).

Clinical Features. Chemotherapy leads to a high incidence of mucositis, which affects the oral, esophageal, gastric, and intestinal mucosa. Patients with mucositis experience considerable pain and discomfort. Other symptoms associated with chemotherapy treatment include nausea, vomiting, stomatitis, anorexia, diarrhea, abdominal pain, and ileus. Chemotherapy-related diarrhea is a common problem. Severe diarrhea affects 15 to 20 percent of patients receiving 5-FU and leucovorin. It can reduce patient compliance and sometimes be a potentially life-threatening disorder. Furthermore, potential alterations in nutritional status can result from inadequate digestion and a decrease in nutrient absorption. Chemotherapy-induced vomiting can lead to Mallory-Weiss tears, intramural hematomas, and esophageal perforation. Duodenal perforations complicate continuous infusion of 5-FU and cisplatin (76). HAIC may result in localized duodenal or gastric ulcers (87). Chemotherapeutic agents such as vinorelbine predispose to bezoar formation (74) secondary to toxic damage to the myenteric plexus or they induce lactose intolerance (80). Malabsorption results from methotrexate or colchicine treatment. Methotrexate can also cause toxic megacolon. Cytosine arabinoside in combination chemotherapy can cause protein-losing enteropathy (85). Paclitaxel has been associated with colonic perforation (82).

Chemotherapy also predisposes patients to mucosal infections, neutropenic enterocolitis, ischemia, hemolytic uremia syndrome, and pseudomembranous colitis. The most common opportunistic organisms include *Candida* sp, herpesvirus, and cytomegalovirus. Some patients develop *C. difficile*-associated colitis. Patients most likely to develop complications due to infection often have late-stage cancers with the compounding effects of malnutrition, ischemia, sepsis, or shock. Bowel perforation can affect those with extensive necrosis. An indirect complication of chemotherapy is erosion by intraperitoneal chemotherapy catheters into the bowel wall.

Gross Findings. Chemotherapeutic agents cause mucositis, ulcers, erosions, strictures, and fistulas anywhere in the gut. The incidence of esophageal injury is high due to the frequent combination of chemotherapy and radiation therapy used in an attempt to aggressively treat tumors arising in the chest. The gross intestinal findings vary considerably from virtually

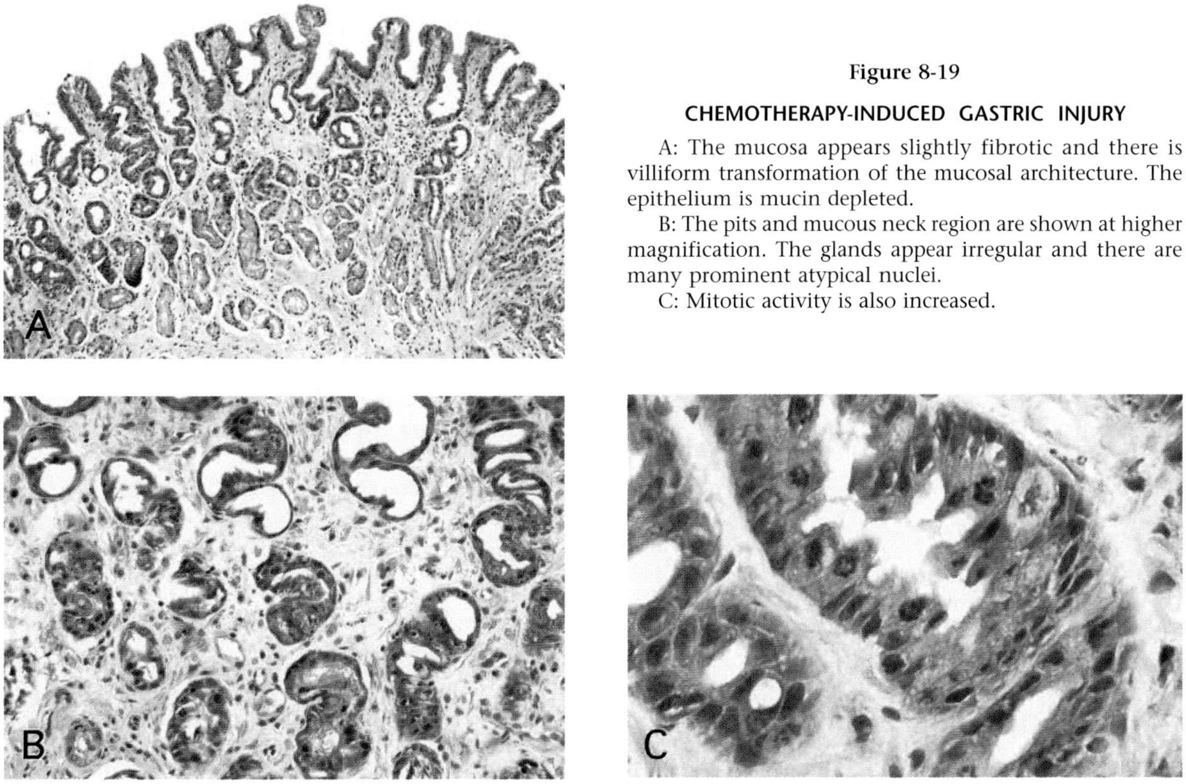

Figure 8-19

CHEMOTHERAPY-INDUCED GASTRIC INJURY

A: The mucosa appears slightly fibrotic and there is villiform transformation of the mucosal architecture. The epithelium is mucin depleted.

B: The pits and mucous neck region are shown at higher magnification. The glands appear irregular and there are many prominent atypical nuclei.

C: Mitotic activity is also increased.

invisible to areas of frank ulceration and perforation. Colonic disease tends to be less severe than small intestinal disease. Chemotherapy-associated ulcers grossly resemble peptic ulcers. In some cases, ischemia or infection complicates the injury induced by the chemotherapeutic agents. The typical gross findings of pseudomembranous colitis or neutropenic enterocolitis may be present (see chapter 10 for a discussion of these entities).

Microscopic Findings. *Esophagus.* Cytotoxic agents damage the esophageal mucosa directly. Nonspecific areas of necrosis, inflammation, and granulation tissue occur in severe injury. In less severe injury, an intact squamous epithelium may contain enlarged, atypical squamous cells. The regenerative basal squamous epithelium may appear atypical, sometimes with atypical mitoses. Underlying stromal cells and submucosal glands also often appear atypical. Chemotherapy with cyclophosphamide, methotrexate, and 5-FU may cause Barrett esophagus.

Stomach. Histologic changes range from reactive glandular atypia to frank mucosal ulceration. Crowded, irregularly shaped glands are lined by mucin-depleted, large, finely vacuolated, cuboidal epithelial cells, sometimes containing pleomorphic nuclei (fig. 8-19). The atypia is accentuated in the mucous neck region and basal gastric glands. Mitoses range from rare or absent to numerous (fig. 8-19) with bizarre configurations (81). The atypia is often more bizarre than that seen in carcinoma; the atypical cells tend to possess abundant cytoplasm (88). The pleomorphism presumably results from interference with nucleic acid metabolism. Pyknotic smudgy nuclei, apoptotic bodies, and necrotic debris lie in both the damaged epithelium and in the glandular lumens. Changes consistent with chemical gastropathy may be present (fig. 8-19). Intestinal metaplasia is usually absent unless the patient has coexisting chronic gastritis.

HAIC can produce gastric ulcers and alarming epithelial regenerative atypia. The atypia is easily confused with carcinoma due to the presence of binucleated or multinucleated cells containing massive nuclei, sometimes with prominent nucleoli (71,77,81,88). The drug-induced cytologic atypia becomes most troublesome when only superficial gastric cells, such as those

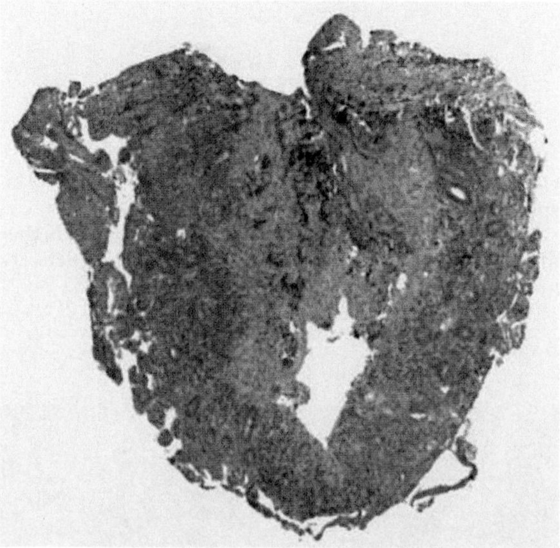

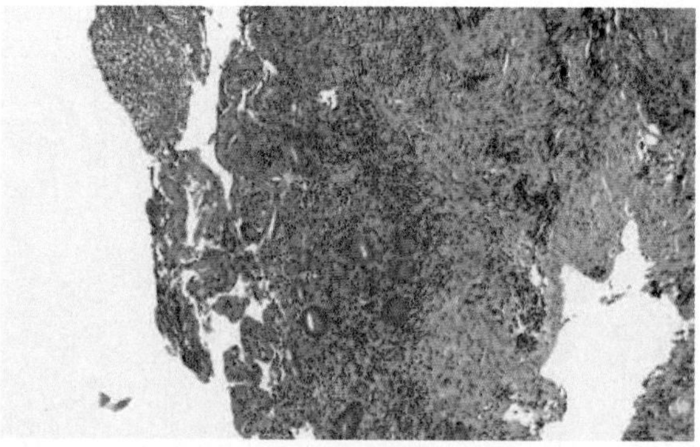

Figure 8-20

ILEAL BIOPSY FROM A PATIENT STATUS POSTCHEMOTHERAPY

The ileal mucosa is almost completely destroyed. The villi are lost; the inflammation is both acute and chronic.

present in superficial gastric mucosal brushings, are examined. The cytologic atypia resembles that seen in severe radiation damage.

Intestines. The mucosa of the small intestine is the region most sensitive to chemotherapeutic injury. Reduced mitoses occur within 3 hours of drug exposure (86,87). Maximum injury occurs after a day and persists for the duration of the treatment. The severity of the changes varies from case to case. Usually, villous damage is patchy in those receiving a single drug. More extensive injury with ulceration (fig. 8-20) affects those receiving a combination of drugs or a combination of chemotherapy and radiotherapy.

Early, the epithelium becomes mucin depleted and the cells appear cuboidal in shape (fig. 8-21). Surface epithelial cells become foamy, and brush borders are lost; the enlarged pleomorphic nuclei contain prominent nucleoli. The nuclei in the crypt bases become pyknotic, lose their polarity, and become karyorrhectic. Often the crypt bases show prominent apoptosis with the production of "popcorn" lesions (fig. 8-22). Eventually, the damage progresses upward, resulting in superficial mucosal necrosis. Within 24 hours, little necrosis remains because the dead cells or dead cell fragments are phagocytosed by neighboring healthy enterocytes and mucosal macrophages (79). After a few days, lymphocytes and eosinophils infiltrate both the epithelium and lamina propria. In cases of severe damage, all crypts are affected and frank erosions or ulcers develop. The degree of villous blunting ranges from mild to complete villous atrophy (fig. 8-20). Macrocytosis may be readily apparent; it is often irregularly distributed from villus to villus or crypt to crypt. The cellular density of the lamina propria decreases. Ulcers may develop. Many glands are cystically dilated and contain cellular debris, apoptotic cells, and numerous granulocytes. Stromal cells also show mild atypia.

Cellular regeneration occurs when therapy is stopped. It is recognizable by a burst in mitotic activity and marked variation in nuclear size. Mitoses are present at all levels of the mucosa, even on the villus surface. These changes usually occur within 2 weeks, but inflammation and telangiectasia persist for longer periods of time (77a). During the resolution phase, the crypt epithelium appears hyperplastic or the crypts appear cystically dilated and lined by bizarre cells. Histiocytic cell infiltrates may become prominent (78). Chemotherapy also severely depletes the normal intestinal lymphoid tissues, producing a hypocellular lamina propria and loss of Peyer patches.

Severe, large, solitary duodenal ulcers or polypoid inflammatory lesions with striking architectural distortion and cellular pleomorphism develop in patients treated with 5-FU HAIC. The changes affect the epithelium, stroma, and endothelial cells (84). The most striking feature in all cases is epithelial cell atypia occurring in glands and in the surface epithelium. Mitoses may be numerous.

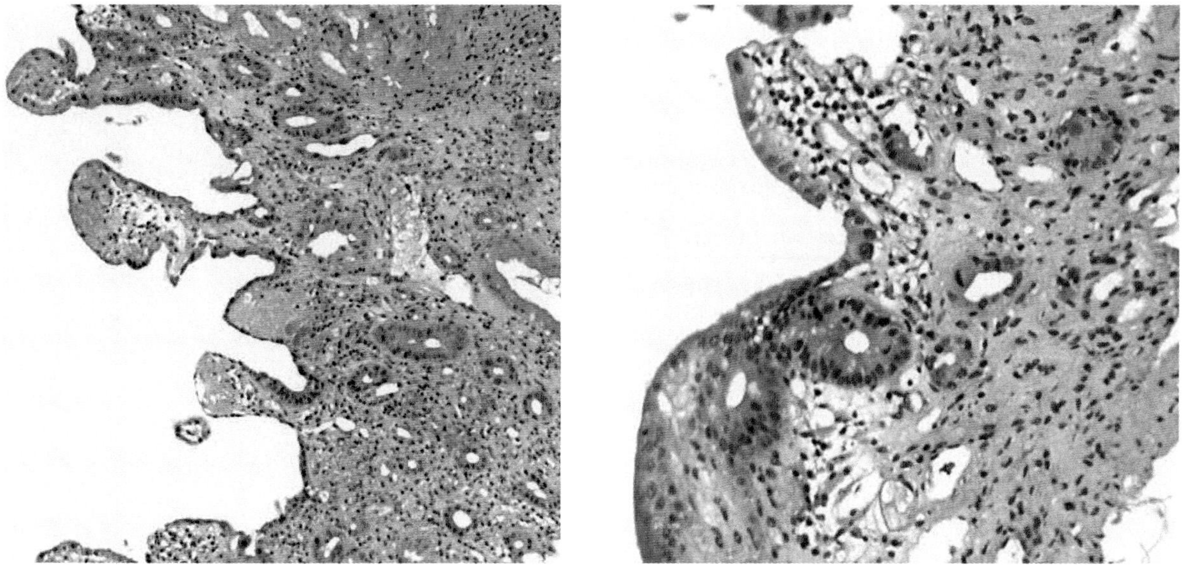

Figure 8-21

CHEMOTHERAPY-INDUCED INJURY IN THE DUODENUM

Left: There is marked deformity of the villi with elongation of the crypts, which have an irregular architecture. Many glands are smaller than normal. The mucosa is edematous and congested.

Right: Another area in the same patient shows glandular dropout as well as glandular regeneration. There is almost complete absence of villi.

The effects of chemotherapeutic agents on the large intestine are best described for 5-FU treatment (75). The earliest recognizable changes affect the crypt bases where the nuclei undergo pyknosis, loss of polarity, karyorrhexis, and apoptosis (fig. 8-22) (75). The lesions may progress to necrosis of the upper mucosa with inflammation in the crypt epithelium and lamina propria. During the resolving phase, the crypt epithelium becomes hyperplastic. Cystic dilatation of crypts lined by bizarre epithelial cells may be present. Colonic biopsies, however, often show only nonspecific colitis with cryptitis, ulcers, and acute and chronic inflammation. Collections of apoptotic cells in the crypt bases, cytologic atypia, and glandular dilatation suggest the diagnosis.

Differential Diagnosis. Erythema, friability, and edematous folds with erosions or ulcerations may occur focally or diffusely in the colon, and may mimic IBD, cytomegalovirus infection, or ischemia. The atypical cytologic features of chemotherapeutic injury may simulate carcinoma. Features that favor the presence of an acute chemotherapeutic effect include the overall preservation of mucosal architecture, recognition of similar atypical changes in nearby stromal cells, the presence of atypia that is more bizarre than that typically seen in carcinomas, the lack of an infiltrative pattern or tumor desmoplasia, the preservation of a low nuclear to cytoplasmic ratio, and late in the regenerative process, a lack of mitoses.

Treatment and Prognosis. The treatment of chemotherapy-related diarrhea is nonspecific, with the aim at reducing the discomfort and inconvenience of frequent bowel movements, avoiding the necessity for oral and parenteral replenishment of fluids and electrolytes, and waiting for recovery from the acute damage of the intestinal mucosa induced by the antineoplastic drugs. Opioid agonists have been a mainstay of the diarrheal treatment. More recently, octreotide is used to manage these manifestations. The epithelium is replaced within several days to 2 weeks following drug cessation. Vascular dilatation and inflammation may continue for several weeks thereafter, leaving the patient with the potential for bleeding.

Long-term gastrointestinal sequelae of chemotherapy are unusual but include the consequences of fissures, fistulas, and strictures. Most

Figure 8-22

CYTOXAN INJURY

A: The crypts have a markedly regenerative appearance. There are apoptotic figures in the base of the crypts creating a "popcorn" lesion.

B: In some areas, the epithelium within the glands has acquired an eosinophilic appearance.

C: The base of the glands shows increased proliferation as well as apoptotic bodies.

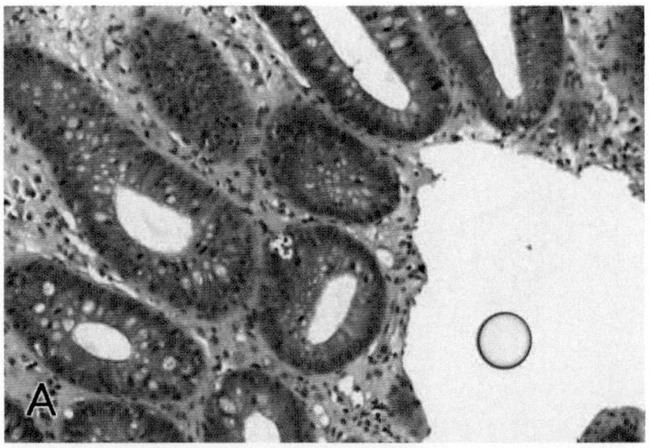

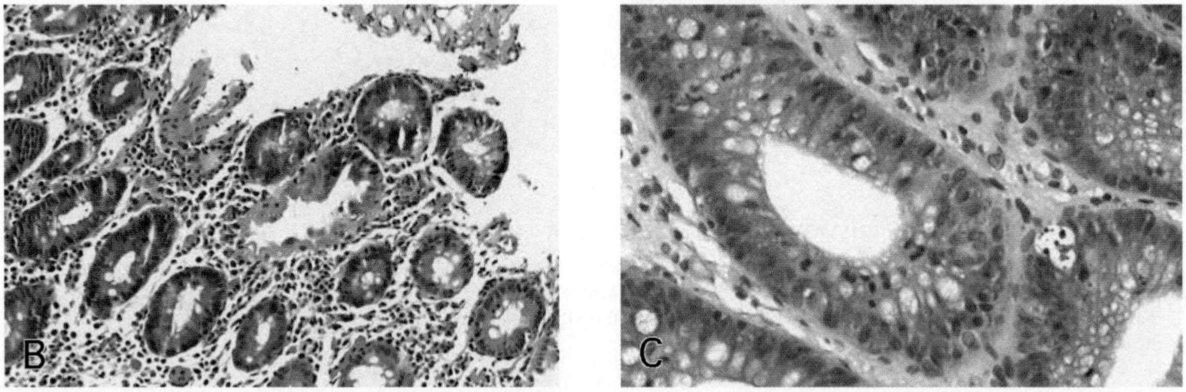

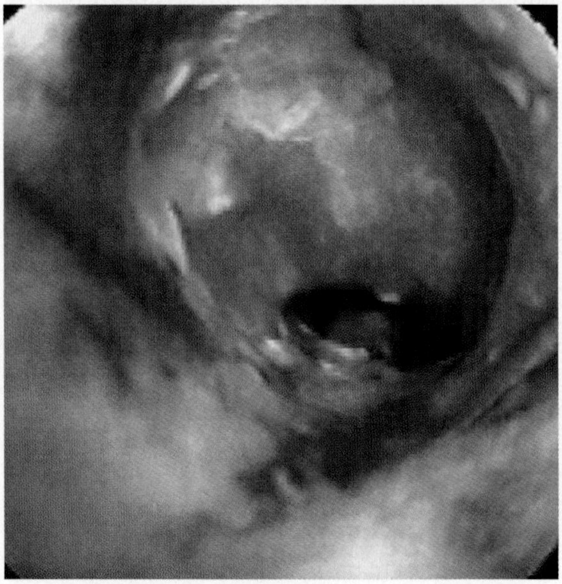

Figure 8-23

ANTIBIOTIC-ASSOCIATED ESOPHAGITIS

Tetracyclines are the most common cause of antibiotic-associated esophagitis, as shown in this endoscopic view.

patients who develop significant problems have been treated with multiple drugs or a combination of chemotherapy and radiotherapy. They may have other complicating illnesses, such as infection, ischemia, perforation, or sepsis.

ANTIMICROBIAL DRUGS

Demography. Antibiotics account for a significant percentage of *drug-associated esophagitis*. They also predispose the esophagus to viral and fungal infection by damaging the esophageal mucosal barrier. Antibiotics are the major cause of *C. difficile-associated colitis*.

Etiology. Tetracyclines, especially doxycycline, are the most common cause of antibiotic-induced esophagitis (fig. 8-23) (92). Numerous antibiotics predispose to *C. difficile* infection. This organism is discussed further in chapter 10. Penicillin and ampicillin cause a right-sided colitis that differs from the antibiotic-associated colitis attributable to *C. difficile*. Tetracycline, neomycin, and erythromycin all cause small intestinal disease. Treatment with erythromycin has recently been associated with hypertrophic pyloric stenosis (92).

Pathophysiology. The pathophysiology of antibiotic-induced injury, particularly in the intestine, varies. Neomycin disrupts micelles and decreases pancreatic lipase secretion, leading to malabsorption of fat. Erythromycin produces diarrhea by increasing motility and inhibiting absorption of intestinal enterocytic neutral amino acids, activity of Na^+K^+-ATPase (90,93), and transport of sodium-dependent sugar. Penicillin, ampicillin, tetracycline, isoniazid, and chloramphenicol all cause vasculitis. Penicillin, ampicillin, tetracycline, and erythromycin can cause Henoch-Schönlein purpura secondary to a drug hypersensitivity reaction. Flucytosine causes ulcerative enterocolitis due to direct mucosal toxicity.

Clinical Features. The major adverse effects of antibiotics include pill-induced esophagitis, malabsorption, diarrhea, and pseudomembranous colitis. Neomycin, erythromycin, some antimalarial agents, and paraaminosalicylate cause malabsorption (92a). The antifungal drugs flucytosine and clofazimine, used to treat leprosy, cause ulcerative enterocolitis. Antibiotics may exacerbate symptoms associated with ulcerative colitis.

Gross Findings. The gross and endoscopic features of antibiotic-related damage reflect the underlying abnormality and the site of damage in the gastrointestinal tract. Drug-induced esophagitis may present with areas of erosion and ulceration. Antibiotic-induced *C. difficile* colitis may be associated with pseudomembrane formation (fig. 8-24). Patients developing hypertrophic pyloric stenosis following erythromycin prophylaxis have a pylorus with the mean thickness and length of a pylorus affected with idiopathic hypertrophic pyloric stenosis (91).

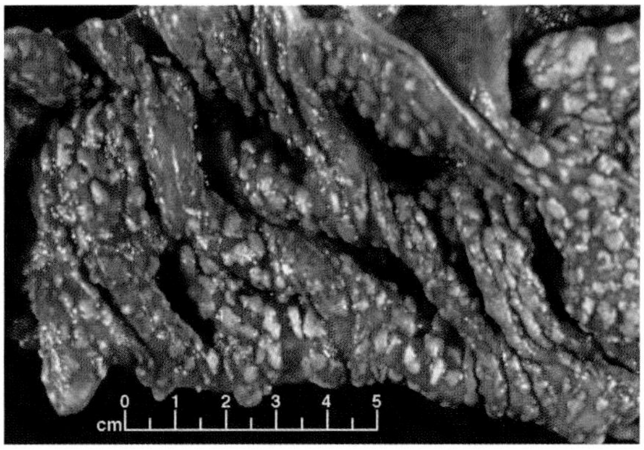

Figure 8-24

PSEUDOMEMBRANOUS COLITIS

The patient was on antibiotic therapy and developed an acute episode of severe colitis necessitating resection. The colonic mucosa was erythematous and covered by discrete and coalescing pseudomembranous lesions.

Microscopic Findings. Neomycin induces villous clubbing, brush border fragmentation, microvillous loss, and ballooning degeneration of the epithelial cells. The small intestinal villi may appear shortened and mitoses are increased. Rarely, the lamina propria becomes infiltrated with plasma cells, neutrophils, eosinophils, and periodic acid–Schiff (PAS)-positive macrophages. The histologic features of *C. difficile*-associated enterocolitis are described in chapter 10.

Differential Diagnosis. The differential diagnosis includes other causes of malabsorption and enterocolitis. The clinician may perform a small bowel biopsy whenever malabsorption is suspected in the absence of an overt pancreatic abnormality. In general, situations associated with villous atrophy (e.g., celiac disease), infiltrations (e.g., amyloidosis), or chronic infections (e.g., giardiasis) are considered. In the colon, the differential diagnosis includes many forms of colitis.

Treatment and Prognosis. Many of the clinical findings resolve upon cessation of the drug therapy. *C. difficile* colitis requires specific treatment.

IMMUNOSUPPRESSIVE AGENTS

Demography. Patients on immunosuppressive therapies who develop gastrointestinal problems are often transplant patients, patients with IBD, or patients with autoimmune diseases. Immunosuppressive agents are now widely used for many "benign conditions" such as asthma, rheumatoid arthritis, IBD, chronic hepatitis, vasculitis, and other conditions with an autoimmune and chronic inflammatory basis, as well as for neoplastic disease.

Etiology. Immunosuppressive agents, including steroids, indomethacin, mycophenolate, azathioprine, tacrolimus, and cyclosporine, all damage the gastrointestinal tract.

Pathophysiology. Controversy exists as to whether steroids directly damage the gastrointestinal tract (98,99,106,109). Steroids do exacerbate underlying gastric mucosal damage by: 1) stimulating G-cell hyperplasia (101); 2) increasing acid production by parietal cells; 3) decreasing epithelial turnover and inhibiting cellular regeneration and fibroblastic repair; and 4) inhibiting mucin secretion. Other immunosuppressive agents directly injure the gut and predispose individuals to gastrointestinal infections, especially those caused by herpesvirus, cytomegalovirus, *Candida, Aspergillus, C. difficile,* and less commonly, *Microsporidia* (96). Indomethacin inhibits mucosal bicarbonate production; induces villous necrosis, hemorrhage, neutrophilic inflammation; and predisposes the duodenal mucosa to peptic ulceration and enhanced bacterial translocation (111). Cyclosporine causes generalized small intestinal microvascular injury (100). Tacrolimus, a potent immunosuppressive drug, decreases mitochondrial adenosine triphosphate (ATP) production, increases intestinal permeability by a mechanism similar to that seen with NSAIDs (104), and predisposes patients to endotoxemia and impaired intestinal absorption (104). Recipients of organ allografts may develop a graft versus host disease–like condition when doses of cyclosporine are tapered off, a phenomenon possibly related to an autoimmune reaction.

Mycophenolate mofetil is a relatively new immunosuppressive drug that inhibits inosine monophosphate dehydrogenase, a key enzyme in the de novo pathway of purine synthesis. It causes lymphocyte-selected immunosuppression. It is used to prevent allograft rejection and is usually administered together with cyclosporin or tacrolimus and corticosteroids. Its major adverse effects are on the gastrointestinal tract (96).

Clinical Features. Patients on immunosuppressive therapies experience various gastrointestinal complications, some of which have an ischemic or infectious basis and others that result from the toxic effects of the drugs themselves. Ulceration, hemorrhage, and perforation may result (94,108). Steroids can suppress clinical symptoms, leading to a delayed diagnosis of either underlying conditions or diseases caused by the steroids themselves. Intestinal side effects of tacrolimus are frequent and include abdominal cramps, distension, nausea, vomiting, diarrhea, and malabsorption (103, 105). Indomethacin in suppositories causes rectal ulceration. Abdominal pain and diarrhea are the most common adverse reactions of mycophenolate therapy (95,96,105). Mycophenolate also causes gastritis, ulcers, gastrointestinal hemorrhage, perforation, esophagitis, and anorexia (96). Neutropenic enterocolitis and toxic megacolon are serious, often life-threatening complications of mycophenolate.

Gross Findings. Immunosuppressive drugs lead to mucosal erosions and ulcerations. Steroid-associated ulcers are usually superficial but deeper ulcerations may lead to perforation. Endoscopically, the mucosa appears edematous, with a decreased vascular pattern. Patchy erythema and erosive changes are frequently observed in the stomach, small intestine, and large intestine. Ulcerative lesions, if present, may be discrete and require biopsy to exclude ischemia, cytomegalovirus, or other opportunistic infections.

Microscopic Findings. Indomethacin causes tissue eosinophilia and cytologic atypia, apparent in gastric brushings (102). Corticosteroids and azathioprine deplete lymphoid tissues, including gut-associated lymphoid tissues (97), causing a decrease in the size of lymphoid follicles (fig. 8-25) and focal small erosions with M-cell necrosis. This predisposes to bacterial invasion and subsequent perforation. The follicular regions become severely B-cell depleted. Steroids also cause inflammation and cellular necrosis (fig. 8-26). They slow mucosal cell renewal and decrease the reparative activity of fibroblasts, further predisposing to perforation. Mycophenolate causes colonic necrosis, secondary regenerative changes (fig. 8-27), and intestinal changes that mimic graft versus host disease (108). High doses of mycophenolate inhibit the proliferation of the basal epithelial cells in the intestinal tract (96).

Treatment and Prognosis. Drug withdrawal usually reverses the gastrointestinal damage, unless severe complications have developed. Steroid-induced ulcers are usually superficial and heal with drug withdrawal, but deeper lesions may perforate. This is particularly a problem in low birth weight neonates receiving high-dose steroids (107,110). Octreotide may resolve the diarrhea associated with mycophenolate therapy.

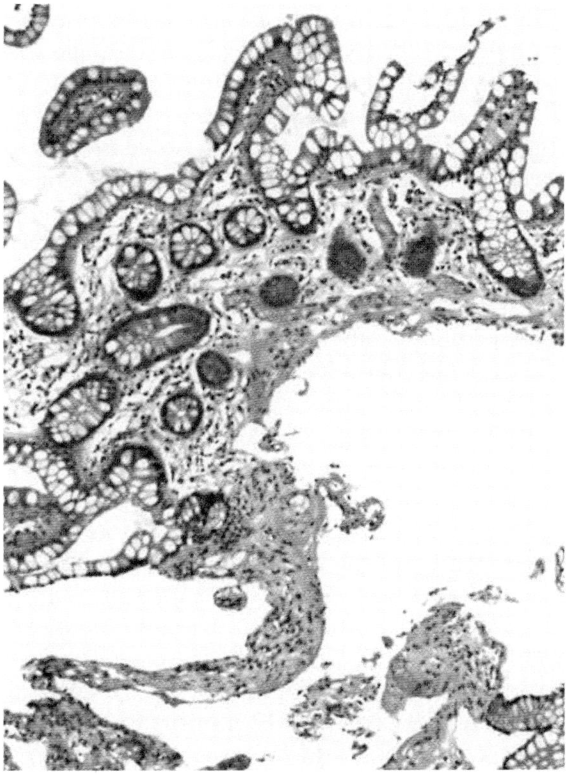

Figure 8-25

TERMINAL ILEAL BIOPSY IN A PATIENT ON LONG-TERM STEROIDS

The biopsy is remarkable for its absence of Peyer patches and for the relative hypocellularity of the lamina propria.

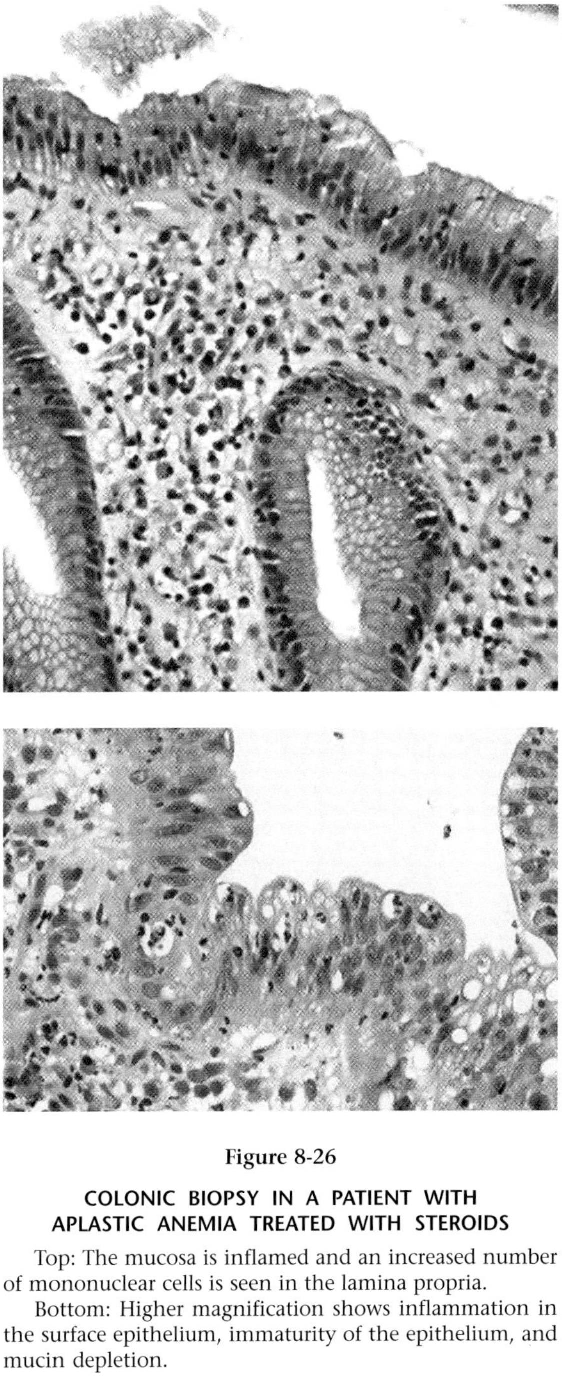

Figure 8-26

COLONIC BIOPSY IN A PATIENT WITH APLASTIC ANEMIA TREATED WITH STEROIDS

Top: The mucosa is inflamed and an increased number of mononuclear cells is seen in the lamina propria.

Bottom: Higher magnification shows inflammation in the surface epithelium, immaturity of the epithelium, and mucin depletion.

LAXATIVE USE

Definitions. *Melanosis coli* is the term used to describe the dark brown mucosal pigmentation that complicates the use of certain laxatives. *Cathartic colon* is the end-stage colon that no longer effectively contracts, presumably due to extensive damage of the myenteric plexus induced by long-term cathartic use (abuse).

Demography. The majority of patients with severe laxative-induced melanosis coli are women who have had chronic constipation and abdominal pain since early childhood and use laxatives long-term. An obsession with bowel movements is common; some patients have a history of sexual abuse. Patients with eating disorders, especially bulimic patients, patients with motility disorders, and laxative abusers constitute other major groups of patients with laxative-induced injury. Bulimic individuals typically consume large amounts of laxatives as part of the binge-purge syndrome (120). Estimates of the incidence of laxative-induced changes is about 5 percent in endoscopic studies based on the presence of melanosis coli. The frequency of melanosis coli at autopsy ranged from 11 to 32 percent in the past, but it appears to be decreasing in incidence.

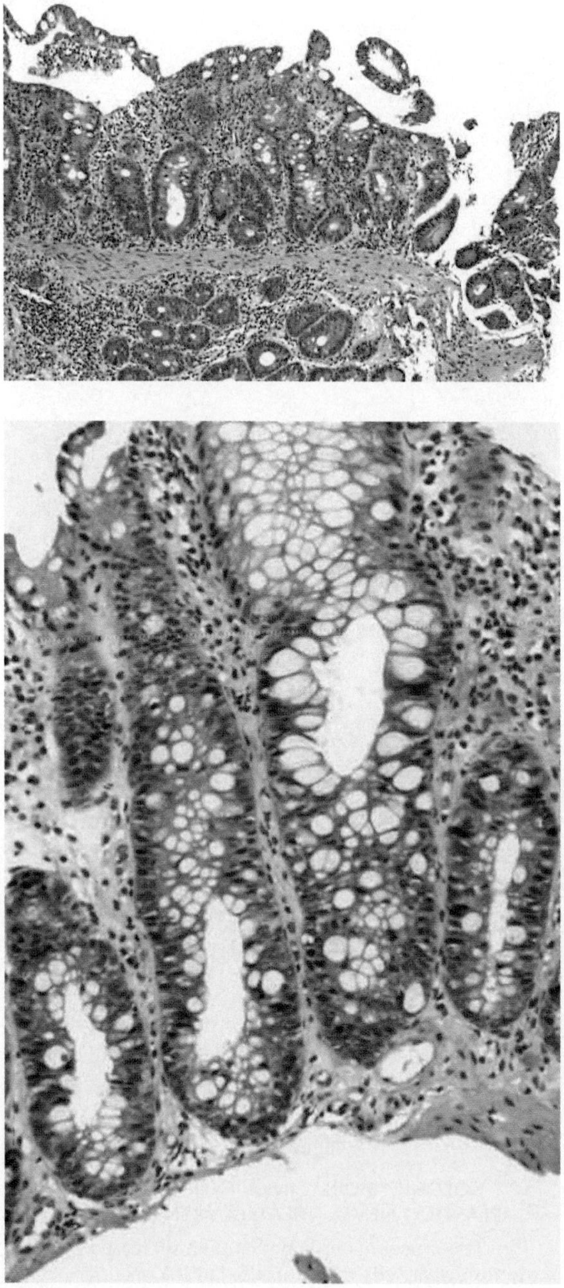

Figure 8-27

MYCOPHENOLATE COLONIC INJURY IN A RENAL TRANSPLANT PATIENT

Top: The mucosa is severely damaged with evidence of chronic changes. The glands are branched and of irregular sizes and the lamina propria contains increased mononuclear cells. There is also evidence of marked cellular regeneration. In some areas, the mucosa appears to have been desquamated.

Bottom: Regenerated glands with dystrophic goblet cells and irregularly shaped tubules.

Etiology. Anthraquinones, bisacodyl phenolphthalein, and magnesium salts all damage the gastrointestinal mucosa. Fleet enemas and bisacodyl may cause sloughing of the rectal surface epithelium; the lesions resolve in 7 days. Melanosis coli results from use of cascara sagrada, aloes, danthron, senna, frangula, and rhubarb. Evidence is beginning to emerge that melanosis coli does not result solely from laxative use. It can also occur in patients with IBD (both Crohn's disease and ulcerative colitis) who have not used laxatives (121) and in individuals with diarrhea unrelated to IBD who have not used laxatives.

Pathophysiology. Anthraquinones concentrate in the colon, particularly in the right colon, where they are potent cellular poisons that cause apoptosis, even when taken in small doses (122, 124). The apoptotic bodies are phagocytized by macrophages and transformed into lipofuscin pigment by lysosomal enzymes (125). The mean apoptotic count is significantly increased in those with melanosis coli compared with a control population. It takes 4 to 12 months for melanosis coli to be visible and the same amount of time for it to disappear. It is possible that any condition associated with increased apoptosis may result in melanosis coli (113,115). When present in small quantities, anthraquinones probably stimulate neural tissues, leading to their purgative actions. But the anthraquinones and other laxatives can also damage the myenteric plexus, causing neuronal loss, Schwann cell proliferation, axonal fragmentation, axonal and dendritic swelling, and smooth muscle damage (122–124). This eventually leads to cathartic colon. Bisacodyl, phenolphthalein, castor oil, and other agents also cause cathartic colon.

Clinical Features. Laxatives are most commonly used by patients with chronic constipation or motility disorders. Laxative abuse occurs in patients with eating disorders. Many patients are symptomless, only to be diagnosed following endoscopic examination for other reasons. Individuals with surreptitious laxative abuse typically present with unexplained chronic diarrhea. Some patients may have an obsession regarding their need to have a bowel "cleansing." In extreme circumstances, individuals using (abusing) laxatives develop protein-losing enteropathy, malabsorption, steatorrhea, hypokalemia or other electrolyte imbalances (118), and cachexia; in

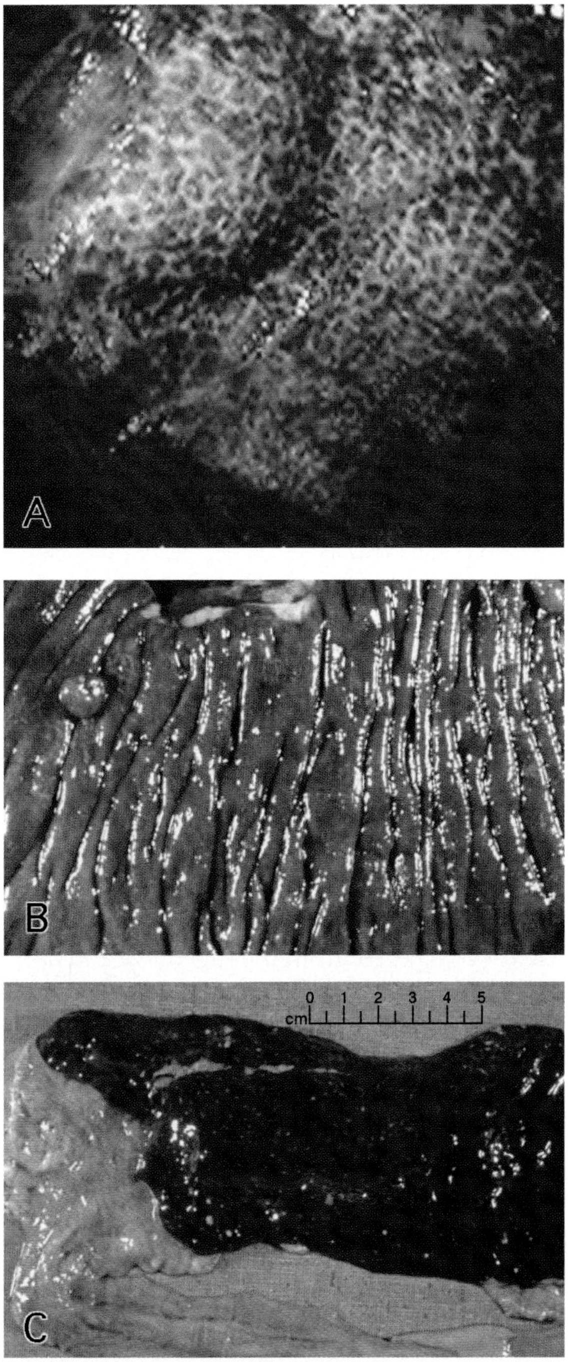

Figure 8-28

MELANOSIS COLI

A: Endoscopic view of the mucosa shows intense brownish pigmentation.

B. Resection specimen shows brownish discoloration of the mucosa. Adenomas appear pink on the brownish background.

C: Intense melanosis coli. The mucosa is very blackened. The changes stop at the ileocecal valve.

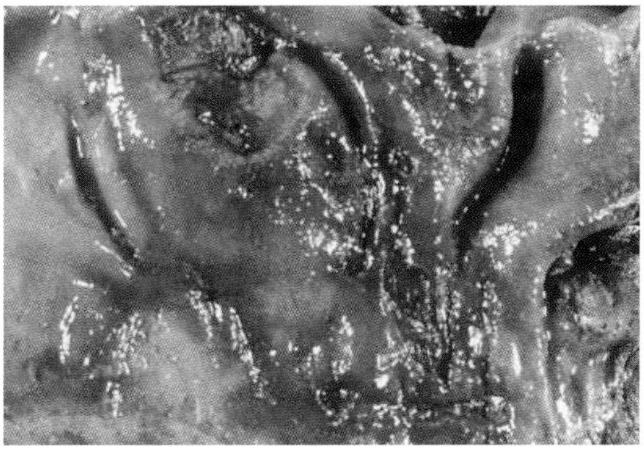

Figure 8-29

CATHARTIC COLON

The bowel is markedly dilated with loss of haustral folds, areas of ulceration, and reddish discoloration.

those with motility disorders, hypogammaglobulinemia (112), chronic constipation, and pseudoobstruction may occur (122).

Patients with cathartic colon present with chronic constipation, a sense of constant abdominal bloating or distension, pseudoobstruction, abdominal pain, and incomplete evacuation. These result from the toxic effects of the drugs on the neural structures in the bowel wall and secondary muscle damage (123). Narcotic use often aggravates the symptoms. Severe constipation leads to the formation of hard fecaliths that can cause local chronic inflammation, acute inflammation, stercoral ulceration, bleeding, and perforation. In patients with stercoral ulcerations it is difficult to determine whether the laxatives are the cause of the changes or are merely associated with them. Concomitant medication use and previous intestinal surgeries complicate the clinical picture.

Gross Findings. The endoscopic features of chronic laxative use depend on whether the patient has only melanosis coli (fig. 8-28) or has a cathartic colon (fig. 8-29). Melanosis coli begins in the right colon and progresses distally as the duration and intensity of cathartic use increases. The pigmentation tends to be heaviest in the right colon, including the appendix. Rectal melanosis coli signifies chronic laxative use. In severe disease, the mucosa appears dark brown or black. The changes typically spare areas occupied by lymphoid follicles, adenomas, and

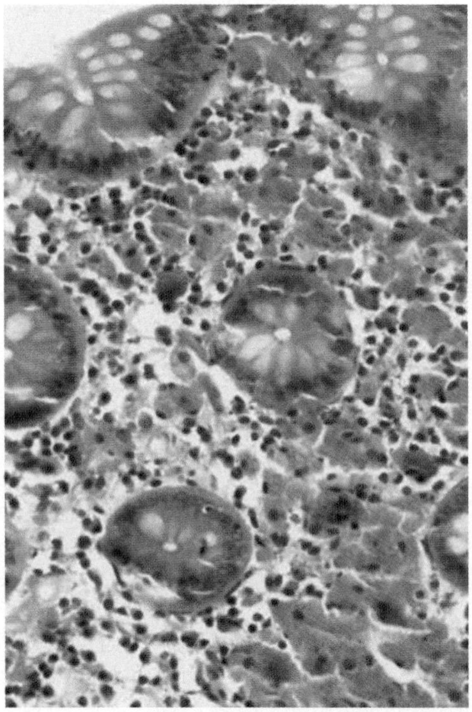

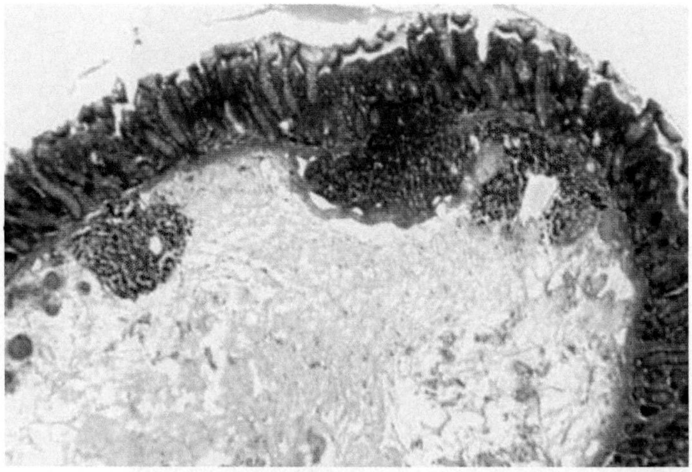

Figure 8-30

MELANOSIS COLI

Left: Numerous pigmented histiocytic cells lie within the lamina propria.

Above: In a case of long-standing laxative abuse, the pigmented melanocytes eventually migrate into the underlying lymphoid follicles at the junction of the muscularis mucosae, submucosa, and mucosa.

carcinomas; these areas usually stand out as lighter areas on an otherwise darkened mucosa.

In patients with cathartic colon, the bowel always shows melanosis coli. The proximal colon tends to develop patchy pigmentation that resembles snakeskin. Eventually, the entire colon and even the terminal ileum become atrophic and atonic. Redundant bowel loops are common. In severe cathartic colon, haustra disappear and the colon is converted into an irregular, focally dilated or sacculated, flattened, atrophic tube (fig. 8-29) (117). The muscularis propria appears thinned and atrophic, and submucosal fat becomes prominent, seeming to bulge from the cut edges of a resected specimen. The ileocecal valve, which is invariably affected, becomes incompetent (122–125).

Microscopic Findings. The histologic features of laxative use range from mild melanosis coli to severe cathartic colon. In early stage disease, pigmented macrophages lie in the superficial mucosa, often associated with nonspecific chronic inflammation and increased numbers of apoptotic bodies. The inflammation probably represents a nonspecific response to an underlying injury or to the stasis that may have been the cause for the laxative ingestion, rather than a direct effect of the laxative consumption. Refractile, golden brown, pigmented macrophages populate the lamina propria (fig. 8-30). The entire mucosa, submucosa, and eventually, mesenteric lymph nodes may contain pigmented macrophages. Pigmented macrophages migrate into regional lymph nodes, resulting in sequential loss of pigment from the superficial and deep lamina propria (125). The pigment may also be found in neurons. The lipofuscin pigment that accumulates is autofluorescent; sudanophilic; acid fast; positive with PAS, Schmorl, and aniline blue sulfate stains; and shows an intense argentaffin reaction that is abolished by bleaching, indicating the presence of a melanic substance. Because the autofluorescent pigment of melanosis coli contains melanin as well as glycoconjugates, it has been suggested that the pigment be termed "melanized ceroid." The ceroid pigment develops from the abundant apoptotic epithelial cells whereas the precursors of the melanic substance may derive from the anthracoids (113). Subluminal microgranulomas, often containing pigment, may form. Magnesium sulfate can cause jejunal mucosal shedding (114), glandular atrophy, thickening of the muscularis mucosae, and atrophy of the muscularis propria. Fatty droplets may be seen within the regional lymph nodes in patients who use mineral oil.

In early cases of cathartic colon, the mucosa appears mildly inflamed and glandular atrophy may develop. Eosinophilic infiltrates may be present. There may also be mucosal ulcers. Abnormalities of the myenteric plexus include neuronal swelling and pallor. Later, there is loss of argyrophilic neurons, marked axonal fragmentation, gliosis of the myenteric plexus, and ganglionic vacuolization. The remaining argyrophilic neurons appear dark and shrunken, with clubbed or swollen processes. Often the myenteric plexus becomes inflamed. Degenerative changes also involve the submucosal plexus and include axonal ballooning, loss of neural tubules and neurosecretory granules, and increased lysosomes. Atrophy of the muscularis propria develops secondary to denervation injury following neural damage. The muscularis mucosae hypertrophies as a compensatory response to the atrophy of the muscularis propria. Although these changes have been ascribed to laxatives, it is possible that they represent a primary disorder of the enteric plexuses that caused the initial constipation and subsequent laxative ingestion.

Special Techniques. Toxicologic analysis of urine or stool for the metabolic byproducts of the drugs detects surreptitious laxative abuse in patients with diarrhea of uncertain origin (116,119). Silver stains or immunostains may highlight the neural changes.

Differential Diagnosis. The differential diagnosis of laxative-induced injury includes an underlying primary or secondary muscular disorder (see chapter 17). Melanosis coli can resemble mucosal hemosiderin, which typically appears as larger, refractile, shiny granules. Iron stains confirm the presence of mucosal iron. Pigment deposition can also be seen in storage diseases and in chronic granulomatous disease, but in those disorders the macrophage collections tend to be larger than those seen in melanosis coli. In addition, with storage diseases other cells are often pigmented as well, including nerve and smooth muscle cells.

Treatment and Prognosis. Treatment consists of modifying the cathartic use and adding bulking and fluid supplements. Psychological support, particularly altering the patient's expectations and treating coexisting depression and obsessive behaviors, is important in laxative abusers. Promotility agents are occasionally successful. Patients who require frequent enemas or who experience fecal impactions need to be considered as having colonic inertia and may benefit from subtotal colectomy.

ENEMAS

Etiology. The various agents used to prepare the colon for endoscopic examination may induce minimal mucosal changes that can be mistaken for mild colitis. Most alterations occur in patients using enemas containing Fleet phosphosoda, bisacodyl (Dulcolax), hydrogen peroxide, and other hypertonic solutions (126, 130–132). Oral sodium phosphate use is becoming increasingly common compared with alternative preparatory agents due to better patient acceptance, superior comparable bowel cleansing effects, and lower cost.

Clinical Features. Soap-containing enemas can cause diarrhea and rectal bleeding. Cleansing enemas can cause a chemical proctosigmoiditis and even a perforation (127,129).

Gross Findings. Both Fleet phosphosoda and bisacodyl produce endoscopic alterations that mimic mild colitis, including obliteration of the vascular pattern with mucosal hyperemia and mucosal friability. The nozzle/tubing may be responsible for localized mucosal trauma. This is generally easily recognized endoscopically as irregular and linear erosions or ulcerations.

Microscopic Findings. Changes associated with enema use differ depending on the preparation (fig. 8-31) (130). Goblet cell mucus is often reduced and there is frequently a mild hyperplasia of the crypt epithelium, nuclear crowding, and mitotic figures higher in the crypt than normal. Hypertonic phosphate enemas may induce surface epithelial vacuolization and subsequent detachment from the basal lamina, subepithelial infiltration by a small number of neutrophils, and edema in the lamina propria. Bisacodyl (Dulcolax) induces more severe changes, with a pale, vacuolated surface and crypt epithelium that extends deep into the mucosa and is associated with a neutrophilic infiltrate of the epithelium and lamina propria. The changes elicited by both of these agents can be mistaken for a mild colitis.

Saline enemas and oral hypertonic solutions usually only cause mild edema of the lamina

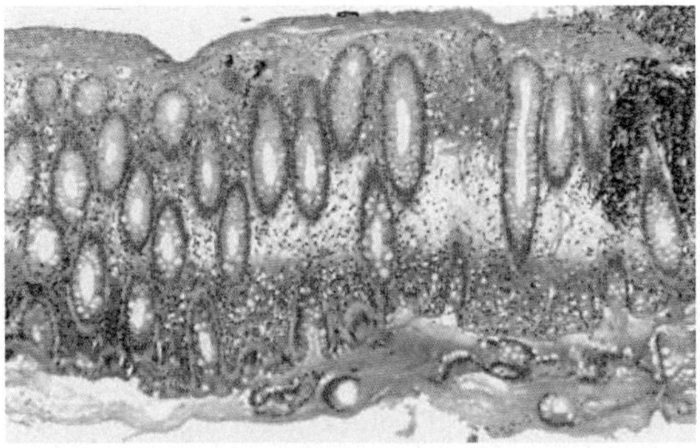

Figure 8-31

LAXATIVE EFFECTS

There is marked edema with minimal inflammation.

propria without epithelial damage. Oral sodium phosphate, a commonly used oral cathartic agent, can cause aphthoid ulcers or a mild focal active colitis in the colon and rectum (135). There may be occasional neutrophilic infiltrates of both the epithelium and the lamina propria. In addition to the presence of aphthous ulcers and inflammation, cell proliferative indices increase. The proliferation rate correlates with the number of apoptotic bodies (126).

Soap-containing enemas or enemas containing alcohol or hydrogen peroxide can cause extensive necrosis, inflammation, and mucosal shedding, and can mimic mild ischemia (128, 132). The changes are usually restricted to the mucosa. Hydrogen peroxide also causes pseudolipomatosis. The gas bubbles in the lamina propria result from the release of nascent oxygen from the peroxide (129,133,134).

Kayexalate-Sorbitol Enema

Demography. Kayexalate-sorbitol enemas are used to treat hyperkalemia in patients with renal insufficiency.

Etiology. The sodium polystyrene sulfonate (Kayexalate/sorbitol) causes the gastrointestinal injury.

Pathophysiology. Kayexalate is a cation exchange resin that releases sodium ions in the large intestine. The sodium ions are replaced by potassium, and the excess potassium is evacuated in the stool. Since kayexalate can cause constipation or impaction, it is administered together with sorbitol, an osmotic laxative. The osmotic load from the sorbitol enema causes vascular shunting, resulting in mild colonic ischemia and colonic necrosis in a subset of uremic patients.

Clinical Features. Patients with intestinal injury present with an abrupt onset of severe abdominal pain within hours of enema administration. Profuse rectal bleeding may occur.

Gross Findings. The endoscopic findings of the upper gastrointestinal tract are abnormal. Esophageal changes mimic esophageal carcinoma, candidial esophagitis, and gastric bezoars. Ulcers and erosions are present in most patients (136). Patients may develop serpiginous ulcers of the stomach, terminal ileum, or large intestine (140). Patients with severe injury may need bowel resection, at which time long segments of (or even the entire) colon and rectum may appear necrotic.

Microscopic Findings. Kayexalate causes esophageal, gastric, and colonic lesions (138, 139). Kayexalate and sorbitol induce localized coagulative necrosis, submucosal edema, and transmural inflammation (138,139). The changes resemble acute ischemia without reperfusion. They also superficially mimic autolysis, although mild neutrophilic infiltrates may be present. These changes occur anywhere in the gastrointestinal tract, although they are most frequent in the stomach or colon. Mucosal dark purple, PAS-positive, acid-fast–positive kayexalate crystals are typically present (fig. 8-32).

Differential Diagnosis. Rhomboid-shaped crystals may also be found within the bowel. They are bright orange-red rather than dark purple, and are red with PAS and bright pink with acid fast stains (137).

Treatment and Prognosis. In some cases, elimination of the kayexalate enema results in resolution of the gastrointestinal manifestations. Treatment is generally supportive, but occasionally, blood transfusion and even hemicolectomy may be necessary.

RADIOGRAPHIC SUBSTANCES

Definitions. Barium causes three types of gastrointestinal problems: 1) barium granulomas, 2) bolus obstruction, and 3) an allergic or anaphylactic reaction from the carboxymethylcellulose component of the barium sulfate suspension. *Barium granulomas* are nodules of

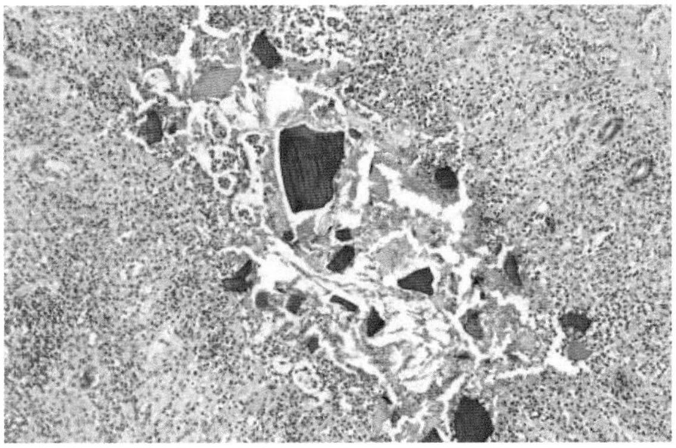

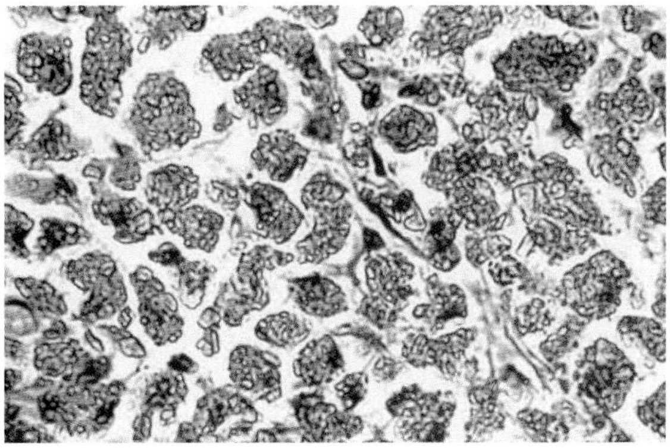

Figure 8-32

KAYEXALATE CRYSTALS ASSOCIATED WITH ACCUTE APPENDICITIS

Left: The basophilic polygonal kayexalate crystals often have a characteristic fish-scale appearance seen here on H&E stain. Right: Higher magnification shows collections of histiocytic cells containing refractile material. (Courtesy of the Division of Gastrointestinal Pathology, Armed Forces Institute of Pathology, Washington, DC.)

histiocytes containing barium sulfate, usually localized to the gastrointestinal submucosa.

Demography. Allergic reactions to barium sulfate affect less than 2 individuals/million (141,142). Perforation is an uncommon complication of contrast media, affecting 1/40,000 patients with barium enemas. When perforation occurs, it does so either following damage caused by previous mucosal disease, such as active colitis or diverticulitis (142,144), or as a result of mechanical damage caused by introduction of enema tips, balloons, and catheters.

Etiology. By far the most common radiographic substance to cause alterations in the gastrointestinal tract is barium. Water-soluble radiographic contrast media may cause an acute colitis (143). Gastrographin may produce a severe colitis, probably due to TWEEN 80, which is used as a wetting agent.

Pathophysiology. Radiologic contrast media cause perforation, granuloma formation, ischemic necrosis, acute appendicitis, bezoars, and masses, as well as mucosal injury. Barium granulomas develop when barium contrast extravasates during the administration of barium enemas via mucosal tears, abrasions, or diverticula. Barium incites an inflammatory reaction that is polymorphic and includes histiocytes and foreign body giant cells.

Clinical Features. Most patients with small barium granulomas remain asymptomatic, and the granulomas are incidental findings. Patients with larger barium granulomas present with masses that cause pain, constipation, and even intestinal obstruction. If the bowel ruptures during a barium enema, the patient may develop barium peritonitis. Many perforations are limited to the retroperitoneum. Intraperitoneal perforation results in acute peritonitis. Shock may occur. Dense intraperitoneal adhesions are a late complication in survivors of the acute event.

Gross Findings. The gross appearance of barium injury differs depending on whether an allergic reaction is present or whether barium has extravasated into the surrounding tissues. Barium granulomas produce brownish green tumorous masses, fibrosis, and strictures that may grossly resemble a carcinoma. Most barium granulomas develop in the rectum, approximately 10 cm proximal to the anal verge, often on the anterior wall. They vary in size, ranging up to 10 cm in diameter, and usually are found in the submucosa. Larger lesions may become centrally umbilicated. Sometimes, the barium forms hard concretions in the bowel lumen. Allergic mucosal changes may be mild.

Microscopic Findings. Barium sulfate is often seen in the gastrointestinal lumen, appearing as fine, greenish, nonrefringent granules, or as larger, birefringent, rhomboid crystals, sometimes located in granulation tissue (fig. 8-32). These findings merely indicate prior use of barium in the patient and does not qualify as a diagnosis of barium granuloma. When barium gains access to the submucosa, it elicits a granulomatous response (fig. 8-33). Barium

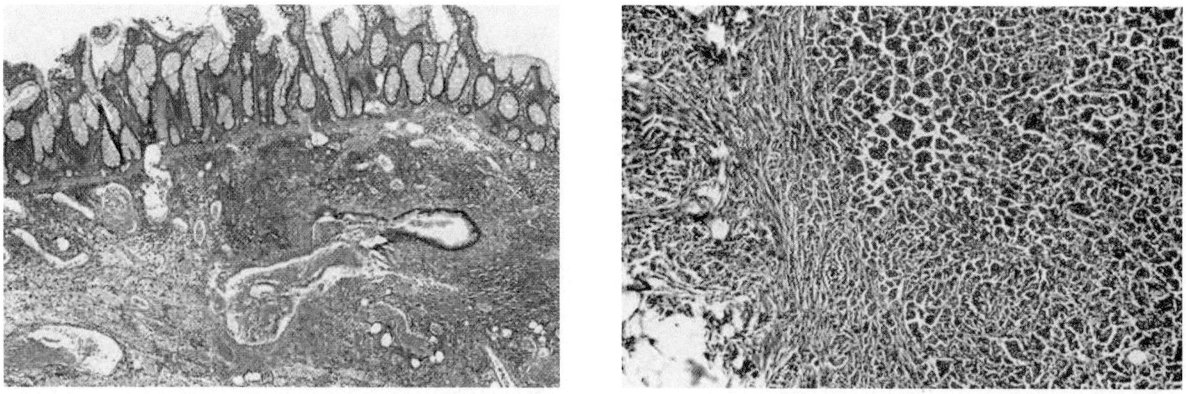

Figure 8-33

BARIUM GRANULOMA

Left: Damaged mucosa overlies an area of displaced glands and a defect within the submucosa surrounded by inflammatory cells.

Right: Higher magnification of the inflammatory response with collections of histiocytes as well as mononuclear cells, all containing refractile barium.

granulomas consist of collections of macrophages containing brownish green-gray barium sulfate crystals, surrounded by typical foreign body giant cells. The barium induces surprisingly little inflammation due to its inert nature. Small granular crystals may be found in clusters. The barium sulfate does not bend polarized light but it is refractile and easily seen when the microscope condenser is lowered. Allergic reactions tend to resemble other forms of allergic gastrointestinal diseases. Eosinophils dominate the histologic picture. The mucosa may be mildly edematous.

Gastrographin does not elicit an inflammatory response. Morphologically, large rectangular or rhomboid, light tan-yellow crystals are found in the bowel lumen, sometimes associated with an occasional giant cell.

Differential Diagnosis. Clinically, other mass lesions of the gastrointestinal tract mimic barium granulomas. The refractile greenish crystals, however, are pathognomonic for barium.

Treatment and Prognosis. Treatment of patients with asymptomatic barium granuloma is usually unnecessary and management generally focuses on excluding other granulomatous disorders. Surgery plays a central role in the treatment of acute perforations and obstructions.

CAUSTIC OR CORROSIVE INJURY

Definition. *Corrosive injury* is mucosal damage resulting from the ingestion of caustic acids, alkalis, or hot liquids. It can also result from instillation of caustic substances per rectum. *Corrosive esophagitis, corrosive gastritis, corrosive colitis,* and *corrosive proctitis* occur depending on the site affected.

Demography. Corrosive ingestion generally results from accidents or suicidal gestures. The amount of corrosive agent ingested tends to be less in accidental consumption than in attempted suicide (152). Corrosive esophagitis most commonly affects young children who accidentally ingest household cleaning agents.

Etiology. The degree and extent of damage induced by corrosive agents depend on the nature of the substances ingested, the morphologic form of the agent, the quantity of the agent, and the intent of the patient. Ingestion of strong alkalis, acids, bleaches and other household cleaning products, or very hot liquids causes corrosive esophagitis. Some of these agents include mineral acids, organic acids such as carbolic acid (phenol) used in many commercial disinfectants, bleach (sodium hypochlorite), liquid drain cleaner, Lysol, acetic acid, ammonia, and sodium acid phosphates used as toilet cleaners. Automatic dishwasher detergents (metasilicates) are also very caustic and can cause serious accidents. Alkalis with a pH of over 12.5 usually injure the esophagus more severely than the stomach; the reverse occurs with acids. Alkalis reaching the stomach are rapidly neutralized by the acid within it.

Liquids tend to produce extensive, geographically continuous erosive esophagitis and gastritis, whereas granular agents produce more proximal and more localized lesions. Crystalline drain cleaners contain more than 50 percent sodium hydroxide and they can produce transmural injury if consumed in sufficient amount but pain usually limits the amount swallowed. Deep ulcers and strictures complicate ingestion of compounds with a pH over 13. Hair relaxers are a common cause of caustic ingestions (146). Heavy metal salts such as zinc or mercuric chloride and ferrous sulfite also cause corrosive injury.

One unique form of corrosive injury results from the ingestion of button batteries used in hearing aids, watches, and calculators. Most of these contain a heavy metal such as mercury and an alkaline electrolyte. Esophageal impaction results in corrosive esophagitis leading to perforation.

Pathophysiology. Alkalis produce liquefaction necrosis with intense inflammation and saponification of the mucosa, submucosa, and muscularis propria (149,150,155). Since alkalis dissolve tissues, they penetrate more deeply than acids. Thrombosis of adjacent vessels leads to ischemic necrosis, followed by bacterial or fungal colonization. Contraction of the lower esophageal sphincter protects the gastric mucosa from injury. Thus, esophageal alkaline-induced injury is most severe in the mid and distal esophagus.

Acids more regularly affect the stomach, presumably due to less esophageal spasm and less esophageal retention of the acids. Acids cause coagulative necrosis, resulting in a firm protective eschar that limits acid penetration and delays injury (147). This results in extensive areas of hemorrhage and ulceration and the potential for perforation and stricture development. Even though the esophageal mucosa is relatively resistant to acid damage, high acid concentrations eventually injure it. In the stomach, both acids and alkalies predominantly damage the antrum due to stasis in this region.

The injury associated with button battery ingestion occurs via four mechanisms: 1) electrolyte leakage from the batteries, 2) alkali produced from external currents, 3) mercury toxicity, and 4) pressure necrosis.

Clinical Features. Ingestion of corrosive substances results in spasm and necrosis of the esophagus and stomach. It also results in drooling and mucosal slough ulcers in the oral cavity (152). Corrosive burns are typically visible on the skin or mucosa around the mouth, oropharynx, esophagus, and stomach when corrosive injury occurs (162). Patients develop systemic leukocytosis. Severe corrosive esophagitis leads to esophageal hemorrhage, perforation, and death. Lye-induced injuries are often complicated by respiratory compromise, esophageal and gastric perforation, sepsis, and death. Ingestion of fuming substances, such as nitric acid or ammonia, causes severe irritation of the upper respiratory passages and bronchi. Burns that are limited to the mucosa resolve rapidly, whereas those that extend into the wall tend to persist (155).

The typical clinical course of uncomplicated caustic ingestion has three phases: acute, latent, and retroactive. In the acute phase, immediate oral burning pain often limits the ingested volume. If enough volume is swallowed, however, chest pain and dysphagia immediately develop. Retching and vomiting follow. Esophageal dysmotility and edema generally subside over the next 3 to 4 days. The acute changes may affect the entire thickness of the wall and may result in perforation (147). The patient usually has no further esophageal symptoms in the latent phase, and both the patient and the physician develop a false sense of security. The esophagus is most likely to perforate during the subacute or latent phase. Perforation is common in corrosive injury. The third phase, scar retraction, begins as early as the 2nd week and lasts months. Clinically apparent strictures develop in 10 to 33 percent of patients. Strictures appear as early as weeks 3 to 8, often progressing rapidly, advancing from mild dysphagia to the inability to handle secretions in only a couple of days. Strictures that appear after the second month progress more slowly (155). Stricture formation is much less common with acid injury than with alkaline-induced damage.

Patient symptoms are unreliable in predicting disease extent or severity. If the patient survives the acute injury, there is still the risk of the development of dysphagia, esophageal rigidity and shortening, gastroesophageal reflux, Barrett esophagus, and even carcinoma (145,160). Benign strictures must be distinguished from

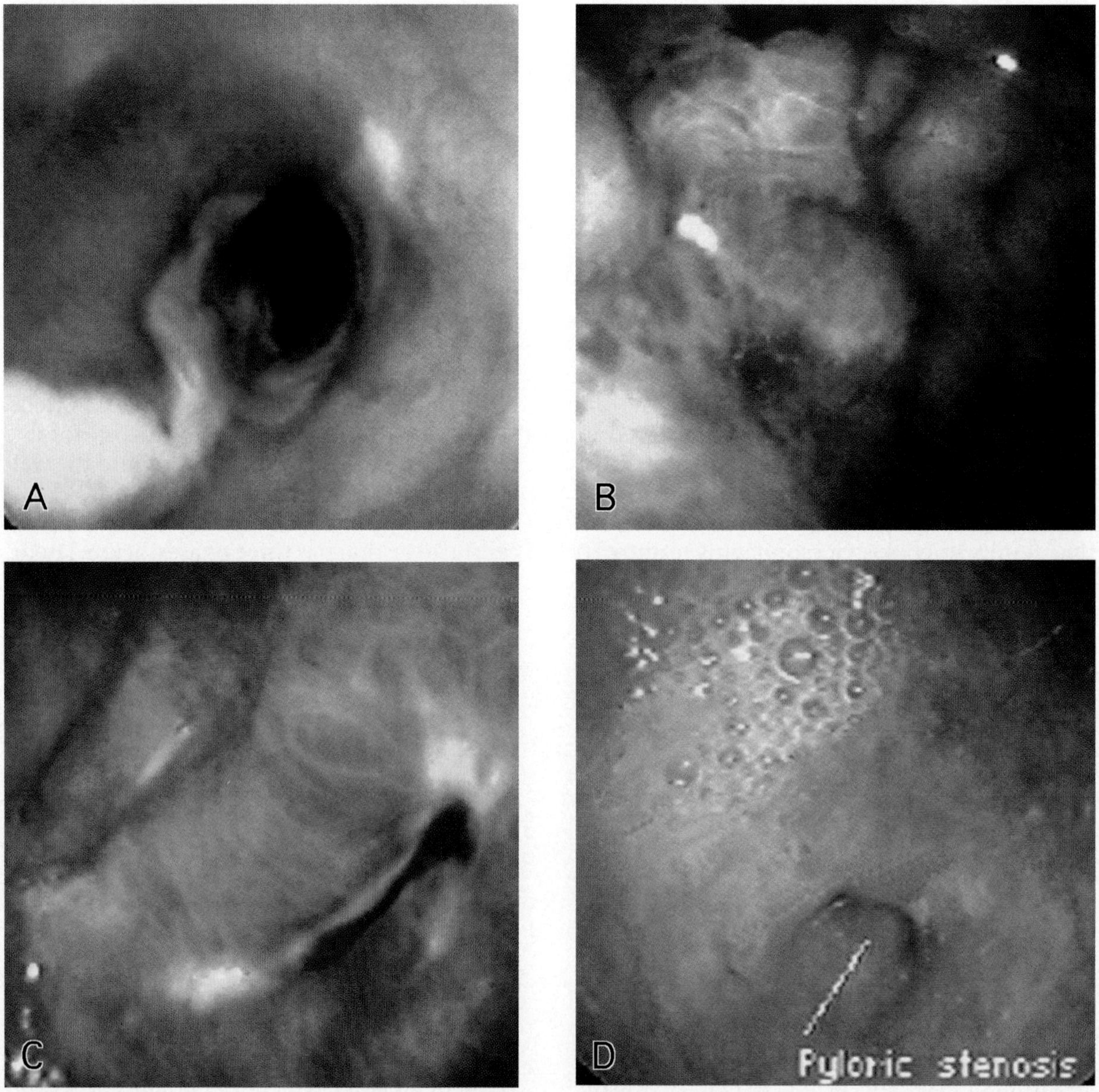

Figure 8-34

ENDOSCOPIC APPEARANCE OF CAUSTIC INJURY

A: Caustic geographic ulcerations of the esophagus.
B: Caustic injury of the stomach with edema and erythema.
C: Another view of the stomach showing the erythema.
D: Pyloric stenosis in a patient with previous caustic ingestion.

carcinoma, particularly when they develop years after the caustic exposure. Endoscopic brushings of the lesional surface should be performed, since densely fibrotic scar tissue may be exceedingly difficult to biopsy. Many recommend periodic surveillance for the detection of malignancy beginning 20 years after caustic ingestion.

Gross Findings. Caustic agents cause burns that remain limited to the mucosa or more diffusely involve the gastrointestinal wall (fig. 8-34). First-degree burns cause superficial mucosal involvement. Second-degree burns cause transmucosal involvement, with or without submucosal involvement but without extension to the surrounding tissues. Third-degree burns cause full-thickness injuries with extension into adjacent tissues. The most severe injury occurs in areas of luminal narrowing such as the area where the aorta or the left main stem bronchus crosses the esophagus at the tracheal bifurcation or in the area of the sphincters.

In the esophagus, the acute injury phase lasts 4 to 5 days and consists of coagulative necrosis variably extending into the esophageal wall. Epithelial sloughing usually follows, sometimes creating deep ulcers. The entire mucosa may also slough in severe burns. Complete separation of the squamous mucosa results in the formation of a mucosal cast that the patient vomits up in a condition referred to as *esophagitis desiccans superficialis* (161). Deep ulcers become fibrotic if the patient survives the acute injury. Strictures (fig. 8-35) cause dilatation and hypertrophy of the esophagus proximal to the narrowed area. Corrosive acids also may induce esophageal intramural pseudodiverticulosis (154). Inflammation of adjacent organs leads to mediastinitis or peritonitis. Severe lesions, involvement of the entire length of the esophagus, hematemesis, and increased serum lactic dehydrogenase are risk factors for the development of strictures induced by caustic ingestion (158). Esophageal strictures may be complicated by the development of Barrett esophagus or carcinoma (145).

Radiologic findings include solitary or multiple strictures of varying lengths, intramural pseudodiverticula, and carcinoma in longstanding corrosive injury (157). Technetium 99M-labeled sucralfate radiography is an accurate technique for assessing the degree of esophageal injury after the ingestion of caustic substances. It may also be used to document healing (156). Radiologic features seen in the stomach include areas of scarring, particularly in the antrum, a linitis plastica type deformity, and multiple pseudodiverticula (157).

The gastric changes tend to be nonuniform, depending largely on the amount of agent ingested and the patient's posture at the time of ingestion. The damage frequently localizes to the prepyloric region (fig. 8-36), because stasis in this area causes a relatively longer mucosal contact time with injurious agents than in other areas of the stomach. If the patient survives, fibrosis causes progressive antral and prepyloric narrowing (fig. 8-37), which can progress to complete gastric outlet obstruction.

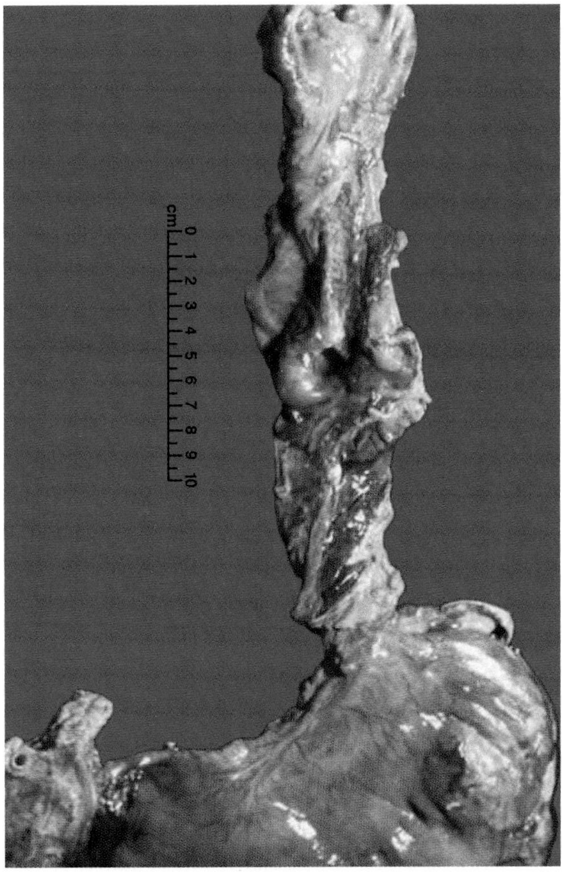

Figure 8-35

LYE INGESTION

Esophageal stricture due to previous lye ingestion.

The mildest form of gastric injury is characterized by mucosal erythema, edema, and friability without necrosis or ulceration. Necrosis, ulceration, mucosal hemorrhage, and exudation are encountered in second-degree injury, while dark necrotic and ulcerated areas and sloughing of mucosa are seen in full-thickness burns. A dark exudate in an aperistaltic and dilated organ suggests a full-thickness, third-degree burn. Sloughing mucosal necrosis often extends into the underlying muscular wall, and may result in perforation.

Charcoal deposits may be present in the esophagus or stomach in patients who survive the acute event, appearing as linear, black, distal esophageal or gastric lesions. These result from

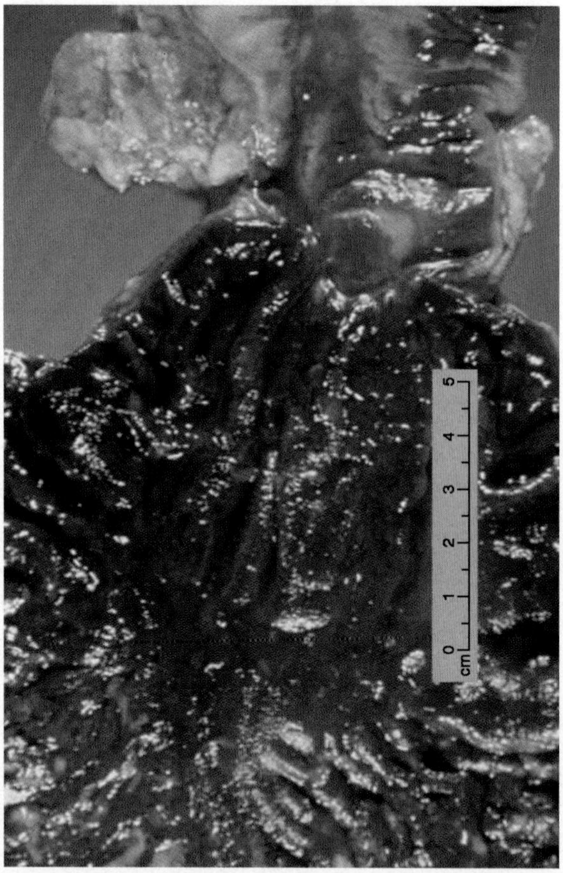

Figure 8-36

LYE INGESTION

Stomach and duodenum in a patient who ingested lye. The most intense changes affect the pyloric region. There is also damage in the duodenum, as evidenced by the reddish discoloration of the mucosa.

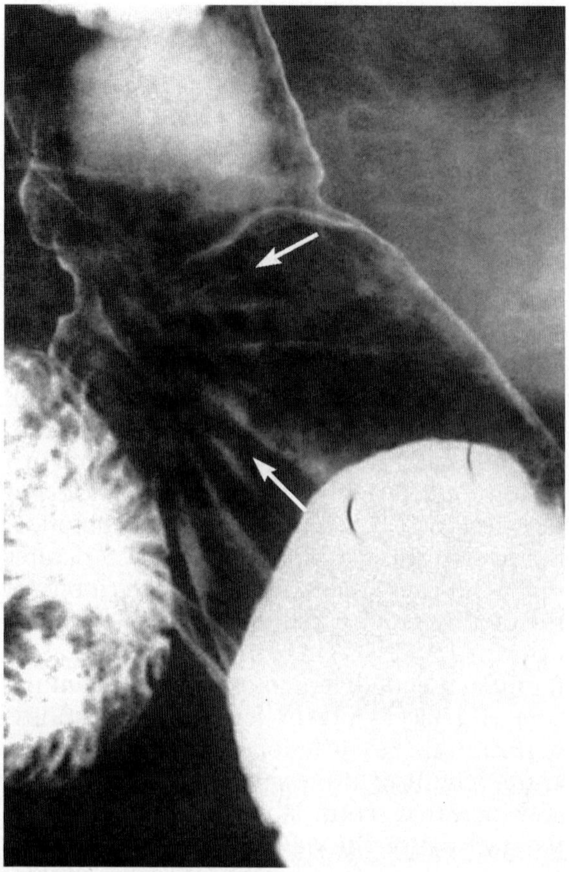

Figure 8-37

LYE INGESTION

X-ray demonstration of an area of healing ulceration following lye ingestion.

the administration of activated charcoal as a therapy for overdoses in patients who have attempted suicide. Mucosal tears from either intubation or vomiting allow the charcoal to gain access into the underlying submucosa, where it persists for decades.

Microscopic Findings. Pathologists most commonly see the acute effects of caustic injury at the time of autopsy, usually in the forensic setting. The overlying surface appears normal, swollen, inflamed, hemorrhagic, ulcerated, hypertrophic, or atrophic, depending on when the tissues are examined in relation to the acute event, and if recurrent damage has occurred.

The acute phase is associated with edema, acute inflammation, and vascular thrombosis. Coagulative necrosis variably extends into the esophageal or gastric wall, with little or no inflammatory response (fig. 8-38). Mural necrosis, ulceration, and inflammation are present. Secondary bacterial infections may complicate the damage. In the subacute phase, the superficial necrotic tissue sloughs off and the mucosa ulcerates, with subsequent repair by granulation tissue that matures into collagenous connective tissue.

During the chronic phase, which lasts from 1 to 3 months, the ulcers reepithelialize and fibrosis begins to develop, sometimes evolving into a stricture. Strictures consist of dense, uniform, mucosal and submucosal fibrosis. Ulceration may be ongoing. Cytologically, the cells usually appear normal without much reactive atypia. The

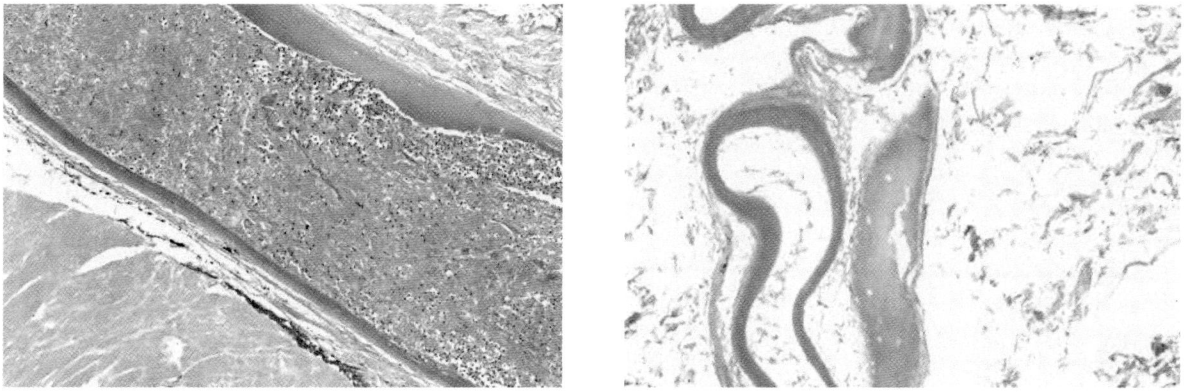

Figure 8-38

LYE INGESTION WITH COAGULATIVE NECROSIS

Left: The mucosa has undergone complete coagulative necrosis so that cellular detail is lost. In addition, the muscularis mucosae is affected.

Right: The changes also affect the submucosa with the complete coagulation necrosis of the submucosal vessels.

charcoal deposits, if present, consist of aggregates of coarse, black, foreign material.

The histologic features of the gastric changes include coagulation necrosis, mucosal hemorrhage, and edema. Early, there is little inflammation. If the patient survives the acute event, emphysematous gastritis may develop due to infection by gas-forming organisms (151).

Treatment and Prognosis. Initial treatment is directed toward the most life-threatening injuries. Perforation, peritonitis, fistula formation, or massive hemorrhage necessitates surgery. In other patients, endoscopic evaluation of the esophagus and stomach determines injury extent. Patients are stratified into four groups: those without injury, those with only gastric injury, those with linear esophageal injuries, and those with circumferential burns. The less severe the injury, the more likely that the patient will survive without sequelae. First-degree injuries generally resolve spontaneously. Patients with second-degree injuries are observed and prophylactically treated with antisecretory agents before eating is allowed. Symptomatic patients without peritonitis are treated with nutritional support, intravenous H2-receptor antagonists (or proton pump inhibitors, if available), and prophylactic antibiotics until liquids can be tolerated. Patients with gastric or linear esophageal burns may require hospitalization for possible transmural extension of the injury. Some patients are treated with steroids in an attempt to limit the edema and reduce stricture formation (159). Patients treated with epidermal growth factor and/or cytokines may have a reduced incidence of subsequent stenosis (148).

Patients developing strictures are treated before the strictures become tight, fixed, and difficult to dilate. Once strictures develop, they are initially treated with dilatation of the esophagus or eventual placement of stents. Many patients do well with periodic dilations. Once well-developed strictures occur, surgical resection may be required. Colonic or jejunal interpositions may be necessary.

Esophageal replacement using the right colon with the terminal ileum allows continuity of peristalsis in the interposed bowel segment with an intact ileocecal valve that decreases the hazard of regurgitation. Patients with gastric outlet obstruction require endoscopic dilatation or surgery. Some patients develop long-term motility disturbances. Esophageal carcinomas may develop, with a latency period of about 30 to 40 years (145). Most tumors develop at the area of the tracheal bifurcation.

PROSTAGLANDIN THERAPY

Prostaglandins are used to treat congenital heart disease in neonates (164) and to maintain patency of the ductus arteriosus in infants with cyanotic congenital heart disease.

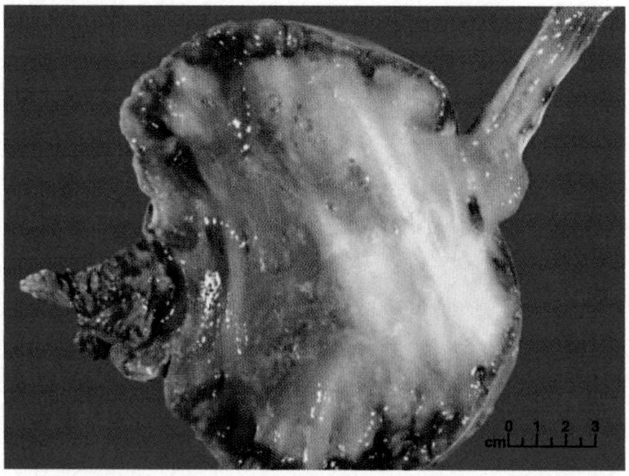

Figure 8-39

PROSTAGLANDIN-INDUCED PYLORIC HYPERTROPHY

This neonatal stomach is completely distended and filled with mucus due to outflow block secondary to mucosal hyperplasia in the pylorus. (Courtesy of Dr. Patrick Lanz, Wake Forest University, NC.)

Prostaglandin E infusions induce mucosal hyperplasia, pyloric stenosis, and gastric outlet obstruction in neonates and adults. Neonates present with feeding problems, vomiting, and abdominal distension.

The stomach appears enlarged and distended, and the intestine has a mucoid appearance (fig. 8-39). Radiographic studies show antral narrowing suggestive of hypertrophic pyloric stenosis. Serial ultrasonograms disclose progressive elongation of the antral pyloric channel without mural thickening (164).

Histologically, the stomach shows foveolar hyperplasia and elongation of the gastric pits, preferentially affecting the antrum. These changes may lead to pyloric stenosis (165). Drug cessation resolves these effects.

BISPHOSPHONATES

Demography. *Bisphosphonate injury* tends to affect older individuals, especially women treated for osteoporosis. Only a fraction of individuals develop severe adverse esophageal reactions to the drug. Patients with serious injury from bisphosphonates are usually taking other medications as well (167).

Etiology. Alendronate (Fosamax), etidronate, and pamidronate are amino bisphosphonates used to treat osteoporosis in postmenopausal women (175) and Paget's disease. These agents are potent inhibitors of bone resorption, suppressing the increased rate of bone turnover and lowering the incidence of fractures (166,173) during the postmenopausal period (176). The drug binds to hydroxyapatite in bone, specifically inhibiting osteoclastic activity without directly affecting bone formation.

Pathophysiology. Alendronate damages the esophagus both by its toxicity and from nonspecific irritation secondary to pill contact with the esophageal mucosa in a manner similar to that seen in other forms of "pill esophagitis" (see below). The esophagitis results from swallowing the medication with little or no water, lying down during or after ingestion of the tablet(s), and continuation of the drug after symptom onset. Because the patients are elderly, many have reduced esophageal motility, predisposing them to the drug injury. Coexisting *H. pylori* infection or the use of NSAIDs to treat arthritis may add to the mucosal toxicity of the bisphosphonates (170). Alendronate causes visible gastric mucosal injury in the majority of patients studied, and is severe in 50 percent. Gastric ulcers are present in 8 percent of patients (170–172).

Clinical Features. Alendronate is well tolerated in most patients but causes severe upper gastrointestinal symptoms in approximately 1.5 percent (174). Patients typically present with dysphagia secondary to midesophageal inflammation or stricture (174,175). In some patients, the ulceration is severe enough to necessitate hospitalization (168,169). Bleeding is rare. Duodenal damage does not appear to occur (170).

Gross Findings. Endoscopy shows an erosive esophagitis with erythema, ulcerations, an inflammatory exudate, and thickening of the esophageal wall (166,169). The esophageal erosions and ulcers may become confluent, developing into multiple deep, large ulcers. Visible gastric mucosal damage resembles that seen with NSAID-induced damage, with the formation of antral ulcers or superficial mucosal erosions (170).

Microscopic Findings. The histologic esophageal changes are those common to many severe ulcerating esophageal disorders. Neutrophilic infiltrates are often present, as is intraepithelial eosinophilia. The squamous epithelium appears reactive, as evidenced by the presence of enlarged and hyperchromatic nuclei. There may also be small intraepithelial vesicles. Clear, refractile, crystalline foreign material is often present in the fibroinflammatory exudate, and is easily seen with polarizing light. The crystals resemble those of crushed alendronate tablets. Scattered, multinucleated giant cells may be associated with the crystals (166). The histologic features of gastric injury resemble those of NSAID injury.

Differential Diagnosis. The differential diagnosis includes other forms of acute and ulcerative esophagitis or gastritis. The diagnosis is made with the appropriate history and sometimes by identifying the alendronate crystals.

Treatment and Prognosis. The changes resolve with drug cessation. The development of late-onset strictures is uncommon.

HEAVY METALS

Definition. Gastrointestinal disease can result from exposure to heavy metals such as copper, gold, and arsenic.

Demography. Many heavy metals are ubiquitous elements in the earth's crust and are transported environmentally by water (178). The distribution of these elements in the environment varies considerably with the geography, and in some places is very high. For example, arsenic toxicity is particularly common in China, Taiwan, Thailand, Mexico, Chile, Bangladesh, and India. Heavy metal injury may occur in those who consume foods stored or cooked in tin, antimony, or copper containers. Children are exposed to lead in lead-containing paint and contaminated food or water. Introduction of lead-free gasoline has dramatically reduced environmental lead poisoning. The majority of patients with gold-salt toxicity are women with rheumatoid arthritis. Exposure to mercury is largely through fish consumption, particularly the consumption of shark, swordfish, and tuna. Certain fish from polluted fresh water, such as pike, walleye, and bass, should be especially avoided.

Etiology. The native forms of heavy metals are generally inert; most damage results from their metallic salts, especially gold and iron salts. The main threats to humans from heavy metals are associated with exposure to lead, iron, cadmium, mercury, arsenic, and gold salts. Gold salt therapy causes most heavy metal–induced enterocolitis (195). Zirconium, silver, zinc, and aluminum (181,182,192) also cause gastrointestinal injury. Lead is toxic by ingestion, inhalation, and transcutaneous exposure. Cadmium emissions have increased due to dumping of batteries with the other household waste into landfills. Cigarette smoking is also a major source of cadmium exposure. Heavy use of calomel can produce watery diarrhea and high mercury levels in the colon (194).

Pathophysiology. Ferrous sulfate pills attach to the mucosa and produce localized ulcers, particularly in the esophagus (188). Ferrous sulfate may also injure the stomach or small intestine. Gold-induced enterocolitis results from either direct mucosal toxicity or an immune-mediated hypersensitivity reaction. The presence of an HLA DRB1*0404 allele increases the risk of developing gold-induced enterocolitis in patients with rheumatoid arthritis (180). Gold salts also predispose to cytomegalovirus infection (195). The gastrointestinal tract is the immediate target organ in cadmium intoxication, since it inhibits enterocyte Na^+K^+-ATPase activity (189). Lead causes small bowel toxicity by modifying the biochemical properties of the enterocyte surface, leading to microvillous damage (193).

Clinical Features. In general, the clinical features of heavy metal gastrointestinal toxicity include nausea, vomiting, abdominal cramps, pain, and severe, watery, bloody diarrhea, a condition sometimes referred to as "welder's fits" when it occurs within this working group due to their occupational exposure to heavy metal. In some situations, the clinical features are typical and provide a clue to the existence of heavy metal toxicity: patients with arsenosis develop hyperpigmentation, hyperkeratosis, and cutaneous malignancies.

The enterocolitis associated with gold therapy usually starts within several weeks of beginning the drug. Patients present with nausea, vomiting, profuse diarrhea, abdominal pain, fever, proteinuria, maculopapular rashes, and hypogammaglobulinemia. Occasionally, the gold-induced enterocolitis progresses to toxic megacolon, perforation, and death (179,181). Twenty-five percent of patients develop peripheral eosinophilia.

The features of acute lead poisoning include severe abdominal pain, vomiting, and diarrhea.

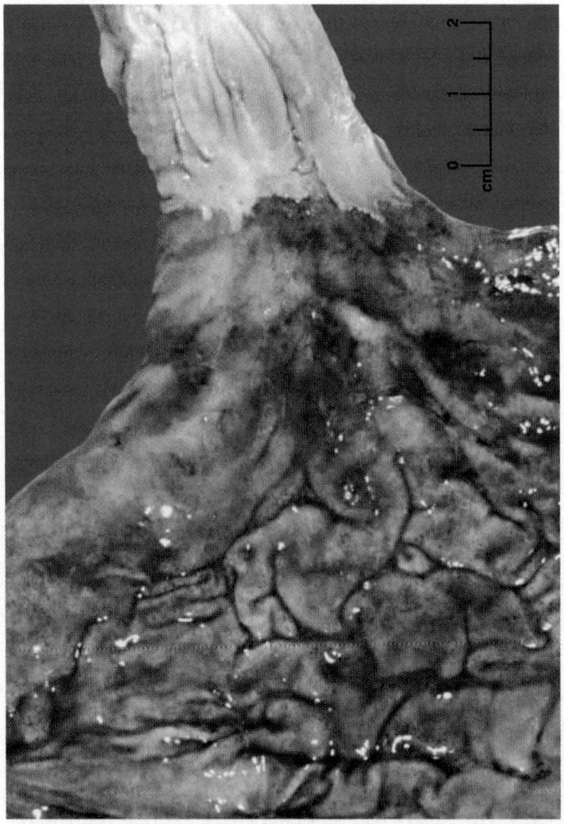

Figure 8-40

MERCURY INGESTION

Opened stomach in an individual who consumed mercury. The mucosa appears reddened and mercury balls lie on the mucosal surface.

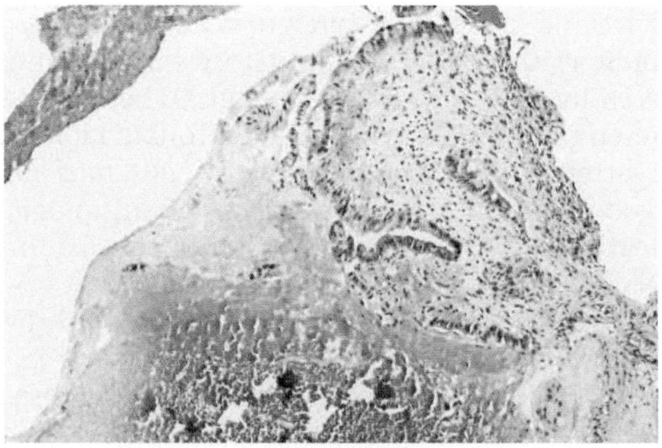

Figure 8-41

GOLD-INDUCED GASTRIC INJURY

This biopsy shows marked edema of the mucosa.

Behavioral disturbances, anorexia, fatigue, and irritability are also seen. Patients may develop ataxia, decreased consciousness, and seizures. Chronic exposure may lead to constipation.

Heavy metal salts such as zinc or mercuric chloride or ferrous or zinc sulfate cause gastritis. Ingestion of large amounts of these substances causes rapid injury which may be severe; such cases are usually only encountered by forensic pathologists. In these patients, there is evidence of corrosive burns in the mouth and esophagus, as well as in the stomach. Oral ferrous sulfate causes transient nausea and induces gastric mucosal edema and erosions (185).

Iron overdose causes gastrointestinal necrosis and strictures. After prolonged contact, intestinal perforation may occur. Patients with aluminum toxicity develop enteropathy, encephalopathy, bone disease, and anemia (185). Patients with chronic renal failure or organ transplants (kidney, liver, bone marrow, heart) who use aluminum-containing antacids or sucralfate drugs may develop gastric mucosal calcinosis. Copper ingestion is associated with diarrhea, with or without abdominal pain and vomiting (190).

Gross Findings. Any patient who has ingested large quantities of a heavy metal will have acute erosive esophagitis or gastritis. Ferrous salts damage any part of the gastrointestinal tract, causing ulcers and hemorrhage. Most ferrous sulfate–induced lesions are superficial but if deeper ulcers develop, fibrous strictures can occur, particularly in the small intestine. Foreign body giant cell reactions may occur. Zinc sulfate may cause gastritis. In those who have ingested mercury, balls of mercury are seen within the gastric lumen (fig. 8-40). Any gastrointestinal site may be damaged by gold salts, although the colon is most commonly affected. The small and large bowel may show hemorrhage, edema, and mural thickening. A focal or extensive, but usually segmental, colitis, sometimes associated with pseudomembrane formation, with erosions and ulcerations simulating IBD, develops in those on gold therapy (186,191,192). Severe gastrointestinal necrosis and strictures develop after iron overdoses.

Microscopic Findings. The stomach shows nonspecific inflammation and edema in gold-associated injury (fig. 8-41). Histologically, the bowel is ulcerated, with diffuse acute and chronic inflammation, sometimes associated with crypt abscesses. The glandular architecture

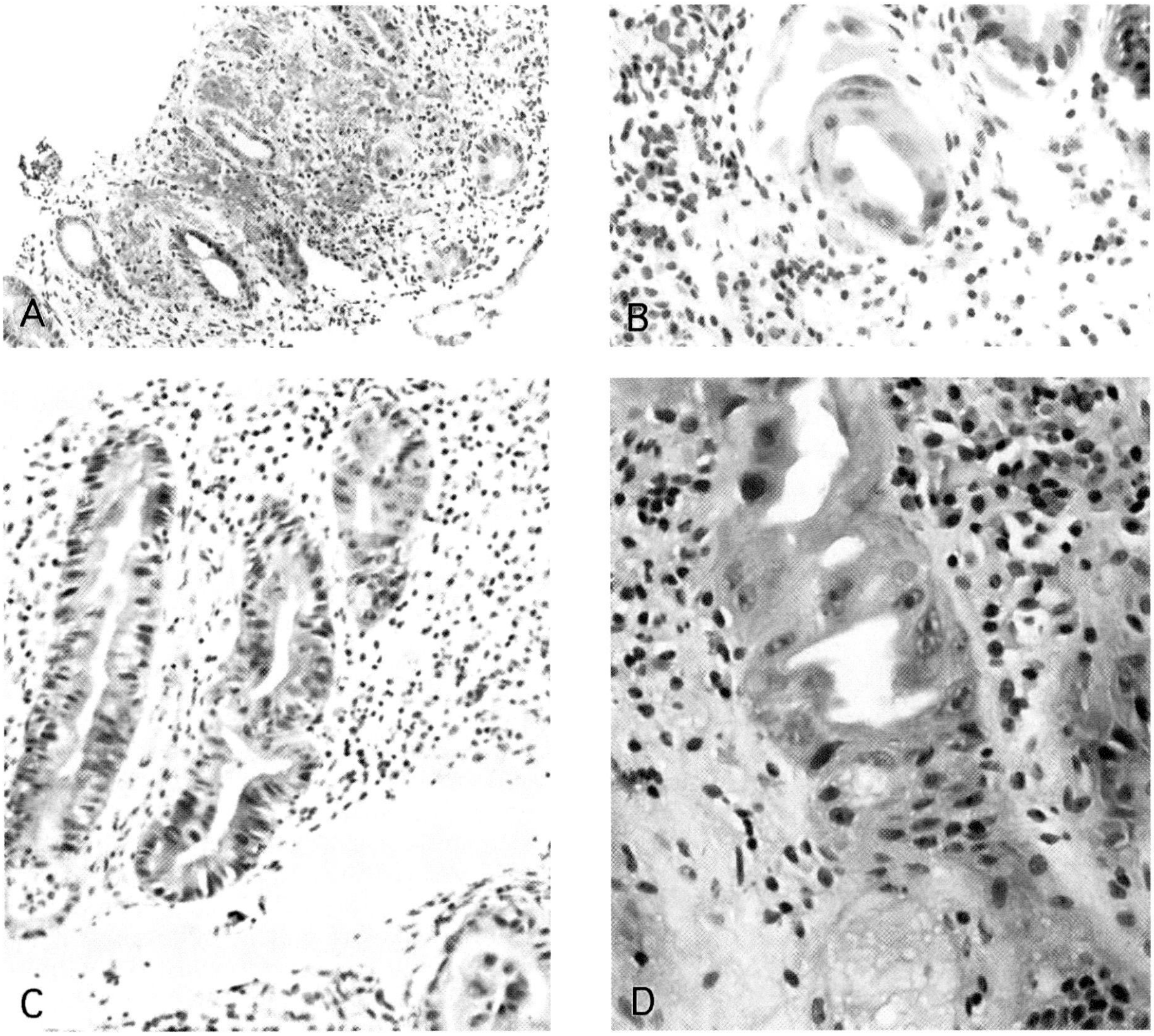

Figure 8-42

GOLD-INDUCED COLONIC INJURY

A: Colonic biopsy shows severe interstitial hemorrhage, edema, and glandular dropout.

B: Some of the glands have started to regenerate and appear more eosinophilic than normal. In this case, the gland in the center shows little cytologic atypia.

C: Another area of regeneration shows cytologic atypia and glandular irregularity.

D: The cytologic changes extend to the surface.

is usually more or less preserved, although individual crypts may drop out (fig. 8-42). Deep ulcers and diffuse mucosal inflammation (179,181), often with a prominent eosinophilic component, characterize the resultant fulminant enterocolitis (183,187,188).

Patients consuming large amounts of iron may have a layer of brownish crystalline iron lining the gastric or esophageal mucosa (177). The iron may be admixed with a luminal fibroinflammatory exudate. Crystalline iron deposits may be present in the lamina propria, covered by an intact epithelium, adjacent to superficial erosions or admixed with granulation tissue. Iron stains show iron covering the epithelial surface in the stomach, and extending into the superficial gastric pits (fig. 8-43). Iron deposits coexist with superficial edema, inflammation, mild epithelial necrosis, and acute inflammation. Ferrous sulfate may cause an

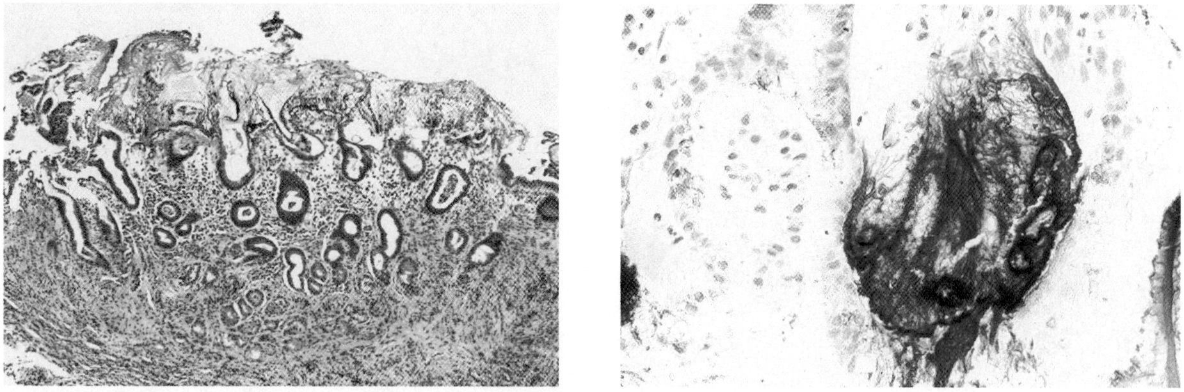

Figure 8-43

IRON DEPOSITS IN THE GASTRIC MUCOSA

A layer of dark pigment covers the surface epithelium. The iron stain (right) is positive.

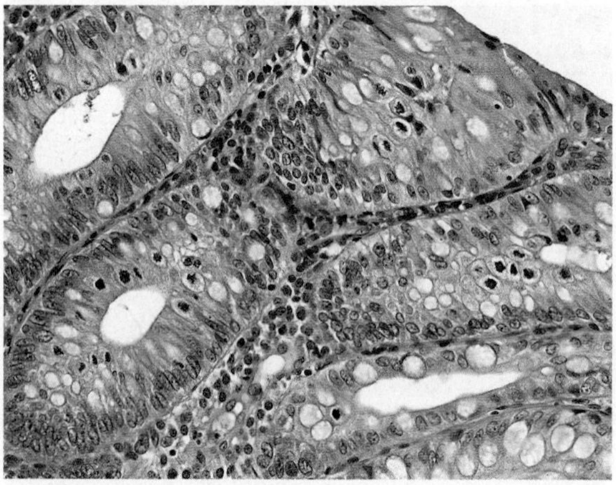

Figure 8-44

CHOLCHICINE TOXICITY

Numerous mitotic figures are arrested in metaphase. Mitoses extend beyond the normal proliferative zone, upward into the superficial half of the crypt.

acute erosive gastritis. Iron-containing thrombi may be found in mucosal blood vessels. Mercury poisoning may cause fibromuscular stenosis of the large intestine (184).

Differential Diagnosis. The enterocolitis associated with gold toxicity mimics IBD. The various entities can be separated based on the clinical history.

Treatment and Prognosis. Mild enterocolitis typically resolves with drug cessation. Patients with severe gold salt enterocolitis have mortality rates as high as 35 to 42 percent (195).

COLCHICINE

Demography. Colchicine is widely used to treat patients with gout. It also has a role as an antifibrosing agent in patients with certain forms of cirrhosis and chronic liver disease.

Pathophysiology. Colchicine leads to malabsorption by depressing intestinal enzyme production and transport, mucosal surface area, and water transport, and by retarding motility (197).

Clinical Features. In most patients, colchicine therapy causes mild nuisance symptoms, including nausea, colicky abdominal pain, vomiting, and diarrhea. In some patients, however, small doses given regularly cause steatorrhea, megaloblastic anemia, and abnormal xylose absorption (196). Some patients develop life-threatening colchicine toxicity with fever, pain, myalgia, lower extremity paresthesias, convulsions, alopecia, and even death (196). Fatal toxicity is rare and characterized by intense diarrhea and dehydration.

Microscopic Findings. The histologic changes accompanying colchicine toxicity include villus atrophy and mitotic arrest with absent mitotic spindles and bizarre chromatin configurations (fig. 8-44). The villi fuse and epithelial cytoplasmic and nuclear swelling develops. Because of the mitotic arrest, the epithelium in the proliferative zone can no longer give rise to new progeny, and villous atrophy and crypt hypoplasia develop (196).

Treatment. The changes disappear upon drug cessation.

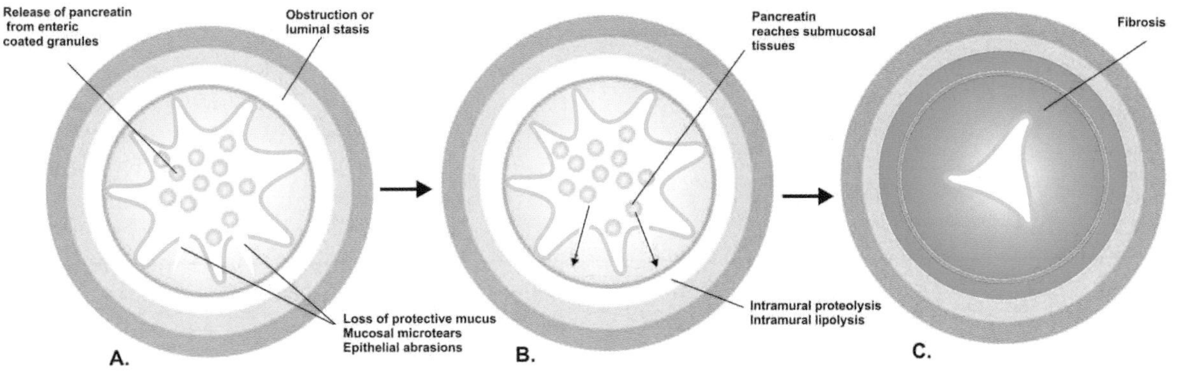

Figure 8-45

DIAGRAM OF PANCREATIC ENZYME–INDUCED INJURY

PANCREATIC ENZYME SUPPLEMENTS AND FIBROSING COLONOPATHY

Demography. High-strength pancreatic enzyme supplements are given to children with cystic fibrosis (CF) to correct their pancreatic insufficiency and control intestinal malabsorption. Patient age at diagnosis varies from 9 months to 13 years (204). The relative risk of developing *fibrosing colonopathy* is 10.9 and 199.5 with doses of 24,000 to 50,000 units of lipase/kg/day and more than 50,000 units/kg/day, respectively. Fibrosing colonopathy has also been described in adults on high doses of pancreatic enzymes in the absence of CF.

Etiology. Pancreatin is an enzyme mixture that supplements defective pancreatic secretion in patients with end-stage pancreatic diseases, enabling effective food digestion. Most preparations are derived from porcine pancreas and consist of amylase, proteases, and lipase. Concomitant use of H2 blockers, corticosteroids, laxatives, or recombinant human DNAase in CF patients increases the risk of developing fibrosing colonopathy (199,200,205–207).

Pathophysiology. It is postulated that delayed disruption of microspheres in the colon or prolonged colonic mucosal contact due to the slower transit times seen in CF patients treated with the pancreatic enzymes exposes the colonic mucosa to nonphysiologic amounts of active enzymes, thereby leading to ulceration, inflammation, and subsequent fibrosis (fig. 8-45) (202). In addition, small intestinal pH is abnormally low in CF patients, possibly delaying dissolution of the enteric coatings until the enzymes reach the distal small intestine or colon. Prolonged colonic exposure could also result from stasis or obstruction. Epithelial abrasions or focal lesions proximal to an obstruction provide intramural or submucosal access to high concentrations of proteolytic and lipolytic enzymes, which then elicit vigorous fibrosing reactions, particularly because the intramural pancreatin is dispersed within the submucosa by peristalsis. Other possible mechanisms of injury include a colon-specific immune-related disorder (201) or primary dysregulated colonic collagen synthesis (200).

Clinical Features. Clinically, patients present with abdominal discomfort and distension due to stricturing and intestinal dilatation. Other findings include ascites, constipation, frequent passage of watery stools, severe anorexia, and weight loss. The changes of fibrosing colonopathy may be restricted to the cecum, ascending colon, or rectum, or they may diffusely affect the entire colon (200,202,203,207). An intense perianal skin irritation affects infants. Clinical recognition of fibrosing colonopathy is complicated by the fact that gastrointestinal obstruction affects up to 15 percent of children with CF without the colonopathy (207).

Gross Findings. The entire colon develops widespread submucosal fibrosis, thickening of the muscularis propria, and subserosal hemorrhages. Maturation and longitudinal contraction of the fibrous tissue further distort and thicken the colon wall and narrow the intestinal lumen, although the external diameter remains normal, especially at the flexures. As the

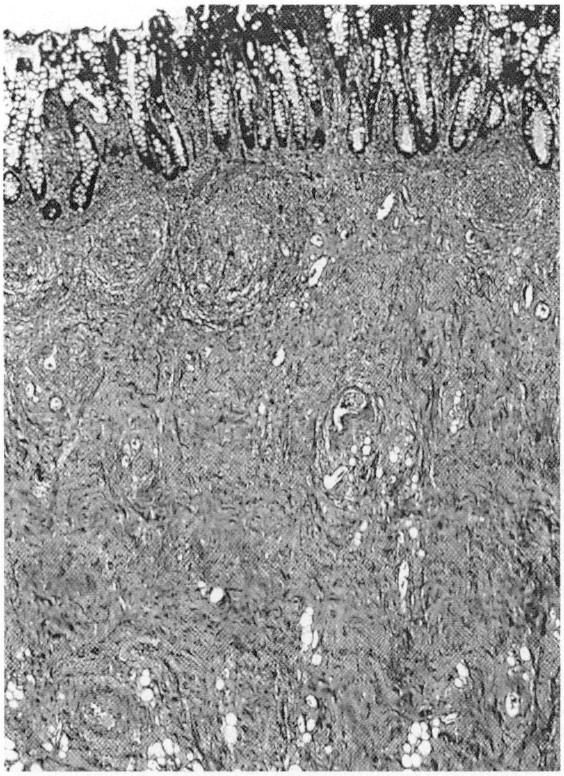

Figure 8-46

FIBROSING COLONOPATHY

Histologic appearance of a dense fibrosing process in the submucosa in a patient receiving pancreatic enzyme supplements. (Courtesy of the Division of Gastrointestinal Pathology, Armed Forces Institute of Pathology, Washington, DC.)

fibrosis continues, the mucosa acquires a cobblestoned appearance with areas of persistent or healing ulceration. The rectum becomes stenotic (199,208). Externally, the colon appears pale and a fusiform band of mature fibrous tissue extends over 10 cm or more in the lamina propria and submucosa.

Microscopic Findings. There may be acute or chronic colitis with active cryptitis (200,202). The lamina propria contains variable amounts of chronic inflammation, usually adjacent to erosions; edema is prominent. The muscle fibers of the muscularis mucosae become frayed, sometimes with complete disintegration and loss of the normal demarcation between the mucosa and submucosa. There is a moderate to severe infiltration of eosinophils and mast cells. The eosinophil count ranges from 26 to 164 per high-power field, with a mean of 64 (202). The submucosa contains dense mature collagen and thick, nearly hyalinized collagen bands, sometimes with a keloidal appearance (fig. 8-46). Ganglion cells are unusually prominent and can usually be found in the deep mucosa near crypt bases. The muscularis propria becomes widened and fibrotic, a process preferentially affecting the inner circular layer. In rare patients, the muscle becomes completely attenuated and both layers of the muscularis propria disappear (202). In some patients, the process distorts the neural plexuses.

Differential Diagnosis. The differential diagnosis of fibrosing colonopathy includes scleroderma, since this disorder is associated with submucosal fibrosis and tissue eosinophilia. Clinical findings separate the two entities.

Treatment and Prognosis. It is recommended that the daily dose of lipase remain below 10,000 units/kg to reduce the incidence of this complication (198). Surgery may be required for mechanically significant stricturing.

ESTROGEN AND PROGESTERONE

Demography. Most individuals with injury due to estrogen or progesterone intake are women over age 50 years. Those with blood type A, cigarette smokers, and hypertensive patients have an increased propensity to develop complications from these hormones. Lesions usually develop in individuals who have taken at least 0.5 g of drug/day for more than a year.

Etiology. Both estrogen and progesterone cause small and large intestinal ischemia but the incidence of damage is low (209–211,213,214).

Pathophysiology. Estrogen, progesterone, and oral contraceptives promote thrombus formation in the mesenteric arteries or veins. This leads to segmental hemorrhage, ischemia, and hemorrhagic infarction (211–213).

Clinical Features. The major clinical features associated with hormone therapy are a result of ischemia. Some patients develop malabsorption. There is a general relationship between the amount of drug ingested and thrombotic sequelae.

Gross Findings. These hormones damage both the small and large bowel. Thrombosis affects the superior mesenteric vein more commonly than the superior mesenteric artery. The gross features of ischemic injury from hormones

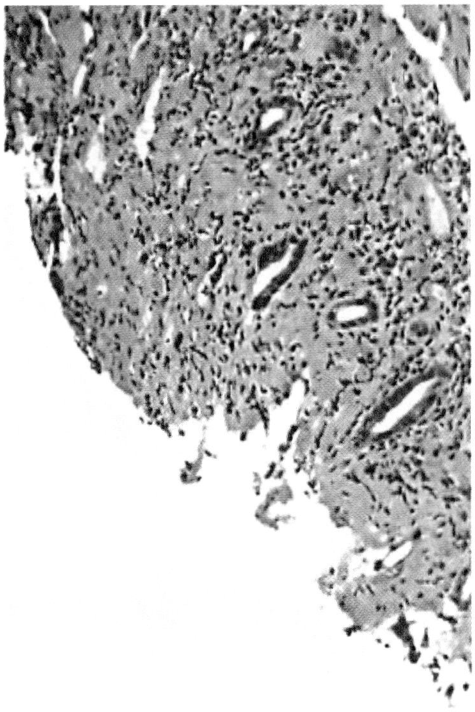

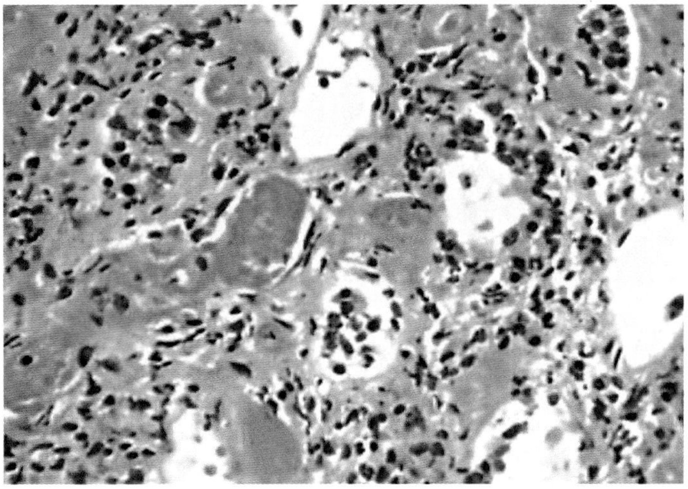

Figure 8-47

ORAL CONTRACEPTIVE INJURY

Colon biopsy in a 27-year-old patient who was on oral contraceptives and presented with rectal bleeding.

Left: The features are consistent with ischemia.

Above: Fibrin thrombi are seen in the vessels.

resemble those of ischemic enterocolitis due to other causes (see chapter 7).

Microscopic Findings. There are two types of histologic findings in patients with injury secondary to estrogen and progesterone: villous atrophy and crypt hypoplasia (214), or ischemia (fig. 8-47). The ischemic changes reflect the size of the thrombosed vessel and typically affect the intestines, sparing other portions of the gastrointestinal tract. In patients with disseminated intravascular coagulation, the changes tend to be mild. Patients with thrombosis of a major vessel may present with widespread transmural ischemic necrosis. Progesterones may also cause pseudodecidual reactions in the serosa or the mesentery that have no clinical consequences (fig. 8-48).

Differential Diagnosis. The differential diagnosis includes other causes of villous atrophy and/or ischemia. Severe disease may mimic IBD.

Treatment and Prognosis. Discontinuation of the hormones cures the problem, but the patient may be left with the sequelae of removed bowel if resection was necessary.

COCAINE

Demography. Gastrointestinal injury from cocaine use is also known as body packer's syndrome (225), which describes the changes that develop in body packers or "mules" who ingest multiple small drug-containing packets that subsequently leak. Affected patients tend to be young males with a long history of cocaine abuse (219,223). Older patients may also be affected, particularly those who use cocaine sporadically.

Etiology. Newer, more toxic forms of cocaine, including crack and "free-base" cocaine, cause acute gastroduodenal perforation and rupture.

Pathophysiology. Cocaine acts at the synaptic level, altering neurotransmitter uptake and potentiating norepinephrine and dopamine effects (216). This results in intense vasoconstriction, focal ischemia, and perforation (219,223).

Clinical Features. Preexisting gastric mucosal damage may predispose to cocaine-induced damage (216). Severe and prolonged ischemic episodes eventually result in bowel necrosis, perforation (215), peritonitis, or abscess formation. Patients develop crampy abdominal pain and varying degrees of nausea, vomiting, anorexia, bloody diarrhea, and abdominal rigidity, especially in those with gastrointestinal perforations (215). Patients may also present with small bowel obstruction caused by ingestion of the packets of cocaine.

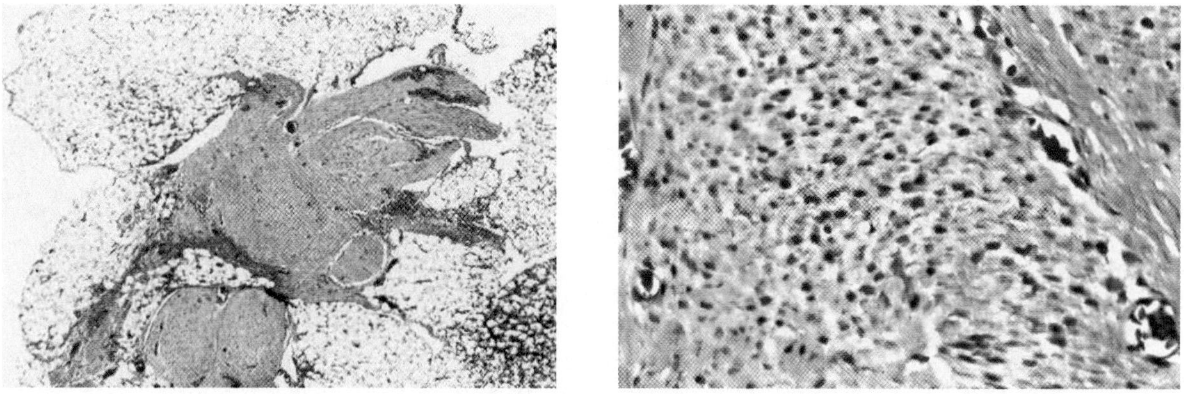

Figure 8-48

PROGESTIN-RELATED PSEUDODECIDUAL NODULES IN THE MESENTERY

Left: Low-power magnification shows the location of the nodules in the mesentery. Right: Higher magnification shows the pseudodecidual response.

Maternal use of cocaine during pregnancy can affect both the mother (228) and the fetus (217,221,222,224). Cocaine is normally detoxified in the plasma and liver by cholinesterase, but plasma cholinesterase levels are very low in fetuses and neonates, predisposing them to high blood drug levels. As a result, the fetus and neonate develop transient or prolonged ischemic episodes, necrotizing enterocolitis, perforation (218), and intestinal atresia (217, 222). Cocaine-induced vasospasm should be considered in those with ischemic bowel who do not have other vascular risk factors. Urinalysis for drugs or their metabolites can establish the diagnosis in patients thought to be body packers or users (226,227).

Gross Findings. Radiologic examination is essential for the diagnosis and management of those with body-packer's syndrome. Plain abdominal radiographs demonstrate the presence of drug packets. They are usually multiple, well-defined, homogeneous, oval or oblong dense packs often surrounded by a crescent of air (the double-condom sign) (220). Grossly, cocaine effects resemble those of ischemia due to other causes.

Microscopic Findings. The gastrointestinal lesions associated with cocaine-induced damage typically show classic ischemic injury. Granulomatous inflammation also affects the stomach of known cocaine addicts, presumably due to the foreign materials that are used to cut the drugs. These substances are sometimes visible within the granulomas (fig. 8-49). The granulomas have the appearance of dense sarcoid granulomas, and usually lack a prominent inflammatory response.

Differential Diagnosis. Other causes of ischemic enterocolitis are in the differential diagnosis.

Treatment and Prognosis. The treatment of cocaine-associated bowel ischemia consists of dealing with the ischemia and the individual's addiction. Ischemic bowel is treated supportively as it is generally reversible unless gangrene and peritonitis supervene. Ischemic involvement of other organs, e.g., cardiac or cerebral, may coexist with mesenteric involvement.

OTHER DRUGS AND CHEMICALS CAUSING ISCHEMIC INJURY

Demography. Most patients who develop ischemic injury from drugs are elderly and have underlying cardiovascular disease (235).

Etiology. A number of drugs cause ischemic injury (Table 8-6). Patients on cardiovascular medications often develop ischemic changes, although it may be difficult to distinguish the damage caused by the drugs and that due to the underlying heart failure. Injury caused by potassium, NSAIDs, and oral contraceptives are the best-documented as chemically induced causes of ischemia. When the slow release form of potassium chloride was introduced, the potassium chloride salt was incorporated into a wax or plastic matrix so that the drug was released at lower

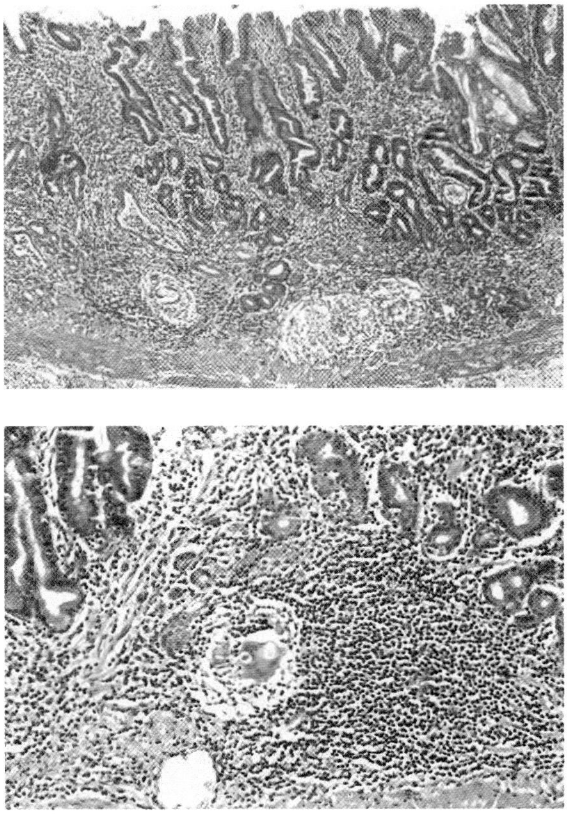

Figure 8-49

FOREIGN BODY GRANULOMAS IN A COCAINE ADDICT

Top: Significant chronic gastritis and nodular aggregates are in the basal part of the mucosa.

Bottom: Higher magnification shows the foreign body response.

Table 8-6

DRUGS AND CHEMICALS CAUSING ISCHEMIA

Induce Thrombosis
DDAVP[a] therapy in diabetes insipidus
Estrogens
Oral contraceptives
Potassium chloride
Progesterone
Induce Autoimmune Vasculitis
Aspirin
Erythromycin
Penicillin
Quinidine
Some NSAIDs
Tetracycline
Thiazide diuretics
Induce Vasospasm and/or Decreased Blood Flow
Alpha-adrenergic vasoconstrictors
Amphetamines
Anesthetics
Cocaine
Cyclosporine
Dialysis
Digitalis
Diuretics
Ergotamine-related drugs
IL2 therapy
Interferon
NSAIDs
Potassium chloride
Sorbital
Vasopressin
Induce Vasculitis
Rutoside

[a]DDAVP = desmopressin; NSAID = nonsteroidal antiinflammatory drug; IL = interleukin.

concentrations. This preparation reduced the incidence of potassium chloride–associated injury but did not eliminate it (230,232).

Scorpion and snake venoms also cause ischemic injury (233,234). Most scorpion and snake venoms contain a mixture of toxic proteins and enzymes that have numerous pharmacologic effects. Desmopressin (DDAVP), used to treat diabetes insipidus, may cause widespread mesenteric venous thrombosis. Vasopressin causes arterial spasm and is used to stop or reduce hemorrhage. It is frequently administered into an artery under radiologic control to reduce gastrointestinal bleeding. Ergot and methysergide also create vasospasm. Ergot compounds, used to treat migraines, may cause ischemic enterocolitis and ergot drugs in suppositories cause a condition resembling solitary rectal ulcer syndrome.

Pathophysiology. Drug-induced ischemia results from: 1) thrombosis or embolism, 2) autoimmune reactions, 3) vasculitis, 4) vasoconstriction or vasospasm, or 5) decreased blood flow (Table 8-6). Potassium chloride causes localized ulceration of the small bowel leading to fibrosis, obstruction, and perforation. Patients who undergo aggressive hemodialysis may develop alterations in blood volume or hyperviscosity that results in decreased peripheral blood flow. This condition preferentially affects the right colon and the damage may be secondary to the generation of oxygen-derived free radicals (231). Venomous bites induce circulatory collapse, hemolysis, coagulation abnormalities, and changes in vascular resistance, all of which contribute to the ischemia.

Table 8-7

CAUSES OF GASTROINTESTINAL STRICTURES

Congenital
Congenital gastrointestinal stenosis
Secondary to Mucosal Inflammation
Diverticulitis
Gastroesophageal reflux disease
Infection
Radiation
Sclerotherapy
Epidermolysis bullosa
Sarcoid (pyloric strictures)
Crohn's disease
Peptic ulcer disease
Ischemia
Neonatal necrotizing enterocolitis
Chronic ulcerative ileojejunitis
Graft versus host disease
Secondary to Chemical Injury
Following caustic injury
Nonsteroidal antiinflammatory drugs (NSAIDs)
Potassium salts
Fibrosing colonopathy secondary to pancreatic enzyme supplements
Secondary to Tumors
Endometriosis

Clinical Features. The clinical features resemble those seen in patients with ischemia due to other causes (see chapter 7).

Gross Findings. The lesions are often impossible to distinguish from other causes of ischemic necrosis, stricture, and ulceration. Enteric-coated potassium chloride preparations cause solitary or multiple, generally small ulcers measuring 1.5 cm in diameter, most commonly located in the jejunum or ileum (229). The mucosa surrounding the ulcers appears edematous and hyperemic (230,236). Submucosal fibrosis leads to stricture formation. The gross features of other cases of drug-induced ischemia are typical of ischemia due to other causes (see chapter 7).

Microscopic Findings. Enteric-coated potassium chloride tablets cause gastrointestinal edema, hemorrhage, erosions, and ischemic infarcts. Enteric-coated potassium chloride is also one of the more common agents to cause deep ulcers and strictures (236). The ulcers resemble the ischemic ulcers caused by other agents. One possible difference is the presence of pyloric metaplasia in the mucosa adjacent to drug-induced lesions. The lesions vary from scattered mucosal petechiae to widespread inflammatory involvement of the small intestine or colon, sometimes simulating active ulcerative colitis. There may be an increase in the number of apoptotic bodies in the crypt bases.

Some drugs cause ischemic injury by inducing widespread venous thrombosis (fig. 8-50). Not surprisingly, the usual histologic features of drug-induced injury resemble those found in patients with ischemia due to other causes (see chapter 7).

Differential Diagnosis. Table 8-7 lists common causes of gastrointestinal strictures.

Treatment and Prognosis. The ischemic bowel is treated supportively, as the damage is generally reversible unless gangrene or perforation occur, in which case resection is necessary.

ANTICOAGULANTS

Demography. Hemorrhages and intramural hematomas affect 30 to 40 percent of patients taking anticoagulants. Significant bleeding affects 1.2 percent of patients taking heparin and 0.2 percent of those taking coumadin (238). The risk of bleeding and other complications increases in those taking other medicines, including NSAIDs, acetaminophen, or corticosteroids (239). Hemorrhage is 3 to 4 times more common in males than in females.

Etiology. Anticoagulants and antiplatelet agents cause the injury. Patients on chemotherapeutic agents may also develop significant bleeding due to reduced numbers of platelets. Submucosal hemorrhages in the esophagus have been detected in patients receiving thrombolytic therapy for myocardial infarction.

Pathophysiology. Since anticoagulants inhibit the clotting mechanisms, patients develop hematomas at sites of trauma.

Clinical Features. Most lesions are small and asymptomatic. When large hematomas form, clinical findings can include pain and signs of obstruction or a mass. Bleeding can occur anywhere in the gastrointestinal tract, but massive bleeding is rare. Clinical symptoms may also arise if the hematoma affects the area of the ampulla of Vater with blockage of the biliary or pancreatic ducts.

Gross Findings. Hematomas can affect any part of the gut. In one series, 59 percent affected the jejunum; 25 percent, the ileum; 9 percent, the duodenum; and 7 percent, the colon (237).

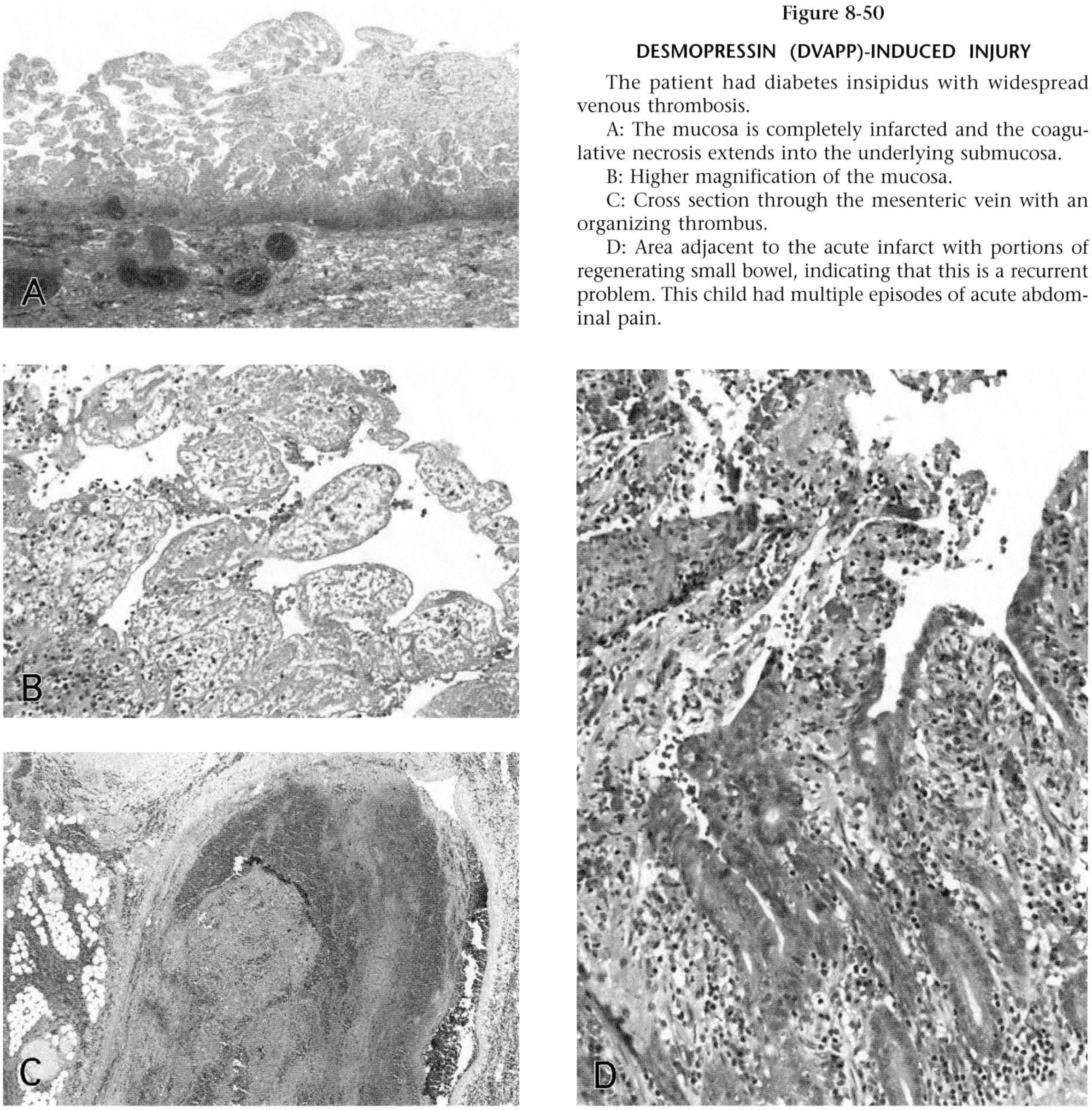

Figure 8-50

DESMOPRESSIN (DVAPP)-INDUCED INJURY

The patient had diabetes insipidus with widespread venous thrombosis.

A: The mucosa is completely infarcted and the coagulative necrosis extends into the underlying submucosa.

B: Higher magnification of the mucosa.

C: Cross section through the mesenteric vein with an organizing thrombus.

D: Area adjacent to the acute infarct with portions of regenerating small bowel, indicating that this is a recurrent problem. This child had multiple episodes of acute abdominal pain.

Microscopic Findings. The hematomas consist of pools of variably clotted, extravasated blood in the gastrointestinal wall (fig. 8-51).

Treatment and Prognosis. Treatment consists of a change of drug dosage or drug cessation. The majority of patients are treated with supportive care. Occasionally, intramucosal hematomas cause luminal obstruction or even track longitudinally and perforate through the serosal or mucosal section of the bowel wall, requiring surgical resection.

CHEMICALLY INDUCED EOSINOPHILIA

Definition. *Chemically induced eosinophilia* is the infiltration of the gastrointestinal tract by eosinophils in response to exposure to or ingestion of various chemical substances.

Etiology. Numerous drugs and chemicals cause gastrointestinal eosinophilia (Table 8-8).

Clinical Features. Trimethoprim-sulfamethoxazole can cause significant eosinophilic esophagitis (243). The eosinophilia-myalgia syndrome usually follows ingestion of L-tryptophan

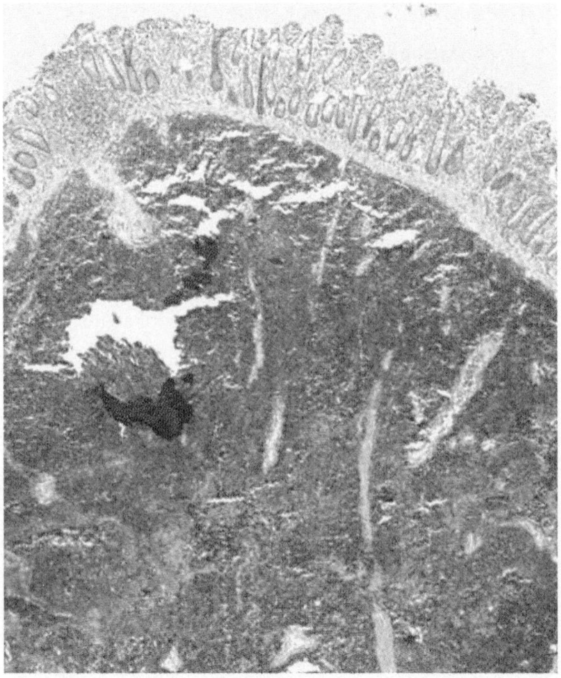

Figure 8-51

ANTICOAGULANT-INDUCED INJURY

Submucosal hematoma in a patient on anticoagulants who had suffered trauma as a result of a motor vehicle accident.

Table 8-8

DRUG- AND CHEMICAL-INDUCED EOSINOPHILIA

Cow's milk intolerance
Food hypersensitivity reactions
Gold
Indomethacin
L-tryptophan
Nonsteroidal antiinflammatory drugs (NSAIDs)
Peritoneal dialysis
Reflux esophagitis
Soy allergen
Toxic oil
Trimethoprim-sulfamethoxazole

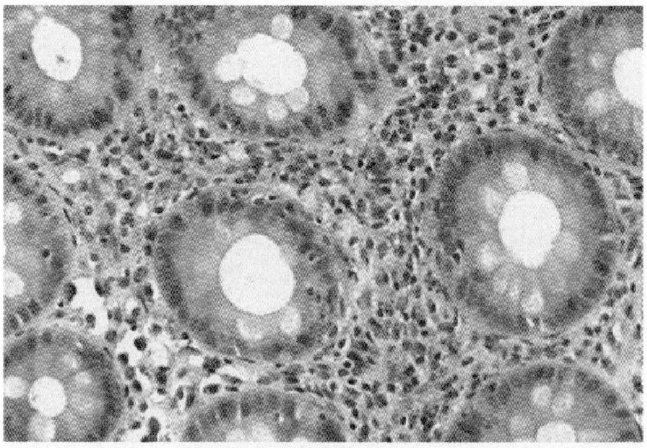

Figure 8-52

MUCOSAL EOSINOPHILIA IN DRUG-INDUCED INJURY

The lamina propria is intensely infiltrated by eosinophils. Some of these enter the glands.

(242,244). Patients present with profound eosinophilia, abnormal hepatic profiles, and myalgias. Some patients develop a connective tissue disease that resembles scleroderma (240,241), with dysmotility and diarrhea. Gastrointestinal involvement leads to significant malabsorption with steatorrhea, hypoalbuminemia, and weight loss. Mucosal eosinophilia also complicates exposure to many drugs, including NSAIDs.

Gross Findings. Usually none.

Microscopic Findings. Histologically, diffuse eosinophilic infiltrates (fig. 8-52) are seen anywhere in the gastrointestinal tract. The number of eosinophils is often quite impressive, numbering more than 25 per high-power field. They are usually seen in the mucosa, but can be present in the other layers of the bowel wall as well. When the eosinophils are present in the lamina propria, we use the term "mucosal eosinophilia." If they also infiltrate the glands, we use the term "eosinophilic gastritis, gastroenteritis, or colitis," depending on the location.

Differential Diagnosis. The differential diagnosis of gastrointestinal eosinophilia usually includes parasitic infections, lymphomas, polyarteritis nodosa, scleroderma, allergic gastroenteritis, eosinophilic gastroenteritis, allergic drug reactions, and IBD. Unfortunately, many times the etiology of the mucosal eosinophilia is not obvious. Also, there appear to be geographic and seasonal variations in the number of eosinophils in general in the gastrointestinal mucosa. The presence of an increased number of apoptotic bodies in the base of the crypts, along with the eosinophilia, suggests chemical (drug) injury, but this finding is not always present.

Treatment and Prognosis. The eosinophilia ceases with removal of the inciting material from the diet or drug regimen.

CHANGES ASSOCIATED WITH UREMIA AND CHRONIC RENAL DISEASE

Definition. Many gastrointestinal abnormalities affect patients with chronic renal disease. *Systemic calciphylaxis* is a rare condition of induced systemic hypersensitivity to appropriate challenging agents, along with calcium deposition (258), that occurs most commonly in patients with end-stage renal disease.

Demography. Duodenal and gastric erosions affect about 17 percent of dialysis patients or patients with renal transplants (257). Up to 60 percent of uremic patients develop mucosal or submucosal hemorrhages, gastric or duodenal erosions, and hemorrhagic vascular ectasias.

Pathophysiology. Patients with chronic renal failure and uremia experience a number of gastrointestinal alterations. The gastrointestinal complications of acute renal failure result from stress, hypotension, and multiple organ failure. Sometimes it is difficult to determine whether these result from the uremia itself or the treatment associated with it, including hemodialysis or transplantation. The cause of gastrointestinal lesions in patients with renal failure is uncertain, but they may result from hypergastrinemia, altered gastric mucosal barrier function, increased gastric acid secretion and mucosal blood flow, and effects possibly mediated by endothelial-derived nitric oxide (258). There may be increased bacterial conversion of urea within the gastric lumen so that there is an increased concentration of ammonia, which may contribute to the mucosal damage. The hypergastrinemia is proportional to the degree of renal dysfunction. Uremia may also negatively impact platelet function, thereby predisposing to mucosal hemorrhage. The use of antiinflammatory or immunosuppressive drugs further aggravates the mucosal damage (246). Patients on chronic dialysis may develop amyloidosis that results in colonic dilatation (252).

Clinical Features. Uremia injures all parts of the gastrointestinal tract. The most commonly affected sites are the stomach, duodenum, ileum, cecum, and colon. The stomach typically develops small petechial mucosal hemorrhages in a pattern simulating acute hemorrhagic or erosive gastritis (251). Patients with uremia may have a more severe gastritis than the usual patient. Peptic ulcer disease worsens during dialysis (251) and delayed gastric emptying is found in patients with chronic renal failure (253). This may contribute to the nausea and vomiting that are common complaints in such patients. Ischemic colitis often complicates chronic uremia. Renal transplant patients also develop mucosal hemorrhages and they have an increased incidence of complications from diverticular disease, an increased incidence of ischemia, and increased use of toxic immunosuppressive drugs. Ischemic injury is known to result from both defective coagulation as well as acute fluid loss. Exacerbation of the diverticulitis may be the result of immunosuppressive therapy (259). Patients also develop pseudomembranous colitis, possibly related to the ischemia.

Systemic calciphylaxis, a phenomenon consisting of severe and progressive ischemic necrosis, involves widespread anatomic regions, including the gastrointestinal tract (245). It most commonly occurs in the setting of chronic renal failure, particularly in patients undergoing renal dialysis, often with secondary or tertiary hyperparathyroidism (254). Calciphylaxis is thought to be due to extensive calcifications that result from increased plasma calcium and phosphorus levels that exceed the solubility end product (245), or possibly from protein C deficiency (256). Medial arterial calcification due to calciphylaxis, along with intimal edema and fibrosis, leads to ischemia and necrosis (255). Rarely, gastrointestinal hemorrhage develops.

Gross Findings. The most commonly observed gross abnormality in uremic patients is the presence of gastroduodenal petechial hemorrhages or stress gastritis. The hemorrhages are frequently multiple and are more common in the stomach and duodenum (257,260). Patients on chronic dialysis often have enlarged, sometimes eroded, gastric mucosal folds. Multiple small ulcers develop in the upper gastrointestinal tract, including the small intestine. In contrast, ulcers in the colon tend to be larger and solitary. Some patients, especially those on chronic dialysis, develop prominent mucosal telangiectasias (248).

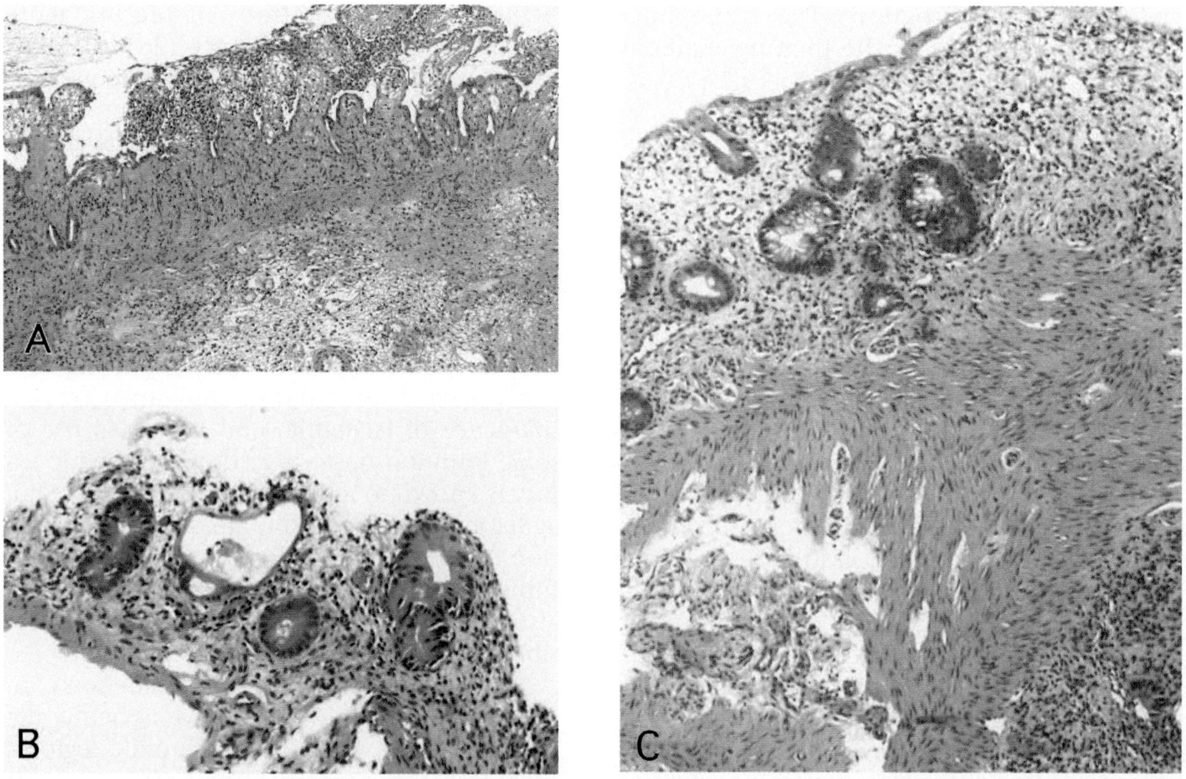

Figure 8-53

GASTROINTESTINAL INJURY IN PATIENTS WITH RENAL DISEASES

Patients with renal disease often have gastrointestinal injury either due to the complications of uremia or as a result of antiinflammatory or immunosuppressive agents used for renal transplants. In some cases, it is difficult to know the exact etiology of the changes that are seen due to the multifactorial nature of the damage.

A: Evidence of ischemia. There is a pseudomembrane covering the mucosal surface.

B: Biopsy from a patient on mycophenolate shows the disappearing glands commonly seen in patients with toxic intestinal injury. The glands become widely dilated and the epithelium appears attenuated, often resembling a dilated vessel.

C: A colonic biopsy in a patient on mycophenolate shows severe damage to the mucosa, with glandular dropout and marked irregularity and distortion of the glands.

Microscopic Findings. Gastroduodenal mucosal and submucosal hemorrhages are sometimes associated with ulceration and bleeding. The stomach shows a superficial gastritis, involving the antrum and fundus. There is foveolar hyperplasia with an increase in the parietal cell mass and changes suggestive of chemical gastropathy. Uremia-associated hypergastrinemia leads to mucosal hyperplasia via the trophic effects of gastrin (250). Patients on regular dialysis may develop multiple mucosal and submucosal telangiectasias, as well as Brunner gland hyperplasia, duodenal mucosal hypertrophy, and peptic duodenitis (250). These changes may regress following transplantation (249). Heterotopic calcification may be seen in patients who develop hyperparathyroidism. Patients with renal disease often undergo transplantation and have secondary changes due to the presence of immunosuppressive agents (see earlier section) or infection. The lesions in the large intestine often resemble those seen in ischemic colitis (fig. 8-53). The calcifications evident in calciphylaxis histologically resemble Mönckeberg's medial calcific sclerosis in the small vessels in the submucosa (247).

Treatment and Prognosis. Many of the gastrointestinal lesions resolve once the uremia and renal failure are treated. Long-term complications include hemorrhage, perforation, or stricture formation.

Table 8-9

DRUGS AND CHEMICALS CAUSING PSEUDOOBSTRUCTION AND SEVERE CONSTIPATION

Alcohol	Phenothiazines	Clonidine
Amanita poisoning	Cimetidine	Theophylline
Anticholinergic drugs	Ganglionic blockers	Nonsteroidal antiinflammatory agents
Antihypertensive drugs	Isoniazid	Rat poisons
Antiparkinsonian drugs	Laxatives	Sympathomimetics
Atropine	Loperamide	Tricyclic antidepressants
Azathioprine (AZT) therapy	Minerals	Vinca alkaloids
Calcium channel blockers	Narcotic analgesics	

DIARRHEIC SHELLFISH POISONING

Demography. *Diarrheic shellfish poisoning* affects individuals who consume shellfish, especially blue mussels that have fed on certain species of marine phytoplankton (261).

Etiology. Toxins from the dinoflagellates of the *Dinophysis* and *Prorocentrum* genera are the main sources of shellfish poisoning (261–265). The major toxin responsible for diarrheic shellfish poisoning is dinophysistoxin 1. It contains okadaic acid, which alters cell function, enhances protein phosphorylation, and increases pericellular intestinal permeability.

Clinical Features. Symptoms, including diarrhea, nausea, vomiting, abdominal pain, and chills, usually start within 4 hours after ingestion and are rare after 12 hours. Occasionally, paraesthesias occur; paralysis is rare. This illness is often misdiagnosed and attributed to fish allergies, gastroenteritis, or nonspecific neurologic disorders.

Microscopic Findings. The toxin causes severe congestion of the villous and submucosal vessels; red blood cells extravasate into the lamina propria. Microvilli degenerate, followed by localized desquamation of cells from the villus tips.

Differential Diagnosis. Other forms of food poisoning.

Treatment and Prognosis. The prognosis for patients with this invariably self-limited illness is excellent.

DRUG-INDUCED NEUROMUSCULAR DISORDERS

Demography. *Drug-induced gastrointestinal dysmotility* is a well-recognized phenomenon (266). Because of the types of medicines that induce pseudoobstruction syndromes, many of the patients have psychiatric diseases or Parkinson's disease.

Etiology. Many drugs cause intestinal pseudoobstruction (Table 8-9), the most common of which are tricyclic antidepressants, phenothiazines, anticholinergic drugs, and vinca alkaloids. It is unclear whether the drugs cause the symptoms or unmask an underlying gastrointestinal motility disorder.

Pathophysiology. Certain foods and drinks and some drugs elevate lower esophageal sphincter (LES) pressure whereas others decrease it.

Clinical Features. The clinical features resemble those present in other motility disorders (see chapter 17). Reflux symptoms may be aggravated or occur de novo. Bowel dysmotility may present with crampy abdominal pain, distension, constipation, and diarrhea associated with bacterial overgrowth. Nausea is common and vomiting may occur.

Gross Findings. When the LES pressure decreases, the gross findings may be those of reflux esophagitis (see chapter 3). If the LES pressure increases, the changes mimic achalasia (see chapter 17). Patients may also develop intestinal pseudo-obstruction and dilation.

Microscopic Findings. It is important to consider a diagnosis of toxic (chemically induced) visceral neuropathy in patients without an obvious cause for their motility disorder, particularly if inflammatory cells are present in the myenteric plexus, in the absence of cancer.

Differential Diagnosis. Other motility disorders (see chapter 17).

Treatment and Prognosis. Treatment consists of withdrawal of the offending agent. Symptoms may persist if another underlying motility disorder is present.

CLOFAZIMINE-INDUCED CRYSTAL-STORING HISTIOCYTOSIS

Demography. Clofazimine is used to treat leprosy and other dermatologic disorders.

Clinical Features. Clofazimine is a riminophenazine compound that is well known for causing reddish discoloration of the skin. Patients may present with epigastric distress and occasional vomiting unrelated to meals, episodic and prostrating abdominal pain, and malabsorption (267).

Gross Findings. Radiologic abnormalities include coarsening of the mucosal pattern and segmentation of barium in the ileum and distal jejunum. Upper gastrointestinal series and abdominal CT scans demonstrate irregular mucosal and submucosal thickening of the jejunal mucosal folds, dilatation of the small intestinal loops, and enlargement of the mesenteric lymph nodes (269).

Microscopic Findings. Clofazimine crystals accumulate in mucosal macrophages, producing infiltrative lesions that radiologically mimic lymphoma and other infiltrative disorders. There is usually an associated lamina propria plasmacytosis that can simulate lymphoplasmacytic lymphoma or multiple myeloma. Both granulomatous enteritis and eosinophilic enteritis may be seen. The crystals also accumulate within nodal macrophages.

Clofazimine crystals appear red in frozen sections, exhibiting a bright red birefringence. They are clear in routinely processed histologic sections because they dissolve in alcohol and organic solvents. They also appear as clear crystalline spaces in ultrastructural studies, but some osmiophilic bodies can be observed. The crystals do not stain with PAS or immunoglobulin immunostains. The clear crystals are several times longer than the macrophage nuclei, and plasma cells and eosinophils are distributed between the crystals.

Treatment and Prognosis. Clofazimine enteropathy regresses after drug withdrawal (268).

DRUG REACTIONS AFFECTING SPECIFIC GASTROINTESTINAL SITES

Drug-Related Esophagitis

Demography. The incidence of *medication-induced esophageal injury* (also termed *pill esophagitis*) is unknown because many cases go unrecognized. In one large study, the incidence was 3.9 cases/100,000 population/year (275). Elderly patients are particularly at risk for developing esophageal drug injury for at least four reasons: 1) they take more medications; 2) they are more likely to have intrinsic or extrinsic esophageal anatomic abnormalities or motility disorders; 3) saliva production decreases with age; and 4) they spend more time in a recumbent position. Injury is facilitated by ingestion of multiple tablets and inadequate liquid consumption. Hiatal hernia, esophageal dysmotility, or strictures also predispose to prolonged esophageal retention of medication and enhance the ability of drugs to damage the mucosa. In patients who have other conditions, such as cardiac enlargement, nodal disease, or an enlarged thyroid gland, the pills may stick at these sites. They also stick at areas of strictures or rings.

Etiology. A large number of drugs cause esophageal damage (Table 8-10). In younger individuals, the injury results from antibiotic therapy, whereas cardiogenic medications and bisphosphonates cause the esophageal injury in the elderly (275). Potassium chloride pills cause severe esophageal injury, including strictures (273) and significant hemorrhages. Reflux esophagitis is a form of chemical injury but it is discussed in chapter 3.

Pathophysiology. Chemical- and drug-induced injury in the esophagus occurs via several mechanisms (Table 8-11). Most esophageal damage results from focal mucosal entrapment that leads to localized burns and ulcerations. Tablets and capsules typically lodge in the midesophagus, giving rise to discrete, multiple, and sometimes serpiginous ulcers. Physical entrapment of undigested medicines especially occurs with drugs that contain a hydrophilic swelling agent or fiber that ensures rapid disintegration when the pills contact water (279). These medicines act as foreign bodies impacting on the esophageal lumen. Pills such as doxycycline, tetracycline, ascorbic acid, ferrous sulfate, and slow-release emepronium bromide produce a pH of less than 3.0 when dissolved in 10 mL of water or saliva thereby injuring the esophagus (270). Esophageal mucosal uptake plays a role in doxycycline-, NSAID-, and alprenolol-induced injury (276). Other postulated mechanisms of injury include local

Table 8-10

EXAMPLES OF DRUG- OR CHEMICAL-INDUCED ESOPHAGEAL INJURY

Alprenol chloride	Ascorbic acid	Ferrous salts
Antibiotics	Barbiturates	Pantogar
Chloramphenicol	Benadryl	Pantozyme
Clindamycin	Bisphosphonates	Phenylbutazone
Cloxacillin	Carbachol	Phenobarbital
Doxycycline	Chemotherapeutic agents	Phenoxymethyl penicillin
Erythromycin	Actinomycin D	Piroxicam
Lincomycin	Adriamycin	Potassium chloride
Minocycline	Cytosine arabinoside	Prednisone and prednisolone
Penicillin	Estramustine phosphate	Quinidine
Sulfa drugs	5-Fluorouracil	Sclerosants for varices
Tetracycline	Chloral hydrate	Serrapeptase
Tinidazole	Clinitest tablets	Sodium amytal
Antiinflammatory agents	Co-trimoxazole	Theophylline
Acetaminophen	Cromolyn sodium	Trimethoprim-sulfamethoxazole
Acetylsalicylic acid	Digoxin, digitoxin	Vasopressin
Ibuprofen	d-Penicillamine	Zidovudine
Indomethacin	Emepronium bromide	
Mefaminic acid		
Naproxen		
Piroxicam		
Sulindac		
Tolmetin		

hyperosmolarity, as with potassium chloride, or induction of reflux, as with theophylline and anticholinergic agents. Most young patients rarely have predisposing factors other than improper pill ingestion.

Clinical Features. Because the histologic features of chemically induced esophagitis are nonspecific, the diagnosis is usually provided by the clinical history. Esophageal chemical injury usually falls into two major groups. One form is transient and self-limiting, as exemplified by tetracycline- and emepronium-induced injury (see fig. 8-23). The second tends to be persistent, leading to stricture formation, as with NSAIDs or in patients with motility disorders in which drugs such as potassium chloride and quinidine injure the mucosa due to delayed transit. Endoscopic examination with biopsy is typically done to determine the extent of the injury and to rule out other causes of esophageal injury such as infection or tumors.

Patients with drug-induced esophageal injury often present with sudden odynophagia or other types of pain (277) and dysphagia. There may be hematemesis, melena, and stricture formation (278,280). The clinical features reflect the patient's age and overall health status as well as the nature of the drug or chemical consumed. Localized esophageal damage, ranging from inflammation to severe hemorrhage and even perforation, develops as the medications dissolve (278).

Table 8-11

MECHANISMS OF CHEMICALLY INDUCED ESOPHAGEAL INJURY

Direct toxicity
Corrosion or acidic injury
Reflux esophagitis
Heat production
Physical entrapment of medication
Allergic reactions
Induction of vasculitis
Altered motility or lower esophageal sphincter function (see Table 8-12)
Predisposition to infection
Induction of ischemia
Mucosal uptake

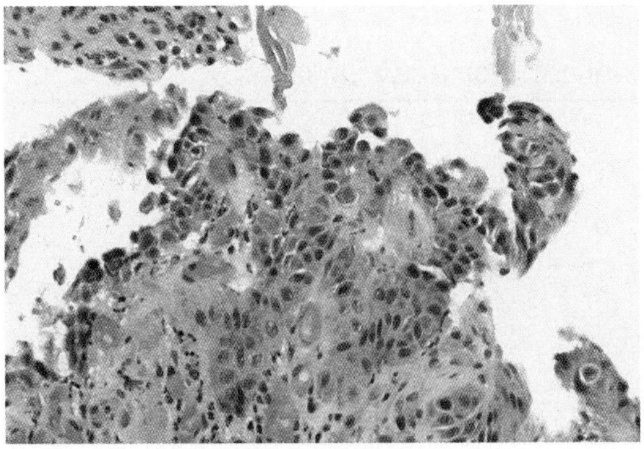

Figure 8-54

PILL-INDUCED ESOPHAGITIS

The esophagitis resulting from medications often resembles that due to reflux. Changes range from mild to severe. In this case, the epithelium is markedly regenerative, congested, and slightly inflamed. In the absence of a history, it would be impossible to make a diagnosis of drug-induced injury.

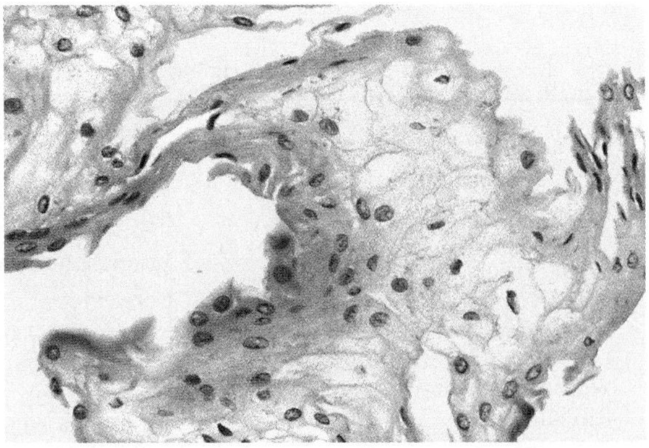

Figure 8-55

ESOPHAGEAL BALLOONING DEGENERATION

Swelling of the superficial epithelium to produce balloon cells is a common response to chemical injury in the esophagus.

Patients frequently have the sensation that a pill is stuck in the esophagus before symptoms develop. Patients with antibiotic injury suddenly develop chest pain after drug administration. Patients on long-term potassium chloride therapy usually present with progressive dysphagia but little pain. Patients with acute quinidine-induced pill injury present with burning pain and dysphagia related to edema and ulcer development. Sulfa drugs and co-trimoxazole are implicated in up to 60 percent of cases of Stevens-Johnson syndrome (274).

Gross Findings. Endoscopy usually shows one or more discrete, shallow, esophageal ulcers; the surrounding mucosa usually appears normal but it may be inflamed or edematous. The ulcers are usually small, pinpoint lesions but large circumferential lesions several centimeters long have also been described (281). Pill remnants are occasionally identified at the injury site (278). Deeper injury results in mediastinitis or hemorrhage due to penetration through the esophageal wall. Extensive and deep penetration may cause circumferential ulcers that may require dilatation or surgical resection. Rarely, medications cause a severe ulcerative esophagitis involving up to 10 cm of the esophageal mucosa, or its entire length. Most ulcers lie in the midesophagus (275,277), usually in areas of normal anatomic narrowing such as the aortic arch or areas narrowed by pathologic processes.

Microscopic Findings. The histologic features of chemically induced esophageal ulcers are nonspecific: subepithelial edema, mucosal hyperplasia, the presence of balloon cells, necrosis, acute inflammation, ulceration, and edema during the acute injury and granulation tissue and regenerative epithelium in the healing phase (fig. 8-54) (271). The presence of balloon cells serves as an early esophageal mucosal marker of chemical injury but it is not specific for any etiology. Balloon cells are recognizable by their distended globoid shape (fig. 8-55). Trimethoprim-sulfamethoxazole as well as other medications cause significant eosinophilic esophagitis. Alendronate is associated with multinucleated giant epithelial cells, which simulate viral cytopathic effects. Stevens-Johnson syndrome is characterized by marked inflammation of the lamina propria with eosinophilia and subepithelial bullae. Resection specimens from patients with long-term damage may show full-thickness fibrosis. If crystals are seen, they may be the result of bisphosphonates or kayexalate and sorbitol. These crystals lie in necrotic areas.

Differential Diagnosis. The differential diagnosis includes other forms of acute esophagitis, especially reflux and viral esophagitis. The endoscopist should suspect drug-induced esophagitis or ulceration when lesions lie proximal to areas where reflux-associated abnormalities occur. The lesions may be circumferential and associated with a significant edematous and erosive reaction. Symptoms may be disproportionate to the endoscopic findings.

Treatment and Prognosis. Most uncomplicated cases of pill-induced esophageal injury heal with symptom resolution in a few days to a few weeks. Antacids, H2-receptor antagonists, and sucralfate are often prescribed, particularly when gastroesophageal reflux exacerbates the injury. Severe odynophagia may necessitate parenteral hydration or gastrotomy with manual disimpaction (272). Acute inflammatory and edematous strictures may resolve spontaneously but chronic strictures may require dilatation or surgical resection. The symptoms of drug-induced esophagitis may continue if gastroesophageal reflux disease is present.

The most dangerous drug-related esophagitis results from potassium chloride. Several patients have died of esophagitis directly related to its ingestion. Complications, such as strictures, usually result from ingestion of caustic substances, such as iron or potassium salts (270).

Table 8-12

CHEMICALLY INDUCED GASTRIC INJURY

Alcohol: chemical gastropathy, ulcers, erosions, chronic gastritis
Alkaline reflux: chemical gastropathy, ulcers, erosions, chronic gastritis
Anticoagulants: gastric hematomas
Bromocriptine: gastric ulcers
Corrosive agents: severe gastric necrosis
Chemotherapeutic agents: gastric necrosis
Corticosteroids: gastritis and ulcers
Ferrous sulfate: gastritis and ulcers
Fluorides: gastric damage
Interleukin 4: acute gastric mucosal injury and hemorrhage
Mercuric chloride: acute gastritis
Methyldopa: autoimmune gastritis
Nonsteroidal antiinflammatory drugs (NSAIDs): chemical gastropathy, ulcers, erosions
Potassium chloride: ulcers, bleeding, perforation, and stricture formation
Omeprazole: chronic atrophic gastritis
Prostaglandins: mucosal hyperplasia
Ticlopidine: lymphocytic gastritis
Tooth bleaching agents: gastric ulcers
Tumor necrosis factor: acute gastric mucosal injury and hemorrhage
Zinc sulfate: gastric ulcers

Chemically Induced Gastric Injury

Demography. *Chemically induced gastric injury* is very common. It appears in two major forms: as *acute gastritis* or as a *chemical* or *reactive gastropathy*. Drug-related gastrointestinal injury accounts for over 33 percent of adverse drug reactions among hospitalized patients (284a); 33 percent of gastric ulcers results from drug use.

Etiology. Almost any drug can irritate the gastric mucosa (Table 8-12). Some gastric injuries result from therapeutic drug interactions whereas others result from accidental or suicidal ingestion of strong alkalis, acids, and other toxic substances. The agents most commonly implicated in gastric injury are aspirin and other NSAIDs, alcohol, potassium chloride, and iron tablets (282,283). Long-term fluoride supplementation also causes gastritis, as do chemotherapeutic agents. Reflux of duodenal contents into the gastric lumen causes chemical injury as well.

Pathophysiology. Some drug-induced and stress-induced ulcers share common pathogenetic events with chemically induced injury, but the factors that lead to the initial cellular damage may differ. The fact that many drugs produce similar changes, whether administered intravenously or orally, suggests that mucosal contact need not occur to produce the damage. Ethanol, NSAIDs, and bile acids are all lipid soluble. They dissolve in the membranes of antral surface foveolar cells, damaging the mucosal mucus-bicarbonate barrier and facilitating back-diffusion of hydrogen ions into the mucosa. The acid in turn causes mucosal injury either due to direct damage or via vasoconstriction and the development of an acute gastritis. These agents also exacerbate preexisting peptic ulcer disease.

H2-receptor antagonists (famotidine [Pepcid], cimetidine [Tagamet], and ranitidine [Zantac]), and proton pump inhibitors such as omeprazole (Prilosec) block gastric acid secretion, significantly decrease the consequences of peptic disease, and promote ulcer healing. Chronic inhibition of gastric acid secretion secondarily leads to G-cell hyperplasia and hypergastrinemia. The degree of antral G-cell hyperplasia occurring secondary to acid blockade varies from patient to patient.

Clinical Features. Patients with acute gastritis typically present with upper abdominal pain, nausea, and vomiting. These may be perceived by the patients as an abrupt onset of acute burning. Patients with skeletal fluorosis, a crippling bone disease caused by excess fluoride ingestion, have gastrointestinal symptoms, the most common being abdominal pain. The discomfort tends to be constant and may be aggravated by food. Pancreatitis or even cholecystitis may need to be considered in the clinical differential diagnosis.

Gross Findings. Endoscopically, gastritis is usually present. Variable changes include edema, erythema, scattered petechiae, and mucosal surface friability. Large areas of hemorrhage may be present, ranging from multiple mucosal streaks to diffuse mucosal involvement with superficial erosions. The endoscopist may diagnose such cases as acute hemorrhagic gastritis or acute erosive gastritis. These lesions are typically confined to the antrum but they may extend more proximally. Associated duodenal changes may be present. Patients with chemical gastropathy are often described as having a nodular antrum or showing erosions.

Microscopic Findings. The histologic features of all of the chemical gastropathies can resemble one another, often making it impossible to determine the exact etiology in the absence of identifiable bile or a pertinent clinical history. Early histologic changes consist of edema, congestion, and patchy hemorrhages in the superficial lamina propria (fig. 8-56). The changes overlap with those of the potential traumatic effects of the biopsy procedure (284). Other changes include surface and foveolar cell hyperplasia (fig. 8-57), gastric pit elongation, minimal degeneration of the foveolar and pit epithelium, a relative paucity of acute inflammation, and regeneration in the mucous neck region (fig. 8-58). Milder lesions remain limited to the upper mucosa and are frequently associated with focal dilatation of gastric pits. The underlying glands are not involved. Vascular congestion is often a prominent feature (fig. 8-56). There may be areas of erosion or ulceration.

Mononuclear cells may be present in the lamina propria, and intestinal metaplasia may be present. Chronic atrophic gastritis may develop. There is a relative paucity of neutrophils despite evidence of mucosal injury. The changes associated with alkaline reflux gastritis resemble those seen in other forms of chemical gastropathy and these lesions cannot be distinguished unless bile is seen in the gastric lumen or gastric pits. Alkaline reflux gastritis is suspected in those patients who have had prior antrectomy and gastrojejunostomy.

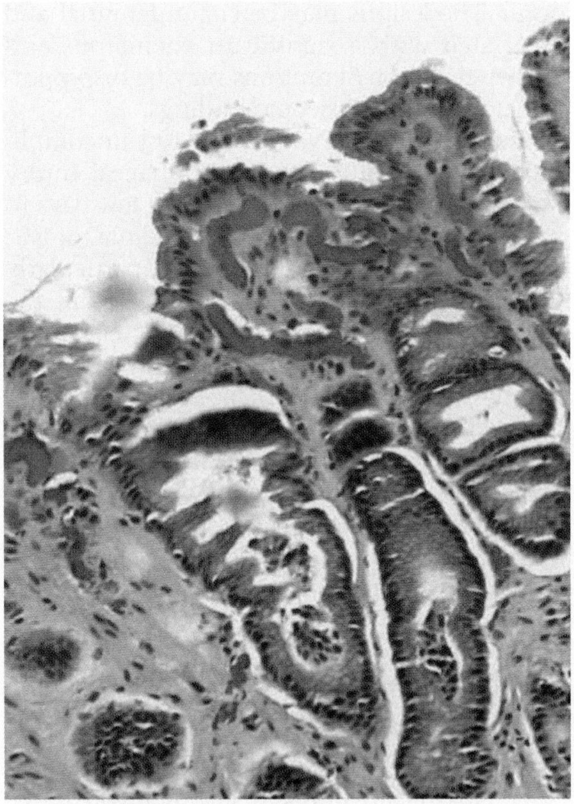

Figure 8-56

CHEMICAL GASTROPATHY

The gastric mucosa shows mild villiform transformation, muscle stranding in the lamina propria, vascular congestion, and mucin depletion of a reactive-appearing epithelium.

Long-term use of antisecretory agents can result in mucosal hyperplasia, sometimes appearing endoscopically as tiny gastric polyps. Histologically, these areas appear as small mucosal cysts lined by flattened parietal and chief cells. A diffuse (fig. 8-59), linear, and/or micronodular hyperplasia of enterochromaffin-like (ECL) cells has been described in patients on long-term treatment with omeprazole. The presence of concomitant *H. pylori* infection is

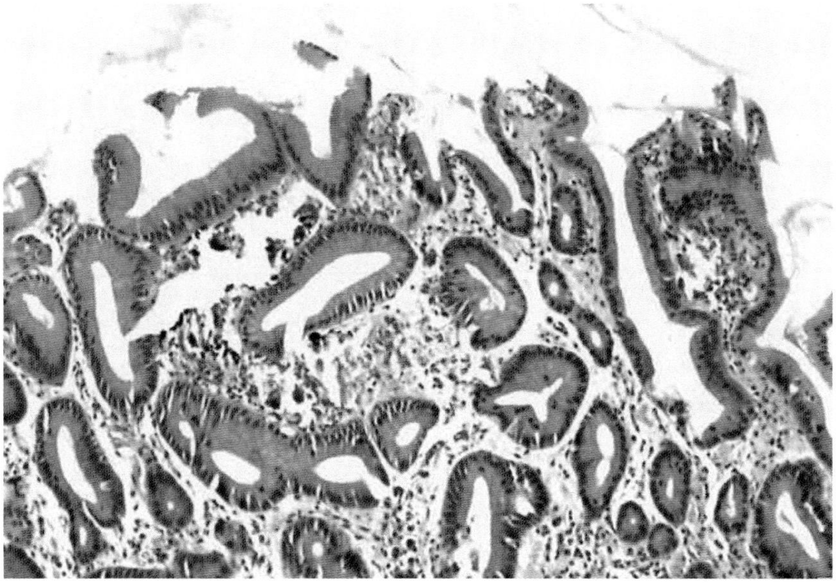

Figure 8-57

BILE REFLUX GASTRITIS

Irregularly shaped glands are lined by foveolar epithelium.

an important factor for the progression of fundic gastritis and the development of argyrophil cell hyperplasia during long-term antisecretory treatment. Patients on proton pump inhibitors also often develop vacuolization of the parietal cells, which occasionally may be quite striking (fig. 8-59). Features suggesting the presence of a chemical gastropathy are listed in Table 8-13.

Differential Diagnosis. The differential diagnosis includes other forms of acute toxic gastritis, including infections, allergic disorders, and chronic active gastritis. The changes also overlap with those of acute stress gastritis.

Treatment and Prognosis. The abnormalities reverse following withdrawal of the offending agent.

Table 8-13

CLUES THAT SUGGEST CHEMICAL INJURY IN THE STOMACH

Pit expansion
Mucus depletion
Superficial edema
No organisms present[a]
No metaplasia
No polyps
No enlarged folds
Muscle fibers extending into the mucosa from the muscularis mucosae
Villiform transformation

[a]*Helicobacter pylori* infection may be superimposed on a chemical gastropathy, confounding the histologic features.

Chemically Induced Intestinal Injury

Demography. Intestinal damage commonly follows drug or chemical exposure. Patient demographics vary depending on the type of injury caused and the agent(s) to which the patient is exposed. Many have been discussed in earlier sections.

Etiology. The most common drugs affecting the intestines are listed in Table 8-14. Probably the most commonly diagnosed drug-induced injury in the colon is pseudomembranous colitis associated with antibiotic use. NSAIDs, gold, potassium chloride, and antibiotics are other common causes of chemically induced intestinal injury. Many of these have already been discussed in previous sections. Penicillin and ampicillin cause *C. difficile*–associated pseudomembranous colitis. In addition, they cause a hemorrhagic right-sided colitis that differs from the antibiotic-associated colitis. The pathogenesis of this form of disease is unknown, but ischemia is thought to play a role. Chemicals, such as alcohol, are injected into the colonic submucosa to facilitate chemical mucosal debridement. 1.0 normal sodium hydroxide produces second-degree colonic mucosal burns within 10 minutes of exposure. It also causes moderate third-degree injury of the underlying muscularis propria (286). Rectal formalin instillation is used

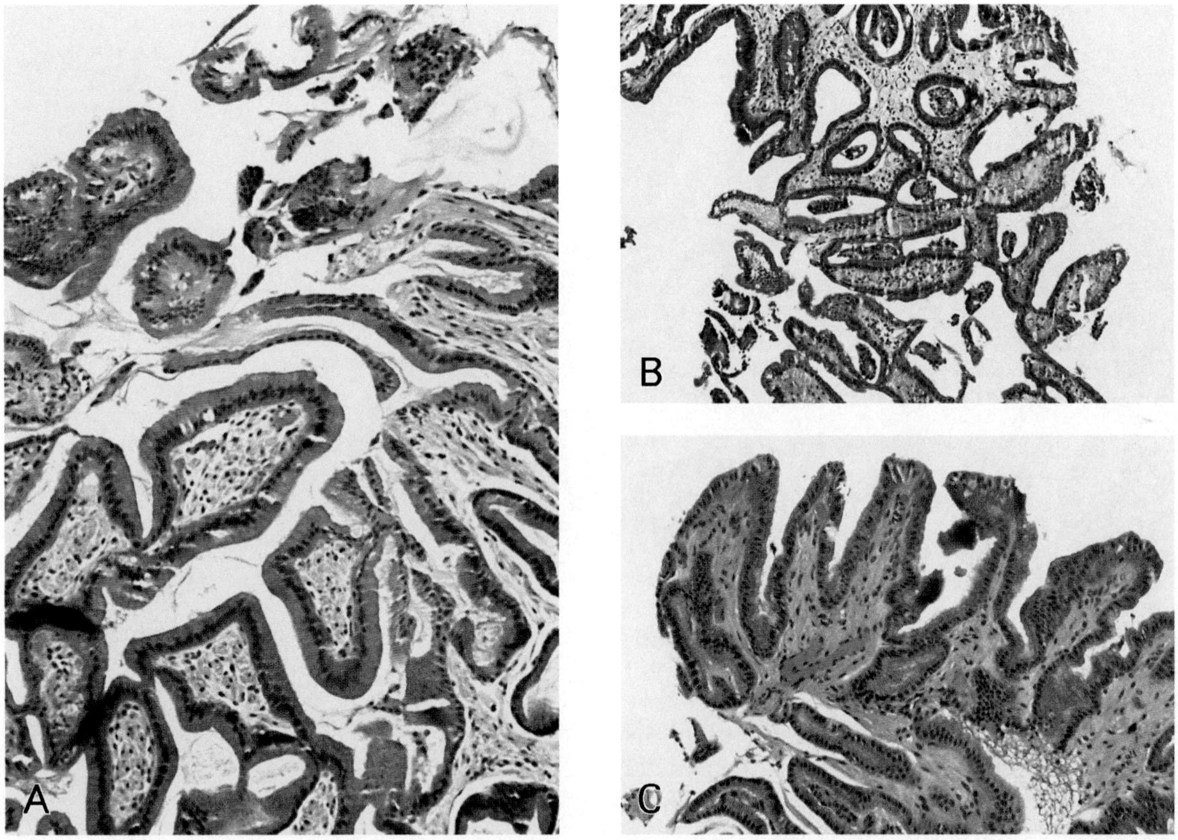

Figure 8-58

CHEMICAL GASTROPATHY

A: Figures A and B show the irregularly shaped glands typical of chemical gastropathy. The patient was a known NSAID user. The superficial mucosa is lined by foveolar cells with abundant mucin.

B: In alkaline reflux gastritis, a basophilic epithelium lines the glands; the epithelium is much more reactive in appearance than in A.

C: Prominent villiform transformation and muscle strands in the lamina propria.

to treat the hemorrhagic proctitis associated with radiation injury (287). Formalin-induced proctitis following instillation of 4 percent formalin in sequential aliquots of a small volume heals within 2 weeks without long-term changes in rectal compliance or collagen content (288). Formalin is used to stop rectal bleeding and is effective in the majority of patients (289). Silver nitrate sticks and 1.25 percent formalin produce first-degree mucosal burns (286).

Isotretinoin (Accutane), a synthetic analogue of 13-cis-retinoic acid, or vitamin A, precipitates IBD. Isotretinoin and acyclovir cause allergic colitis; toxic megacolon complicates methotrexate use. Ergotamine tartrate sometimes causes solitary rectal ulcer formation. Aluminum hydroxide gel causes constipation and bowel distension. Long-term use of the phlebotonic drug, cyclo-3-FORT, causes lymphocytic colitis. Enalapril (Vasotec) causes angioedema of the small bowel, which presents as abdominal pain, nausea, vomiting, and diarrhea.

Granulomatous reactions develop when oils are inserted into anal fistulas or abscess cavities. These reactions result from the escape of oily substances used to soften the feces. Oils are also used to inject hemorrhoids. The degree of the reaction depends on the type of oil used. Vegetable oils produce less severe reactions than animal fats; mineral oils cause the most damage.

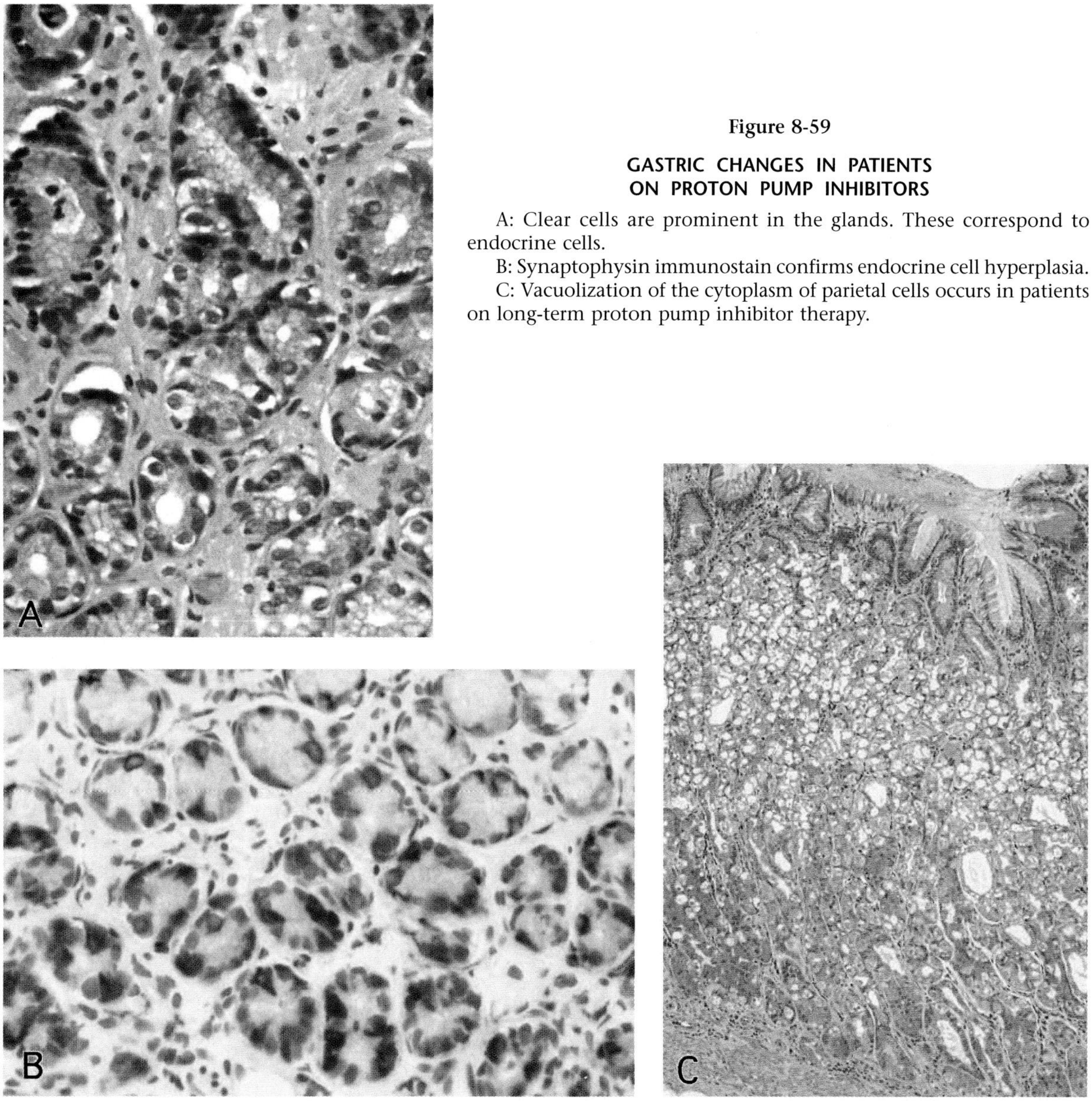

Figure 8-59

GASTRIC CHANGES IN PATIENTS ON PROTON PUMP INHIBITORS

A: Clear cells are prominent in the glands. These correspond to endocrine cells.

B: Synaptophysin immunostain confirms endocrine cell hyperplasia.

C: Vacuolization of the cytoplasm of parietal cells occurs in patients on long-term proton pump inhibitor therapy.

Pathophysiology. Drugs injure the intestine in various ways. They cause apoptosis, exacerbate preexisting intestinal lesions, lead to neuromuscular damage, and predispose to infections or ischemia.

Clinical Features. The clinical features vary depending on the pathogenesis of the injury. Patients with anorectal granulomas may present with masses easily mistaken for cancer. Patients exposed to glutaraldehyde develop a self-limited syndrome of cramps, abdominal pain, tenesmus, and rectal bleeding within 48 hours of uncomplicated sigmoidoscopy or colonoscopy (285). The diagnosis should be suspected in individuals developing hemorrhagic colitis immediately after undergoing colonoscopy. Patients with oil granulomas present with pain, constipation, or bleeding.

Gross Findings. The gross appearance of drug- or chemical-induced injury varies depending on the type of damage produced. Most agents causing disease in the intestine have already been discussed in previous sections. Endoscopic or radiographic features of glutaraldehyde injury tend to show a left-sided distribution. Patients with drug-induced strictures have lesions that can be

Table 8-14
CAUSES OF INTESTINAL CHEMICAL INJURY
Chemotherapeutic agents: damage replicating cells causing mucositis; predisposition to infection
Nonsteroidal antiinflammatory drugs (NSAIDs): erosions, ulcers, diaphragms, focal enterocolitis
Methotrexate: crypt hypoplasia and villous atrophy
Neomycin: malabsorption, minimal histologic damage to villous atrophy and mucosal inflammation
Drugs causing ischemia (see Table 8-6)
Laxatives and bowel-cleansing agents: mild inflammation
Enemas and cathartics: mild inflammation
Isotretinoin: acute colitis
Heavy metals: enterocolitis
Agents causing strictures (see Table 8-7)
Oily liniments: granulomatous inflammation, usually in anorectal area
Agents causing motility disorders (see Table 8-9)
Agents causing eosinophilia (see Table 8-8)
Caustic agents: mucosal burns
Antibiotic-associated colitis: colitis with or without pseudomembranes
Drugs or chemicals causing hypersensitivity reactions
Immunosuppressive agents: inflammation, predisposition to infection

short or long, single or multiple. Oil granulomas present as rounded, annular or ulcerated, submucosal anorectal tumors, occurring as high as the rectosigmoid junction. The tumorous masses may become fixed to other structures. They consist of firm, yellowish gray masses of dense fibrotic tissue containing entrapped globules of oil that ooze from their cut surfaces.

Microscopic Findings. Most drugs and chemicals produce a nonspecific histologic picture easily confused with idiopathic IBD, ischemia, or infectious colitis. Many drugs are implicated in the production of intestinal malabsorption but they do not usually result in histologic abnormalities. The presence of cystically dilated glands adjacent to reactive-appearing glands suggests the presence of chemical or toxic injury in the intestines (fig. 8-60). Localized, nonspecific proctitis results from suppository insertion or sulfasalazine enemas. Drugs such as methyldopa and penicillamine cause a diffuse colitis. Long-term therapy with immunosuppressive agents or corticosteroids may result in cytomegalovirus infections, thrombus formation, and ischemia.

Oil-based granulomas (oleogranulomas) found in the anorectal region exhibit a characteristic histology that varies with the stage of

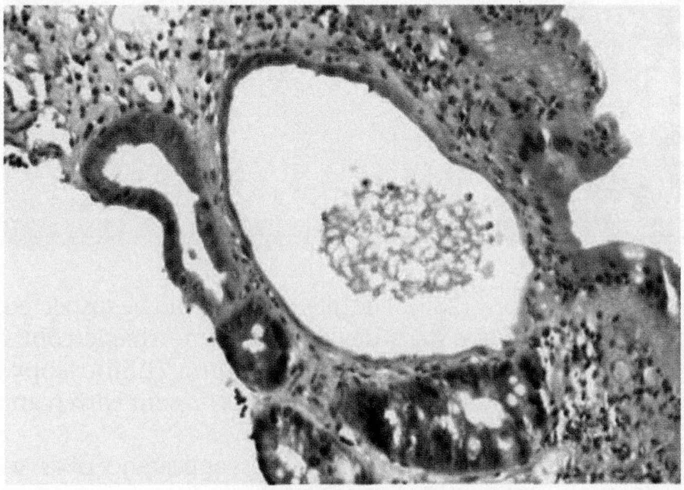

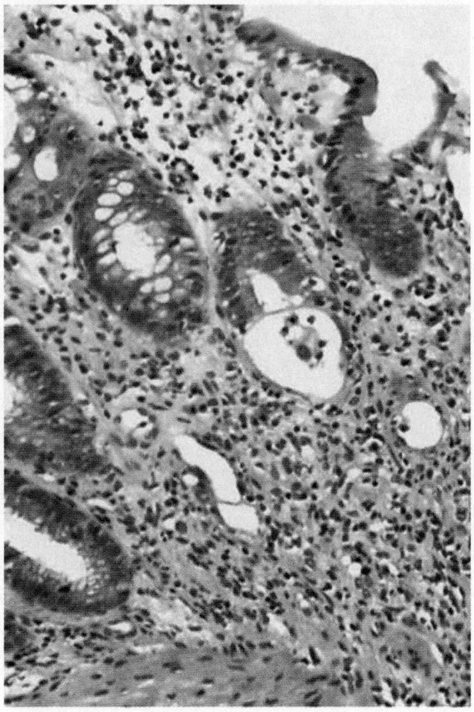

Figure 8-60

CHEMICAL INJURY OF THE COLON

Above: The mucosa has a distorted glandular architecture with glandular dilatation and thinning of the epithelium.

Right: There is prominent apoptosis in the base of the crypts, with inflammation and edema.

development. Characteristically, irregular spaces are surrounded by macrophages with prominent fibrosis. Giant cells are usually sparse. Sarcoid type granulomas are absent. In some cases, there is significantly more inflammation, perhaps reflecting the nature of the oily substance or the time in the evolution of the lesion, with changes being more acute than normally seen. The spaces that are present result from lipid extraction during slide preparation. In the early stages, there is acute inflammation with many eosinophils. Increasing fibrosis and zones of mononuclear phagocytes, epithelioid cells, giant cells, and a peripheral boundary of proliferating fibrous connective tissue gradually replace the acute inflammation. Round spaces are lined by mononuclear cells or multinucleated histiocytes. Prominent fibrosis may be present. Variable numbers of eosinophils and lymphocytes are associated with the reactive tissues. Fat is not easily identified in tissues that have undergone routine processing but can easily be identified in frozen sections using fat stains. This is generally not necessary, however, since the morphology is so distinctive.

Differential Diagnosis. The foreign body giant cell reaction associated with oleogranulomas distinguishes them from the granulomas seen in Crohn's disease or those associated with certain infections, such as *Yersinia* or tuberculosis. Oleogranulomas lack the compact epithelioid appearance seen in Crohn's disease. In addition, there is often fat necrosis associated with oleogranuloma that helps distinguish this lesion from granulomas associated with infections or Crohn's disease. The histologic features of oleogranulomas can also be confused with those of lymphangiomas or pneumatosis intestinalis.

REFERENCES

General

Riddell RH. The gastrointestinal tract. In: Riddell RH, ed. Pathology of drug-induced and toxic diseases. New York: Churchill Livingstone; 1982:515–606.

Introduction

1. Beaugerie L, Luboinski J, Brousse N, et al. Drug induced lymphocytic colitis. Gut 1994;35:426–8.
2. Beaugerie L, Patey N, Brousse N. Ranitidine, diarrhoea, and lymphocytic colitis. Gut 1995;37:708–11.
3. Lewis JH. Gastrointestinal injury due to medicinal agents. Am J Gastroenterol 1986;81:819–34.
4. Pirmohamed M, James S, Meakin S, et al. Adverse drug reactions as cause of admission to hospital: prospective analysis of 18,820 patients. BMJ 2004;329:15–9.
5. Price AB. Pathology of drug-associated gastrointestinal disease. Br J Clin Pharmacol 2003;56:477–82.

Nonsteroidal Antiinflammatory Drugs

6. Agrawal NM Roth S, Graham WC, et al. Misoprostol compared with sucralfate in the prevention of nonsteroidal anti-inflammatory drug-induced gastric ulcer: a randomized, controlled trial. Ann Intern Med 1991;115:195–200.
7. Allison MC, Howatson AG, Torrance CJ, Lee FD, Russell RI. Gastrointestinal damage associated with the use of nonsteroidal antiinflammatory drugs. N Engl J Med 1992;327:749–54.
8. Ament PW, Childers RS. Prophylaxis and treatment of NSAID-induced gastropathy. Am Fam Phys 1997;55:1323–6, 1331–2.
9. Armstrong CP, Blower AL. Nonsteroidal anti-inflammatory drugs and life-threatening complications of peptic ulceration. Gut 1987;28:527–32.
10. Baert F, Hart J, Blackstone MO. A case of diclofenac-induced colitis with focal granulomatous change. Am J Gastroenterol 1995;90:1871–3.
11. Barrier CH, Hirschowitz BI. Controversies in the detection and management of nonsteroidal antiinflammatory drug-induced side effects of the upper gastrointestinal tract. Arthritis Rheum 1989;32:926–32.
12. Baum C, Kennedy DL, Forbes MB. Utilization of nonsteroidal antiinflammatory drugs. Arthritis Rheum 1985;28:686–92.
13. Bjarnason I, Hayllar J, MacPherson AJ, Russell AS. Side effects of nonsteroidal anti-inflammatory drugs on the small and large intestine in humans. Gastroenterology 1993;104:1832–47.
14. Bjarnason I, Macpherson A. Intestinal toxicity of non-steroidal anti-inflammatory drugs. Pharmac Ther 1994;62:145–57.

15. Bjarnason I, Price AB. The small and large intestinal pathologies of non-steroidal anti-inflammatory drug ingestion. Ann Pathol 1994; 14:326–32.
16. Bjarnason I, Price AB, Zanelli G, et al. Clinicopathological features of nonsteroidal antiinflammatory drug-induced small intestinal strictures. Gastroenterology 1988;94:1070–4.
17. Bjarnason I, Williams P, Smethurst O, Peters TJ, Levi AJ. The effects of non-steroidal anti-inflammatory drugs and prostaglandins on the permeability of the human small intestine. Gut 1986;27:1292–7.
18. Bombardier C, Laine L, Reicin A. Comparison of upper gastrointestinal toxicity of rofecoxib and naproxen in patients with rheumatoid arthritis. N Engl J Med 2000;343:1520–8.
19. Chan FK, Graham DY. Review article: prevention of non-steroidal anti-inflammatory drug gastrointestinal complications—review and recommendations based on risk assessment. Aliment Pharmacol Ther 2004;19:1051–61.
20. Cortina G, Wren S, Armstrong B, Lewin K, Fajardo L. Clinical and pathologic overlap in nonsteroidal anti-inflammatory drug-related small bowel diaphragm disease and the neuromuscular and vascular hamartoma of the small bowel. Am J Surg Pathol 1999;23:1414–7.
21. Cryer B, Feldman M. Effects of very low dose daily, long-term aspirin therapy on gastric, duodenal, and rectal prostaglandin levels and on mucosal injury in healthy humans. Gastroenterology 1999;117:17–25.
22. Davies NM. Review article: non-steroidal anti-inflammatory drug-induced gastrointestinal permeability. Aliment Pharmacol Ther 1998;12: 303–20.
23. Dickman A, Ellershaw J. NSAIDs: gastroprotection or selective COX-2 inhibitor? Palliat Med 2004;18:275–86.
24. Donnelly MT, Hawkey CJ. COX-II inhibitors—a new generation of safer NSAIDS? Aliment Pharmacol Ther 1997;11:227–36.
25. El-Zimaity HM, Genta RM, Graham GY. Histological features do not define NSAID-induced gastritis. Hum Pathol 1996;27:1348–54.
26. Fellows IW, Clarke JM, Roberts PF. Non-steroidal anti-inflammatory drug-induced jejunal and colonic diaphragm disease: a report of two cases. Gut 1992;33:1424–6.
27. Fries JF, Murtagh KN, Bennett M, Zatarain E, Lingala B, Bruce B. The rise and decline of nonsteroidal antiinflammatory drug-associated gastropathy in rheumatoid arthritis. Arthritis Rheum 2004;50:2433–40.
28. Gabriel SE, Haakkimainen L, Bombardier C. Risk of serious gastrointestinal complications related to the use of nonsteroidal anti-inflammatory drugs: a meta analysis. Ann Intern Med 1991;115:787–96.
29. Gardner G, Furst DE. Disease-modifying antirheumatic drugs. Potential effects in older patients. Drugs Aging 1995;7:420–37.
30. Gibson GR, Whitacre EB, Ricotti CA. Colitis induced by nonsteroidal anti-inflammatory drugs. Report of four cases and review of the literature. Arch Intern Med 1992;152:625–32.
31. Gizzi G, Villani V, Brandi G, Paganelli GM, DiFebo G, Biasco G. Ano-rectal lesions in patients taking suppositories containing non-steroidal anti-inflammatory drugs (NSAID). Endoscopy 1990;22:146–8.
32. Going JJ, Canvin J, Sturrock R. Possible precursor of diaphragm disease in the small intestine. Lancet 1993;341:638–9.
33. Haber MM, Lopez I. Gastric histologic findings in patients with nonsteroidal anti-inflammatory drug-associated gastric ulcer. Mod Pathol 1999;12:592–8.
34. Hawkey CJ. Non-steroidal anti-inflammatory drug gastropathy: causes and treatment. Scand J Gastroenterol 1996;220:124–7.
35. Hawkey CJ, Naesdal J, Wilson I, et al. Relative contribution of mucosal injury and *Helicobacter pylori* in the development of gastroduodenal lesions in patients taking non-steroidal anti-inflammatory drugs. Gut 2002;51:336–43.
36. Hayllar J, Smith T, Macpherson A, Price AB, Gumpel M, Bjarnason I. Nonsteroidal antiinflammatory drug-induced small intestinal inflammation and blood loss. Effects of sulfasalazine and other disease-modifying antirheumatic drugs. Arthritis Rheum 1994;37:1146–50.
37. Keenan GF, Giannini EH, Athreya BH. Clinically significant gastropathy associated with nonsteroidal antiinflammatory drug use in children with juvenile rheumatoid arthritis. J Rheumatol 1995;22:1149–51.
38. Konturek SJ, Konturek JW. Gastric adaptation: basic and clinical aspects. Digestion 1994;55: 131–8.
39. Laine L. Nonsteroidal anti-inflammatory drug gastropathy. Gastrointest Endosc Clin N Am 1996;6:489–504.
40. Lanas A, Serrano P, Bajador E, Esteva F, Benito R, Sainz R. Evidence of aspirin use in both upper and lower gastrointestinal perforation. Gastroenterology 1997;112:683–9.
41. Lang J, Price AB, Levi AJ, Burke M, Gumpel JM, Bjarnason I. Diaphragm disease: pathology of disease of the small intestine induced by nonsteroidal anti-inflammatory drugs. J Clin Pathol 1988;41:516–26.

42. Langman MJ. Epidemiologic evidence on the association between peptic ulceration and antiinflammatory drug use. Gastroenterology 1989;96:640–6.
43. Lee FD. Importance of apoptosis in the histopathology of drug-related lesions in the large intestine. J Clin Pathol 1993;46:118–22.
44. Lee M, Feldman M. Age-related reductions in gastric mucosal prostaglandin levels increase susceptibility to aspirin-induced injury in rats. Gastroenterology 1994;107:1746–50.
45. Malagelada JR, Rodriguez de la Serna A, Dammann HG, et al. Sucralfate therapy in NSAID bleeding gastropathy. Clin Gastroenterol Hepatol 2003;1:51–6.
46. Mason JC. NSAIDs and the oesophagus. Eur J Gastroenterol Hepatol 1999;11:369–73.
47. Mitchell JA, Akarasereenont P, Thiemermann C, Flower RJ, Vane JR. Selectivity of nonsteroidal antiinflammatory drugs as inhibitors of constitutive and inducible cyclooxygenase. Proc Natl Acad Sci USA 1993;90:11693–7.
48. Park RH, Mills PR, Russell RI, Lee FD, McArdle C. Acute mucosal ulceration of the entire small intestine. Postgrad Med J 1989;65:45–8.
49. Quinn CM, Bjarnason I, Price AB. Gastritis in patients on non-steroidal anti-inflammatory drugs. Histopathology 1993;4:341–8.
50. Robinson MH, Wheatley T, Leach IH. Nonsteroidal antiinflammatory drug-induced colonic stricture: an unusual cause of large bowel obstruction and perforation. Dig Dis Sci 1995; 40:315–9.
51. Semble EL, Wu WC, Castell DO. Nonsteroidal antiinflammatory drugs and esophageal injury. Semin Arthritis Rheum 1989;19:99–109.
52. Silverstein FE, Faich G, Goldstein JL, et al. Gastrointestinal toxicity with celecoxib vs. nonsteroidal anti-inflammatory drugs for osteoarthritis and rheumatoid arthritis: the CLASS study: a randomized controlled trial. Celecoxib Longterm Arthritis Safety Study. JAMA 2000;284: 1247–55.
53. Silverstein FE, Graham DY, Senior JR, et al. Misoprostol reduces serious gastrointestinal complications in patients with rheumatoid arthritis receiving nonsteroidal anti-inflammatory drugs. A randomized, double-blind, placebo-controlled trial. Ann Intern Med 1995;123:241–9.
54. Simon LS, Weaver AL, Graham DY, et al. Antiinflammatory and upper gastrointestinal effects of celecoxib in rheumatoid arthritis. JAMA 1999;282:1921–8.
55. Szabo S, Spill WF, Rainaford KD. Non-steroidal anti-inflammatory drug-induced gastropathy: mechanisms and management. Med Toxicol Adverse Drug Exp 1989;4:77–94.
56. Vane JR, Botting RM. Mechanism of action of nonsteroidal anti-inflammatory drugs. Am J Med 1998;104:2S–8S.
57. Wallace JL, Keenan CM, Granger DN. Gastric ulceration induced by nonsteroidal anti-inflammatory drugs is a neutrophil-dependent process. Am J Physiol 1990;259:G462.
58. Wilcox CM, Shalek KA, Cotsonis G. Striking prevalence of over-the-counter nonsteroidal antiinflammatory drug use in patients with upper gastrointestinal hemorrhage. Arch Intern Med 1994;154:42–6.
59. Wilkens RF. An overview of the long-term safety experience of nabumetone. Drugs 1990;40:34–7.
60. Zvaifler N. A review of the antiarthritic efficacy and safety of etodolac. Clin Rhematol 1989;8: 43–53.

Alcohol

61. Baraona E, Pirola RC, Lieber CS. Small intestinal damage and changes in cell population produced by ethanol ingestion in the rat. Gastroenterology 1974;66:226–34.
62. Dinda PK, Buell MG, Morris O, Beck IT. Studies on ethanol-induced subepithelial fluid accumulation and jejunal villus bleb formation. An in vitro video microscopic approach. Can J Physiol Pharmacol 1994;72:1186–92.
63. Dinoso VP, Ming S, McNiff J. Ultrastructural changes of the canine gastric mucosa after topical application of graded concentrations of ethanol. Am J Dig Dis 1976;21:626–32.
64. Draper LR, Gyure LA, Hall JG, Robertson D. Effect of alcohol on the integrity of the intestinal epithelium. Gut 1983;24:399–404.
65. Keshavarizan A, Polepalle C, Iber FL, Durkin M. Esophageal motor disorder in alcoholics: result of alcoholism or withdrawal? Alcohol Clin Exp Res 1990;14:561–7.
66. Kvietys PR, Twohig B, Danzell J, Specian RD. Ethanol-induced injury to the rat gastric mucosa. Role of neutrophils and xanthine oxidase-derived radicals. Gastroenterology 1990;98:909–20.
67. Laine L, Weinstein WM. Histology of alcoholic hemorrhagic "gastritis": a prospective evaluation. Gastroenterology 1988;94:1254–62.
68. Persson J. Alcohol and the small intestine. Scand J Gastroenterol 1991;26:3–15.
69. Simanowski UA, Suter P, Stickel F, et al. Esophageal epithelial hyperproliferation following long-term alcohol consumption in rats: effects of age and salivary gland function. J Natl Cancer Inst 1993;85:2030–3.

Chemotherapeutic Agents

70. Anilkumar TV, Sarraf CE, Hunt T, Alison MR. The nature of cytotoxic drug-induced cell death in murine intestinal crypts. Br J Cancer 1992;65: 522–8.
71. Becker SN, Sass MA, Petras RE, Hart WR. Bizarre atypia in gastric brushings associated with hepatic arterial infusion chemotherapy. Acta Cytol 1986;30:347–50.
72. Cunningham D, Morgan RJ, Mills PR, et al. Functional and structural changes of the human proximal small intestine after cytotoxic therapy. J Clin Pathol 1985;38:265–70.
73. Fata F, Ron IG, Kemeny N, O'Reilly E, Klimstra D, Kelsen DP. 5-Fluorouracil-induced small bowel toxicity in patients with colorectal carcinoma. Cancer 1999;86:1129–34.
74. Ferrero JM, Francois E, Frenay M, Namer M. Occurrence of a gastric phytobezoar after chemotherapy with vinorelbine. Presse Med 1993;22:638.
75. Floch MH, Hellman L. The effect of 5-fluorouracil in rectal mucosa. Gastroenterology 1965;48: 430–7.
76. Houghton JA, Houghton PJ, Wooten RS. Mechanism of induction of gastrointestinal toxicity in the mouse by 5-fluorouracil, 5-fluorouridine, and 5-fluoro-2'-deoxyuridine. Cancer Res 1979;39: 2406–13.
77. Kwee WS, Wils JA, Schlangen J, Nuyens CM, Arends JW. Gastric epithelial atypia complicating hepatic arterial infusion chemotherapy. Histopathology 1994;24:151–4.

77a. Lewis JH. Gastrointestinal injury due to medicinal agents. Am J Gastroenterol 1986;81:819–34.

78. Miller SS, Muggia AL, Spiro HM. Colonic histologic changes induced by 5-fluorouracil. Gastroenterology 1962;43:391–8.
79. Moore JV. Ablation of murine jejunal crypts by alkylating agents. Br J Cancer 1979;39:175–81.
80. Parnes HL, Fung E, Schiffer CA. Chemotherapy-induced lactose intolerance in adults. Cancer 1994;74:1629–33.
81. Petras RE, Hart WR, Bukowski RM. Gastric epithelial atypia associated with hepatic arterial infusion chemotherapy. Its distinction from early gastric carcinoma. Cancer 1985;56:745–50.
82. Rose PG, Piver MS. Intestinal perforation secondary to paclitaxel. Gynecol Oncol 1995;57:270–2.
83. Rubin P. Late effects of chemotherapy and radiation therapy. Radiation Oncol Biol Phys 1984;10:5–34.
84. Schuger L, Peretz T, Goldin E, Durst AL, Okon E. Duodenal epithelial atypia: a specific complication of hepatic arterial infusion chemotherapy. Cancer 1988;61:663–6.
85. Slavin RE, Dias MA, Sarai R. Cytosine arabinoside induced gastrointestinal toxic alterations in sequential chemotherapeutic protocols. A clinico-pathologic study of 33 patients. Cancer 1978;42:1747–59.
86. Trier JS. Morphologic alterations induced by methotrexate in the mucosa of the human proximal intestine. I. Serial observations by light microscopy. Gastroenterology 1962;42:295–305.
87. Trier JS. Morphologic alterations induced by methotrexate in the mucosa of the human proximal intestine. II. Electron microscopic observations. Gastroenterology 1962;43:407–24.
88. Weidner N, Smith JG, LaVanway JM. Peptic ulceration with marked epithelial atypia following hepatic aterial infusion chemotherapy. A lesion initially misinterpreted as carcinoma. Am J Surg Pathol 1983;7:261–8.
89. Wu K, Leighton JA. Paclitaxel and cell division. N Engl J Med 2001;344:815.

Antimicrobial Agents

90. Bill AH. Malrotations and failures of fixation of the intestinal tract. In: Holder TM, Ashcraft KW, eds. Pediatric surgery. Philadelphia: WB Saunders; 1980.
91. CDC. Hypertrophic pyloric stenosis in infants following pertussis prophylaxis with erythromycin—Knoxville, Tennessee, 1999. MMWR 1999;48:1117–20.
92. Kikendall JM, Friedman AC, Oyewole MA, Fleischer D, Johnson LF. Pill-induced esophageal injury. Case reports and review of the literature. Dig Dis Sci 1983;28:174–82.

92a. Lewis JH. Gastrointestinal injury due to medicinal agents. Am J Gastroenterol 1986;81:819–34.

93. Navarro H, Arruebo MP, Alcalde A, Sorribas V. Effect of erythromycin on D-galactose absorption and sucrase activity in rabbit jejunum. Can J Physiol Pharmacol 1993;71:191–4.

Immunosuppressive Agents

94. Aabakken L, Osnes M. Gastroduodenal lesions induced by naproxen: an endoscopic evaluation of regional differences and natural causes. Scand J Gastroenterol 1990;25:1215–22.
95. Akioka K, Okamoto M, Nakamura K, et al. Abdominal pain is a critical complication of mycophenolate mofetil in renal transplant recipients. Transplant Proc 2003;35:300–1.
96. Behrend M. Adverse gastrointestinal effects of mycophenolate mofetil: aetiology, incidence and management. Drug Safety 2001;24:645–63.
97. Bowen DL, Fauci AS. Adrenal corticosteroids. In: Gallin JI, Goldstein M, Sondermen R, eds. Inflammation: basic principles and clinical correlates. New York: Raven Press; 1988:877.

98. Conn HO, Blitzer BL. Nonassociation of adrenocorticosteroid therapy and peptic ulcer. N Engl J Med 1976;294:473–9.
99. Conn HO, Poynard T. Corticosteroids and peptic ulcer: meta-analysis of adverse events during steroid therapy. J Intern Med 1994;236:619–32.
100. Crane PW, Clark C, Sowter C, et al. Cyclosporine toxicity in the small intestine. Transplant Proc 1990;22:2432.
101. Delaney JP, Michel HM, Bonsack ME, Eisenberg MM, Dunn DH. Adrenal corticosteroids cause gastrin cell hyperplasia. Gastroenterology 1979;76:913–6.
102. Drake M. Gastric cytology. Normal and abnormal. In: Orell SR, ed. Monographs in clinical cytology, vol. 10. Gastroesophageal cytology. Basel, Switzerland: Karoger; 1985:120.
103. Fisher A, Schwartz M, Mor E, et al. Gastrointestinal toxicity associated with FK506 in liver transplant recipients. Transplant Proc 1994;26:3106–7.
104. Gabe SM, Bjarnason I, Tolou-Ghamari Z, et al. The effect of tacrolimus (FK506) on intestinal barrier function and cellular energy production in humans. Gastroenterology 1998;115:67–74.
105. Maes BD, Dalle I, Geboes K, et al. Erosive enterocolitis in mycophenolate mofetil-treated renal-transplant recipients with persistent afebrile diarrhea. Transplantation 2003;75:665–72.
106. Messer J, Reitman D, Sacks HS, Smith H Jr, Chalmers TC. Association of adrenocorticosteroid therapy and peptic-ulcer disease. N Engl J Med 1983;309:21–4.
107. O'Neil EA, Chwals WJ, O'Shea MD, Turner CS. Dexamethasone treatment during ventilatory dependency: possible life-threatening gastrointestinal complications. Arch Dis Child 1992;67:10–1.
108. Papadimitriou JC, Cangro CB, Lustberg A, et al. Histologic features of mycophenolate mofetil-related colitis: a graft-versus-host disease-like pattern. Int J Surg Pathol 2003;11:295–302.
109. Prillaman WW, Hurst DC, Gall GV, Bennett JC. Intestinal complications in rheumatoid arteritis and their relationship to corticosteroid therapy. J Chronic Dis 1974;27:475–81.
110. Remine SG, McIlrath DC. Bowel perforation in steroid-treated patients. Ann Surg 1990;192:581–6.
111. Selling JA, Hogan DL, Aly A, Koss MA, Isenberg HI. Indomethacin inhibits duodenal mucosal bicarbonate secretion and endogenous prostaglandin E_2 output in human subjects. Ann Int Med 1987;106:368–71.

Laxative Use

112. Badiali D, Marcheggiano A, Pallone F, et al. Melanosis of the rectum in patients with chronic constipation. Dis Colon Rectum 1985;28:241–5.
113. Benavides SH, Morgante PE, Monserrat AJ, Zarate J, Porta EA. The pigment of melanosis coli: a lectin histochemical study. Gastrointest Endosc 1997;46:131–8.
114. Bretagne JF, Vidon N, L'Hirondel C, Bernier JJ. Increased cell loss in the human jejunum induced by laxatives (ricinoleic acid, dioctyl sodium sulphosuccinate, magnesium sulphate, bile salts). Gut 1981;22:264–9.
115. Byers RJ, Marsh P, Parkinson D, Haboubi NY. Melanosis coli is associated with an increase in colonic epithelial apoptosis and not with laxative use. Histopathology 1997;30:160–4.
116. Bytzer P, Stokholm M, Andersen I, Klitgaard NA, Schaffalitzky de Muckadell OB. Prevalence of surreptitious laxative abuse in patients with diarrhoea of uncertain origin: a cost benefit analysis of a screening procedure. Gut 1989;30:1379–84.
117. Heilbrun N, Bernsteon C. Roentgen abnormalities of the large and small intestine associated with prolonged cathartic ingestion. Radiology 1955;65:549–56.
118. Heizer WD, Warshaw AL, Waldkman TA, Laster L. Protein-losing gastroenteropathy and malabsorption associated with factitious diarrhea. Ann Intern Med 1968;68:839–52.
119. Kacere R, Srivatsa S, Tremaine W, Ebnet LE, Batts KP. Chronic diarrhea due to surreptitious use of bisacodyl: case reports and methods for detection. Mayo Clin Proc 1993;68:355–7.
120. Killen J, Taylor B, Telch M, Saylor KE, Maron DJ, Robinson TN. Self-induced vomiting and laxative and diuretic use among teenagers. Precursors of the binge-purge syndrome? JAMA 1986;255:1447–9.
121. Pardi DS, Tremaine WJ, Rothenberg HJ, Batts KP. Melanosis coli in inflammatory bowel disease. J Clin Gastroenterol 1998;26:167–70.
122. Smith B. Effect of irritant purgatives on the myenteric plexus in man and the mouse. Gut 1968;9:139–43.
123. Smith B. Pathologic changes in the colon produced by anthraquinone purgatives. Dis Colon Rectum 1973;16:455–8.
124. Smith B. Pathology of cathartic colon. Proc R Soc Med 1972;65:288.
125. Walker NI, Bennett RE, Axelsen RA. Melanosis coli: a consequence of anthraquinone-induced apoptosis of colonic epithelial cells. Am J Pathol 1988;131:465–76.

Enemas

126. Driman DK, Preiksaitis HG. Colorectal inflammation and increased cell proliferation associated with oral sodium phosphate bowel preparation solution. Hum Pathol 1998;29:972–8.
127. Hardin RD, Tedesco FJ. Colitis after Hibiclens enema. J Clin Gastroenterol 1986;8:572–5.
128. Herreiras JM, Muniain MA, Sanchez S, Garrido M. Alcohol-induced colitis. Endoscopy 1983; 15:121–2.
129. Jonas G. Mahoney A, Murray J, Gertler S. Chemical colitis due to endoscopic cleansing solutions: a mimic of pseudomembranous colitis. Gastroenterology 1988;95:1403–8.
130. Leriche M, Devroede G, Sanchez G, Rossano J. Changes in the rectal mucosa induced by hypertonic enema. Dis Colon Rectum 1978;21: 227–36.
131. Meisel JL, Bergman D, Graney D, Saunders DR, Rubin CE. Human rectal mucosa: proctoscopic and morphological changes caused by laxatives. Gastroenterology 1977;72:1274–9.
132. Meyer CT, Brand M, DeLuca VA, Spiro HM. Hydrogen peroxide colitis: a report of three patients. J Clin Gastroenterol 1981;3:31–5.
133. Snover DC, Bond J. Mucosal plaques seen at colonoscopy: chemical colitis or mucosal pseudolipomatosis? Gastroenterology 1989;96: 1626–7.
134. Snover DC, Sandstad J, Hutton S. Mucosal pseudolipomatosis of the colon. Am J Clin Pathol 1985;84:575–80.
135. Zwas FR, Cirillo NW, el-Serag HB, Eisen RN. Colonic mucosal abnormalities associated with oral sodium phosphate solution. Gastrointest Endosc 1996;43:463–6.

Kayexalate Enemas

136. Abraham SC, Bhagavan BS, Lee LA, Rashid A, Wu TT. Upper gastrointestinal tract injury in patients receiving kayexalate (sodium polystyrene sulfonate) in sorbitol: clinical, endoscopic, and histopathologic findings. Am J Surg Pathol 2001;25:637–44.
137. Fogt F, Vortmeyer AO, Senderowicz AM. Sodium polystyrene sulfonate damage. Am J Surg Pathol 1998:22;379–81.
138. Gardiner GW. Kayexalate (sodium polystyrene sulphonate) in sorbitol associated with intestinal necrosis in uremic patients. Can J Gastroenterol 1997;11:573–7.
139. Rashid A, Hamilton SR. Necrosis of the gastrointestinal tract in uremic patients as a result of sodium polystyrene sulfonate (Kayexalate) in sorbitol: an underrecognized condition. Am J Surg Pathol 1997;21:60–9.
140. Roy-Chaudhury P, Meisels IS, Freedman S, Steinman TI, Steer M. Combined gastric and ileocecal toxicity (serpiginous ulcers) after oral kayexalate in sorbitol therapy. Am J Kidney Dis 1997;30:120–2.

Radiographic Substances

141. Gelfand DW, Sowers JC, DePonte KA, Sumner TE, Ott DJ. Anaphylactic and allergic reactions during double-contrast studies: is glucagon or barium suspension the allergen? Am J Roentgenol 1985;144:405–6.
142. Janower ML. Hypersensitivity reactions after barium studies of the upper and lower gastrointestinal tract. Radiology 1986;161:139–40.
143. Lutzger LG, Factor SM. Effects of some water-soluble contrast media on the colonic mucosa. Diagn Radiol 1976;118:545–8.
144. Stringer DA, Hassall E, Ferguson AC, Cairns R, Nadel H, Sargent M. Hypersensitivity reaction to single contrast barium studies in children. Pediatr Radiol 1993;23:587–8.

Corrosive or Caustic Injury

145. Appleqvist P, Salmo M. Lye corrosion carcinoma of the esophagus: a review of 63 cases. Cancer 1980;45:2655–8.
146. Aronow SP, Aronow HD, Blanchard T, Czinn S, Chelimsky G. Hair relaxers: a benign caustic ingestion? J Pediatr Gastroenterol Nutr 2003;36:120–5.
147. Ashcraft KW, Padula R. The effect of dilute corrosives on the esophagus. Pediatrics 1974;53: 226–32.
148. Berthet B, di Costanzo J, Arnaud C, Choux R, Assadourian R. Influence of epidermal growth factor and interferon gamma on healing of oesophageal corrosive burns in the rat. Br J Surg 1994;81:395–8.
149. Butler C, Madden JW, Davis WM. Morphologic aspects of experimental lye strictures. I. Pathogenesis and pathophysiologic correlations. J Surg Res 1974;17:232–44.
150. Citron BP, Pincus IJ, Geokas MC, Haverback BJ. Chemical trauma of esophagus and stomach. Surg Clin North Am 1968;48:1303–11.
151. Clearfield HR, Shin YH, Schreibman BK. Emphysematous gastritis secondary to lye ingestion. Am J Dig Dis 1969;14:195–9.
152. Havanond C. Clinical features of corrosive ingestion. J Med Assoc Thai 2003;86:918–24.
153. Kikendall JW. Caustic ingestion injuries. Gastroenterol Clin North Am 1991;20:847–57.
154. Kochhar R, Mehta SK, Nagi B, Goenka MK. Corrosive acid-induced esophageal intramural pseudodiverticulosis. A study of 14 patients. J Clin Gastroenterol 1991;13:371–5.

155. Leape LL, Ashcraft KW, Scarpelli DG, Holden TM. Hazard to health—liquid lye. N Engl J Med 1971;284:578–81.
156. Millar AJ, Numanoglu A, Mann M, Marven S, Rode H. Detection of caustic oesophageal injury with technetium 99m-labelled sucralfate. J Pediatr Surg 2001;36:262–5.
157. Nagi B, Kochhar R, Thapa BR, Singh K. Radiological spectrum of late sequelae of corrosive injury to upper gastrointestinal tract. A pictorial review. Acta Radiol 2004;45:7–12.
158. Nunes AC, Romaozinho JM, Pontes JM, et al. Risk factors for stricture development after caustic ingestion. Hepatogastroenterology 2002;49:1563–6.
159. Ramasamy K, Gumaste VV. Corrosive ingestion in adults. J Clin Gastroenterol 2003;37:119–24.
160. Song HY, Han YM, Kim HN, Kim CS, Choi KC. Corrosive esophageal stricture: safety and effectiveness of balloon dilation. Radiology 1992;184:373–8.
161. Stevens AE, Dove GA. Esophageal cast: esophagitis dessicans superficialis. Lancet 1960;ii: 1279–81.
162. Tewfik TL, Schloss MD. Ingestion of lye and other corrosive agents—a study of 86 infants and child cases. J Otolaryngol 1980;9:72–7.
163. Zargar SA, Kochhar R, Nagi B, Mehta S, Mehta SK. Ingestion of corrosive acids. Spectrum of injury to upper gastro-intestinal tract and natural history. Gastroenterology 1989;97:702–7.

Prostaglandins

164. Mercado-Dean MG, Burton EM, Brawley AV, Hatley R. Prostaglandin-induced foveolar hyperplasia simulating pyloric stenosis in an infant with cyanotic heart disease. Pediatr Radiol 1994;24:45–6.
165. Peled N, Dagan O, Babyn P, et al. Gastric-outlet obstruction induced by prostaglandin therapy in neonates. N Eng J Med 1992;327: 505–10.

Bisphosphonates

166. Abraham SC, Cruz-Correa M, Lee LA, Yardley JH, Wu TT. Alendronate-associated esophageal injury: pathologic and endoscopic features. Mod Pathol 1999;12:1152–7.
167. Aki S, Eskiyurt N, Akarirmak U, et al. Gastrointestinal side effect profile due to the use of alendronate in the treatment of osteoporosis. Yonsei Med J 2003;44:961–7.
168. Bauer DC, Black D, Ensrud K, et al. Upper gastrointestinal tract safety profile of alendronate. Arch Intern Med 2000;160:517–25.
169. de Groen PC, Lubbe DF, Hirsch LJ, et al. Esophagitis associated with the use of alendronate. N Engl J Med 1996;335:1016–21.
170. Graham DY, Malaty HM. Alendronate gastric ulcers. Aliment Pharmacol Ther 1999;13:515–9.
171. Lanza FL, Evans DG, Graham DY. Effect of *Helicobacter pylori* infection on the severity of gastroduodenal mucosal injury after the acute administration of naproxen or aspirin to normal volunteers. Am J Gastroenterol 1991;86: 735–7.
172. Lanza FL, Graham DY, Davis RE, Rack MF. Endoscopic comparison of cimetidine and sucralfate for prevention of naproxen-induced acute gastroduodenal injury. Effect of scoring method. Dig Dis Sci 1990;35:1494–9.
174. Liberman UA, Weiss SR, Broll J, et al. Effect of oral alendronate on bone mineral density and the incidence of fractures in postmenopausal osteoporosis. The Alendronate Phase III Osteoporosis Treatment Study Group. N Engl J Med 1995;333:1437–43.
173. Liberman UI, Hirsch LJ. Esophagitis and alendronate. N Engl J Med 1996;335:1069–70.
175. Lilley LL, Guanci R. Avoiding alendronate-related esophageal irritation. Am J Nursing 1997;97:12–4.
176. Rodan GA, Fleisch HA. Bisphosphonates: mechanisms of action. J Clin Invest 1996;97: 2692–6.

Heavy Metal Injury

177. Abraham SC, Yardley JH, Wu TT. Erosive injury to the upper gastrointestinal tract in patients receiving iron medication. Am J Surg Pathol 1999;23:1241–7.
178. Chen CJ, Lin LJ. Human carcinogenicity and atherogenicity induced by chronic exposure to inorganic arsenic. In: Nriagu JO, ed. Advances in environmental science and technology, vol. 27. Arsenic in the environment. Part II: Human health and ecosystem effects. New York: John Wiley & Sons; 1994:109–31.
179. Eaves R, Hansky J, Wallis P. Gold-induced enterocolitis: case report and a review of the literature. Aust N Z J Med 1982;12:617–20.
180. Evron E, Brautbar C, Becker S, et al. Correlation between gold-induced enterocolitis and the presence of HLA-DRB1*0404 allele. Arthritis Rheum 1995;38:755–9.
181. Fam AG, Paton TW, Shamess CJ, Lewis AJ. Fulminant colitis complicating gold therapy. J Rheumatol 1980;7:479–85.
182. Huston GJ. Gold colitis, therapy and confirmation of mucosal recovery by measurement of rectal potential difference. Postgrad Med J 1980;56:875–6.

183. Kaplinsky N, Pras M, Frankle O. Severe enterocolitis complicating chrysotherapy. Ann Rheum Dis 1973;32:574–7.
184. Kim SK, Gerle RD, Rozanski R. Cathartic colitis. Am J Roentgenol Radium Ther Nucl Med 1978;131:1079–81.
185. Laine L, Bentley E, Chandrasoma P. The effects of oral iron therapy on the upper gastrointestinal tract. A prospective evaluation. Dig Dis Sci 1988;33:172–7.
186. Langer HE, Hartmann G, Heinemann G, Richter K. Gold colitis induced by auranofin treatment of rheumatoid arthritis: case report and review of the literature. Ann Rheum Dis 1987; 46:787–92.
187. Martin DM, Goldman JA, Gillian J, Nasrallah SM. Gold-induced eosinophilic enterocolitis. Response to oral cromolyn sodium. Gastroenterology 1981;80:1567–70.
188. Mason SJ, O'Meara TF. Drug-induced esophagitis. J Clin Gastroenterol 1981;3:115–20.
189. Mesonero JE, Rodriguez Yoldi MC, Rodriguez Yoldi MJ. Effect of cadmium on enzymatic digestion and sugar transport in the small intestine of rabbit. Biol Trace Elem Res 1993;38:217–26.
190. Pizarro F, Olivares M, Araya M, Gidi V, Uauy R. Gastrointestinal effects associated with soluble and insoluble copper in drinking water. Environ Health Perspect 2001;109:949–52.
191. Reinhart WH, Kappeler M, Halter F. Severe pseudomembranous and ulcerative colitis during gold therapy. Endoscopy 1983;15:70–2.
192. Schofl C, Sanchez-Bueno A, Dixon CJ, et al. Aluminium perturbs oscillatory phosphoinositide-mediated calcium signaling in hormone-stimulated hepatocytes. Biochem J 1990;269: 547–50.
193. Tomczok J, Grzybek H, Sliwa W, Panz B. Ultrastructural aspects of the small intestinal lead toxicology. Exp Pathol 1988;35:49–55.
194. Wands JR, Weiss SW, Yardley JH, Maddrey WC. Chronic inorganic mercury poisoning due to laxative abuse. Am J Med 1974;57:92–101.
195. Wong V, Wyatt J, Lewis F, Howdle P. Gold induced enterocolitis complicated by cytomegalovirus infection: a previously unrecognised association. Gut 1993;34:1002–5.

Colchicine

196. Stemmermann GN, Hayashi T. Colchicine intoxication. A reappraisal of its pathology based on a study of three fatal cases. Hum Pathol 1971;2:321–32.
197. Venho VM, Koivuniemi A. Effect of colchicine on drug absorption from the rat small intestine in situ and in vitro. Acta Pharmacol Toxicol 1978;43:251–9.

Pancreatic Enzyme Supplements

198. Fitzsimmons SC, Burkhart GA, Borowitz D, et al. High-dose pancreatic-enzyme supplements and fibrosing colonopathy in children with cystic fibrosis. N Engl J Med 1997;336:1283–9.
199. Freiman J, Fitzsimmons SC. Colonic strictures in patients with cystic fibrosis: results of a survey of 114 cystic fibrosis care centres in the US. J Pediatr Gastroenterol Nutr 1996;22:153–6.
200. Knabe N, Zak M, Hansen, et al. Extensive pathological changes of the colon in cystic fibrosis and high-strength pancreatic enzymes. Lancet 1994;343:1230.
201. Lee J, Ip W, Durie P. Is fibrosing colonopathy an immune mediated disease? Arch Dis Child 1997;77:66–77.
202. Pawel BR, de Chadarevian JP, Franco ME. The pathology of fibrosing colonopathy of cystic fibrosis: a study of 12 cases and review of the literature. Hum Pathol 1997;28:395–9.
203. Pettei MJ, Leonidas JC, Levine JJ, Gorvoy JD. Pancolonic disease in cystic fibrosis and high-dose pancreatic enzyme therapy. J Pediatr 1994; 125:587–9.
204. Powell CJ. Colonic toxicity from pancreatins: a contemporary safety issue. Lancet 1999;353: 911–5.
205. Schwartzenberg SJ, Wielinski CL, Shamieh I, et al. Cystic fibrosis-associated colitis and fibrosing colonopathy. J Pediatr 1995;127:565–70.
206. Smyth RL, Ashby D, O'Hea U, et al. Fibrosing colonopathy in cystic fibrosis: results of a case-control study. Lancet 1995;346:1247–51.
207. Smyth RL, van Velzen D, Smyth AR, Lloyd DA, Heaf DP. Strictures of ascending colon in cystic fibrosis and high-strength pancreatic enzymes. Lancet 1994;343:85–6.
208. Van Velzen D, Ball LM, Dezfulian AR, Southgate A, Howard CV. Comparative and experimental pathology of fibrosing colonopathy. Postgrad Med J 1996;72:S39–48.

Estrogen and Progesterone

209. Brennan MF, Clarke AM, MacBeth WA. Infarction of the midgut associated with oral contraceptives: report of two cases. N Engl J Med 1969;279:1213–4.
210. Cotton PB, Thomas ML. Ischemic colitis and the contraceptive pill. Br Med J 1971;3:27–8.
211. Gelfand MD. Ischemic colitis associated with a depot synthetic progesterone. Dig Dis Sci 1972;17:275–7.
212. Hoyle M, Kennedy A, Prior AL, Thomas GE. Small bowel ischemia and infarction in young women taking oral contraceptives and progestational agents. Br J Surg 1977;64:533–7.

213. Tedesco FJ, Volpicelli NA, Moore FS. Estrogen- and progesteron-associated colitis: a disorder with clinical and endoscopic features mimicking Crohn's colitis. Gastrointest Endosc 1982; 28:247–9.
214. Watson WC, Murray D. Lactase deficiency and jejunal atrophy associated with administration of Conovid. Lancet 1966;1:65.

Cocaine

215. Abramson DL, Gertler JP, Lewis T, Kral JG. Crack-related perforated gastropyloric ulcer. J Clin Gastroenterol 1991;13:17–9.
216. Cregler LL, Mark H. Medical complications of cocaine abuse. N Engl J Med 1986;315:1495–500.
217. Downing G, Horner S, Kilbride H. Characteristics of perinatal cocaine-exposed infants with necrotizing enterocolitis. Am J Dis Child 1991; 145:26–7.
218. Endress C, Gray DG, Wollschlaeger G. Bowel ischemia and perforation after cocaine use. Am J Roentgenol 1992;159:73–5.
219. Escobedo LG, Ruttenber J, Agocs MM, Anda RF, Wetli CV. Emerging patterns of cocaine use and the epidemic of cocaine overdose deaths in Dade County, Florida. Arch Pathol Lab Med 1991;115:900–5.
220. Greenberg R, Greenberg Y, Kaplan O. 'Body packer' syndrome: characteristics and treatment—case report and review. Eur J Surg 2000;166:89–91.
221. Hall TR, Zaninovic A, Lewin D, et al. Neonatal intestinal ischemia with bowel perforation: an in utero complication of maternal cocaine abuse. Am J Roentgenol 1992;158:1303–4.
222. Hoyme HE, Jones KL, Dixon SD, et al. Prenatal cocaine exposure and fetal vascular disruption. Pediatrics 1990;85:743–7.
223. Lee HS, LaMaute HR, Pizzi WF, Picard DL, Luks FI. Acute gastroduodenal perforations associated with use of crack. Ann Surg 1990;211:15–7.
224. Lipshultz SE, Frassica JJ, Orav EJ. Cardiovascular abnormalities in infants prenatally exposed to cocaine. J Pediatr 1991;118:44–51.
225. McCarron M, Wood MA. The cocaine "body packer" syndrome. Diagnosis and treatment. JAMA 1983;250:1417–20.
226. Meatherall RC, Warren RJ. High urinary cannabinoids from hashish body packer. J Anal Toxicol 1993;17:439–40.
227. Nihira M, Hayashida M, Ohno Y, Inuzuka H, Yamamoto Y. Urinalysis of body packers in Japan. J Anal Toxicol 1988;22:61–5.
228. Rosenak D, Diamant YZ, Yaffe H, et al. Cocaine: maternal use during pregnancy and its effect on the mother, the fetus and the infant. Obstet Gynecol Surg 1990;45:348–59.

Other Drugs and Chemicals Causing Ischemic Injury

229. Baker DR, Schrader WH, Hitchcock CR. Small bowel ulceration apparently associated with thiazide potassium therapy. JAMA 1964;90: 586–90.
230. Barloon T, Moore SA, Mitros FA. A case of stenotic obstruction of the jejunum secondary to slow-release potassium. Am J Gastroenterol 1986;81:192–4.
231. Dahlberg PJ, Kisken WA, Newcomer RL, Yutue WR. Mesenteric ischemia in chronic dialysis patients. Am J Nephrol 1985;5:327–32.
232. Leijonmarck CE, Raf L. Gastrointestinal lesions and potassium chloride supplements. Lancet 1985;1:57–8.
233. Tu AT. The mechanism of snake venom actions: Rattlesnakes and other crotalids. In: Simpson LL, ed. Neuropoisons: their pathophysiological actions. New York: Plenum Press; 1971:87.
234. Wallace JF. Disorders caused by venoms, bites and stings. In: Petersdorf RG, Adams RD, Braunwald E, et al, eds. Harrison's principles of internal medicine, 10th ed. New York: McGraw-Hill; 1983:1241.
235. Wayte DM, Helwig EB. Small bowel ulceration—iatrogenic or multifactorial origin. Am J Clin Pathol 1968;49:26–40.
236. Weiss SM, Rutenberg HL, Paskin DL, Zeren HA. Gut lesions due to slow-release KCl tablets. N Engl J Med 1977;296:111–2.

Anticoagulant-Induced Injury

237. Herbert DC. Anticoagulant therapy and the acute abdomen. Br J Surg 1968;55:353–7.
238. Jick H, Porter J. Drug-induced gastrointestinal bleeding. Report from The Boston Collaborative Drug Surveillance Program, Boston, University Medical Center. Lancet 1978;2:87–9.
239. Johnsen SP, Sorensen HT, Mellemkjoer L, et al. Hospitalisation for upper gastro-intestinal bleeding associated with use of oral anticoagulants. Thromb Haemost 2001;86:563–8.

Chemical-Induced Eosinophilia

240. Clauw DJ, Nashel DJ, Umhau A, Katz P. Tryptophan-associated eosinophilic connective-tissue disease. A new clinical entity? JAMA 1990;263:1502–6.
241. De Schryver-Kecskemeti K, Bennert KW, Cooper GS, Yang P. Gastrointestinal involvement in L-tryptophan (L-Trp) associated with eosinophilia-myalgia syndrome (EMS). Dig Dis Sci 1992;37:697–701.

242. Gresh JP, Vasey FB, Espinoza LR, Adelman HM, Germain BF. Eosinophilia-myalgia syndrome in association with L-tryptophan ingestion. J Rheumatol 1990;17:1557–8.
243. Landres RT, Kuster GC, Strum WB. Eosinophilic esophagitis in a patient with vigorous achalasia. Gastroenterology 1978;74:1298–1301.
244. Varga J, Heinman-Patterson TD, Emmery DL. Clinical spectrum of the systemic manifestations of the eosinophilia-myalgia syndrome. Semin Arthritis Rheum 1990;19:313–28.

Changes Associated with Uremia and Chronic Renal Disease

245. Adrogue HI, Frazier MR, Zeluff B, Suki WN. Systemic calciphylaxis revisited. Am J Nephrol 1981;1:177–83.
246. Boyle JM, Johnston B. Acute upper gastrointestinal haemorrhage in patients with chronic renal disease. Am J Med 1983;75:409–12.
247. Brown DF, Denney CF, Burnes DK. Systemic calciphylaxis associated with massive gastrointestinal hemorrhage. Arch Pathol Lab Med 1998;122:656–9.
248. Cunningham JT. Gastric telangiectasias in chronic hemodialysis patients: a report of six cases. Gastroenterology 1981;81:1131–3.
249. Franzin G, Musola R, Mencarelli R. Changes in the mucosa of the stomach and duodenum during immunosuppressive therapy after renal transplantation. Histopathology 1982;6:439–49.
250. Franzin G, Musola R, Mencarelli R. Morphological changes of the gastroduodenal mucosa in regular dialysis uraemic patients. Histopathology 1982;6:429–37.
251. Goldstein H. Murphy D, Sokol A, Rubina ME. Gastric acid secretion in patients undergoing chronic dialysis. Arch Intern Med 1967;120: 645–53.
252. Ikegaya N, Kobayashi S, Hishida A, Kaneko E, Furuhashi M, Maruyama Y. Colonic dilatation due to dialysis-related amyloidosis. Am J Kidney Dis 1995;25:807–9.
253. Kao CH, Hsu YH, Wang SJ. Delayed gastric emptying in patients with chronic renal failure. Nucl Med Commun 1996;17:164–7.
254. Khaffif RA, DeLima C, Silverberg A, Frankel R. Calciphylaxis and systemic calcinosis: collective review. Arch Intern Med 1990;150:956–9.
255. Massry SG, Gordon A, Coburn JW, et al. Vascular calcification and peripheral necrosis in a renal transplant recipient. Am J Med 1970;49:416–22.
256. Mehta RL, Scott G, Sloand JA, Francis CW. Skin necrosis associated with acquired protein C deficiency in patients with renal failure and calciphylaxis. Am J Med 1990;88:252–7.
257. Musola R, Franzin G, Mora R, Manfrini C. Prevalence of gastroduodenal lesions in uremic patients undergoing dialysis and after renal transplantation. Gastrointest Endosc 1984;30:343–6.
258. Quintero E, Guth PH. Renal failure, increased gastric mucosal blood flow and acid secretion in rats: role of endothelium-derived nitric oxide. Am J Physiol 1992;263:G75–G80.
259. Scheff RT, Zuckerman G, Harter H, Delmez J, Koehler R. Diverticular disease in patients with chronic renal failure due to polycystic kidney disease. Ann Intern Med 1980;92:202–4.
260. Tani N, Harasawa S, Suzuki S, et al. Lesions of the upper gastrointestinal tract in patients with chronic renal failure. Gastroenterol Jpn 1980;15:480–4.

Diarrhetic Shellfish Poisoning

261. Edebo L, Lange S, Li XP, Allenmark S. Toxic mussels and okadaic acid induce rapid hypersecretion in the rat small intestine. APMIS 1988;96:1029–35.
262. Edebo L, Lange S, Li P, et al. Seasonal, geographic and individual variation of okadaic acid content in cultivated mussels in Sweden. APMIS 1988;96:1036–42.
263. Gago-Martinez A, Rodriguez-Vazquez JA, Thibault P, Quilliam MA. Simultaneous occurrence of diarrheic and paralytic shellfish poisoning toxin in Spanish mussels in 1993. Natural Toxins 1996;4:72–9.
264. Morrow J, Margolies G, Rowland B, Roberts L. Evidence that histamine is the causative toxin of scombroid-fish poisoning. N Engl J Med 1991;324:716–20.
265. Yasumoto T, Oshima Y, Sugawara W, et al. Identification of *Dinophysis fortii* as the causative organism of diarrhetic shellfish poisoning. Bull Jpn Soc Sci Fish 1980;46:1405–12.

Drug-Induced Neuromuscular Disorders

266. Faulk DL, Anuras S, Christensen J. Chronic intestinal pseudoobstruction. Gastroenterology 1978;74:922–31.

Clofazimine-Induced Crystal-Storing Histiocytes

267. Atkinson AJ Jr, Sheagren JN, Rubio JB, Knight V. Evaluation of B-663 in human leprosy. Int J Lepr 1967;35:119–27.
268. DeMicco C, Routboul R, DeVaux J, et al. Enteropathie a la clofazimine. Une observation avec etude ultrastructurale. Ann Pathol 1982; 2:149–53.
269. Sukpanichnant S, Hargrove NS, Kachintorn U, et al. Clofazimine-induced crystal-storing histiocytes producing chronic abdominal pain in a leprosy patient. Am J Surg Pathol 2000; 24:129–35.

Drug-Related Esophagitis

270. Bonavina L, DeMeester TR, McChesney L, Schwizer W, Albertucci M, Bailey RT. Drug-induced esophageal strictures. Ann Surg 1987;206:173–83.
271. Brewer AR, Smyrk TC, Bailey RT Jr, Bonavina L, Eypasch EP, Demeester TR. Drug-induced esophageal injury, histopathological study in rabbit model. Dig Dis Sci 1990;35:1205–10.
272. Brown DC, Doughty JC, George WD. Surgical treatment of oesophageal obstruction after ingestion of a granular laxative. Postgrad Med J 1999;75:106.
273. Collins FJ, Mathews HR, Baker SE, Strakova JM. Drug-induced oesophageal injury. Br Med J 1979;1:1673–6.
274. Elias PH, Fritsch PO. Erythema multiforme. In: Pitzpatrick TB, Eisen AZ, Wolff K, Freedberg JM, Austen KF, eds. Dermatology in general medicine, 2nd ed. New York: McGraw Hill; 1979:295–303.
275. Kikendall JW. Pill-induced esophageal injury. Gastroenterol Clin North Am 1991;20:835–46.
276. Olovson SG, Havo N, Regardh CG, et al. Oesophageal ulcerations and plasma levels of different alprenolol salts: potential implications for the clinic. Acta Pharmacol Toxicol 1986;58: 55–60.
277. Ovartlarnporn B, Kulwichit W, Hiranniramol S. Medication-induced esophageal injury: report of 17 cases with endoscopic documentation. Am J Gastroenterol 1991;86:748–50.
278. Schreiber JB, Covington JA. Aspirin-induced esophageal hemorrhage. JAMA 1988;259:1647–8.
279. Seidner DL, Roberts IM, Smith MS. Esophageal obstruction after ingestion of a fiber-containing diet pill. Gastroenterology 1990;99:1820–2.
280. Stein MR, Thompson CK, Sawicki JE, Martel AJ. Esophageal stricture complicating Stevens-Johnson syndrome. Am J Gastroenterol 1974; 62:435–9.
281. Stoschus B, Allescher HD. Drug-induced dysphagia. Dysphagia 1993;8:154–9.

Chemical-Induced Gastric Injury

282. Carne-Ross IP. Pyloric stenosis and sustained-release iron tablets. Br Med J 1976;2:642–3.
283. Filpi RG, Majd M, LoPresto JM. Reversible gastric stricture following iron ingestion. South Med J 1973;66:845–6.
284. Laine L, Weinstein WM. Subepithelial hemorrhages and erosions of human stomach. Dig Dis Sci 1988;33:490–503.
284a. Lewis JH. Gastrointestinal injury due to medicinal agents. Am J Gastroenterol 1986;81:819–34.

Chemical-Induced Intestinal Injury

285. Birnbaum BA, Gordon RB, Jacobs JE. Glutaraldehyde colitis: radiologic findings. Radiology 1995;195:131–4.
286. Kojima Y, Sanada Y, Fonkalsrud EW. Evaluation of techniques for chemical debridement of colonic mucosa. Surg Gynecol Obstet 1982; 155:849–54.
287. Mall J, Pollmann C, Myers JA. Rectale formalininstillation-eine praktikable und sichere Therapie der hamorrhagischen Proktitis. Chirug 1999;70:700–4.
288. Myers JA, Hollinger EF, Mall JW, Jakate SM, Doolas A, Saclarides TJ. Mechanical, histologic, and biochemical effects of canine rectal formalin instillation. Dis Colon Rectum 1998;41:153–8.
289. Saclarides TJ, King DG, Franklin JL, Doolas A. Formalin instillation for refractory radiation-induced hemorrhagic proctitis. Dis Colon Rectum 1996;39:196–9.

9 PHYSICAL INJURY

RADIATION-INDUCED INJURY

Definition. *Gastrointestinal radiation injury* is the damage that develops anywhere in the gastrointestinal tract either as a result of acute radiation toxicity or as a long-term consequence of the vascular disease that develops in response to radiation injury. Ionizing radiation may be characterized by the way that the energy is emitted, propagated, and absorbed. Radiant energy absorbed from a source outside the body is known as external radiation. Correspondingly, energy from a source located inside the body, such as a radionuclide, is termed internal radiation, and the source is referred to as an internal emitter. By convention, radiation pathology is divided into early and delayed effects. Early effects are those that occur within the initial 60 days postexposure; delayed effects are those occurring thereafter. Types of gastrointestinal radiation injury include *radiation esophagitis, radiation gastritis, radiation enteritis, radiation colitis, radiation proctitis*, and *radiation enteropathy*.

Demography. Two seminal events in the 19th century changed our thinking with respect to radiation injury. The first was the discovery of X rays and the other was the demonstration of naturally occurring radioactive materials in the earth's crust. Add to this knowledge of the long-term effects of nuclear warfare and nuclear accidents in the following century, and we have an increased understanding of the long-term effects of this form of physical injury.

Energy that results in human irradiation is predominantly derived from two sources: natural or background radiation and technologically induced or enhanced radiation. The relative degree to which these two sources contribute to an individual's annual exposure depends primarily on where the person lives, the individual's occupation, and the degree of technological development in the local environment. Most patients who develop radiation injury have received the radiation as a consequence of cancer therapy or through imaging studies. Radiation is also used as a conditioning agent for bone marrow transplants. Individuals are also exposed to radiation during warfare or nuclear accidents.

Etiology. The effects of radiotherapy depend on the duration of the therapy and the particle type. Radiation comes in two forms: electromagnetic waves and particle radiation (Table 9-1). Radiation particles have variable charges, and include beta-particles (electrons), protons, alpha-particles, and neutrons. The most common type of radiation injury results from X rays containing low or moderate energy photons with a relatively high tissue penetrance.

The effects of radiation differ not only by its type but also by its energy. Radiation that causes dense ionization along its tract, such as alpha-particles and neutrons, is called high linear energy transfer (LET) radiation, a physical parameter to describe average energy release per unit length of the tract. In contrast, low LET transfer radiation produces sparse ionization along its tract. High LET is more destructive than low LET radiation at the same dose. The localized DNA damage caused by dense ionization from high LET radiation is more difficult to repair than the diffuse DNA damage caused by sparse ionization from low LET radiation.

Table 9-1

TYPES OF RADIATION

Type	Major Source	Tissue Penetration
Electromagnetic Waves		
Gamma rays	Isotope	Deep
X rays	Diagnostic machine	Deep
Particulate Matter		
Beta	Isotope	Intermediate
Proton	Isotope	Intermediate
Alpha	Isotope	Superficial
Neutron	Isotope	Superficial

Table 9-2

FACTORS THAT ENHANCE RADIATION INJURY

Radiation doses of ≥4,500 rads
The way radiation is given (accelerated fractionation increases the incidence of late radiation enteropathy)
Presence of other diseases
Diabetes
Hypertension
Severe atherosclerosis
Previous intestinal injury
Cardiovascular disease
Prior surgery
Prior radiation
Drugs
Adriamycin and other chemotherapeutic agents
An empty intestinal lumen during radiation therapy

The degree of radiation damage is determined by many factors (Table 9-2) (1,6,16,46,51,52,95). Certainly the radiation dose rate influences the degree of damage. Injuries seldom occur at doses less than 4,200 rads. There is a 1 to 5 percent risk of gastrointestinal ulceration, perforation, fibrosis, and obstruction at 4,500 rads. At 6,000 rads, the risk increases to 25 to 50 percent (68). A single whole body dose of external radiation is more lethal than regional fractionated doses with shielding. Total body exposure in the range of 1,000 to 2,000 rads is fatal within 10 days due to the extensive gastrointestinal injury, which results in severe loss of water, electrolytes, and proteins, as well as hemorrhage and sepsis (92). Fractionated doses allow time for cellular repair. Delayed enteric injury follows fractional radiation doses above 4,000 rads (44).

Pathophysiology. None of the morphologic events that result from radiation injury is unique. Each of the alterations encountered in irradiated cells is found with other forms of gastrointestinal injury, such as those caused by ischemia, heat, cold, or toxic substances.

Radiation injury causes two types of gastrointestinal damage. One is the radiation damage itself; the second is the long-term consequence of radiation, i.e., ischemic changes or cancer development. Radiation-induced gastrointestinal damage is associated with loss of barrier function and inflammatory responses. Radiation injury affects all parts of the gastrointestinal tract, from the esophagus to the anus, and the pathologic effects are similar in all areas. Epithelial and vascular injuries are common.

The frequency of gastrointestinal lesions varies as a result of local radiosensitivity and radiation dose. Varying sensitivity of different parts of the gastrointestinal tract results from the fact that radiation preferentially affects intermitotic cells with short reproductive cycles. The most severe damage occurs in areas of intestinal fixation, such as in the duodenum, terminal ileum, or in bowel loops fixed by adhesions.

Radiation damages DNA, impairs cell replication, and results in cell death, either by necrosis or apoptosis; it also causes mutations. Ionizing irradiation rapidly generates oxygen radicals by water radiolysis (22,58,70), yielding superoxide, hydrogen peroxide, and hydroxyl radicals (36). Endothelial cells are very sensitive to these molecules (23). Recent evidence suggests that microvascular endothelial apoptosis represents a major lesion in gastrointestinal radiation-induced damage. A close correlation exists between crypt dysfunction and the intensity of the microvascular endothelial apoptosis (61). The damaged endothelium produces proinflammatory mediators (41) and upregulates adhesion molecule expression, causing leukocytes to roll, become activated, and adhere to the endothelial cells. The activated leukocytes then produce a second oxygen radical burst, inducing further microvascular dysfunction (57,58). If the cells undergo extensive damage or if they are unable to repair the damage, they enter apoptosis. Apoptotic cells remain confined to stem cells at the crypt bases (64). Free radical scavengers and antioxidants protect against radiation injury.

Microvascular function regulates expression of radiation-induced crypt stem cell clonogen damage in the evolution of radiation injury to the gastrointestinal mucosa (48). Beta-fibroblast growth factor (β-FGF) is radioprotective by preventing crypt shrinkage. The protection afforded by β-FGF results in an increased number of surviving crypts, thus improving the likelihood of restitution of the intestinal mucosa (48). The pericryptal myofibroblast sheaths may also be a critical determinant in the type of injury. Crypt luminal cells return to normal at the end of treatment, but the effects of radiation on the pericryptal sheaths are longer lasting (65,97).

Transforming growth factor-beta (TGF-β) is a differential growth factor for intestinal epithelium and is synthesized in part by the myofibroblast sheaths. Increased levels have been reported in intestinal tissue following radiation (8). Also following radiation, members of the WNT signaling pathway are lost from the luminal cells and the surrounding fibroblasts, including E-cadherin and beta-catenin (85). Additionally, cytokines are activated during radiation-induced damage (39); cytokines are proinflammatory in nature.

Other changes to the gastrointestinal tract include loss of intestinal barrier integrity, with increased leakage of proteins, and alterations in intestinal absorption due to the immaturity of the cells or due to motility defects as a result of damage to the enteric nervous system. Damage to the ileum, which is particularly sensitive to radiation injury, may result in the impaired absorption of vitamin B12 and bile acids. Both of these are absorbed in the terminal ileum by specific transporters located within the villous epithelial cells.

Our understanding of the acute consequences of whole body exposure in humans is primarily derived from Japanese atomic bomb survivors, victims of nuclear accidents, and patients irradiated therapeutically. The acute effects of ionizing radiation range from frank necrosis at high doses, death of proliferating cells at intermediate doses, and no histologic effects at doses of less than 50 rads (88). Radiation injury eventually leads to mucosal atrophy. Acute cell death, especially of endothelial cells, causes delayed organ dysfunction months to years after the radiation exposure. In general, this delayed injury results from a combination of parenchymal cell atrophy, ischemia due to vascular damage, and fibrosis. Malabsorption results from radiation-induced dysmotility that leads to bacterial overgrowth–related radiation enteropathy (37,38) and impaired ileal function with defective lactose and bile acid absorption.

Many patients receiving radiotherapy also receive drugs with radiosensitizing effects (30). These drugs are directly toxic to the mucosa (see chapter 8), predisposing it to further radiation damage. Factors that increase the incidence of radiation injury are listed in Table 9-2.

Table 9-3

RADIATION-INDUCED CARCINOGENESIS

Mutation (direct effects)
Oncogene activation
Tumor suppressor gene inactivation
Genetic Instability (indirect effects)
Chromosome instability (aneuploidy, breaks, deletion, amplification)
Minisatellite mutation (germ cell mutation)
Microsatellite instability (replication error)

Mechanisms of radiation-induced carcinogenesis are summarized in Table 9-3. Radiation-induced ionizations act directly or indirectly via water-derived radicals, thereby injuring cellular components. The major damage in single cells is single- or double-strand DNA breaks. Double-strand breaks are more difficult to repair by non-homologous enjoining or homologous recombination. Erroneous rejoining of broken ends may occur, resulting in cell death or the induction of mutations that activate proto-oncogenes or inactivate tumor suppressor genes.

Clinical Features. The clinical manifestations of radiation injury depend on whether an individual has experienced an acute whole body exposure or has received small doses of radiation targeted to a particular area. Most patients who receive small radiation doses experience early acute symptoms of bowel injury, including tenesmus, urgency, bleeding, diarrhea, and incontinence. These symptoms usually resolve within 2 to 3 months following cessation of the radiation exposure, although a small percentage of patients develop chronic problems.

The most common problem following pelvic radiation is proctitis followed by enteritis, anorectal stricture, and fibrosis (63). Neural, muscular, or neuromuscular damage results in localized or generalized gastrointestinal dysmotility, esophageal dysmotility, gastroparesis, or intestinal pseudoobstruction. Radiation alters mucosal barrier function and causes malabsorption. The gastrointestinal tract of patients who receive radiotherapy for primary gastrointestinal malignancies may perforate due to tumor necrosis. Most moderate to severe intestinal injuries develop within 2 to 5 years after radiation, with a cumulative 10-year incidence of 8 percent for moderate injuries and 3 percent for severe injuries.

Table 9-4

CLINICAL FEATURES OF THE ACUTE RADIATION SYNDROME

Category	Whole-Body Dose (rem)	Symptoms	Prognosis
Subclinical	<200	Mild nausea and vomiting Lymphocytes <1,500/mm^3	100% survival
Hematopoietic	200-600	Intermittent nausea and vomiting Petechiae, hemorrhage Maximum neutrophil and platelet depression in 2 weeks	Infections May require bone marrow transplant
Gastrointestinal	600-1,000	Nausea, vomiting, diarrhea Hemorrhage and infection in 1 to 3 weeks Severe neutrophil and platelet depression Lymphocytes <500/mm^3	Shock and death in 10 to 14 days even with replacement therapy
Central nervous system	>1,000	Intractable nausea and vomiting Confusion, somnolence, convulsions Coma in 15 min to 3 hours Lymphocytes absent	Death in 14 to 36 hours

Mucosal biopsies are generally performed in cases of suspected radiation injury in order to confirm the presence of a radiation effect or to exclude the presence of recurrent tumor, the reemergence of a new tumor, or the presence of an opportunistic infection. The endoscopist must exercise caution whenever utilizing large biopsy devices to obtain tissue from areas with poor vascularity or suboptimal healing potential as perforation or fistulization constitute possible complications.

Progressing and unrelenting fibrosis, particularly in the small bowel, results in part from vascular insufficiency. It also results from persistent functional loss of mucosal cells that lack the appropriate nutrients for healing. There is also increased expression of TGF-β in the area of radiation injury. There may also be alterations in the coagulation cascade that may contribute to the progression of delayed injury.

Acute Whole Body Exposure. Whole body irradiation is potentially lethal; the clinical manifestations are dose dependent. They are typically described as *acute radiation syndrome* or *radiation sickness*. In radiation accidents and atomic warfare, single radiation exposures in the range of 1,000 to 2,000 rads may cause death. Acute radiation syndrome or radiation sickness is characterized by three successive phases: 1) prodromal phase: this transient period generally develops within a few hours of exposure. The severity and duration of symptoms are dose dependent. The most frequent prodromal symptoms are anorexia, nausea, and vomiting; 2) latency period: the prodromal stage rarely exceeds 24 hours. This is then followed by an asymptomatic period, the duration of which is inversely proportional to the radiation dose. In patients with large radiation exposures (those in excess of 1,000 rads), the prodromal phase often merges with either gastrointestinal or acute incapacitation syndrome. These are generally fatal, so that the latency period may not be apparent. At lower doses, the duration of the latency period primarily reflects the time required for the untoward consequences of cell depletion to become clinically evident. This specifically affects mitotically active cells; and 3) principal phase: during the third and principal phase, the syndrome can be subcategorized on the basis of the mode of death and the organ system most conspicuously involved. These include hematopoietic syndrome, gastrointestinal syndrome, or central nervous system syndrome (Table 9-4).

Localized Exposure. Esophagus. The esophagus was initially thought to be radioresistant, but it has now been shown that esophageal squamous epithelium, stroma, and blood vessels all have sufficient radiosensitivity to result in early and delayed complications after exposure to therapeutic doses of radiation. The radiosensitivity of the esophagus is comparable to that of other regions of the gastrointestinal tract. Radiation doses of 4,500 to 5,000 rads or more administered to a previously normal esophagus produce significant esophageal injury.

Radiation esophagitis follows radiation therapy for cancers arising in the head and neck, thyroid, thymus, lung, mediastinum, and esophagus. Symptoms of radiation esophagitis begin about 2 weeks after the initiation of radiation therapy. They tend to occur earlier and be more severe with increasing radiation dose and decreasing time of the dosage spread. Patients with radiation esophagitis present with dysphagia, odynophagia, substernal burning, and esophageal dysmotility. Motility disturbances are common, especially in those receiving over 4,500 rads over a 6- to 8-week period. The dysphagia results from interruption of primary peristaltic waves. The symptoms may subside on their own, they may persist for a short period of time, or they may persist for up to 2 to 3 months and require analgesic therapy. Ulcers can develop at the end of the therapy or shortly thereafter and may persist but they usually heal spontaneously (44). Late esophageal effects manifest clinically by difficulty swallowing secondary to fibrosis and stricture formation, and motility disturbances. Rare complications include pseudodiverticula development and fistula formation.

Medical conditions associated with increased radiation sensitivity include collagen vascular diseases, diabetes, ataxia-telangiectasia, Bloom's syndrome, and acquired immunodeficiency syndrome (AIDS) (13). These all constitute contraindications to high-dose radiation to the esophagus due to an increased risk for the development of late complications (12). The clinical situation is often complicated by the presence of esophageal superinfection as a result of immune suppression due to the underlying disease, or concomitant administration of chemotherapy, other myelosuppressive agents, and other medications that may have local topical erosive effects. The clinician and pathologist, therefore, often have to determine whether more than one pathologic process is present and which factor is predominant in increasing clinical disease, namely radiation, opportunistic infection, acid reflux, or drug-induced inflammation.

Stomach. Acute gastric lesions (gastritis) follow total body irradiation or local gastric irradiation (25,27). Gastric glandular necrosis can follow as little as 1,200 rads of therapy. Fifty percent of patients with gastric doses of 5,500 or more rads develop clinical evidence of gastric mucosal injury (70). It is not unusual for the stomach to receive doses of radiation ranging from 4,000 to 6,000 rads during treatment of lower esophageal tumors and tumors of the biliary tract, pancreas, and the stomach itself. The stomach may also be in radiation fields for treatment of lymphomas or Hodgkin's disease involving periaortic lymph nodes.

Irradiation causes direct mucosal damage as well as capillary endothelial cell abnormalities and acute thromboses. Gastric ulcers are the most important complication of gastric radiation exposure. Ulcers may occur as early as 9 weeks following therapy completion. They are indistinguishable from ordinary peptic ulcers. The ulcers are usually solitary, measuring 0.5 to 2.0 cm in diameter. Since gastric acid and peptic secretion is reduced, the ulcers do not respond to dietary or antacid treatment. They may heal spontaneously but the accompanying submucosal fibrosis can produce antral fibrosis.

Other nonacute clinical syndromes complicating gastric radiation are: 1) dyspepsia, arising 6 months to 4 years after radiation exposure without clinical or radiographic signs and 2) gastritis, arising 1 to 12 months from the completion of radiation, accompanied by evidence of antral spasm or stenosis. Gastroscopy reveals smooth mucosal folds and mucosal atrophy. Fistulas sometimes complicate radiation therapy for gastric cancer (18).

Small Intestine. The small intestine is very sensitive to radiation; abdominal radiotherapy results in chronic gastrointestinal complaints in 10 to 30 percent of patients (15,32,34,42). Fixed portions of the small bowel sustain a greater degree of injury than mobile ones. The duodenum has a particularly low tolerance to radiation because of its fixed position. The irradiated duodenum may be further injured by exposure to gastric juice, bile, and pancreatic digestive enzymes. The lower small intestine is frequently exposed during treatment of neoplasms involving the bladder, prostate, and female reproductive tract as well as the lower large intestine.

Because of the frequency of neoplasms in this area, radiation injury involving the distal small intestine is one of the most common radiation injuries seen in the gastrointestinal tract. The radioresponsiveness of the small intestine often results in modification of radiotherapy plans for other diseases.

At 4,500 rads, there is a 1 to 5 percent risk of ulceration, perforation, fibrosis, and obstruction. In the range of 5,000 to 6,000 rads, 20 to 50 percent of patients develop clinical enteritis (66), mainly in the terminal ileum or in bowel loops fixed by adhesions. Acute radiation enteropathy is usually self-limited, but up to 31 percent of patients require surgery. Over 6,000 rads, about 75 percent of patients develop clinical symptoms, usually by the middle of the 2nd week of therapy. Patients often have acute but temporary diarrhea during, and immediately after, a course of abdominal radiation. Nausea, vomiting, and abdominal cramps also develop. The acute manifestations usually subside within weeks, due to rapid mucosal regeneration. At this dose, the risk of perforation is 25 to 50 percent (69).

Chronic radiation enteropathy develops months, years, or decades following treatment. Patients present with diarrhea, crampy abdominal pain, nausea, and cachexia. Villous atrophy results in malabsorption. Late complications tend to persist (19,42,83). A small percentage of patients experience a chronic deteriorating disease, referred to as *severe late radiation enteropathy*. It is characterized by diarrhea, pain, malabsorption, small bowel obstruction, acute or chronic gastrointestinal bleeding, intestinal perforation, and pseudoobstruction (42). Strictures predispose to intestinal stasis and blind loop syndrome.

Late changes develop secondary to intramural vasculitis, with resultant ulcer, stricture, and fistula formation. Chronic radiation injury is a major cause of intestinal ischemia. Small intestinal ischemia with perforation or fistula formation accounts for 16 percent of late intestinal complications of radiotherapy (19). Patients may also develop radiation-induced intestinal obstruction or pseudoobstruction (59). In these situations the clinician is often confronted with the task of excluding other disease processes affecting the small bowel, including Crohn's disease, mycobacterial infections, lymphoma, and other infiltrative disorders. As the radiologic features invariably overlap, the clinician is dependent on the pathologist to confirm the diagnosis.

Large Intestine. The large intestine has a radiosensitivity as great as that of the small intestine and is exposed to radiation just as frequently, yet diffuse radiation injury occurs less commonly. Nevertheless, there is a high incidence of radiation damage because of the frequent use of radiation to treat pelvic tumors and the fixed position of the rectosigmoid. Between 75 to 90 percent of all intestinal complications affect the distal colon (2), with the rectum being most commonly involved (16,55).

Acute, symptomatic rectosigmoid lesions are very common and are almost invariably due to therapy for pelvic neoplasms with doses of 3,000 to 4,000 rads delivered within a 3- to 4-week period. Transient diarrhea accompanied by tenesmus, incomplete evacuation, mild abdominal cramps, and a mucoid or bloody discharge can be expected as a result of acute mucosal cellular injury (45). Pain, alterations in bowel habits, and bleeding are also prominent symptoms (45). Bleeding is due to the underlying vascular changes (76). Severe proctosigmoiditis follows radiation therapy in 2.4 to 5.0 percent of patients; it is more common in patients treated with over 6,000 rads over 6 weeks. Restricted function of the internal anal sphincter is important in causing intestinal disease. Diffuse pancolitis may develop, as may ulcerations, stenosis, necrosis, and fistulas, all caused by progressive intramural vasculitis with submucosal and subserosal fibrosis.

Delayed lesions resemble those seen in the small intestine, and include strictures, perforation, intestinal pseudoobstruction (91), vascular obliteration, and mural fibrosis (28,91). The frequency of chronic radiation damage varies from 0.5 to 30.0 percent (77). Delayed proctosigmoiditis with intermittent bleeding of mild to moderate severity occurs 6 months to 5 years following therapy but can be delayed for as many as 30 years. Other intestinal symptoms include a mucoid rectal discharge, tenesmus, abdominal distension, and abdominal pain. Radiation also induces solitary rectal ulcers (14).

Anus. Radiation-induced changes often affect the anus because the common therapy for advanced cervical or prostate cancer includes radiotherapy. Secondary changes as a result of soiling and fungal skin infections are common.

Gross Findings. *Esophagus*. The location of radiation esophagitis depends on what part of the esophagus was exposed to the radiation.

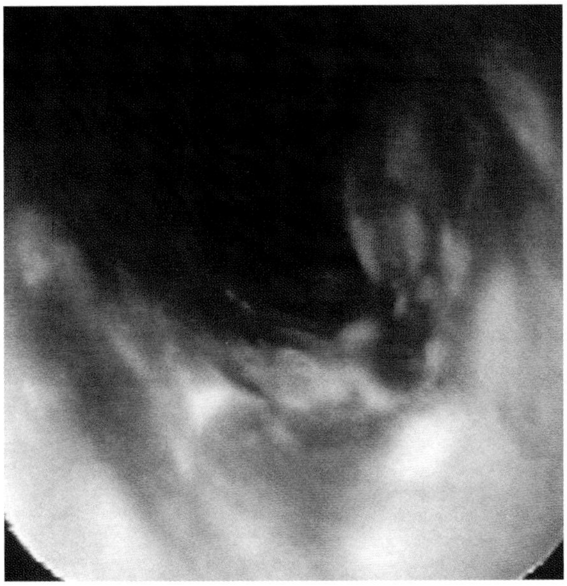

Figure 9-1

RADIATION ESOPHAGITIS

Endoscopic appearance of the eroded reddened mucosa in a patient with radiation esophagitis.

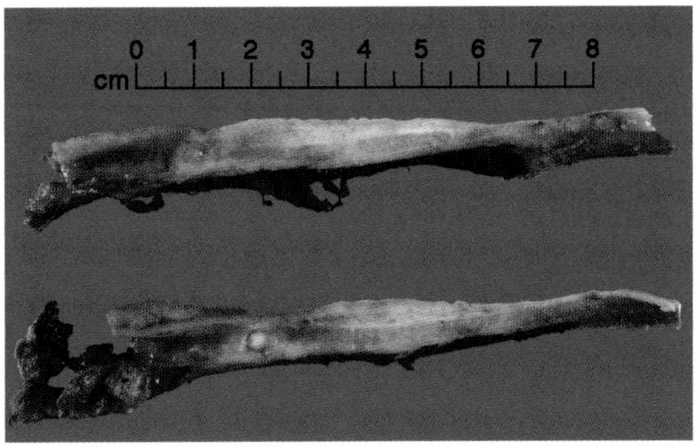

Figure 9-2

RADIATION-INDUCED ESOPHAGEAL INJURY

Cross section through the esophageal wall of a patient with esophageal cancer who was treated with preoperative radiotherapy. No residual tumor was present in the resected specimen. The wall of the esophagus shows an area of fibrosis. The small white nodule just to the left is a small leiomyoma.

Radiation esophagitis presents as areas of erosion, ulceration (fig. 9-1), fibrosis, and/or stricture. Esophageal ulcers and esophageal fistulas develop during the subacute phase. The ulcers may become quite large, measuring up to 5 cm in diameter; these may perforate into adjacent structures causing hemorrhage (71). Esophageal strictures, mucosal webs, and mucosal stromal bridges (60) develop during chronic radiation injury, usually 13 to 21 months after the initiation of therapy. Stricture length depends on the size of the radiation field. The most consistent radiologic finding is abnormal motility; esophageal strictures or ulcers occur less frequently (29). Late changes include mural fibrosis (fig. 9-2).

Stomach. Patients receiving radiation in doses over 4,000 rads demonstrate both acute and chronic gastritis, with areas of epithelial necrosis and shallow ulcers (17), many of which involve the antrum and pylorus. Radiographic changes include irregular antral contractions and gastric ulcerations (29). If sufficient peptic acid secretion persists, the ulcers resemble usual peptic ulcers, with a necrotic base over a prominent fibrinoid layer, beneath which are successive layers of chronic active granulation tissue and dense fibrosis (see chapter 5).

Computerized tomography (CT) of radiation-induced gastritis shows nonspecific gastric thickening. In the acute phase, small ulcers may be visible and the mucosa may appear shaggy. Narrowing and deformity of the antrum and pylorus, without ulceration, are more frequent during chronic injury (7).

Small Intestine. Both early and delayed complications develop. The delayed complications are responsible for many of the changes related to radiation injury in the small bowel. Delayed complications result from fibrosis and vascular injury; these changes are progressive and often relentless. Patients also develop acute ulcers with underlying granulation tissue containing prominent vessels. In acute and subacute radiation-induced enteritis, barium studies often show nodular filling defects or thumbprinting. These features result from arteriolar obliteration. The mucosa has a marked regenerative ability and erosions heal rapidly, the edema subsides, and mucosal integrity is rapidly restored. Some injury, however, may remain, altering the underlying mucosal histology and function. Additionally, the microvasculature develops telangiectasias and endothelial cell functions can be lost.

Late radiation injury results in bleeding, fistula formation, and obstruction. The bowel and its mesentery shorten; mucosal ulceration and submucosal fibrosis are present. In late stage disease, mucosal atrophy is invariably present. Eventually, the serosa acquires a matte-white appearance as adhesions develop; the bowel appears markedly thickened and fibrotic (29). When the bowel is resected, it often appears mottled red and gray with a markedly thickened serosa. The changes are identical to those seen in ischemia. The fatty tissue of the mesentery does not extend over the surface of the small intestine as it does in Crohn's disease. Mesenteries are thickened and indurated. The valvulae conniventes may be irregular and thickened, with focal erosions in the central areas. The submucosa appears whitened. The muscularis propria becomes hypertrophic. Dense adhesions, with kinking of loops of small bowel, are often present. The bowel proximal to strictures distends. Often, the abnormal bowel merges imperceptibly with the noninjured bowel, making it difficult to identify the exact junction of the injured and uninjured bowel. This can cause problems at the time of resection because the surgeon may place an anastomosis in a damaged part of the intestine that grossly appears normal. If this occurs, postoperative anastomotic leaks can develop. Frozen section monitoring helps determine whether the resection margins are histologically normal or whether they, too, are affected by underlying radiation damage.

CT provides useful information regarding the extent of the bowel wall thickening and mesenteric fibrosis. Separation of bowel loops results from mural fibrosis. Long segment strictures may be present. In cases of moderate radiation damage, CT shows the affected small bowel loops as accurately as barium studies. CT is accurate also for detecting fistulas and abscesses. On CT, a thickened intestinal wall, configured with a middle layer of low attenuation surrounded on each side by layers of higher attenuation, has been termed the "target sign." Fat density target sign is useful in identifying patients with chronic radiation enteritis (10).

Large Intestine. Early colorectal changes include mucosal edema, mucosal discoloration or duskiness, and loss of normal mucosal vascular patterns (fig. 9-3). Pallor, loss of mucosal folds, and irregular shallow ulcers may be present. Strictures develop late in the disease (fig. 9-4).

On CT, radiation-induced proctitis has regular and symmetrical rectal wall thickening as-

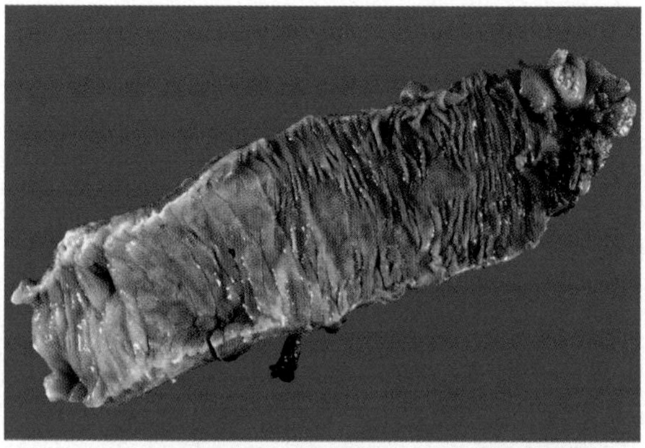

Figure 9-3

RADIATION PROCTITIS

The right half of the specimen shows mucosal discoloration whereas the left half shows loss of mucosal folds.

sociated with inflamed perirectal fat. An increase in the presacral space of more than 1 cm in anteroposterior diameter and a thickening of the perirectal fascia typify chronic radiation-induced proctitis and create the so-called halo effect. Complications such as fistulas and abscesses are seen on CT scan.

Barium studies of acute radiation-induced colitis often demonstrate spasm, mucosal irregularity, and nodular submucosal thickening, which results in a cobblestoned pattern. Effacement of the valves of Houston and interhaustral folds is observed. Chronic radiation-induced colitis often manifests as strictures that may be long or short, and generally have tapered and smooth margins. In some cases, ulcers, fistulas, and sinus tracts are seen (9). Radiation changes in patients who have received treatment for pelvic malignancies are invariably confined to that area of the bowel within the pelvis.

Microscopic Findings. *General Features.* Radiation damage occurs within several hours of administration and mucosal loss occurs within 1 to 2 days. Acute ulceration, edema (fig. 9-5), and vascular fibrinoid necrosis are seen in the acute period. Chronic effects include mucosal atrophy, telangiectasia (fig. 9-6), atypical stromal cells (fig. 9-7), fibrosis (fig. 9-8), submucosal neuronal proliferations, and degeneration of the muscle fibers of the circular layer of the muscularis propria. Vascular injury affects all gastrointestinal sites (fig. 9-9). Following the initial

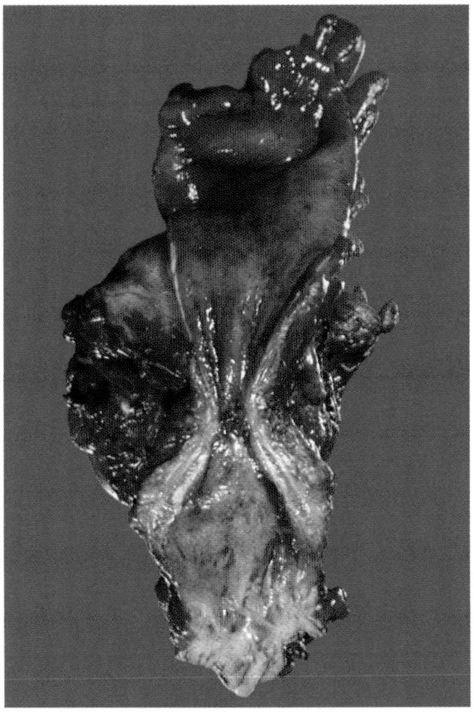

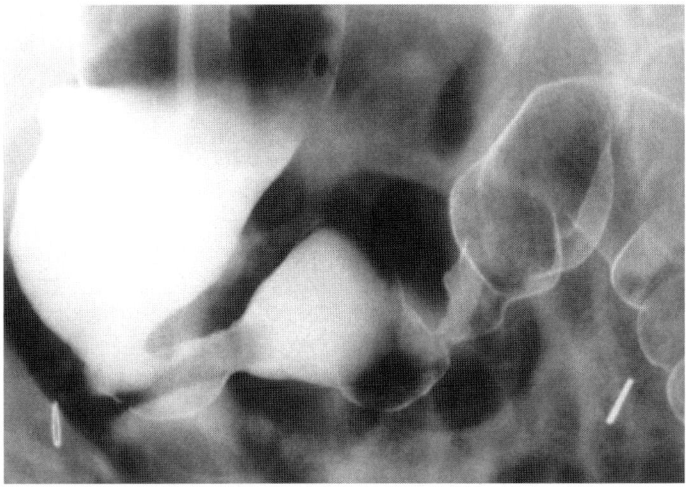

Figure 9-4

RADIATION-INDUCED STRICTURE

Left: There is marked thickening of the intestinal wall with narrowing of the lumen. The gross appearance resembles that of certain types of adenocarcinoma.

Above: Radiographically, an area of narrowing is seen.

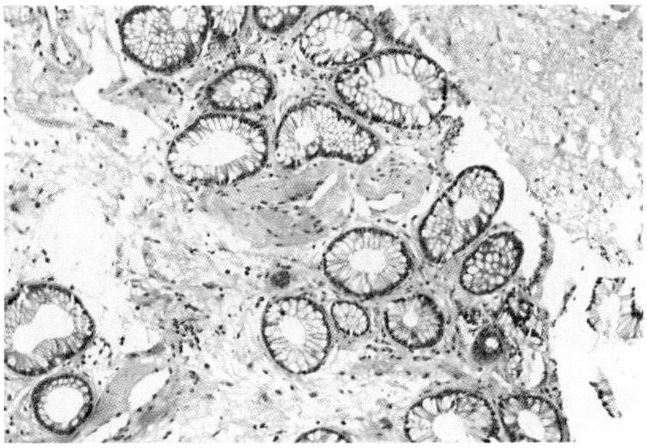

Figure 9-5

ACUTE RADIATION DAMAGE AFFECTING THE RECTUM

Acute changes in the rectal mucosa in a patient receiving radiation. Mucosal edema is prominent.

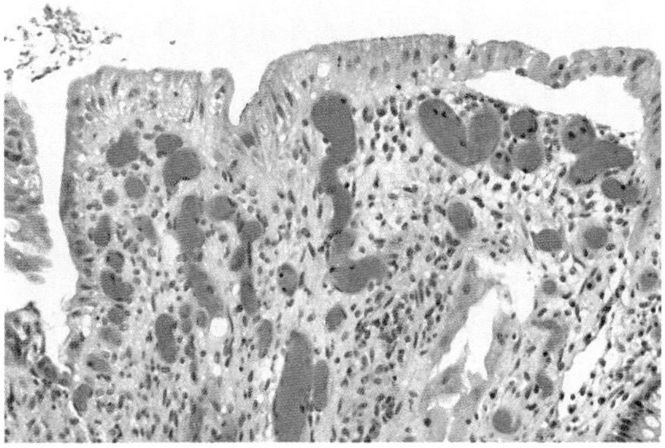

Figure 9-6

ACUTE RADIATION INJURY IN THE COLON

Mucosal telangiectasia is characteristic of early radiation-induced lesions.

vascular injury, the blood vessels develop subintimal fibrosis and fibrosis of the muscle wall, degeneration of the internal elastic lamina, and severe luminal narrowing. Capillaries may become thrombosed and obliterated or ectatic. The organs supplied by these damaged vessels become ischemic, atrophic, and fibrotic. Other vascular changes include subendothelial accumulations of lipid-laden macrophages, calcification, and thrombosis. The likelihood of finding arteriolar damage with severe myointimal thickening and lipophages depends on the time following radiation exposure rather than the dose. In chronic radiation damage, the vasculature of the bowel is markedly compromised by progressive endarteritis. Late radiation effects include progressive hyalinization of vascular walls, obstruction of vascular lumens, ischemia,

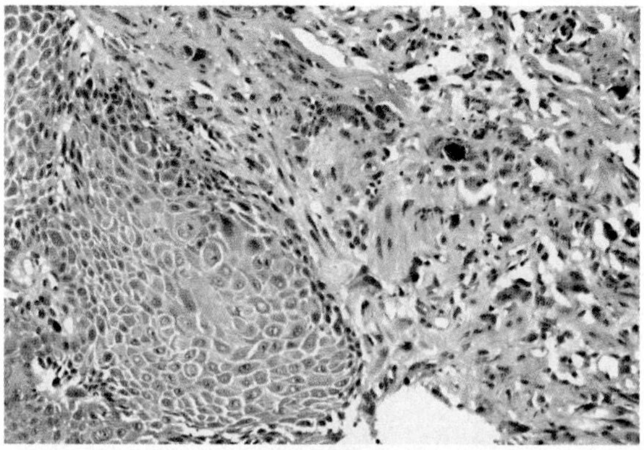

Figure 9-7

RADIATION-INDUCED ESOPHAGEAL INJURY

Prominent atypical cells are in the stroma in this esophageal biopsy from a patient receiving radiation therapy. These atypical cells can be quite striking. The esophageal squamous epithelium shows some disorganization, intercellular edema, nuclear enlargement, and loss of polarity.

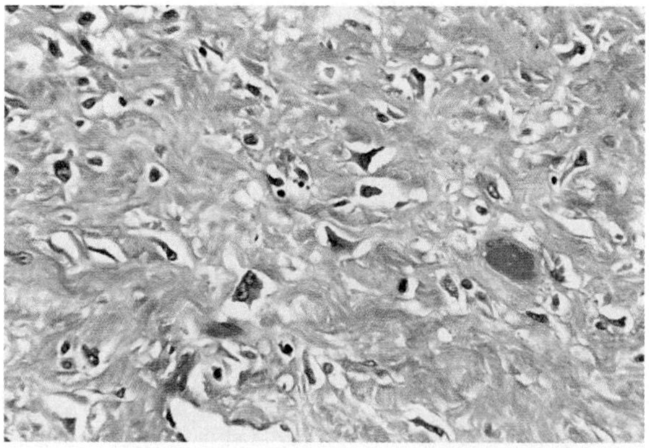

Figure 9-8

RADIATION-INDUCED INJURY

Dense submucosal fibrosis with swallow-tailed radiation fibroblasts distributed throughout.

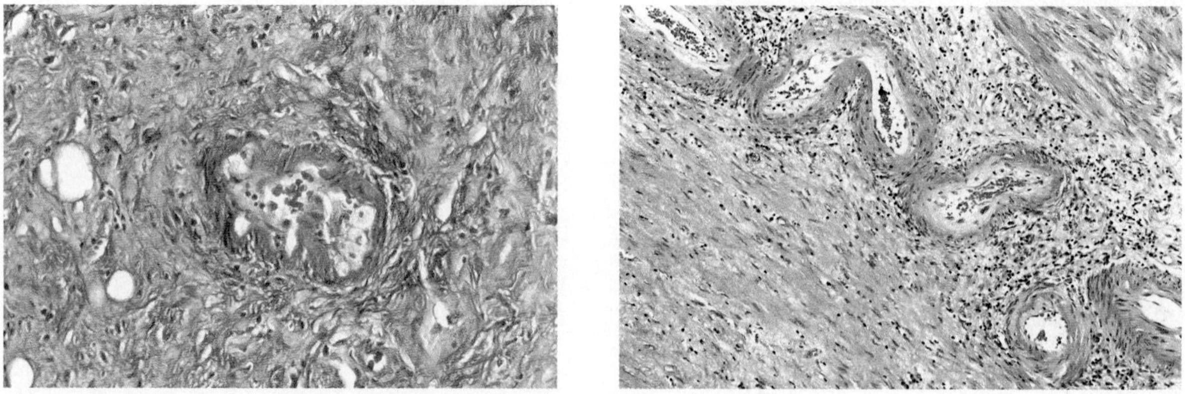

Figure 9-9

RADIATION-INDUCED VASCULAR INJURY

Left: Fibrinoid necrosis of the vascular wall.

Right: Long-standing radiation-induced obliterative endarteritis. There is a marked proliferation of fibrous tissue within the intima. An inflammatory response surrounds the damaged vessels.

and tissue necrosis. Atypical stromal cells surround the damaged vessels. Stromal changes persist longer than epithelial changes, although the mucosal damage is usually more obvious.

Esophagus. Early changes in the esophageal mucosa include epithelial swelling and vacuolization, an absence of mitoses in the basal layer, thinning of the squamous cell layer, and focal basal epithelial cell necrosis (apoptosis). The tissues appear edematous, erythematous, and friable, with superficial erosions coalescing to form larger superficial ulcers. Prominent endothelial cells lie in the edematous granulation tissue. Degenerated epithelial cells show cytoplasmic enlargement, vacuolization, and multinucleation. Both radiation- and chemotherapy-associated esophagitis result in large, bizarre-appearing, squamous epithelial cells with increased cytoplasmic volume and increased nucleoplasm (fig. 9-7). Nucleoli are usually not prominent. Dead or dying tumor cells may be seen. Fibrin-platelet thrombi may be visible in capillaries and small veins.

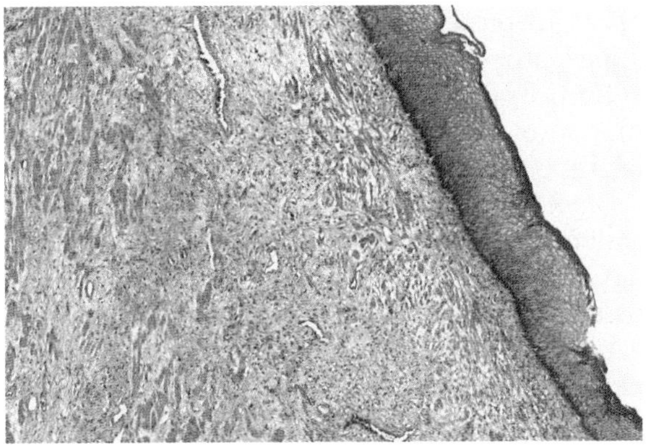

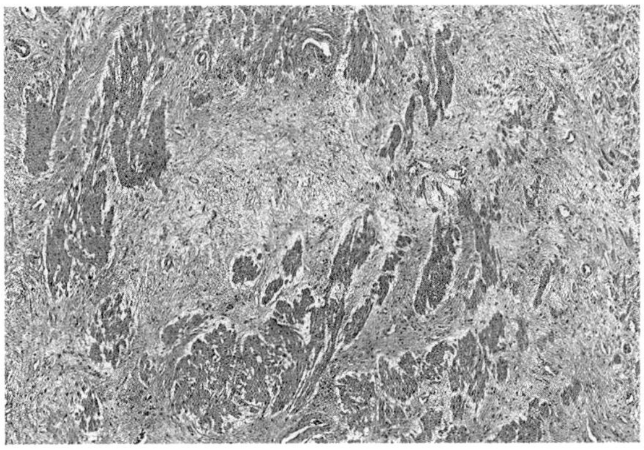

Figure 9-10

RADIATION-INDUCED ESOPHAGEAL FIBROSIS

Left: Dense fibrosis in the submucosa, with atypical stromal cells. Right: Fibrosis of the muscularis propria.

Patients who develop odynophagia and/or dysphagia typically have discrete ulcers. If ulcers develop, there is often acute and chronic inflammation, fibrosis, and numerous fibroblasts containing large hyperchromatic nuclei. Bizarre (radiation) fibroblasts and vascular changes suggest the diagnosis. Epithelial hyperplasia develops in an effort to reepithelialize the mucosal surface. Mitotic figures may appear more numerous in the mucosa than normal. The regenerating epithelium may show features simulating dysplasia. Nuclear membrane irregularities and multinucleation may be present. The chromatin usually remains finely granular. If bizarre epithelial or stromal cells are found in an area of unexplained esophagitis or fibrosis, it is always wise to query the clinician concerning a history of previous radiation exposure if this history has not already been provided. Eventually, the epithelial lining regenerates, with an increase in the basal cell layer and a possible increase in the overall epithelial thickness.

Histologic examination in the late period discloses the presence of acanthosis, parakeratosis, hyperkeratosis, hyalinized blood vessels, submucosal and muscular fibrosis (fig. 9-10), and muscular degeneration. The myenteric plexus becomes inflamed and fibrotic. The muscularis propria appears degenerated (fig. 9-11); the muscularis mucosae may appear normal or fibrotic. The mucosa may be thrown up into folds by scarring and contraction of the underlying tissue, especially in areas of stricture.

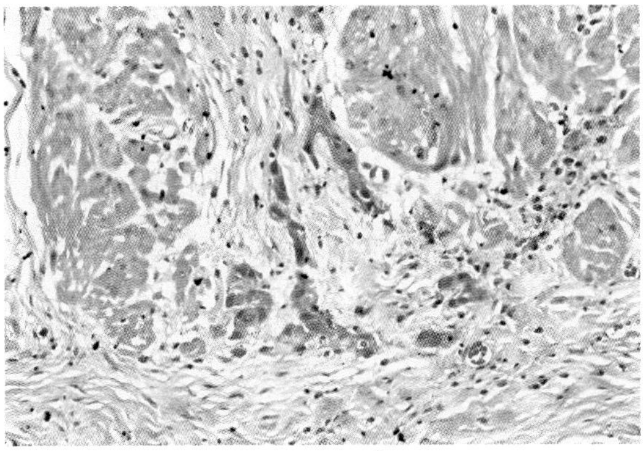

Figure 9-11

RADIATION-INDUCED MUSCULAR CHANGES

Changes of the muscularis propria in a patient radiated for esophageal carcinoma. The muscle cells appear to be degenerating. In the center are some residual viable tumor cells.

There may also be smooth muscle fiber fragmentation. Atypical fibroblasts may be embedded in dense collagenous tissue. Submucosal glands become atrophic, with acinar loss and dilatation, and inspissation of the ductular contents. A mild inflammatory infiltrate may be present. Patients who receive brachytherapy in addition to external beam therapy develop more severe mucosal injury. If a boost of 1,000 to 1,500 rads of brachytherapy is added to 5,000 rads of external beam therapy, the mucosa that was previously normal adjacent to the carcinoma being treated can develop severe erosions,

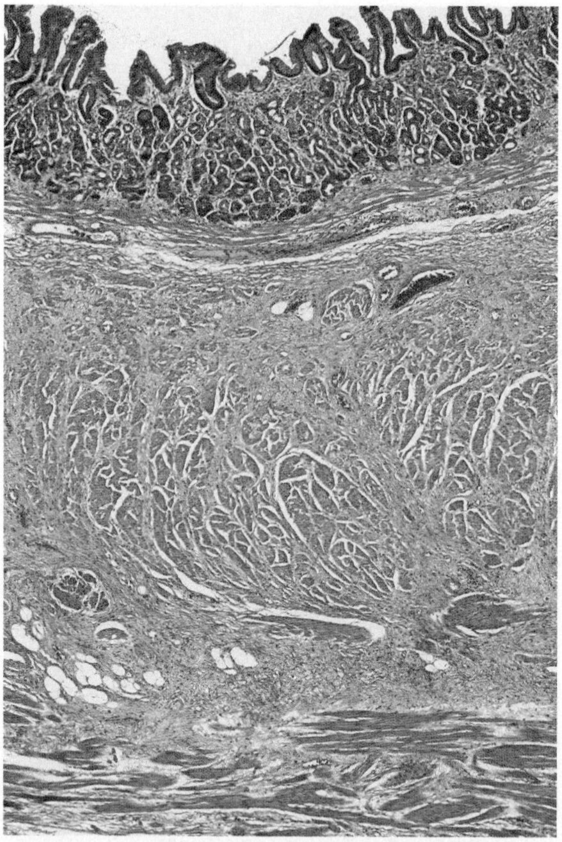

Figure 9-12

RADIATION-INDUCED GASTRIC INJURY

The gastric pits are elongated and the glands are mildly atrophic. The submucosa is densely fibrotic and there is also fibrosis of the muscularis propria.

which may be circumferential. These may heal spontaneously, but they may also progress to chronic ulcers or even strictures.

Patients develop motility abnormalities following radiation, usually within 4 to 12 weeks after exposure. The ganglion cells of the submucosal and myenteric plexuses, however, generally appear normal. This does not rule out the possibility of abnormal function.

The most common long-term complication of radiation therapy is stricture formation. The wall is thickened, and the epithelium appears atrophic with parakeratosis, although the epithelial layer may also be thickened. The submucosa appears fibrotic and there may be irregular bundles of eosinophilic and hyaline collagen. Numerous atypical, swallow-tail fibroblasts are present and the arterioles and venules appear thick-walled and hyalinized or fibrotic. Submucosal esophageal glands and their ducts may show atypical squamous metaplasia, mimicking early carcinoma.

Stomach. Gastric radiation injury assumes several forms. *Acute radiation gastritis* develops a few days to a few months following radiation exposure. Patients develop erosive and ulcerative gastritis characterized by extensive glandular necrosis and superficial ulceration. Chief and parietal cells are damaged first; the surface epithelium is damaged later. By the 8th day of therapy, karyopyknosis develops within the gastric pits, with loss of secretory granules in the chief cells and parietal cells. Acute vascular changes develop. The connective tissue in the mucosa and submucosa develops edema, congestion, telangiectasia, swelling of the collagen bundles, and fibrin exudates. Lymphocytes and plasma cells infiltrate the lamina propria in the 2nd and 3rd weeks. Glandular atypia develops by 21 days. The degree of epithelial and stromal atypia resembles that found in patients receiving chemotherapy via intraarterial hepatic infusion (see chapter 8).

When the epithelium sloughs, it is replaced from the mucous neck region. As the mucosa heals, it regenerates and the gastric pits elongate, but variable degrees of atrophy, fibrosis, edema, and endarteritis persist (fig. 9-12). The regenerating glands are surrounded by a mononuclear cell infiltrate. Gastric ulcers may develop due to desquamation and erosion of the damaged mucosa as well as alterations in the underlying vasculature.

Eventually, *severe atrophic gastritis* develops. The intensity of the inflammation diminishes and the submucosa develops capillary telangiectasia and arterial wall hyalinization with intimal fibrosis. Bizarre endothelial cells and "radiation fibroblasts" develop. Some patients develop a deep *acute ulcer* 1 to 2 months following radiation exposure, which usually walls off before perforation occurs. The ulcer represents the long-term effects of vascular damage and has an ischemic etiology. The only clues to its etiology are the clinical history, an unusually prominent antral fibrosis with obliterative endarteritis (fig. 9-13) involving the submucosal blood vessels, and the presence of radiation fibroblasts (see fig. 9-8). Biopsies in late-stage

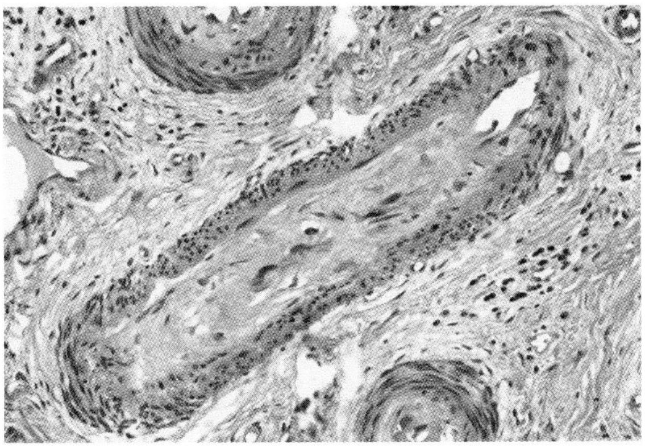

Figure 9-13

RADIATION-INDUCED OBLITERATIVE ENDARTERITIS IN THE SUBMUCOSA

The vascular lumen is almost completely obstructed by a proliferation of intimal fibrous tissue.

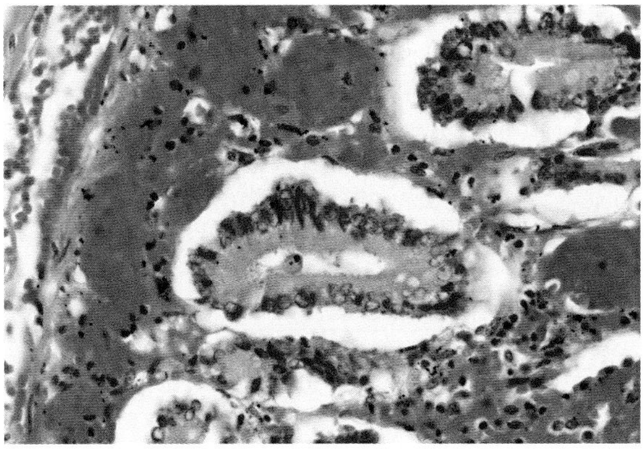

Figure 9-14

ACUTE RADIATION CHANGES IN THE SMALL INTESTINE

The lamina propria is edematous and contains scattered inflammatory cells. The nuclei appear to have inclusions within them and are extremely hyperchromatic. There is early apoptosis and cells are megaloblastic.

radiation gastritis show an atrophic mucosa with scar tissue, thick-walled blood vessels, and distended lymphatics. Some patients develop arteriovenous malformations.

Healing can result in scarred and sclerosed gastric segments that are sometimes difficult to distinguish from tumor. Rarely, sharply defined submucosal or muscular areas become densely hyalinized (81).

Small Intestine. Acute radiation effects range from barely visible epithelial damage to massive intestinal necrosis. Morphologic changes include loss of enterocyte columnar shape and nuclear polarity, epithelial degeneration, ulceration with mucosal denudation, nuclear pyknosis and karyorrhexis, crypt disintegration, mucosal edema, enlarged bizarre nuclei (fig. 9-14), absent mitoses, mucin depletion, crypt abscesses with prominent eosinophilic and neutrophilic infiltrates, and numerous apoptotic bodies in the crypt bases (87).

During acute injury, the damaged epithelium sheds into the crypt lumen. Cell loss from the villus tips exceeds cellular replacement from the crypts, leading to surface erosions, ulcers, alterations in the crypt to villus ratio, and severe villous atrophy with crypt hyperplasia or crypt hypoplasia. Decreased mitotic activity indicates defective cellular replication. The total epithelial surface decreases by almost 50 percent in 2 to 4 weeks. During this period of time, absorption of fat, protein, carbohydrates, and bile salts is abnormal. A macrocytosis develops that may be irregularly distributed, varying from crypt to crypt or villus to villus. Paneth cells often are unusually prominent. The lamina propria becomes infiltrated by neutrophils and other inflammatory cells. Plasma cells increase in number in the lamina propria and radiosensitive lymphocytes decrease. The capillary endothelium swells and the vessels become telangiectatic. Increases in vascular permeability immediately following radiation lead to edema and fibrin deposition in the interstitial spaces and blood vessel walls. These changes tend to disappear within 1 to 2 months.

Radiation changes may revert to normal depending upon the degree of damage. Complete structural recovery usually occurs within 2 to 3 weeks of therapy cessation but villous atrophy and abnormal crypts may result in subclinical malabsorption. Disordered glandular proliferation and persistent ulceration ultimately result in prominent fibrosis, radiation fibroblasts, and ectatic vessels in the lamina propria. Distorted villi and ulcerations are characteristic of advanced injury. Fibrosis causes secondary lymphangiectasia. Patients with systemic sclerosis may exhibit exaggerated fibrosis in irradiated areas (78).

Patients who have undergone total lymphoid radiation treatment in preparation for bone marrow transplantation may show depletion of lymphoid follicles in Peyer patches. As a result, Peyer patches appear smaller than usual, but with a normal architecture. The follicular cells are reduced to a very small number of cells; T cells are almost completely absent. The lamina propria throughout the intestine appears hypocellular.

Acute lesions develop shortly after high-dose radiation exposure and usually affect individuals exposed during radiation accidents or atomic warfare. During the first few weeks following exposure there are aggressive mucositis, epithelial swelling, cytoplasmic vacuolization, and atypical multilobated nuclei and prominent nucleoli (47). If the exposure involves the entire body, including the bone marrow, then a neutrophilic response is often conspicuously absent (47). In the first 8 hours there is extensive cell death in the proliferative segment of the bowel and mitotic activity ceases. Maximum karyopyknosis and cellular sloughing occur in 6 to 8 hours. A transient proliferative burst, sometimes with atypical mitoses, occur between 8 and 24 hours. This ceases and the cells continue to migrate and desquamate without being replaced; this results in a progressive loss of the epithelial covering of the villi. Compensatory crypt hyperplasia develops, the villi become shorter, and the cells are retained longer before being desquamated (99). In spite of the compensatory mechanisms, the villi are denuded by 5 to 7 days and the individual dies of sepsis, hemorrhage, protein loss, and electrolyte loss (25).

Late effects of gastrointestinal radiation injury lead to *chronic irradiation enteritis*. This progressive disease results from underlying progressive fibrosis and vascular damage. Villi appear short and broad; there is atrophy of the muscularis propria with interstitial fibrosis. Characteristic changes of chronic radiation damage include the presence of telangiectasia and hyalinized blood vessels. Enterocyte nuclei appear larger than normal and exhibit atypical features such as stratification; there may be a relative increase in the number of endocrine cells (62). The submucosa appears irregularly fibrotic, and occasionally, there is distinct hypereosinophilic hyalinization of the collagen that may resemble amyloid (52,54). As the lesions evolve, the lamina propria and submucosa become increasingly fibrotic and the muscularis mucosae becomes hypertrophic (87). Fibrosis and parenchymal atrophy subsequently replace the tissues. Lymphangiectasia develops secondary to lymphatic obstruction, presumably due to the submucosal fibrosis. Epithelial displacement into the submucosa produces enteritis cystica profunda. Radiation fibroblasts are present in the deeper layers of the bowel wall. Neuronal proliferation and muscular changes are prominent in patients presenting with pseudoobstruction; the ganglion cells may appear bizarre.

Vascular alterations, which are random and focal and often require multiple sections to be seen, characterize late lesions. Vascular damage ranges from isolated endothelial cell injury to complete capillary and venule obliteration. Thrombosis can be seen as well as areas of fibrinoid necrosis. Focal acute vasculitis involves small arterioles, which may be heavily infiltrated with lymphocytes and neutrophils. Muscular arteries demonstrate marked intimal thickening, with fibrosis and luminal narrowing leading to endarteritis obliterans. Abnormal cell proliferation as well as the fibrosis of the vascular intima and media narrow the lumen and reduce blood flow to the bowel. Smaller vessels exhibit marked hyaline sclerosis and obliterative vasculitis. Progressive vascular damage, with increasing intimal fibrosis, leads to ischemia. The complications of the ischemia include strictures, perforation, fistulas, malabsorption, and pseudoobstruction (95).

Large Intestine. Large intestinal changes resemble small intestinal lesions. During acute injury, the characteristic changes usually remain confined to the mucosa. They include crypt cell damage, crypt abscesses, inflammatory cell infiltrates, nuclear atypia, reduced mitotic activity, loss of nuclear polarity, crypt loss, and mucosal sloughing (fig. 9-15). Eosinophils are often prominent. Other acute effects are cryptitis (fig. 9-16), prominent submucosal edema, ulcers, inflammatory polyps, mucosal telangiectasia, and sometimes ischemia. There may be glandular proliferation with mild cellular atypia. The changes may simulate dysplasia. Most of the changes resolve within a month, and although mild atrophy and inflammatory cells may remain up to 3 months following treatment cessation (74), they eventually regress.

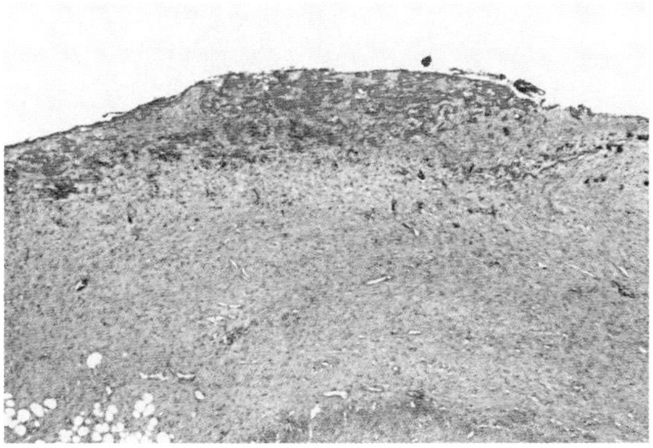

Figure 9-15

ACUTE RADIATION DAMAGE INVOLVING THE APPENDIX

The entire mucosa has sloughed, making the tissue completely unrecognizable.

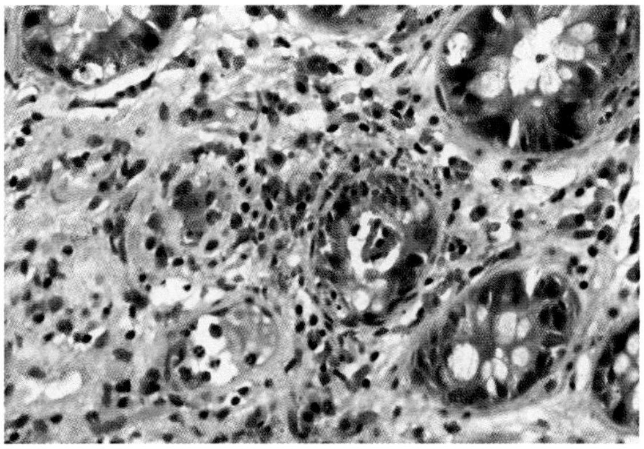

Figure 9-16

ACUTE RADIATION PROCTITIS

Individual crypts are disappearing while others have a heavy infiltration of acute inflammatory cells. Acute inflammation is also present in the lamina propria.

Mucosal lesions that develop in the delayed period include erosions, ulcers, perforations, fistulas, cytologic atypia, and neoplasia. Vascular changes include petechiae, hemorrhages, hyalinized arterioles, areas of healed necrosis in the vessels, thrombi, and fibrous intimal plaques. Stromal changes include submucosal fibrosis, leading to strictures, interstitial fibrosis of the muscularis propria, serosal fibrosis, and loss of sphincter control.

Chronic features include crypt architectural distortion with variable atrophy (fig. 9-17), goblet cell loss, shortened crypts, a thickened and distorted muscularis mucosae, epithelial atypia, intestinal wall fibrosis (fig. 9-18), serosal thickening, vascular sclerosis (fig. 9-19), lymphangiectasia, and thickening of the collagen layer beneath the surface and crypt epithelium (16,33). The changes may mimic collagenous colitis. Paneth cell metaplasia may be present. Marked hyalinization of the submucosal vessels (fig. 9-18) may mimic amyloidosis. Variable distortion of the intestinal wall results in glandular entrapment deep in the bowel wall, causing colitis cystica profunda, focal discontinuity of the muscularis mucosae, mucosal erosions, deep ulcers, vascular ectasia, and serosal thickening (24,26,54). The atypical nuclei in the displaced glands may simulate an invasive carcinoma. Submucosal neuronal proliferations and muscular degeneration also develop.

Biopsy features that suggest a diagnosis of radiation damage include the patchy nature of the process, marked telangiectasia, enlarged nuclei in either the epithelium or the stroma, and, if one is lucky enough to have submucosa in the biopsy, typical vascular changes sometimes associated with characteristic radiation fibroblasts. In other cases, the tissue appears nonspecifically chronically damaged. The lamina propria contains excessive numbers of chronic inflammatory cells. The fibroblasts have enlarged nuclei and the cytoplasm tends to become basophilic. The cells may acquire a swallow-tailed appearance. The arterioles often show intimal proliferation, sometimes with foamy endothelial cells, particularly earlier in the disease.

Late effects of radiation damage include mucosal, submucosal, and muscular fibrosis with stricture formation (fig. 9-20). Biopsies of the strictures typically show portions of distorted colorectal mucosa with fibrosis in the lamina propria and vascular dilatation.

Differential Diagnosis. The gross appearance of chronic radiation damage may resemble that of Crohn's disease but without fissures and without the creeping growth of the mesenteric fat. The gross appearance can also mimic a carcinoma. Histologic changes of radiation enteritis may mimic those seen in other diseases (Table 9-5). Radiation colitis mimics other large intestinal inflammatory disorders, including

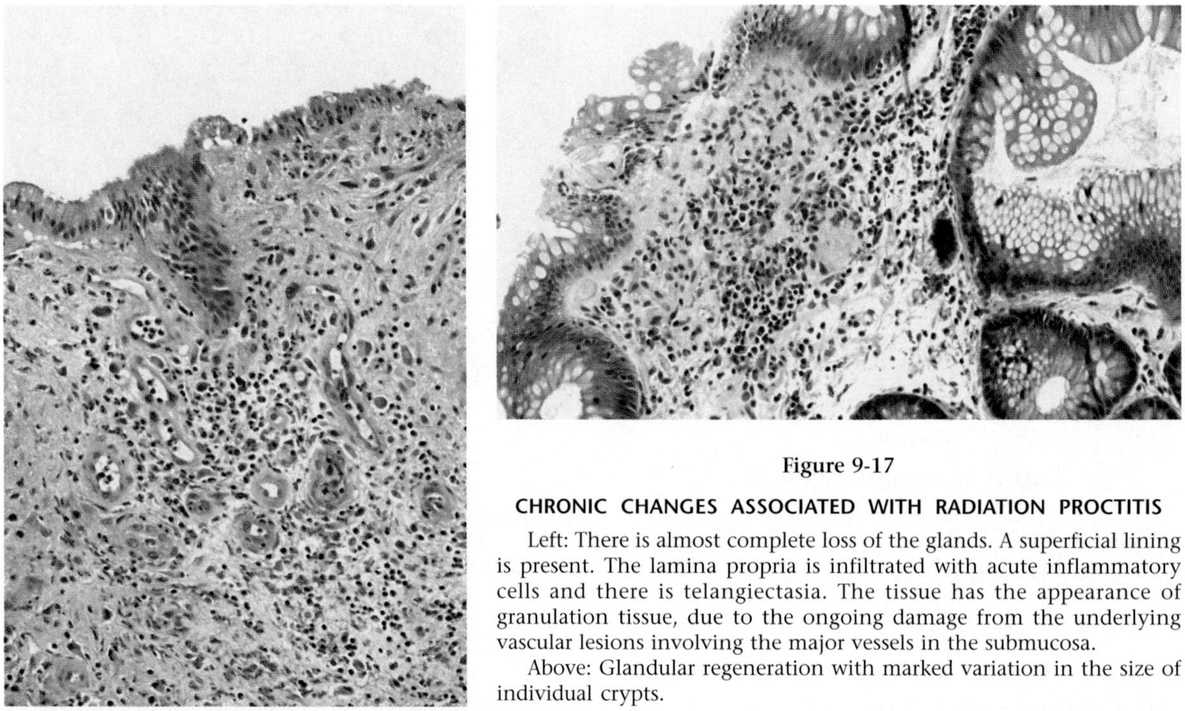

Figure 9-17

CHRONIC CHANGES ASSOCIATED WITH RADIATION PROCTITIS

Left: There is almost complete loss of the glands. A superficial lining is present. The lamina propria is infiltrated with acute inflammatory cells and there is telangiectasia. The tissue has the appearance of granulation tissue, due to the ongoing damage from the underlying vascular lesions involving the major vessels in the submucosa.

Above: Glandular regeneration with marked variation in the size of individual crypts.

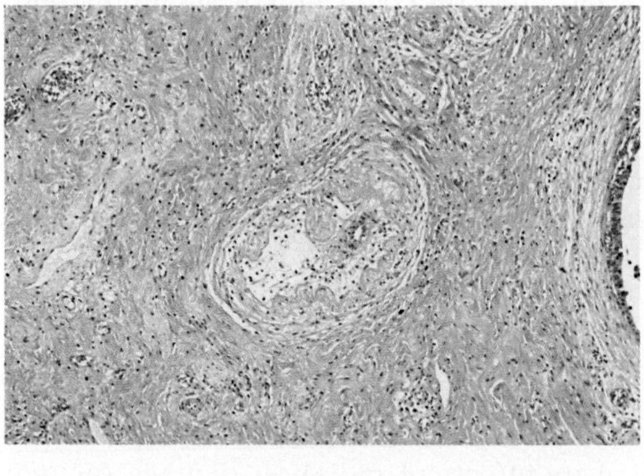

Figure 9-18

RADIATION-INDUCED SUBMUCOSAL FIBROSIS WITH MARKED VASCULAR CHANGES

The portion of an epithelial-lined structure on the right represents epithelium displaced into the submucosa. No lamina propria surrounds it.

infectious, microscopic, ischemic, or drug-induced colitis, as well as idiopathic inflammatory bowel disease, particularly if only a superficial biopsy is examined. The presence of macrocytosis can also be seen in patients with folic acid or vitamin B12 deficiency, or in patients receiving chemotherapy. If the collagen table underlying the large intestinal surface epithelium thickens, the differential diagnosis includes collagenous colitis. Tumors arising in radiation strictures sometimes mimic areas of colitis cystica profunda. The vascular damage to arterioles, myointimal hyperplasia, and subintimal collections of foamy macrophages may be seen in radiation damage, chronic allograft rejection with medial sclerosis, fibrinoid necrosis, and thrombosis in varying degrees and combinations (78). Because the mechanisms of radiation injury resemble those seen in ischemia and reperfusion injury, it is not surprising that the histologic features of both ischemia and radiation injury resemble one another.

Treatment and Prognosis. Given the recent surge in terrorist activities, which could involve the use of radioactive material, scenarios have been developed for dealing with such acts. A consensus document was developed by the Strategic National Stockpile Radiation Working Group (96) to provide a framework for physicians in medical subspecialties for evaluation and management of large-scale radiation injuries. Since this is not the major emphasis of this text, the reader is referred to the document prepared by this group for further details.

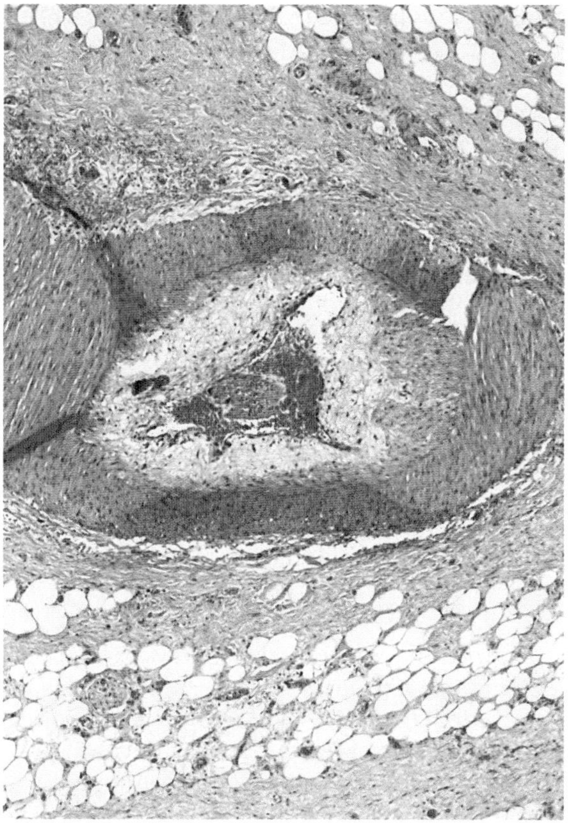

Figure 9-19

RADIATION-INDUCED VASCULAR DAMAGE

Radiation-induced vascular damage affects not only the vessels of the submucosa but also the perirectal tissues. Marked fibroblastic proliferation and edema affect the intima and media.

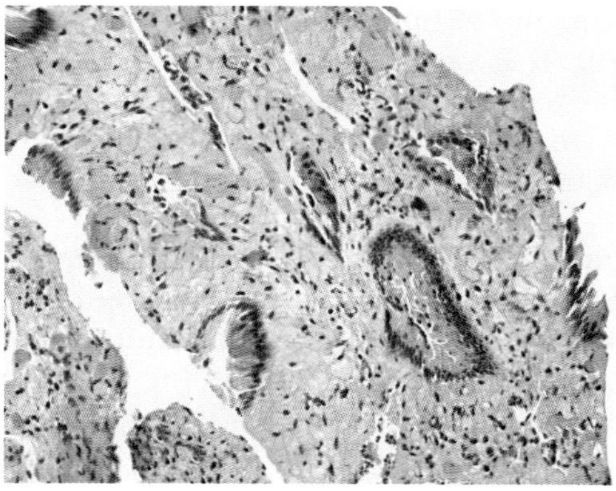

Figure 9-20

LATE EFFECTS FOLLOWING RADIATION

Biopsy from a rectal stricture in a patient who had received radiotherapy for prostate cancer many years previously. The lamina propria is completely fibrotic.

A tremendous amount of effort has been directed at reducing the harmful effects of radiation. These include careful planning of radiation fields, surgical procedures to elevate and keep the small bowel away from radiation fields, and the use of substances such as prostaglandin inhibitors and sulfhydryl and thiol compounds, an emphasis on diets high in polyunsaturated fats, and attempted reduction of bile and/or pancreatic enzymes in the intestinal contents. These efforts sometimes are helpful, but sometimes they contribute to further injury. Therefore these strategies are under continual investigation, particularly the surgical interventions.

Numerous agents, including antimicrobials, local and systemic analgesics, antiinflammatory drugs, antidiarrheal drugs, and mucosal protectives (11), alone or in combination with dietetic care, have been used or are being evaluated for the palliation of radiation-induced gastrointestinal symptoms. Argon plasma coagulation may play a role in control of hemorrhagic

Table 9-5

CONDITIONS THAT MIMIC RADIATION ENTEROPATHY

Celiac disease
Infectious gastroenteritis
Cow's milk intolerance
Soy or soy protein sensitivity
Malnutrition
Kwashiorkor
Microvillous inclusion disease
Familial enteropathy
Collagenous sprue
Graft versus host disease
Common variable immunodeficiency
Acquired immunodeficiency syndrome (AIDS) enteropathy
Crohn's disease
Eosinophilic gastroenteritis
Zollinger-Ellison syndrome
Dermatitis herpetiformis
Lymphoma
Ischemic enteritis
Drug effects
Autoimmune enteritis

lesions in the setting of radiation-induced injury (86). These agents often increase the quality of life for patients subjected to radiotherapy. The mainstay of medical therapy has been sulfasalazine, steroids applied orally and per rectum, and bile acid sequestering resins.

Sucralfate, an aluminum hydroxide complex of sulfated sucrose used in the treatment of gastric ulcers, prevents some radiation-induced bowel discomfort or rectal bleeding (11,35). Sucralfate is also useful in treating radiation-induced mucositis (35,50,82,90). Topical sucralfate induces lasting remissions in many patients (43). Octreotide is often used to manage radiation-induced diarrhea in cancer patients (3). It reduces the acute mucosal changes and markedly ameliorates acute mucosal injury as well as subsequent chronic structural alterations (94). Growth hormone is sometimes used to modify the response of the intestinal mucosa to radiation through its effect on the cell cycle or by increasing cell mass (66). Supplemental dietary arginine accelerates intestinal mucosal regeneration (31). Glutamine administration is currently under investigation in clinical trials (72). Formalin instillation and endoscopic obliterative therapy are sometimes used to control the bleeding that results from radiation-induced telangiectasias (21). Symptomatic strictures may be amenable to endoscopic dilation, and stent placement may have a role for those who experience frequent restricturing and those with unremitting fistulas. Radiation strictures in the colon and elsewhere (esophagus, small bowel) are particularly resistant to endoscopic dilation, often requiring repeat interventions that result in a significant perforation rate.

Surgical treatment of large bowel radiation injury can cause substantial morbidity but can be successful in patients with strictures, perforations, or fistulas. The success rates are worst after fistula repair (67). Arteriodigestive fistulas may complicate intraoperative and external beam therapy following surgery for gastric cancer.

A long-term consequence of radiation exposure is cancer development. An excess in cancer-related deaths was first noted in victims of atomic bomb exposure (80). Most of these effects are non-gastrointestinal but cancer can develop at any gastrointestinal site that has been irradiated, including the esophagus (5,20,40,79), stomach (40), or colon (49,73,79,89). The cancers include adenocarcinomas, squamous cell cancers (92), and sarcomas, including malignant fibrous histiocytoma or angiosarcoma (4,12,53,56,75,84,93,100). The neoplasms follow exposure to both low and medium radiation doses, and they develop after a long latency period (40,66). Women radiated for gynecologic cancers have a relative risk of subsequent colorectal cancer of 2.0 to 3.6 (68). Diagnostic criteria to establish a radiation-induced tumor include the following: 1) the tumor must arise in the irradiated field; 2) it must be histologically different from the tumor that was radiated; and 3) there must be a latency period of at least 2 years. The latency period ranges from 37 months to 50 years (4,9,53,100). Malakoplakia may also develop in previous radiation fields.

THERMAL INJURY

Definition. *Thermal injury* follows exposure to temperature extremes. Most examples of gastrointestinal thermal injury result from exposure to excessive heat. Burn victims develop gastrointestinal *mucosal stress ulcers* (*Curling ulcers*).

Demography. Thermal injury to the gastrointestinal tract results from two major categories of exposure: gastrointestinal damage that occurs in burn victims and localized damage to the gastrointestinal tract from the consumption of hot fluids, as a result of therapeutic interventions using cautery, or along bullet tracks sustained from gunshot wounds (113,115). Gauchos, the original cattle herders of Argentina, were particularly fond of drinking hot maté in a way that burned the esophageal mucosa, thereby leading to the development of esophagitis and eventually esophageal carcinoma (113,115). There is an increasing possibility of gastrointestinal thermal injury from the use of laparoscopic procedures to remove gastrointestinal tissues or to perform other forms of pelvic or intra-abdominal procedures.

Pathophysiology. During the shock that follows severe burns, the blood volume decreases and blood flow shunts away from the gastrointestinal tract. When burns involve more than 20 percent of the total body surface area, the diversion of the blood flow causes gastrointestinal functions to diminish or stop entirely, leading to ileus and gastrointestinal dysmotility.

The gastrointestinal erosions seen in severely burned patients have an ischemic basis and their pathophysiology resembles that of stress ulcers. They occur within 5 hours of injury (107) and result in enterocyte membrane disruption and mucosal barrier breakdown (109). This is mediated in part by transient intestinal hypoperfusion and increased intestinal permeability with increased transcellular permeability (103,107). The damaged mucosal barrier allows macromolecules to be absorbed (101,103,104,106) and bacteria to translocate from the gut. Bacterial and luminal endotoxins gain access to the systemic circulation (104,115,116). Systemic infections may also alter the integrity of the bowel and make the patient less tolerant of enteral feedings (111). Gastric distension is common due to delayed gastric emptying.

Clinical Features. Gastrointestinal disorders, including gastric and duodenal ulcers (see fig. 9-22), ileus, constipation, and diarrhea (110), are common in burn patients. Severe burns lead to a disruption in the gastrointestinal mucosal integrity and facilitate bacterial translocation. Patients with hypotensive episodes and sepsis are at risk for developing ischemic bowel disease. Those who develop ischemia have a statistically significant larger percentage of total burned surface area compared to those with other gastrointestinal complications. Hemorrhage results from the ulcers and ischemic bowel and rarely, perforations also develop. Curling ulcers develop in 11 to 86 percent of patients who do not receive ulcer prophylaxis.

Acute pseudoobstruction is a rare complication of burns. Factors implicated in its pathogenesis include bed rest, the use of narcotic medications, hypokalemia, sepsis, and surgery (108). Early diagnosis, the use of prokinetic and cathartic agents, and attempts at decompression are essential in patients who develop acute pseudoobstruction. There is an increased risk of sepsis and thrombotic complications from parenteral hyperalimentation in burn patients. The severely elevated intraabdominal pressure associated with pseudoobstruction sometimes requires surgical treatment by laparotomy to avert cardiac, respiratory, and renal compromise (112).

Gross Findings. Curling ulcers are large, dark, irregular, geographic mucosal defects (fig. 9-21).

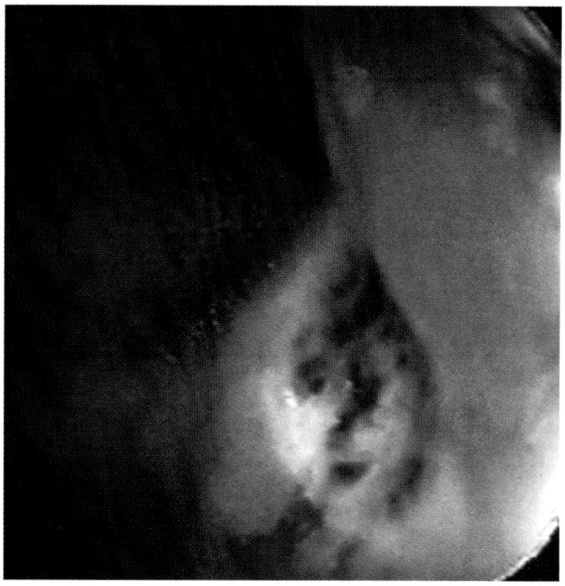

Figure 9-21

CURLING ULCER

A well-circumscribed, punched-out defect is in the duodenal mucosa. The surrounding mucosa is hyperemic.

Smaller punctate ulcers are also present. The duodenal mucosa is markedly hyperemic.

Microscopic Findings. The microscopic features of Curling ulcers resemble those of peptic ulcers, stress ulcers, or ischemic ulcers, depending upon the stage of development.

Probably the most common form of thermal injury that pathologists encounter is that secondary to cautery. Cautery may be part of the biopsy procedure itself or may represent secondary effects from inadvertent injury during laparoscopic procedures. Typically, there is evidence of coagulation necrosis (fig. 9-22).

Treatment and Prognosis. Enteral nutritional support is the primary mode of treatment in patients with severe surface burns. Prophylactic introduction of antacids, mucosal protective agents, and nutritional supplements, as well as H2 blockers may help prevent the gastric injury. Intravenous proton pump inhibitors may become the standard of care in the future. Surgery may be necessary in patients with ischemia, intractable hemorrhage, perforation, or pseudoobstruction (108). Treatment with bombesin helps restore the mucosal barrier of the burned gut by increasing biliary secretory IgA levels and

Figure 9-22

CAUTERY DAMAGE

A: Mild cautery damage to the gastrointestinal mucosa. The epithelium tends to be preferentially affected and the cells become elongated, with nuclei appearing to stream like a school of fish.

B: Another area of injury due to cautery with marked edema.

C: Intense coagulation necrosis of the submucosa at the base of a mucosal biopsy.

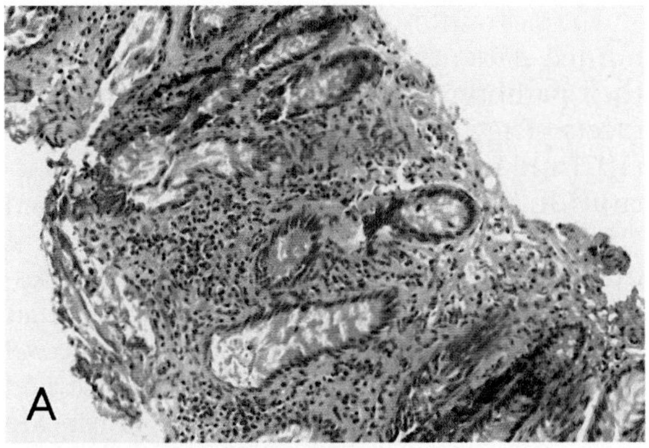

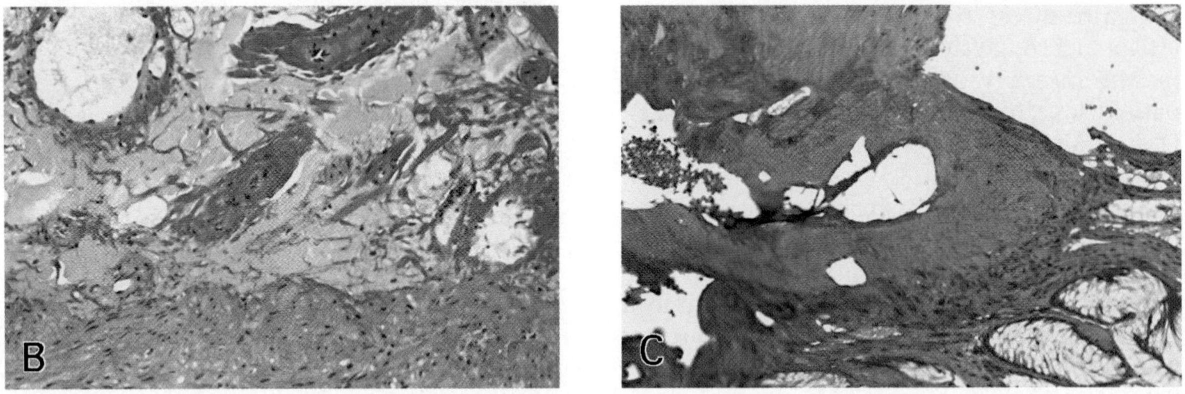

increasing mucosal height (105). Butyrate also hastens the restoration of barrier function (114).

Animal Models. Administration of epidermal growth factor in burned rodents attenuates the internal organ damage. It significantly reduces intestinal necrosis (102).

Electrical Injury

Definition. *Electrical injury* is a unique form of thermal damage. The extreme heat generated by tissue resistance to the passage of a high voltage electrical current (1,000 volts or more), the unpredictable course of electricity through the body, and the variation in response of individual tissues separates these injuries from other types of thermal injury.

Demography. Major electrical burns constitute approximately 3 percent of all admissions to major burn centers (117). Approximately one third of high voltage injuries affect electrical workers, one third occur in construction workers, and the remainder result from nonworker home accidents. An exceptional case of death from electrocution complicated autoerotic stimulation (119). Thermal injury also results from lightning strikes.

Pathophysiology. Electrical injuries cause disruption of cardiac rhythm and breathing, burns, gastrointestinal injury, vascular damage, disseminated intravascular coagulation, and peripheral and spinal cord injury. Some of the gastrointestinal damage occurs directly and some occurs indirectly. Damage to the central or peripheral nervous system can cause pseudoobstruction. Massive gastrointestinal hemorrhage may result from duodenal or gastric ulcers. Segmental esophageal aperistalsis may follow esophageal injury (120).

Clinical Features. Many electrical injuries involve the skin so that treatment requires attention to these direct wounds. The complications of electrical injuries can also affect almost every organ, including the gastrointestinal tract. There may be direct injury to intraabdominal structures from abdominal contact points. In both lightning and high voltage injuries, impaired mental status often means that the patient cannot complain of the abdominal pain.

Transient segmental aperistalsis may develop in the distal esophagus (122). There may also be abdominal wall and gastric perforation (121). Intraabdominal injury is ruled out by peritoneal lavage, CT scan, laparotomy, or ultrasonography. Ileus can lead to abdominal distension, vomiting, and aspiration. Patients may have long-term gastrointestinal functional abnormalities, which include increasing stool frequency and urgency. Inner anal sphincter control may remain abnormal (118).

Gross Findings. The presence of submucosal hemorrhages scattered throughout the gastrointestinal tract is the most frequent finding in electrical injury. Curling ulcers may be present. Other injuries include gastric necrosis with general intestinal necrosis and intestinal perforation (119,121). If the thermal injury causes disseminated intravascular coagulation, then ischemia may affect any part of the gastrointestinal tract.

Microscopic Findings. The histologic findings often resemble those of ischemic injury.

Treatment and Prognosis. The residual effects of electric injury are frequent and often unapparent for months. Late complications often result in recurrent dysfunction of the gastrointestinal tract. A nasogastric tube is useful in preventing distension, vomiting, and aspiration. Use of antacids and H2 blockers decreases the incidence of duodenal and gastric stress ulcers. Bleeding gastrointestinal lesions are managed in a similar manner to other stress-related mucosal lesions.

TRAUMA AND HEMATOMAS

Definition. Physical injuries are classified as penetrating and blunt injuries. *Perforations* are defects involving less than 20 percent of the luminal circumference, *lacerations* involve between 20 and 70 percent of the luminal circumference, and *disruptions* involve over 70 percent of the luminal circumference (128).

Demography. Hollow visceral injuries are far less common with blunt abdominal trauma than with penetrating abdominal trauma: more than 95 percent of intestinal injuries are penetrating. The nature of the penetrating agent varies and includes gunshot and stab wounds, iatrogenic injuries, automobile accidents, and war wounds, in a decreasing order of incidence. Blunt trauma injury to the small bowel is most common, followed by injury to the colon and stomach. Colonic trauma accounts for only 3 to 5 percent of blunt abdominal injuries (129); most affect the descending colon, ascending colon, or cecum (129,135).

Blunt abdominal injuries usually result from motor vehicle or athletic accidents, falls, physical abuse, or cardiopulmonary resuscitation (130, 132). Hemophiliacs, patients with von Willebrand's disease, and patients with idiopathic thrombocytopenic purpura, as well as those on drugs that decrease the number of platelets such as chemotherapeutic agents, are at increased risk for hematomas following trauma. Blunt abdominal trauma causes rupture of hollow gastrointestinal organs in 11 to 18 percent of patients (136). The midabdomen is particularly vulnerable to direct blows and results in compression injuries to viscera anatomically fixed against the spine. The most common mechanism of traumatic bowel or mesenteric injury in children is motor vehicle accidents. Children are particularly prone to lap belt injuries (124). Other common mechanisms of pediatric injury include being hit by a car, bicycle handlebar injuries, and child abuse. Visceral trauma is the second leading cause of death in child abuse after central nervous system injury.

Gastrointestinal hematomas most commonly result from trauma or occur in patients with underlying coagulopathies or who are on anticoagulation therapy (131). In the esophagus, hematomas complicate esophageal tears (Mallory-Weiss tears) and perforation of the esophageal wall (Boerhaave's syndrome). Other predisposing factors include recurrent vomiting and episodes of food impaction (126). Hematomas also result from surgical or endoscopic intervention.

Trauma may also result from the use of enema tubes or the insertion of various objects into the rectum for sexual gratification. Lacerations, abrasions, and perforations lead to exsanguinating hemorrhage, especially if the foreign bodies are inserted when the patient is under the influence of illicit psychoactive drugs or excessive alcohol consumption. Lacerations also occur in severe impactions.

Tubes or foreign bodies in the esophagus cause local irritation, ulceration, and acute inflammation. Pill esophagitis occurs when medications

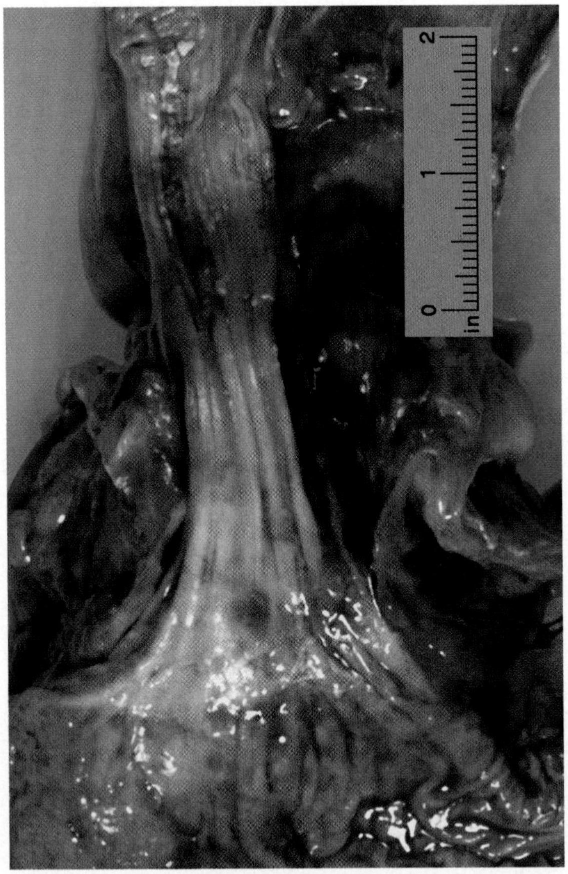

Figure 9-23

ESOPHAGEAL LACERATION

Esophageal laceration in an individual who was involved in a motor vehicle accident. It extends down into the submucosa. The upper muscularis propria was involved but it was not a full-thickness injury.

become stuck in the esophagus (see chapter 8). Diaphragmatic eventrations also result from trauma, as in automobile accidents. Some runners develop an entity called cecal flap syndrome, which is repeated microtrauma to the cecum as it hits against a hypertrophic muscular wall.

Pathophysiology. The extent of gastrointestinal damage varies with the cause. The pathologic spectrum ranges from hematomas to full-thickness lacerations that, if not repaired, lead to fistulas, perforation, and peritonitis.

Clinical Features. Patients with esophageal hematomas may present with pain high in the epigastrium or retrosternal region, which is aggravated by swallowing. The pain may be accompanied by vomiting or hematemesis. Larger hematomas cause dysphagia, occasionally in the absence of pain (126). These hematomas may follow instrumentation.

Most alert patients have physical findings suggestive of mediastinal or peritoneal irritation, with tenderness or guarding. Symptoms of peritoneal irritation include abdominal pain, tenderness, and rigidity, and usually occur following rupture. Vomiting due to obstruction occurs in patients with large hematomas. A palpable mass may be found. The clinical features depend on the size of the hematoma and include acute or chronic pain, obstruction, bleeding, anemia, and hemoperitoneum (123,125). The most accurate and safest abdominal assessment methods in hemodynamically unstable individuals with suspected abdominal injuries following blunt trauma are immediate laparotomy and diagnostic peritoneal lavage, and CT evaluation (134). Trauma may also lead to acute pseudoobstruction.

Rare spontaneous retroperitoneal or mesenteric hemorrhage involves the root of the small bowel mesentery. It is characterized by severe bleeding into the retroperitoneum or intraperitoneum. Its clinical presentation depends on the exact site of the bleeding. In most cases, hemorrhage from large vessels follows an acute course and patients have abrupt abdominal pain with severe blood loss or hemorrhagic shock. Such hemorrhages usually resolve spontaneously or they may go undetected. The etiology of these lesions is uncertain. Predisposing factors include hypertension, arteriosclerosis, arterial malformations, inflammation, and anticoagulant therapy or underlying coagulation disorders.

Gastrobronchial or esophagobronchial fistulas complicate trauma. Esophageal rupture or laceration sometimes complicates motor vehicle accidents (fig. 9-23). Gastric rupture is an unusual catastrophe following blunt trauma or cardiopulmonary resuscitation. The lesser curvature of the stomach is the most frequent site of traumatic rupture because of its fixed character and its position anterior to the vertebral bodies. The antrum is also in danger because of its intermediate position between the mobile body and fundus and the fixed pylorus (130). Tears tend to be larger on the serosal side than on the mucosal side because the initial disruption, even in blunt trauma, is the muscular coat and the mucosa is only secondarily involved

(130). The anterior wall is more often affected than the posterior wall (132,136).

Gross and Radiologic Findings. CT scans are useful in demonstrating esophageal hematomas, which are viewed as esophageal masses with a density similar to that of blood. A typical barium contrast study usually shows an indentation into the esophageal lumen, but occasionally may reveal a false lumen. CT findings in children with bowel or mesenteric trauma include free intraperitoneal air, free retroperitoneal air, extraluminal oral contrast material, free intraperitoneal fluid, bowel wall defect, bowel wall thickening, mesenteric stranding, fluid at the mesenteric root, focal hematoma, active hemorrhage, and mesenteric pseudoaneurysm. Occasionally, angiography is required to identify the responsible vessel should hematomas enlarge or reaccumulate following initial evacuation. Some radiologic findings, such as free intraperitoneal air and focal bowel wall thickening, are associated with a strong likelihood that the bowel injury will require surgical repair.

The seromuscular tear is the hallmark of intestinal injury due to seatbelt syndrome and is an unambiguous lesion similar in all segments of the bowel. It is caused by a tear that separates the inner muscularis from the submucosa. It is characterized by a wedge that strips the mucosa from the inner circular muscle; a bending retraction of the torn muscularis toward the uninvolved bowel; and mucosal-submucosal fold effacement causing the mucosal-submucosal bridge spanning the tear to become paper thin. The vulnerability of this bridge to ischemia is such that 35 percent of tears culminate in incipient or frank perforations or gangrene (133). Large seromuscular tears, particularly the circumferential degloving type, are most prone to these complications. Tears cluster in three major sites: the ileocecal region, the sigmoid, and the jejunum. Perforations are the principal lesion in the jejunum and seromuscular tears at the other locations. Multiple sites are commonly affected in individual patients. This suggests the simultaneous action of different traumatic mechanisms on the bowel and its mesenteries in seatbelt injuries sustained during motor vehicle accidents (133).

Hematomas complicate blunt trauma if a blood vessel is damaged and the blood does not

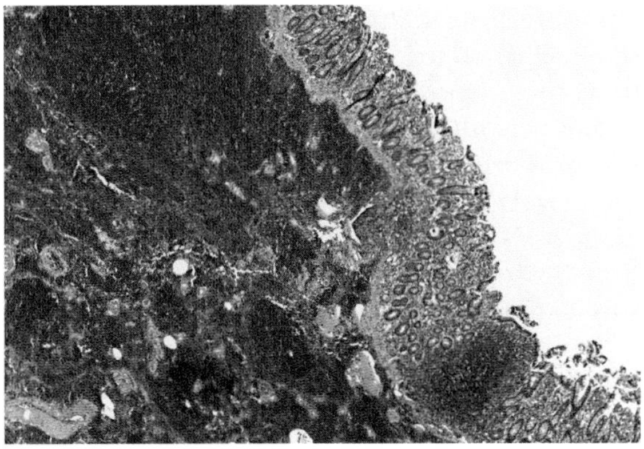

Figure 9-24

SUBMUCOSAL HEMATOMA

Submucosal hematoma in a patient injured in a motor vehicle accident. Large amounts of extravasated red blood cells are within the submucosa. There is no evidence of organization.

gain access to the bowel lumen. The diagnosis of a hematoma is suggested radiographically by mass effects or unusual fold patterns. CT shows the presence of a high-density intramural mass. If the blood gains access to the bowel lumen, then the bowel wall appears grossly normal but contains large amounts of fresh blood. Patients with gunshot wounds have lacerations in the tissue and hemorrhage.

Microscopic Findings. The histologic changes associated with trauma depend on whether the tissue is examined during an acute phase or after repeated traumatic episodes. Acutely, there is hemorrhage and possibly inflammation, depending on the age of the injury. If repeated trauma has occurred, mucosal distortion may be present. The tissue along bullet paths demonstrates coagulation injury. Patients who have prolonged intubation may show esophageal hyperkeratosis or parakeratosis. Patients with hematomas typically have collections of extravasated red blood cells in the submucosa (fig. 9-24). Patients with lacerations often have mucosal tears that variably extend through the wall of the affected gastrointestinal segment.

Treatment and Prognosis. As endoscopists are loath to biopsy bleeding lesions, endoscopic biopsies are seldom performed in the acute setting. Those patients who continue to experience significant bleeding despite therapeutic endoscopic intervention may require radiologic embolization or surgery. Unfortunately, endoscopic interventions may result in trauma to bowel, e.g., postpolypectomy hemorrhage or bowel perforation. Fortunately, the majority of the bleeding complications are managed conservatively or endoscopically, and perforations diagnosed early before peritoneal contamination has occurred may be treated by primary surgical closure.

Perforation as a result of blunt abdominal trauma is usually treated by simple closure followed by resection and anastomosis, or simple closure plus the creation of a proximal ostomy (127). Surgical evacuation is necessary only for large hematomas; smaller hematomas resolve spontaneously. Surgical intervention is required if rupture occurs. Mortality is influenced by the time interval between the injury and the surgical intervention. Complications include fistulas, obstruction, sepsis, and peritonitis. Antibiotics are used in patients with penetrating wounds. In patients with multiorgan trauma, as in automobile accidents or other severe injuries, death may not be the result of gastrointestinal wounds but of central nervous system injury or injuries to other vital organs, such as liver, spleen, and pancreas.

Management of esophageal hematoma is conservative. Intravenous fluids and analgesics usually cause symptoms to remit within a few days. Surgery is occasionally required for late perforation or uncontrolled bleeding.

REFERENCES

General References

Fajardo LF, Berthrong M, Anderson R. Radiation pathology. New York: Oxford University Press; 2001.

Radiation-Induced Injury

1. Anseline PF, Lavery IC, Fazio VW, Jagelman DG, Weakley FL. Radiation injury of the rectum: evaluation of surgical treatment. Ann Surg 1981;194:716–24.
2. Anderson RE, Witkowski LJ, Pontius GV. Radiation stricture of the small intestine. Surgery 1955;38:605–9.
3. Baillie-Johnson HR. Octreotide in the management of treatment-related diarrhoea. Anticancer Drugs 1996;1:11–5.
4. Ben-Izhak O, Kerner H, Brenner B, Lichtig C. Angiosarcoma of the colon developing in a capsule of a foreign body. Report of a case with associated hemorrhagic diathesis. Am J Clin Pathol 1992;97:416–20.
5. Biological effects of ionizing radiation: the effects on populations of exposure to low levels of ionizing radiation. Washington DC: National Academy of Sciences; 1980:431.
6. Black WC, Gomez LS, Yuhas JM, Kligerman MM. Quantitation of the late effects of x-radiation on the large intestine. Cancer 1980;45:444–51.
7. Boudiaf M, Soyer P, Pelage JP, et al. CT of radiation-induced injury of the gastrointestinal tract: spectrum of findings with barium studies correlation. Eur Radiol 2000;10:920–5.
8. Canney PA, Dean S. Transforming growth factor beta: a promotor of late connective tissue injury following radiotherapy? Br J Radiol 1990;63:620–3.
9. Chen KT, Hoffman KD, Hendricks EJ. Angiosarcoma following therapeutic irradiation. Cancer 1979;44:2044–8.
10. Chen S, Harisinghani MG, Wittenberg J. Small bowel CT fat density target sign in chronic radiation enteritis. Australas Radiol 2003;47:450–2.
11. Chun M, Kang S, Kil HJ, Oh YT, Sohn JH, Ryu HS. Rectal bleeding and its management after irradiation for uterine cervical cancer. Int J Radiat Oncol Biol Phys 2004;58:98–105.
12. Coia LR, Myerson RJ, Tepper JE. Late effects of radiation therapy on the gastrointestinal tract. Int J Radiat Oncol Biol Phys 1995;31:1213–36.
13. Costleigh BJ, Miyamoto CT, Micaily B, Brady LW. Heightened sensitivity of the esophagus to radiation in a patient with AIDS. Am J Gastroenterol 1995;90:812–4.
14. Crowe J, Stellato TA. Radiation-induced solitary rectal ulcer. Dis Colon Rectum 1985;28:610–2.
15. Danielsson A, Nyhlin H, Persson H, Stendahl U, Stenling R, Suhr O. Chronic diarrhoea after radiotherapy for gynaecological cancer: occurrence and aetiology. Gut 1991;32:1180–7.
16. DeCosse JJ, Rhodes RS, Wentz WB, Reagan JW, Dworken HJ, Holden WD. The natural history and management of radiation induced injury of the gastrointestinal tract. Ann Surg 1969;170:369–84.

17. De Sagher LI, Van den Heule B, Van Houtte P, Engelholm L, Balikdjan D, Bleiberg H. Endoscopic appearance of irradiated gastric mucosa. Endoscopy 1979;3:163–5.
18. De Villa VH, Calvo FA, Bilbao JI, et al. Arteriodigestive fistula: a complication associated with intraoperative and external beam radiotherapy following surgery for gastric cancer. J Surg Oncol 1992;49:52–7.
19. Deitel M, Vasic V. Major intestinal complications of radiotherapy. Am J Gastroenterol 1979; 72:65–70.
20. Doll R. Radiation hazards: 25 years of collaborative research. Br J Radiol 1981;54:179–86.
21. Donner CS. Pathophysiology and therapy of chronic radiation-induced injury to the colon. Dig Dis 1998;16:253–61.
22. Dubner D, Gisone P, Jaitovich I, Perez M. Free radicals production and estimation of oxidative stress related to gamma irradiation. Biol Trace Element Res 1995;47:265–70.
23. Dunn MM, Drab EA, Rubin DB. Effects of irradiation on endothelial cell-polymorphonuclear leukocyte interactions. J Appl Physiol 1986;60:1932–7.
24. Epstein SE, Ascari WQ, Ablow RC, Seaman WB, Lattes R. Colitis cystica profunda. Am J Clin Pathol 1966;45:186–201.
25. Fajardo LF. Pathology of radiation injury. Paris, New York: Masson; 1982.
26. Gardiner GW, McAuliffe N, Murray D. Colitis cystica profunda occurring in a radiation-induced colonic stricture. Hum Pathol 1984;15: 295–8.
27. Goldgraber MB, Rubin CE, Palmer WL, Dobson RL, Massey BW. The early gastric response to irradiation. Gastroenterology 1954;27:1–20.
28. Goldman H, Szabo S. Chemical and physical disorders. In: Ming SC, Goldman H, eds. Pathology of the gastrointestinal tract. Philadelphia: WB Saunders; 1992:141.
29. Goldstein HM, Rogers LF, Fletcher GF, Dodd GD. Radiological manifestations of radiation-induced injury to the normal upper gastrointestinal tract. Radiology 1975;117:135–40.
30. Greco FA, Brereton HD, Kent H, Zimbler H, Merrill J, Johnson RE. Adriamycin and enhanced radiation reaction in normal esophagus and skin. Ann Intern Med 1976;85:294–8.
31. Gurbuz AT, Kunzelman J, Ratzer EE. Supplemental dietary arginine accelerates intestinal mucosal regeneration and enhances bacterial clearance following radiation enteritis in rats. J Surg Res 1998;74:149–54.
32. Harling H, Balslev I. Long-term prognosis of patients with severe radition enteritis. Am J Surg 1988;155:517–9.
33. Hasleton PS, Carr N, Schofield PF. Vascular changes in radiation bowel disease. Histopathology 1985;9:517–34.
34. Hauer-Jensen M. Late radiation injury of the intestine. Clinical, pathophysiological and radiobiological aspects. A review. Acta Oncol 1990;92:401–15.
35. Henriksson R, Bergstrom P, Franzen L, Lewin F, Wagenius G. Aspects on reducing gastrointestinal adverse effects associated with radiotherapy. Acta Oncol 1999;38:159–64.
36. Holahan EV. Cellular radiation biology. In: Conklin JJ, Walker RI, eds. Military radiobiology. New York: Academic Press; 1987:87.
37. Husebye E, Hauer-Jensen M, Kjorstad K, Skar V. Severe late radiation enteropathy is characterized by impaired motility of proximal small intestine. Dig Dis Sci 1994;39:2341–9.
38. Husebye E, Skar V, Hoverstad T, Iversen T, Melby K. Abnormal intestinal motor patterns explain enteric colonization with gram-negative bacilli in late radiation enteropathy. Gastroenterology 1995;109:1078–89.
39. Indaram AV, Visvalingam V, Locke M, Bank S. Mucosal cytokine production in radiation-induced proctosigmoiditis compared with inflammatory bowel disease. Am J Gastroenterol 2000; 95:1221–5.
40. Kato H, Schull WJ. Studies of the mortality of A-bomb survivors. 7. Mortality, 1950-1978: Part I. Cancer mortality. Radiat Res 1982;90:395–432.
41. Kimura H, Wu NZ, Dodge R, et al. Inhibition of radiation-induced up-regulation of leukocyte adhesion to endothelial cells with the platelet-activating factor inhibitor, BN52021. Int J Radiat Oncol Biol Phys 1995;33:627–33.
42. Kinsella TJ, Bloomer WD. Tolerance of the intestine to radiation therapy. Surg Gynecol Obstet 1980;151:273–84.
43. Kochhar R, Sriram PV, Sharma SC, Goel RC, Patel F. Natural history of late radiation proctosigmoiditis treated with topical sucralfate suspension. Dig Dis Sci 1999;44:973–8.
44. Konturek SJ, Konturek JW. Gastric adaptation: basic and clinical aspects. Digestion 1994;55: 131–8.
45. Radiation-induced proctosigmoiditis. Lancet 1983;1:1082–3.
46. Langberg CW, Waldron JA, Baker ML, Hauer-Jensen M. Significance of overall treatment time for the development of radiation induced intestinal complications. An experimental study in the rat. Cancer 1994;73:2663–8.
47. Liebow AA, Warren S, DeCoursey E. Pathology of atomic bomb casualties. Am J Pathol 1949; 25:853–1028.
48. Maj JG, Paris F, Haimovitz-Friedman A, Venkatraman E, Kolesnick R, Fuks Z. Microvascular function regulates intestinal crypt response to radiation. Cancer Res 2003;63:4338–41.

49. Martins A, Sternberg SS, Attiyeh FF. Radiation-induced carcinoma of the rectum. Dis Colon Rectum 1980;23:572–5.
50. Meredith R, Salter M, Kim R, et al. Sucralfate for radiation mucositis: results of a double-blind randomised trial. Int J Radiat Oncol Biol Phys 1997;37:275–9.
51. Moore JV, Broadbent DA. Survival of intestinal crypts after treatment by adriamycin alone or with radiation. Br J Cancer 1980;42:692–6.
52. Mulholland MW, Levitt SH, Song CW, Potish RA, Delaney JP. The role of luminal contents in radiation enteritis. Cancer 1984;54:2396–402.
53. Nanus DM, Kelsen D, Clark DG. Radiation-induced angiosarcoma. Cancer 1987;60:777–9.
54. Ng W, Chan K. Postirradiation colitis cystica profunda. Case report and literature review. Arch Pathol Lab Med 1995;119:1170–3.
55. Novak JM, Collins JT, Donowitz M, Farman J, Sheahan DH, Spiro HM. Effects of radiation on the human gastrointestinal tract. J Clin Gastroenterol 1979;1:9–39.
56. Ordonez NG, del Junco GW, Ayala AG, Ahmed N. Angiosarcoma of the small intestine: an immunoperoxidase study. Am J Gastroenterol 1983;78:218–21.
57. Panès J, Anderson DC, Miyasaka M, Granger DN. Role of leukocyte-endothelial cell adhesion in radiation-induced microvascular dysfunction in rats. Gastroenterology 1995;108:1761–9.
58. Panès J, Granger DN. Neutrophils generate oxygen free radicals in rat mesenteric microcirculation after abdominal irradiation. Gastroenterology 1996;111:981–9.
59. Perino LE, Schuffler MD, Mehta SJ, Everson GT. Radiation induced intestinal pseudoobstruction. Gastroenterology 1986;91:994–8.
60. Papazian A, Capron JP, Ducroix JP, Dupas JL, Quenum C, Besson P. Mucosal bridges of the upper esophagus after radiotherapy for Hodgkin's disease. Gastroenterology 1983;84:1028–31.
61. Paris F, Fuks Z, Kang A, et al. Endothelial apoptosis as the primary lesion initiating intestinal radiation damage in mice. Science 2001;293:293–7.
62. Pietroletti R, Blaauwgeers JL, Taat CW, Simi M, Brummelkamp WH, Becker AE. Intestinal endocrine cells in radiation enteritis. Surg Gyn Obstet 1989;169:127–30.
63. Perez CA, Lee HK, Georgiou A, Lockett MA. Technical factors affecting morbidity in definitive irradiation for localized carcinoma of the prostate. Int J Radiat Oncol Biol Phys 1994;28:811–9.
64. Potten CS, Merritt A, Hickman J, Hall P, Faranda A. Characterization of radiation-induced apoptosis in the small intestine and its biological implications. Int J Radiat Biol 1994;65:71–8.
65. Powell DW, Mifflin RC, Valentich JD, Crowe SE, Saada JI, West AB. Myofibroblasts. II. Intestinal subepithelial myofibroblasts. Am J Physiol 1999;277:C183–201.
66. Prieto I, Gomez de Segura IA, Garcia Grande A, Garcia P, Carralero I, de Miguel E. Morphometric and proliferative effects of growth hormone on radiation enteritis in the rat. Rev Esp Enferm Dig 1998;90:163–73.
67. Pricolo VE, Shellito PC. Surgery for radiation injury to the large intestine. Dis Colon Rectum 1994;37:675–84.
68. Quirke P, Dixon MF, Day DW, Fozard JB, Talbot IC, Bird CC. DNA aneuploidy and cell proliferation in familial adenomatous polyposis. Gut 1988;29:603–7.
69. Roswit B, Malsky SJ, Reid CB. Severe radiation injuries of the stomach, small intestine, colon, and rectum. Am J Roentgenol Radiol Ther Nucl Med 1972;114:460–75.
70. Rubin P, Casarett GW. Clinical radiation pathology, vol I. Philadelphia: WB Saunders; 1968:153–240.
71. Sandler RS, Sandler DP. Radiation-induced cancers of the colon and rectum: assessing the risk. Gastroenterology 1983;84:51–7.
72. Savarese DM, Savy G, Vahdat L, Wischmeyer PE, Corey B. Prevention of chemotherapy and radiation toxicity with glutamine. Cancer Treat Rev 2003;29:501–13.
73. Schottenfeld D. Radiation as a risk factor in the natural history of colorectal cancer. Gastroenterology 1983;84:186–7.
74. Sedgwick DM, Howard GC, Ferguson A. Pathogenesis of acute radiation injury to the rectum: a prospective study in patients. Int J Colorectal Dis 1994;9:23–30.
75. Seki K, Inui Y, Kariya Y, et al. A case of malignant hemangioendothelioma of the stomach. Endoscopy 1985;17:78–80.
76. Shackelford RT, Zuidema R. Radiation injuries of the rectum. In: Shackleford RT, Zuidema GD, eds. Surgery of the alimentary tract, 2nd ed, vol 3. Philadelphia: WB Saunders; 1982:650–61.
77. Sher ME, Bauer J. Radiation-induced enteropathy. Am J Gastroenterol 1990;85:121–8.
78. Sheehan JF. Foam cell plaques in the intima of irradiated small arteries one hundred to five hundred microns in external diameter. Arch Pathol 1944;37:297–308.
79. Sherrill DJ, Grishkin BA, Galal FS, Zajtchuk R, Graeber GM. Radiation associated malignancies of the esophagus. Cancer 1984;54:726–8.
80. Shimizu Y, Pierce DA, Preston DL, Mabuchi K. Studies of the mortality of atomic bomb survivors. Report 12, part II. Noncancer mortality: 1950-1990. Radiat Res 1999;152:374–89.
81. Smith JC, Bolande RP. Radiation and drug induced hyalinization of the stomach. Arch Pathol 1965;79:310–6.
82. Solomon MA. Oral sucralfate suspension for mucositis. N Engl J Med 1986;315:459–60.

83. Summers RW, Glenn CE, Flatt AJ, Elahmady A. Does irradiation produce irreversible changes in canine jejunal myoelectric activity. Dig Dis Sci 1992;37:716–22.
84. Taxy JB, Battifora H. Angiosarcoma of the gastrointestinal tract. A report of three cases. Cancer 1988;62:210–6.
85. Thiagarajah JR, Gourmelon P, Griffiths NM, Lebrun F, Naftalin RJ, Pedley KC. Radiation induced cytochrome c release causes loss of rat colonic fluid absorption by damage to crypts and pericryptal myofibroblasts. Gut 2000;47: 675–84.
86. Toyoda H, Jaramillo E, Mukai K, et al. Treatment of radiation-induced hemorrhagic duodenitis with argon plasma coagulation. Endoscopy 2004:36:192.
87. Trier JS, Browning TH. Morphologic response of the mucosa of human small intestine to x-ray exposure. J Clin Invest 1966;45:194–204.
88. Upton AC. Ionizing radiation. In: Craighead JE, ed. Pathology of environmental and occupational disease. St. Louis: Mosby; 1996:205.
89. Valiulis AP, Gardiner GW, Mahoney LJ. Adenocarcinoma and colitis cystica profunda in a radiation-induced colonic stricture. Dis Colon Rectum 1985;28:128–31.
90. Vallis A, Algara M, Domenech M, Llado A, Ferrer E, Marin S. Efficacy of sucralfate in the prophylaxis of diarrhoea secondary to acute radiation induced enteritis. Preliminary results of a double-blind randomised trial. Med Clin (Barc) 1991;96:449–52.
91. Varga J, Haustein UF, Creech RH, Dwyer JP, Jimenez SA. Exaggerated radiation-induced fibrosis in patients with systemic sclerosis. JAMA 1991;265:3292–5.
92. Vatistas S, Hornsey S. Radiation induced protein loss into the gastrointestinal tract. Br J Roentgenol 1966;39:547–50.
93. Vrind HM, Becker AE. Multiple malignant angioendotheliomas of the stomach and small intestine. Arch Chir Neerl 1970;22:15–23.
94. Wang J, Zheng H, Sung CC, Hauer-Jensen M. The synthetic somatostatin analogue, octreotide, ameliorates/acute and delayed intestinal radiation injury. Int J Radiat Oncol Biol Phys 1999;45:1289–96.
95. Warren SL, Whipple GH. Roentgen ray intoxication. J Exp Med 1922;35:187–193.
96. Waselenko JK, MacVittie TJ, Blakely WF, et al. Strategic National Stockpile Radiation Working Group. Medical management of the acute radiation syndrome: recommendations of the Strategic National Stockpile Radiation Working Group. Ann Intern Med 2004;140:1037–51.
97. Weisbrot IM, Liber AF, Gordon BS. The effects of therapeutic radiation on colonic mucosa. Cancer 1975;36:931–40.
98. White DC. An atlas of radiation histopathology. Technical Information Center, Office of Public Affairs, US Energy Research and Development Administration. 1975:75–92.
99. Wiernick G, Perrins D. The radiosensitivity of a mesenchymal tissue. The pericryptal fibroblast sheath in the human rectal mucosa. Br J Radiol 1975;48:382–9.
100. Wolov RB, Sato N, Azumi N, Lack EE. Intraabdominal "angiosarcomatosis" report of two cases after pelvic irradiation. Cancer 1991;67: 2275–9.

Thermal Injury

101. Alexander JW, Boyce ST, Babcock GF, et al. The process of microbial translocation. Ann Surg 1991;212:496–510.
102. Berlanga J, Lodos J, Lopez-Saura P. Attenuation of internal organ damages by exogenously administered epidermal growth factor (EGF) in burned rodents. Burns 2002;28:435–42.
103. Carter EA, Gonnella A, Tompkins RG. Increased transcellular permeability of rat small intestine after thermal injury. Burns 1992;18:117–20.
104. Carter EA, Udall JN, Kirkham SE, Walker WA. Thermal injury and gastrointestinal function I. Small intestinal nutrient absorption and DNA synthesis. J Burn Care Rehabil 1986;7: 469–74.
105. Chen LW, Hsu CM, Huang JK, Chen JS, Chen SC. Effects of bombesin on gut mucosal immunity in rats after thermal injury. J Formos Med Assoc 2000;99:491–8.
106. Epstein MD, Tchervenkov JI, Alexander JW, Johnson JR, Vester JW. Increased gut permeability following burn trauma. Arch Surg 1991;126: 198–200.
107. Horton JW. Bacterial translocation after burn injury: the contribution of ischemia and permeability changes. Shock 1994;1:286–90.
108. Ives A, Muller M, Pegg S. Colonic pseudo-obstruction in burns patients. Burns 1996;22:598–601.
109. Jones WG 2nd, Minei JP, Barber AE, et al. Bacterial translocation and intestinal atrophy after thermal injury and burn wound sepsis. Ann Surg 1990;21:399–405.
110. Kirksey TD, Moncrief JA, Pruitt BA Jr, O'Neill JA Jr. Gastrointestinal complications in burns. Am J Surg 1968;116:627–33.
111. Kowal-Vern A, McGill V, Gamelli RL. Ischemic necrotic bowel disease in thermal injury. Arch Surg 1997;132:440–3.
112. Mayes T, Gottschlich MM, Warden GD. Nutrition intervention in pediatric patients with thermal injuries who require laparotomy. J Burn Care Rehabil 2000;21:451–6.
113. Muñoz N, Victora CG, Crespi M, Saul C, Braga NM, Correa P. Hot *maté* and precancerous lesions of the oesophagus: an endoscopic survey in southern Brazil. Int J Cancer 1987;39:708–9.

114. Venkatraman A, Ramakrishna BS, Pulimood AB. Butyrate hastens restoration of barrier function after thermal and detergent injury to rat distal colon in vitro. Scand J Gastroenterol 1999;34: 1087–92.
115. Victora CG, Munoz N, Day, NE, Barcelos LB, Peccin DA, Braga NM. Hot beverages and oesophageal cancer in southern Brazil: a case-control study. Int J Cancer 1987;39:710–6.
116. Zapata-Sirvent RL, Hansbrough JF, Wolf P, Grayson LS, Nicolson M. Epidermal growth factor limits structural alterations in gastrointestinal tissues and decreases bacterial translocation in burned mice. Surgery 1993;113:564–73.

Electrical Injury

117. Baxter CR, Zedlitz WH, Shires GT. High output acute renal failure complicating traumatic injury. J Trauma 1964;4:567–71.
118. Buniak B, Reedy DW, Caldarella FA, Bales CR, Buniak L, Janicek D. Alteration in gastrointestinal and neurological function after electrical injury: a review of four cases. Am J Gastroenterol 1999;94:1532–6.
119. Fish RM. Electric injury, part II: specific injuries. J Emerg Med 2000;18:27–34.
120. Klintschar M, Grabuschnigg P, Beham A. Death from electrocution during autoerotic practice. Am J Forensic Med Pathol 1998;19:190–3.
121. Kumar S, Thomas S, Lehri S. Abdominal wall and stomach perforation following accidental electrocution with high tension wire: a unique case. J Emerg Med 1993;11:141–5.
122. Rubin BM, Doman DB, Goldberg HJ, Golding MI. "Deathgrip" esophagus: segmental aperistalsis following electrical injury. Dig Dis Sci 1998;43:1970–2.

Trauma and Hematomas

123. Altner PC. Constrictive lesions of the colon due to blunt trauma to the abdomen. A critical review of management of right colon injuries. Surg Gynecol Obstet 1964;118:1257–64.
124. Argan PF, Dunkle DE, Winn DG. Injuries to a sample of seatbelted children evaluated in a hospital emergency room. J Trauma 1987;27: 58–64.
125. Chilmindris C, Boyd DR, Carson LE, et al. A critical review of management of right colon injuries. J Trauma 1971;11:651–60.
126. Chao M, Xu H, Yang G, Yang B. Spontaneous hematoma in root of the small bowel mesentery: imaging findings. Chin Med J 2003;116: 954–6.
127. Ciftci AO, Tanyel FC, Salman AB. Gastrointestinal tract perforation due to blunt abdominal trauma. Pediatr Surg Int 1998;13:259–64.
128. Flint LM, McCoy M, Richardson JD, et al. Duodenal injury. Analysis of common misconceptions in diagnosis and treatment. Ann Surg 1981;19:697–701.
129. Jeffrey RB, Federle MP, Stein SM, Crass RA. Intramural hematoma of the cecum following blunt trauma. J Comp-Assist Tomogr 1982;6: 404–5.
130. Richardson G, Schiller WR, Shuck J. Gastric rupture from blunt trauma. Rocky Mt Med J 1979;76:309–10.
131. Santoro R, Iannaccaro P. Spontaneous intramural intestinal haemorrhage in a haemophiliac patient. Br J Haematol 2004;125:419.
132. Semel L, Frittelli G. Gastric rupture from blunt abdominal trauma. NY State J Med 1981;81: 938–9.
133. Slavin RE, Borzotta AP. The seromuscular tear and other intestinal lesions in the seatbelt syndrome: a clinical and pathologic study of 29 cases. Am J Forensic Med Pathol 2002;23:214–22.
134. Talton DS, Craig MH, Hauser CJ, Poole GV. Major gastroenteric injuries from blunt trauma. Am Surg 1995;61:69–73.
135. Westcott JL, Smith JR. Mesentery and colon injuries secondary to blunt trauma. Radiology 1975;114:597–600.
136. Yajko RD, Seydel F, Trimble C. Rupture of the stomach from a blunt abdominal trauma. J Trauma 1975;15:177–83.

10 GASTROINTESTINAL INFECTIONS

INTRODUCTION

The gastrointestinal mucosa acts as a major interface between the individual and the environment. As a result, mucosal barrier defenses have evolved to protect against pathogen invasion. A continuous monolayer of columnar epithelial cells, sealed by circumferential tight junctions, covers a surface area of nearly 200 m^2, protecting it from passive diffusion of small and large solutes, particles, microorganisms, and cells. The epithelial cells composing the lining function together in terminal digestion, solute and water transport, host defense, and barrier function. Proper barrier function is required for efficient transport of water and solutes and for host defense. Mucosal barrier damage predisposes individuals to gastrointestinal infections.

Epidemiologic Settings in which Infections Occur

There has been a relatively recent change in the types of gastrointestinal infections that people now develop. This change is attributable to a number of factors, including the fact that individuals live longer and travel more extensively. In addition, there is an increasing incidence of chronic disease, an increasing incidence of immunodeficiency due to tissue transplantation and acquired immunodeficiency syndrome (AIDS), and globalization of food products (Table 10-1).

Worldwide, diarrhea is second only to cardiovascular disease as a cause of death (2,6). In the United States alone, an estimated 211 to 375 million episodes of acute diarrheal illness occur each year, accounting for approximately 73 million doctors' office visits, 1.8 million hospital admissions, and 3,100 deaths (3–5). Worldwide, intestinal infections are responsible for the deaths of 3 to 4 million individuals annually, the majority of whom are preschool-aged children. The World Health Organization (WHO) estimates that 70 percent of diarrheal episodes result from biologically contaminated food (6). The Center for Disease Control (CDC) recently reported that in the United States, foodborne pathogens or contaminants account for 76 million illnesses, 325,000 hospitalizations, and 5,000 deaths annually (1).

Table 10-1

FACTORS ASSOCIATED WITH CHANGES IN THE SPECTRUM OF INFECTIOUS DISEASE

Globalization of the food supply with many fruits and vegetables being grown in developing countries
Increased travel to endemic areas of infection
Increased immunodeficiency secondary to increasing age of the population, transplantation surgery, and acquired immunodeficiency syndrome (AIDS)
Emergence of drug-resistant infections
Large scale food production, distribution, and retailing (fast food chains)

Diagnosis of Gastrointestinal Infections

If the patient undergoes endoscopic examination and has features that suggest an infectious process, the endoscopist may submit tissue for bacterial, mycobacterial, and viral cultures, as well as for parasitologic, toxicologic, or molecular examination. The pathologic diagnosis of gastrointestinal infection depends on the recognition of several factors, including specific pathogens, specific tissue reactions, and specific cytopathic effects of the infection.

The recognition of specific pathogens results from several factors, one of which is their localization to specific tissue sites, including the epithelial apical surfaces, intestinal lumen, lamina propria, submucosa, muscularis propria, or myenteric plexus (Table 10-2). Special stains performed on tissue sections, particularly Gram, acid fast, fungal, and Giemsa, can confirm the presence of infections, particularly in the setting of diffuse histiocytic infiltrates or granulomas (Table 10-3). More specialized studies help identify specific pathogens. For example, the use of immunohistochemical reagents or in situ hybridization reactions may identify specific

Table 10-2

LOCALIZATION OF GASTROINTESTINAL INFECTIONS

Attachment to epithelial luminal surfaces	
	Helicobacter pylori
	Cryptosporidium
	Spirochetes
	Giardia
	Enteroadherent *Escherichia coli*
	Ascaris
Intraepithelial localization	
	Isospora
	Microsporidia
	Candida
	Cytomegalovirus
	Herpes simplex virus
	Adenovirus
Localization in the lamina propria	
	Cytomegalovirus
	Strongyloides
	Mycobacterium
	Tropheryma whipplei
	Histoplasma
	Microsporidia
	Leishmaniasis
	Schistosomiasis
Localization in the submucosa or in areas of ulceration	
	Candida
	Histoplasma
	Aspergillus
	Zygomycosis
	Entamoeba
	Balantidium
	Schistosoma
Localization in the muscularis propria or myenteric plexus	
	Chagas' disease
	Cytomegalovirus

Table 10-3

SPECIAL STAINS USED TO IDENTIFY MICROORGANISMS

Acid-fast stain	
	All acid-fast bacteria
Alcian yellow	
	Helicobacter pylori
Giemsa	
	H. pylori
	Microsporidia
	Cryptosporidium
Gram stain	
	Gram-negative and Gram-positive bacteria
	Microsporidia
Grocott methenamine silver	
	Fungi
Periodic acid–Schiff	
	Tropheryma whipplei
	Amoebae
	Fungi
Trichrome	
	Escherichia coli
	Giardia
Warthin-Starry	
	Spirochetes
	Campylobacter species
	H. pylori

bacterial or viral products. In some cases, such as with microsporidiosis, ultrastructural examination facilitates the diagnosis. Genetic tests identify specific organisms by finding specific microbial DNA, and differentiate among several strains of the same organism, as in *Escherichia coli* enterocolitis. Finally, serologic tests confirm the presence of some infections.

General Pathologic Features

The endoscopic findings of gastrointestinal infections include mucosal granularity, erosions, ulcers, bleeding, friability, mass lesions, and pseudomembranes. The changes usually resolve rapidly and spontaneously.

It is difficult to generally characterize the histopathology of intestinal infections given the multiple types of microbial agents that can infect the gut, their differing degrees of invasiveness, and the variety of their virulence factors. At one extreme, some infections cause dramatic or even lethal physiologic derangements but produce no significant pathologic alterations, as in cholera infections. Conversely, diseases associated with significant histopathologic lesions do not always have clinical features that correlate with the degree of inflammation.

The histologic features of bacterial infections differ depending on the mechanism of bacterial virulence. Many pathologists have learned to recognize the classic features of invasive bacterial infection when a lesion known as acute self-limited colitis (ASLC) is produced (fig. 10-1). The most important histologic changes occur in the first 4 days following the onset of clinical disease. There is a prominent neutrophilic infiltrate within the crypts and lamina propria, sometimes with adherent pseudomembranes. Cryptitis occurs more commonly than crypt abscesses. Lamina propria edema and hemorrhage are often present, whereas architectural

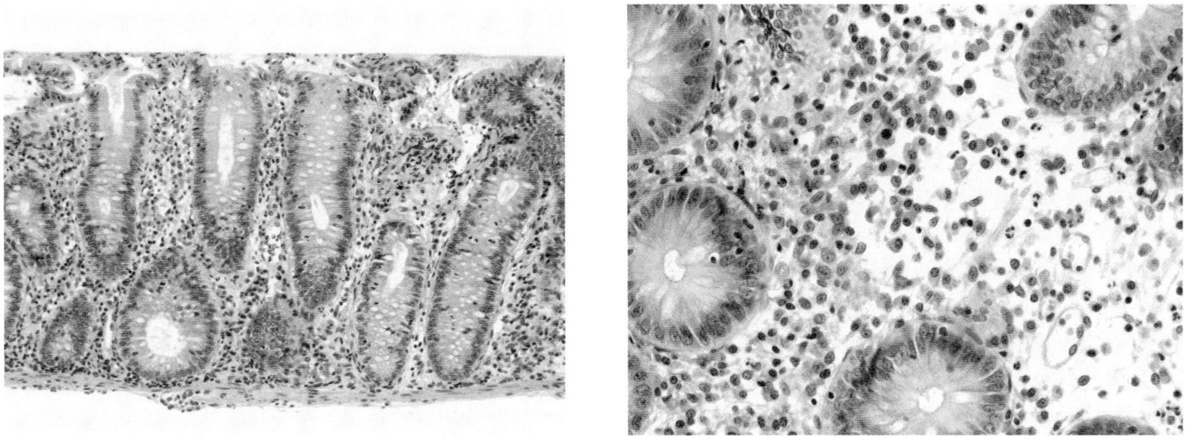

Figure 10-1

ACUTE SELF-LIMITED COLITIS

Left: The overall architecture of the colonic mucosa is preserved. The lamina propria is mildly edematous and contains an increased number of inflammatory cells.

Right: Higher-power view demonstrates mucosal edema and scattered neutrophils in the lamina propria.

abnormalities, including glandular distortion, granulomas, and giant cells, are usually absent or inconspicuous. Later, the colonic mucosa appears regenerative and lymphoplasmacytic infiltrates may be seen in the lamina propria.

Many viruses cause gastrointestinal infections. Rotavirus, Norwalk virus, and enteric adenoviruses are characterized by invasion of mature small intestinal enterocytes. Mucosal injury leads to villous atrophy, crypt hyperplasia, and increased cellularity of the lamina propria. Viral infections are associated with a chronic inflammatory cell infiltrate and sometimes with eosinophils. Some viruses, such as cytomegalovirus (CMV), herpesvirus (HSV), and adenovirus, are identified because they produce characteristic inclusions.

Parasites often cause prominent mucosal eosinophilia. The organisms or their ova may be found in the tissues. Fungal infections are usually recognized by the identification of the specific organism on hematoxylin and eosin (H&E)-, periodic acid–Schiff (PAS)-, or Grocott-stained sections.

BACTERIAL INFECTIONS

Escherichia Coli

Infections are caused by any of the pathogenic species of *Escherichia coli*. These organisms are classified into enteropathogenic, enteroaggregative, enterohemorrhagic, enterotoxigenic, and enteroinvasive types (Table 10-4).

Enteropathogenic *E. Coli*

Demography. *Enteropathogenic E. coli* (EPEC) was the first group of the genus to be identified as a causal agent of diarrhea. These organisms do not produce toxins and do not invade cells (43). The incidence of EPEC infection has declined in industrialized countries and routine serotyping has been discontinued in many laboratories. In developing countries, however, it remains an important cause of infantile diarrhea.

Pathophysiology. EPEC organisms do not produce classic toxins, but do possess a number of virulence factors. The organisms adhere to host enterocytes or M cells causing localized destruction of the brush border microvilli and distortion of the apical cytoplasmic membrane. This initial contact is probably mediated by plasmid-encoded bundle-forming pili (34). Attachment results in rearrangement of the actin cytoskeleton of the cell with formation of a cup-like indentation at the site of bacterial contact ("attaching and effacing lesion") (55). Formation of these attaching-effacing lesions is mediated by a group of approximately 40 genes contained within a pathogenicity island on the bacterial chromosome (30). The formation of the attaching-effacing lesion results in the introduction of bacterial products into the host cell, resulting

Table 10-4

ESCHERICHIA COLI INFECTIONS

Organism	Disease	Epidemiology
Enteropathogenic *Escherichia coli* (EPEC)	Severe fatal diarrhea in newborns Traveler's diarrhea	Spread by ingestion of contaminated food or water Neonates and adults infected
Enterohemorrhagic *E. coli* (EHEC)	Hemorrhagic colitis Hemolytic uremia syndrome Thrombotic thrombocytic purpura	*E. coli* O157:H7 infections occur sporadically and in outbreaks Affects the oldest and youngest in the population Spread by ingestion of contaminated water and person-to-person contamination
Enterotoxigenic *E. coli* (ETEC)	Traveler's diarrhea Infant diarrhea in developing world	Acquired by ingestion of contaminated food and water; person-to-person transmission
Enteroaggregative *E. coli* (EAEC)	Persistent diarrhea in infants in the developing world	Affects mainly infants and children, but also adults and travelers to endemic areas

in disruption of the integrity of the cell membrane, and leading to diarrhea (53).

Pathologic Findings. In EPEC infections, *E. coli* organisms are intimately attached to the apical epithelial cell membrane, effacing the brush border microvilli.

Treatment and Prognosis. Risk factors for death from EPEC infections include young patient age and bacterial virulence. Almost all deaths occur in patients younger than 2 years of age (16). Treatment is supportive: replacement of fluids and electrolytes lost as a result of diarrhea. In addition, antibiotic treatment with trimethoprim-sulfamethoxazole or a fluoroquinolone is recommended (37).

Enteroaggregative *E. Coli*

Demography. *Enteroaggregative E. coli* (EAEC) is a recent addition to the diarrheagenic classes of *E. coli*. The name comes from the "stacked-brick like" adherence to cultured epithelial cells (29). These organisms are a significant cause of diarrhea in developing countries and are most notably associated with prolonged, chronic diarrheal illness in children (50,57). EAEC outbreaks, however, are increasingly being recognized in developed countries (40,48,64). EAEC is a cause of traveler's diarrhea in countries where the organism is endemic (33). Many individuals may be asymptomatic carriers of these organisms (50).

Pathophysiology. EAEC produces several toxins including the enteroaggregative heat stable enterotoxin (29) and two heat labile toxins (9,31). Their aggregative adherence is mediated by at least two fimbriae (21).

Clinical Features. EAEC characteristically produces watery, often protracted, diarrhea. Diarrhea may be associated with abdominal cramping, borborygmi, and low-grade fever (12,40,62). Occasionally, gross mucus or blood is present in the stool (20,74). EAEC also causes intestinal inflammation in the absence of diarrhea. Children with such infections develop malnutrition and have impaired growth (74).

Pathologic Findings. EAEC causes moderate to severe small and large intestinal mucosal damage, irregularity of the surface epithelium, and subnuclear vacuolization of the crypt epithelium. Clumps of bacteria adhere to the mucosal cells, especially in immunocompromised patients. Heavily colonized cells show marked cytologic changes (70). The lamina propria is populated by increased numbers of lymphocytes, plasma cells, and eosinophils, but neutrophils are generally not seen. Rarely, villous atrophy results.

Treatment and Prognosis. Eradication of EAEC is desirable because of the risk that the organism may cause protracted diarrhea. Most strains of EAEC are susceptible to ciprofloxacin, but antibiotic susceptibility testing should be performed in all cases, since many EAEC strains are resistant to multiple antibiotics (25,38,59). In patients with persistent diarrhea, nutritional support may be necessary.

Enterohemorrhagic *E. Coli*

Demography. In 1982, two outbreaks of hemorrhagic colitis associated with consumption of improperly cooked hamburgers took place in the United States (68). Investigation into these incidents led to the discovery of a novel *E. coli* phenotype, now known as *enterohemorrhagic E. coli* (EHEC). *E. coli* O157:H7 is the most common EHEC serotype seen in the United States. The mean annual infection rates range from 2.0 to 12.1/100,000 population (61). The infections are now sufficiently prevalent that the American Gastroenterologic Association termed the infection "an emerging national health crisis" (19). Populations most susceptible to the infection are the very young and the very old, or those with immunodeficiency states.

EHEC outbreaks are established through three principal routes of transmission: 1) contaminated food and contaminated drinking or swimming water, 2) person-to-person transmission, and 3) animal contacts. Outbreaks develop from the ingestion of infected common food sources or organism exposure in communities, nursing homes, daycare centers, kindergartens, and children's wading pools (11,14,44).

Cattle are the principal reservoir of *E. coli* O157:H7. Overall, the prevalence of this organism in cattle feces and hides is 28 percent and 11 percent, respectively (28). Epidemiologic surveys have revealed that EHEC strains are also prevalent in the gastrointestinal tracts of domestic animals, including dogs and cats (7,81). Other sources of infection are other meat products, butter, unpasteurized milk, cheese, vegetables, and fruits (8,13,22,23,26,47,56,67,68,71), especially in the setting of mass food production. The mortality and morbidity associated with several recent large disease outbreaks highlight the threat that EHEC poses to public health (36).

Pathophysiology. The main virulence factors of *E. coli* O157:H7 result from the production of Shiga-like toxins, some of the most potent human toxins. *E. coli* O157:H7 organisms possess one or two cytotoxin genes encoding verotoxin 1 and verotoxin 2, both of which are nearly identical to the Shiga toxin, the principal extracellular cytotoxin of *Shigella dysenteriae* (45,75). This toxin binds to host cells and is internalized through endocytosis. Within the cell, the toxin disrupts the integrity of ribosomes, resulting in cessation of protein synthesis and cell death (69). Interestingly, intestinal enterocytes are partially resistant to the effects of the toxin, but endothelial cells are susceptible to it. This results in intravascular coagulation, not just in the gut, but also in other organs including the kidney, pancreas, heart, and brain (60). The metabolic events leading to intravascular coagulation may also lead to thrombocytopenia, microangiopathic hemolytic anemia, erythrocyte fragmentation, and renal failure characteristic of hemolytic uremic syndrome (63).

Disease-producing strains of EHEC usually also produce virulence factors other than Shiga toxins. These include adhesins similar to those seen in enteropathogenic *E. coli* (32).

Clinical Features: Infection with EHEC is associated with a range of symptoms. Most patients initially present with abdominal cramps and watery diarrhea. Within 2 to 3 days, bloody diarrhea develops (42). The passage of gross blood or clots occurs in severely affected patients. The diarrhea is more prolonged in children than in adults (9.1 versus 6.6 days) (65). Generally, however, the illness is self-limited (63,70,79). In the most severe cases, ischemic colitis or perforation may develop (49). Approximately half of the patients also experience nausea and vomiting. Fever is uncommon, and when present, is usually low grade. The infectious dose of EHEC has been estimated to be fewer than 100 organisms (57). As a result, family members of affected individuals frequently have evidence of concurrent infection, although they are commonly asymptomatic (51). The incubation period is usually 1 to 6 days, but may be as long as 14 days (18).

Not all strains of EHEC carry a risk for the development of hemolytic uremic syndrome (HUS). HUS develops in 5 to 8 percent of patients with EHEC infection (58). High white blood cell counts, elevated C-reactive protein, and fever early in the course of the disease are indicators of risk for the development of HUS (10,15,24,41,46).

Gross Findings. EHEC causes marked hemorrhagic mucosal necrosis with mucosal congestion, erythema, and patchy ulceration, usually with surface exudates and occasional pseudomembranes. Blood may ooze from the mucosal surfaces. Submucosal edema causes radiologic thumbprinting. The gross and endoscopic changes may be indistinguishable from those of ischemic colitis. A gradient of injury is present, with the most severe disease in the

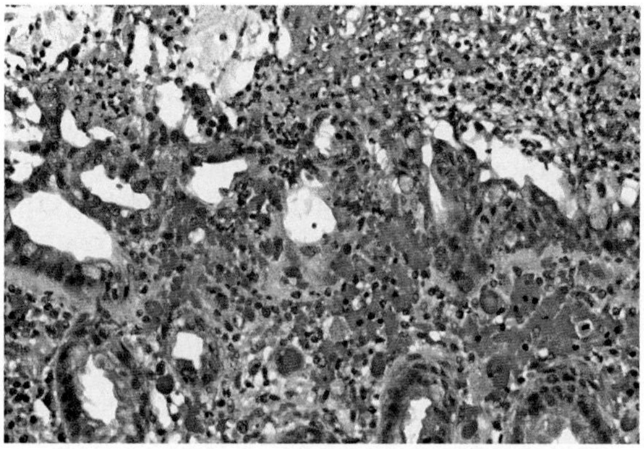

Figure 10-2

ESCHERICHIA COLI O157:H7 INFECTION

The colonic mucosa shows prominent epithelial injury; the superficial epithelium is lost in a pattern similar to that seen in ischemia. The lamina propria contains numerous extravasated red blood cells and inflammatory cells. An acute inflammatory exudate is present overlying the eroded mucosal surface.

proximal colon and less severe disease in the rectum (35), a distribution mimicking Crohn's disease. The entire colon may be involved, particularly in children.

Microscopic Findings. *E. coli* O157:H7 causes the most severe histologic changes of all *E. coli* infections. The histologic patterns of ischemia and infectious colitis overlap due to the presence of both epithelial and endothelial injury (fig. 10-2). Microscopic features associated with an infectious histologic pattern include prominent neutrophilic infiltrates within the crypts and lamina propria and adherent pseudomembranes. Cryptitis occurs more commonly than crypt abscesses and in all cases the neutrophilic infiltrates are focally accentuated rather than uniform in appearance. Features associated with ischemia include focal marked submucosal edema, hemorrhage, pseudomembranes, bland mucosal necrosis, ulcers, abundant intramural fibrin deposits, and thrombi. The ischemia leads to extensive mucosal necrosis, leaving ghosts of crypts filled with neutrophilic infiltrates. The necrosis may extend into the submucosa or even transmurally. The mucosa between the ulcerated areas shows a range of changes from mucus depletion and occasional neutrophils to epithelial dropout, fibrin deposition, and hemorrhage.

In patients with HUS, the histologic findings include marked endothelial cell injury, with swollen vascular lining cells pulling away from the basement membrane, and the presence of fluffy deposits and thrombotic microangiopathy. Renal changes include swollen and detached glomerular endothelial cells with deposition of fibrin and platelets in the renal microvasculature, particularly in the glomerulus (66). Thrombotic lesions also occur in the microvasculature of the bowel, brain, and pancreas.

Treatment and Prognosis. Complications associated with *E. coli* O157:H7 infection include end-stage renal disease, hypertension, and central nervous system (CNS) damage. CNS complications include lethargy, severe headache, seizures, cerebral edema, encephalopathy, stroke, and coma. Rare and unusual complications of EHEC infections are rhabdomyolysis, pancreatic necrosis with subsequent diabetes mellitus, and acute intestinal obstruction from intestinal hematomas (63).

The objectives of therapeutic strategies are 3-fold: 1) to limit the severity and/or duration of the gastrointestinal symptoms; 2) to prevent life-threatening systemic complications such as HUS; and 3) to prevent infection spreading to close contacts. Since patients affected by EHEC may progress to HUS, close observation following the onset of diarrhea for symptoms of HUS leads to earlier intervention and improved initial management (73). Treatment of *E. coli* O157:H7 infection consists of rehydration during the hemorrhagic colitis, monitoring for blood loss, and patient support during the multiple systemic complications of HUS. Antimotility drugs should be avoided (37). Antibiotics are not beneficial, and may in fact increase the risk of HUS (80). Improved clinical management and renal dialysis have reduced the mortality associated with HUS in recent decades. Nonetheless, some individuals develop chronic renal insufficiency, hypertension, and neurologic deficits.

Preventive approaches include educating the public on the danger of eating undercooked meat, increasing physician awareness of the signs and symptoms of *E. coli* O157:H7 infection, mandating case reporting (76), and promoting safe food preparation and food handling practices (77).

Enterotoxigenic *E. Coli*

Demography. *Enterotoxigenic E. coli* (ETEC) was first identified as a cause of diarrhea in 1970, and is now known to be a major cause of diarrhea worldwide (39). ETEC infections are associated with poor sanitation and hygiene, and are therefore of most importance in developing countries. Transmission is through ingestion of contaminated food or water. Outbreaks also occur secondary to person-to-person spread (18).

Pathophysiology. Once the bacteria colonize the small intestine, they produce two toxins: a heat labile toxin (LT) resembling cholera toxin, and a heat stable toxin (ST) that activates guanylate cyclase and impairs colonic water resorption (54). These structurally and functionally different enterotoxins bind to different membrane receptors and induce active fluid secretion without injuring the enterocytes. Special toxin assays are required to differentiate ETEC from normal flora *E. coli*.

Clinical Features. ETEC infections are the most common cause of traveler's diarrhea (17,52,78) and are an important cause of secretory infantile diarrhea in developing countries. The incubation period is 24 to 48 hours. The disease often begins with upper intestinal distress followed by watery diarrhea. The clinical course may be extremely mild or it may be very severe, mimicking cholera and producing severe dehydration and rice-water stools. Symptoms, including the sudden onset of abdominal cramps, nausea, borborygmi, and malaise, are generally most severe on the first day of the infection. The acute watery diarrhea may be accompanied by low-grade fever and chills. The diarrhea is usually self-limited, lasting only 3 to 4 days.

Gross Findings. Toxigenic *E. coli* infections occur throughout the colon, usually inducing mucosal edema. Ulcers are usually absent. Pseudomembranes are rare.

Microscopic Findings. ETEC infections cause mucosal edema, sometimes with extravasation of red blood cells (fig. 10-3). *E. coli* can sometimes be seen adhering to the epithelium without inducing structural mucosal damage.

Treatment and Prognosis. ETEC infection is usually self-limited and therefore requires mainly supportive care. Trimethoprim sulfamethoxazole or fluoroquinolones may be used for treatment (37).

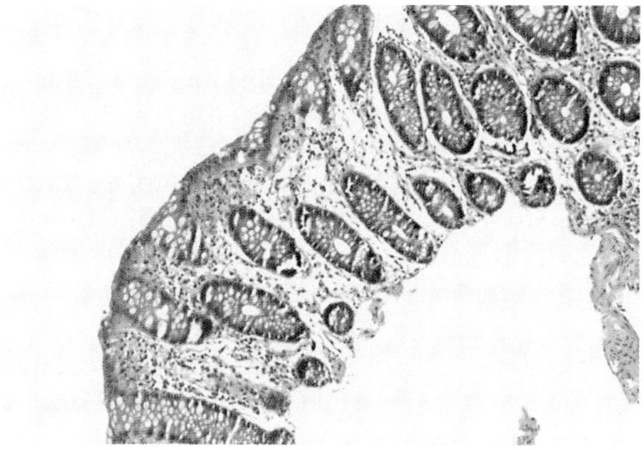

Figure 10-3

ENTEROTOXIGENIC *E. COLI* INFECTION

The colonic mucosa appears edematous, but there is no significant inflammatory cell infiltration.

Enteroinvasive *E. Coli*

Demography. *Enteroinvasive E. coli* (EIEC) is a significant cause of morbidity and mortality in children in both developing and developed countries (18).

Pathophysiology. The central pathogenetic mechanism of EIEC is the ability to invade epithelial cells. This invasive capability correlates with the presence of a 140-MDa plasmid also found in *Shigella* organisms (39,72).

Clinical Features. The symptoms of EIEC infection generally begin 2 to 3 days following ingestion of contaminated food (42). The organisms invade the colonic mucosa and cause a dysentery-like illness. The presenting symptoms include watery diarrhea, tenesmus, cramps, and low-grade fever. The diarrhea may be associated with the passage of small amounts of blood and mucus. White blood cells are usually found in the stool. The clinical symptoms resemble those found in patients with *Shigella* infection.

Pathologic Findings. EIEC penetrates the intestinal epithelium, producing acute inflammation and ulceration of the mucosa in a manner similar to that seen with *Shigella* infection.

Treatment and Prognosis. Antibiotics (trimethoprim-sulfamethoxazole or a fluoroquinolone) may be administered in addition to supportive care (37).

Special Techniques for Identifying *E. Coli*

Techniques that identify specific *E. coli* organisms or their toxins include serotyping, tissue culture, immunochemical methods, DNA hybridization studies, and polymerase chain reactions (PCR). Stool samples should be examined for *E. coli* by both culture and toxin detection methods in order to identify the specific type of *E. coli* and to differentiate disease-causing *E. coli* from the normal colonic flora. It is particularly important to detect EHEC organisms in stool.

EIEC organisms are difficult to identify using standard microbiologic techniques and most microbiologists overlook lactose nonfermenting organisms if they are not of the *Salmonella*, *Shigella*, or *Yersinia* genus. EIEC can be identified with DNA technology (27).

Differential Diagnosis of *E. Coli* Infection

The clinical differential diagnosis of *E. coli* infections includes other infections, inflammatory bowel disease (IBD), intussusception, acute appendicitis, pseudomembranous colitis, and ischemic enterocolitis. Antibodies to *E. coli* O157:H7 distinguish this infection from other causes of ischemic enterocolitis (76). The histologic changes of EHEC infection may resemble those seen in *Campylobacter, Salmonella,* and early amoebic infections. Toxicologic and microbiologic assays help to differentiate these entities. Other Enterobacteriaceae can produce Shiga toxins that cause serious gastrointestinal disease and HUS. The most notable of these is *S. dysenteriae* type I, the cause of bacillary dysentery.

Salmonella Infections

Definition. *Salmonella* infection leads to two forms of disease affecting the gastrointestinal tract. *Typhoid fever*, a protracted systemic disease, results from the translocation of *Salmonella* from the intestinal or renal epithelium to the reticuloendothelial system. In the latter, the bacteria multiply within phagocytes in the liver, spleen, lymph nodes, and Peyer patches. *Salmonella food poisoning* or *gastroenteritis* is usually a mild self-limited disease that develops 3 to 48 hours following organism ingestion (132).

Demography. *Salmonella* infections are a global health problem with a devastating social impact in developing countries. The number of cases of salmonellosis has been increasing steadily during the past decade. In the United States, *Salmonella* has been estimated to be responsible for 18,000 annual hospital admissions, 500 deaths, and $50 million in medical costs (97). More than 95 percent of *Salmonella* infections are foodborne, and salmonellosis accounts for approximately 30 percent of deaths from foodborne illness in the United States (117a). Outbreaks of *Salmonella* gastroenteritis have been linked to ingestion of contaminated fish, poultry, eggs, cheese, dry cereal, ice cream, fresh sprouts, juice, cantaloupes, and a variety of fresh vegetables (90,91,96,110,127). Less commonly, the infection is acquired from household pets (reptiles and birds), direct personal contact with other infected individuals, nosocomial sources, contaminated water, and contaminated drugs or solutions (86,92,93,110).

Poultry serve as the major reservoir for infection with nontyphoidal *Salmonella* strains (127). The northeast United States, parts of Europe, South America, and Africa have experienced a marked increase in food poisoning due to *S. enterica* serotype *enteritidis* (128,132). The increase relates to increased consumption of infected eggs and poultry. Widespread antibiotic use to improve animal growth has contributed to the emergence of multiple antibiotic-resistant *Salmonella* strains that cause serious human disease and the increase in occurrence of symptomless excreters. The incidence of salmonellosis has steadily increased as *Salmonella* organisms have become antibiotic resistant.

The peak incidence of infection occurs in infancy, although all individuals at the extremes of age appear to be at risk. Other risk factors include alteration of the endogenous bowel flora as a result of either antibiotic therapy or surgery, diabetes, malignancy, rheumatologic diseases, altered function of the reticuloendothelial system (as occurs in malaria, sickle cell disease, or some infections), and immunocompromise (110,130). AIDS patients have a 20-fold higher incidence of recurrent nontyphoidal *Salmonella* infections, with or without clinical enteritis.

Etiology. Salmonellae are Gram-negative, nonspore-forming, highly motile rods that belong to the family Enterobacteriaceae. Homologous genes in *Salmonella* and *E. coli* average 85 percent sequence identity, suggesting that the lineages split over 100 million years ago (123). However, the *Salmonella* genome also consists of material that is absent in *E. coli* (113,122). The *Salmonella* species that cause gastrointestinal disease in humans are listed in Table 10-5.

Pathophysiology. Following oral ingestion, *Salmonella* organisms colonize the intestines and invade the intestinal mucosa. The organisms have the ability to penetrate, invade, and multiply in many cell types. One of the hallmarks of systemic infection is the ability of the bacteria to spread from intestinal tissues via lymphatics into the blood stream and to multiply within macrophages of the liver and spleen (89,101).

The disease pattern reflects species virulence, the number of organisms ingested, and the presence of normal flora in the upper intestinal tract. Plasmids integrated into the bacterial genome encode virulence factors involved in the adherence to, invasion of, and growth within epithelial cells. *Salmonella* organisms are the only species of bacteria that contain two type III secretion systems, encoded by two distinct gene clusters, referred to as *Salmonella* pathogenicity islands-1 and -2 (SPI-1 and SPI-2). These two type III secretion systems play different roles in *Salmonella* pathogenesis. SPI-1 is required for invasion of host cells, while SPI-2 is necessary for the subsequent systemic stages of infection (111).

Invasion of intestinal epithelial cells is a characteristic feature of *Salmonella* infection. When injected into ligated ileal loops of calves, *Salmonella* invades enterocytes and M cells within minutes (102). Upon contact with host cells, the organisms induce degeneration of surface microvilli (134). Next, they elicit apical membrane ruffles on both M cells and enterocytes, a change that results in their uptake into membrane-bound vesicles.

The invasion of epithelial cells is dependent on secretion of type III secretion system-1 (TTSS-1) proteins. Many of these TTSS-1 proteins are encoded on SPI-1, but some components are encoded elsewhere in the bacterial genome. TTSS-1 proteins can be loosely divided into two groups, the translocators and the translocated effectors. The translocator proteins are essential for movement of the protein effectors across the eukaryotic cell membrane and into the host cell. Translocator proteins include SipB, SipC, and SipD (98). TTSS-1 effector proteins include a group of *Salmonella* outer proteins (Sop) (136) including SopA, SopB, SopD, and SopE. SopE, for example, is required for efficient bacterial entry into cells. It functions to directly stimulate actin cytoskeletal rearrangements in the host cells, allowing bacterial entry (107).

Table 10-5

SALMONELLA SPECIES THAT CAUSE INFECTIONS IN HUMANS

S. typhimurium	*S. agona*
S. typhi	*S. javiana*
S. paratyphi	*S. oranienburg*
S. enteritidis	*S. schottmuelleri*
S. choleraesuis[ab]	*S. amatum*

[a]Most likely to affect patients with acquired immunodeficiency syndrome (AIDS).

[b]Cause bacteremia with localized infections; ileitis rare.

TTSS-1 also plays a major role in the induction of intestinal secretory and inflammatory responses. SopB (also known as SigD in *S. typhimurium*) is an inositol phosphate phosphatase that is capable of hydrolyzing several inositol phosphates (121). This results in transient elevation of intracellular levels of inositol 1,4,5,6-tetrakisphosphate which antagonizes closure of chloride channels, resulting in fluid secretion. *Salmonella*-infected epithelial cells secrete chemokines and prostaglandins that act to recruit inflammatory cells to foci of infection. This is probably mediated, at least in part, by Sop proteins (103).

In the lymphoid tissue underlying infected epithelial cells, *Salmonella* organisms are phagocytosed by resident macrophages. The organisms are able to survive and replicate inside the phagocytic vacuoles in these cells, and in this way are able to use the macrophages as a vehicle for dissemination to other organs (82, 101,114,118). Survival and proliferation within host cells may be mediated by genes encoded on SPI-2 (108). The bacteria then replicate in the liver, spleen, and bone marrow, leading to bacterial sepsis, organ failure, and possibly death of the host. SPI-1 proteins mediate a cytotoxic effect on macrophages, leading to apoptosis and cell death (94).

Clinical Features. *Salmonella* organisms produce five clinical syndromes: 1) gastroenteritis (70 percent of infections); 2) bacteremia, with or without gastrointestinal involvement; 3) typhoid or enteric fever; 4) localized infections in bones, joints, and meninges; and 5) a carrier state. Typically, *Salmonella* gastroenteritis is a mild, self-limited illness that develops 8 to 48 hours after ingestion of the organism, but 2 to 5 percent of infected individuals develop bacteremia and sepsis-associated complications (84). Signs and symptoms of *Salmonella* gastroenteritis vary widely, but most patients present with nausea, vomiting, abdominal cramps, fever, and diarrhea that sometimes becomes bloody. Symptoms usually last for 3 to 12 days. The duration of the carrier state, however, depends on the age of the infected patient. Children under 5 years of age carry nontyphoidal strains for approximately 12 weeks, whereas adults clear the organism after 4 weeks (85). Chronic carriers are individuals who continue to excrete organisms in their stool for a year or more after the symptoms of *Salmonella* gastroenteritis or enteric fever have passed. *Salmonella* is also a cause of traveler's diarrhea (116a).

Infections with *S. enterica* serotype *typhi* and, to a lesser extent, *S. enterica* serotypes *paratyphi*, *schottmuelleri*, and *hirschfeldii*, follow an enteric fever pattern. Dissemination is common and ileal lymphoid proliferation at the site of invasion is prominent during the first 1 to 2 weeks of infection. Patients with typhoid fever remain relatively asymptomatic during a 1- to 2-week incubation period. The onset of bacteremia is heralded by fever and malaise. Other signs and symptoms include nausea, vomiting, vague abdominal discomfort, headache, cough, myalgia, and reactive bradycardia (83,87,133). Physical examination typically shows abdominal tenderness and hepatosplenomegaly. Complications occur in 10 to 15 percent of patients (124). Gastrointestinal complications include massive intestinal hemorrhage, perforation, intussusception, mesenteric lymphadenitis, peritonitis, fistulas, toxic megacolon, and paralytic ileus (100,112). The bleeding results from ulceration of Peyer patches. The stool acquires a "pea soup" appearance because of the purulent material shed from the ulcerated mucosa. A prolonged convalescent stage of 3 months is usual. Relapse occurs in 5 to 10 percent of patients and is usually milder than the original attack (124). Bacterial shedding may be prolonged, with 1 to 4 percent of patients becoming long-term carriers.

Salmonella infections in the elderly, AIDS patients, or immunosuppressed individuals may be unusually severe and these patients have a poorer prognosis than do younger, immunocompetent individuals. These patients have a higher incidence of bacteremia, disseminated extraintestinal infections, and relapse than immunocompetent patients. Recurrent bacteremia occurs despite treatment and the relative paucity of gastrointestinal manifestations.

Gross Findings. Because the major portal of entry for bacteria causing gastroenteritis is in the area of Peyer patches, the lymphoid follicles become hyperplastic, swollen, congested, and ulcerated, often resulting in typical longitudinally oriented ulcers and areas of hemorrhage (115,119). Edema, fibrinous exudation, and vascular thrombosis precede the ulceration. Aphthous ulcers sometimes develop (99).

In typhoid fever, bacterial sequestration in the reticuloendothelial system causes lymphoid hyperplasia, lymphadenopathy, and splenomegaly. The disease primarily affects intestinal lymphoid tissues of the ileum, appendix, and colon. Four sequential stages of the disease have been described, each of which lasts a week: hyperplasia, necrosis, ulceration, and healing (131). Hyperplasia develops during the incubation period with the onset of fever. The Peyer patches enlarge and become elevated and hyperemic. The necrotic stage corresponds to the phase of maximal fever. The necrosis begins in Peyer patches as isolated, localized foci with fibrinous exudates in the surrounding mucosa. The ulceration stage begins when the necrotic tissue sloughs. This event occurs approximately the same time as the lysis of the fever. The ulcer bases typically lie on the muscularis propria but they occasionally penetrate the entire thickness of the bowel wall. They are oval, longitudinal, and located on the antimesenteric borders. With progressive disease, the bowel wall becomes paper thin and susceptible to perforation (100).

Microscopic Findings. Nontyphoidal *Salmonella* organisms cause acute infectious ileocolitis indistinguishable from other infectious colitides (117). The changes are self-limited and the mucosa returns to normal in approximately 2 weeks.

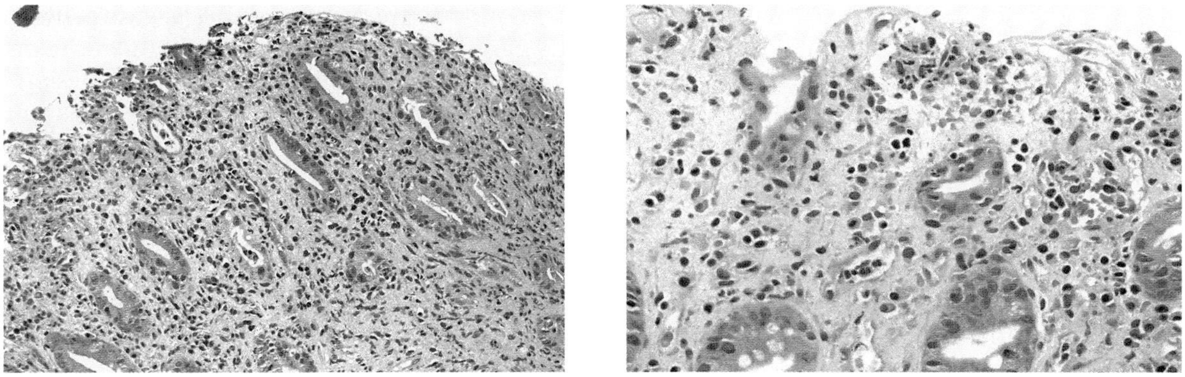

Figure 10-4

SALMONELLA COLITIS

Left: Low-power view shows preservation of the mucosal architecture. The lamina propria is somewhat edematous and contains an increased number of inflammatory cells. Most of the crypts are lined by flattened, regenerative epithelium.

Right: Higher-power view shows regenerative glands and inflammatory cells within the lamina propria.

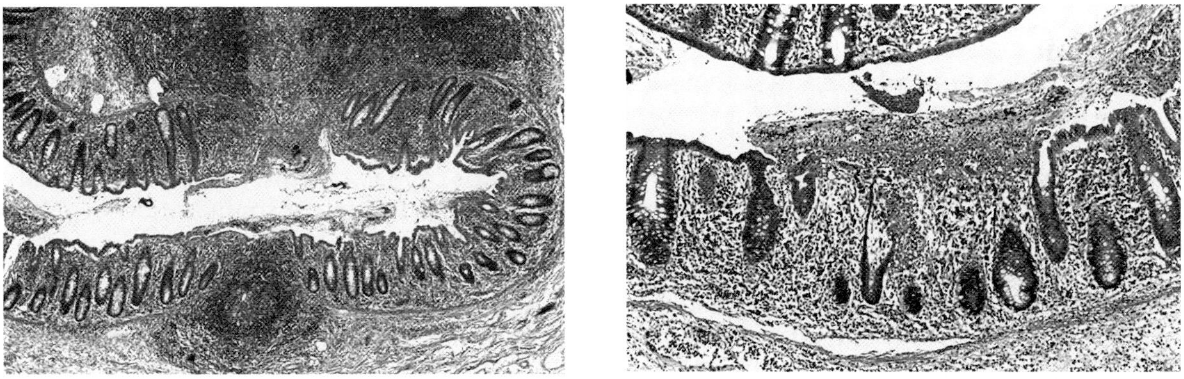

Figure 10-5

SALMONELLA COLITIS

Left: The mucosa overlying the lymphoid follicles is ulcerated.

Right: Higher magnification shows changes resembling those of acute self-limited colitis. The mucosal architecture is preserved. There is evidence of mucosal erosion associated with lamina propria edema and inflammation. Some crypts contain infiltrating neutrophils and a crypt abscess is present. (Courtesy of the Division of Gastrointestinal Pathology, Armed Forces Institute of Pathology, Washington, DC.)

Histologically, mild cases of *Salmonella* gastroenteritis show nonspecific changes including edema, congestion, and focal inflammation (fig. 10-4). More severe cases show crypt abscesses with prominent neutrophilic infiltrates in degenerating crypts. The neutrophilic infiltration is more intense in the lamina propria than in the glands. Areas of hemorrhage and ulceration are also present (fig. 10-5). Microthrombi fill small vessels in the mucosa and submucosal venules, simulating the features of acute ischemic colitis. Occasional patients, especially those with persistent diarrhea, have mild crypt distortion and branching.

During the hyperplastic phase of typhoid fever, the mucosa appears intact but contains foci of neutrophilic cryptitis. The germinal centers, mantle zones, and interfollicular areas of the lymphoid follicles become progressively infiltrated by macrophages, and have prominent erythrophagocytosis and tingible bodies. The follicles eventually are obliterated by this process. Plasma cells and immunoblasts increase and infiltrate into the underlying submucosa.

The lymphatics at the edges of the Peyer patches appear dilated and contain numerous lymphocytes, monocytes, and immunoblasts.

During the necrotic phase of the disease, variable portions of the Peyer patches remain viable. Areas of ulceration develop in the mucosa (fig. 10-5). A fibrinous exudate on the peritoneal surface may underlie these deep ulcers. During the healing stage, the ulcers are covered by a thin layer of granulation tissue and a layer of intestinal epithelium. Healing occurs rapidly, usually with little fibrosis or stricturing.

Special Techniques. The gold standard for diagnosis of typhoid fever is culture of *S. enterica* serotype *typhi* from blood, stools, or urine. New enzyme-linked immunoabsorbent assay tests and rapid antigen detection methods are being developed to meet the need for inexpensive and reliable diagnostic techniques in underdeveloped countries (126). Once *Salmonella* is identified, it is important to determine whether the isolate is *S. enterica* serotype *typhi* because antibiotics are efficacious for typhoid fever.

Differential Diagnosis. A substantial overlap of clinical symptoms exists between enteric fever and other gastrointestinal inflammatory conditions. Colonic infections generally mimic ulcerative colitis or other forms of infectious colitis (116). The changes of salmonellosis differ from those of IBD by the relative scarcity of chronic inflammatory cells in the former and their frequency in the latter. In severe cases of salmonellosis, giant cells or histiocytic aggregates are present. When these coexist with transmural inflammation, a diagnosis of Crohn's disease might be entertained. The giant cells, however, do not form compact granulomas, as seen in Crohn's disease. The differential diagnosis of the histiocytic aggregates includes mucin granulomas as well as other bacterial infections, including those caused by *Campylobacter*, *Yersinia*, *Shigella*, *E. coli*, and mycobacteria.

The lesions in the bowel and mesenteric lymph nodes may also mimic Kikuchi-Fujimoto disease and Rosai-Dorfman disease, as well as infections caused by non-*Salmonella* bacteria.

Treatment and Prognosis. In the absence of systemic infection, no treatment other than supportive care is warranted. In fact, studies suggest that antibiotic treatment in patients with mild to moderate *Salmonella* gastroenteritis may result in prolonged shedding of the organism (110,120). Since the intestinal lesions heal with minimal fibrosis, stricture formation is unusual. Antimicrobial therapy should be instituted in patients with severe gastroenteritis, or in those at risk for developing disseminated disease. Usually 3 to 7 days of treatment with fluoroquinolones, trimethoprim-sulfamethoxazole, ampicillin, or a third generation cephalosporin is adequate (110). Resistance to antibiotics by these organisms is becoming increasingly common.

Typhoid fever is a chronic systemic illness with a mortality rate that can reach 50 percent in untreated individuals in some parts of the world (109,125,129). Treatment reduces the mortality rate to less than 1 percent. There is strong evidence that fluoroquinolones such as ciprofloxacin are the most effective drugs for the treatment of typhoid fever (88,95,104,106, 135). Quinolone-resistant *Salmonella* strains have emerged. These are often resistant to multiple drugs, and are usually treated with azithromycin or cephalosporins. A subset of patients with severe infection or complications requires surgical intervention.

The most important infection control measure for salmonellosis is awareness that the organism is present in many foods and recognition of the postsymptomatic and asymptomatic carrier states. Food should be cooked well to kill organisms and hands and utensils should be washed thoroughly after coming in contact with uncooked foods. More prudent use of antimicrobial agents in farm animals and more effective disease prevention on farms are necessary to reduce the dissemination of multidrug-resistant strains and to slow the emergence of resistance to additional agents in this and other strains of *Salmonella* (105).

Shigella Infections

Demography. *Shigella* infections are an important cause of morbidity and mortality in developing countries, especially in areas with poor hygiene and overcrowding. Person-to-person transmission and consumption of contaminated food and water cause the disease (143, 149). Children and young adults are the main victims, with over 500,000 deaths occurring as a result worldwide (144,146,156,160). *Shigella* infections are also a significant problem among institutionalized children in nurseries and mental hospitals, and the organism is implicated as a cause of traveler's diarrhea (156).

Etiology. *Shigella* organisms are nonmotile, Gram-negative bacilli that are among the more virulent human enteropathogens. The *Shigella* species (*dysenteriae, flexneri, boydii,* and *sonnei*) cause colitis, diminishing in severity from the first type to the last (147). Cases of mixed infection with both *S. boydii* and *S. sonnei* have been described (139). Multiple drug-resistant strains are a common characteristic in the epidemic form of the disease.

Pathophysiology. *Shigella* gains access to the intestinal epithelium through invasion of M cells (154). The ability to invade epithelial cells represents a property that is required for the organism's virulence (151). As many as 27 genes are required for entry of the bacteria into host cells. Most of these genes are located in two operons in the *Shigella* virulence plasmid. One operon, termed *mxi-spa*, encodes a specialized activatable type III secretory apparatus similar to that found in enteropathogenic *E. coli* or *Salmonella* (139b). After a complex signaling process, these proteins cause major rearrangements of the actin and microtubular cytoskeletal network, thereby allowing bacterial entry by a macropinocytotic event (139b,157,158).

Epithelial signaling caused by apical bacteria induces adherence and transmigration of basal neutrophils, further facilitating bacterial invasion (153). Once inside the epithelial cell, they lie in phagocytic vacuoles, multiplying, causing mucus secretion, goblet cell depletion, and inducing neutrophilic infiltrates. The neutrophils further injure the epithelium, facilitating *Shigella* invasion (148). The bacteria lyse their phagocytic vacuole and initiate intracytoplasmic movement due to polar assembly of actin filaments caused by a bacterial surface protein, IcsA. The bacteria move within the cell and spread laterally into adjacent cells and into the adjacent lamina propria (153). This allows very efficient colonization of the host cell cytoplasm and passage to adjacent cells via protrusions that are engulfed by a cadherin-dependent process. This cycle of intracellular and intercellular infection allows colonization of large epithelial surfaces while the bacteria remain protected from host immune surveillance mechanisms. Eventually, microulcers develop in the surface epithelium. Endotoxin absorption leads to thrombosis, hemorrhage, and vascular insufficiency, causing further crypt damage.

The severe diarrhea that develops in patients with *Shigella* results from the bacterial induction of macrophage apoptosis (161). Dying macrophages infected with the organism release interleukin-1 (159). The cytokine elicits a strong inflammatory response that is a central component to the pathogenesis of shigellosis (152).

Clinical Features. *Shigella* causes a range of symptoms varying from mild watery diarrhea to bacillary dysentery. The usual disease incubation period ranges from 1 to 3 days. The typical clinical presentation of bacillary dysentery is crampy abdominal pain, rectal burning, and fever, accompanied by small-volume, bloody, mucoid bowel movements. This presentation, however, occurs in only a few patients. The most common symptoms are abdominal pain and diarrhea. Fever is present in 40 percent of patients, and the typical dysenteric mucoid stool is present in less than one third. Many patients have a biphasic illness that begins with fever, abdominal pain, and watery, nonbloody diarrhea. This is followed within 3 to 5 days by tenesmus, typical dysenteric bowel movements, and lower abdominal pain.

Patients with prolonged diarrhea often develop severe complications, including anal or perianal disease that causes fissures, fistulas, hemorrhoids, or mucosal prolapse. Other complications include malnutrition, pneumonia, and septicemia (139). Extraintestinal manifestations include convulsions, disturbances of consciousness, shock, disseminated intravascular coagulopathy, nerve paralysis, severe anemia, and HUS (141). Dysentery can be a life-threatening illness in infants, elderly, or malnourished individuals. In patients with fatal infections, particularly children, death results from severe colitis often complicated by septicemia, concomitant malnutrition, and pneumonia (139). Factors that predict mortality include younger age, decreased serum protein, altered consciousness, and thrombocytopenia (138).

Gross Findings. Gastrointestinal changes caused by *Shigella* infection range from relatively mild mucosal inflammation with contact bleeding, edema, and hyperemia to ragged ulcerations, sometimes associated with pseudomembrane formation (137,145,155). Serpiginous ulcers develop on the free edges of mucosal folds. The intervening mucosa appears granular and hemorrhagic; aphthous ulcers may be present. The continuous, diffuse lesions begin in the rectosigmoid, with the intensity of inflammation decreasing as one moves proximally. In fatal cases, pancolitis is common (140).

Microscopic Findings. Biopsy evaluation of patients with shigellosis shows the typical features of other forms of acute self-limited colitis. The earliest lesions occur at the portal of entry and consist of small aphthous ulcers overlying lymphoid follicles. Extensive ulceration is associated with invasion of epithelial cells by the organism. There is marked mucus depletion of the epithelium and crypt hyperplasia. Other changes include acute inflammation with neutrophilic infiltrates, occasional superficial crypt abscesses, goblet cell depletion, edema, vascular congestion, and minimal lymphocyte and plasma cell infiltrates (150). Eventually, the mucosa reverts to normal (142), although some residual distortion of the crypt architecture may persist (137,139).

Special Techniques. The definitive diagnosis depends on demonstrating the organism in stool cultures or by genetic analysis of the tissues or stool specimens.

Differential Diagnosis. The gross findings resemble those present in *Campylobacter* and *Salmonella* infections or ulcerative colitis. When pseudomembranes form, the differential diagnosis includes *Clostridium difficile*–associated colitis, ischemia, amebiasis, and other disorders associated with pseudomembranes. The histologic features usually allow the disease to be distinguished from ulcerative colitis due to the lack of architectural distortion and other chronic changes. Distinction from other acute infectious diseases is generally not possible based solely on the histologic appearance. Definitive diagnosis requires organism identification and clinical correlation.

Treatment and Prognosis. Therapy for *Shigella* gastroenteritis is not always necessary. Mild disease is usually self-limited and a prolonged carrier state virtually never occurs. Moderate to severe disease, however, should be treated with antibiotics and systemic support, especially oral rehydration. Treatment with fluoroquinolones or trimethoprim-sulfamethoxazole is often effective (139a). *Shigella* susceptibility testing should be performed, since resistance to antibiotics is common. Patients who develop megacolon require surgery (138).

Staphylococcal Infections

Demography. Staphylococci are a common cause of food poisoning worldwide. *Staphylococcal food poisoning* accounted for 16 percent of outbreaks of foodborne illness in France between the years 1999 and 2000 (164).

Etiology. Most cases of staphylococcal food poisoning are due to toxin-producing *Staphylococcus aureus*. Enterotoxins are also produced by *S. cohnii, S. epidermidis, S. xylosus,* and *S. haemolyticus* (162). *S. intermedius* is the only non-*S. aureus* species that has clearly been linked to outbreaks of staphylococcal food poisoning (166).

Pathophysiology. Staphylococcal food poisoning results from consumption of food contaminated with preformed toxins. Fourteen different, but related, *S. aureus* enterotoxins have been described (167). These toxins cause disease in several ways. Toxin binding to class I histocompatibility antigens on macrophages or mast cells may stimulate these cells to release large amounts of soluble mediators, such as interleukin 1 and tumor necrosis factor (165), which induce diarrhea and vomiting (168). Alternatively, the toxins may stimulate proliferation and lymphokine production by T lymphocytes. This occurs as a result of cross-linking of the T-cell receptor with the major histocompatability complex (MHC) class II molecule of an antigen presenting cell, leading to nonspecific T-cell activation and massive secretion of interleukins (169).

Clinical Features. Staphylococcal food poisoning is an explosive, but self-limited, gastroenteritis associated with ingestion of infected food. Patients develop nausea, vomiting, and watery, nonbloody diarrhea, usually within 30 minutes to 8 hours after ingesting contaminated food. The symptoms usually remit within 24 hours (167).

Pathologic Findings. In most cases, the disease resolves before endoscopy and biopsy are necessary. In severe cases, however, patients present with nonspecific enterocolitis with intense mucosal congestion, necrosis, and ulceration (163). The histologic features resemble those seen with other intestinal bacterial infections.

Treatment and Prognosis. Because the disease results from ingestion of a preformed toxin and is self-limited, no treatment is necessary.

Campylobacter Infections

Demography. *Campylobacter* species are widespread in mammals and birds, and they survive well in the environment. As a result, sources of human infection include animal contact, food, milk, and water. *Campylobacter* is one of the most frequently isolated stool pathogens (172,195), and its incidence differs from country to country. In the United States and other industrialized countries, *Campylobacter* is responsible for 2 to 7 times as many cases of diarrhea as is *Salmonella, Shigella,* or *E. coli* (174,197). *C. jejuni* is a common cause of bacterial gastroenteritis (185a), with approximately 1 percent of the population of the United States becoming infected each year (171). *Campylobacter* infections affect persons of all ages, but they peak in incidence in infancy, with a smaller peak between 15 and 30 years of age (175,196). *Campylobacter* outbreaks are associated with consumption of unpasteurized milk and contaminated water, meat, vegetables, and especially, poultry. Person-to-person transmission also occurs (173). Household pets may serve as reservoirs for the infection (172,174,198).

In developing countries, *Campylobacter* infections are hyperendemic among young children, especially those younger than 2 years of age (170). In underdeveloped countries, asymptomatic infection is common in both children and adults, whereas in developed countries, asymptomatic infection is uncommon.

Etiology. *Campylobacter* organisms (from the Greek "curved rod") are Gram-negative, spiral, highly motile bacteria. Numerous *Campylobacter* species exist, however, the vast majority of cases (over 95 percent) are caused by *C. jejuni* and *C. coli* (180,187,188). A number of additional species cause disease in humans (183,184,186–189,199).

Pathophysiology. Once ingested, organisms that survive the gastric acid reach the bile-rich microaerobic upper small intestine, an environment that promotes their growth. *Campylobacter* organisms are thought to produce diarrheal illness by two mechanisms: 1) intestinal adherence and toxin production and 2) bacterial invasion and proliferation within intestinal epithelial cells. The bacteria attach to and invade enterocytes (177–179,185). When the organisms contact the cell surface, the epithelium becomes damaged and bacteria invade the cells (177–179,185).

C. jejuni strains produce an enterotoxin and at least one cytotoxin, the cytolethal distending toxin (CDT) (191). Although the role of this toxin in the pathogenesis of diarrhea in humans is not yet clear, in vitro studies have demonstrated that this protein causes eukaryotic cells to become arrested in the G_2 phase of the cell cycle (200). In vivo, this could affect the rapidly dividing cells of the intestinal crypts, leading to loss of function and erosion of the epithelial lining of the gut. Some strains of *C. jejuni* may elaborate additional toxins (192,194). *C. jejuni* organisms are more often enterotoxigenic and possibly more virulent than *C. coli* and *C. laridis.*

Clinical Features. *Campylobacter* organisms cause both gastrointestinal and extragastrointestinal illnesses. The incubation period ranges from 1 to 7 days. The clinical features of the infection are not specific enough to allow distinction from other enteric infections. Typically, *C. jejuni* infection results in an acute, self-limited gastroenteritis characterized by diarrhea, fever, and abdominal cramps. A prodrome of headache, myalgias, chills, and fever may precede the diarrhea. The abdominal pain may be severe enough to mimic acute appendicitis. The diarrhea may be watery or bloody. White blood cells are identifiable in the stool. Symptoms usually resolve within a week, with or without treatment, but they persist from 1 to 3 weeks in about 20 percent of patients. Recurrences or chronic symptoms occur, particularly in infants (181).

Human immunodeficiency virus (HIV)-infected patients typically develop persistent, severe *C. jejuni* infections that require prolonged antimicrobial therapy; these patients are more likely to develop bacteremia than non-HIV patients. The organism fails to clear because of the underlying immunodeficiency and the bacteria tend to become antibiotic resistant (176,190).

Local complications of *Campylobacter* infections occur as a result of direct spread of the organisms from the gastrointestinal tract, and include cholecystitis, pancreatitis, and peritonitis. Massive gastrointestinal hemorrhage may occur. Extraintestinal disease is rare, but includes meningitis, endocarditis, septic arthritis, osteomyelitis, and sepsis. Postinfectious Guillain-Barre syndrome develops in 1 to 2 infected persons/100,000 in the United States (170).

Gross Findings. *Campylobacter* causes both small and large intestinal disease. Jejunal lesions are more common than those occurring in the ileum or colon. In fatal cases, the jejunum and ileum are always affected. A patchy, bloody, edematous, erythematous enterocolitis develops, characterized by multiple, superficial ulcers measuring up to 1 cm in diameter. The ulcers sometimes develop over the Peyer patches. The normal vascular pattern disappears. The appendix and lymph nodes may also be involved. Severe cases resemble severe ulcerative colitis with pancolitis, toxic megacolon, and colonic perforation (182).

Microscopic Findings. The histologic features of *Campylobacter* infection resemble those seen in other infections and range from mild mucosal edema and increased cellularity of the lamina propria to full-blown acute colitis (175,193). In the small intestine, mucosal congestion, inflammation, edema, neutrophilic infiltrates, goblet cell depletion with cryptitis, crypt abscesses, and hemorrhagic necrosis are seen. The ulcer bases are acutely inflamed, with granulation tissue and prominent vascularity but little fibrosis. Architectural villous changes include broadening, distortion, flattening, and atrophy. The histologic features of *Campylobacter* appendicitis and colitis are mucosal infiltration by polymorphonuclear leukocytes and eosinophils, crypt abscesses, mucosal edema, and histiocytic collections that may resemble granulomas. The Warthin-Starry stain may highlight the curved rods of *Campylobacter*.

Special Techniques. Since biopsy findings are nonspecific, bacterial culture or other diagnostic techniques are necessary to establish the exact diagnosis. The diagnosis of *Campylobacter* infection is usually established by isolating the organism from the stool. A simple rapid, specific, and sensitive approach to strain differentiation is DNA hybridization.

Differential Diagnosis. *Campylobacter* infections clinically mimic appendicitis, IBD, and other forms of bacterial enterocolitis. Unlike chronic ulcerative colitis, the changes tend to be segmental in nature. Poorly formed mucosal granulomas may be present, suggesting the diagnosis of Crohn's disease, however, suppurative foci in the granulomas distinguish *Campylobacter* infection.

Treatment and Prognosis. Complications, including sepsis, meningitis, toxic megacolon, pseudomembranous colitis, massive gastrointestinal hemorrhage, arthritis, endocarditis, and genital and urinary infections occur rarely and tend to affect debilitated persons. *Campylobacter* infections occurring during pregnancy are associated with spontaneous abortions, stillbirths, prematurity, and neonatal sepsis.

Guillain-Barre syndrome complicates *Campylobacter* infections and results from cross-reactivity between neural and *C. jejuni* antigens (201). The bacterial gene *NeuB* encodes a surface molecule on *C. jejuni* that is antigenically similar to a ganglioside found in high concentrations in the nervous system. This close resemblance tricks the immune system into attacking nervous tissue as well as the invading bacteria. The immune system produces antibodies that cross-react with peripheral nerves, thereby damaging them.

Most patients recover fully from their infection, either spontaneously or after antibiotic therapy. When antibiotics are indicated for the treatment of *Campylobacter* enteritis, erythromycin or a fluoroquinolone such as ciprofloxacin is the drug of choice (170).

Clostridium Difficile Infections

Demography. *Clostridium difficile* is present in normal colonic flora in 2 to 5 percent of the general population, but its prevalence increases in hospitalized individuals (224). Colonization rates increase in the elderly, and are probably dependent on the use of antibiotics and the amount of time spent in institutions such as nursing homes or hospitals (223). *C. difficile* is the most frequent cause of nosocomial diarrhea, developing in as many as 1 percent of hospitalized patients receiving antibiotics (212,218). The hospital environment is variably contaminated with the organism (20 to 70 percent of sampled sites) (224). Heat-resistant *C. difficile* spores persist in the environment for months, so that the organism can be cultured from many items commonly used in hospital rooms or wards where patients with *C. difficile*-associated diarrhea have been recently treated. *C. difficile* organisms have also been isolated from domesticated animals including horses, cows, pigs, dogs, and cats, although no evidence exists to suggest that *C. difficile* infection represents a zoonosis.

Etiology. *C. difficile* is a Gram-positive, spore-forming, anaerobic bacillus that causes a spectrum of diseases ranging from an asymptomatic carrier state to full-blown pseudomembranous colitis. *C. difficile*-associated diarrhea usually follows antibiotic use. Clindamycin, ampicillin, and the cephalosporins are most commonly associated with the disease, but virtually any antibiotic may produce it. Chemotherapeutic agents cause *C. difficile*-associated colitis (209).

Pathophysiology. The colon normally contains a lush commensal bacterial population that keeps pathogenic bacteria at bay. Agents such as antibiotics, which alter the normal ecological balance, predispose the colon to *C. difficile* infection. Factors that determine whether or not a patient develops the infection include: 1) the nature of the fecal flora; 2) whether the flora is disrupted by antibiotics, other medications, or medical procedures; 3) the size of the *C. difficile* population (a reflection of a loss of the mucosal protective barrier of normal flora); 4) cytotoxin production; 5) the presence of virulence factors; 6) other organisms that affect *C. difficile* toxin expression or activity; 7) the presence of predisposing host risk factors, such as advanced age, severe underlying illness, immune status, and a prolonged hospital stay; and 8) the use of enemas, gastrointestinal stimulants, and stool softeners (217).

C. difficile produces two exotoxins, classically referred to as A and B, which cause both the diarrhea and the colitis. Nontoxigenic bacterial strains are not pathogenic. The two toxins are encoded on a pathogenicity locus on the bacterial DNA. Both toxins A and B are large, single-chain peptides, measuring 308 kDa and 270 kDa, respectively (202). The two toxins are 50 percent homologous at the amino acid level, and have similar primary structures. Both toxins bind to cells, entering them by endocytosis (222). Toxin A binds to a glycoprotein receptor on brush border membranes, causing direct epithelial cell damage. After binding to the cell, toxin A is internalized, causing secondary cytoskeletal changes of cell contraction, rounding, and nuclear migration (211). The cellular rounding enhances the permeability of the mucosal barrier, exposing the deeper cell layers to the luminal toxins. The cellular injury results in recruitment of neutrophils to the site. Toxin A binding also triggers mediator release from the basolateral aspects of the enterocytes thereby altering tight junction permeability and cytoskeletal structure, and damaging the mucosal barrier. Toxin B also binds to specific enterocyte receptors and stimulates chemokine release from macrophages, leading to hemorrhagic necrosis, fluid secretion, and altered smooth muscle function. Toxin B is approximately 1,000 times more potent than toxin A (205). Both ultimately induce apoptosis in infected cells (210,216).

Clinical Features. Patients with *C. difficile* infections exhibit various clinical manifestations ranging from an asymptomatic carrier state to fulminant colitis with bloody diarrhea, transmural inflammation, and necrosis. The most severe forms of the disease are the least common. In adults, *C. difficile* infection usually causes mild to moderate diarrhea, sometimes accompanied by lower abdominal cramps. The average symptom duration is 8 to 10 days (204) and the incubation period in early onset disease ranges from 1 to 10 days after the inciting antibiotic is started. More frequently, symptoms may be delayed for 2 to 6 weeks following antibiotic discontinuance (late onset disease). *C. difficile* toxins are present in the stool at this time, but endoscopic and histologic findings are frequently normal in patients with mild disease.

In severe cases, diarrhea can occur 20 to 30 times/day and can last up to 2 to 3 months if not treated. Patients with severe colitis without pseudomembrane formation present with profuse debilitating diarrhea, abdominal pain, abdominal distension, and toxic megacolon. Common systemic manifestations include fever, nausea, anorexia, malaise, and dehydration. Peripheral leukocytosis and increased numbers of fecal leukocytes are common (213,224). Patients may experience occult colonic bleeding; rarely, frank hematochezia develops.

The most dramatic form of the disease, pseudomembranous colitis, clinically resembles

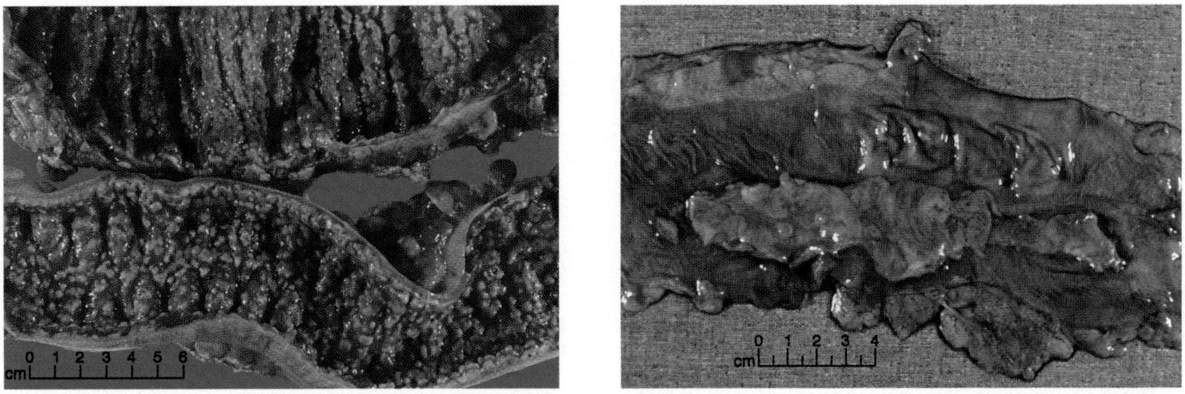

Figure 10-6

PSEUDOMEMBRANOUS COLITIS

Left: Multiple foci of adherent yellow-green pseudomembrane in a patient with *C. difficile* pseudomembranous colitis. Right: In another patient, a large area of the mucosa is covered by an attached pseudomembrane.

C. difficile colitis without pseudomembranes except that the diarrhea, abdominal tenderness, and systemic manifestations are more severe. Megacolon develops as intestinal muscular tone disappears, resulting in a paradoxical decrease in the diarrhea. Other changes that can occur with *C. difficile* infection include protein-losing enteropathy and HUS.

Gross Findings. The gross and endoscopic features of *C. difficile* colitis reflect disease severity. Patients with mild disease may lack gross abnormalities or show only a patchy colitis. Patients with early pseudomembranous colitis have 2- to 10-mm, raised, yellowish white plaques with erythematous bases that are separated by a normal or only mildly edematous or erythematous mucosa (fig. 10-6). Patients with severe disease may have coalescing mucosal plaques covering large mucosal areas. Edema, blurring of the vascular pattern, and thickening and blunting of the haustral folds develop. The lesions are most prominent in the large intestine but the distal small bowel (214) and even the appendix (207) occasionally become involved.

Microscopic Findings. The histologic features of *C. difficile* colitis reflect the disease stage. *C. difficile* can produce a wide range of mucosal appearances, sometimes exhibiting only congestion and edema or nonspecific colitis. Only slightly more than 50 percent have classic pseudomembranous lesions (220).

Type I lesions of pseudomembranous colitis (the earliest lesions) show focal epithelial necrosis, neutrophilic infiltrates, and an edematous lamina propria. Pseudomembrane formation is initiated by epithelial breakdown and eruption of the exudate into the intestinal lumen. The linear deposition of neutrophils and Gram-positive sporulating bacilli within the fibrin strands and mucus imparts an almost pathognomonic appearance (fig. 10-7).

Type II lesions are better developed and consist of well-demarcated groups of disrupted crypts that lose their superficial epithelial lining and become distended by mucin, neutrophils, and eosinophils. The epithelial damage extends into the lower crypts as the process continues. The changes resemble those found in ischemic colitis. Fibrin thrombi may be found in superficial mucosal capillaries. Focal mushroom-shaped or volcanic pseudomembrane eruptions attach to the necrotic mucosa. The pseudomembranes contain epithelial debris, red blood cells, fibrin, mucus, and inflammatory cells. The changes are patchy in nature and the mucosa between the individual pseudomembranes often appears normal.

Type III lesions show complete structural mucosal necrosis with only a few surviving glands covered by cellular inflammatory debris, mucin, and fibrin. The edematous, congested, and hemorrhagic lamina propria bulges into the intestinal lumen. Marked mural edema extends into the muscularis propria. There may be transmural colonic inflammation with massive mural edema and even toxic megacolon (206).

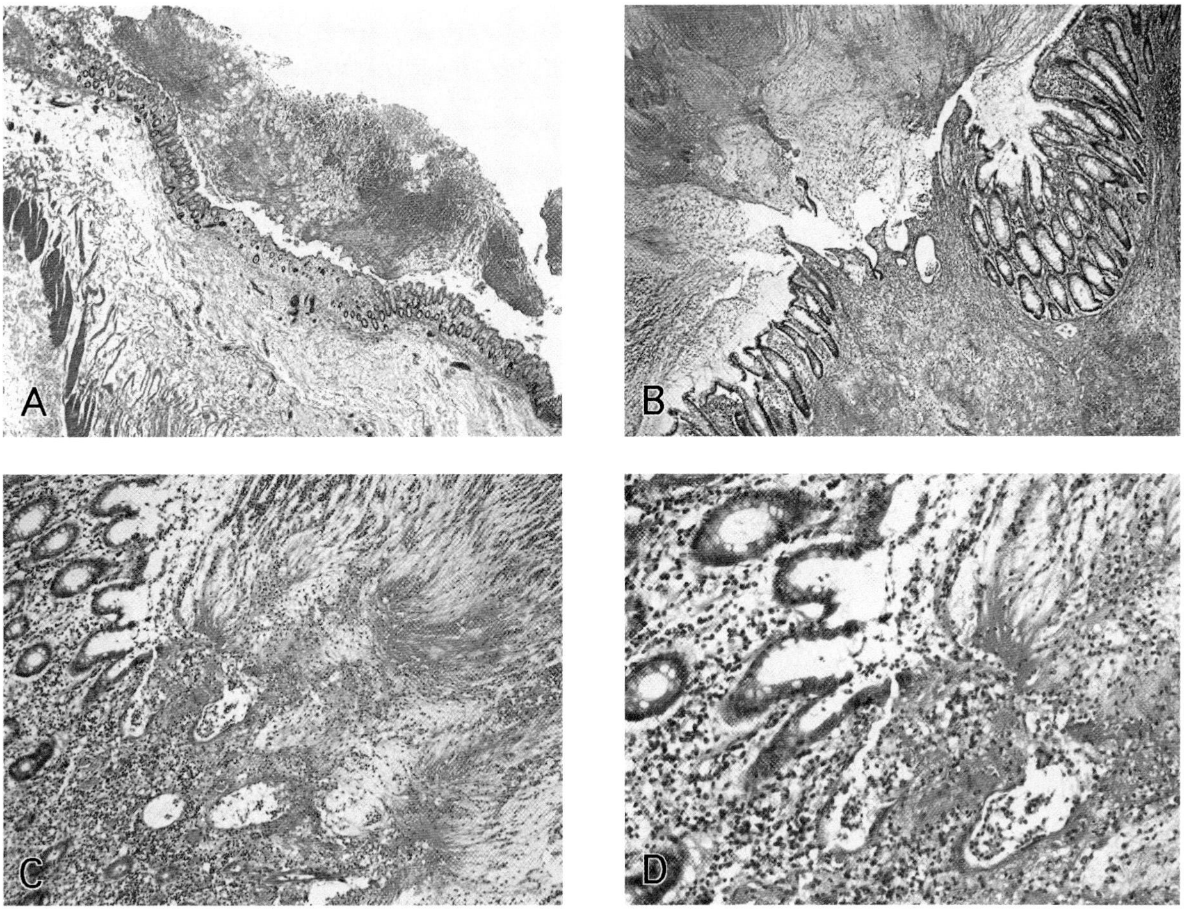

Figure 10-7

PSEUDOMEMBRANOUS COLITIS

A: A thick pseudomembrane adheres to the colonic mucosa.

B: The exudate erupts from areas of mucosal erosion in a pattern that has been described as resembling lava erupting from a volcano.

C: Neutrophils and fibrin form the pseudomembrane that covers the mucosal surface. The neutrophils demonstrate a linear alignment within the fibrin that exudes from areas of erosion.

D: On higher power, the crypt damage resembles ischemic injury. The epithelium lining some crypts is flattened and regenerative. The lamina propria is edematous and contains numerous acute inflammatory cells. Cryptitis and crypt abscesses are present.

Rarely, signet ring cells are found in colonic biopsies of patients with toxic megacolon resulting from pseudomembranous colitis (219, 221). These degenerating cells are usually confined within the basement membrane of the crypts without infiltrating other tissues, a feature that can be highlighted with pancytokeratin immunostains. The nuclei of the signet ring cells are not enlarged but have uniform chromatin and inconspicuous nuclei.

Special Techniques. The laboratory diagnosis of *C. difficile* is based on microbiological isolation of the organism and detection of the specific bacterial toxins. *C. difficile* is a fastidious anaerobic bacterium that must be cultured in anaerobic conditions quickly. Failure to culture *C. difficile* organisms from individuals who are infected may result from delays in specimen transport and processing. Since bacterial cultures detect all *C. difficile* colonies irrespective of their pathogenicity, the colonies must be tested for their toxin production. If pseudomembranes are identified endoscopically, stool specimens should be sent for *C. difficile* toxin

Table 10-6

DIFFERENCES BETWEEN ISCHEMIA AND BACTERIAL ENTEROCOLITIS

Feature	Ischemia	Bacterial Enterocolitis
Focal process	Often	Sometimes
Pseudomembranes	Common	Present in *Clostridium difficile* infection
Mucosal changes of chronicity	Sometimes	No
Hemosiderin-laden macrophages in lamina propria	Common	No
Inflammation extending into submucosa	Common	Common
Crypt abscesses	No	Sometimes
Glandular ghosts	Yes	Yes
Granulomas	No	Usually no, but are seen in *Yersinia* infection
Atrophic microcysts	Common	No
Lamina propria fibrosis	Common	No
Basal plasmacytosis	No	No
Mesenteric vessels	May be abnormal	Normal

analysis and biopsies should be obtained in order to confirm the diagnosis. Testing for either toxin A or B results in misdiagnosis more frequently than testing for both toxins (215).

Differential Diagnosis. Clinically, other diseases that may mimic *C. difficile* colitis include other infections, an acute episode of a chronic condition, drug reactions, or complications of procedures. Infections that clinically resemble *C. difficile* colitis include those caused by *Shigella, Salmonella, Campylobacter, Candida, E. coli* (O157:H7), amoebae, fungi, and viruses. Patients with chronic conditions such as Crohn's disease, diverticulitis, and ischemia have acute episodes of diarrhea that clinically resemble *C. difficile* infection.

Histologically, the two major entities in the differential diagnosis are ischemic colitis and severe IBD. When mucosal necrosis becomes confluent, it may be impossible to distinguish *C. difficile* colitis from other forms of severe colitis associated with extensive necrosis. Pseudomembranous colitis due to *C. difficile* exhibits a more patchy distribution than ulcerative colitis and the rectum may be spared. Secondary infections can complicate ischemic injury and, conversely, bacterial toxins may cause thrombosis and secondary ischemic damage, so that it may be impossible to differentiate between ischemia and bacterial toxin-induced injury. Ways to differentiate the two are listed in Table 10-6.

Treatment and Prognosis. A number of strategies have been used to treat or prevent *C. difficile*-associated disease: 1) discontinuation of the inducing agent; 2) use of antibiotic therapy directed against *C. difficile;* 3) use of resin to bind the toxins; 4) replacement of the normal colonic flora; and 5) use of probiotics to prevent the initial infection. For uncomplicated diarrhea, a conservative approach is recommended, including cessation of the inciting antibiotic and oral rehydration to compensate for fluid loss. In patients with moderate diarrhea, metronidazole or vancomycin may eradicate the organism. Vancomycin therapy, however, is associated with disease relapse and there is increasing vancomycin resistance. Metronidazole may be preferred to reduce the risk of vancomycin resistance among other organisms in hospitals. Anion exchange resins (colestipol) and cholestyramine can bind toxins A and B but estimates of the effectiveness of these agents are currently unclear (203). When severe, pseudomembranous or fulminant colitis requires surgical resection to avoid perforation. Some studies suggest that concurrent antibiotic and probiotic treatment may prevent the development of antibiotic-associated diarrhea (208).

Symptoms recur in 7 to 20 percent of patients due to both relapse and reinfection. Over 90 percent of first recurrences can be treated successfully in the same manner as initial cases. Combination treatment with vancomycin plus rifampin or the addition of the yeast *Saccharomyces boulardii* to vancomycin or metronidazole treatment may prevent subsequent diarrhea in patients with recurrent disease (212).

Prevention. An important aspect of the treatment and prevention of *C. difficile* infection is infection control using measures designed to prevent horizontal transmission. The prevention of nosocomial spread requires patient isolation and enforced hand washing. It also includes the use of gloves in handling body substances and replacement of electronic thermometers with disposable devices. The most successful control measure directed at reduction in symptomatic disease is antimicrobial restriction.

Clostridium Septicum Infections

Demography. *C. septicum* infections are rare but are often associated with serious if not fatal outcomes. They are not associated with a single specific defect in cellular or humoral immunity, but can be seen in patients with multiple medical problems, including leukemia, solid tumors, cyclic neutropenia, diabetes mellitus, and severe arteriosclerosis (225,228,231). The incidence of neutropenic enterocolitis is increasing, particularly in patients with acute myelogenous leukemia who undergo high-dose cytosine arabinoside chemotherapy.

Etiology. *C. septicum* is a rod-shaped, spore-forming, saprophytic, anaerobic, Gram-positive bacterium that grows well on devitalized tissues with a low pH because the latter provide the perfect environment for clostridial spore germination (227). They also grow well in the cecum.

Pathophysiology. The marked pathogenicity of the organism is related to its lethal alpha-toxin. It becomes pathogenic during neutropenia when protease levels are too low to neutralize the toxin (226). The production of bacterial exotoxins or other bacterial virulence factors further damages the mucosa and leads to necrosis of the bowel wall. The organism also produces a number of enzymes, including fibrinolysin, deoxyribonuclease, and several hemolysins that increase its ability to aggressively invade tissues (229). This also leads to bowel wall necrosis and ischemia.

Other factors that play a role in the pathogenesis of the disease are neutropenia and mucosal barrier damage due to chemotherapy. Chemotherapy damages the gastrointestinal mucosa by destroying the rapidly dividing epithelium. Alternatively, neoplastic infiltrates may cause breaks in the mucosal barrier. Loss of mucosal integrity, when coupled with the neutropenia, allows bacteria to invade the bowel wall and sepsis to develop. Ischemia also undoubtedly plays a role in the genesis of the lesion. Ischemia likely results from vascular invasion by bacteria and the development of disseminated intravascular coagulopathy. Other causes of ischemia include perivascular neoplastic infiltrates, episodes of hypotension following sepsis, and mucosal hemorrhage complicating severe thrombocytopenia.

Clinical Features. Neutropenic enterocolitis affects both children and adults. Most patients are profoundly neutropenic (less than 1,000 cells/mm^3). Patients are typically neutropenic for at least a week before symptom onset (232). Patients usually present with a dramatic onset of fever, watery or bloody diarrhea, right upper quadrant pain, abdominal distension, rebound tenderness, nausea, and vomiting. The presence of fever, rigors, and shock suggest the development of sepsis or colonic perforation. The disorder is often fatal unless aggressively treated, usually by resection of the involved bowel segment. Because infected patients receive antibiotic therapy, they may have a coexisting *C. difficile* antibiotic-associated colitis. Mortality rates range from 5 to 100 percent and average 40 to 50 percent (233). Death results from cecal perforation, bowel necrosis, and sepsis.

Gross Findings. The lesions of neutropenic enterocolitis center around the terminal ileum and right colon, and consist of patchy areas of transmural edema and necrosis. The process preferentially involves the cecum due to the luminal stasis that occurs at this site. Rarely, other bowel segments become involved. Some patients develop pneumatosis intestinalis.

Abdominal computerized tomography (CT) and ultrasound are not only useful in evaluating patients with neutropenic colitis, but are preferable to contrast enemas, since the bowel is often massively dilated, very fragile, and likely to perforate if contrast medium is inserted into its lumen. CT findings include symmetrical bowel wall thickening, pericecal inflammation, and, if perforation has occurred, a mass.

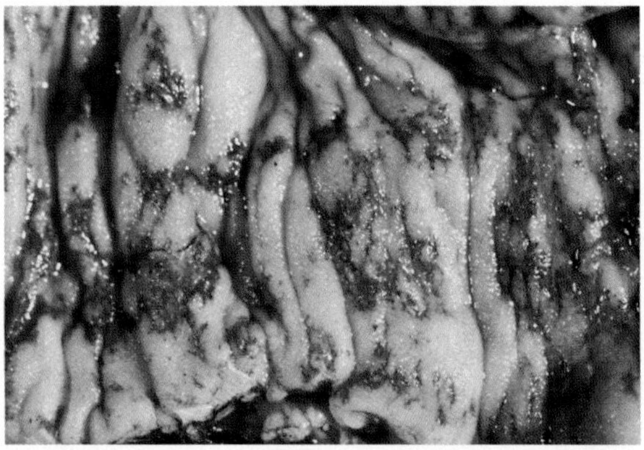

Figure 10-8

COLONIC RESECTION SPECIMEN FROM A PATIENT WITH NEUTROPENIC ENTEROCOLITIS

The colonic mucosal surface appears ulcerated and focally hemorrhagic. There is marked edema.

The gross features of neutropenic enterocolitis vary due to the influence of the multiple etiologic factors. The changes range from areas of mucosal erythema and hemorrhagic necrosis with moderate degrees of edema to severe transmural edema and diffuse hemorrhagic necrosis (fig. 10-8). In some patients, the hemorrhagic features predominate, whereas in others, the edema predominates. Usually, the bowel appears markedly thickened, edematous, and dusky, with scattered serosal ecchymoses. The mucosa often appears beefy red, eroded, and ulcerated. Pseudomembranes develop, probably from the accompanying ischemia.

Microscopic Findings. Histologically, there is evidence of transmural edema, necrosis, and microbial invasion with a minimal cellular response (fig. 10-9). Severe necrotizing colitis is associated with marked edema, vasculitis, and stromal hemorrhage with patchy to complete epithelial necrosis. Degenerated epithelial cells detach from the basement membrane and lie within dilated glandular lumens. This process starts superficially and progressively involves the remainder of the crypt, frequently extending to the base and producing the glandular dropout typical of ischemia. The mucosa becomes variably ulcerated and a pseudomembrane containing fibrin and necrotic cellular debris covers the luminal surface. In severe cases, the bowel exhibits transmural necrosis and degeneration of the muscularis propria (fig. 10-10). Vascular damage produces subtle or profuse intramural and intraluminal hemorrhages, and fibrin thrombi are often present in the submucosal vessels. Additionally, changes characteristic of chemotherapeutic injury, including prominent apoptosis in the crypts, focal crypt dropout, and glandular regeneration, are often present (fig. 10-9). There is a striking paucity of inflammatory cells, despite the degree of mucosal damage, and neutrophils are absent. The absence of neutrophils in the face of significant cell injury confirms the diagnosis of neutropenic enterocolitis.

Differential Diagnosis. *C. septicum* is the major cause of neutropenic enterocolitis; however, other organisms can cause the disease. In children, the infections usually result from *Pseudomonas* or *E. coli*, whereas in adults *C. septicum* is the usual infecting organism. The histologic features overlap with those of *C. difficile*-associated pseudomembranous colitis. Unlike the traditional pseudomembranous colitis associated with *C. difficile* in which there are large numbers of neutrophils present in the exudate, patients with neutropenic enterocolitis lack a neutrophilic infiltrate. The features also overlap with ischemic enterocolitis and infectious enterocolitis, but the absolute lack of neutrophilic infiltrates only occurs in ischemia prior to reperfusion injury.

Treatment and Prognosis. Mortality approaches 100 percent if care is not rendered within 12 to 24 hours (230). Patients may develop secondary infections that complicate the histologic picture; the most common are infections due to *C. difficile*, *Candida*, or CMV.

Clostridium Perfringens and *Clostridium Welchii* Infections

Demography. *C. perfringens* is a widely occurring pathogenic bacterium readily found in soil and in the intestines of humans and animals (242). It is associated with outbreaks of foodborne diarrhea, as well as with antibiotic-associated diarrhea (234,235,245,248,254,259). *C. perfringens* infections tend to affect the elderly, and often result in hospitalization (234,245,259).

In Papua, New Guinea and several other developing countries, *C. perfringens* and *C. welchii* cause a segmental, necrotizing enteritis sometimes

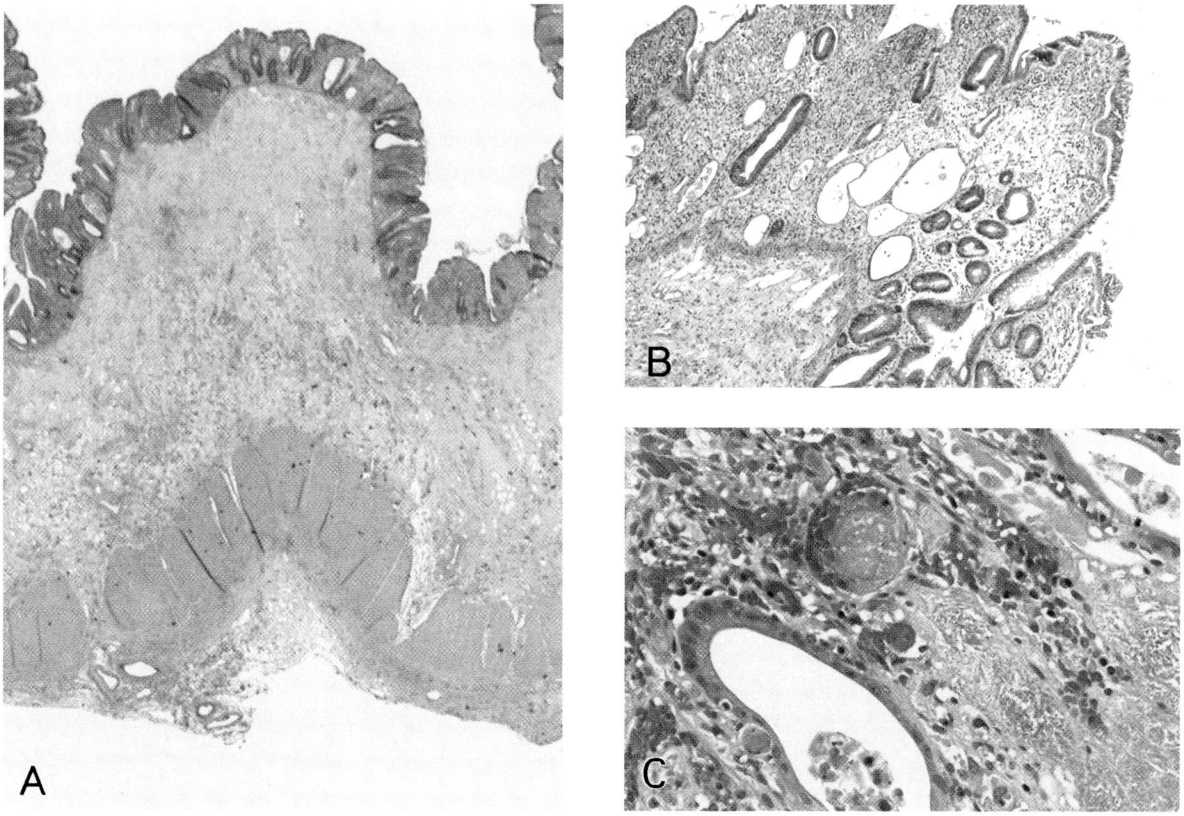

Figure 10-9

NEUTROPENIC ENTEROCOLITIS IN A PATIENT UNDERGOING TREATMENT FOR LEUKEMIA

A: Prominent submucosal edema.

B: The colonic mucosa is also edematous, and shows gland dropout secondary to chemotherapy for leukemia.

C: Higher-power magnification depicts the regenerative glands and lamina propria. A fibrin thrombus occludes a mucosal vessel. No neutrophils are identifiable.

referred to as "pigbel." This disease affects children who are chronically malnourished, and is commonly associated with ingestion of large quantities of contaminated protein-rich foods as occurs at feasts. In rare instances, it is encountered in developed countries, where the infection is generally confined to individuals with severe chronic illnesses (240,250,252,260).

Etiology. *C. perfringens* is a Gram-positive, nonmotile, straight rod with blunt ends, that occurs singly or in pairs. *C. perfringens* can produce over 13 different toxins, although each bacterial strain produces only a subset of the total (251). The production of four major lethal toxins, designated α, β, ε, and ι, are used to type isolates A to E (Table 10-7) (237,244,257,258).

C. perfringens type A is associated with self-limited foodborne diarrhea. The disease occurs following consumption of food contaminated with enterotoxin-producing *C. perfringens*. The contaminated food is almost always heat-treated, which kills competing bacteria but not the spores of *C. perfringens*. Type C *C. perfringens* causes necrotizing enteritis. The disease is mainly due to production of the β-toxin with contribution from δ- and θ-toxins (239,243).

Pathophysiology. Food poisoning due to *C. perfringens* results from the action of the clostridial enterotoxin (CPE). CPE is capable of forming cation-permeant pores in the apical cell membranes of intestinal epithelial cells in culture (241). This action most likely accounts for the diarrheagenic properties of the toxin.

Necrotizing enteritis results from ingestion of organisms capable of producing the *C. perfringens* β-toxin. This toxin is inactivated

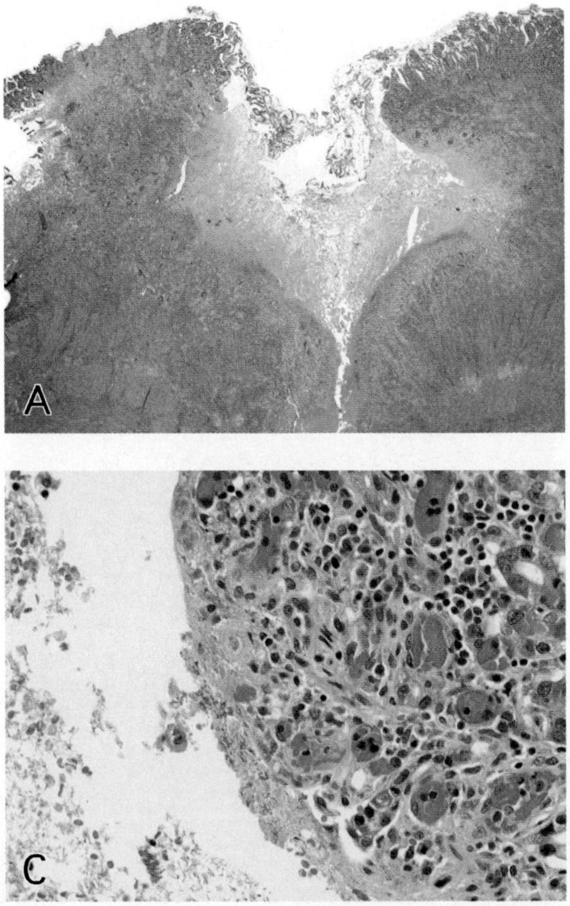

Figure 10-10

NEUTROPENIC ENTEROCOLITIS IN A PATIENT WITH RHEUMATOID ARTHRITIS AND FELTY'S SYNDROME

A: The transmural area of necrosis led to small bowel perforation.

B: Higher-power view taken from the edge of the ulcer. Numerous bacteria lie in the luminal debris and invade the necrotic tissues.

C: There is an absence of neutrophils in the ulcerated area.

Table 10-7

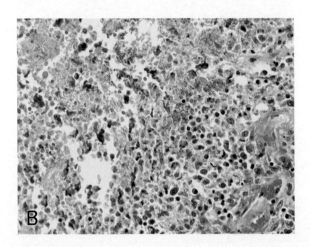

TOXINS PRODUCED BY *CLOSTRIDIUM PERFRINGENS*

C. Perfringens Type	α-Toxin	β-Toxin	ε-Toxin	ι-Toxin	Enterotoxin
A	+	–	–	–	+
B	+	+	+	–	+
C	+	+	–	–	+
D	+	–	+	–	+
E	+	–	–	+	+
Gene	*plc*	*cpb1, cpb2*	*etx*	*iap, ibp*	*cpe*
Genetic location	Chromosome	Plasmid	Plasmid	Plasmid	Plasmid/chromosome

rapidly in the gastrointestinal tract by trypsin. Therefore, another important factor in the pathogenesis of the disease is the presence of trypsin inhibitors that prevent intestinal degradation of the toxin and reduce intestinal motility, thereby favoring stasis and local toxin accumulation (257). Protein malnutrition, a factor that is commonly associated with the development of necrotizing enteritis, is associated with decreased trypsin activity and further predisposes to the disease (238,246,247, 250,255,257). In addition, sweet potatoes, an important dietary staple in areas where pigbel is endemic, contain trypsin inhibitors that further contribute to disease development (246, 247,253).

Clinical Features. *C. perfringens* type A food poisoning develops 8 to 12 hours after eating contaminated food. Symptoms include abdominal pain, nausea, and diarrhea. The disease is generally self-limited, lasting approximately 24 hours. Elderly or very young patients may die of the disease, usually secondary to dehydration (236).

Patients with necrotizing enteritis present with severe, progressive abdominal pain, vomiting, diarrhea, progressive dehydration, blood-stained feces, and finally, constipation lasting for several days. The necrotic bowel predisposes to midgut volvulus, jejunal and ileal ileus, and other forms of small bowel strangulation (249,250). Occasionally, *C. perfringens* is responsible for the genesis of suppurative gastritis or pneumatosis intestinalis.

Gross Findings. Clostridial necrotizing enterocolitis variably affects the upper jejunum, ileum, and colon. The duodenum is only minimally involved. In approximately 25 percent of cases, one or more yellowish serosal patches are present, corresponding to areas of full-thickness infarction. These areas are paper thin and friable, and balloon outward; therefore, they tend to perforate. The affected bowel becomes dilated, edematous, thickened, rigid, and markedly congested, with a reddened serosal surface. The small intestinal valvulae conniventes become very prominent, imparting a "washboard" appearance to the mucosal surface. As the necrotic mucosa sloughs, extensively ulcerated areas remain that may extend into the underlying muscularis propria.

Microscopic Findings. In resection specimens, the histologic features of necrotizing enterocolitis resemble those found in ischemic injury. The small intestine from the duodenum to the cecum shows segmental ischemic necrosis, starting at the villus tips and progressing toward the base. The mucosa appears severely necrotic and hemorrhagic. Mural thickening results from marked submucosal edema. Fibrin thrombi are often present in the inflamed areas. The mucosa lying between the thickened valvulae may appear variably normal, whereas the surface of the valvulae appears damaged. A clearly defined junctional zone exists between the necrotic and non-necrotic tissues, as in other forms of ischemic injury. The mucosa becomes infiltrated with polymorphonuclear leukocytes, mononuclear cells, and eosinophils. Arterial walls appear edematous and infiltrated by inflammatory cells, and demonstrate fibrinoid necrosis. If the patient survives, areas of scarring develop due to extensive and deep disease. Pneumatosis and pseudomembranes may be present.

Special Techniques. *C. perfringens* organisms may be identified as a result of their ability to reduce nitrate; ferment glucose, lactose, maltose, sucrose, and other sugars; and liquefy gelatin. Primers specific for the clostridial *cpa* and *cpb* genes can help diagnose the infection (252).

Differential Diagnosis. The histologic features of clostridial infection overlap with those seen in neutropenic enterocolitis and ischemia. Neutropenic enterocolitis can be distinguished from necrotizing enteritis by the absence of neutrophils in the former and their presence in the latter. The changes cannot be distinguished from ischemia purely on histologic examination.

Treatment and Prognosis. Clostridial food poisoning requires no specific treatment since the disease is usually self-limited. Fluid and electrolyte replacement should be provided as needed. Necrotizing enteritis often requires surgical intervention for resection of necrotic segments of bowel. Even with treatment, as many as one quarter of patients die of the disease (256).

Vibrio Infections

Demography. *Vibrio* is a motile, Gram-negative, curved, rod-shaped bacterium that lives in marine or brackish water. *Vibrio*-associated illnesses, therefore, tend to occur in coastal areas in the summer and fall when the water is warm and bacterial counts are highest (261–263). Cholera occurs in relatively localized epidemics, usually in developing countries. The disease is endemic in southern Asia, parts of Africa, and Latin America. Cholera is also becoming endemic along the Gulf Coast (274) and Chesapeake Bay area of the United States. It is estimated that 5 to 7 million cases of cholera occur each year worldwide, resulting in over 100,000 deaths (272). In the United States, cholera is associated with the consumption of raw oysters and clams, or improperly cooked seafood (262,271). In other countries, cholera is associated with drinking contaminated water or eating contaminated shrimp, cockles, mussels, clams, and dried fish.

Etiology. Cholera is caused by the Gram-negative bacterium *Vibrio cholerae*. The species includes at least 206 different serogroups, of which only the O1 or O139 serogroups cause the disease (265). Other *Vibrio* species also cause gastrointestinal disease including *V. vulnificus* and *V. hollisae*.

Pathophysiology. Pathogenic *V. cholerae* organisms carry a set of virulence genes that is required for pathogenesis in humans. These genes include those encoding the cholera toxin, a colonization factor referred to as toxin coregulated pilus (TCP), and a regulatory protein, ToxR, that coregulates the expression of cholera toxin and TCP (266). The genes for the cholera toxin reside within a lysogenic phage (CTx) integrated into the bacterial chromosome (276). The CTx phage is capable of horizontal transfer to nontoxin producing *V. cholerae* strains provided the recipient bacterium expresses TCP, which acts as the phage receptor. Other potential virulence factors have been identified and include HA protease, RTX toxin, Vac a-like toxin, and the CTxϕ structural proteins, Ace and zonula occludens toxin (270).

Vibrio organisms enter the small intestine where they begin to express low levels of TCP, presumably in response to an as yet unidentified luminal factor. Expression of TCP allows the organism to adhere to the intestinal epithelium. A second environmental signal induces increased expression of TCP, increased colonization of the intestinal mucosa, and production of the cholera enterotoxin (269).

Cholera enterotoxin, the prototype for secretory enteritis and toxigenic diarrhea, has a direct secretory effect on crypt cells. This results in the most overwhelming feature of cholera, extreme fluid loss resulting in "rice-water" stools. The toxin enters the intestinal epithelial cell through the apical cell membrane by means of a complex mechanism, and ultimately activates adenylyl cyclase on the basolateral cell membrane. This results in massive salt and water efflux from the intestinal mucosa with resultant watery diarrhea (270).

Clinical Features. *V. Cholerae Infection.* Incubation periods range from 6 to 48 hours; most patients recover in 2 to 7 days. The clinical spectrum of cholera varies from asymptomatic carriers to patients with voluminous diarrhea that kills within hours of onset. In the acute phase of the disease, the water secretion from the small intestine is greater than the ability of the colon to absorb the water loss. Daily outputs of 15 to 20 L of fluid have been observed when adequate fluid replacement is given. The severity of the disease is related to many factors including inoculum size, biotype of the infecting organism, and absence of preexisting immunity (272).

V. Vulnificus Infection. Three major clinical syndromes result from infection with *V. vulnificus*: primary septicemia, wound infections, and gastrointestinal illness without septicemia or wound infection (268). Acute diarrhea is the usual symptom of gastrointestinal illness. The disease is characterized by a 24-hour incubation period followed by the sudden onset of septicemia, fever, chills, hypotension, nausea, vomiting, bloody diarrhea, and rash. The symptoms and duration are not as severe as in cholera. The skin lesions consist of large hemorrhagic bullae that progress to necrotic ulcers. Although the infection is uncommon, the mortality rate is as high as 50 percent.

V. Hollisae Infection. V. hollisae causes severe gastroenteritis (264).

Gross Findings. Gross specimens are usually only seen at the time of autopsy in those who die of cholera. The bowel appears slightly edematous and only mildly abnormal. The intestinal mucosa appears intact.

Microscopic Findings. Because most cases are examined at the time of autopsy, autolysis can be confused for cholera-induced effects. Biopsy results show that the mucosa remains intact, even during the active stages of the disease (267). Histologic changes include damage to the surface and/or crypt epithelium, epithelial regeneration, altered mucin secretion, and mucosal hyperemia and edema. Dilated intestinal crypts appear mucus depleted and if goblet cells are present, they appear empty. The lamina propria exhibits mild edema and vascular dilatation. Occasional inflammatory cells are present but significant inflammation is absent. The mildness of the histologic features is in marked contrast to the clinical features. Correlation with microbial, immunological, and clinical information is critical to establishing the appropriate diagnosis.

Treatment and Prognosis. Cholera is a leading cause of death in some parts of the world. The large volume fluid depletion associated with the massive diarrhea leads to acidosis and renal failure. Death can occur within 3 to 4 hours of disease onset, with fecal outputs exceeding 1L/hour at the height of the disease. Untreated, the mortality rate ranges between 50 and 75 percent (272,275). Proper rehydration decreases the mortality rate to less than 1 percent (273).

Aeromonas Infections

Demography. *Aeromonas* is ubiquitous in fresh and brackish water; soil; foods including meats, fish, and vegetables; and in the intestines of apparently healthy humans (289). Infections usually occur during the summer months (278) and are acquired via consumption of infected water (288,291), trauma involving soil exposure, or minor trauma sustained while cleaning aquariums, snorkeling, or handling fish (292). Transmission of infection via infected food as well as human-to-human transmission probably also occur (280,293,298). The organism most commonly affects young children (302), and has been isolated from acute diarrheal outbreaks in daycare centers (285). The organism can also be isolated from patients with traveler's diarrhea (286,301). *Aeromonas* species are also commonly isolated from healthy humans, and therefore their role in the causation of diarrheal illness remains somewhat controversial. The difficulty in definitively determining their pathogenic role results from the fact that so many species and subgroups of the organism exist, and only a small proportion represent pathogens (295).

Pathophysiology. *Aeromonas* is a facultative anaerobic, Gram-negative bacillus with a single polar flagellum. The three species that most commonly infect man are *A. hydrophila*, *A. veronii* biovar *sobria*, and *A. caviae* (281,283,290, 295,296). *Aeromonas* produces a number of potential virulence factors including enterotoxins, cytotoxins, hemolysins, aerolysins, hemagglutinins, and proteases (277,279,284,285,287,291, 299,304). In addition, the organism is able to adhere to and invade intestinal epithelial cells in culture (294,303).

Clinical Features. Children with *Aeromonas* infection present with severe diarrhea commonly containing mucus and blood (302). In contrast, adults tend to present with a more chronic disease associated with vomiting and abdominal cramps (282,297,304). The mean duration of illness and length of hospitalization is longer in infants aged 2 to 6 months than at other ages. The spectrum of gastrointestinal diseases ranges from a self-limited diarrhea to acute persistent dysentery (291,300). The most common symptom is diarrhea, followed by abdominal cramps and pain, fever, and vomiting. The disease may result in dehydration, acidemia, and azotemia. The duration of the illness is usually more than 10 days (302).

Gross Findings. The gross findings of *Aeromonas* infection resemble those of other forms of bacterial enterocolitis. Sigmoidoscopy reveals a friable mucosa, sometimes with frank ulceration, associated with acute proctosigmoiditis.

Microscopic Findings. Histologic changes range from alterations that resemble celiac disease, to edema and a plasmacytosis of the lamina propria, to the presence of a full-blown enterocolitis with acute and chronic inflammatory cells in the lamina propria and frank abscesses. The changes resemble those found in other forms of bacterial colitis.

Special Techniques. The diagnosis is made by microbial culture of the stool or tissues.

Differential Diagnosis. The differential diagnosis includes other acute colitides, including infections and ulcerative colitis.

Treatment and Prognosis. Treatment with sulfamethoxazole and trimethoprim results in clinical improvement.

Plesiomonas Infections

Demography. *Plesiomonas* is an increasingly recognized cause of diarrhea around the world, but it is especially common in Asian countries (306,309,312–314). It is associated with eating uncooked fish or seafood, and with foreign travel. The causative organism, *Plesiomonas shigelloides,* is a facultative anaerobic, Gram-negative, rod-shaped bacterium.

Pathophysiology. *P. shigelloides* produces a cholera enterotoxin-like protein (305), as well as thermostable and thermolabile enterotoxins (311). In addition, the organisms may produce cytotoxins and β-hemolysins (307,308). The exact mechanism by which the organism produces diarrheal illness, however, is not yet understood.

Clinical Features. Children with *Plesiomonas* infection most commonly present with watery diarrhea and fever, while adults usually present with diarrhea and abdominal pain (313). The symptoms are most commonly mild and self-limited. Occasionally, chronic diarrhea is reported (310,314). Rarely, severe enterocolitis, pseudoappendicitis, osteomyelitis, and bacteremia develop. The changes mimic those of other forms of severe bacterial enterocolitis.

Pathologic Findings. The gross and microscopic findings resemble those found in other forms of bacterial enterocolitis.

Special Techniques. The diagnosis is established by cultures.

Differential Diagnosis. Other forms of acute colitis.

Treatment and Prognosis. The disease is usually self-limited without complications. Patients with severe or prolonged symptoms may be treated with antibiotics.

Yersinia Infections

Demography. The incidence of *Yersinia* infection is highest in cold months and in cold climates. The disease is more common in Canada and Europe than in the United States. There is a high incidence of the disease in Scandinavia, Japan, and Belgium (343). The geographic distribution of the infection may reflect differences in culinary practices or host reservoirs, or it may simply reflect more intensive surveillance in some countries. Belgium has the highest disease incidence, probably strongly correlating with Belgium's consumption of raw pork (343). Infections are more common in patients who have had gastrectomies, suggesting that gastric acid normally protects against *Yersinia* infection (323). Immunosuppressed patients often develop severe, fatal *Yersinia* bacteremia.

Infection usually follows ingestion of contaminated meat, vegetables, water, and milk (315,330), and pigs are an important reservoir for infection (320,323–325). *Yersinia* infections are an occupational health risk to hog slaughterers (332). The organism has also been isolated from numerous other animals, including dogs, cats (319,326), birds, amphibians, fish, insects, and crustaceans (326,339,340). Transmission can occur via person-to-person contact and by blood transfusions (342). Infants, children, and young adults are most often affected.

Etiology. *Yersinia enterocolitica* is a facultative, anaerobic, nonlactose-fermenting, Gram-negative coccoid bacillus in the genus Enterobacteriaceae. Over 30 serotypes and several biotypes have been identified. In Europe, sporadic infections result from serotypes O:3 and O:9. In the United States, outbreaks are associated with multiple serotypes, the most common of which is O:8 (319). Recently, Lamps et al. (331) sought to determine the presence or absence of *Y. enterocolitica* and *Y. pseudotuberculosis* in patients diagnosed with granulomatous appendicitis. Overall, 25 percent of their cases were positive for pathogenic *Yersinia*: 50 percent for *Y. enterocolitica* and 50 percent for *Y. pseudotuberculosis*.

Pathophysiology. The pathogenicity of *Yersinia* species is determined by a number of virulence factors encoded by the bacterial chromosome or by the virulence plasmid pYV (316–318,338). These factors include various adhesins, invasin and attachment-invasion locus. In addition, the pYV proteins make up a type III secretion system similar to that seen in pathogenic *E. coli* and *Salmonella*.

Bacteria in the lumen of the small bowel or colon adhere to M cells or absorptive cells in areas of the follicle-associated epithelium. *Y. enterocolitica* penetrates into the lamina propria by passing through the enterocyte cytoplasm in a manner similar to that exhibited by *Salmonella*. Chromosomally encoded proteins facilitate bacterial intestinal attachment, mucosal penetration, survival, and proliferation (327, 329,333,334,336). Once inside the cell, the bacteria become enclosed by membranous vesicles (344). Only potentially pathogenic strains invade the lamina propria. *Y. enterocolitica* organisms subsequently multiply within lymphoid follicles in Peyer patches, then drain into the mesenteric lymph nodes, eventually giving rise to systemic infections.

Clinical Features. *Yersinia* causes a wide spectrum of clinical changes that ranges from asymptomatic infection to self-limited enterocolitis or even potentially fatal systemic infection. Patients present with gastroenteritis, acute diarrhea, low-grade fever, pharyngitis, abdominal pain, ileocolitis, diffuse mesenteric lymphadenitis, sepsis, and endocarditis (322,323,328,335,341,345). Diarrhea is the most common symptom, but fever and crampy abdominal pain are also frequent. Occasionally, the abdominal pain localizes to the right lower quadrant, mimicking acute appendicitis. In patients under age 5, the usual disease pattern is a mild, self-limited gastroenteritis indistinguishable from other gastrointestinal infections (321). Typically, the disease lasts 2 to 3 weeks; infrequently, infants develop chronic diarrhea lasting for months. Older children and adults develop mesenteric lymphadenitis and have a syndrome that mimics acute Crohn's disease or tuberculosis. Intestinal perforation occurs rarely (337)

Gross Findings. Because *Yersinia* organisms preferentially invade the area around Peyer patches, *Yersinia* infections typically affect the terminal ileum, appendix, and proximal colon. The rectosigmoid may also be involved, but this is uncommon. The bowel wall appears thickened, inflamed, congested, and edematous. Patients develop aphthous, diffuse, or focal ulcers. Even though the ulcers may be numerous, they are rarely very deep. CT scans demonstrate mesenteric lymphadenopathy. The enlarged mesenteric lymph nodes may become matted and contain yellowish microabscesses. Fistulas and ileal stenosis are unusual.

Microscopic Findings. The affected bowel appears congested, edematous, and ulcerated. A characteristic microscopic feature is sharply demarcated lymphofollicular hyperplasia; microabscesses and prominent germinal centers are in the mesenteric lymph nodes and bowel wall. Small, punctate aphthoid ulcers, covered by fibrinopurulent exudates and measuring 1 to 2 mm in diameter, overlie the hyperplastic lymphoid follicles (322,328). Large numbers of Gram-negative coccobacilli may be present. Epithelioid granulomas with central necrosis, polymorphonuclear cells, and microabscesses are seen (fig. 10-11). The granulomas can be found throughout the bowel wall. The changes superficially resemble those found in cat-scratch fever. The muscularis propria and serosa become infiltrated by pleomorphic cellular infiltrates that often include eosinophils.

Mesenteric lymphadenitis is common. The characteristic lesion consists of necrotizing paracortical epithelioid granulomas, B-cell hyperplasia, and neutrophilic infiltrates with irregular areas of necrosis. The lymph nodes may contain large collections of macrophages, imparting a "starry sky" appearance.

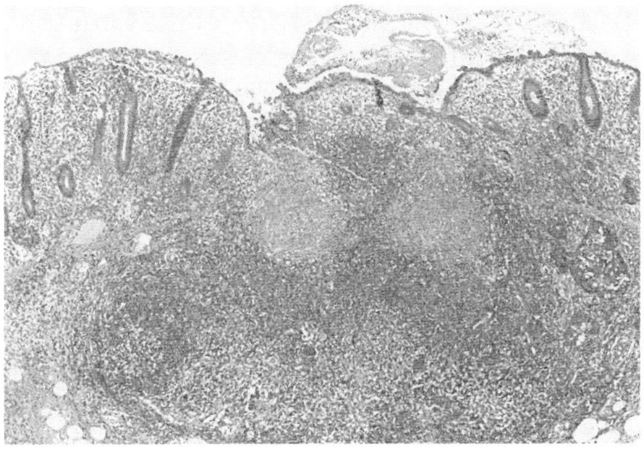

Figure 10-11

YERSINIOSIS

Numerous necrotizing granulomas are located within the mucosa and submucosa. The adjacent mucosa is edematous and the colonic glands appear regenerative.

Special Techniques. The organism can be cultured from lymph nodes and intestinal tissue. If the pathologic specimen is received fixed, the presence of *Yersinia* can be confirmed serologically. PCR-based assays distinguish between pathogenic and nonpathogenic strains of the organism.

Differential Diagnosis. Clinically, radiographically, and grossly, *Yersinia* infections mimic tuberculosis and Crohn's disease because the most severe disease centers around the ileocecal region and the organism produces nodularity of the bowel wall, mucosal thickening, and aphthous ulcers. *Yersinia* infections seldom thicken the bowel wall to the same degree that Crohn's disease does nor does it usually cause fistula formation. The absence of well-formed granulomas in *Yersinia* infections differentiates them from brucellosis and mycobacterial infections. Granulomas may also be seen in *Shigella* or *Salmonella* enteritis, although they are seldom a dominant histologic feature, and when present, are small and lack necrosis.

The differential diagnosis of the mesenteric lymph node lesions includes tuberculosis, brucellosis, tularemia, histoplasmosis, and cat scratch fever. Similar changes in the lymph nodes are seen with *Y. pseudotuberculosis,* but in the latter case, a distinct granulomatous component surrounds the microabscesses in the lymphoid tissues (322).

Treatment and Prognosis. Antibiotic treatment is usually unnecessary, as the illness is typically self-limited. Patients with severe infection or bacteremia, and those who are immunocompromised, may be treated using combination antibiotic therapy including doxycycline, aminoglycosides, trimethoprim-sulfamethoxazole, or fluoroquinolones (328a).

Mycobacterium Tuberculosis Infections

Demography. The tuberculosis bacterium, *Mycobacterium tuberculosis*, has been called the world's most effective pathogen, since it kills an estimated 2 million people each year and lurks in one third of the world's population. Globally, *M. tuberculosis* causes more deaths than any other infection (354). Until recently, tuberculosis was uncommon in North America and Europe, but was endemic in Asia where it represented a major health problem. During the last several decades, however, it has emerged as a worldwide problem, not just restricted to underdeveloped or Asian countries (351,352,356). The number of cases diagnosed in Western countries has dramatically increased due to the appearance of AIDS and the migration of many people from areas with a high tuberculosis incidence to areas with a lower incidence.

Pathophysiology. Transmission of the infection occurs by inhalation of aerosolized droplet nuclei containing the organism, ingestion via the gastrointestinal tract, or infection through a skin lesion. Mycobacteria are intracellular pathogens that reside almost exclusively within macrophages of infected individuals. They are opsonized via complement (C)3 or the complement receptors CR1, CR3, and CR4 (357). Internalization into macrophages requires the association of the complement cleavage product C2A with mycobacteria to form C3 convertase (358). Pathogenic mycobacteria initiate long-term infections by causing extensive remodeling of their vacuolar environment to prevent vacuolar acidification and lysosomal fusion (346,347). Replication in macrophages is crucial for pathogenic mycobacteria. Normally, macrophages phagocytize and destroy the organisms. Certain genes, particularly those encoding virulence proteins from the glycine-rich PE-PGRS family, play a key role in mycobacteria viability within macrophages (355). Infected macrophages then migrate to the regional lymph nodes where they stimulate cell-mediated immunity and eventual granuloma formation.

Tuberculous gastroenteropathy presumably follows swallowing organisms from pulmonary sites of infection. Another probable pathogenetic mechanism involves rupture of, or disease extension from, tuberculous lymph nodes. Intestinal lesions can spread to the serosa by direct extension or hematogenously from the lung.

Clinical Features. The signs and symptoms associated with enteric tuberculosis vary considerably. The signs and symptoms of gastrointestinal and peritoneal tuberculosis are nonspecific and the diagnosis is easily missed or delayed unless there is a high index of suspicion. Gastrointestinal tuberculosis may be limited to the abdomen or it may be part of a systemic disorder. Only 15 to 20 percent of patients have concomitant active pulmonary disease (353).

Esophageal tuberculosis manifests with dysphagia, odynophagia, and bronchial aspiration due to tracheoesophageal fistulas (349,361). Compression of the esophagus from enlarged mediastinal lymph nodes may cause dysphagia.

Symptoms of gastric tuberculosis are usually nonspecific and may mimic a resistant ulcer, gastric outlet obstruction, or fistula (349). Pyloric ulcers or tuberculomas may result in obstruction in a manner similar to that caused by malignancy or peptic ulcers. Although unusual in most communities, tuberculosis is a common cause of pyloroduodenal obstruction among South African blacks (349).

Patients with abdominal disease present with abdominal lymphadenopathy, splenomegaly, hepatomegaly, ascites, and intrasplenic or intrahepatic masses (350). Massive lymphadenopathy may exist without bowel involvement (349). Central lymph nodes along the mesentery and nodes around the ileocecal and pyloroduodenal region are usually involved. Patients may have recurrent abdominal pain, palpable abdominal masses, subacute intestinal obstruction, and the effects of compression on major organs. Chronic nonspecific abdominal pain is the most common complaint. Other symptoms include diarrhea, hemorrhage, and severe wasting.

Intestinal tuberculosis causes fever, weight loss, malaise, severe enterocolitis, massive hemorrhage, perforation, obstruction, fistula formation, strictures, malabsorption, a right lower quadrant mass, and severe secretory diarrhea. The most common form of gastrointestinal disease is ulcerative ileocecal tuberculosis. Patients with primarily ulcerating disease have a virulent course and a high mortality rate. Patients with primarily stenosing changes present with signs and symptoms of bowel obstruction or malabsorption. The malabsorption is due to villous atrophy, lymphatic obstruction, stagnation of luminal contents, blind loops, and fistula formation.

Perirectal tuberculosis often presents as anorectal fissures and fistulas. Anal tuberculosis may result in the development of abscesses and fistulas between the abscesses.

Gross Findings. Tuberculosis can involve any part of the gastrointestinal tract from the tongue to the anus. Ileocecal involvement affects 90 percent of patients and results in ileocecal valve distortion. Other affected locations in decreasing order of frequency are the ascending colon, appendix, jejunum, duodenum, stomach, esophagus, sigmoid, and rectum (349,361).

Esophageal tuberculosis usually represents extension from mediastinal disease into the esophagus. This may result in the formation of fistulas between the tracheobronchial tree and the esophagus. Radiographic findings of tuberculous esophagitis range from focal ulcerated lesions to stricture and fistula formation.

Gastric lesions are usually multiple, ulcerated, and infiltrated, and situated along the lesser curvature. The edge of the ulcer is ragged, thickened, edematous, and undermined, differentiating it from carcinoma (361). The lesions can be serpiginous with violaceous edges or consist of superficial tubercles in the vicinity of ulcers.

Typically, intestinal disease is transmural, consisting of confluent necrotizing granulomas with overlying ulceration (fig. 10-12). Intestinal tuberculosis assumes one of three gross forms: 1) *ulcerating*: characterized by the presence of multiple ulcers; 2) *hypertrophic*: characterized by the presence of scarring, fibrosis, and heaped up mass lesions; and 3) *ulcerohypertrophic*: characterized by thickening and ulceration of the intestinal wall associated with an inflammatory mass, stricture, or an apple-core lesion centering around the ileocecal valve that can clinically mimic cecal carcinoma.

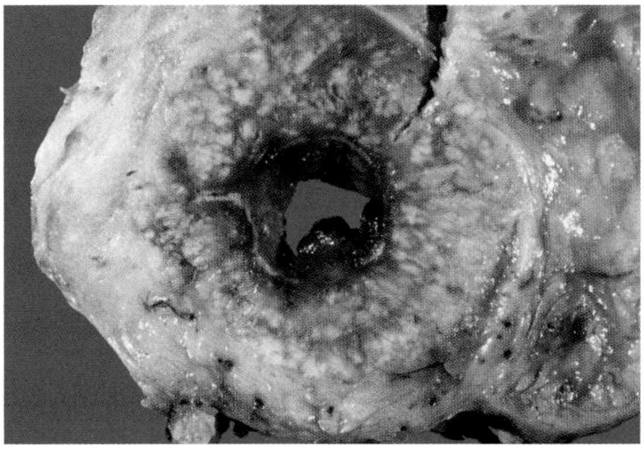

Figure 10-12

TUBERCULOSIS

The wall of the cecum (cut in cross section) is diffusely thickened, and numerous whitish foci of necrosis, which correspond to caseating granulomas, can be seen throughout the full thickness of the colonic wall.

Ulcerating disease appears as ragged, undermining ulcers that may be single, multiple, large, or small. The intestinal wall in these ulcerated areas becomes thickened and fibrotic. Granulomas typically stud the serosa and regional mesenteric lymph nodes are involved. The hypertrophic form is thought to be the result of an exuberant fibroblastic reaction to the infection and may produce a mass lesion that clinically and grossly mimics a carcinoma. The ulcerohypertrophic form is an intermediate lesion with features of ulceration, nodularity, hyperplasia, and stricture formation. The wall of the colon may be so extensively damaged by the inflammatory process that the small intestine is indistinguishable from the colon in an ileocolectomy specimen. Necrotizing granulomas are easily appreciated on the cut surface of the thickened bowel wall or in enlarged regional mesenteric lymph nodes. The normally smooth visceral and parietal peritoneal surfaces become studded with miliary tubercles. Mesenteric nodes may also become infected and hypertrophic. In patients with severe disease, there may be widespread studding of the peritoneal surface with thousands of individual nodules and matting of individual loops of bowel.

Tuberculous disease of the anorectal region appears in four types: ulcerative, varicose, lupoid,

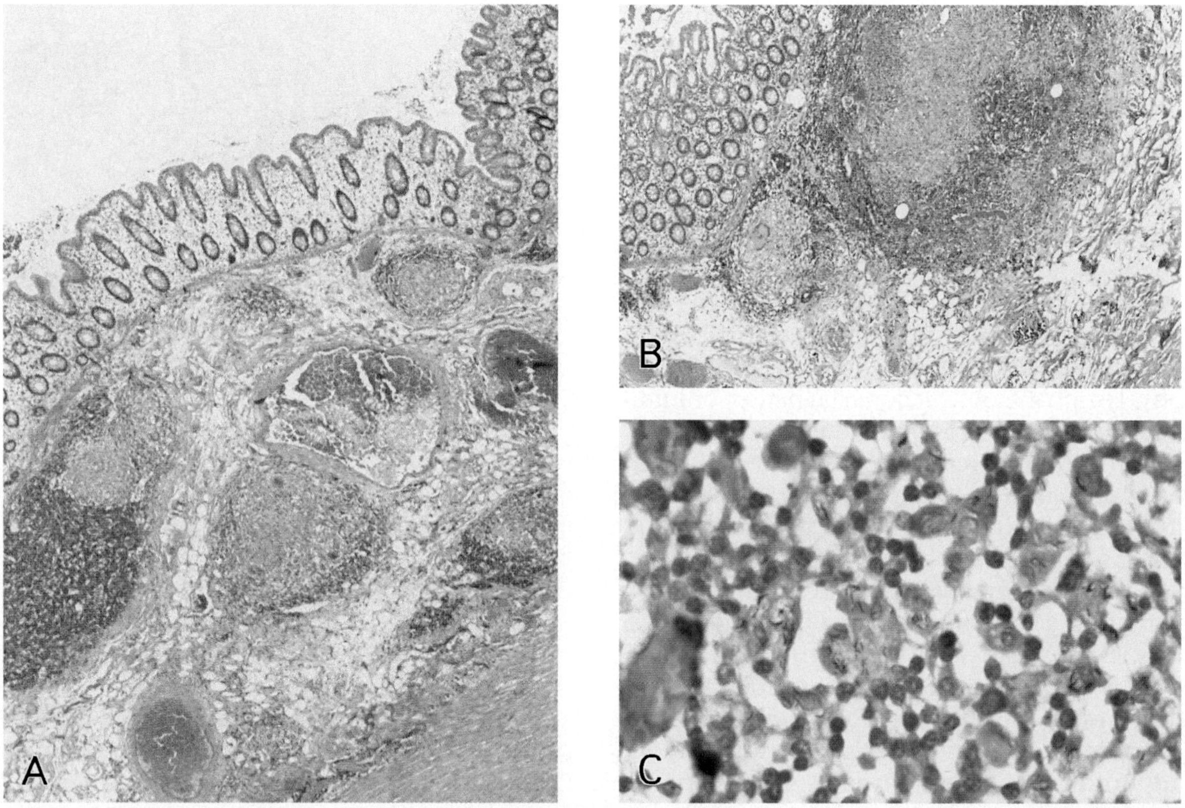

Figure 10-13

TUBERCULOSIS

A: At low power, scattered large, well-formed, submucosal granulomas are seen.
B: A caseating granuloma and an adjacent granuloma with a multinucleated giant cell.
C: Scattered acid-fast organisms are within the necrotic center of a granuloma (Ziehl-Neelsen stain).

or miliary. Ulcers are the most common. They are bluish, resemble amoebic colitis, and produce a thick mucopurulent discharge. Varicose forms are rare, presenting as warty growths. Lupoid forms are infrequent, nodular, and ulcerated, and cause lower abdominal pain, proctitis, ischiorectal abscesses, fistulas, and perianal lesions (359,360).

Microscopic Findings. Biopsies are often not helpful in establishing the diagnosis. Gastrointestinal tuberculosis occurs anywhere in the gut, and typically manifests with caseating granulomas that may be isolated or, in more severe disease, confluent (fig. 10-13). Noncaseating granulomas or disorganized collections of macrophages may also be present.

The granulomas consist of histiocytes aggregated around an area of central necrosis. Macrophages may take the form of epithelioid histiocytes and Langerhans cells. Langerhans giant cells typically have nuclei marginated at the cell membrane. Granulomas may be intact or display several types of central necrosis. They are often large and irregular, producing an appearance of stellate necrosis. Caseation consists of eosinophilic material in which the ghosts of cells are still visible. The bacteria are highlighted by the Ziehl-Neelsen stain (fig. 10-13); they may be extremely difficult to find or may be numerous.

In the intestine, granulomas usually begin in the Peyer patches or lymphoid follicles, imparting a cobblestoned appearance to the mucosal surface. As the disease progresses, they tend to encircle the entire bowel wall, and multiple granulomas may stud the serosa and mesentery. Confluent necrotizing granulomas can completely destroy the underlying architecture of the bowel wall and extend into the pericolonic or periilcal fatty tissues. Giant cell granulomas with obvious caseation occur more frequently in ulcerative than in hyperplastic lesions. They lie throughout the entire thickness of the intestinal wall. Ulcers may contain acid-fast bacteria, even in the absence of granulomas. The nonulcerated mucosa usually appears markedly edematous and focally hemorrhagic. Perirectal fissures and fistulas may contain giant cells; granulomas are not always present.

In order to establish the diagnosis of tuberculosis, multiple deep biopsies of the ulcer bed and its margins must be performed. In some instances, the lymph nodes are completely replaced by confluent necrotizing granulomas and there may be small granulomas on the serosal surface.

Tuberculous peritonitis consists of granulomatous inflammation involving both the visceral and parietal peritoneum. Ascites is often present, with an increase in peritoneal fluid protein concentration and a lymphocyte predominance in the differential count. The diagnosis is made by culturing the ascitic fluid.

Special Techniques. The first step in the detection of acid-fast bacteria is suspicion of the disease so that an acid-fast–stained preparation can be examined. Granulomas or disorganized collections of macrophages are the usual clues. Isolated acid-fast bacilli can be seen in the tubercles and lymph nodes with the use of special stains or they are recoverable by culturing the tissue. The measurement of adenosine deaminase levels in ascites may represent a major diagnostic advance in tuberculous peritonitis, particularly in underdeveloped areas where the disease is common and laparoscopy may not be available (353). It is useful in distinguishing tuberculosis from other causes of exudative ascites.

Differential Diagnosis. The clinical differential diagnosis of tuberculosis anywhere in the gut includes carcinoma and other causes of granulomatous inflammation. In the intestines, it mimics Crohn's disease, *Yersinia* colitis, and fungal infection. Crohn's disease and *Yersinia* infection tend to concentrate around the ileocecal valve and all three diseases produce granulomatous ileocolitis with strictures, aphthous ulcers, and fistulas. In contrast to Crohn's disease, tuberculous ulcers tend to be circumferential, with their long axis perpendicular to the lumen, without fissuring. The granulomas of tuberculosis are more florid and numerous than those of Crohn's disease and caseation is found in larger granulomas. Even when necrosis is not especially prominent in the intramural lesions of tuberculosis, the associated lymph nodes usually show evidence of caseation.

Treatment and Prognosis. Mortality has fallen from 50 to 3 percent with the introduction of antituberculous treatment and supportive nutritional therapy (348). Factors that still contribute to the death of patients are complications, late presentation, a delay in institution of antituberculous therapy due to failure to diagnose the disease early, and coexisting factors such as cirrhosis, alcoholism, diabetes, immunocompromise, and gross debilitation. If the small bowel is seriously affected, parenteral nutrition may be needed. Successful treatment of patients with extrapulmonary tuberculosis requires the use of multiple antibiotic agents for long periods of time. Multidrug-resistant strains of mycobacteria have recently emerged. Surgery is reserved for patients with complications such as obstruction or fistulas or for those in whom uncertainty exists in the diagnosis.

Other Mycobacterial Infections

Mycobacterium avium complex infections are predominantly seen in AIDS patients. Therefore, they are discussed in chapter 11.

Neisseria Gonorrhoeae Infections

Demography. *Neisseria gonorrhoeae* is a cause of proctitis in those engaging in anal intercourse or in those with urogenital infections. The disease affects both men and women. The prevalence of gonococcal infections in sexually abused children in North America ranges from 0 to 11 percent (365). *N. gonorrhoeae* probably represents the most common cause of acute and chronic proctitis in AIDS patients.

Etiology. *N. gonorrhoeae* is the causative organism. The most obvious route of inoculation is direct implantation by rectal intercourse, but in women, the infectious vaginal discharge from genital gonorrhea may also infect the anorectal mucosa everted during defecation (362). Risks of sexual transmission and acquisition include unprotected anal intercourse and oral-fecal contact.

Pathophysiology. Stratified squamous epithelium resists bacterial invasion, while the columnar and transitional epithelia of the anal canal and rectum are more easily penetrated by bacteria. This explains the preferential localization of the infection to the rectal rather than the anal mucosa. The neutrophils associated with gonococci are often packed with intact, seemingly viable, intracellular bacteria or have gonococci bound to their surfaces. This suggests that neutrophils are unable to kill the infecting bacteria. The massive influx of neutrophils that accompanies a gonococcal infection is in part generated by complement components that serve as strong chemotactic factors. An outer membrane protein I (PI), produced by the bacteria, is inserted into the cytoplasmic membrane of neutrophils causing depolarization of the cell (363). This may inhibit intracellular killing of gonococci by inhibiting the release of granule proteins. A second mechanism by which phagocytosis can be impeded involves the attachment of gonococci to the neutrophilic surface in a manner that inhibits their ingestion. Gonococcal surface components appear to be involved in this process.

Clinical Features. Two thirds of patients with anorectal *Neisseria* infections remain asymptomatic (362). Patients with severe symptoms develop anorectal discomfort, copious purulent anal discharge, burning or stinging rectal pain, blood or mucus in the stools, and tenesmus. Milder cases may be characterized by the presence of perianal itching or burning with some purulent staining of underwear. Physical examination shows a moist or stained perianal area; a large percentage of patients have coexisting condyloma acuminata (362). In symptomatic patients, an extremely florid proctitis is present and the patient often has difficulty tolerating the examination due to the pain. Inflammation may extend high into the rectum. Deep perirectal ulcers or abscesses develop that may contain large numbers of bacteria.

Gross Findings. The rectal mucosa appears normal in a large percentage of patients (364); others present with the gross features of proctitis. The disease does not involve the bowel more proximally than the rectum. In severe cases, the mucosa appears reddened and edematous. It bleeds easily when touched with a swab or an instrument. A copious amount of purulent exudate overlies the mucosal changes (362).

Microscopic Findings. Smears taken from purulent exudates of patients with gonorrhea demonstrate numerous neutrophils, many of which, but not all, are packed with cytoplasmic gonococci. Histologically, biopsies of the anorectal region show acute or subacute proctitis affecting the upper anal canal, including the area of the anal crypts and ducts. Although not common, epithelial ulceration and disorganization may be seen (364). Plasma cells of the IgA-secreting type and lymphocytes may also be present within the infiltrate, as may neutrophils. Histologic features resemble those found in IBD, stressing the importance of culture or Gram stain on the tissues in order to identify the organism. The histologic findings reflect the clinical and gross findings. Many patients with culture-proven rectal gonorrhea lack any histologic abnormalities. Mildly symptomatic disease often only manifests as a slight increase in lymphocytes and plasma cells within the lamina propria (364,366).

Special Techniques. The diagnosis is best made using a Gram stain prepared from a rectal swab or by microbial culture of a distal rectal mucosal swab, rather than by biopsy. Gram stains demonstrate the presence of Gram-positive intracellular diplococci. Not all patients with the disease have a positive smear.

Differential Diagnosis. Sexually transmitted gastrointestinal diseases result in proctitis, proctocolitis, and enteritis due to one or multiple pathogens. Evaluation should include appropriate diagnostic procedures such as endoscopy or sigmoidoscopy, stool examination, and culture. Empirical therapy for acute proctitis in persons who have recently practiced receptive anal intercourse should be chosen to treat *N. gonorrhoeae* and *Chlamydia trachomatis* infections. The differential diagnosis includes IBD, usually as ulcerative colitis. Biopsies help distinguish between the two lesions.

Treatment and Prognosis. Penicillin is the drug of choice. In the United States, antimicrobial resistance in *N. gonorrhoeae* continues to evolve and coinfection with *C. trachomatis* is a serious problem. Gonococci are capable of prolonged survival in untreated areas and they frequently reinfect patients with considerable mucosal and systemic immune responses to the infection. Multiple mechanisms account for the high reinfection rate: 1) variations in surface antigen expression; 2) production of an extracellular IgA protease by the organism; 3) presence of an antigen that preferentially stimulates the host production of antibodies that block the killing activity of other antibodies; 4) masking of critical epitopes by chemical modifications of surface structures; 5) molecular mimicry of host antigens; 6) shedding of antigens in the form of outer membrane blebs; and 7) subversion of certain nonimmunologic antimicrobial defenses by the bacterium. Moreover, gonococci are capable of considerable phenotypic adaptation to changing environmental conditions in vivo.

Treponemal Infections

Demography. The venereal infection *syphilis* was considered to be a primary public health concern in the United States for a long period of time but with the development of effective antibiotic treatment, prevalence decreased dramatically. Recently, the rates have again increased with the emergence of the AIDS epidemic. Rates of primary and secondary syphilis have been declining in the United States since the last national epidemic in 1990 (367). The rate of syphilis is higher in the South than in the rest of the country; it is highest in blacks and lowest in Asians and Pacific Islanders.

Clinical Features. In the primary phase of the infection, *Treponema pallidum* enter the body through the skin or mucous membranes and invade the blood or lymphatic vessels, eventually accumulating in the regional lymph nodes. Several weeks later, a firm, relatively painless ulcerating nodule or chancre forms at the site of initial invasion. If this infection remains untreated, it progresses to secondary syphilis, which is characterized by rash, fever, lymphadenopathy, and mucocutaneous inflammation. If patients develop gastritis, symptoms of vomiting and abdominal pain occur. Patients with tertiary syphilis develop a variety of extragastrointestinal lesions, including the classic findings of aortitis, parenchymal or skeletal gumma formation, and tabes dorsalis associated with neuropathic joint disease. At this stage, a mass or gumma may form in the gastrointestinal wall.

Gastrointestinal syphilitic involvement occurs either from direct infection from the anorectal region or from acquisition of the disease from the mother. The latter is uncommon today, at least in Western populations. Syphilitic involvement of the gastrointestinal tract presents as gastritis, enteritis, or anorectal disease. Esophageal syphilis is rare. In the past, when syphilis was more common, esophageal gummas, diffuse ulceration, and esophageal strictures could be seen in patients with tertiary syphilis. Additionally, syphilitic aortic aneurysms could rupture into the esophagus. Unless they are secondarily infected, the lesions usually remain painless. Patients may have coexisting sexually transmitted rectal infections, including herpesvirus, *N. gonorrhoeae*, or *C. trachomatis*.

Gross Findings. The radiographic features of gastric syphilis vary depending on the stage of the disease. In early disease, there are no radiologic manifestations. During the secondary phase, a small percentage of patients develop acute gastritis that radiographically appears nonspecific, with diffusely thickened folds that become nodular with or without detectable ulcers (fig. 10-14). In late stage disease (tertiary syphilis), a number of extragastrointestinal manifestations are present and a mass or gumma may develop in the gastric wall. The changes may evolve into a fibrotic narrowing of the stomach, leading to the development of a funnel-shaped deformity (fig. 10-14) (368). Gastric syphilis usually presents as endoscopically visible gastritis, but may simulate the appearance of gastric lymphoma (369).

In the small bowel, involvement consists of multiple ulcers, gummatous plaques, or diffuse fibrosis with scarring and stenosis. The latter sometimes exhibits an annular infiltrative pattern grossly simulating a carcinoma. Depending on disease stage, the anorectal lesions can appear as either proctosigmoiditis or a mass lesion. Large, papular perianal skin lesions, referred to as condylomata lata, may be seen in patients with secondary syphilis.

Microscopic Findings. The histologic features of syphilis include perivascular lymphoplasmacytic infiltrates and obliterative endarteritis (fig. 10-15). Crypt abscesses and granulomas may also be present.

Special Techniques. In tissue sections, Warthin-Starry silver, immunofluorescent, or

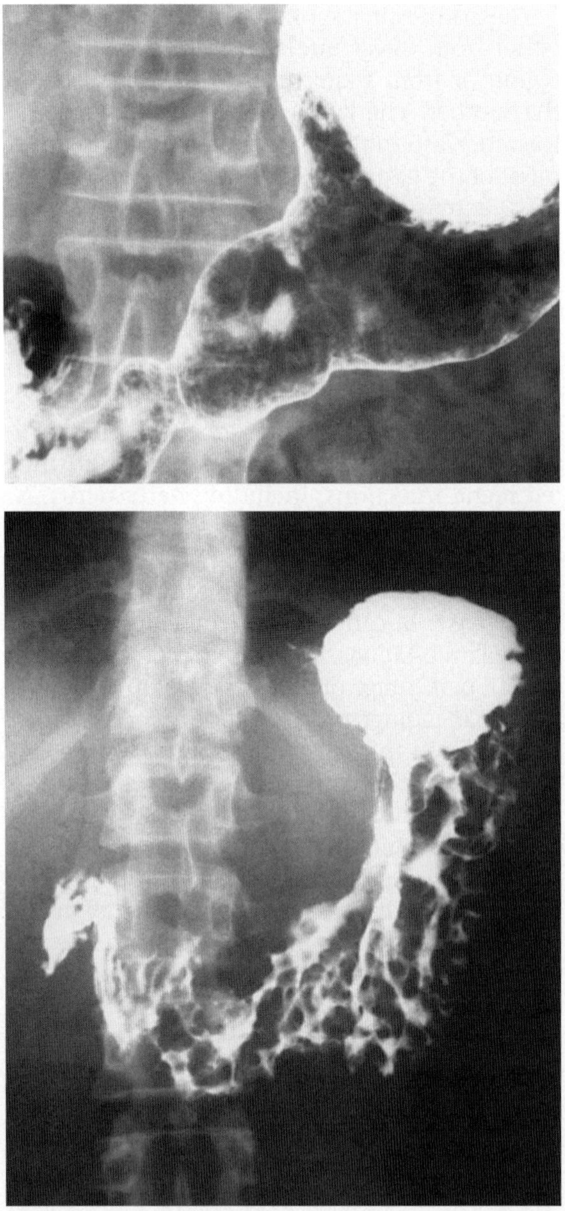

Figure 10-14

GASTRIC SYPHILIS

Top: Acute syphilitic gastritis. Single contrast upper gastrointestinal image of a 33-year-old woman with postprandial vomiting. The gastric rugal folds are markedly thickened and irregular in the body and antrum.

Bottom: Antral deformity after treatment of tertiary syphilis. Radiograph from a double-contrast upper gastrointestinal study shows smooth antral tapering and foreshortening extending distally from the midportion of the study. The classic deformity of the antrum and proximal duodenum has been compared to the appearance of a ram's horn. (Figs. 5 and 1A from Jones BV, Lichtenstein JE. Radiographic manifestations of gastric syphilis: pictorial essay. AJR 1993:160;59–61.)

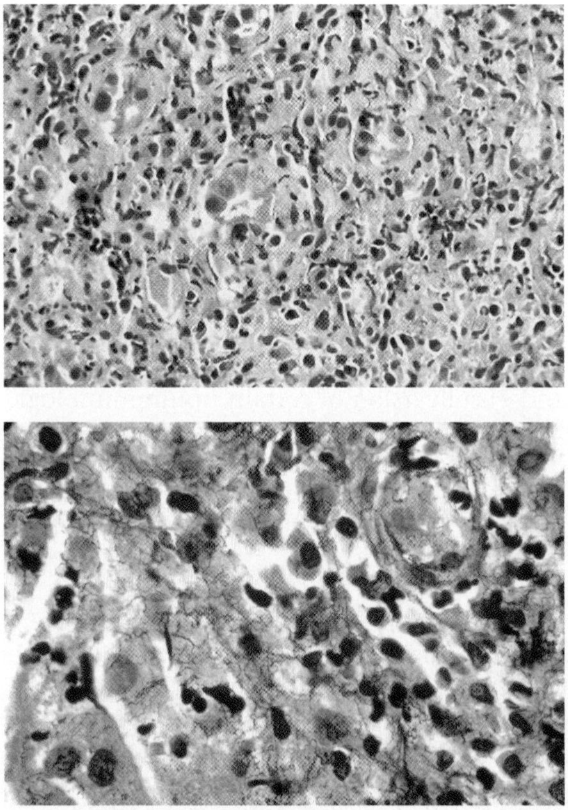

Figure 10-15

GASTRIC SYPHILIS

Top: Almost complete mucosal destruction by an infiltrate that consists of mononuclear cells and neutrophils is seen with the hematoxylin and eosin (H&E) stain. Remnants of glands are present.

Bottom: Warthin-Starry stain demonstrates numerous spirochetes. (Courtesy of Dr. D. Schwartz, Atlanta, GA.)

immunoperoxidase stains identify the organism. Warthin-Starry and other silver-based stains are hard to read and the immunoperoxidase stain offers an attractive alternative. Most often the diagnosis is established by conventional serologic tests.

Differential Diagnosis. Gastric syphilis can mimic a wide range of lesions, including gastritis and benign ulcer disease, as well as gastric carcinoma and lymphoma. The differential diagnosis includes other causes of gastritis or chronic intestinal inflammation. In the small intestine or proximal colon, the differential diagnosis includes Crohn's disease, *Yersinia* infection, or tuberculosis.

Treatment and Prognosis. Syphilis is treated with penicillin.

Intestinal Spirochetosis

Homosexual men have the highest prevalence of spirochetosis, and the disease is commonly seen in the HIV-positive population. This entity is discussed further in chapter 11.

Granuloma Inguinale (Donovanosis)

Demography. *Granuloma inguinale (donovanosis)* is a highly contagious, venereally transmitted, chronically progressive, autoinoculable ulcerating disease that involves the skin, mucosa, and lymphatics of the perianal and genital area. The disease is endemic in the tropics, but has a patchy geographic distribution. It is relatively common in Papua New Guinea and parts of South Africa, India, Australia, and Brazil (375). The disease is uncommon in the United States.

Etiology. The disease results from an intracellular Gram-negative microorganism identifiable morphologically as the Donovan body. The causative bacterium is *Calymmatobacterium granulomatis,* which is antigenically related to the *Klebsiella* species. In fact, there has been a recent proposal to rename the organism *Klebsiella granulomatis* (371).

Clinical Features. The incubation period is usually 1 to 4 weeks, but longer periods are common (374,376). The anorectum, particularly in females, is most commonly affected. The infection consists of inflammatory nodules, fissures, fistulas, and extensive fibrosis. The fibrosis causes obstruction of the lymphatics and perianal elephantiasis.

Pathologic Findings. Inflammatory nodules may be present and feel like firm tumors in the bowel wall. The scarring fibrosis leads to deformity and strictures. Chronic ulceration and scarring may resemble that of lymphogranuloma venereum. Perianal granuloma inguinale also resembles the condylomata lata of secondary syphilis. Locally destructive lesions and secondary infections may lead to severe morbidity or even death.

Histologic studies reveal the presence of marked acanthosis and pseudoepitheliomatous hyperplasia of the squamous mucosa. The lamina propria contains collections of histiocytes, monocytes, and plasma cells. Capillaries and blood vessels appear prominent. Inclusion bodies, or Donovan bodies, are present in enlarged histiocytes. The organisms are best seen in air-dried smears made by crushing biopsy tissue between the slides, fixing the slides in methanol, and staining them with the Wright-Giemsa or Warthin-Starry stain. Using this method, Donovan bodies appear as rounded coccobacilli lying within cystic cytoplasmic spaces in the mononuclear cells. They resemble bluish black safety pins due to bipolar chromatin condensations.

Differential Diagnosis. Clinically, the differential diagnosis includes syphilis, amoebiasis, chancroid, and lymphogranuloma venereum. Histologically, donovanosis must be distinguished from rhinoscleroma, leishmaniasis, and histoplasmosis. The diagnosis is confirmed with the use of special stains.

Treatment and Prognosis. Complications of the disease include deep ulcers, chronic scarring, lymphedema, and exuberant epithelial proliferations grossly resembling carcinoma. Squamous cell carcinoma may complicate long-standing disease. Patients may also develop disseminated disease involving bone and other organs. Disseminated disease frequently leads to debilitation and death.

Granuloma inguinale is treated with antibiotics. Doxycycline is most commonly used in developed countries, but trimethoprim-sulfamethoxazole, chloramphenicol, erythromycin, and azithromycin are also effective (373). Penicillin is not an effective treatment (372,377). Patients with severe fissures and fistulas unresponsive to medical therapy may require surgical intervention (370).

Chancroid

Demography. *Chancroid* results from infection by *Haemophilus ducreyi.* It is the most common cause of genital ulcer disease in many developing countries (392), and has recently become established as a significant sexually transmitted disease in the United States (382, 389,390,396). The disease affects both males and females, although the male to female ratio in one study was 27 to 1 (397).

Etiology. *H. ducreyi* is a Gram-negative, short, slender organism with blunt ends. In smears, the organisms are typically seen in pairs or in short or long chains, the appearance of which has been likened to a "school of fish" (398).

Pathophysiology. *H. ducreyi* produces a number of potential virulence factors including pili, extracellular toxins, and hemolysin (379,380, 384,395,399). The organism enters the skin or mucosa through microabrasions that develop during sexual intercourse. After a variable incubation period, an erythematous papule arises at the affected site. This papule evolves to a pustule that, after 2 to 3 days, undergoes necrosis, forming a pathognomonic, tender, nonindurated ulcer with undermined margins. Inflammation spreads to the draining lymph nodes (386,397).

Clinical Features. The incubation period for chancroid is short, varying between 3 and 5 days; this period may be longer in patients with HIV infection (397). Tender ulcers with a tendency to bleed on touch develop at the site of infection. Unilateral, regional lymphadenopathy commonly accompanies the ulcer. The lymph nodes are tender, swollen, and matted together, ultimately forming a single fluctuant aggregate. Spontaneous rupture may result in a single discharging sinus in the inguinal region (385,388,391).

Gross Findings. The organism produces single or multiple, painful anal ulcers; abscesses form in the draining lymph nodes. The ulcers develop at the inoculation site. When multiple ulcers are present, they often differ in their stage of development. The ulcer begins as a macule that rapidly becomes pustular and ruptures, leaving a shallow, saucer-shaped ulcer surrounded by a narrow erythematous margin. The ulcers have ragged edges and a base covered by a grayish necrotic exudate (397).

Microscopic Findings. Histologic sections of well-developed chancroid ulcers reveal three distinct layers. The superficial layer consists of red blood cells, polymorphonuclear leukocytes, histiocytes, fibrin, necrotic debris, and intracellular and extracellular Gram-negative coccobacilli (*H. ducreyi*) at the ulcer base. Vascular proliferations and edema characterize the middle layer. Thrombosis with subsequent tissue necrosis and ulceration may result from endothelial swelling. The deep layer contains a dense infiltrate of plasma cells, lymphocytes, and polymorphonuclear leukocytes (383).

Special Studies. Gram stains of the exudate obtained from ulcerations are unreliable (378), and isolation of the causative bacterium, *H. ducreyi*, is difficult because the organism is fastidious and the media required for primary isolation are extensive (386). By using a single, enriched, selected medium in optimal cultural conditions, the isolation rate of *H. ducreyi* from presumptive chancroidal ulcerations is estimated to be between 60 to 70 percent, with higher rates achieved if two media are employed (393). More recently, PCR-based tests have been used to diagnose the infection (381,394,400).

Treatment and Prognosis. The disease is treated with antibiotics including erythromycin, azithromycin, ceftriaxone, ciprofloxacin, and spectinomycin. Resistance to other commonly used antibiotic agents has been reported (387).

Actinomyces Infections

Demography. Although *Actinomyces* is a normal commensal inhabitant of the digestive tract, especially in the oropharyngeal region, *A. israelii* infections do develop. These infections are more common in patients with impaired immune defenses. Occasionally, the organisms are encountered in otherwise normal individuals.

Etiology. *A. israelii* is a filamentous, Gram-positive bacterium that is part of the normal flora of the oral cavity. Abdominal infections usually result when swallowed organisms escape destruction in the stomach. Other cases of invasive abdominal actinomycosis result from appendiceal or colonic perforations following acute appendicitis, diverticulitis, or abdominal trauma, including surgery.

Clinical Features. *A. israelii* can cause serious small intestinal and colonic infections, often at the ileocecal valve or in the rectum (403,406). Changes in bowel habits, low-grade fever, malaise, weight loss, abdominal pain, and a palpable abdominal mass may lead to a misdiagnosis of carcinoma. *Actinomyces* infections also present as sinuses that drain to the abdominal wall. Rectal lesions demonstrate areas of induration, with or without ulceration, fistulas, or strictures.

Gross Findings. In patients with severe disease, the affected bowel appears thickened with multiple suppurative foci, sinus tracts, and scar tissue. Thick-walled abscesses with tough fibrous walls enclosing loculi and filled with yellow or white pus can be found along the sinus tracts. Ulceration may be minimal, but fistulas can develop, resulting in full-thickness intestinal involvement and extension into surrounding tissues.

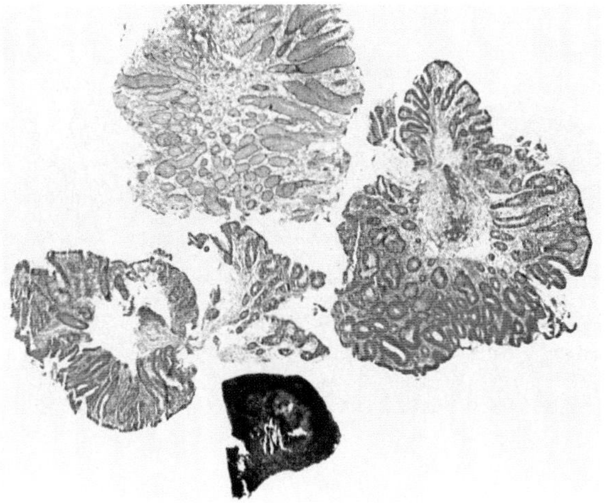

Figure 10-16

ACTINOMYCOSIS

Fragments of colonic mucosa are admixed with a large colony of *Actinomyces* (bottom center).

Microscopic Findings. The characteristic microscopic lesion is an abscess, which is often multiloculated, surrounded by a zone of vascular granulation and scar tissue with extensive fibrosis. Large, foamy macrophages surround the suppurative centers of the lesions and scattered lymphocytes and plasma cells are in the granulation tissue (401). Fistulous tracts often extend into the surrounding tissues. The diagnosis is based on finding the distinctive-appearing organisms usually floating in the pus (fig. 10-16). They consist of rounded masses of branching filaments measuring approximately 300 µm in diameter, readily seen with Gram or H&E stain. A radial corona of eosinophilic material, called Splendore-Hoeppli fibers, surrounds the bacterial masses, producing the characteristic sulfur granules. The Gram-positive bacterial colonies have a club-shaped Gram-negative edge.

Occasionally, the organisms are encountered in the absence of any inflammation. If they are seen in the esophagus or stomach in the absence of significant inflammation, it is unlikely that the organisms are causing disease. They are likely to be the result of swallowing organisms from the tonsillar region or passage on the endoscope. The significance of organisms in the absence of inflammation in large intestinal biopsies is less clear.

Special Procedures. In Brown-Brenn–stained sections, Gram-positive, slender, branching, beaded bacilli can be demonstrated tangled in the center of the granules.

Differential Diagnosis. Based on gross findings, the differential diagnosis includes other stenosing and fistula-producing infections, such as Crohn's disease, tuberculosis in the intestine, or *Chlamydia* in the anorectal region. Some cases clinically and grossly resemble carcinoma (404,405). The differential diagnosis is easily resolved by finding the characteristic organisms on histologic examination. The differential diagnosis also includes *Nocardia* infection, which also forms loose masses without the club-shaped peripheral edge and, unlike *Actinomyces,* is acid fast.

Treatment and Prognosis. Abdominal actinomycosis can be successfully treated with penicillin (402,404).

Tropheryma Infections

Demography. *Whipple's disease,* the common term for *Tropheryma* infection, is a rare disorder that is most commonly encountered in Caucasians living in mid-Europe or the United States. It tends to affect middle-aged individuals (mean age at diagnosis is 50 years), and is eight times more common in men than women (420,438). Several familial cases have been reported, but most analyzed cases do not suggest a familial component (413,424,441). The HLA B27 haplotype is found in 26 percent of infected patients (418); however, this characteristic is not found in all populations (408,440).

Etiology. Whipple's disease results from infection with the bacterium *Tropheryma whipplei.* The habitat of the organism is unknown. It has been cultured from sewage in Germany, and from feces of patients without evidence of Whipple's disease (411,425,430). In addition, PCR-based studies have shown that bacterial DNA sequences can be amplified in saliva, gastric fluid, and duodenal biopsy samples from healthy patients (412,416,431). The ability to amplify bacterial DNA from these sites appears to be dependent on the geographic region in which the individual lives (411).

Pathophysiology. It is thought that patients who develop Whipple's disease may have some form of persistent monocyte or macrophage dysfunction that predisposes to the infection. Although numerous immunologic abnormalities have been described in patients with Whipple's disease, it is likely that the defect is subtle and specific for the causative organism, *T. whipplei*, since these patients do not show an increased susceptibility to other infections (435). Only a few reports suggest an increased frequency of Whipple's disease in immunodeficient individuals (immunosuppressed or AIDS patients) (426,429,432,437).

Populations of T cells in the lamina propria and in the circulation of patients with active Whipple's disease show a shift toward a mature T-cell population, and a decreased CD4/CD8 T-cell ratio (414,433,434). In addition, peripheral T cells show a reduced proliferative response to a number of factors (418,423). Some patients have an inhibitory serum factor that down-regulates the T-cell response (423,434).

Macrophages in infected patients show decreased intracellular degradation (409) and a decrease in phagocytosis (428). In addition, with active disease, the macrophages show decreased expression of CD11b, a molecule that facilitates microbial phagocytosis (415); they may also show defects in the production of interleukin 12, a cytokine important in the regulation of cell-mediated immunity (433,434).

Clinical Features. In most cases, the initial manifestation of Whipple's disease is a chronic, migratory, nondestructive polyarthropathy that affects mainly the peripheral joints (435). The arthropathy may precede the diagnosis of Whipple's disease by as many as 8 years (436). At the time of diagnosis, intestinal disease with diarrhea and malabsorption dominate the clinical picture. The diarrhea is usually watery and malodorous, often associated with steatorrhea. The diarrhea is frequently accompanied by abdominal pain and distension, and may contain occult blood (420). Weight loss is invariably present.

Systemic manifestations include polyserositis, low-grade fever, pericarditis, cardiac valvular stenosis or insufficiency, mesenteric and peripheral lymphadenopathy, hepatosplenomegaly, and CNS disease (417,420,422,435,438, 442–444). Lymphadenopathy, the most common physical sign, affects approximately 50 percent of patients. The enlarged lymph nodes are typically firm, nontender, and freely movable. A periumbilical mass representing enlarged mesenteric lymph nodes is sometimes palpable. Whipple's disease of the CNS may be the primary manifestation (407,445).

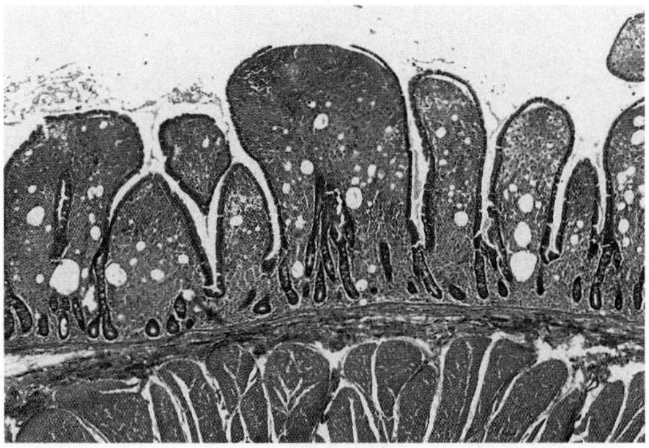

Figure 10-17

WHIPPLE'S DISEASE

The lamina propria is distended with histiocytes. The villi are distorted by the infiltrate. Clear lipid globules lie in dilated lacteals and in the lamina propria. (Fig. 3-56 from Emory TS, Carpenter HA, Gostout CJ, Sobin LH. Atlas of gastrointestinal endoscopy & endoscopic biopsies. Washington D.C.: Armed Forces Institute of Pathology; 2000:202.)

Gross Findings. Whipple's disease typically involves the small intestine. Endoscopically, the small intestinal mucosa has areas that appear pale yellow and shaggy alternating with areas that appear erythematous, eroded, or friable (421,439). In some cases, whitish yellow plaques with a patchy distribution are seen.

Grossly, the bowel wall is thickened and rigid. Yellowish subepithelial and peritoneal plaques and massive infiltration of the mesenteric fat are characteristic. Mesenteric thickening and lymphadenopathy characterize advanced disease, with lymph nodes sometimes measuring as much as 3 to 4 cm in diameter.

Microscopic Findings. Whipple's disease is characterized by collections of foamy histiocytes, sometimes accompanied by lymphocytes, neutrophils, and eosinophils, infiltrating the lamina propria, distorting the mucosal architecture, and pushing the crypts and villi apart (fig. 10-17). Subtotal or total villous atrophy characterizes severe disease. Finely granular, grayish histiocytes are most numerous just beneath the luminal epithelial basement membrane; they decrease in number as one

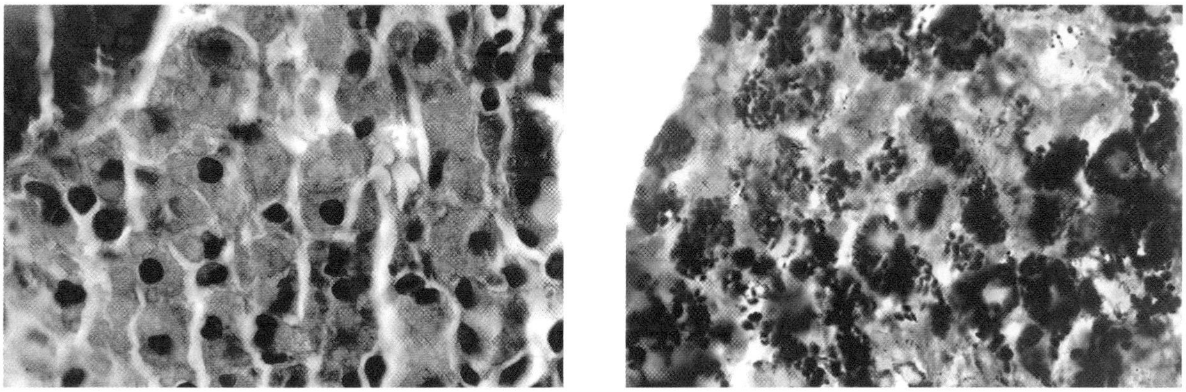

Figure 10-18

WHIPPLE'S DISEASE

Left: The lamina propria contains numerous histiocytes with foamy cytoplasm.

Right: Characteristic periodic acid–Schiff (PAS)-positive bacilli are in the histiocyte cytoplasm. (Figs. 3-57 and 3-58 from Emory TS, Carpenter HA, Gostout CJ, Sobin LH. Atlas of gastrointestinal endoscopy & endoscopic biopsies. Washington D.C.: Armed Forces Institute of Pathology; 2000:203.)

progresses toward the submucosa. The enterocytes appear relatively normal, although there may be patchy vacuolization. Rarely, necrosis and fibrosis are seen. Lymphangiectasia is characteristically present. It results from lymphatic obstruction due to massive histiocytic collections in the enlarged lymph nodes.

The diagnosis depends on the demonstration of multiple, rounded or sickle-shaped, PAS-positive, diastase-resistant bacterial fragments in the infiltrating histiocytes, smooth muscle cells, endothelium, and fibroblasts (fig. 10-18). Widespread fatty deposits and lipogranulomas are present in both the mucosa and in the intra-abdominal lymph nodes, reflecting lymphatic obstruction with fatty extravasation. Regional lymph nodes lose their normal architecture and become fibrotic.

Special Techniques. Ultrastructurally, the histiocytes contain bacteria in various stages of degeneration (410). Today, a PCR test diagnoses Whipple's disease in intestinal biopsies. Testing of cerebrospinal fluid in patients with Whipple's disease yields a high rate of positive results, even in patients without neurologic symptoms (446). The recent cultivation of the bacterium of Whipple's disease may allow the development of a serologic test for the disorder (443).

Differential Diagnosis. The differential diagnosis of the PAS-positive, diastase-resistant lamina propria histiocytes includes mucosal xanthomas, collections of muciphages, infection with *Mycobacterium avium*, histoplasmosis, storage diseases, and macroglobulinemia. Although the histiocytes may resemble one another in these diseases, fatty deposits and lipogranulomas are usually only present in Whipple's disease.

Treatment and Prognosis. The disease was uniformly fatal prior to the use of antibiotic therapy. Most patients respond well and rapidly to treatment with antibiotics such as trimethoprim-sulfamethoxazole, but some patients have chronic relapsing disease (419,427). Antibiotics should be administered for at least 1 year (419). The prognosis of patients with CNS Whipple's disease is much less favorable than of patients with involvement limited to the bowel (427).

Chlamydia Infections

Definition. *Lymphogranuloma venereum* (LGV) is a tropical and subtropical, chronic scarring disease transmitted sexually, caused by certain serogroups of *Chlamydia trachomatis*. Infections caused by LGV strains of *C. trachomatis* affect travelers from endemic areas or individuals with sexual contacts from endemically infected populations.

Demography. LGV has a worldwide distribution. Its prevalence varies from country to country; it is most common in tropical and subtropical countries (448).

Etiology. Both LGV and non-LGV chlamydial serotypes cause gastrointestinal disease

(449). LGV results from an organism that is biologically and serologically distinct from the *C. trachomatis* strains that cause trachoma or the more common sexually transmitted chlamydial diseases such as cervicitis and urethritis. Infection by both LGV and non-LGV chlamydial serotypes results from direct anal inoculation by infected partners or secondary to lymphatic spread from a penile lesion or from infected vaginal secretions. In women, anorectal infections with LGV or non-LGV strains of *C. trachomatis* can also arise from contiguous spread of infected secretions along the perineum or by spread via the pelvic lymphatics. Patients may have other associated diseases, including genital herpes or syphilis (450).

Clinical Features. The spectrum of intestinal chlamydial infections ranges from asymptomatic infection to severe granulomatous proctocolitis. Some patients with proven infection remain asymptomatic, while at the opposite extreme, patients can present with significant pain, bleeding, and mucopurulent discharge. The clinical manifestations and histopathologic features of chlamydial infections depend on organism serotype, host immune status, and the presence or absence of concurrent infections. LGV chlamydial infections produce much more severe inflammation than non-LGV chlamydial infections.

Clinically, LGV infection is divided into three stages. Primary lesions develop 3 to 30 days after the initial infection. The primary lesion is transient, often imperceptible, and painless, and may heal rapidly with subsequent scarring. Lymphadenitis with suppurative inflammatory reactions, known as buboes, characterizes the secondary stage. The tertiary stage usually affects the gastrointestinal tract, often presenting as rectal strictures, rectovaginal or rectovesical fistulas, or perirectal abscesses. LGV proctitis causes diarrhea, a bloody or mucopurulent discharge, fever, and inguinal and perirectal lymphadenopathy.

Gross Findings. The lesions begin as a papule that ulcerates and develops into a painless elevated area of beefy red granulation tissue. In chronic cases, the ulcers are large and irregularly shaped, with serpiginous extensions. The rectal mucosa in LGV loses its haustral folds, appearing ulcerated, friable, nodular, hemorrhagic, and edematous, with fibrosis of the underlying tissues. The fibrosis causes mural thickening, rigidity, and stenosis. The rectal strictures usually have an abrupt line of demarcation with the uninvolved, more proximal large intestine. The inflammatory changes may extend proximally as far as to the transverse colon, although the disease tends to remain confined to the distal bowel. Fistulas are common. Endoscopic findings range from mild erythema and friability to severe mucosal disease with ulceration and fistula formation.

Microscopic Findings. The histologic findings are as variable as the clinical features. Early inflammatory reactions of LGV consist of neutrophilic infiltrates particularly involving the superficial epithelium, sometimes associated with pseudomembranes (fig. 10-19). Crypt abscesses, superficial ulcers, stellate abscesses, and granulomas develop. As the ulcers enlarge, the mucosa is completely replaced by granulation tissue. After a short period of time, the inflammation evolves into a mixed or predominantly mononuclear cell response with large numbers of histiocytes. Lymphoid follicles form. Late-stage disease is associated with fistula development and marked fibrosis.

Special Techniques. The diagnosis is established by isolation of the organism in culture, direct immunofluorescence testing of biopsies or rectal swabs, application of genetic probes to the tissues, or by a positive serologic test.

Differential Diagnosis. The disease mimics Crohn's disease because of the presence of proctitis associated with fibrosis, strictures, deep fissures, ulcers, granulomas, and sometimes skip lesions. The lesions associated the LGV, however, are rarely seen proximal to the mid-portion of the descending colon, contrasting with Crohn's disease (447). The disease also mimics herpetic or gonorrheal proctitis and other causes of infective colitis/proctitis.

Treatment and Prognosis. Complications of untreated anorectal infection include perirectal abscesses, fistula-in-ano, and rectovaginal, rectovesical, and ischiorectal fistulas. Secondary bacterial infection contributes to the complications. Anorectal strictures are a late complication, usually occurring 2 to 6 cm from the anal orifice. Strictures may be mistaken for carcinoma. There is the possibility of the late development of adenocarcinoma or squamous carcinoma.

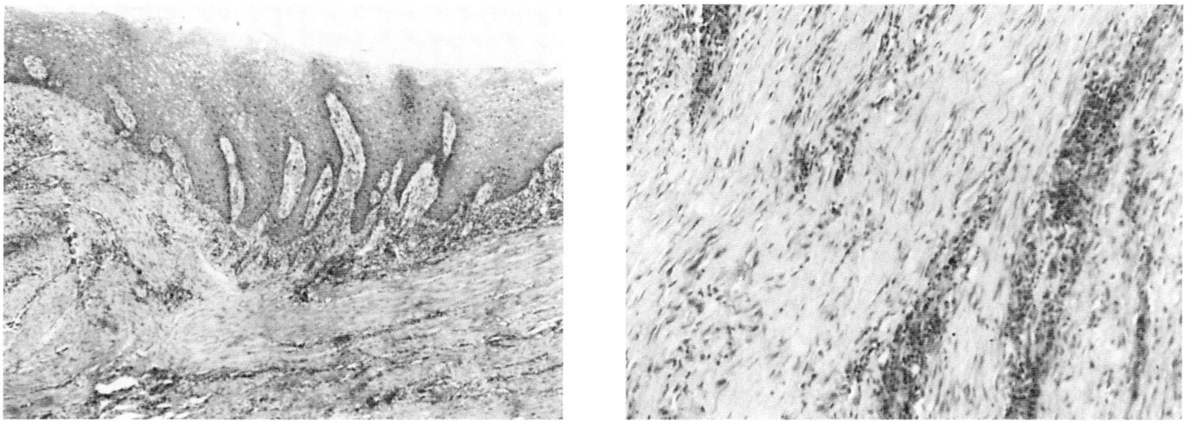

Figure 10-19

LYMPHOGRANULOMA VENEREUM

Left: Nonspecific submucosal inflammation of the anus.

Right: Higher-power view of the inflammatory infiltrate shows numerous neutrophils and scattered lymphocytes and plasma cells.

Anthrax

Definition. *Anthrax* is an often fatal infection that occurs when *Bacillus anthracis* enters the body through abrasions in the skin or by inhalation or ingestion. It is the zoonosis to which most mammals, especially grazing herbivores, are considered susceptible.

Demography. *Anthrax* is a particular problem in tropical environments in Africa, Asia, South and Central America, and the Caribbean. *B. anthracis* is ubiquitous and the infection occurs in semi-arid rural agricultural countries where animal husbandry is economically important. It is also a problem in locations where veterinary services are lacking and traditions and economic conditions lead to the use of meat, hide, and wool from animals that die suddenly (451, 452,456,460). The infection is usually acquired from sick animals or from infected urban laborers who deal with contaminated hides and bone meal. Recently, exposure to anthrax has resulted from biological terrorism.

Etiology. *B. anthracis* is a large, spore-forming, encapsulated, aerobic, nonmotile, toxin-producing, Gram-positive rod. It measures 1 x 3 to 10 µm in size. Anthrax spores are formed in the soil and in dead animal tissues. Human infections result from contact with contaminated animals or animal products. There are no known cases of human-to-human transmission.

The bacterial endospores do not divide, have no measurable metabolism, and are resistant to drying heat, ultraviolet light, gamma radiation, and many disinfectants (461). Endospores introduced into the body are carried to regional lymph nodes. These germinate inside macrophages and become vegetative bacteria (459). They are then released from the macrophages and multiply in the lymphatics. They then enter the bloodstream, eventually creating massive septicemia (453).

The major virulence factors of *B. anthracis* are encoded on two virulence plasmids, pXO1 and PCO2. The toxin bearing pXO1 encodes genes that produce secreted exotoxins. The toxin gene complex consists of a protective antigen, lethal factor, and edema factor (457).

Pathophysiology. Gastrointestinal anthrax is thought to result from penetration of the mucosa by bacterial spores, with subsequent germination to the vegetative form. The portal of entry is considered to be either in the stomach, the cecum, or the terminal ileum.

Clinical Features. The four clinical forms of human anthrax—cutaneous, oral-oropharyngeal, gastrointestinal, and inhalational—are determined by the portal of entry. The vast majority of cases are of the cutaneous type. Gastrointestinal anthrax is rare and contracted by eating contaminated meat (451,452,460). The signs and symptoms are similar to many other causes of gastroenteritis: fever, diffuse abdominal pain, and rebound tenderness. There may also be constipation and diarrhea and the stools may be blood-tinged or exhibit melena. Ascites develops with concomitant reduction of abdominal pain, 2 to 4 days after symptom onset. The ascites fluid may be clear to purulent and often yields colonies of *B. anthracis* if cultured (453). Ulceration of the gastrointestinal tract and invasion of regional lymphatics are common, and hemorrhagic gastritis or ileocolitis may cause obstruction or perforation. Death results from electrolyte imbalance, fulminant diarrhea, and progressive ascites.

Gross Findings. The stomach and/or intestines appear phlegmonous and hemorrhagic, and contain serpiginous ulcers. The pathologic findings of the ileocecal lesion include a solitary, hemorrhagic, necrotic, edematous mucosa and hemorrhagic mesenteric lymphadenitis.

Microscopic Findings. Histologically, bacilli are seen microscopically in the mucosal and submucosal lymphatics and there is evidence of mesenteric lymphadenitis (454). Ulceration always occurs. There is also massive edema and mucosal necrosis (455). The stomach or intestines show massive edema and moderate perivascular hemorrhage. Intramural lymphatics contain anthrax bacilli. Involvement of regional lymphatics parallels that seen in the mediastinum.

Special Techniques. The diagnosis is confirmed by culturing the organism or through the use of serologic or immunologic tests. In addition, newer molecular diagnostic techniques focus on the use of PCR to amplify markers specific to *B. anthracis*.

Treatment and Prognosis. Patients with systemic infection resulting from inhalation of the organism have a mortality rate approaching 100 percent, with death usually occurring within a few days after the onset of symptoms (458). High-dose penicillin G is the treatment of choice; streptomycin, erythromycin, and tetracycline have also been used. Intensive supportive care is often necessary. Other potential new treatments include the administration of antitoxins (453).

Listeria Infections

Demography. *Listeria monocytogenes* causes approximately 2,500 cases of serious illness, and 500 deaths per year in the United States (462,474,477,477a). Most commonly, *Listeria* causes severe systemic illness in immunocompromised persons (471,475), including sepsis, meningitis, and encephalitis. It also affects previously healthy people. Less commonly, *Listeria* causes gastroenteritis.

Etiology. *L. monocytogenes*, a Gram-positive bacterium, grows at low temperatures and causes several illnesses in humans and animals. Acquisition of the organism has been described following consumption of infected coleslaw, hot dogs, delicatessen meats, seafood, fresh vegetables, milk, and cheese (463,464,467,472,482, 484,485). In a recent outbreak, 72 percent of people exposed to infected corn reported symptoms and 19 percent were hospitalized due to the severity of the symptoms (463).

Pathophysiology. The major portal of entry of *Listeria* in humans is thought to be the intestinal tract. The bacteria likely enter through Peyer patches (480,481). *Listeria* is able to penetrate many cell types, including enterocytes and M cells (478). Entry into host cells is mediated by two bacterial surface proteins belonging to the internalin family, In1A and In1B (469, 473). These proteins interact with receptors on the host cell, E-cadherin and c-met (478,486). This interaction leads to receptor-mediated internalization of the bacteria into the host cell.

Once the *Listeria* organisms are inside the cell, they manufacture a pore-forming protein called listeriolysin O, which tunnels into phagosome membranes, dissolving them, and setting the microbes free within the cytoplasm. A *Listeria* PEST (P, Prog; E, Glu; S, Ser; T, Thr) sequence prompts the protein degrading machinery of the bacteria's host macrophages to eliminate the pore-forming protein. The PEST tag ensures that, once freed from the vacuoles, the proteins are destroyed or disabled before they damage the host cell membrane, killing the cell in which the *Listeria* organisms reside (468).

Following their release into the cytoplasm, the bacteria proliferate and polymerize cellular actin (465,466). Bacteria move from cell to cell via membranous extensions of the host cell plasma membranes. These extensions protrude into adjacent cells where they are lysed by two bacterial toxins, PlcA and PlcB, allowing the organisms to enter the cytoplasm of the neighboring cell (466). *Listeria* produces no known enterotoxins.

Clinical Features. Unlike other foodborne infections, the clinical manifestations of *L. monocytogenes* infection usually result from sepsis or involvement of the CNS, often in immunocompromised persons. Sometimes, however, gastrointestinal symptoms are produced, including diarrhea, nausea, vomiting, and abdominal cramps, often accompanied by fever (463,467,483,485). The organism requires a brief incubation period of 24 hours to cause disease with gastrointestinal symptoms and fever (463); some have reported shorter incubation times of 18 and 20 hours (467,483).

Pathologic Findings. No gross lesions associated with listeriosis have been described. Histologically, *Listeria* organisms are associated with localized acute inflammation of the small intestine and appendix (470,476,479)

Differential Diagnosis. The differential diagnosis includes all other forms of foodborne gastroenteritis.

Treatment and Prognosis. In immunocompetent patients, *Listeria* produces a mild, self-limited gastroenteritis. No antibiotic treatment is warranted in such individuals. In immunocompromised patients, however, *Listeria* may produce a severe invasive enteritis with a high risk for systemic dissemination of the organism. These patients should be treated aggressively with antibiotics. *Listeria* is generally susceptible to a wide range of antibiotic agents (476).

Tropical Sprue

Definition. A working definition of *tropical sprue* that is supported by most investigators is "malabsorption of two unrelated test substances by a patient from an appropriate geographic area with exclusion of other diseases such as those of parasitic origin and nontropical sprue" (488,490,493).

Demography. Tropical sprue is a major health problem among natives of, visitors to, and expatriates from selected countries largely located between the Tropic of Cancer and the Tropic of Capricorn. The disorder is well documented in Asia, parts of Central and South Africa, the Philippines, the East Indies, the West Indies, and parts of central and northern South America. It also occurs in India (487,488,492).

Etiology. Most believe that tropical sprue results from infection by toxigenic bacteria. Several microorganisms are suspected pathogens including *Escherichia coli*, *Klebsiella pneumoniae*, and *Enterobacter cloacae*, but no one organism is common to all patients.

Clinical Features. For tropical sprue to develop, a person must reside in or visit a country in which the disease is endemic. Characteristic clinical features of severe tropical sprue include malabsorption, nutritional deficiencies, anorexia, abdominal distension, and persistent diarrhea. Symptoms of nutritional deficiency include pallor, weakness, edema, and night blindness. Severe vitamin B12 malabsorption can cause neurologic signs; the malabsorption occurs secondary to mucosal damage. Chronic tropical sprue occurs if the acute phase does not completely resolve. When the disease develops in expatriates, its initial manifestations may appear in temperate countries, sometimes years after emigration from an area where it is endemic (489). Jejunal biopsies are necessary to establish the presence of the characteristic morphologic abnormalities and to exclude other disorders such as Whipple's disease, parasites, or lymphoma.

Gross Findings. The major changes affect the jejunum and the ileum. Radiographic abnormalities are nonspecific and include small intestinal thickening, coarsening of the mucosal folds, and barium segmentation.

Microscopic Findings. The early changes of tropical sprue resemble those seen in celiac disease. The jejunal mucosa appears normal or only slightly abnormal, with increased numbers of intraepithelial lymphocytes. Later, villous atrophy and crypt hyperplasia develop (fig. 10-20). A marked mononuclear infiltration with lymphocytes and plasma cells develops in the lamina propria and epithelium. Eosinophils may be present. Less than 10 percent of patients develop a completely flattened mucosa. Nuclei of crypt enterocytes appear megaloblastic. Paneth cells are normal in number and endocrine cells are increased. The basement membrane underlying the surface epithelium is thickened.

Differential Diagnosis. The histologic features completely mimic those seen in celiac disease. Therefore, clinical correlation is required. Serologic tests specific for celiac disease may exclude tropical sprue. Additionally, the symptoms of tropical sprue do not remit when the patient adheres to a gluten-free diet. Diagnostic

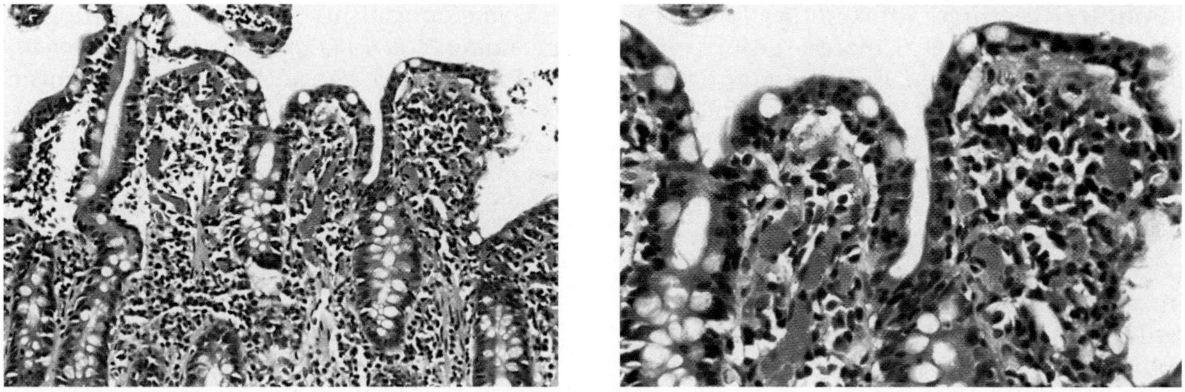

Figure 10-20

TROPICAL SPRUE

Left: Mild to moderate villous atrophy of the small intestine. There is an increase in intraepithelial lymphocytes similar to that seen in celiac disease.

Right: Higher-power view shows the intraepithelial lymphocytosis and prominent lymphoplasmacytic infiltrate within the lamina propria.

Table 10-8

FACTORS PREDISPOSING TO BACTERIAL OVERGROWTH

Gastric hypochlorhydria or achlorhydria
Atrophic gastritis
Partial gastrectomy
Vagotomy
Proton pump inhibitor therapy
Surgical factors
Resection of ileocecal valve
Billroth II
Surgical blind loop
Anatomic factors
Intestinal obstruction
Duodenal-jejunal diverticulosis
Gastrocolic or enterocolic fistula
Dysmotility syndromes
Scleroderma
Idiopathic intestinal pseudoobstruction
Diabetic autonomic neuropathy
Others
Other medical conditions
Crohn's disease
Chronic pancreatitis
Cirrhosis
Immunodeficiency
End-stage renal disease

evaluation of tropical sprue also requires its differentiation from parasitic diarrheal diseases. In contrast to bacterial or viral infections, which are short-lived, tropical sprue usually fails to improve after returning to a temperate climate.

Treatment and Prognosis. Treatment for 6 months with a poorly absorbed sulfonamide (sulfaguanidine) or sulfasuxidine is very effective (491).

Bacterial Overgrowth Syndromes

Definition: *Bacterial overgrowth syndromes* are characterized by excessive numbers of bacteria in the proximal small intestine. Patients who typically develop bacterial overgrowth syndromes are those who have had surgical procedures that create an anastomotic blind loop, those with underlying motility disorders, or those with multiple small intestinal diverticula. Certain medical conditions and advanced age may also predispose to bacterial overgrowth (Table 10-8).

Pathophysiology. Bacterial overgrowth alters normal gastrointestinal function via direct mucosal injury or through disturbed brush border function. A number of functional consequences of this damage occur, including decreased disaccharidase activity; decreased transport of monosaccharides, amino acids, fatty acids; and protein-losing enteropathy.

Fat malabsorption occurs because bacteria of the small intestine deconjugate bile salts, resulting in impaired transport of lipids through the damaged epithelium. Water soluble, conjugated bile salts form mixed micelles with partially digested dietary lipids. When bile salts are deconjugated by the action of bacteria, micelle formation is impaired, leading to fat malabsorption. In addition, the free bile salts formed in this process may be directly toxic to the small intestinal epithelium, leading to further mucosal damage (501).

Carbohydrate malabsorption also occurs in bacterial overgrowth syndromes. This is likely the result of a combination of factors including intraluminal degradation of carbohydrates by luminal bacteria, impaired disaccharidase activity, and damage to the brush border of the epithelium. Luminal bacteria metabolize malabsorbed carbohydrates to form short-chain organic acids that increase the osmolarity of the luminal contents, thus contributing to diarrhea. Protein malabsorption may also occur secondary to impaired absorption of amino acids, utilization of luminal protein by bacteria, or as a result of a protein-losing enteropathy that may occur as a result of damage to enterocytes (495,498,499).

A classic manifestation of bacterial overgrowth is vitamin B12 deficiency that cannot be corrected by replacement of intrinsic factor. Anaerobic bacteria competitively absorb vitamin B12 bound to intrinsic factor, leading to diminished availability of this vitamin to the host (502).

Another factor that may contribute to diarrhea in bacterial overgrowth is the formation of bacterial metabolites that stimulate water and electrolyte secretion from enterocytes. Such products include free bile acids, hydroxylated fatty acids, and other organic acids. Experimental evidence suggests that bacterial overgrowth may induce dysmotility in the small intestine, predisposing to further bacterial proliferation (497).

Clinical Features. The symptoms experienced by patients with bacterial overgrowth depend on the predisposing small bowel abnormality. Patients with small intestinal strictures, obstruction, dysmotility, or surgically formed blind loops usually complain of vague abdominal discomfort, periumbilical cramping pain, and bloating, followed later by diarrhea and malabsorption. The symptoms of bacterial overgrowth in patients with Crohn's disease, chronic intestinal pseudoobstruction, and short bowel syndrome may be masked by symptoms attributable to the primary diagnosis. Weight loss may occur in association with steatorrhea in any of these patients. Hypoproteinemia is common, and may be of sufficient severity to cause edema.

Vitamin B12 deficiency accompanying bacterial overgrowth syndrome results in macrocytic and megaloblastic anemia. In severe cases, neurologic damage occurs, including peripheral neuropathy and cognitive defects. Malabsorption of fat-soluble vitamins may lead to night blindness, osteomalacia, coagulopathy, or vitamin E deficiency syndromes (499). Iron deficiency anemia may occur as a result of chronic occult blood loss from the damaged mucosa (496).

Pathologic Findings. In mild cases, focal, mild, patchy histologic abnormalities may be easily missed by a single random biopsy or easily overlooked in the specimen. In severe cases, the spectrum of changes ranges from patchy, villous broadening and flattening to complete villous atrophy with crypt hyperplasia or hypoplasia. Numerous microorganisms adhere to the mucosa or embed in the unstirred mucus layer overlying the epithelium.

Special Techniques. The diagnosis of bacterial overgrowth relies on three criteria: 1) presence of increased intestinal volume; 2) the demonstration of increased bacterial concentrations; and 3) a positive response to antibiotic therapy. Bacterial overgrowth syndromes can also be diagnosed by jejunal culture, gas-liquid chromatography of jejunal fluid, and ^{14}C-D xylose or hydrogen breath tests. Of these, the most sensitive is jejunal culture.

Differential Diagnosis. The differential diagnosis of bacterial overgrowth includes other entities leading to malabsorption (see chapter 12).

Treatment and Prognosis. The main objectives in the treatment of bacterial overgrowth syndrome are correction of the underlying small intestinal abnormality if possible, elimination of the bacteria through the use of antibiotics, and treatment of any coexisting dysmotility syndrome with prokinetic agents. Nutritional deficiencies should also be corrected.

In most patients, a single course of antibiotic treatment results in marked improvement in symptoms. In some, however, cyclic treatment is necessary because of recurrent symptoms. Numerous antibiotics are effective including amoxicillin-clavulanic acid (494), cephalexin and metronidazole, colistin and metronidazole, ciprofloxacin, and trimethoprim-sulfamethoxazole (500).

FUNGAL INFECTIONS

Fungi are ubiquitous in nature, since they are associated with plants, animals, and insects. Humans are continually exposed to many fungal types by various routes, but particularly, by ingestion of food, allowing colonization of the gastrointestinal tract. Depending on the interaction between the host mucosal defense mechanisms and fungal virulence factors, colonization may be transient or persistent, or local disease may develop. Of the various pathogenic fungi, yeasts of the *Candida* species are the most frequent fungi responsible for human gastrointestinal infections.

Candida Infections

Demography. Typically, candidiasis affects patients on antibiotics, hemodialysis, or chemotherapeutic agents; immunocompromised individuals; immunocompetent patients with serious postoperative complications, cancer, severely debilitating diseases, and penetrating abdominal trauma; and patients with indwelling vascular access devices. Increasing numbers of cases are acquired in the hospital setting. *Candida* organisms also commonly colonize blind loops, sites of bacterial stasis, and necrotic tissue. Candidiasis develops in three stages: colonization by the organism, followed by epithelial infection, then deeper invasion. The degree of underlying immune suppression is the most important determinant of the prevalence and consequences of *Candida* infection (504).

Etiology. The most common species of *Candida* are *C. albicans*, *C. tropicalis*, *C. glabrata*, *C. parapsilosis*, and *C. lausei*. *C. glabrata* is responsible for approximately 15 percent of mucosal and systemic candidiasis. In the immunocompromised host, there is a higher frequency of disseminated *C. tropicalis* than *C. albicans*.

Pathophysiology. *C. albicans* expresses a number of adhesion molecules capable of interacting with ligands on a variety of different cell types. These adhesins recognize and bind to proteins such as fibronectin, vitronectin, and laminin, among others (506,509,514–516). *C. glabrata* organisms also avidly adhere to epithelial cells via an adhesin encoded by the *EPA-1* gene, which recognizes a specific carbohydrate molecule (505). Despite the presence of this adhesion molecule, *Candida* has difficulty colonizing nonsquamous cell sites such as the small intestine. In the small bowel, the rapid passage of luminal contents due to peristalsis and the prevention of *Candida* mucosal interactions by bacterial antagonism reduce the likelihood of fungal colonization. The normal gastrointestinal flora profoundly antagonizes and suppresses *Candida* growth in a variety of ways (512,513). Symptoms due to *Candida* infection in the gut relate primarily to tissue invasion, although hypersensitivity mechanisms and, possibly, byproducts of fungal growth, may induce functional abnormalities.

The ability of *Candida* to form hyphae under certain environmental conditions is considered an additional virulence factor. Transcription factors that are activated during morphogenesis may induce expression of genes involved not only in the formation of hyphae, but those that also encode virulence factors (510). In addition, *Candida* organisms secrete a variety of proteinases and phospholipases, which contribute to their ability to invade tissues (510,514).

Clinical Features. *Esophagus*. Patients with *Candida* esophagitis are frequently asymptomatic, especially when immunologically intact, and have only scattered adherent plaques within the esophagus. Asymptomatic patients seldom undergo endoscopy and the prevalence of fungal esophagitis among patients with minor abnormalities of motility or immunity is probably under reported. When symptomatic, patients with C*andida* esophagitis present most commonly with dysphagia, odynophagia, and retrosternal pain. Constitutional symptoms, including fever, occasionally occur. Vomiting and bleeding are rare. In some patients, epigastric pain is the dominant symptom. Most patients have underlying hematologic malignancies or AIDS, or have undergone transplantation.

In AIDS patients, there may be a complete lack of symptoms (504). In those who are particularly prone to esophageal *Candida* infection, the diagnosis can often be derived from a careful history and physical examination. The presence of both esophageal symptoms and oral candidiasis has a positive predictive value for esophageal candidiasis of 100 percent; the absence of symptoms and oral candidiasis has a negative predictive value of 96 percent (517).

Stomach. The role of acid in influencing gastric carriage rates of *Candida* is controversial, since the yeast thrive in a wide pH range and can proliferate and germinate at low pH. Nonetheless, *Candida* infections in the stomach occur far less frequently than those in the esophagus. For this reason, the stomach appears to be intrinsically more resistant to *Candida* infections. Generally, the organism only invades preexisting gastric lesions, particularly gastric ulcers (benign and malignant), as well as sites of gastric resection. The extent of gastric *Candida* infection ranges from colonization only, to superficial overgrowth of the surface of an ulcer, to histologically confirmed mucosal invasion. Most frequently, the yeast are seen in superficial exudates, especially overlying ulcers.

It is difficult to determine the exact symptoms associated with gastric candidiasis because it usually coexists with another medical problem, such as a gastric ulcer. When symptoms are present, they include epigastric pain, nausea, and vomiting.

Small Intestine and Colon. Autopsy surveys of adults with hematologic malignancies and other debilitating diseases, including AIDS, show that enteric and colonic mucosal invasion by *Candida* occurs (511). Infection of the small bowel is found at autopsy in 20 percent of patients with gastrointestinal candidiasis (507). These patients generally have an ulcerated mucosa. Patients with intestinal candidiasis have watery and sometimes explosive diarrhea, occasional cramps, mild diffuse abdominal tenderness, and weight loss. Multiple, variably sized ulcers with heaped-up edges and necrotic bases are distributed throughout the colon. They grossly resemble CMV infection. In some cases, an allergic reaction to the fungi may be responsible for the associated diarrhea (503).

Gross Findings. *Esophagus.* Candida esophagitis is characterized by adherent, white or tan mucosal plaques (fig. 10-21). Additional findings include hyperemia, areas of ulceration, a cobblestoned appearance of the mucosal surface, and disordered motility. There is occasional narrowing of the esophageal lumen. Rare complications include perforation and fistula formation. A reliable diagnosis is only made by histologic evidence of tissue invasion in biopsy material.

Stomach. Plaque-like lesions can be seen endoscopically in the stomach, and when found, are usually superimposed on preexisting gastric ulcers or gastritis.

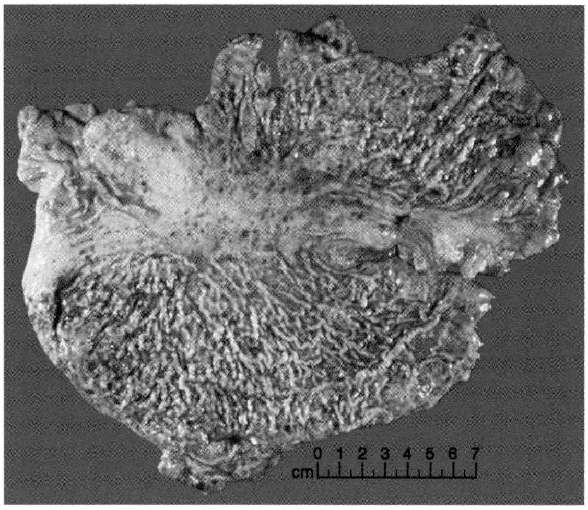

Figure 10-21

GASTRIC *CANDIDA*: GROSS APPEARANCE

Fungi colonize areas of erosion or ulceration.

Intestine. *Candida* enteritis may involve multiple intestinal sites, and multiple candidal ulcers or perforations can be seen.

Microscopic Findings. Endoscopy with brushings and biopsy is currently the gold standard technique for diagnosis of esophageal infections because the sensitivity and specificity are superior to those of radiography in the diagnosis of *Candida* esophagitis. Histologically, *Candida* organisms are 4- to 6-μm, budding, yeast-like forms admixed with nonseptate pseudohyphae that stain positively with PAS and silver stains (fig. 10-22).

Candida infections may be classified as either noninvasive or invasive. In noninvasive disease, the fungi grow in devitalized tissues without invading underlying intact tissues, as commonly occurs in tissues overlying gastric ulcers (fig. 10-23). In invasive infections, the organisms are seen within viable tissues. The organism often invades the vasculature, leading to ischemia and candidal sepsis. If the patient has preexisting ischemia, the disease may worsen.

Special Techniques. Fungal stains highlight organismal structure and allow assessment of the extent of tissue or vascular invasion.

Differential Diagnosis. Other opportunistic infections in immunocompromised patients.

Treatment and Prognosis. The decision whether to use topical therapy, oral systemic

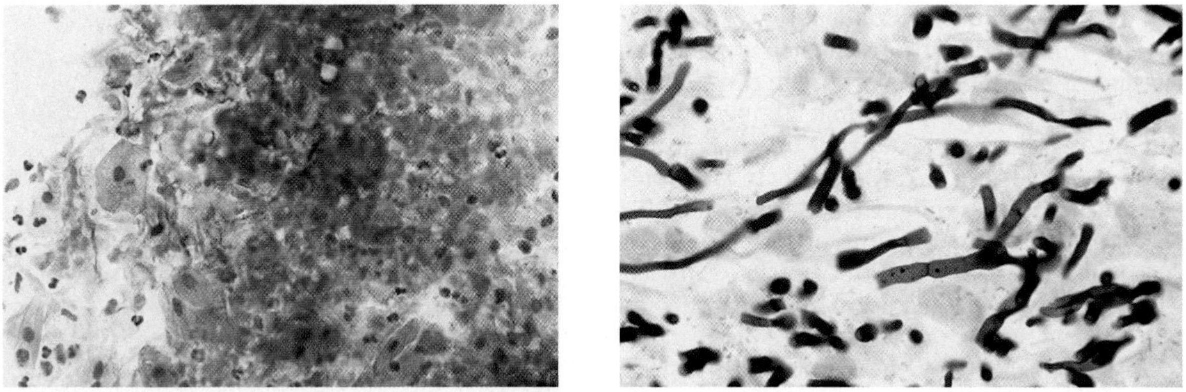

Figure 10-22

CANDIDA ESOPHAGITIS

Left: Esophageal brush specimen shows numerous squamous cells with admixed fungi. Both yeast forms and pseudohyphae are present.

Right: A methenamine silver stain highlights the fungal organisms.

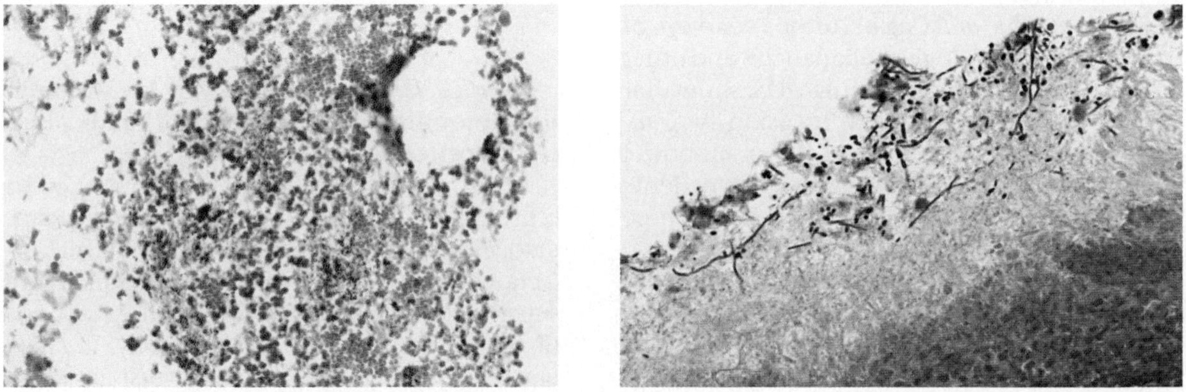

Figure 10-23

CANDIDA

Left: *Candida* spores are present in the exudate overlying an ulcer (ulcer not shown).

Right: Fungal hyphae grow in the devitalized tissue.

therapy, or intravenous therapy to treat *Candida* infections is based on the degree of immunocompromise present in the affected patient, and whether or not there is invasive disease. For patients with a normal immune system, nystatin suspension or clotrimazole is effective. Immunocompromised patients require systemic therapy with agents such as fluconazole. Caspofungin is also effective (518). Prophylaxis is not recommended. Severe infections may require treatment with amphotericin B. Mere colonization of gastric ulcers does not require therapy. Esophageal resection with antifungal therapy is sometimes necessary in patients with severe invasive esophageal candidiasis with transmural necrosis and perforation (508). After therapy with antifungal drugs, patients generally recover with no persistent sequelae. Patients who present with severe fungal esophagitis complicated by fistula formation, perforation, or stricture may have residual anatomic defects following the antifungal therapy. Granulocytopenic patients with severe esophagitis may succumb from disseminated fungal infection or from changes of renal toxicity due to amphotericin B therapy.

Histoplasma Infections

Demography. *Histoplasma capsulatum* has a worldwide distribution, occurring in the central region of the United States from the Gulf Coast to the Great Lakes, including a broad area along the Ohio and Mississippi River Valleys. It is the most common endemic systemic mycosis in the United States. It is also endemic in the Caribbean, and in Central and South America. Skin testing reveals that most people living in endemic areas become infected. The fungus grows in soil with a high nitrogen content, particularly that enriched by bird and bat guano. Even a brief exposure to the fungus may result in infection. Disseminated histoplasmosis is rare and predominantly affects immunocompromised individuals. It also affects some patients without an identifiable immunological defect. Immunosuppressed patients develop particularly severe infections.

Etiology. *H. capsulatum* is a dimorphic ascomycete with a saprophytic infectious, but nonpathogenic, mold morphotype, and host-adapted pathogenic yeast morphotype. Three variants within the species exist: *H. capsulatum* var. *capsulatum*, *H. capsulatum* var. *duboisii*, and *H. capsulatum* var. *farciminosum*. The first two variants infect humans and other mammals, while the third does not (535). The morphologic features of the fungus depend on the temperature. In the soil at 25°C, it exists as a mold (hyphae or mycelia) and asexual spores, whereas at 37°C (in the mammalian host) it exists as a budding yeast. Temperature switches are sufficient to induce the change in the morphology.

Pathophysiology. *H. capsulatum* is an effective intracellular parasite of macrophages. The organism is acquired by inhalation of spores or mycelial fragments. Once inside the host, the organism converts to its pathogenic yeast form, which survives and multiplies within macrophages. It is thought that in most cases the host mounts a fungistatic, rather than fungicidal, response, leading to the establishment of persistent inactive infection. The infection can later be reactivated if the host pathogen balance becomes disrupted (535,545,547). It is thought that the organism remains quiescent within the reticuloendothelial system and perhaps in endothelial cells as well. Organisms can also be found in calcified granulomas that remain following the initial infection. This may also represent a source of reactivation in the event that the patient becomes immunocompromised.

Macrophages ingest the yeast after opsonization with antibody or complement, or following direct binding of the organism to the beta-2 or CD18 integrins on the surface of phagocytes (523) via the fungal adhesin HSP60s (532). The organism is internalized via a phagosome that subsequently fuses with lysosomes within the macrophage cytoplasm.

Once inside the lysosome, *Histoplasma* employs several mechanisms to escape destruction. The major *Histoplasma*-secreted antigen, the M antigen, is thought to be a hydrogen peroxide–degrading catalase (548). This catalase may neutralize the harmful effect of host cell–generated hydrogen peroxide. Survival of intact viable fungus in the hostile environment of phagolysosomes within the macrophages requires *Histoplasma* protein synthesis (534,546), indicating an active role of the organism in promoting its own survival. It may accomplish this by moderating the microenvironmental pH, reducing its acidity. This function may occur through a fungal protein pump (537). Additionally, the mode of entry of the organism into macrophages via alternative nonopsonophagocytic mechanisms may help the organism avoid or suppress host defenses against it (544).

Hosts also defend against pathogens via sequestration of essential nutrients, such as free iron, that are necessary for pathogen survival. Most iron in the mammalian host is not freely available, but is bound to host proteins such as transferrin. The host response to microbial infection may include reduction of the iron saturation level of transferrin and downregulation of host cell transferrin receptors (524). *Histoplasma* acquires iron through several mechanisms. The organism secretes low molecular weight, iron-chelating siderophores that scavenge ferric iron (528,529,540). *H. capsulatum* also has the ability to reduce ferric iron, allowing the organism to utilize ferric salts as a source of usable iron (539).

Histoplasma is resistant to calcium deprivation as occurs in phagolysosomes. A low calcium concentration within the phagolysosome acts as an environmental signal for expression of the fungal proteins necessary for intracellular survival. The organisms secrete a calcium-binding protein, CBP1, that allows them to grow in this calcium-poor environment (519,520).

H. capsulatum also has defense machinery that interferes with the fusion of phagosomes and lysosomes and blocks acidification of phagolysosomes, a step that may be necessary for activation of lysosomal enzymes (525). This may be accomplished in part by exclusion of the host vacuolar ATPase/proton pump from phagocytic vacuoles in which the organisms are located (538).

Clinical Features. The fungi usually gain access to the body through the lungs. Inhaled spores reach the bronchioles or alveoli and germinate within 48 to 72 hours, producing the yeast form of the fungus. If only a few or a moderate number of spores are inhaled, the pulmonary lesions are asymptomatic. Heavy spore inhalation causes symptomatic illness, even in immunocompetent individuals. In a small percentage of individuals, a more severe form of progressive pulmonary infection or disseminated disease occurs. These patients often have some form of immunocompromise.

The clinical syndromes associated with *H. capsulatum* include acute self-limited syndrome, disseminated histoplasmosis, chronic pulmonary histoplasmosis, mediastinal granulomata, and fibrosing mediastinitis. The acute syndrome in the normal host is generally mild, manifested by fever, headaches, chills, cough, and chest pain in at least two thirds of patients (527). Gastrointestinal histoplasmosis usually appears as part of disseminated disease and is acquired by the hematogenous route. Isolated gastrointestinal histoplasmosis may also occur (530).

Gastrointestinal involvement by *Histoplasma* may affect any site, including the esophagus, stomach, small bowel, and large bowel. Manifestations include nausea, vomiting, diarrhea, fever, hepatosplenomegaly, gradual weight loss, fatigue, and weakness. Terminal ileum involvement predominates in one third of the cases. In severe disease, perforation and peritonitis may occur (522). Masses or ulcers in the gastrointestinal tract often mimic IBD or carcinoma (526). AIDS patients with disseminated histoplasmosis often have acute severe symptoms associated with shock, respiratory failure, and disseminated intravascular coagulation (543).

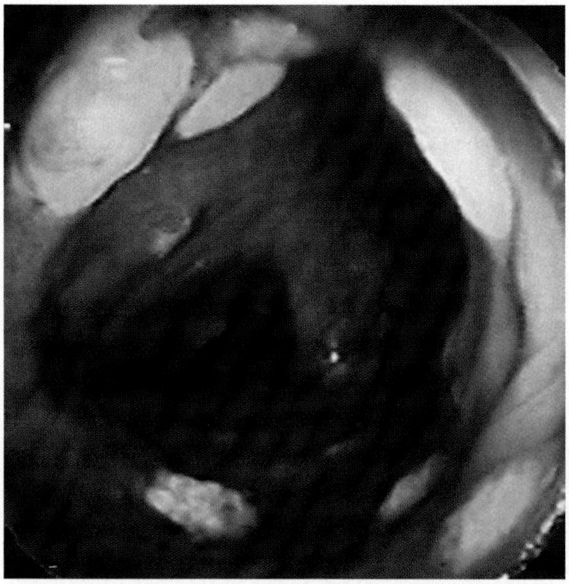

Figure 10-24

COLONIC HISTOPLASMOSIS

Endoscopic photograph demonstrates yellowish plaque-like lesions in the colon of a patient with disseminated histoplasmosis.

In patients with mediastinal granuloma syndrome, the enlarged lymph nodes obstruct and encroach upon the esophagus producing obstruction, motility problems, and sometimes, perforation. Patients with sclerosing mediastinitis have similar features.

Gross Findings. A spectrum of gross findings may be seen in patients with gastrointestinal histoplasmosis. The most common is mucosal ulceration; other findings are submucosal plaques or nodules (fig. 10-24), foci of hemorrhage, and obstructive mass lesions. The mucosa may appear normal in up to one quarter of cases (531). Extensive disease leads to widespread tissue destruction and even perforation.

Microscopic Findings. Histoplasmosis is predominantly an intracellular mycosis of reticuloendothelial cells. Histologically, mucosal plaques consist of diffuse histiocytic collections filled with organisms that expand the lamina propria. Small particulate bodies are seen within the histiocytes, even in H&E-stained preparations. The yeast-like phase is a round to oval spore with rigid cell walls from which the cytoplasm has often retracted, measuring 2 to 4 µm in diameter (fig. 10-25). It reproduces by budding.

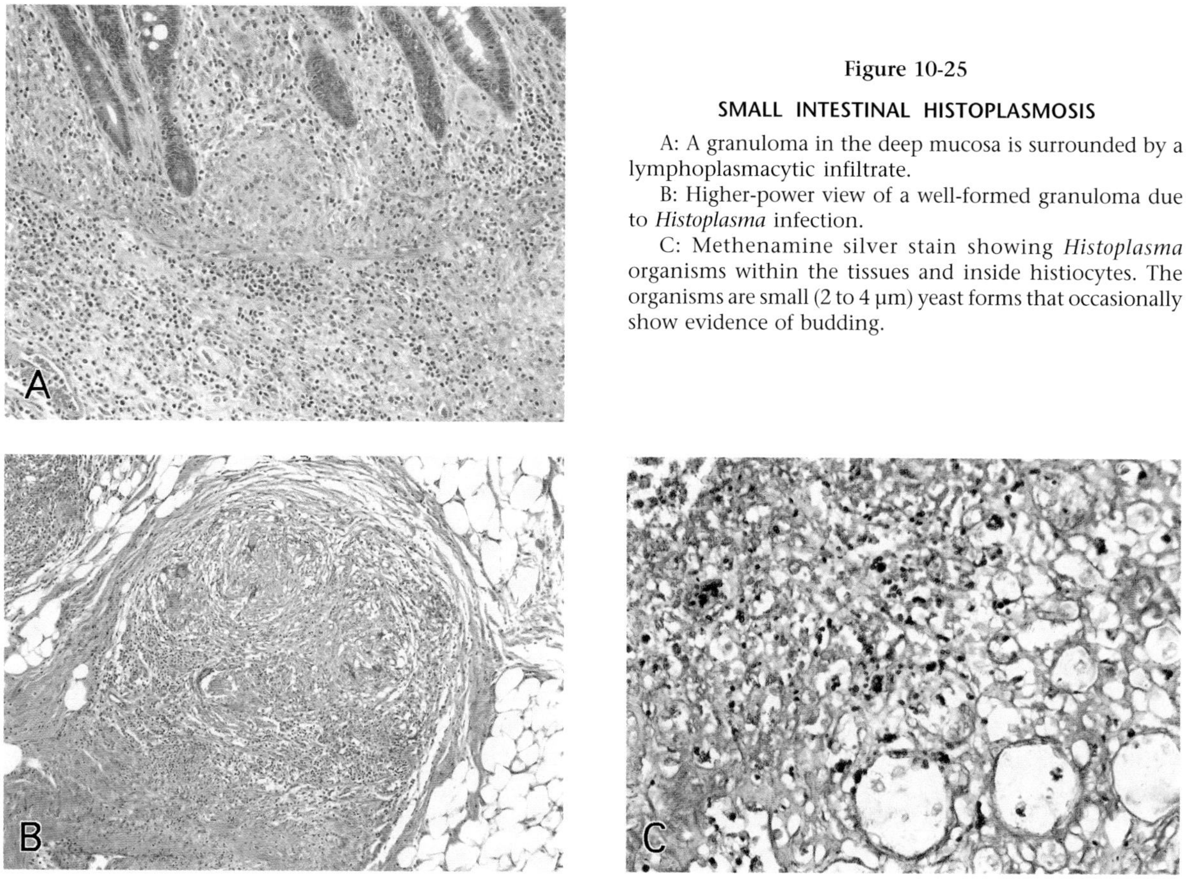

Figure 10-25

SMALL INTESTINAL HISTOPLASMOSIS

A: A granuloma in the deep mucosa is surrounded by a lymphoplasmacytic infiltrate.

B: Higher-power view of a well-formed granuloma due to *Histoplasma* infection.

C: Methenamine silver stain showing *Histoplasma* organisms within the tissues and inside histiocytes. The organisms are small (2 to 4 µm) yeast forms that occasionally show evidence of budding.

In severe disease, fungi fill the macrophages. The organisms are easily visualized with PAS and other fungal stains. Although occasionally the organism lies within well-formed granulomas, more often, diffuse histocytic infiltrates are present (531). Following therapy, degenerating and dead organisms are seen. Long after disease remission, there may be fungal cell wall remnants within macrophages.

Special Techniques. The diagnosis of disseminated disease is usually accomplished by demonstrating the fungus in cultured material from blood, urine, liver, bone marrow, or other affected tissues. In patients with limited disease, however, cultures are frequently negative (542). Patients with systemic histoplasmosis and AIDS have positive blood cultures in 83 percent of cases and positive bone marrow cultures in 71 to 75 percent, making these tissues the best sources of *Histoplasma* organisms for microbiologic study (549). Serologic testing may be helpful in detecting *Histoplasma* antigens. Recently, molecular testing methods for the diagnosis of infection have become available (521,533,536).

Differential Diagnosis. Histologically, the fungus-containing histiocytic infiltrates morphologically resemble those seen in various disorders, including Whipple's disease and mycobacterial infections. The characteristic organisms are easily distinguishable from Whipple's bacilli or *Mycobacteria* with special stains. Other entities in the differential diagnosis are other fungi with yeast-like forms (Table 10-9). If well-formed granulomas are present, the differential diagnosis includes xanthoma, tuberculosis, yersiniosis, Crohn's disease, and foreign body granulomas.

Treatment and Prognosis. Therapy is required for disseminated disease, since the mortality rate for untreated patients is extremely high. Amphotericin B is the drug of choice for fulminant disease and patients receive at least 35 mg/kg total dose for 3 to 4 months. Over 90 percent of AIDS patients relapse, and therefore, maintenance therapy with oral itraconazole is

Table 10-9

MORPHOLOGIC FEATURES OF FUNGI THAT OCCUR AS YEAST-LIKE CELLS IN TISSUE

	Histoplasma capsulatum var *capsulatum*	*Blastomyces dermatitidis*	*Paracoccidioides brasiliensis*	*Candida* sp.	*Torulopsis glabrata*
Size (µm)	2-4	7-15	5-60	3-6	2-5
Shape	Spherical or oval	Spherical	Spherical	Spherical or oval	Spherical or oval
Number of buds	Single	Single	Multiple; "steering wheel" forms	Single; chains	Single
Attachment of buds	Narrow	Very broad	Narrow	Narrow	Narrow
Thickness of cell wall	Thin	Thick	Variable	Thin	Thin
Pseudohyphae and/or hyphae	Rare	Rare	Rare	Present	Absent
Number of nuclei	Single	Multiple	Multiple	Single	Single
Mucicarmine reaction	–	±	–	–	–

recommended indefinitely. In non-AIDS patients, amphotericin B treatment should be followed by oral itraconazole for 6 to 18 months (542). Itraconazole is an excellent alternative to amphotericin B in patients with mild or moderately severe infections (541). If the patients have developed sclerosing mediastinitis as part of the disease and the fibrosing process compromises the esophagus, surgical resection may be required. Esophageal complications from histoplasmosis are generally treated with surgery.

Aspergillus Infections

Demography. *Aspergillus* species are ubiquitous, rapidly growing, environmental pathogens that occur worldwide. Risk factors for acquiring the infection include granulocytopenia and the use of immunosuppressive drugs, cytoreductive agents, broad-spectrum antibiotics, and steroids (557,559,560). Patients with chronic granulomatous disease may present with invasive *Aspergillus* because of the inability of their phagocytes to generate microbicidal substances.

Inhalation of spores from the environment is believed to be the most frequent route of infection. Accordingly, upper respiratory tract, sinus, and pulmonary diseases are the major sequelae of *Aspergillus* infection. There may also be invasion from cutaneous sources, such as central venous catheters. *Aspergillus* infections pose particular problems in hospitalized populations when patients are exposed to organisms present in the ventilation system or in areas near construction or renovation sites.

Etiology. Approximately 600 species of *Aspergillus* are recognized. The most frequent disease-causing species are *A. fumigatus*, *A. flavus*, *A. niger*, and occasionally, *A. terreus*. Aspergilli are molds that reproduce by means of spores, termed conidia.

Pathophysiology. As with other molds, *Aspergillus* organisms have a tendency toward vascular invasion, producing thrombosis, ischemia, infarction, and tissue necrosis. Most infections originate in the lungs and then spread to other organs.

Clinical Features. *Aspergillus* is primarily a pulmonary pathogen that infects patients with preexisting pulmonary disease. Invasiveness is promoted by factors that suppress granulocyte function such as high-dose corticosteroid therapy in patients with obstructive airway disease. In profoundly immunocompromised hosts, *Aspergillus* behaves aggressively, affecting many organs. *Aspergillus* infection is particularly severe in patients with cancer and AIDS where it may cause deep mucosal lesions in the esophagus that can lead to tracheoesophageal fistula formation (556). Patients typically present with symptoms of painful or difficult swallowing, weight loss, and concurrent mucosal candidiasis. Colonic involvement may also occur, in which case the affected patients usually present with lower gastrointestinal bleeding. Perforation may occur secondary to angioinvasion by the fungi, with resultant ischemia.

Gross Findings. Although most infections involve the esophagus, gastric, small intestinal and colonic disease also occur. Vascular invasion by the organisms results in thrombosis and infarction, leading to ulceration, hemorrhage, and perforation (550,554). Aspergillus is rare in the stomach but may produce pseudomembranous gastritis (558,561); colonic lesions are characterized by submucosal ulcers and confluent necrosis (555).

Microscopic Findings. The diagnosis of invasive aspergillosis depends on the histologic demonstration of typical *Aspergillus* hyphae in the tissues. The organism tends to invade vessels, causing vasculitis, thrombosis, ischemia, and infarction. Often, the organisms are visible on routine H&E-stained material. Methenamine silver and PAS stains demonstrate the dichotomously branched septate hyphae of aspergilli and occasionally show the characteristic conidiophores.

Special Techniques. Endoscopic brushings and biopsies are essential for an accurate diagnosis of *Aspergillus* esophagitis. The fungi are easily demonstrated using fungal stains.

Differential Diagnosis. The differential diagnosis of *Aspergillus* infection includes other fungi that exhibit hyphal forms in tissue. They are distinguished from one another by examining the length and width of the hyphae, the presence or absence of septation, the frequency of septa, the pattern of branching and the orientation of the branches, the uniformity of the size and shape of the hyphae, the presence or absence of natural brown pigmentation, and the presence of blastoconidia or arthroconidia. The lesion somewhat resembles mucormycosis which also tends to penetrate blood vessels and disseminate through the vasculature.

Treatment and Prognosis. Therapy for invasive disease is inadequate. Mortality rates range from 50 to 100 percent, depending on the underlying disorder (551). Pulmonary or cerebral *Aspergillus* in bone marrow transplant patients is associated with a 95 percent mortality rate, regardless of therapy (551). The mainstay of therapy for invasive *Aspergillus* organisms is still intravenous amphotericin B, with doses ranging from 0.6 to 1.5 mg/kg/day for the duration of the neutropenia, for a total dose of 1.5 to 4.0 g. This is because *Aspergillus* are resistant to the commonly used imidazoles, ketoconazole and fluconazole. Itraconazole, an absorbable imidazole derivative, is active against *Aspergillus* organisms and may be useful in the treatment of mucosal *Aspergillus* infection (552,553). Surgical therapy alone or in combination with antifungal chemotherapy is used in patients with localized disease. A critical factor in optimizing therapy is removal of the immunosuppression, if possible (555).

Blastomyces Infections

Demography. *Blastomyces dermatitidis* infections occur worldwide but are endemic in certain geographic regions. In the United States, blastomycosis occurs in the same areas as histoplasmosis: along the Mississippi and Ohio River Valleys.

Etiology. *B. dermatitidis* is a species of dimorphous, round, budding yeast. It grows in tissues as a thick-walled, round cell measuring 8 to 15 µm in diameter and reproduces by broad-based budding. Multiple nuclei are seen in well-fixed sections. The organism spreads in the intestine by invading submucosal lymphoid tissue, with subsequent erosion into the mucosa and gastrointestinal lumen.

Clinical Features. The infection begins with the inhalation of spores into the lung, followed by control of the infectious process by lung macrophages (562). Gastrointestinal involvement is rare and usually manifests with lesions in the mouth or oropharynx. Disease distal to the oropharynx is very rare and usually due to disseminated infection (562).

Gross Findings. Endoscopically, mucosal friability or erythema is seen.

Microscopic Findings. The typical histologic picture consists of granulomatous inflammation with superimposed pyogenic inflammation. Lesions without secondary infections resemble the epithelioid granulomas of sarcoidosis. The organism is demonstrable with fungal stains.

Treatment and Prognosis. Ketoconazole is used to treat mild to moderate infections and amphotericin B severe infections (563).

Paracoccidioides Infections

Demography. *Paracoccidioides* infection (also known as *South American blastomycosis*) is an important public health problem in South America; it does not usually extend further north

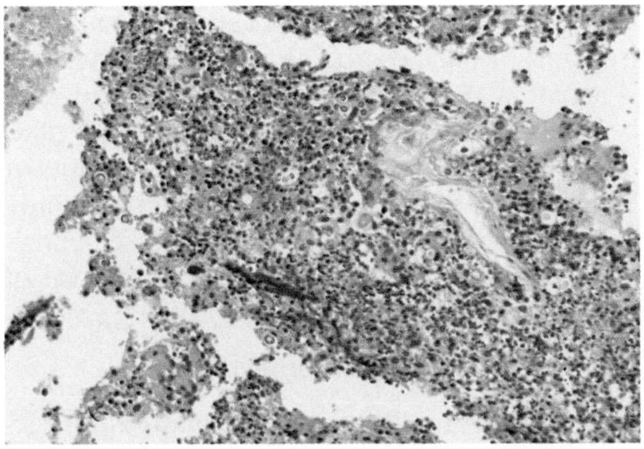
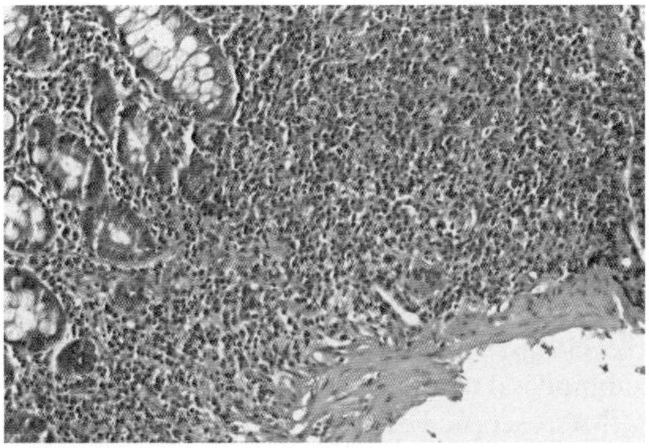

Figure 10-26

PARACOCCIDIOIDES INFECTION

Left: Low-power view of the inflammatory exudate from an ulcer due to paracoccidioidomycosis. The exudate contains numerous eosinophils, neutrophils, macrophages, and scattered large fungal organisms.

Right: The intestinal mucosa contains a dense inflammatory infiltrate of eosinophils, neutrophils, macrophages, and scattered multinucleated giant cells.

than Central America and Mexico, unless an infected person travels into a nonendemic area. Brazil is the center of the endemic region.

Etiology. In tissue, *Paracoccidioides* grows to be a large, round, oval cell measuring 5 to 15 µm in diameter that reproduces by single or multiple budding. Budding cells can measure up to 20 µm or more. The disease has a long latency period of up to 30 years (565). The infection is acquired when conidia are inhaled into the lungs. This results in a chronic granulomatous process that begins with an asymptomatic pulmonary infection. When the organisms disseminate outside the lungs, they form ulcerating granulomas.

Clinical Features. Paracoccidioidomycosis is a systemic disease that disseminates to several organ systems. The portal of entry is the lung. From there it disseminates to other organs, including the gastrointestinal tract. Paracoccidioidomycosis infects both the large and small intestines. Recently, the organism has been shown to be associated with ascites and colonic malakoplakia (566).

Gross Findings. The ulcerative lesions of paracoccidioidomycosis have a characteristic rolled border with a white exudative base and small hemorrhagic dots. These lesions are due to the formation of multiple granulomas. The draining lymph nodes are often involved.

Microscopic Findings. The fungi are easily seen in H&E-stained sections because of their large size (fig. 10-26), but they also can be highlighted by fungal stains. The fungi are often surrounded by a granulomatous reaction combined with pyogenic inflammation. The distinctive feature of the fungus in tissue is an occasional large cell that, when hemisected, reveals peripheral buds protruding from a thin-walled, round, mother cell, a pattern that sometimes looks like a ship's wheel.

Differential Diagnosis. Clinically, intestinal paracoccidioidomycosis simulates idiopathic IBD, but finding the organisms resolves the differential diagnosis.

Treatment and Prognosis. Ketoconazole is usually given for prolonged periods of time, usually 12 to 18 months (564). The triazoles, itraconazole and fluconazole, are extremely successful in producing disease remission with less toxicity than ketoconazole (564). Sulfadiazine or long-acting sulfonamides can also be used.

Zygomycosis

Demography. Zygomycetes are ubiquitous and generally saprophytic, rarely causing disease in immunocompetent hosts. They have a propensity to affect acidotic, usually diabetic patients, but they also affect patients with acidosis secondary to uremia, diarrhea, or aspirin use (aspirin abuse). The most prevalent underlying conditions are kwashiorkor, amebiasis, uremia, typhoid fever, and gastric neoplasms.

Etiology. The most common infectious zygomycete is *Rhizopus arrhizus* (*R. oryzae*), which tends to produce an acute and rapidly fatal infection, *mucormycosis*, despite early diagnosis and treatment.

Pathophysiology. The major defect leading to gastrointestinal tract zygomycosis is the disruption of mucosal integrity as occurs in peptic ulcers. The organisms have a predilection for invading major blood vessels and causing ischemia, infarction, and necrosis of adjacent tissues.

Clinical Features. Zygomycosis has five major clinical forms: rhinocerebral, pulmonary, abdominopelvic and gastric (gastrointestinal), primary cutaneous, and disseminated. Each is associated with various abnormalities and host defense mechanisms (568).

Gastrointestinal zygomycosis is uncommon and results from ingestion of the organism by malnourished individuals, individuals with chronic renal failure, or those with underlying gastrointestinal tract disease. The infection usually affects the stomach and colon, producing necrotic ulcerations, ischemia, and gangrene (567). Occasionally, the organisms colonize benign gastric ulcers without invading further. More frequently, they cause mucosal infiltration and vascular invasion. The presence of the mucosal infiltration and tissue invasion may simulate malignancy.

Infections also occur in the ileum. In most cases, dyspepsia, abdominal pain, and diarrhea are present. There may be vomiting and gastrointestinal bleeding. Perforation may occur, resulting in peritonitis. The fungal pathogens may then extend from the gut lumen to the gallbladder, liver, pancreas, and spleen. Gastrointestinal involvement is usually rapidly progressive, resulting in death within a few days.

Gross Findings. Zygomycosis shows a predilection for the stomach and colon. Patients develop mucosal ulcers that lead to bloody diarrhea. The organism produces discrete mucosal erosions and deep ulcers, causing hemorrhage, necrosis, and perforation as the infection spreads into the bowel wall. Transmural hemorrhage and necrosis may also be present.

Microscopic Findings. The organisms of zygomycosis are ordinarily recognized in large numbers in the lesions. The organisms have characteristic pleomorphic, broad, aseptate, irregularly right-angled, branched hyphae measuring 10 to 20 µm in diameter that are well seen in H&E-stained sections (fig. 10-27). They can also be highlighted by PAS and methenamine silver stains. They invade the surrounding tissues and blood vessels, causing local tissue destruction, vascular thrombosis, and ischemic necrosis. Histologically, the ulcer bases contain necrotic tissue with a surrounding rim of acute polymorphonuclear leukocytes and occasional giant cells, unless patients are on chemotherapeutic drugs, in which case the inflammatory response may be negligible.

Treatment and Prognosis. Successful treatment of zygomycosis requires a high index of clinical suspicion for rapid diagnosis. Mortality rates as high as 85 percent have been documented. Treatment requires reversal of the underlying condition, possible surgical removal of the infected tissue, and intravenous amphotericin B. The fungus is relatively resistant; high doses are needed to treat it and the prognosis remains poor.

Cryptococcus Infections

Demography. *Cryptococcus neoformans*, a yeast-like fungus, occurs worldwide, and is seen with increased frequency in immunocompromised patients. It is a life-threatening fungal infection in HIV-infected patients. The most important environmental source of infection is soil contaminated by bird droppings. Gastrointestinal cryptococcal infections are rare, occurring either as part of disseminated disease or as an isolated finding (571) that complicates AIDS and hematologic malignancies, or in patients on corticosteroids (570,573).

Clinical Features. The most common clinical forms of the disease are subacute progressive meningitis followed by pulmonary infection. Esophageal infections have been seen primarily in HIV-positive patients (572). Gastrointestinal involvement is rare (569,570,573).

Pathologic Findings. *Cryptococcus* may involve the stomach, duodenum, and colon. Grossly, the mucosa may have a nodular or ulcerated appearance. Histologically, yeast cells are visualized in affected tissues.

Special Techniques. Fungal cultures should exclude other fungal pathogens.

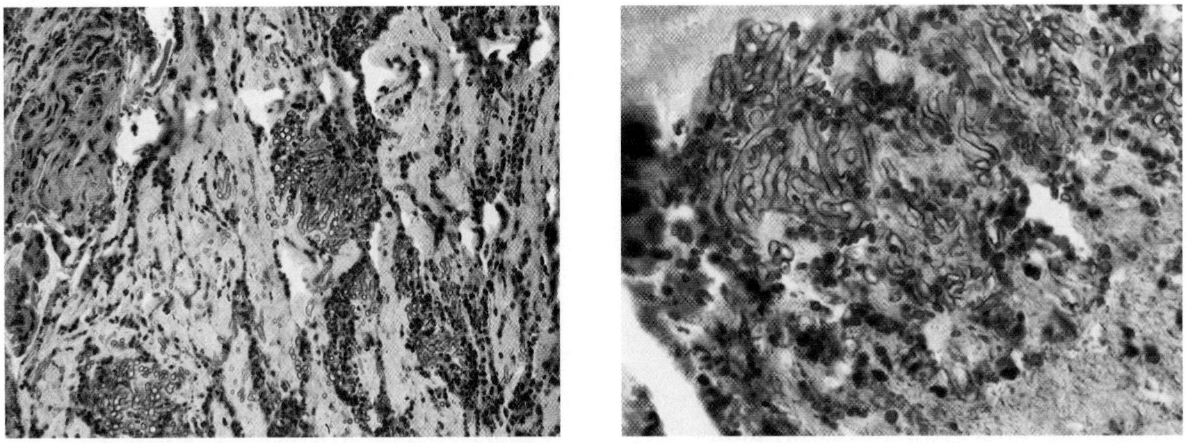

Figure 10-27

MUCOR COLONIZING A GASTRIC ULCER

Left: Numerous ribbon-like hyphae are in the inflammatory debris overlying the ulcer.
Right: Higher-power view of the organisms.

Treatment and Prognosis. The standard therapeutic regimen for acute cryptococcal infection is a combination of amphotericin B plus flucytosine. Optimal treatment for gastrointestinal disease is unknown.

Coccidioides Infections

Demography. *Coccidioides immitis* is a dimorphic fungus found predominantly in the southwestern United States and northern Mexico. Predisposing factors that lead to dissemination and infection include pregnancy, age under 5 years and over 50 years, and Hispanic, Asian, or African descent (574,577,578). Gastrointestinal coccidioidomycosis is rare.

Etiology. Infection is acquired by inhalation of arthroconidia. In the host, these enlarge and form spherules containing endospores.

Clinical Features. Weisman et al. (579) described a gastrointestinal infection with massive chylous ascites and extensive abdominal and lymphatic involvement. Coccidioidal peritonitis also occurs (576).

Pathologic Findings. Histologic examination may show the presence of necrotizing granulomatous inflammation surrounding the organisms (575).

VIRAL INFECTIONS

Gastrointestinal viral infections are common causes of diarrhea worldwide. Since most infections in immunocompetent patients are short-lived and self-limited, biopsy is rarely required to make the diagnosis. Immunocompromised patients frequently develop viral infections, most notably infection with HSV or CMV. In such patients, biopsy is necessary to make the correct diagnosis.

Rotavirus and Rotavirus-Like Particle Infections

Demography. *Rotaviruses* are the most common cause of infantile gastroenteritis worldwide, accounting for an estimated 140 million cases of diarrhea, 1 million deaths in young children, and the most hospital admissions for diarrhea in children under 2 years of age (589,593, 606,628). Most affected patients are between 5 months and 4 years of age, although individuals of any age may become infected. Each year in the United States rotavirus infections account for an estimated 3.5 million cases of diarrhea, 500,000 physician visits, 50,000 hospitalizations, and 20 deaths among children less than 5 years of age (593).

In children in temperate climates, rotavirus infections are acquired more frequently in winter months, but such seasonal variation does not occur in adults (584,602,606,616). Geographic variation influences the frequency of rotavirus infection, with the higher rates of infection being reported in Japan, Australia, Indonesia, and

Mexico relative to those reported in the United States and Europe (587,588,591,603,611,612, 618,620). Rotavirus infections also affect travelers (often to Mexico or the Caribbean), immunosuppressed patients, and the elderly (580, 582,585,598,610,619,623).

Etiology. Rotaviruses are members of the Reoviridae family of RNA viruses. Intact infectious rotaviruses measure approximately 100 nm in diameter and consist of three protein layers surrounding a viral genome composed of 11 segments of double-stranded RNA (581). The RNA encodes six viral proteins that compose the viral capsid, and six nonstructural proteins.

Pathophysiology. Rotavirus most commonly spreads from person to person via a fecal-oral route. Rarely, the virus may be foodborne or waterborne (583,600). Once acquired, the infection usually spreads from the proximal small bowel to the ileum over a period of 1 to 2 days. Rotaviruses have very specific cell tropism, infecting mature enterocytes on the villus tips and differentiated enterocytes in the dome epithelium overlying Peyer patches. Interaction of the virus with the host enterocyte is probably a multistep process involving the binding of more than one cell surface receptor (581). The virus enters the cell either via calcium-dependent endocytosis or via direct entry. Once inside the enterocyte, the virus replicates. The new viral particles may then infect additional downstream enterocytes, or may be excreted in the feces.

The mechanisms by which rotaviruses cause diarrhea are not yet fully understood. Potential mechanisms include reduction of the absorptive surface of the intestine through damage to the villi, impaired absorption due to decreased brush border transport functions (597,609,615), altered epithelial permeability (590,604,617), stimulation of the enteric nervous system (614), or direct enterotoxigenic effects of the rotavirus protein NSP4 (601).

Clinical Features. Primary rotavirus infection typically occurs in infants and children between the ages of 6 months and 2 years. Infection may occur in younger children, usually in a hospital setting. The classic presentation is fever and vomiting for 2 to 3 days followed by the onset of watery, nonbloody diarrhea (595). The diarrhea may be profuse, with 10 to 20 bowel movements per day being common. Repeat infections are generally less severe than primary infections (622).

In adults, rotavirus infection may or may not be symptomatic (594,607,627). Symptoms begin 2 to 6 days following contact with the virus, and last for 1 to 4 days. When symptoms do occur, they include fever, headache, malaise, nausea, cramping pain, and diarrhea (608,624–626).

Microscopic Findings. Viral replication within the enterocytes leads to enterocyte lysis, epithelial shedding, crypt hyperplasia, and inflammatory cell infiltration of the lamina propria (586,599). The ratio of the crypt depth to villous height increases. Severe infection causes gross destruction of the villous architecture.

Special Techniques. The diagnosis of a rotavirus infection is usually made by examining the stool for the presence of the virus. Negative contrast electron microscopy demonstrates characteristic 70-nm wheel-like particles, and was the technique initially used for diagnostic purposes (592). Enzyme-linked immunosorbent assay (ELISA) and enzyme-interface immunoassay (EIA) are now commercially available and commonly used. These techniques require the presence of large numbers of virions to generate a positive result (628,629). PCR is a more sensitive technique that is currently being used in a research capacity for detection of the virus (628).

Differential Diagnosis. There are four major subclassifications of gastroenteritis-causing viruses: rotavirus and rotavirus-like viruses, enteric adenoviruses, caliciviruses (including Norwalk and Norwalk-like viruses), and astrovirus. These entities are usually distinguished from one another using ultrastructural, microbiologic, or serologic tests. Rotavirus infections destroy villous epithelial cells, contrasting with parvovirus infections which destroy crypt epithelial cells.

Treatment and Prognosis. Because the diarrhea is more severe than that seen in many other gastrointestinal infections, rotavirus causes a disproportionate number of deaths (589). Treatment is symptomatic and consists of fluid replacement and supportive care. Severe cases of rotavirus diarrhea have been successfully managed with administration of oral human immunoglobulins directed against the virus (596, 605,613). A rotavirus immunization would be capable of preventing over 1 million cases of diarrhea in the first 5 years of life (621). In 1999, shortly after approval of a rotavirus vaccine, an excess of cases of intussusception was noted among recently vaccinated infants, and the vaccine was withdrawn from the market.

Norwalk and Norwalk-Like Virus Infections

Demography. *Norwalk-like viruses* cause more than 96 percent of outbreaks of acute nonbacterial gastroenteritis in the United States and Europe (637,640,649). The degree to which the infection is endemic is unknown, because most individuals who are affected do not seek medical care. Norwalk and Norwalk-related viruses have a cosmopolitan distribution, infecting both adults and children. Outbreaks occur in a variety of settings, including military installations, nursing homes, restaurants, schools, daycare facilities, summer camps, and cruise ships (635–638,640). The infection is most commonly acquired through consumption of food directly contaminated by an infected food handler (638). As a result, cold foods such as salads, sandwiches, and bakery products are most frequently implicated in outbreaks (634). Food may also be contaminated at its source; for example, oysters harvested from contaminated water are commonly associated with Norwalk virus outbreaks (631,639,648). In addition, the virus may be spread by person-to-person contact (630,641). Airborne transmission likely also occurs (642,643,646).

Etiology. Norwalk-like viruses are small (27 to 32 nm), single stranded RNA viruses that constitute one genus in the family Caliciviridae. Multiple strains of these viruses circulate at any given time, although at certain times, one strain may predominate (633).

Clinical Features. Norwalk-like viruses have an incubation period of 12 to 48 hours (632), and the resulting disease usually runs its course in 1 to 3 days, although symptoms may persist for longer, especially in children (633,645). The most common symptoms of the infection are diarrhea and vomiting. Patients may also experience low-grade fever, abdominal pain or cramping, nausea, malaise, myalgia, and headache (633,645). Vomiting is more common among children, while diarrhea tends to predominate in adults. In temperate regions, the disease is more prevalent in winter months, although Norwalk-like virus–associated gastroenteritis occurs year round (644). Viral shedding may occur for as many as 3 weeks after the onset of symptoms (645).

Microscopic Findings. Volunteers who experimentally receive Norwalk virus develop histologic abnormalities in the small intestine within 12 to 48 hours. The abnormalities include mucosal inflammation, enterocyte changes, villous shortening, and crypt hyperplasia with increased epithelial cell mitoses. Mononuclear cells and neutrophils infiltrate the lamina propria. The changes persist for at least 4 days and clear by 6 to 8 weeks after the acute illness (647).

Special Techniques. Diagnostic tests include immunoelectron microscopy, enzyme immunoassay, and reverse transcriptase (RT)-PCR for detection of the virus.

Sapporo and Sapporo-Like Virus Infections

Demography. *Sapporo-like viruses* are another genus in the Caliciviridae family of viruses. These viruses occur worldwide, and affect predominantly infants and young children (650, 650a). Rarely, Sapporo virus gastroenteritis occurs in the elderly. Older children and adults are virtually never affected (650a).

Etiology. Sapporo-like viruses are antigenically distinct from Norwalk and Norwalk-like viruses.

Clinical Features. Sapporo virus causes gastroenteritis in young children and infants. Ninety-five percent of patients develop diarrhea, and vomiting occurs in 60 percent (650a). These symptoms are often accompanied by abdominal pain, cramps, nausea, and fever. The stools may contain mucus, but are not bloody. The median duration of symptoms is 6 days (645). Viral shedding is of shorter duration than for Norwalk viruses.

Enteric Adenovirus Infections

Demography. Enteric *adenovirus* infections account for up to one sixth of cases of viral diarrhea in children in Britain and the United States (653,654a,655,667). Adenoviral illnesses usually affect children under age 2, particularly those in the first year of life (654a,661,665). The infections do not demonstrate seasonality. Severe infections affect immunodeficient individuals and bone marrow transplant recipients, sometimes causing death (651,669). Adenovirus can be

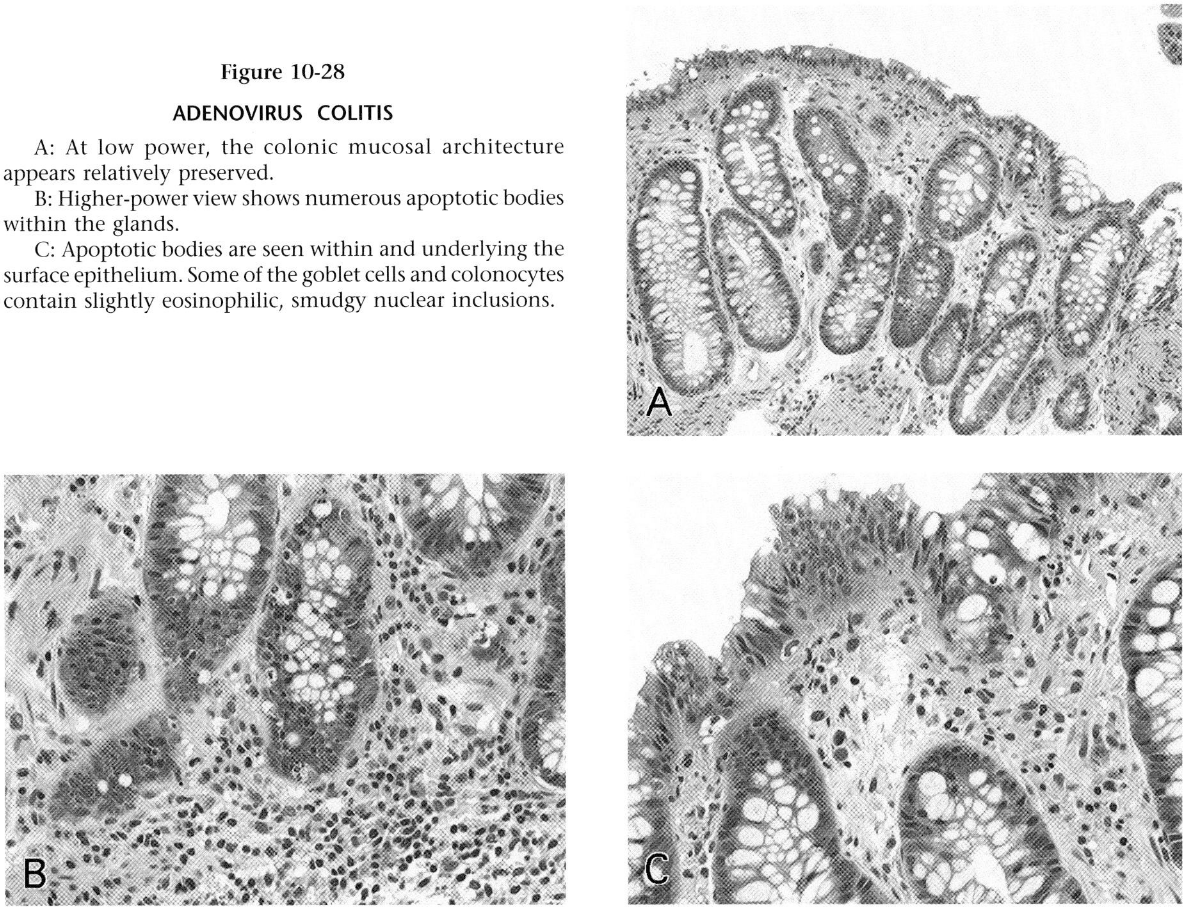

Figure 10-28

ADENOVIRUS COLITIS

A: At low power, the colonic mucosal architecture appears relatively preserved.

B: Higher-power view shows numerous apoptotic bodies within the glands.

C: Apoptotic bodies are seen within and underlying the surface epithelium. Some of the goblet cells and colonocytes contain slightly eosinophilic, smudgy nuclear inclusions.

isolated from the stool of from 4 to 18 percent of HIV-infected patients (656,659,662,664,666).

Etiology. Some adenoviruses, in particular serotypes 40 and 41, produce gastroenteritis, but unlike conventional adenoviral serotypes, enteric adenoviruses do not primarily produce nasopharyngitis or keratoconjunctivitis.

Clinical Features. Adenovirus infections affect the stomach, small intestine, and colon. The clinical features of adenovirus infection in children are diarrhea, fever, vomiting, and mild dehydration (661). Vomiting and fever are less prominent than with rotavirus infection (663). Affected children may also complain of associated abdominal pain and respiratory tract infection (661). Adenovirus infections in HIV-infected patients typically last from 5 to 12 days, producing protracted, watery, nonmucoid, nonbloody diarrhea and weight loss (659). The diarrhea results from extensive epithelial sloughing. Intussusception may occur in some patients as a result of terminal ileal lymphoid hyperplasia accompanying nonenteric adenovirus infection (654,657,658).

Gross Findings. The endoscopic appearance of the colonic mucosa is either normal or shows erythematous raised lesions measuring several millimeters in diameter.

Microscopic Findings. The histologic changes of adenovirus infection are relatively nonspecific and include villous atrophy and inflammation. The diagnosis relies on finding the nuclear viral inclusions. Adenovirus-infected cells have characteristic amphophilic or eosinophilic nuclear inclusions, predominantly affecting the goblet cells in the epithelium and the upper parts of the crypts (fig. 10-28) (668). The enlarged nuclei sometimes have a smudgy appearance or appear crescenteric; they lie at the cell bases. Other changes include budding of the epithelium and shedding of the epithelium into the lumen. Rare glands become necrotic and inflamed. The infection often spares cells in the lamina propria, such as endothelial cells or smooth muscle cells. In AIDS patients, adenovirus infection may coexist with CMV infection.

Special Techniques. The diagnosis can be established by ultrastructural examination of the stool, viral cultures, monoclonal antibody-based immunoassays, PCR, or in situ hybridization reactions. Ultrastructurally, pathognomonic viral particles are seen in the nuclei of the mucosal epithelium. The cells contain irregular, hexagonal paracrystalline arrays of virions averaging 73 to 80 mm in diameter (652).

Differential Diagnosis. The differential diagnosis depends on the clinical presentation. If the patient presents with intussusception, then the various causes of intussusception come into the differential diagnosis, including an adenovirus infection with lymphoid hyperplasia. If, on the other hand, viral inclusions are seen, then the differential diagnosis is that of other viral infections that cause nuclear inclusions, especially CMV infection (660).

Treatment and Prognosis. There is no effective therapeutic agent for adenovirus. As a result, treatment is supportive.

Astrovirus Infections

Demography. *Astrovirus* infection is the second most common cause of gastroenteritis in children (672,686,688). The viruses affect children below the age of 7 years much more frequently than older children and adults. Infants under 2 years of age are particularly vulnerable. Astrovirus infections are more common in the winter and spring than in the summer in temperate climates (672,683,686). They are associated with diarrheal outbreaks in newborn nurseries and pediatric wards, in community settings, and in nursing homes (673–676,680,682, 687). Most children acquire antibodies to the virus by 5 years of age (673,679). Immunocompromised patients are also susceptible to astrovirus infection (671,677).

Etiology. Astrovirus is a 28-nm, single-stranded RNA virus that belongs to the family Astroviridae. Astrovirus infections are acquired through ingestion of contaminated foods, often shellfish or raw fish (681), and potentially through contaminated water or fomite transmission (670,684,685).

Clinical Features. Clinically, astrovirus infection causes diarrheal disease resembling rotaviral illness, although the disease is less severe (672,688). Patients may experience fever and vomiting. The median duration of the disease is 3 days (688).

Microscopic Findings. The changes resemble those found in other pediatric viral diseases.

Special Techniques. Ultrastructural viral identification relies on identifying the characteristic viral morphology. Astroviral antibodies are detectable using indirect fluorescence. The organism is detected with RT-PCR (678).

Herpesvirus Infections

Demography. Neonates, children, and adults all suffer from herpetic infections. In the case of neonates, the disease is acquired as an intrauterine, intrapartum, or postnatal infection. Herpes simplex virus type I (HSV-I) is a frequent cause of esophagitis in patients who have underlying malignancies, diabetes, previous radiation therapy, or HIV disease, or have been treated with steroids or other cytotoxic agents. Herpes esophagitis is found in the same clinical settings as esophageal candidiasis. It may also occur in otherwise healthy individuals without underlying immunologic problems. Herpetic esophagitis is especially common following trigeminal nerve surgery. Two possible interrelated predisposing conditions may account for this association: 1) oropharyngeal shedding of HSV frequently follows trigeminal surgery, and 2) esophageal intubation during the surgery produces secondary mucosal trauma. Reactivation of a latent herpetic infection should be considered when patients develop odynophagia following esophageal instrumentation (705).

Colonic herpes infections are extremely rare, and usually occur in the setting of immunocompromise (689,691,693,696,701,703). They have also been found in patients with IBD (698) and in neonates (695). Herpetic proctitis often results from HSV-II infections, but HSV-I proctitis may also occur (709). Disease transmission requires direct contact with infectious lesions or secretions.

Etiology. Two distinct types of herpes simplex virus exist, HSV-I and HSV-II. Each is composed of numerous distinctive viral strains. HSV-I predominantly causes nasal, labial, oropharyngeal, and esophageal infections, while HSV-II causes genital and perianal herpes. Both viruses are acquired through close personal contact with infected individuals.

Pathophysiology. The virus enters the host via the mucous membranes. It replicates locally within epithelial cells, leading to cell destruction and resultant formation of vesicular and ulcerated lesions. The virus can invade peripheral neural tissues where it may remain latent within sensory nerve ganglia. During primary infection, an immune response evolves but usually matures only after neuronal invasion. This immune response eliminates the local mucous membrane infection but cannot eliminate the latent virus residing within the sensory nerve root ganglion. Reactivation of latent virus within a ganglion leads to a recrudescence of viral replication at a mucous membrane site innervated by the nerve root. Reactivation of HSV from its latency in nerve and ganglion cells leads to viral DNA replication, transcription, translation, encapsulation, and viral shedding, features that depend on host-virus interactions. In healthy individuals, reactivation episodes are milder than the initial infection due to the presence of partial immunity. In contrast, in immunocompromised patients, activations are more frequent and more severe. Thus, the prime determinants of disease severity are the immunocompetence of the host and whether the infection is primary or recurrent (699).

Clinical Features. Typical herpetic esophagitis is seen in immunocompromised patients but also develops in immunocompetent individuals (697,706), especially following trigeminal nerve surgery (705). Herpes esophagitis usually manifests clinically by the sudden onset of severe odynophagia and/or dysphagia, fever, heartburn, and retrosternal pain (706). Nonspecific findings include epigastric pain, nausea, and vomiting. Constant retrosternal pain may be present as well as hematemesis. When severe, herpetic esophagitis may cause hemorrhage (707). Intestinal bleeding can be the presenting sign, especially if platelet counts are low. Clinically, esophageal herpes infections remain underdiagnosed unless there is a high degree of suspicion for the virus because the patient is in a high-risk group. The presence of herpetic vesicles (blisters) on the lips may suggest the diagnosis.

Herpes colitis is uncommon, but may occur in patients with disseminated disease. Symptoms include fever, bloody diarrhea, and dehydration. The colon may perforate (695).

Anogenital herpes infections may occur in immunocompetent or immunocompromised patients. Herpetic ulceration is probably the most common anal manifestation of AIDS (711). The clinical presentation usually begins with itching and soreness in or around the anus. Severe anorectal pain follows. The pain may be so intense that the patient becomes reluctant to have a bowel movement and develops constipation and impaction. Patients also present with fever, inguinal adenopathy, tenesmus, anorectal discharge, and bleeding. Neurologic symptoms develop in the distribution of the sacral roots in some patients. Abdominal pain can simulate a bowel obstruction. The disease often resolves within a couple of weeks but recurrences are common.

Gross Findings. The middle and distal thirds of the esophagus are the most commonly affected portions of the gastrointestinal tract (692,704), followed by the anus. Small vesicles are the earliest endoscopically identifiable esophageal lesions. These vesicles subsequently rupture to form discrete, superficial ulcers of the esophageal mucosa. These discrete "punched out" ulcers have white exudates in their bases and erythematous or yellow raised margins. Typically, the ulcers appear shallow, even in extensive disease, and they do not extend through the muscularis mucosae. Large areas of denuded mucosa develop in severe disease. Herpetic ulcers usually stop at the gastroesophageal junction, although rare cases of herpetic gastritis occur (fig. 10-29). The changes of herpetic esophagitis occur alone or they develop superimposed on preexisting tissue damage resulting from nasogastric tubes, caustic esophageal burns, or reflux esophagitis. The presence of preexisting damage may obscure the classic pathologic features of the viral infection.

Colonic involvement is rare, and usually presents as diffuse colitis, typically most severe in the sigmoid colon. Colonoscopy shows erythema and friability of the mucosa, aphthous ulcers, inflammatory polyps, and areas of ulceration (696). Sigmoidoscopic features of herpetic proctitis include mucosal friability and distal rectal ulcers or vesicles.

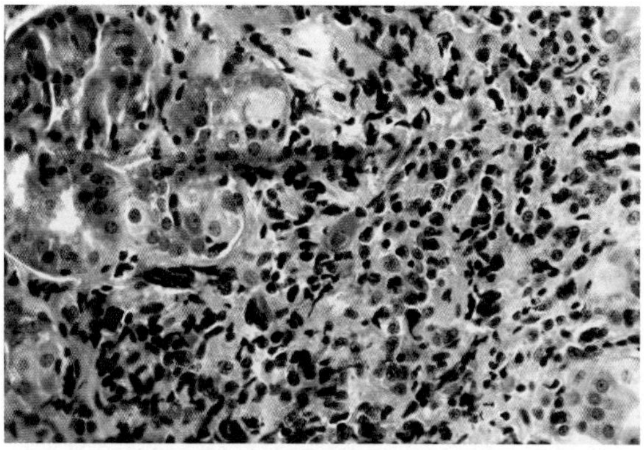

Figure 10-29

HERPES GASTRITIS

The stomach contains an intense mononuclear cell infiltrate. A single viral inclusion is in a gastric glandular remnant in the center.

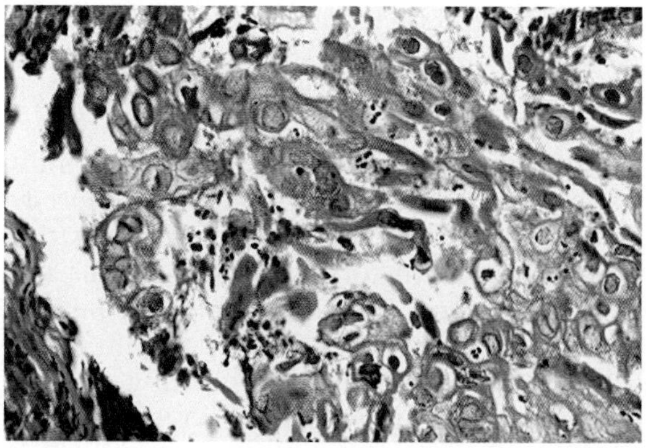

Figure 10-30

HERPES ESOPHAGITIS

The squamous epithelial cells contain characteristic inclusions. The nuclei appear glassy, with marginated chromatin. Multinucleated giant cells have molded nuclei that also contain typical viral inclusions. (Courtesy of the Division of Gastrointestinal Pathology, Armed Forces Institute of Pathology, Washington, DC.)

Microscopic Findings. Herpesviruses usually infect squamous mucosa, although they can infect enterocytes as well. The virus penetrates the epithelium, causing cytolysis and a localized inflammatory reaction. In over 50 percent of cases, characteristic viral inclusions are present (706). Herpetic esophagitis is usually easy to recognize if a biopsy is taken at the edge of the herpetic ulcer. The squamous epithelial cells at the margin of the ulcer contain Cowdry type A inclusions (fig. 10-30). A clear zone with an outer dark margin of condensed chromatin at the nuclear membrane surrounds large, intranuclear, eosinophilic inclusions. Multinucleated syncytial squamous cells containing molded nuclei and a typical "ground-glass" appearance are also common. In immunocompetent patients, only a small number of viral inclusions are present, contrasting with a large number present in immunosuppressed patients. Occasionally, there is histologic evidence of herpetic infection in the ducts and acini of the submucosal glands underlying areas of ulceration. Biopsies taken from the base of herpetic ulcers only reveal the presence of nonspecific inflammation, necrosis, granulation tissue, and desquamated epithelial cells.

The diagnosis of herpetic esophagitis may be difficult in AIDS patients, since the characteristic nuclear inclusions and multinucleated giant cells may be absent. Instead, aggregates of large mononuclear cells that contain convoluted nuclei are adjacent to the infected epithelium. The presence of such aggregates of macrophages highly suggests an inflammatory response to herpetic esophagitis.

Histologic examination of biopsy material in patients with colonic herpes simplex infections demonstrates lamina propria edema, lymphoplasmacytic infiltrates, and areas of ulceration. Typical viral inclusions and multinucleated cells may be seen, but may be small in number and patchy in distribution (696).

Histopathologic findings in herpetic proctitis are often nonspecific, with crypt abscesses and increased numbers of neutrophils in the lamina propria. Some patients have more characteristic findings, including perivascular lymphocytic cuffing in the submucosa, intranuclear inclusions, and multinucleated giant cells with ground-glass nuclei in the submucosa. The viral inclusions occur alone or in a setting of diffuse necrosis.

Special Techniques. The diagnosis is often made clinically and confirmed by cultures or biopsy of the ulcer. Viral culture not only increases the diagnostic yield on the tissues but distinguishes among viral infections with overlapping histologic and cytologic features. The virus grows readily in diploid fibroblasts or

Table 10-10

FEATURES OF GASTROINTESTINAL VIRAL INFECTIONS

Virus	Gross Features	Location	Histology
HSV[a] VZV	Multiple discrete shallow ulcers	Esophagus (HSV) common site although in severe infection both can be found in the esophagus	Biopsy of ulcer base: only granulation tissue; inflammation; necrosis; epithelial ballooning; inclusions in epithelium at ulcer edge
CMV	Resembles HSV	Involves the stomach and intestines more frequently than esophagus	Cytopathic effects involve submucosal glands, endothelium, stromal fibroblasts; infection of squamous cells is rare
HIV	May resemble HSV and CMV	Esophageal involvement hard to document	No specific changes
HPV	Normal or papillomas	Esophagus and anorectum	Koilocytosis, condyloma or normal-appearing; virus found by antigenic or molecular biologic tests
EBV	Deep, linear ulcers	Midesophagus	Resembles oral leukoplakia

[a]HSV = herpes simplex virus; VZV = varicella zoster virus; CMV = cytomegalovirus; HIV = human immunodeficiency virus; HPV = human papillomavirus; EBV = Epstein-Barr virus.

rabbit kidney cells, and cytopathic changes are usually evident within 24 to 96 hours (694). The use of immunohistochemistry or in situ hybridization for HSV nucleic acids confirms the diagnosis if the exact nature of the viral inclusions is uncertain. In addition, immunohistologic stains may highlight infected cells that do not show the morphologic changes characteristic of HSV.

Differential Diagnosis. The differential diagnosis includes other infections and acute causes of esophagitis, enteritis, colitis, and proctitis. The differential diagnosis of herpetic esophagitis includes drug-induced esophagitis, reflux esophagitis, caustic esophagitis, and radiation esophagitis. These conditions are almost always differentiated from herpetic esophagitis by the clinical history and presentation. It is important to distinguish herpetic esophagitis from other forms of infectious esophagitis, particularly other forms of viral esophagitis, because specific drugs exist to treat each of the diseases. The features that differentiate HSV and CMV infections are summarized in Table 10-10.

Treatment and Prognosis. Complications from herpetic esophagitis include hemorrhage, fistula formation, and viral dissemination. Submucosal fibrosis can lead to subsequent esophageal stricture. Some patients die of herpes pneumonia or hepatitis. Another complication is superinfection of the denuded esophagus with fungi and bacteria. *Candida albicans* is the most common coexisting infection; other opportunistic infections include *Mucor*, *Aspergillus*, or *Torula*. Another infectious agent that may coinfect the esophageal mucosa, particularly in the immunocompromised host, is CMV.

Herpes esophagitis in immunocompetent patients requires only symptomatic treatment with analgesics, viscous lidocaine, and antacids, because the illness is self-limited and complete resolution of symptoms occurs in 1 to 2 weeks (699, 710). Specific treatment with acyclovir is required in patients who are debilitated, immunocompromised, or have severe odynophagia (700,702). Acyclovir is recommended in a dose of 5 mg/kg intravenously every 8 hours for 7 to 10 days. Intravenous hydration may be necessary for patients to maintain adequate fluid intake because of the painful swallowing. The prodrugs famciclovir and valacyclovir are also effective (700).

Resistance to acyclovir is uncommon in herpetic infections occurring in immunocompetent hosts. In immunocompromised patients, however, resistance is frequent, occurring in 4 to 7 percent of patients (690,708). Resistance occurs in viral strains with mutations in the thymidine kinase gene, a gene required for phosphorylation of the drug to its active form. Foscarnet inhibits viral DNA polymerase and does not require phosphorylation and is therefore recommended for resistant strains.

Varicella Zoster Virus Infections

Demography. On rare occasions, *varicella zoster virus* (VZV) infects the esophagus in children with severe disseminated chickenpox. It has also been reported to infect the small intestine in immunocompromised individuals (718). In addition, it has been hypothesized that VZV is responsible for some motility disorders such as achalasia and Ogilvie's syndrome (712,713a,717).

Etiology. VZV is a double-stranded DNA virus morphologically identical to HSV. Fatal VZV infections usually affect children with cancer or those who are otherwise immunocompromised (713,716). Adults who develop symptomatic infections usually have reactivation of a viral infection acquired during childhood as occurs with HSV infections.

Clinical Features. Primary VZV infection in children causes the characteristic generalized vesicular eruptions of chickenpox. The disease is more severe in immunocompromised children, 20 to 30 percent of whom exhibit visceral dissemination and a mortality rate of 7 to 30 percent (711a). Symptomatic esophageal involvement in children with chickenpox is uncommon but does occur, usually in severely immunocompromised or very ill patients.

Gross Findings. Esophageal lesions consist of necrotizing esophagitis with superficial and deep esophageal ulcerations. The endoscopic features of VZV are indistinguishable from those of HSV.

Microscopic Findings. The histologic features of VZV are characterized by edema, ballooning degeneration, and vesicles lined by multinucleated giant cells with intranuclear eosinophilic inclusions (fig. 10-31). Intranuclear eosinophilic inclusion bodies can be seen in the epithelium, endothelium, and stromal cells. Immunohistochemical staining with monoclonal antibodies to VZV antigens confirms the diagnosis.

Differential Diagnosis. The differential diagnosis of VZV infection mainly includes HSV, but also includes other infectious etiologies.

Treatment and Prognosis. Treatment is accomplished with acyclovir or famciclovir (714,715).

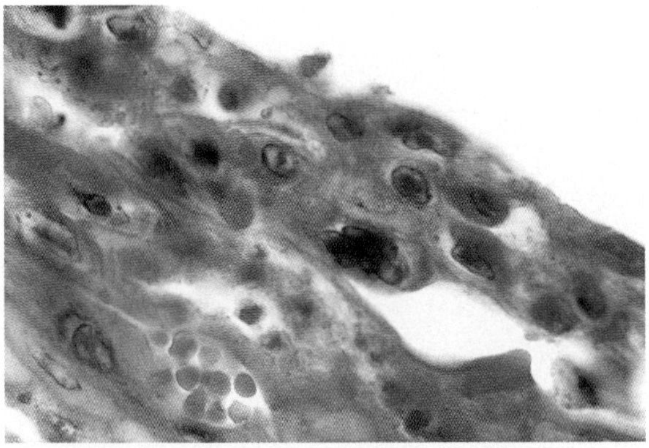

Figure 10-31

VARICELLA ZOSTER VIRUS INFECTION IN THE ESOPHAGUS

The squamous epithelial cells are spongiotic. A multinucleated cell is in the center. Eosinophilic inclusions are in the multinucleated cell, as well as in scattered individual squamous cells.

Cytomegalovirus Infections

Demography. *Cytomegalovirus* (CMV) is a ubiquitous herpesvirus whose incidence varies significantly by geographic location but results in a positive serology in approximately 80 percent of the world's adult population (719a). Like HSV, CMV exhibits a tendency to affect debilitated, elderly, or immunocompromised individuals. Populations at highest risk for disseminated gastrointestinal infection are neonates, allograft recipients, HIV-infected individuals, pregnant women, malnourished patients, those with malignancy, or the elderly. CMV infection is also seen in immunocompetent patients as well as in patients with IBD.

Pathophysiology. CMV infection is classified as primary infection, reactivation infection, and superinfection. CMV is usually not eliminated from the body after a primary infection. Rather, it persists as a low-grade chronic infection or it remains in a latent state. This allows reactivation or increased viral excretion at a later time and further viral transmission to new hosts. The macrophage serves as the infection reservoir during latent periods (724).

A number of host and viral factors determine the outcome of CMV infection. The most important is a shift in favor of the virus when the host's immune system becomes compromised or is immature. The determinants of acquisition of CMV infection vary among newborns, organ or bone marrow transplant recipients, HIV-infected persons, or blood transfusion recipients. CMV is transmitted to neonates transplacentally, by passage through a contaminated birth canal, or by ingestion of infected breast milk. In adults, CMV is sexually transmitted or transmitted via infected organs, blood, or needles (723).

Analysis of tissues by in situ hybridization shows that latent CMV affects most organs in the body (728). The predominant tissue site remains unknown, but circulating lymphocytes, monocytes, neutrophils, and endothelial cells all probably contain latent virus (727). Both humoral and cellular immune responses function to control CMV infection and, therefore, primary CMV infections in immunosuppressed patients tend to be more severe than those occurring in immunocompetent patients.

The underlying pathogenic mechanism relates in part to CMV infection of the vasculature. Immunocompromised individuals develop CMV viremia, endothelial viral infection followed by endothelialitis, submucosal ischemia, and secondary ulceration. CMV-associated vasculitis in the gastrointestinal tract is especially well documented in the AIDS population, where it preferentially involves the colon in up to 67 percent of patients. Both arteries and veins are affected and undergo segmental necrosis, perivascular hemorrhage, and possible thrombosis (725,734).

Clinical Features. Diverse symptoms are the result of CMV infection in many organ systems. The presence of CMV organisms does not always equate with clinical disease, and virologic evidence of CMV must be interpreted within the clinical context before treatment is considered. Immunocompetent individuals with primary infections usually remain asymptomatic, but may have a mononucleosis-type illness.

Symptoms of gastrointestinal CMV infection generally depend on the location and severity of the infection and the immune status of the patient. CMV infects the esophagus, stomach, small intestine, appendix, colon, and anal region, often appearing as an erosive or ulcerative process. The onset of symptoms of CMV esophagitis is more gradual than that seen in herpes infection. Nausea, vomiting, fever, epigastric pain, diarrhea, and weight loss are usual, whereas painful, difficult swallowing and retrosternal pain occur less often than is seen with HSV infections (726,735).

Patients with CMV gastritis also present with epigastric pain, nausea, and vomiting. Complications include bleeding, gastric outlet obstruction, and perforation. Unusual presentations include gastrocolic fistula (719), recurrent stomal ulcer with afferent limb obstruction in the postgastrectomy patient, submucosal antral mass, and acute self-limited gastropathy associated with a protein-losing enteropathy and pediatric forms of Menetrier's disease (729).

CMV enterocolitis causes nausea, vomiting, and crampy abdominal pain, often accompanied by profuse persistent or intermittent fever, weight loss, and severe wasting. A typical colitis pattern of bowel movements develops, including tenesmus, bloody stool, hematochezia, and small volume movements with regular frequency. The cecum and right colon become infected more commonly than distal locations (721), although the rectum and sigmoid colon may also be affected (732). Malabsorption, protein-losing enteropathy, perforation, and peritonitis may also occur (720,730). Additionally, CMV infection may affect the gastrointestinal innervation, possibly leading to motility disturbances.

Patients with disseminated CMV infections often demonstrate circulating cytomegalic inclusion–containing cells in the peripheral blood. These are endothelial in origin and contain viral capsids within the nucleus, and virus particles and dense bodies in the cytoplasm. The circulating cytomegalic cells can disseminate the infection throughout the body (722).

Gross Findings. In CMV esophagitis, discrete superficial ulcers occur in the mid- or distal esophagus. In some patients, one or more large, relatively flat, serpiginous or oval ulcers, surrounded by a radiolucent rim of edematous mucosa, develop. These coalesce to form giant ulcers, particularly in the distal esophagus. The presence of one or more giant esophageal ulcers suggests the diagnosis of CMV. Fistulas may also form.

In CMV gastritis the stomach appears variably congested and atrophic. The entire small bowel may be involved by CMV infection, although some patients have disease limited to the ileocecal region. The organism characteristically causes colonic ulcers that tend to localize in the ileocecal region. Rare patients develop CMV pancolitis. Colonoscopy shows ulcers or

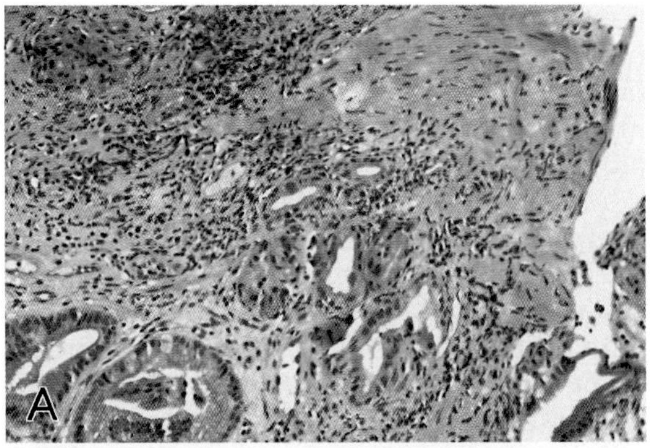

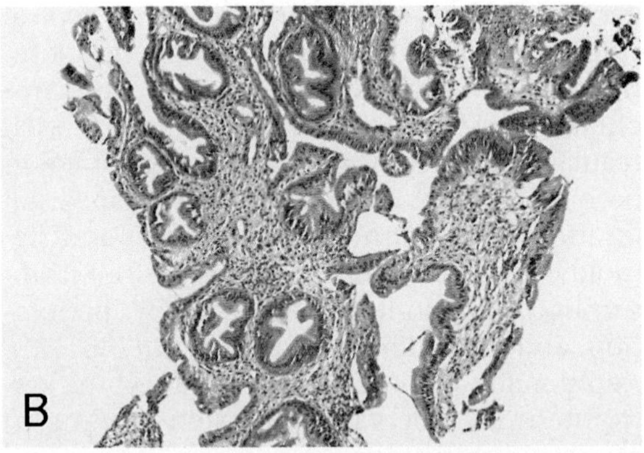

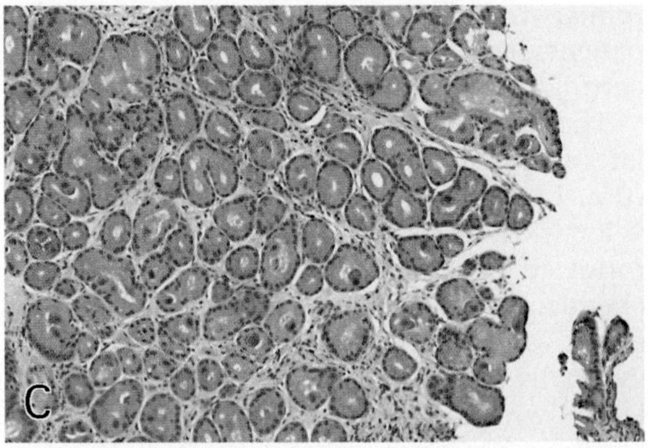

Figure 10-32

CYTOMEGALOVIRUS GASTRITIS

A: Eosinophilic inclusions are within the glandular epithelium. There is a patchy increase in the number of mononuclear cells in the lamina propria.

B: The gastric epithelium appears regenerative and the lamina propria contains viral inclusions.

C: Cytomegalovirus (CMV) infection in another patient with less obvious gastritis but more numerous viral inclusions.

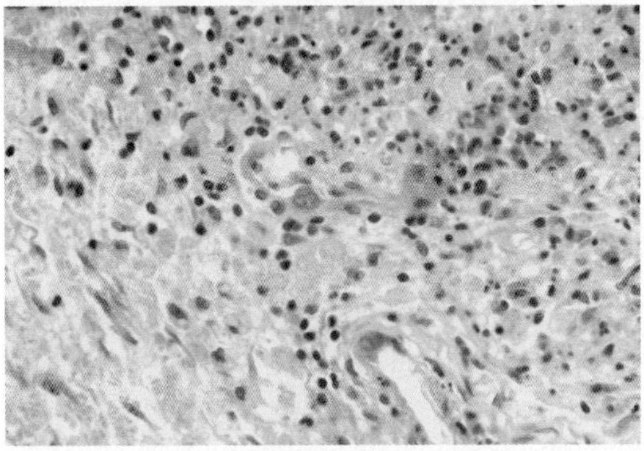

Figure 10-33

CYTOMEGALOVIRUS INFECTION

The endothelial cell is enlarged and contains a large intranuclear CMV inclusion surrounded by a clear halo.

dark violaceous lesions resembling Kaposi's sarcoma. A mildly abnormal intervening mucosa separates discrete ulcers in many patients. In its most severe form, multiple ulcers and perforations occur throughout the gut. The gross appearance may resemble ischemic colitis.

Microscopic Findings. The characteristic cytopathic effects of CMV infection include prominent eosinophilic, intranuclear inclusions; cellular enlargement; and occasional granular basophilic cytoplasmic inclusions. The affected cells differ from those seen in HSV infections in that CMV cytopathic effects typically develop in the glandular epithelium (as opposed to the squamous cells), submucosal endothelial cells, macrophages, and fibroblasts in the granulation tissue of the ulcer bases (fig. 10-32). The cells in the stroma often appear enlarged or cytomegalic, with conspicuous intranuclear inclusions.

CMV is notorious for its ability to invade muscle cells, ganglion cells, and endothelial cells (fig. 10-33). Endothelial infections may lead to the development of venulitis. Additionally, the virus causes endothelial proliferation and secondary vascular occlusion by swollen, plump endothelial cells, particularly small vessels. The vascular damage predisposes the vessels to thrombosis. Other lesions form, including a granulomatous-like lesion characterized by histiocytic collections without giant cells, which surrounds the vascular wall. Viral

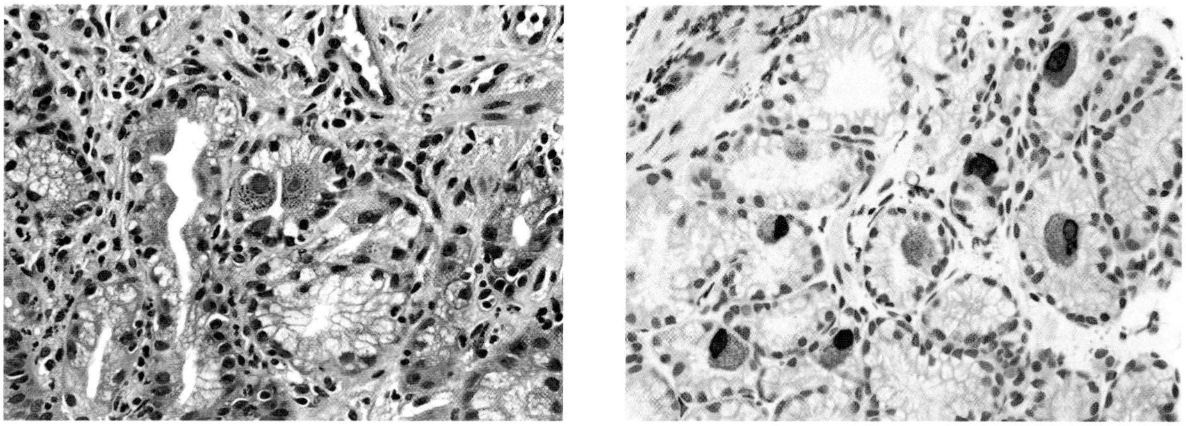

Figure 10-34

CYTOMEGALOVIRUS ESOPHAGITIS

Left: CMV inclusions in esophageal submucosal glands. The nuclei of the affected cells contain eosinophilic, glassy inclusions as well as basophilic cytoplasmic inclusions. (Both figures courtesy of the Division of Gastrointestinal Pathology, Armed Forces Institute of Pathology, Washington, DC.)

Right: The immunohistochemical stain for CMV shows strong nuclear positivity.

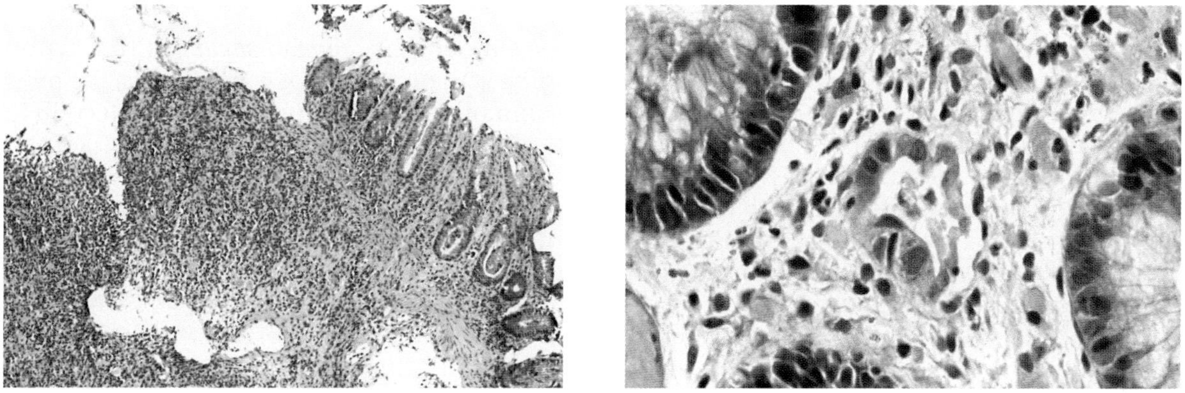

Figure 10-35

CYTOMEGALOVIRUS COLITIS

Left: Colonic mucosa with an area of ulceration (left).

Right: On high power, an enlarged cell with a characteristic nuclear inclusion lies within a vessel in the lamina propria.

inclusions are not always identifiable within the endothelium of the affected vessels, probably due to sampling problems; however, they are present in the nearby vicinity.

Histologically, CMV esophagitis is characterized by large cells in the subepithelial layer and in areas of ulceration. These cells contain amphophilic and intranuclear inclusions and may also have cytoplasmic inclusions (fig. 10-34). The presence of the virus is confirmed by either immunohistochemical staining or in situ hybridization for CMV DNA (fig. 10-34).

In the intestinal tract, CMV is associated with hemorrhage and ulceration. The virus appears to have a special affinity for cells in and around small vessels (fig. 10-35). The infected cells are often significantly enlarged (cytomegalic), with an increase in both nuclear and cytoplasmic volume, although these changes are not always present. Typical nuclear and cytoplasmic inclusions may be seen. CMV infection of the duodenum may cause papillary stenosis and sclerosing cholangitis in AIDS patients (733).

In the colon, the histologic changes range from isolated inclusions with no accompanying tissue reaction to the presence of discrete ulcers to more diffuse inflammatory changes characterized by edema, erythema, mucosal erosions, pseudomembranous colitis, toxic megacolon, and perforation. The diagnosis of a CMV infection in mucosal biopsies is often not difficult. In severely immunosuppressed patients, numerous CMV-infected cells are easily identified by the presence of both nuclear and cytoplasmic inclusions. Inclusion-bearing cells are most numerous in ulcerated areas, especially in the ulcer bases and the endothelium. They also occur in granulation tissue, pseudopolyps, and the intervening mucosa in both stroma and epithelial cells. More subtle infection requires an awareness of, or high suspicion for, the possibility that the infection might exist so that multiple sections can be carefully examined to find the characteristic inclusion-bearing cells.

In severe cases, ischemia causes many of the pathologic features because viral infection of small vessels results in endothelialitis, stimulating the formation of microthrombi and secondary ischemic damage. The nonendothelial cells surrounding the infected vessels are also commonly infected. Occasional CMV infection involves medium-sized arteries, resulting in endothelial inclusions, inflammation, panarteritis, necrosis, and large mucosal ulcerations.

Special Techniques. CMV is detected by direct viral isolation from clinical specimens via growth in conventional tissue culture or rapid viral culture systems. The virus is also detected using serologic methods for CMV-specific IgG antibodies. Direct histologic and immunohistochemical techniques detect viral particles and CMV antigens, respectively, in fixed tissue sections, or in cytologic or cytospin preparations. The virus may also be detected via various DNA detection systems, including in situ hybridization, dot blot hybridization, or PCR.

Differential Diagnosis. The clinical differential diagnosis of CMV infection includes various entities, depending on the organ system. In the esophagus, the differential diagnosis includes herpes esophagitis, *Candida* esophagitis, and gastroesophageal reflux disease. In the intestines and colon, the differential diagnosis includes many forms of infectious enterocolitis. Identification of the characteristic cytomegalic inclusions rules out other entities.

Treatment and Prognosis. Progressive intestinal disease and death are frequent in immunocompromised patients. In one study, however, mortality from CMV infections was significantly greater in normal patients than in transplant, HIV-positive, or other immunosuppressed patients (731). Mortality is also greater in individuals over 65 years of age and when time to institution of therapy is great. The site of infection in the gut has no impact on prognosis (731). Ganciclovir and foscarnet are effective drugs for treating CMV infection.

Prevention. Screening of blood products for CMV antibodies significantly decreases the morbidity and mortality from primary CMV infection among CMV-seronegative organ transplant recipients. Ganciclovir can also be used as prophylactic treatment.

Human Papilloma Virus Infections

Demography. *Human papilloma virus* (HPV) is the causative agent of genital warts, the most common sexually transmitted viral infection in the United States (745). Anorectal and perianal condylomata frequently develop in individuals who have engaged in anal intercourse, and their incidence has increased by about 50 percent in the past several decades (737,740). Most affected patients are male, many of whom admit to homosexual lifestyles. Men with advanced HIV disease have a high prevalence of anal HPV infections and potentially precancerous anal disease. An increased incidence of anal and perianal condylomata also exists in women with cervical and/or vulvar warts.

Etiology. *Condyloma acuminatum* results from infection by double-stranded DNA-containing HPV. HPV 6 and 11 are the usual HPV types found in genital warts (738,741,748,749). HPV infects the basal cells of the squamous epithelium, although it can infect transitional and cuboidal epithelia as well. The infection is thought to occur after trauma to the epithelium and it results in cellular hyperplasia of the basal cells (747). Infectious viral particles are produced only by completely differentiated cells of the upper epithelium, because cellular differentiation is required for the HPV growth cycle (736). Infection with HPV can lead to clinical, subclinical, or latent infection, as well as the development of dysplasia and cancer. Subclinical or latent HPV infections are common and may persist for long periods of time (746). Squamous cell carcinomas of the anus are strongly associated with genital or anal warts; HPV types 16, 18, and 31 are found in these lesions (739,742).

Clinical Features. HPV infections may or may not result in clinically apparent lesions. Perianal condylomas are the most common visible manifestation of anal HPV infection (743). These lesions are raised and often papillary, and are seen on physical examination in the perianal region. They are often multifocal and may grow to a large size. Subclinical lesions often occur within the internal anal canal or rectal mucosa.

Gross Findings. The gross features of condylomata vary widely, with the spectrum of lesions ranging from single to multiple growths and from small benign tumors to extensive superficial lesions covering large mucosal areas. Patients with anal condylomas frequently have lesions on the penile mucosa, perineum, perianal area, anorectal junction, cervix, or vulva. Condylomas assume a characteristic soft, grayish pink to purple, papillary, warty, cauliflower-like appearance. Occasional lesions are pigmented. Areas of erosion may be present and may distort these features.

Microscopic Findings. Histologically, condylomata are acanthotic, papillomatous squamous growths showing variable thickening of the stratum corneum, superficial parakeratosis, and dyskeratosis. The superficial cells appear large and contain clear cytoplasm with a central hyperchromatic nucleus and perinuclear halo, features known as koilocytosis. These koilocytotic features are the histologic hallmark of HPV infection. Anisokaryosis, nuclear hyperchromasia, and the presence of binucleate cells correlate with the presence of HPV, as detected by in situ hybridization (fig. 10-36) (744). Scattered mitotic figures, some of which may appear bizarre, may be present in the acanthotic epithelium. The stroma contains a chronic inflammatory cell infiltrate, and the tissue may appear edematous and show vascular dilatation.

Some condylomas grow in a flat pattern similar to that seen in the cervix. Such lesions, sometimes referred to as *condyloma planum*, show koilocytosis and other cytologic features of condylomas but lack the prominent acanthotic growth pattern typical of the more common condyloma acuminatum. Venereal warts treated with podophyllin may appear histologically alarming and mimic dysplasia.

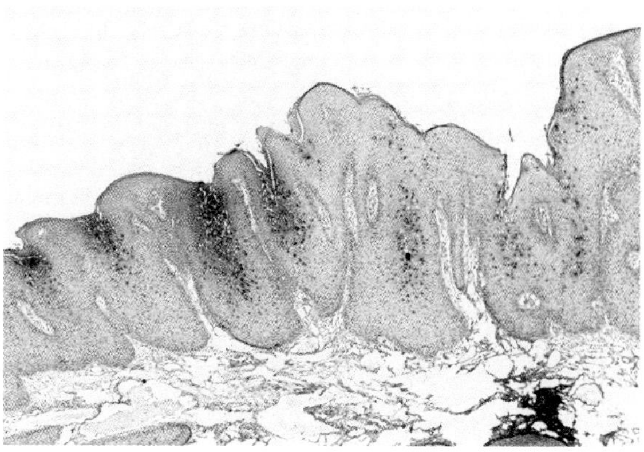

Figure 10-36

HUMAN PAPILLOMA VIRUS

In situ hybridization for human papilloma virus (HPV) types 6 and 11 in an anal condyloma. The viral DNA is stained blue, and can be seen within nuclei of squamous cells in the upper half of the epithelium.

Molluscum Contagiosum

Molluscum contagiosum, a contagious disease resulting from a viral infection, is characterized by the appearance of multiple, small, waxy papules that have characteristic umbilicated centers. The most common sites of involvement are the abdominal skin and the skin of the perineum thigh, penis, scrotum, and vulva; the buttock and perianal regions are sometimes affected. Histologically, the lesions consist of a lobular epidermal proliferation that extends into the dermis. Prominent inclusion bodies are characteristic of the lesion (fig. 10-37).

PARASITIC INFECTIONS

Giardia Infections

Demography. *Giardia* is found worldwide and infects domestic as well as wild animals (776,786). *Giardiasis* is the most commonly diagnosed intestinal parasitic infection in public health laboratories in the United States and around the world. Worldwide, it is estimated that 1.5 to 20.0 percent of humans are infected with *Giardia* (764,772). There is an approximately

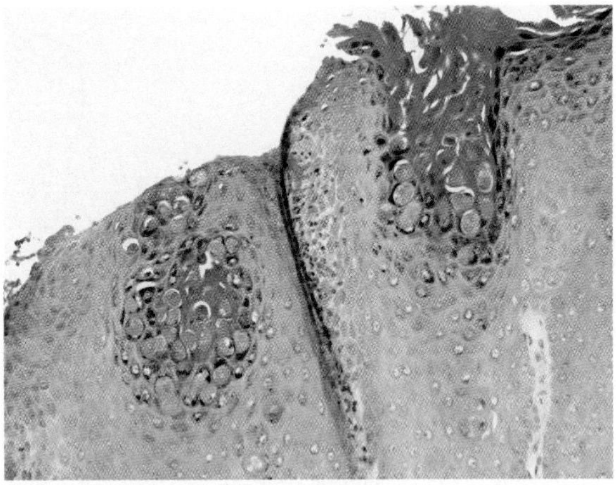

Figure 10-37

MOLLUSCUM CONTAGIOSUM

Characteristic eosinophilic molluscum bodies are present in the superficial squamous epithelium.

equal sex distribution. Rates of infection are the highest among children under 5 years of age, followed closely by persons aged 31 to 40 years. Most cases are reported during late summer and early fall.

Giardiasis occurs sporadically, although outbreaks also occur. *Giardia* infection is most commonly spread through contact with contaminated water. This may occur as a result of drinking contaminated tap water or through recreational exposure in lakes, rivers, and swimming pools (768,771,774,781). Person-to-person spread also occurs, and has been documented in daycare centers (780) and among male homosexuals (758,773,782). The organism may additionally be transmitted through contaminated food (777,779).

Etiology. *Giardia* exists in two morphologic forms: the motile trophozoite and the infective cyst. The pear-shaped trophozoite measures 12 to 15 µm in length and 5 to 9 µm in width. A pair of nuclei is located in the anterior half of the organism, with basal bodies lying between the anterior poles of the nuclei. Four pairs of flagella originate from the basal bodies: one pair on the ventral surface and three pairs on the periphery. The elliptical cyst measures 6 to 12 x 6 to 10 µm. It contains two to four nuclei and the flagellae are retracted into axonemes. A median body and curved fibrils may also be present. Cysts remain viable in cold or tepid water for several months and can survive the chlorine concentrations usually present in municipal water systems (769).

Pathophysiology. Cysts are ingested and excystation begins in the stomach. Trophozoites emerge in the duodenum and upper jejunum where they colonize the intestines. Bile salts stimulate their excystation, growth, and replication, perhaps accounting for the fact that the duodenum and proximal jejunum represent their favorite habitat (760). They lie in the intestinal fluid phase, attach to mucus strands in the lumen, or penetrate the mucus gel layer and attach to the epithelial microvilli via their ventral suction disc. Attachment of the microorganism to the epithelial cells leads to alterations in brush border enzyme activity, with resultant malabsorption (752,759,785). In addition, the organism may cause rearrangements in F-actin and alpha-actinin in cells in the duodenum, resulting in abnormalities in electrical resistance across the cell membrane (787). Villous blunting and shortening may occur (775). Epithelial damage may develop as a result of toxin production by the organisms (766). Other factors that may play a role in the pathogenesis of the diarrhea induced by *Giardia* include bacterial overgrowth, bile salt deconjugation, and bile salt uptake by the organism.

Variations in the clinical manifestations of *Giardia* infection result from differences in virulence among organisms or from immune or nonimmune host factors in the intestinal microenvironment. An intact immune system plays an important role in eradicating the infection and in the development of protective immunity. Immunosuppression increases infection severity (775). IgA-deficient individuals develop persistent infections (753). There may also be a genetic predisposition to infection (783).

Clinical Features. *Giardia* infections may remain self-limited and asymptomatic or they may persist for years, causing diarrhea, malabsorption, weight loss, and failure to thrive in children (750,784). The most common presentation is the acute onset of diarrhea lasting 5 to 7 days following an incubation period of 1 to 3 weeks. The acute illness varies in severity. Some patients experience an abrupt, explosive onset of frequent, watery, foul-smelling stools while others have only a few loose bowel movements.

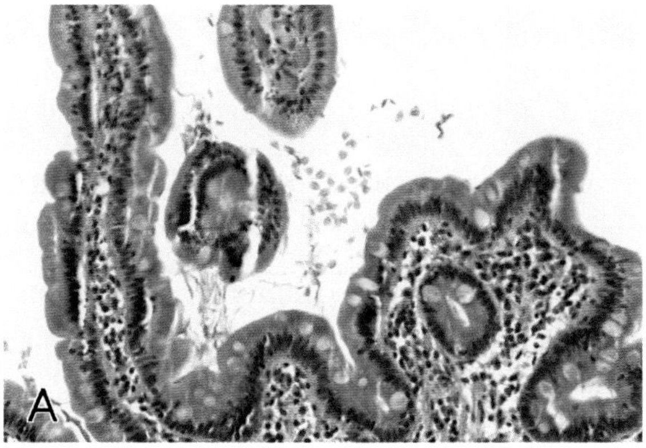

Figure 10-38

GIARDIA

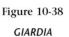

A: At low power, the villous architecture of the small intestinal mucosa is preserved and there is no increase in inflammatory cells in the lamina propria. Clusters of pale pink *Giardia* organisms can be seen within the lumen.

B: Higher-power view shows grayish pink, pear-shaped *Giardia* within the small intestinal lumen. The organisms are approximately the size of an epithelial cell nucleus.

C: Occasional organisms adhere to the small intestinal epithelium. No significant inflammatory reaction can be appreciated in this case, as is typical of *Giardia* infestations.

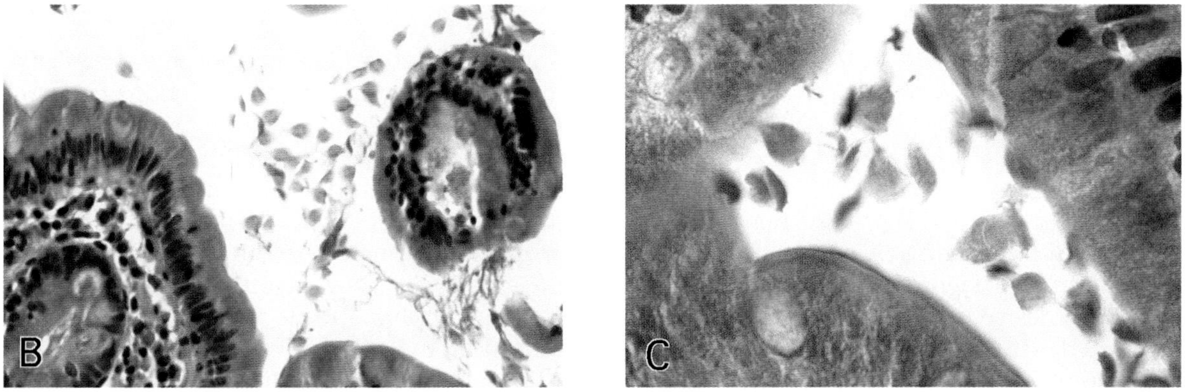

Some patients present with abdominal cramps, abdominal pain, flatus, lassitude, malabsorption, and progressive weight loss. Less often, fever and vomiting occur.

Patients with chronic giardiasis develop intermittent diarrhea that is less severe than that seen in the acute illness. Occasionally, allergic and other inflammatory phenomena develop (756). Chronic diarrhea may lead to rectal prolapse. *Giardia* cysts can be excreted in the stool intermittently for weeks or months, resulting in a protracted period of communicability (780). One possible sequela of *Giardia* infection is reactive arthritis or synovitis (770).

Microscopic Findings. In H&E-stained biopsy material, *Giardia* organisms appear pear-shaped, about the size of an epithelial cell nucleus, with two nuclei (fig. 10-38). The organisms are gray or faintly basophilic. They have an elliptical shape, with one nucleus visible when seen in profile. When present, they are often numerous. *Giardia* organisms, however, often have a patchy distribution, and are therefore not always seen on biopsy material, even in symptomatic patients.

One of three mucosal patterns is seen histologically in association with *Giardia* infection. In some patients there are no alterations present. In others, the villous architecture is normal, but increased numbers of intraepithelial lymphocytes and immunoglobulin-containing cells are in the lamina propria, with a relative increase in the number of IgA- and IgG-containing cells. Still others show partial or complete villous atrophy and crypt hyperplasia associated with variable degrees of inflammation, large numbers of intraepithelial lymphocytes, and IgA- and IgM-containing cells in the lamina propria. Villous height tends to be low in patients with large numbers of trophozoites. Focally, neutrophils may infiltrate the mucosa.

Special Techniques. Traditionally, the diagnosis of *Giardia* infection is made by the direct detection of characteristic cysts in the stool (fig. 10-39). However, stool examinations are only diagnostic in a portion of patients with known infection. In recent years, numerous rapid immunologic detection assays have been developed for the detection of *Giardia* antigens in stool. These tests are highly sensitive and specific for

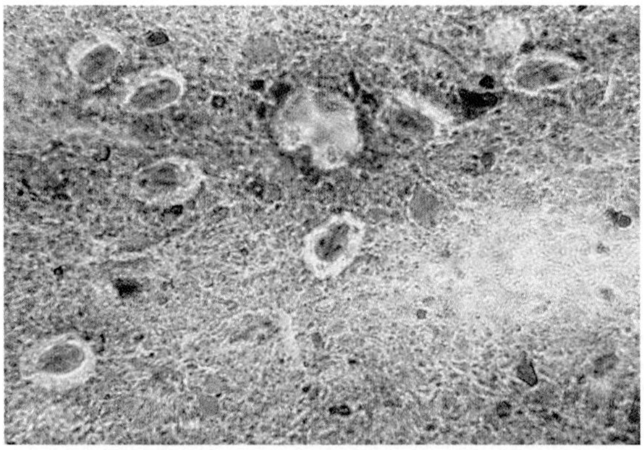

Figure 10-39

GIARDIA TROPHOZOITES IN A FECAL SMEAR

The organisms are pear shaped, and have a central axostyle straddled by two nuclei, which give the organisms an "owl's eye" appearance.

the organisms (761,762,767,788). There is also a PCR assay for detecting *Giardia* in stool (765).

Differential Diagnosis. The differential diagnosis includes celiac disease or other disorders associated with intraepithelial lymphocytosis. Immunohistochemical findings help distinguish giardiasis from celiac disease, since a relatively high number of IgG- and IgA-containing cells are present in giardiasis as compared with the large number of IgM-containing cells in celiac disease.

Treatment and Prognosis. Many effective treatment alternatives are available for symptomatic patients. Metronidazole is the treatment of choice in the United States. Other effective agents include tinidazole (750) and ornidazole (778), neither of which is available in the United States. Albendazole has been reported to be as effective as metronidazole with fewer side effects in children (754,757,763). Nitazoxanide has recently been approved in the United States for the treatment of the diarrhea caused by *Giardia* in patients 1 to 11 years of age (751). A recent study suggests that in some patients *Giardia* infection may trigger functional irritable bowel disease, leading to prolonged symptoms not amenable to anti-*Giardia* therapy (755).

Amoeba Infections

Demography. *Amebiasis* has a worldwide distribution. It is more prevalent in the tropics than in temperate climates, in areas with primitive or nonexistent sanitation, or where human feces are used as fertilizer. In these areas, patients most commonly acquire the organism by ingestion of infected water, although contaminated food is also a source. Spread within households is common as a result of direct fecal-oral contact. Individuals at the highest risk for infection are travelers to endemic regions, immigrants or migrant workers, immunocompromised persons, and institutionalized patients (798).

Etiology. Amebiasis results from infection with *Entamoeba histolytica.* A recently recognized species of *Entamoeba, E. dispar,* is morphologically similar to *E. histolytica,* but does not produce invasive disease (789,791,796). It is now thought that this species is responsible for most of the asymptomatic infections formerly attributed to *E. histolytica* (792).

E. histolytica has two life forms: the invasive motile trophozoite, which measures 12 to 60 µm in size, and the 10- to 20-µm cyst. Amoebae propagate through cysts, the resistant form in their life cycle. They are immediately infectious and can survive outside the host for weeks to months in moist environments. Cysts resist the chlorine concentrations used in sewage systems.

Pathophysiology. Ingested *E. histolytica* cysts resist gastric digestion and pass to the ileocecal region where they excyst and divide, giving rise to trophozoites that then colonize the colon. The organisms are able to degrade the mucus barrier overlying the colonic mucosa through secretion of a number of enzymes, including glycosidase, galactosidase, mannosidase, fucosidases, xylosidase, glucosidase, amylase, and hyaluronidase (797,807,809). The organisms then attach to the epithelial cells by means of a multifunctional adherence lectin that is also involved in signaling cell lysis, and that also protects the organism from the attack complex of complement (792, 802,804). Proteases secreted by the organism degrade the extracellular matrix and aid in lysis of target epithelial cells (790,799, 801). The result is an erosion of the mucosal surface into which the organisms invade. Once within the ulcerated tissue, the organisms appear to modulate the host immune response, predominantly through interaction with neutrophils and macrophages. Macrophage migration to areas of infection may be inhibited by elaboration of a macrophage locomotion-inhibitory factor produced by the organism (794).

It is not known why some infected patients are predisposed to develop severe amebiasis whereas others are not. Both host and parasite factors probably play a role in determining the ultimate outcome of exposure to the organism. Factors that may be essential for initiating the infection and promoting severe disease include poor nutrition, a tropical climate, decreased host immunocompetence, the integrity of the mucosal barrier, altered colonic bacterial flora, trauma, and other host immune or genetic factors. Different zymodemes (enzyme populations or patterns) characterize different populations of *E. histolytica* and they may be markers of pathogenicity (795,806). Additionally, there may be genetic differences in a cysteine protease that also serves as a virulence factor (808).

Clinical Features. Amebiasis affects individuals of all ages, including infants. Many individuals remain asymptomatic but fulminant amebic colitis and even death may occur. The infection may remain limited to the gastrointestinal tract or it may extend to the liver and other organs. Intestinal amebiasis presents in four clinically recognized forms: 1) as a typical dysenteric infection with intermittent bloody diarrhea and lower abdominal cramps; 2) as fulminant amebic colitis; 3) as amebic appendicitis; and 4) as a localized mass lesion in the colon, the *ameboma* (792). Extraintestinal lesions may also occur, most commonly in the liver as abscesses.

Mild cases of amebiasis are characterized by mild diarrhea, cramps, or abdominal discomfort, often with mucus in the stool and perhaps some blood. Malaise and anorexia may be present. Low-grade fever is uncommon.

Patients with the dysenteric form of the disease experience gradually increasing lower abdominal discomfort, loose stools, malodorous flatus, and recurrent bouts of diarrhea. Intermittent constipation also occurs. Within a period of 3 to 4 days, the number of stools may increase to 25 per day, causing weakness and prostration. Nausea, vomiting, and right-sided cramps are usual. Amebic colitis often persists for weeks, months, or years. Patients with chronic diarrhea may develop rectal prolapse. Patients may have mild anemia or a mildly elevated white blood cell count. The dysenteric form affects less than 10 percent of patients in temperate zones.

Patients with fulminant disease develop dehydration, severe abdominal pain, and hypotension. Localized or generalized peritonitis and toxic megacolon are sometimes seen. Amebomas cause numerous symptoms, including alternating diarrhea and constipation, weight loss, and low-grade fever. In endemic areas, cramping, lower abdominal pain, and a palpable mass suggest the diagnosis.

Laboratory findings are nonspecific. There may be a mild elevation of the white count in patients with severe disease. Eosinophilia is usually absent.

Gross Findings. Asymptomatic or mildly symptomatic patients seldom show any specific endoscopic findings. Colonoscopy allows assessment of the entire colon for the presence of ulcerating disease or amebomas. Ulcerating changes are most often seen in the cecum followed by the sigmoid and descending colon and rectum. The appendix may also be affected, but it is rare for the terminal ileum to become involved. The transverse colon is commonly spared.

Developing ulcers have irregular, hyperemic mucosal outlines with markedly undermined, overhanging edges, producing a characteristic flask-like shape. The ulcers generally are discrete, smooth, and round, with only a slight elevation of the borders. The intervening mucosa appears relatively normal. Ulcers vary in size from a couple of millimeters to several centimeters in diameter. They may be few in number or so prevalent as to be confluent. In the most severe circumstances, the ulcers extend through the entire colonic wall to the serosa.

Amebomas present as localized, often circumferential areas of bowel wall thickening, strictures, mucosal excrescences, or large tumor-like masses. They result from persistent ulceration and granulation tissue formation, with fibroblastic proliferation and inflammation, and may be up to 15 cm in diameter.

Microscopic Findings. The only specific diagnostic finding is the identification of the organism in either the trophozoite or cyst form (fig. 10-40). Typical trophozoites are large, round to ovoid structures, varying from 6 to 40 µm in diameter. They contain voluminous pinkish purple cytoplasm with a distinctive foamy, vacuolated, or granular appearance. The cytoplasm is PAS positive and, unlike nonpathogenic amoebae,

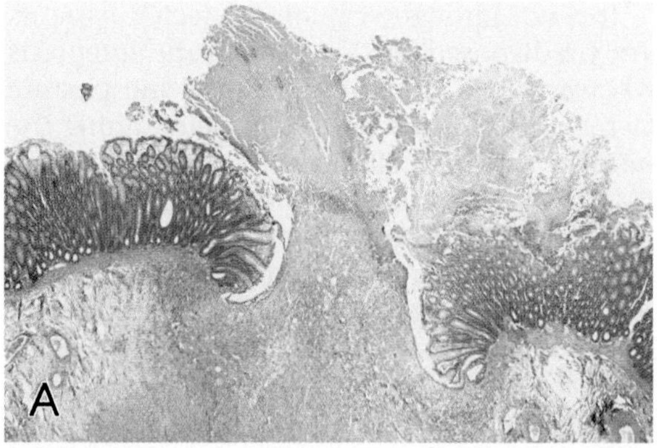

Figure 10-40

AMEBIC COLITIS

A: Low-power view of a large ulcer with slightly undermined edges. Necrotic debris exudes from the ulcer surface.

B: On higher power, numerous large, round organisms are seen within the necrotic debris.

C: The amoeba trophozoites have abundant eosinophilic cytoplasm and a single nucleus. Some organisms are surrounded by a clear halo, a fixation artifact that is commonly seen.

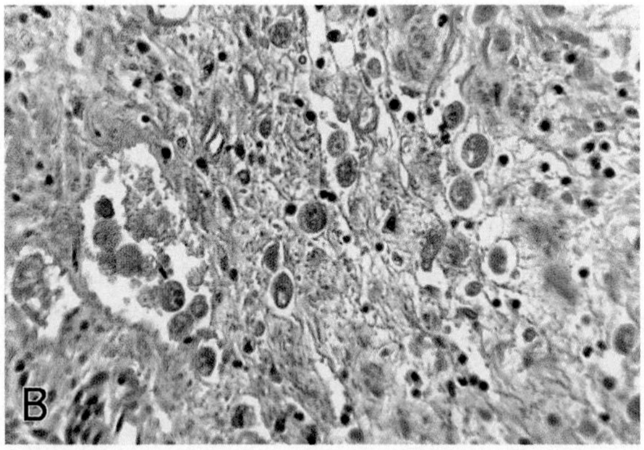

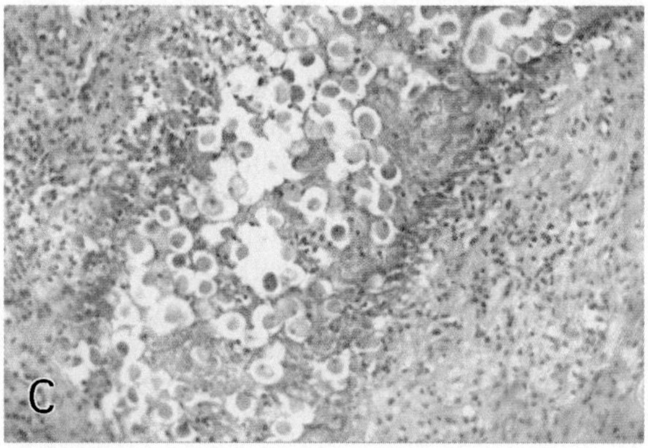

contains ingested red blood cells. Erythrophagocytosis is easily demonstrated with the Heidenhain iron hematoxylin stain. In tissue sections, the amoeba may be surrounded by a clear space, a fixation-induced shrinkage artifact.

Amebic colitis is an ulcerating disease that begins with small areas of necrosis in the colonic mucosa, presumably due to the enzymatic activity of the trophozoites (fig. 10-40). A few amoebae may lie in the lamina propria, surrounded by a mild inflammatory response (803). Early amebic lesions appear as small, yellow mucoid elevations containing necrotic material and the parasite. The lesions rupture, undermining the adjacent intact mucosa and creating discrete, oval-shaped ulcers with overhanging edges. As the ulcers enlarge, they produce the characteristic flask shape that extends into the underlying submucosa. Necrotic cellular debris and fibrin cover the base of the ulcer. The mucosa between ulcers appears normal, although some areas may appear polypoid due to the presence of hyperemia and edema adjacent to areas of ulceration.

Minimal inflammation surrounds superficial mucosal ulcers, whereas a dense fibrotic inflammatory response often accompanies submucosal penetration into the circular or longitudinal muscles. Prolonged inflammation leads to the production of inflammatory pseudopolyps and strictures. Extensive undermining leads to widespread ulceration and perforation. As the ulcers extend, the organisms are found in tissue spaces and small vessels, usually in groups in areas of necrosis and tissue disruption. In patients with severe disease, trophozoites may extend through the bowel wall to lie free in the abdominal cavity or serosal fat.

Because amebic ulcers develop slowly, fibrosis occurs, often protecting against perforation. Some lesions eventually heal without significant scarring, but others progress to chronic fibrosis with persistent or recurrent focal ulceration.

Patients with long-standing infections and exuberant tissue reactions develop tumorous, exophytic, cicatricial, inflammatory masses known as amebomas. These can develop anywhere in the colon, and usually occur in untreated or inadequately treated patients years after the last recognized dysenteric attack. Histologically, amebomas consist of granulation tissue with round cell infiltration and giant cells. Fibrous tissue is absent or uncommon.

Special Techniques. Stool examination is the usual way of demonstrating *E. histolytica*. Cysts, trophozoites, and Charcot-Leyden crystals are seen. Three stools are collected over a several-day period, since amebic cysts are shed intermittently. Since the trophozoites only survive a short time outside the intestines, the specimen should be examined within 30 minutes or a preservative should be added to it. The use of supravital stains, such as buffered methylene blue, facilitates recognition of trophozoite nuclear detail. In fixed stool specimens, the trichrome or iron hematoxylin stain identifies the trophozoites. Repeatedly negative stool examinations do not rule out the disease.

PAS stains and the use of direct fluorescent antibodies on ethanol-fixed material are more sensitive for recognizing amoebae in biopsies than the three conventional detection methods (H&E, trichrome, and phosphotungstic acid hematoxylin [PTAH]) (793).

Serologic tests have superior sensitivity and predictive value in recognizing invasive disease than do biopsies (800). They also are unaffected by substances that may have been used to treat the symptoms, such as antibiotics, antacids, or enema products, which may decrease the viability of the trophozoites. A DNA hybridization probe recently has been developed (805) but it has not been used extensively.

Differential Diagnosis. In severe cases, the symptoms of patients with amebiasis mimic those of ulcerative colitis and toxic megacolon, especially in geographic areas where amoebiasis is not endemic. Like IBD, chronic amebic colitis may begin insidiously and exhibit cyclic remissions. In the United States, the symptoms in younger individuals suggest Crohn's disease or appendiceal abscess; in older individuals, colonic cancer or diverticulitis are suggested. If pseudomembranes are present, the differential diagnosis includes antibiotic-associated colitis due to *C. difficile* ischemia and shigellosis, among others.

Histologically, amoebae can easily be mistaken for white blood cells or other protozoa. *Balantidium coli* infections produce similar histologic changes. *Balantidium coli,* however, is a larger organism, measuring 30 x 150 x 40 µm in contrast to *Entamoeba* which measures 30 to 40 µm in largest diameter. The trophozoites must also be distinguished from histiocytes. Histiocytes tend to be smaller, less intensely PAS positive, and contain a clearly identified nucleus.

Treatment and Prognosis. Complications of amebiasis often occur as a result of the hematogenous dissemination of organisms to distant sites. Trophozoites may migrate to the liver to form an amebic abscess. They may also invade adjacent structures including the pulmonary parenchyma, peritoneum, and pericardium. Amoebae also disseminate to the brain (798).

A number of drugs are available for treating amebiasis and the treatment regimen depends on the clinical state of the patient, the availability of drugs, and physician experience. The Infectious Disease Society of America's recommended treatment guidelines for amebiasis include metronidazole plus either diiodohydroxyquin or paromomycin (793a).

Balantidium Infections

Demography. *Balantidiasis* has a cosmopolitan distribution, but most infections occur in tropical and subtropical regions. The infection is uncommon, accounting for less than 5 percent of cases of acute diarrhea in countries where the organism is endemic (811,814,816). Balantidiasis is usually contracted through ingestion of contaminated water, but the disorder may also be transmitted from person to person. Since pigs serve as reservoirs for the infection (811–813), the infection is most often seen where pigs and humans are in close contact.

Etiology. *Balantidium coli,* the largest protozoan to infect man, has both a cyst and trophozoite form. It is the only ciliated protozoan known to infect humans. The oval to spherical, refractile cysts represent the infectious form of the organism, and measure 40 to 65 µm in diameter. Young cysts are covered by cilia that disappear as they age. Trophozoites are liberated from the cysts in the small intestine and invade the large intestine. They continue to excyst as they descend through the large intestine. The oval trophozoites contain a characteristic large

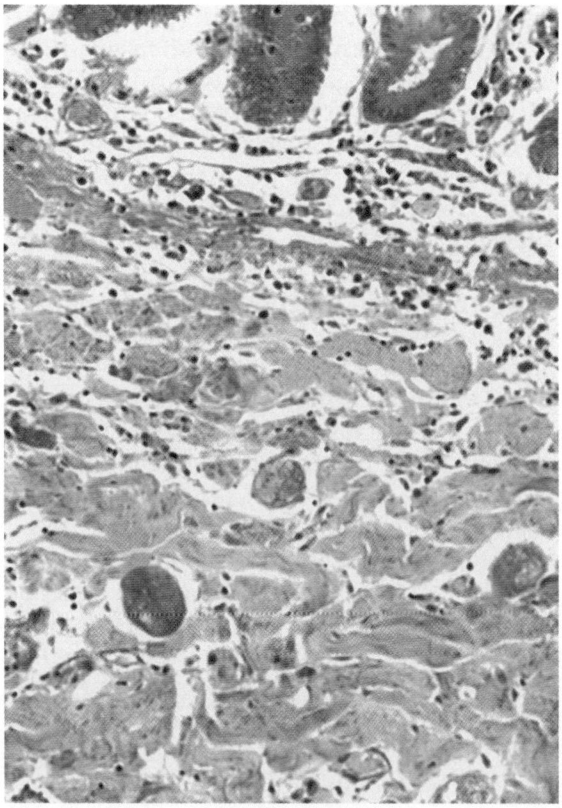

Figure 10-41

BALANTIDIUM COLI

Scattered large trophozoites are in the submucosa of the colon. The organisms contain a characteristic kidney-shaped macronucleus.

kidney-shaped macronucleus with a small or round micronucleus. The cytoplasm contains two contractile vacuoles and numerous food vacuoles. The pointed anterior end contains a funnel-shaped cytosome.

Clinical Features. *B. coli* infections are associated with a range of presentations from asymptomatic cyst passage to chronic diarrhea and fulminant colitis. When patients are symptomatic, the most common clinical pattern is chronic disease, characterized by alternating diarrhea and constipation. The symptoms can last from days to months; patients have up to 15 bowel movements per day. In contrast, patients with severe acute disease exhibit nausea, vomiting, anorexia, abdominal pain, and up to 30 bloody, mucus-filled bowel movements per day. Perforation and hemorrhage are rare complications. Symptoms may persist for years (815,817).

Gross Findings. The right half of the colon and cecum are most commonly involved, but the rectum, sigmoid, and appendix can also become infected. Endoscopically, shallow ulcers and pseudomembranes are present (810). Most ulcers are superficial and multiple, but when deep ulcers develop, they may perforate, particularly in fulminant disease.

Microscopic Findings. Invasion of the colon by *B. coli* produces mucosal ulcers containing numerous trophozoites and demonstrating prominent submucosal inflammation (fig. 10-41). The histologic features mimic those of amebiasis, including the presence of flask-shaped ulcers containing trophozoites separated by intervening normal mucosa. The intervening mucosa may also appear edematous or hemorrhagic. Pseudomembranes containing neutrophils and fibrin cover the ulcers. The diagnosis rests on identifying the parasite.

Special Techniques. The diagnosis of balantidiasis is made by finding the parasite in the stool. It is almost always present in the trophozoite form.

Differential Diagnosis. The disease mimics amebiasis but the two diseases are distinguished by finding the large ciliated protozoan.

Treatment and Prognosis. *Balantidium coli* is sensitive to tetracycline and iodoquinol. Metronidazole is also effective (813).

Cryptosporidium Infections

Demography. Since the first reported case of human *cryptosporidiosis* in 1976, *Cryptosporidium* has become one of the most common enteric pathogens in both immunocompetent and immunocompromised patients worldwide (845). In developed countries, cryptosporidial infection accounts for 2.2 percent of cases of diarrhea in immunocompetent adults and 7 percent of cases in children (832). The rate of infection is higher in developing countries where cryptosporidiosis occurs in 6.1 percent of adults and 12.0 percent of children with diarrhea. The rates in all geographic regions are higher for immunocompromised patients, especially those with AIDS (832).

Cryptosporidial infections are frequently acquired through the ingestion of contaminated water including untreated surface water, filtered swimming pool water, and even chlorinated or filtered drinking water (845). In 1993, an outbreak of cryptosporidiosis occurred in Milwaukee, Wisconsin as a result of contamination of the municipal water supply. As many as 403,000 people were infected, representing 52 percent of those individuals served by the contaminated water supply (840). *Cryptosporidium* may also be spread through contaminated foods (845). Human-to-human transmission also occurs by means of either a direct fecal-oral route, or indirectly through fomites (820). Zoonotic transmission from infected animals (cattle and sheep) has also been documented (842,844).

Etiology. Cryptosporidia are intracellular protozoal parasites. Most cases of human cryptosporidiosis are attributable to infection with *Cryptosporidium parvum,* although *C. meleagridis, C. felis,* and a dog genotype of *C. parvum* have also been identified in stools of infected HIV-positive patients, as well as in apparently immunocompetent children in Peru (846,848,857).

Pathophysiology. Infection in humans occurs following ingestion or inhalation of cryptosporidial oocysts. The life cycle of the organism is depicted in figure 10-42. Once inside the host, each oocyst excysts in the gastrointestinal tract, releasing four infective sporozoites. Excystation is thought to be facilitated through contact with bile salts, and possibly small bowel enzymes (837). Sporozoites attach to intestinal epithelial cells via Gal/GalNAC-specific lectins (821), disrupting the microvilli on the host cell surface. Attachment of the organism to the enterocyte induces reorganization of the host cell cytoskeleton, and protrusion of the host cell cytoplasmic membrane around the sporozoite to form a vacuole around the organism (821,823,855). The internalized organism undergoes asexual reproduction to produce merozoites. The merozoites are then released into the intestinal lumen. Merozoites may infect other intestinal epithelial cells, or they may mature into gametocytes, the sexual form of the parasite. Fertilization of gametocytes results in oocyst formation. Oocysts are then passed into the environment in the feces. Oocysts may also sporulate, releasing more sporozoites and producing cycles of autoinfection, leading to persistent infection with a heavy parasite burden (845,847).

The mechanisms by which cryptosporidia produce diarrheal illness are not fully understood.

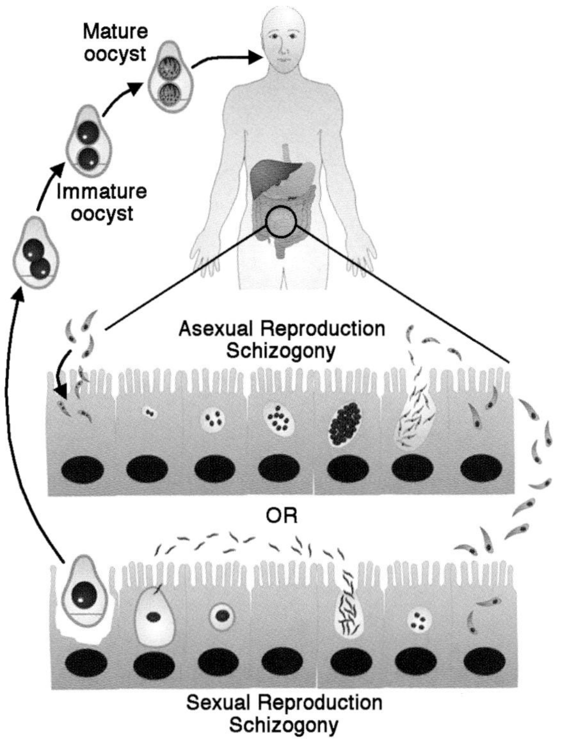

Figure 10-42

DIAGRAM OF THE LIFE CYCLE OF *CRYPTOSPORIDIUM*

An enterotoxin-like activity has been detected in stool extracts, but no actual enterotoxin has been identified. Attachment of the parasite to intestinal epithelial cells does result in some alterations in cell function (828). In in-vitro cultures, the initial encounter of the organism with a host intestinal epithelial cell results in expression of neutrophil- and lymphocyte-targeted chemokines (838,841). In addition, infection with *Cryptosporidium* triggers the apoptotic machinery of the host cell; however, parasite-mediated activation of the nuclear factor-kappa B (NF-kappa B) system has been demonstrated in infected biliary epithelial cells, a function that may circumvent the apoptotic signal within the host cell (822). The organism does appear to induce apoptosis in neighboring uninfected cells through activation of the Fas receptor-Fas ligand death pathway (819).

Clinical Features. Diarrhea is the key clinical feature of cryptosporidiosis. In immunocompetent individuals, the disease usually

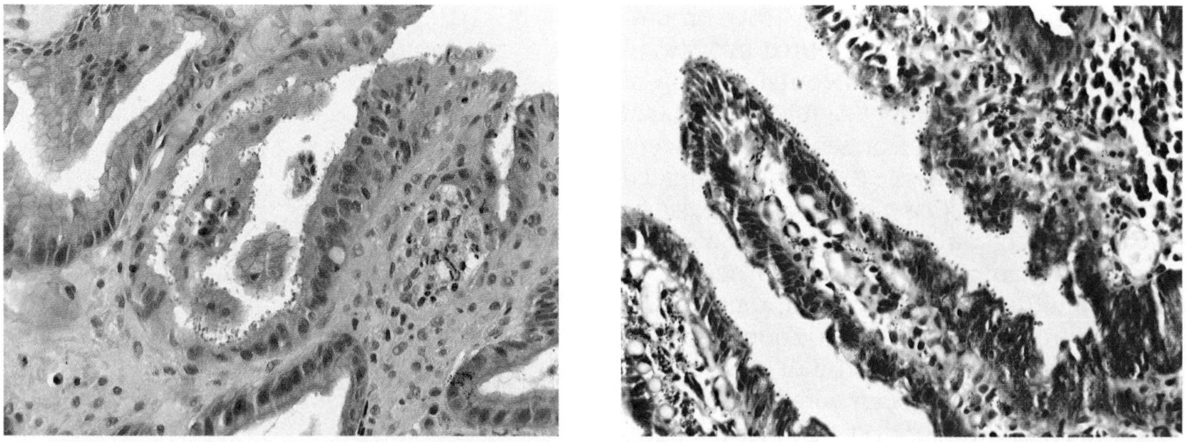

Figure 10-43

CRYPTOSPORIDIUM

Left: H&E stain demonstrates numerous round blue organisms that appear attached to the surface epithelium. Right: Giemsa-stained section shows numerous blue-stained organisms on the surfaces of the villi.

presents as an acute, mild to moderate, self-limited illness usually lasting 3 to 4 days (825), although it may persist for longer periods. Patients experience nonspecific clinical manifestations including passage of watery, nonbloody stools, vomiting, anorexia, abdominal cramps and pain, and possibly malabsorption. Most patients with a fully functional immune system are free of symptoms within a few weeks and of parasites in a few months (835,852). Immunocompetent patients who acquire symptomatic cryptosporidiosis may secrete oocytes for 8 to more than 50 days, with a mean duration of 16.5 days (852, 853). Oocyst secretion may persist despite resolution of the patient's symptoms.

Symptoms of cryptosporidiosis in immunocompromised patients depend in part on the degree of immunocompromise present. Four clinical syndromes have been described in AIDS patients with *Cryptosporidium* infection: 1) chronic diarrhea (36 percent of patients), often with severe weight loss; 2) cholera-like disease (33 percent of patients); 3) transient diarrhea (15 percent of patients); and 4) relapsing illness (15 percent of patients) (843). AIDS patients with CD4 counts of less than 50/mm^3 may develop a fulminant diarrheal illness with passage of more than 2 L of stool per day (818). In addition, immunocompromised patients may show atypical disease presentations with involvement of unusual anatomic sites including the stomach, esophagus, pancreas, and respiratory tract (824,829,836,839,849,856).

Pathologic Findings. The diagnosis of cryptosporidial infection requires close scrutiny of all epithelial surfaces, including those in the lumens of intestinal or gastric glands, for the presence of the characteristic organisms. The organisms appear as spherical or ovoid basophilic or golden brown bodies attached to the luminal surface of the epithelium (fig. 10-43). The organisms measure 2 to 4 µm in diameter, and can easily be overlooked or mistaken for mucus droplets. Conversely, cellular debris and mucus clinging to the epithelium can be mistaken for cryptosporidia. Unlike the apical mucin droplets that they resemble, however, cryptosporidia are mucicarmine negative. Instead, the organisms stain deep blue with Giemsa and Gram stains, are positive with PAS stains, and are negative with the Grocott methenamine silver (GMS) stain (fig. 10-43). In esophageal cryptosporidiosis, organisms attach to the superficial squamous mucosa and the luminal borders of the submucosal glands and ducts.

A spectrum of intensity of infection exists. Low-intensity infections are usually associated with normal intestinal or colonic histology, whereas severe inflammation and villous atrophy complicate high-density infections (830, 831). The mucosa may show an acute inflammatory reaction and an apparent increase in intraepithelial lymphocytes. The infected cells show a range of changes, from only minimal injury and fragments of organisms in the cells to focal necrosis. A variable degree of villous and crypt atrophy may be present.

Special Techniques. Most cases of cryptosporidiosis are diagnosed by the detection of oocysts in stool samples stained with a modified acid-fast stain. Other methods of diagnosis include direct and indirect fluorescence microscopy and ELISA (833,854). PCR-based assays are also used to detect the organisms (827,834).

Treatment and Prognosis. There is no routinely effective antiparasitic therapy for cryptosporidiosis. Nonspecific, supportive treatment, including rehydration and nutritional support, remains the mainstay of management. A number of compounds have been used with variable responses. Antimicrobial drugs that have been employed with some success include paromomycin (854), paromomycin plus azithromycin (851), and nitazoxanide (826,850).

Cyclospora Infections

Demography. *Cyclospora cayetanensis*, a coccidian protozoan, is a recently recognized cause of waterborne and foodborne diarrhea. The organism affects many animal species, including man. It occurs widely in Europe, Asia, North Africa, and Central and South America (875). In most developed countries, the disease is most commonly associated with foodborne outbreaks or in travelers to developing countries. *Cyclospora* outbreaks in the United States have been reported in association with consumption of contaminated berries imported from Central America and with contaminated water (858,863,865,876).

Etiology. There are 17 species of *Cyclospora*. Currently, humans are the only known hosts for *Cyclospora cayetanensis*, and an environmental source of infection or animal model has not yet been identified (861).

The infective form of the organism is the oocyst. Within the sporulated oocyst, two sporocysts can be identified, each of which yields two sporozoites. Oocysts excyst in the small intestine, typically the jejunum, and sporozoites are released. The sporozoites invade intestinal epithelial cells where they undergo asexual reproduction to produce two generations of merozoites (870). Merozoites enter the intestinal lumen from which they may either invade other intestinal cells, or mature into either microgametocytes or macrogametocytes. Fertilization of gametocytes results in the development of oocysts, which are shed into the environment in the feces. Oocysts leave the host in an unsporulated, noninfective form. They must undergo sporulation, in which the oocyst differentiates into a sporocyst containing two sporozoites, prior to becoming infectious. The environmental conditions that induce sporulation are not yet understood (870).

Clinical Features. Symptoms of cyclosporiasis develop 1 to 7 days after suspected exposure, and include diarrhea associated with nausea, anorexia, malaise, and abdominal cramping. Symptomatic periods alternate with periods of apparent remission (859). The diarrhea is watery, and may last 3 to 7 weeks in immunocompetent individuals and may continue for up to 4 months in HIV-infected patients (868,870). With prolonged illness, weight loss is severe (874). Patients can also be asymptomatic excreters of oocysts, although this is not common (864,866,871,875).

Microscopic Findings. *Cyclospora* organisms can be seen in duodenal aspirates but they have not been seen in biopsies of the distal duodenum (860). The jejunal histology of *Cyclospora* infection varies from essentially normal to changes resembling tropical sprue. Jejunal biopsies show partial villous atrophy, villous blunting and fusion, lymphocytic infiltration of the lamina propria, crypt hyperplasia, and increased numbers of intraepithelial lymphocytes. The epithelial cells show both focal vacuolization and disruption of the brush border. The enterocytes change their shape from columnar to cuboidal.

Special Techniques. The diagnosis relies on detecting the organism or its DNA in stool samples. Almost all cases are diagnosed by detecting oocysts in stool samples or jejunal or duodenal aspirates (871). Because *Cyclospora* oocysts may be passed intermittently, sporadically, or in small numbers, techniques to concentrate oocytes are used as part of the routine diagnostic procedure (862). Acid-fast stains, such as the Ziehl-Neelsen, enable detection of oocysts 8 to 10 µm in diameter (870); however, some ova do not pick up the stain and appear as glassy, wrinkled spheres (862).

Table 10-11

COMPARISON OF MICROSCOPIC APPEARANCE OF *CYCLOSPORA, ISOSPORA,* AND *CRYPTOSPORIDIUM*

Feature	*Cyclospora*	*Isospora*	*Cryptosporidium*
Size range (µm)	8-10	20-33 x 10-19	4-6
Appearance in formol-ether concentration	Spherical refractile, greenish central morula; unsporulated when passed in feces	Oval; usually unsporulated when passed in feces	Not usually seen
Sporulated oocyst	2 oval sporocysts, each containing 2 sporozoites	2 spherical sporocysts, each containing 4 sporozoites	Spherical or slightly ovoid; 4 sporozoites
Appearance in modified Ziehl-Neelsen stain	Acid fast, variable staining; some do not stain and appear as glassy, wrinkled spheres	Acid fast; sporoblasts stain deep red; oocyst wall outlined by stain precipitate	Acid fast; staining variable; "erythrocyte" staining common
Appearance under ultraviolet light	Bright blue autofluorescence	No effect	No effect
Fluorescence with auramine	Poor	Variable	Good; bright yellow discs, often with erythrocyte pattern
Fluorescence with monoclonal antibody to *Cryptosporidium*	Absent	Absent	Good; often shows suture line on surface of oocyst

Depending on the degree of staining, the oocysts range from colorless to light pink to an intense, deep reddish purple. Staining also varies in different parts of the smear. More recently, a safranin staining procedure has been developed, which includes heating in a microwave, that appears to be superior for identifying the organism (862,869).

Size is an important criterion in the identification of the protozoan cysts and the measurement of the oocyst helps establish the correct diagnosis. Unstained, oocysts appear as spherical bodies containing a refractile, greenish central morule. The organisms autofluoresce bright blue when examined with ultraviolet (UV) epifluorescence microscopy. Ultrastructural examination of the parasite provides confirmatory evidence.

A PCR assay recently has been developed to detect *Cyclospora*. It takes advantage of amplification of a small subunit ribosomal RNA coding region (872).

Differential Diagnosis. *Cyclospora* infections clinically resemble cryptosporidiosis, microsporidiosis, and isosporiasis. *Cyclospora, Isospora,* and *Cryptosporidia* are compared in Table 10-11.

Treatment and Prognosis. The disease appears to be self-limited. The mainstay of treatment is oral rehydration and appropriate supportive measures. The drug of choice is trimethoprim-sulfamethoxazole. Cotrimoxazole is beneficial in some cases (867). Guillain-Barre syndrome may be a late complication (873).

Leishmania Infections

Demography. *Visceral leishmaniasis* is endemic in 62 countries, but over 90 percent of cases occur in India, Bangladesh, Nepal, Sudan, and northeastern Brazil (883). The population at risk totals 350 million people with 0.5 to 2.0 million new cases diagnosed per year (881,882) and 41,000 resultant deaths (892). In endemic areas, leishmaniasis is transmitted by sandflies, but the disease is also transmitted via blood transfusions, congenital infections, person-to-person contact, hypodermic needles, or sexual contact. Risk factors for the development of the disease include malnutrition, treatment with immunosuppressive drugs, and HIV infection (877,878,880).

Etiology. Most cases of visceral leishmaniasis are caused by *Leishmania donovani*, an obligate intracellular protozoan. In the Mediterranean area and South America, two other species of *Leishmania* also cause the disease, *L. infantum* and *L. chagasi,* respectively. Humans are the only known reservoir for *L. donovani*, but *L. infantum* and *L. chagasi* may be carried by canines, particularly domestic and stray dogs (883).

Leishmania organisms have a dimorphic life cycle. The infection is acquired through bites of infected, blood-sucking, female sandflies of either the genus *Phlebotomus* (Old World) or *Lutzomyia* (New World). In the insect vector, *Leishmania* appears as a motile, spindle-shaped promastigote, measuring 2 to 4 µm x 15 to 20 µm, that possesses a single anterior flagellum. After mononuclear phagocytosis in humans, the promastigotes lose their flagella and multiply as small, round or oval, intracellular amastigotes measuring 2 to 4 µm in diameter.

Clinical Features. Visceral leishmaniasis consists of a complex constellation of clinical manifestations that follow chronic infection with *L. donovani* and related members of this genus. Clinically, leishmaniasis manifests as visceral, cutaneous, and mucosal syndromes. Visceral leishmaniasis, particularly in the Indian subcontinent, may result in enteric infections. Gastrointestinal symptoms include diarrhea, odynophagia, esophagospasm, dysphagia, abdominal pain, malabsorption, and incontinence (885,890, 891). The disease affects the esophagus, stomach, small intestine, colon, rectum, and anus, as well as regional lymph nodes and extragastrointestinal sites such as the bone marrow, oral mucosa, liver, lungs, spleen, brain, and skin (884).

Gross Findings. Radiologic examination of the upper gastrointestinal tract and small bowel shows thickening of the small intestinal folds and increased separation of the bowel loops due to edema. Endoscopy is normal in half of patients (885).

Microscopic Findings. The *Leishmania* amastigotes are often detected in biopsies of what macroscopically appears to be normal small or large intestine. Alternatively, the lamina propria of the intestines and stomach can be obliterated by an infiltration of macrophages containing abundant cytoplasmic *Leishmania* amastigotes. In immunocompetent hosts, granulomas form and an inflammatory response with increased numbers of histiocytes, plasma cells, and lymphocytes occurs in affected organs. The granulomas are absent or poorly formed in immunocompromised individuals.

The intracellular amastigotes are readily seen on either H&E- or Giemsa-stained sections (fig. 10-44). The organisms are round to oval, measure 1 to 3 µm in diameter, and have two characteristic black dots corresponding to the nucleus and the kinetoplast. The organisms appear blue in Wright-Giemsa–stained preparations. At high magnification, a dark red, slightly flattened, eccentrically placed nucleus and a rod-shaped kinetoplast may be discerned. The enterocytes lining the crypts and villi appear normal and do not contain organisms.

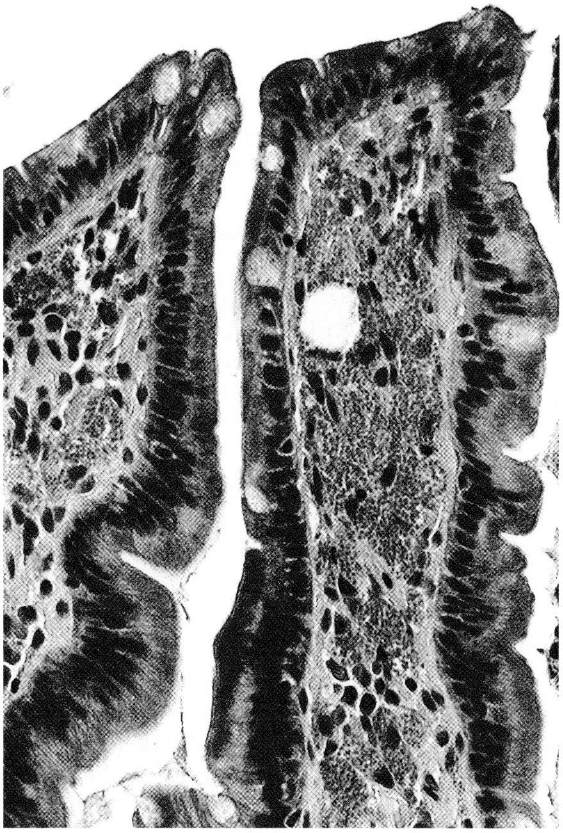

Figure 10-44

LEISHMANIASIS

Discrete, round, uniform blue *Leishmania* organisms fill histiocytes within the lamina propria. (Fig. 3-59 from Emory TS, Carpenter HA, Gostout CJ, Sobin LH. Atlas of gastrointestinal endoscopy & endoscopic biopsies. Washington D.C.: Armed Forces Institute of Pathology; 2000:204.)

Special Techniques. The diagnosis requires microscopic identification of characteristic *Leishmania* amastigotes in smears, touch preparations, or biopsy specimens; culture of the organism; or serologic positivity for the protozoan. Microscopic diagnosis is usually carried out on aspirates or biopsies of bone marrow, spleen, liver, or lymph nodes (883). PCR techniques are highly sensitive for detecting infection (879,889)

Differential Diagnosis. Digestive leishmaniasis must be differentiated from other opportunistic protozoal, bacterial, and fungal infections. The only organism that may contain a characteristic kinetoplast similar to that found in *Leishmania* is *Trypanosoma*. Leishmaniasis must also be differentiated from other infections predominantly resulting in histiocytic infiltrates including disseminated histoplasmosis, *Mycobacterium avium-intracellulare* infection, and cryptococcosis. *Histoplasma* and *Cryptococcus* stain with silver methenamine stains, and *M. avium-intracellulare* stains with acid-fast stains, contrasting with the staining reactions of *Leishmania*. In AIDS patients, intracellular organisms that need to be differentiated from *Leishmania* amastigotes are *Penicillium marneffei* and *Toxoplasma gondii*.

Treatment and Prognosis. Pentavalent antimonials (sodium stibogluconate and meglumine antimoniate) are the mainstays of therapy for patients with leishmaniasis in most of the world. Parasite resistance to these drugs, however, does occur (887). Other drugs that may be used include amphotericin B and pentamidine (881,883). Treatment of immunocompromised patients with leishmaniasis is difficult, and relapse rates approach 60 percent (886,888).

Chagas' Disease

Demography. *Chagas' disease*, or *American trypanosomiasis*, is a zoonosis resulting from human infection by the protozoan *Trypanosoma cruzi*. The chronic form of the disease is endemic in all Central and South American countries, where it is a major cause of morbidity and mortality among poor people. According to the World Health Organization estimates, approximately 25 percent of the Latin American population is at risk for the disease and 16 to 18 million people are infected (892). Of these, 30 percent are likely to develop severe clinical symptoms, and 10 percent will die (895). Males are affected more than females. Chagas' disease is also found in parts of the southern United States.

Etiology. The organism parasitizes over 100 species of mammals, including domestic animals, rodents, and humans. Triatomid insects act as the main disease vector. The insects prefer to inhabit mud huts with cracked walls and thatched roofs. Thus, infections most commonly affect poor socioeconomic classes who inhabit such dwellings. Parasites occasionally pass from the mother to the fetus and cause spontaneous abortion or congenital Chagas' disease. Rarely, the disease is transmitted by blood transfusions. Laboratory workers may also become accidentally infected.

Adult insects ingest trypomastigotes (trypanosomes) when taking blood from infected animals or humans. The life cycle of *T. cruzi* involves a reproductive phase in the host as well as in the insect. *T. cruzi* trypomastigotes are ingested by the insect, and transformed in its gut into epimastigotes, flagellate forms with an anterior kinetoplast. Epimastigotes multiply by binary fission, then migrate to the hindgut where they change to infective, metacyclic trypomastigotes. These are excreted in the insect feces. The human host is infected by rubbing the triatomid insect bite, thereby assisting penetration of the metacyclic trypomastigotes through the skin. The protozoans penetrate the skin, enter the bloodstream, and circulate, invading smooth muscles and the myocardium. Inside the host cells, they form small (3-µm) amastigotes. These amastigotes multiply by binary fission, enlarging the cell and leading to its rupture. New circulating trypomastigotes then invade other cells and the cycle is repeated. In this way, a cycle is established that alternates asynchronously between intracellular multiplying forms and nondividing but infective forms that circulate in the bloodstream.

Pathophysiology. The mechanisms by which *T. cruzi* infection damages the gastrointestinal system are poorly understood. Several lines of evidence suggest that immunologic mechanisms, including possible autoimmune cross-reactivity between antibodies to *T. cruzi* and mammalian nervous tissues, are of significance (893,896,899).

Clinical Features. Chagas' disease comprises a variety of clinical and pathologic manifestations ranging from severe, such as cardiomyopathy, to insignificant (893). Acute illness occurs in childhood. Initial spread of the parasites from the site of entry and their multiplication may be accompanied by fever, malaise, and edema of the face and lower extremities, as well as generalized lymphadenopathy and

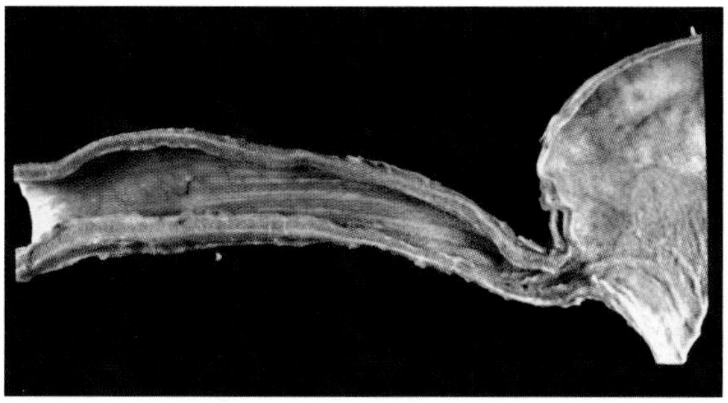

Figure 10-45

MEGAESOPHAGUS IN A PATIENT WITH CHAGAS' DISEASE

The esophagus is markedly dilated in this patient with long-standing Chagas' disease. The gross appearance mimics that of achalasia. (Courtesy of the Division of Gastrointestinal Pathology, Armed Forces Institute of Pathology, Washington, DC.)

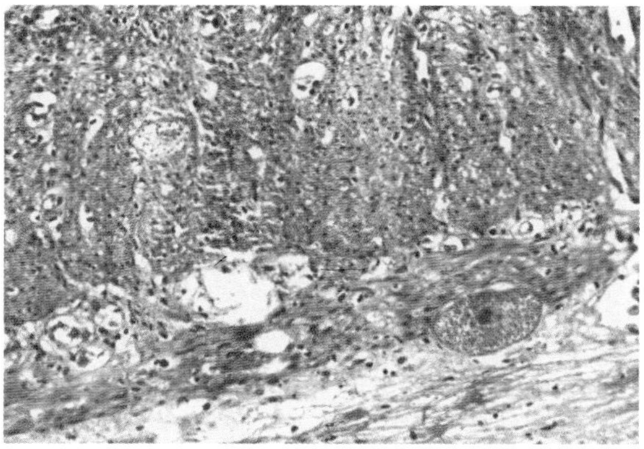

Figure 10-46

ACUTE CHAGAS' DISEASE INVOLVING THE INTESTINE

An organism is adjacent to the myenteric plexus.

hepatosplenomegaly. The muscles, including the heart, are often heavily parasitized and severe myocarditis develops in a small proportion of patients (897). In rare cases, the organism invades the CNS causing meningoencephalitis (897). The acute illness resolves spontaneously over 4 to 6 weeks in most patients.

Approximately 10 to 20 percent of patients develop chronic disease, which may become manifest as long as 10 or more years after the initial infection (897). Gastrointestinal involvement is common at this time. Gastrointestinal dysfunction in the form of megaesophagus or megacolon is a major problem for many patients with chronic Chagas' disease. Patients with colonic involvement complain of constipation, abdominal distension, and pain. Megacolon can be complicated by fecal impaction, volvulus, enterocolitis, or toxic megacolon. Clinical signs and symptoms of the latter include pain, progressive abdominal distension accompanied by fever, severe toxemia, and shock.

Gross Findings. Both megaesophagus and megacolon develop in patients with chronic Chagas' disease (fig. 10-45). Chest radiographs show cardiomegaly and a dilated esophagus with air-fluid levels. The gross features of the esophagus resemble those seen in achalasia. The colon can reach immense proportions, with a length of over 2 m and a capacity of 30 to 40 L (898).

Microscopic Findings. The process of nerve destruction usually develops insidiously over many years and varies considerably in terms of its extent in individual patients as well as in different segments of the gastrointestinal tract. The histologic features of Chagas' disease reflect the stage of the disease. During the acute infection, the organism lies in or near the myenteric plexus (fig. 10-46). Early degenerative changes involve the muscularis propria and the myenteric plexus. In late-stage disease, the myenteric plexus becomes fibrotic and neurons disappear. Histologic examination of the wall of the colon shows depletion of the neural cells in the myenteric plexus, with fibrous tissue replacing the plexus. Focal inflammation and hypertrophy of the muscularis propria occur.

Special Techniques. A complement fixation test for *T. cruzi* infection is usually positive in patients with chronic Chagas' disease. Esophageal manometry studies confirm the absence of peristalsis in the body of the esophagus and failure of coordinated relaxation of the lower esophageal sphincter in response to swallowing.

Differential Diagnosis. Clinically, the disease mimics any of the chronic idiopathic intestinal pseudoobstruction syndromes and achalasia. Histologically, late-stage disease may resemble scleroderma.

Treatment and Prognosis. Two drugs are available for the treatment of Chagas' disease, benznidazole, the drug of choice, and nifurtimox (894). Prevention of the disease is of primary importance. Once the neurons of the myenteric plexus are destroyed, progressive dilatation of the gastrointestinal tract is inevitable. Medical therapy for gastrointestinal symptoms includes stool softeners and laxatives for chronic constipation, and antireflux measures for gastroesophageal reflux. Surgery may be necessary for medically nonresponsive symptoms, for patients with massive dilatation of aperistaltic gastrointestinal segments, or for volvulus.

Blastocystis Infections

Demography. In many studies, *Blastocystis hominis* represents the most commonly encountered intestinal parasite in humans (902,915). Organism prevalence ranges from 2 to 18 percent in the United States, 3 to 13 percent in Canada, and 3 to 7 percent in Great Britain (912,918). The prevalence is as high as 50 percent in the developing world (913,914). *B. hominis* infection is particularly common among immunocompromised patients (902). Travelers to tropical locales are at risk (906).

Etiology. *B. hominis* is a protozoan in the subphylum Sporozoa. This strict anaerobe reproduces by binary division or sporulation. It exhibits three major morphologic forms: vacuolar, granular, and ameboid (913). The vacuolar form is variable in size, measuring from 2 to 200 µm (917,922), with an average diameter of 2 to 15 µm (920). This form of the organism contains a single nucleus at the edge of the cytoplasm and a large, central, optically empty body surrounded by the peripheral cytoplasm containing other cellular organelles. If two nuclei are present, they are at opposite poles of the cell. Sometimes, four nuclei line up at the edges of the protozoan. The granular form is spherical and has a diameter of 10 to 60 µm (921). It contains reproductive granules that correspond to the offspring, round or tubular-like lipidic cytoplasmic bodies, and a central body. The ameboid form has a diameter of 10 to 25 µm and measures up to 100 µm in length. It has irregular edges and its pseudopodia extend and retract as it feeds on bacteria.

Clinical Features. *B. hominis* is found in asymptomatic patients, and in those presenting with symptoms of acute or chronic gastroenteritis. Because the organism is so commonly identified in asymptomatic individuals, the pathogenicity of *Blastocystis* is debated. When present, symptoms are nonspecific and include abdominal pain, cramps, diarrhea, anorexia, nausea, vomiting, flatulence, and weight loss (903, 904,909,910,912,916,919,923,924). In acute forms of the illness, diarrhea may be profuse (919).

Pathologic Findings. Grossly, the colonic mucosa usually appears normal, although rarely it appears erythematous and friable (901,905, 907). Biopsies from infected persons also often appear normal. When abnormal, they may exhibit only mild nonspecific inflammation (907). Rarely, the organism causes colonic mucosal destruction and invasion of tissues (900,920).

Special Techniques. The parasite is directly identifiable by immediate examination of feces. Rarely, the organism is identified in the duodenal secretions obtained by string tests.

Treatment and Prognosis. Treatment with metronidazole or trimethoprim-sulfamethoxazole is effective in eradicating the organism (908,911).

Ascaris Infections

Demography. *Ascaris* is the most prevalent intestinal helminth infecting humans, affecting as much as 25 percent of the population in some areas (934). These parasites have profound health, social, and economic implications for developing countries and certain regions of developed nations. The worms exhibit a worldwide distribution, although they are most commonly encountered in tropical and subtropical regions of Asia, Africa, and South America. In the United States, *Ascaris* is prevalent in rural areas of the south. Infection may also be seen in travelers and migrants from endemic areas.

Ascaris infection is most common in areas with overcrowding and poor sanitation (931). It occurs at all ages but is seen more often in preschool and young school-aged children, especially in the 5- to 9-year-old group. Transmission usually occurs by a hand-to-mouth route. Children acquire the infection by ingesting mature eggs from contaminated soil where they play; ova may also be ingested in fecally contaminated food and water. In endemic areas, the ova are recovered from many surfaces including utensils, furniture, money, door handles, food items, and fingers (933). There are also rare reports of neonatal transmission (929). The balance between exposure rate and rate of loss of the infection due to host immune defenses determines the intensity of infection (927). Some of these factors may be genetically determined (935).

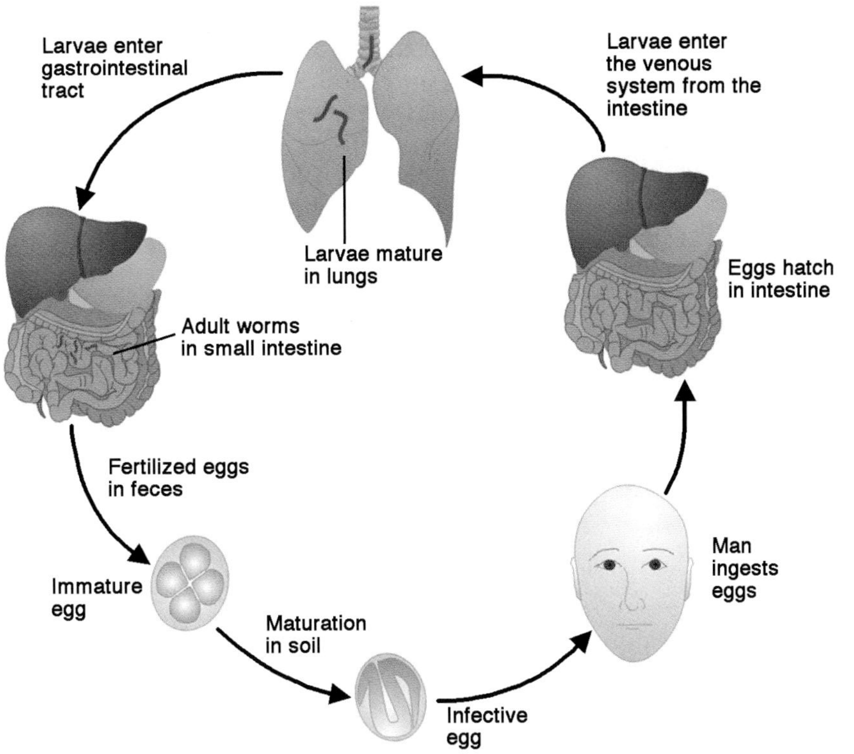

Figure 10-47

DIAGRAM OF THE LIFE CYCLE OF *ASCARIS*

Etiology. *Ascaris lumbricoides* is the largest human nematode, measuring up to 40 cm in length. The worm is elongated, cylindrical, and tapered at both ends. Females measure 20 to 35 cm in length and 3 to 6 mm in diameter; males are 15 to 30 cm and 2 to 4 mm in diameter (933). The male posterior end is curved and has a copulatory spicule. The cuticle or outer skin is striated with two lateral lines. The color of the parasite varies from yellow to white with a pinkish hue. It is characterized by a constricted area known as a vulvar waist (genital girdle) located at the junction of the anterior and middle thirds of the body.

After mating, the female worms deposit eggs that are excreted from the host in the feces. Females may release over 200,000 ova per day (937). Fertile eggs are ovoid, measure 6 to 40 µm, and acquire a golden brown color due to bile staining. The outer shell of a fertilized egg appears mammillated, while unfertilized eggs are smooth. Eggs become infective in soil 3 to 4 weeks after excretion. Survival of such infective ova is variable, although some survive for up to 15 years (939).

Eggs ingested by humans hatch into first-stage larvae within a few hours in the jejunum due to the action of larval enzymes with assistance from gastric and duodenal digestion. They molt into second-stage larvae that penetrate the jejunal mucosa and pass to the liver via the portal system, and then to the heart and lungs. It takes 2 to 3 weeks following ingestion for infective larvae to develop in the intestine, penetrate the mucosa, and reach the portal venous system. Migration to the lungs takes 3 to 4 days and after 2 to 3 weeks the larvae penetrate from the capillary bed into the alveoli where they molt into third-stage larvae. The latter migrate up the tracheobronchial tree, are coughed up and swallowed again. Fourth-stage larvae reach the small intestine and develop into adults where they copulate and reproduce (940). Following migration, the adult worms (one to several hundred) develop in the small intestine (usually mid-jejunum) where they anchor themselves to the mucosal surface. Adult worms live 12 to 18 months. The life cycle of *Ascaris* is summarized in figure 10-47.

Clinical Features. Three phases of disease may be present: first, a larval migration phase; second, a migration/oviposition phase; and third, a complications phase (933). In many cases, the infection is asymptomatic. Patients with low worm burdens may experience only

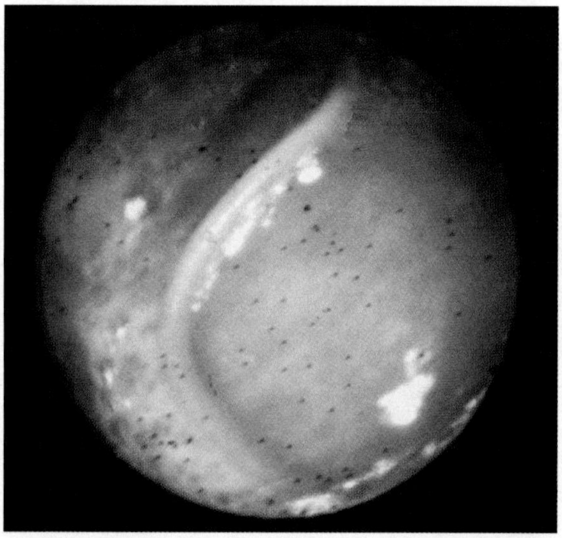

Figure 10-48

ASCARIS

Endoscopic photograph of *Ascaris* in the lumen of the stomach of a patient who had abdominal pain and vomiting.

vague abdominal pain. In patients with heavy worm burdens, more severe symptoms occur including intestinal obstruction, perforation, and peritonitis (928,930,932,941). Masses of worms may obstruct the common bile and pancreatic ducts, producing cholangitis and pancreatitis. In severe cases, the liver may be involved. Repeat infection can sometimes lead to serious hypersensitivity reactions in sensitized individuals. Such patients develop urticaria, angioneurotic edema, and bronchospasm, as well as elevated IgE levels.

Gross Findings. As adults, most *Ascaris* parasites reside in the jejunal lumen where they are grossly and endoscopically evident (fig. 10-48). Radiographic examination of the intestine may reveal parallel cylindrical filling defects that show a string-like shadow of barium in the worm's intestine. In cases of bowel obstruction, abdominal films may show the outline of interlocking worms.

Microscopic Findings. The cross section of the worm may be seen in histologic sections. Once the infection clears, there are only residual traces of their presence. The organisms are seen as small polypoid structures lying within the submucosa and surrounded by fibrotic reactive tissue. Granulomas may also be present. They can develop in any organ, including the intestines, or on the peritoneal surfaces.

Special Techniques. The diagnosis of ascariasis is usually made by detecting eggs in the feces. Three types of eggs are found: the typical fertilized egg, the unfertilized egg, and the decorticated fertilized egg. Regular fertilized eggs measure 55 to 75 x 35 to 50 µm and have thick shells with a bile stained, prominent, outer albuminoid, mamillated coat. Decorticated fertilized eggs measure 30 to 40 µm in diameter and lack mammillation. Eggs are usually abundant so that only direct microscopic examination of a fecal smear is necessary. Concentration techniques, such as flotation, sedimentation, formalin ethyl acetate, centrifugation, or the Kato-Katz technique are useful in mild infections.

Differential Diagnosis. Other helminthic infections are the entities in the differential diagnosis.

Treatment and Prognosis. A number of antihelminthics are available for treating intestinal ascariasis. The drug of choice is mebendazole (Vermox) or a single dose of pyrantel pamoate (Antiminth) or albendazole (Zentel) (926,936–938). *Ascaris* cure rates are over 97 percent (925). In endemic areas, where multiple helminthic infections are common, the initial treatment can be followed by 100 mg of mebendazole taken orally. Retreatment is often necessary, especially in endemic areas. Cases of complete obstruction due a worm bolus with signs of an acute abdomen require surgery.

Hookworm Infections

Demography. *Hookworms* infect an estimated 1.3 billion people worldwide (943). They are particularly common in moist, tropical, rural areas where there are inadequate hygiene and lack of footwear, and where crops provide shade or are cultivated under tall trees. Most heavy infestations occur in people who live where coconuts, cocoa, coffee beans, tea, sugar cane, sweet potatoes, or mulberry trees are grown (945). *Necator americanus* is more common in Asia, the Americas, Africa, Australia, and the Pacific islands; *Ancylostoma duodenale* is found in Africa, India, China, Japan, and parts of Australia and South America. Both species coexist in several parts of the world. Zoonotic ancylostomiasis (*A. caninum*) can be acquired from domestic pets in developed urban communities (948).

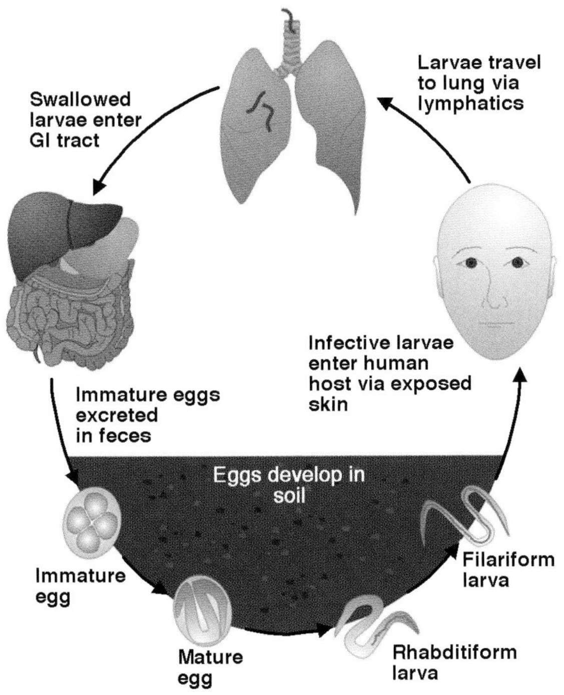

Figure 10-49

DIAGRAM OF THE LIFE CYCLE OF THE HOOKWORM

Etiology. The most significant human parasites in the hookworm group are *A. duodenale* and *N. americanus*. *A. duodenale* sometimes is referred to as the old-world hookworm, whereas *N. americanus* is referred to as the new-world hookworm; however, the geographic distribution of these two species overlaps.

The principal mode of human infection is through percutaneous penetration by the larvae. Infectious filariform larvae invade the skin through bare feet or other exposed skin surfaces. A purpuric, papular, or vesicular eruption develops at the entry site. Adult hookworms live in the small intestine of human beings (fig. 10-49). Under optimal conditions, the eggs in the feces hatch in moist, warm soil within 24 hours to release first-stage larvae. Second-stage larvae develop 3 days later. One week after hatching, the filariform larvae develop, migrate to the surface of the soil, and remain viable for weeks. The filariform larvae then penetrate the skin of the host and enter the venous or lymphatic system where they are carried to the lung. The larvae emerge in the alveolar spaces. They then migrate through the bronchi and trachea to the esophagus where they are swallowed.

In the small intestine, the larvae mature into adult worms. The adult worms attach themselves to the intestinal epithelium via a buccal capsule that is armed with teeth (*Ancylostoma*) or cutting plates (*Necator*). Large, anterior glands secrete proteases and anticoagulants that act to digest host tissues. Worms change position every 4 to 6 hours, possibly in response to tissue depletion or the onset of local inflammation (946). Adult *Ancylostoma* probably survive in the host for only 6 to 12 months, although individual infections may persist for years as a result of intermittent reactivation of hypobiotic larvae. In contrast, adult *Necator* organisms survive an average of 5 years, although survival for as long as 18 years has been recorded (947).

The nematodes measure approximately 0.7 to 1.3 cm in length. Males are slightly smaller than females and *Necator* is smaller than *Ancylostoma*. They are cream to gray-white and possess a distinctive oral or buccal capsule in which is situated a bilateral pair of fused teeth in *A. duodenale* and a ventral and dorsal pair of semilunar cutting plates in *N. americanus*. The posterior tip of the male forms a distinctive broad, transparent, umbrella-like structure, the copulatory bursa, used to hold the female during insemination. The female deposits immature eggs in a fecal stream that are usually in a 2- to 8-cell stage when seen in fresh stool specimens. The eggs of the two species are indistinguishable from one another.

Pathophysiology. The invasive stage of the nematode releases hyaluronidase, metalloproteinases, and cysteine proteinases, which serve as potential allergens and induce an eosinophilic enteritis via a type I hypersensitivity response (942,944). These enzymes also degrade glycoproteins and play a role in tissue breakdown and mucosal invasion (945).

Clinical Features. Once filariform larvae penetrate the skin, a pruritic, erythematous, papular, or vesicular urticarial rash may occur at the entry point. Secondary pyogenic infections commonly develop at these sites. This is accompanied by intense itching, edema, erythema, and neutrophilic and eosinophilic infiltration of the site. The skin eruption may last for several weeks. Pulmonary manifestations of the disease are

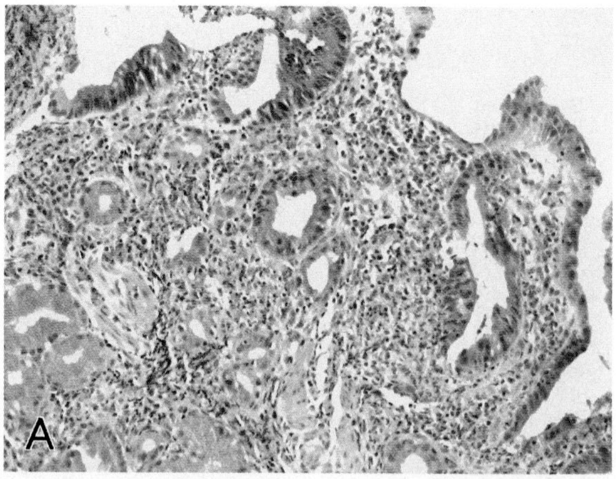

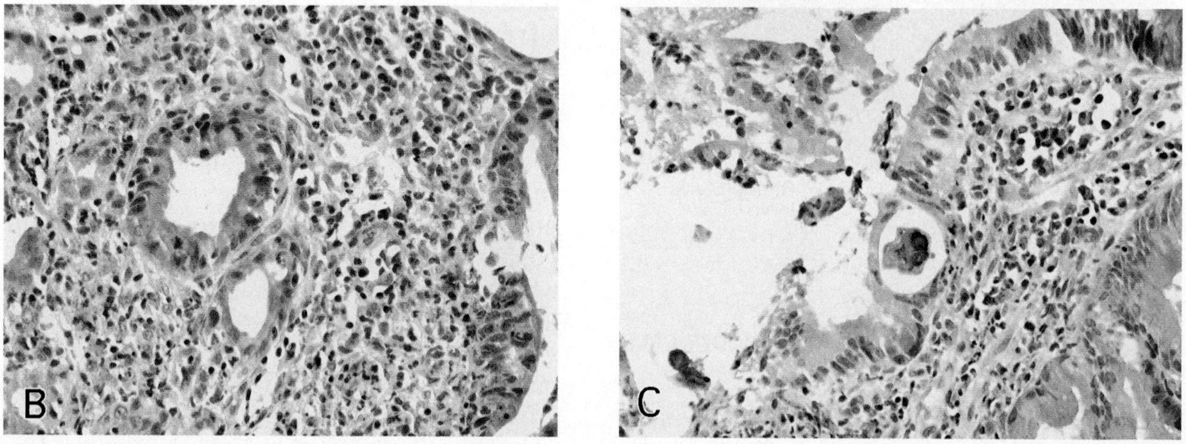

Figure 10-50

HOOKWORM INFECTION

A: A duodenal biopsy specimen shows villous blunting and increased inflammatory cells within the lamina propria.

B: The inflammatory infiltrate contains numerous eosinophils and occasional neutrophils.

C: A cross section of a hookworm is near the opening of a duodenal crypt.

similar to those seen with ascariasis. Patients may develop a mild transient cough. Many patients remain asymptomatic after the larvae reach the small intestine. Dyspepsia, nausea, and epigastric discomfort may occur early in the disease. In untreated patients, symptoms progress, with anemia, constipation, or diarrhea developing. In severe cases and chronic infections, malnutrition, hypoproteinemia, and profound anemia with cardiac decompensation may be seen. The severity of the symptoms depends on the number of worms present and the host's nutritional and immune status. Laboratory examination typically shows peripheral eosinophilia and elevated IgE levels.

Gross Findings. Radiographic studies usually demonstrate nonspecific changes, such as excessive peristalsis and "puddling" changes, particularly in the proximal jejunum.

Microscopic Findings. Small erosive lesions, hemorrhages, tissue cytolysis, and neutrophilic responses may result from the attachment of the worms to the intestinal mucosa. Worms suck blood and plasma vigorously, and often abandon one site and move to another, leaving the old site oozing blood and plasma. *A. caninum* is often diagnosed by identifying the 1-cm–long worm in gastrointestinal biopsies or duodenal aspirates, especially in patients with heavy parasitic infections. The mucosa may appear hemorrhagic, eroded, congested, and edematous. Focal or diffuse eosinophilic infiltrates are commonly seen (fig. 10-50). Increased numbers of eosinophils in the lamina propria are particularly prominent near areas of parasitic attachment. Charcot-Leyden crystals and eosinophil degranulation are often present. Granulomas may sometimes be seen. Some patients develop focal crypt hyperplasia and villous atrophy.

Special Techniques. Stool examination usually reveals the presence of hookworm eggs. The eggs are thin-shelled, ovoid, and measure 65 x

40 μm. Direct fecal smears examined microscopically usually reveal the eggs, but in light infections a concentration technique is needed. Rhabditiform larvae measuring 0.3 to 17.0 μm may be found in the feces if the stool specimen is stored in the laboratory for hours prior to examination. The larvae can be differentiated from those of *Strongyloides stercoralis* by the presence of a long buccal capsule and the indistinct genital primordia. *S. stercoralis* larvae have a short buccal cavity and large genital primordia. *A. caninum* can be diagnosed by total serum IgE assay and serologic testing with ELISA and Western blot assay using the excretory secretory antigens of *A. caninum*.

Differential Diagnosis. The edema, eosinophilic infiltration of the gut wall, ascites, and regional lymphadenopathy are identical to that seen in eosinophilic gastroenteritis, which falls within the differential diagnosis (949).

Treatment and Prognosis. Antihelminthic therapy is necessary to eradicate the adult intestinal worms. The infection is treated with mebendazole, albendazole, or pyrantel pamoate. Anemia should be treated with 50 to 100 mg of ferrous sulfate daily along with a high protein diet and vitamins. This regimen is continued until the hemoglobin levels stabilize for several months. In patients with severe anemia, blood transfusions and intravenous iron supplements may be required.

Schistosoma Infections

Demography. *Schistosomiasis* is one of the world's most prevalent diseases, ranking second only to malaria as a cause of serious global morbidity. It is estimated to afflict as many as 200 million people worldwide (953): 120 million of these are symptomatic and 20 million suffer from serious disease. Eighty to 85 percent of cases of schistosomiasis occur in sub-Saharan Africa, where the estimated mortality reaches 280,000 per year (962). The disease is also endemic in the Middle East, Brazil, Venezuela, the Caribbean, China, Indonesia, the Philippines, Cambodia, and Laos. Environmental changes resulting from the development of water resources, population growth, and migration have facilitated the spread of the disease to new areas (960).

Etiology. Schistosomiasis is an infection caused by trematodes in the genus *Schistosoma*. Three schistosomal species cause most human infections: *S. mansoni, S. japonicum*, and *S. haematobium*. *S. mansoni* is endemic throughout Africa and is also found in many areas of Latin America, the West Indies, Puerto Rico, and the Middle East. *S. japonicum* is confined to Asia, with most cases found in China, especially along river basins. The parasite is also found in scattered areas of Taiwan and the Philippines. *S. haematobium* is endemic in Africa and the Middle East. Rare infections with *S. intercalatum*, *S. mekongi*, and *S. mattheei* also occur. *S. intercalatum* infections occur in Africa and *S. mekongi* is found along the Mekong River and adjacent parts of Southeast Asia, including Indochina. *S. mattheei* is found in South Africa.

All schistosomes have similar life cycles (fig. 10-51). Eggs are passed by urine or stool into fresh water where they hatch. Ciliated larvae, called miracidia, are released and penetrate into appropriate snails. Sporocysts develop in each snail from which thousands of daughter sporocysts form. These forms emerge from the snail in 3 to 5 weeks as fork-tailed, free-swimming organisms called cercariae. As many as 100,000 may develop from a single miracidium. The cercariae penetrate the human skin on contact and enter the venous circulation, terminating in various places. Larvae of *S. mansoni* terminate in the venules of the inferior mesenteric venous system; *S. haematobium* terminates in the inferior, hemorrhoidal, and vesicle plexuses; and larvae of *S. japonicum* primarily reside in the inferior mesenteric system, with some larval worms terminating and developing in the superior mesenteric veins (951). The worms are slender, being 0.5 mm in diameter and about 6 to 20 mm in length. The female lies in the longitudinal body cleft of the male and both reside within their predetermined venous system in a copulatory position. To lay eggs, the females migrate peripherally to terminal venules over the bowel and bladder walls. Eggs subsequently laid generally move through the venules to the bowel or bladder wall and many are swept to the liver or lungs by venous drainage. The eggs work their way through the bowel and bladder tissue to their respective lumens. After reaching the lumen, the eggs are passed to the outside world and the cycle is complete. Eggs are first detected 6 to 10 weeks after cercarial penetration.

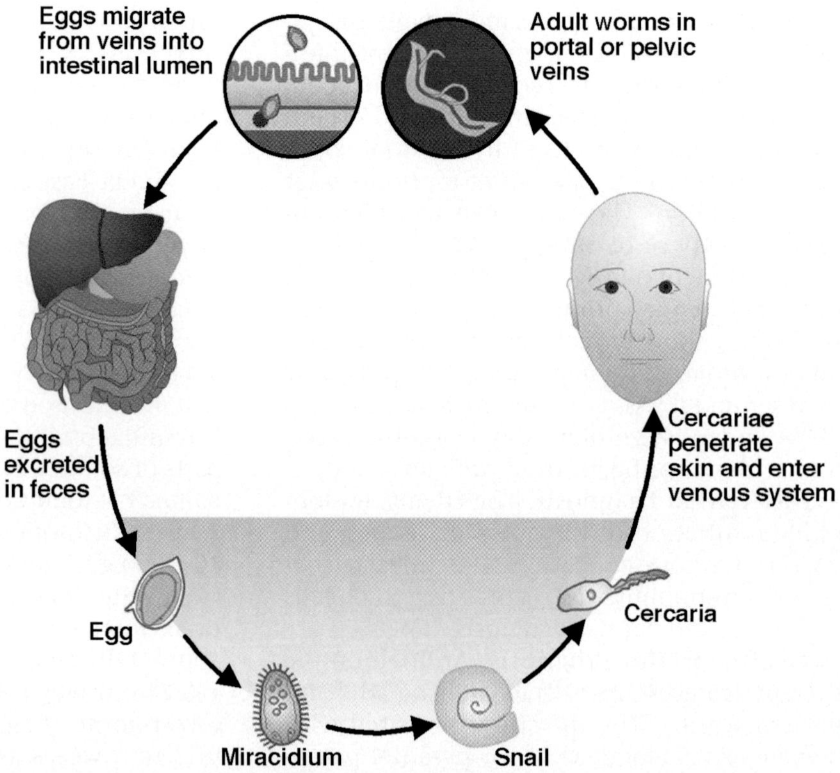

Figure 10-51

DIAGRAM OF THE LIFE CYCLE OF *SCHISTOSOMA*

Clinical Features. Schistosomiasis occurs in three stages: initial penetration, an acute condition known as *Katayama fever*, and chronic disease. In the initial penetration stage, cercarial penetration of the skin results in a maculopapular eruption at the site. In unsensitized individuals, the faint red macules appear within 12 hours; in others, the skin reactions appear up to 1 week later (961).

The acute stage, also called stage II or Katayama fever after a valley in Japan where the disease was endemic, generally starts 4 to 6 weeks and sometimes as late as 10 weeks or more following infection. It coincides with the initial egg production of the newly acquired worms. This stage is seen commonly in areas with high transmission rates (961). Symptoms are thought to be mediated by immune complexes that form in response to egg deposition. Patients most frequently present with fever, headache, generalized myalgias, right upper quadrant pain, and bloody diarrhea. Respiratory symptoms occur in up to 70 percent of patients infected with *S. mansoni*, but are less common in patients infected with other *Schistosoma* species (950,954,955). The liver is enlarged and tender to palpation. Splenomegaly is frequent. Laboratory studies show eosinophilia and elevated IgG and IgE levels. The syndrome usually lasts days to weeks.

Many patients in the chronic phase are asymptomatic, particularly if the infection is mild. With heavier infection, mild chronic diarrhea develops, sometimes associated with hypogastric or left iliac fossa pain. Mucus and small amounts of blood may be present in the stool but gross hemorrhage is unusual. Iron deficiency anemia can result from persistent blood loss. There may be mild weight loss or difficulty maintaining weight, as well as fatigue. Severe chronic disease may result in colonic or rectal stenosis. *S. mansoni* infections may result in colonic polyposis associated with diarrhea and protein-losing enteropathy (957,959). Chronic deposition of eggs in the liver via the portal system leads to portal hypertension, splenomegaly, and esophageal varices.

Gross Findings. In the early stages of the infection, acute proctitis and colitis are accompanied by edema and hemorrhage as ova are discharged into the bowel lumen. Morphologic features of chronic infection include localized or

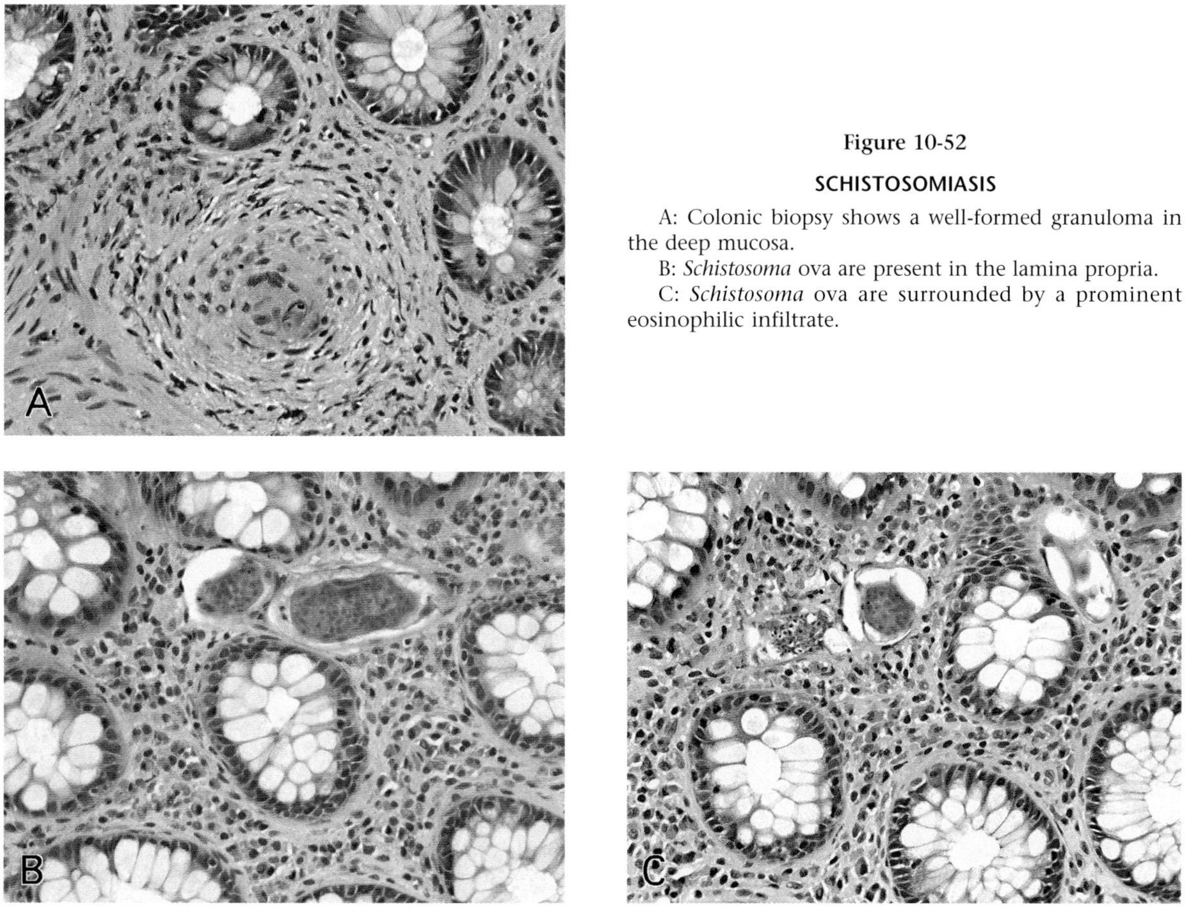

Figure 10-52

SCHISTOSOMIASIS

A: Colonic biopsy shows a well-formed granuloma in the deep mucosa.

B: *Schistosoma* ova are present in the lamina propria.

C: *Schistosoma* ova are surrounded by a prominent eosinophilic infiltrate.

diffuse mucosal ulcers, pronounced submucosal thickening due to fibrosis and lymphoid hyperplasia, strictures due to extensive granulomatous or fibrous reactions, pericolic masses, polyposis, and masses of granulation tissue. Schistosoma-associated polyps range from small to quite large, may be pedunculated, and may bleed. They are most common in the distal colon and rectum. Granulomas may be seen grossly as sandy patches or small yellow nodules on the serosal surfaces.

Microscopic Findings. The diagnosis depends on the histologic recognition of *Schistosoma* eggs and the granulomas and colitis they induce (fig. 10-52). The eggs measure 100 to 180 µm in length and about 70 µm in width. Those of *S. mansoni* are marginally longer than *S. japonicum* and have a distinctive subterminal lateral spine. The shell has a light brown, translucent appearance, and in the case of *S. mansoni*, contains acid-fast material. This feature is diagnostically helpful if only the shell fragments are present. Eosinophils and histiocytes surround the ova. A sarcoid-like reaction eventually envelops the eggs, which become embedded in a granulomatous focus of epithelial histiocytes and giant cells. As the disease becomes more chronic, concentric fibrosis develops around the ova.

Histologic examination of schistosomal polyps usually demonstrates an inflammatory polyp containing *Schistosoma* ova surrounded by dense infiltrates of eosinophils and lymphocytes. The surfaces of the lesions become eroded.

Special Techniques. The diagnosis of schistosomiasis is usually made through identification of the characteristic ova in the stool or urine. The shedding of eggs may be intermittent, and therefore, examination of multiple specimens may be required in some patients. Stool examination by direct smear or concentration may be used. The greatest sensitivity is achieved using a formalin-ether concentration method (956).

Differential Diagnosis. The disease may grossly mimic Crohn's disease or carcinoma.

Treatment and Prognosis. Praziquantel is the schistosomal drug of choice. Praziquantel cures 60 to 90 percent of patients and substantially decreases worm burden in those who are not cured of the disease. A second course of the drug is usually successful in treating these patients. Resistance to praziquantel has been reported (958,963). Alternative treatments include oxamniquine for *S. mansoni* infections and metrifonate for *S. haematobium*, although the latter drug is no longer available commercially.

Patients with colonic or rectal stenosis or those with large inflammatory masses may require surgical resection. Some patients develop colonic carcinoma, presumably due to continuing mucosal inflammation and proliferation in a manner analogous to that seen with ulcerative colitis (952).

Anisakis Infections

Demography. *Anisakidosis* is a parasitic infection caused by anisakid nematodes belonging to the family Ascaridoidea. The infection is zoonotic, acquired following ingestion of parasitized marine fish. The causative organisms (*Anisakis simplex*, and less commonly, *Pseudoterranova decipiens*) are widely distributed geographically, affecting fish in many different oceans and seas (973,974,976–978,989). Over 95 percent of cases of anisakidosis occur in Japan, where 2,000 cases are reported annually (972,983). The incidence is lower in North America and Europe, but is increasing as the popularity of sushi and sashimi rises in these areas (966). In North America, the disease is most frequently associated with eating salmon and rockfish. The prevalence of *Anisakis* larvae in wild coho and chum salmon in the Pacific Northwest is as high as 100 percent (979,980, 982,991). Cooking the fish to a temperature of 60°C for a few minutes, however, is sufficient to kill infective larvae (984). Freezing also eliminates the risk of infection. Larvae are able to survive cold smoking, brining, and marination (967,968,992).

Etiology. Anisakidosis is transmitted to humans by ingestion of seafood products harboring the infective third-stage larvae of the anisakid nematodes. Adult anisakids infect sea mammals, including seals, sea lions, whales, porpoises, and dolphins. Ova are released into the seawater where they undergo one or two molts, then hatch, releasing the first- or second-stage larvae into the water. Second-stage larvae are eaten by small pelagic crustaceans in which they molt again, developing into third-stage larvae (969). The infected crustaceans are then ingested by susceptible marine fish or squid. In these hosts, the larvae migrate into the peritoneal cavity, viscera, and musculature where they encapsulate without undergoing further development (970). The life cycle is completed when infected fish or squid are eaten by marine mammals in which the parasite matures. Human beings are accidental or unsuitable hosts and no maturation takes place in human tissues. When humans eat raw fish contaminated by the larvae, the latter attach to the mucosa of the stomach or the intestines, causing local ulceration, penetration, and perforation. The organism usually invades the gastric wall. Intestinal anisakidosis occurs less commonly.

Clinical Features. The majority of cases of anisakidosis involve the stomach (97 percent), although small intestinal involvement is also seen (987,988). Both invasive and noninvasive forms of infection occur. Infection with *P. decipiens* is usually localized to the stomach, and is a noninvasive disease (965). These infections produce mild or no symptoms. Some patients report a "tingling" sensation in the throat. Expectoration of worms may occur days or weeks following infection (986).

Infection with *A. simplex* may result in more serious disease, with invasion of the gastric or intestinal mucosa, and larval migration to extragastric sites (971,986). Patients with gastric involvement develop intense epigastric pain, nausea, and vomiting 2 to 5 hours after ingestion of raw fish. The pain is generally self-limited. Intestinal anisakidosis presents as lower abdominal pain that generally subsides after several days. Some patients develop acute abdominal signs and symptoms that mimic acute appendicitis and result in laparotomy due to their potential seriousness; bowel obstruction may occur (985). Slight fever and leukocytosis with eosinophilia may occur in both forms of the disease.

In invasive disease, the parasite may penetrate the gastric or intestinal wall, migrating to the peritoneum, mesenteric lymph nodes, greater omentum, liver, and gallbladder. The prognosis of

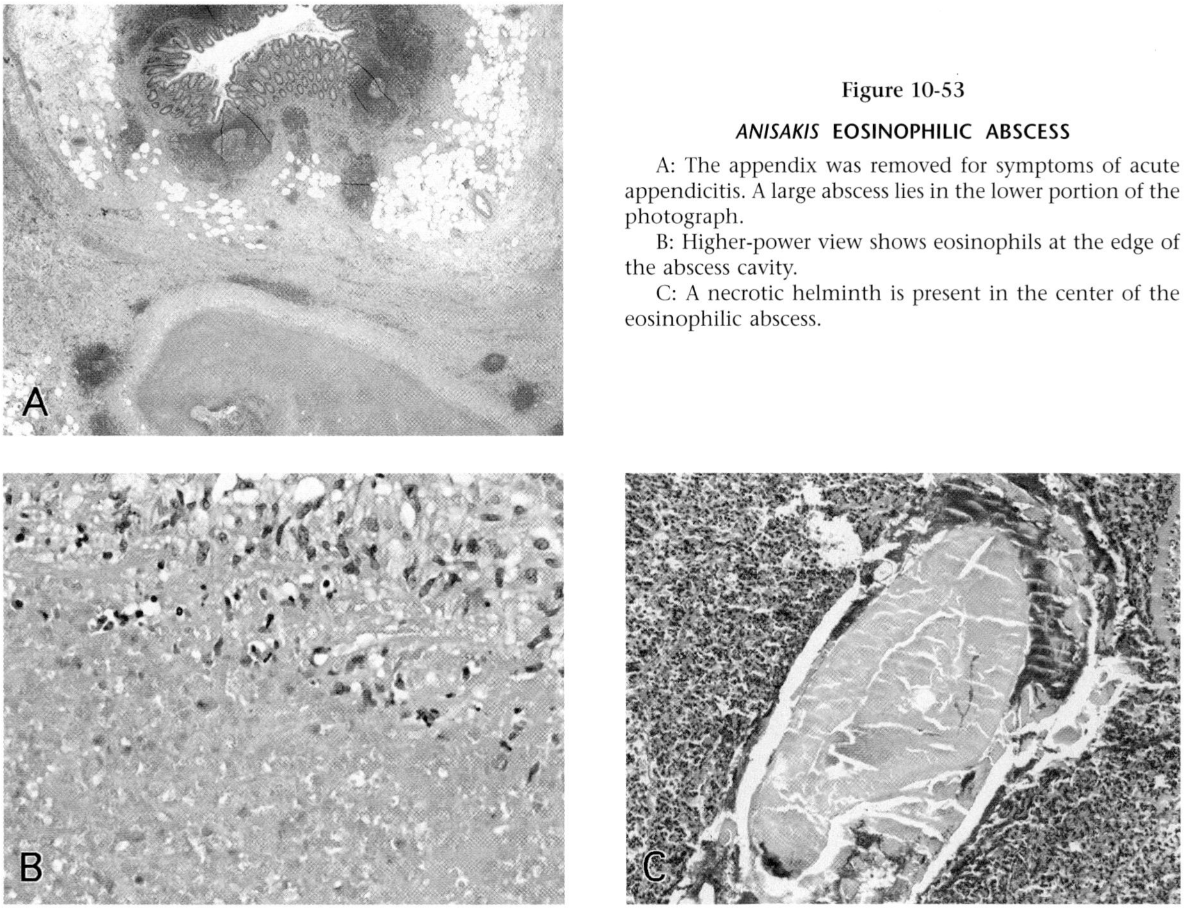

Figure 10-53

***ANISAKIS* EOSINOPHILIC ABSCESS**

A: The appendix was removed for symptoms of acute appendicitis. A large abscess lies in the lower portion of the photograph.

B: Higher-power view shows eosinophils at the edge of the abscess cavity.

C: A necrotic helminth is present in the center of the eosinophilic abscess.

patients with this form of infection is usually worse than for those with other forms.

Allergic reactions to the organisms may occur, with patients developing systemic allergic symptoms ranging from urticaria to anaphylactic shock. These symptoms result from an allergic reaction to the heat-stable antigen of the parasite that is conserved even when fish is frozen or cooked (964,981).

Gross Findings. Anisakidosis usually involves the stomach and small intestine; only rarely does it involve the colon or regional lymph nodes (975). The gastric or small intestinal wall appears thickened due to edema and inflammation. Indurated nodules that may be identified on the mucosal surfaces mimic benign or malignant tumors or Crohn's disease, particularly when regional lymph nodes are involved. Superficial ulcers or patchy hemorrhages may be seen. When colonic involvement does occur, it is usually right-sided. The diagnosis is sometimes made by seeing the worm at the time of endoscopy or on radiographs (989).

Microscopic Findings. Larval entrance into intestinal mucosa elicits a granulomatous reaction around the worm, with infiltration of neutrophils, eosinophils, and histiocytic giant cells. Several days later, the submucosa becomes edematous and there is massive infiltration of eosinophils, lymphocytes, monocytes, neutrophils, and plasma cells. Eventually, an abscess develops that is characterized by necrosis, hemorrhage, and eosinophilic infiltrates (fig. 10-53). Worms are often found in the early lesions but they are eventually destroyed by the inflammation.

When larvae are identified, they are typically surrounded by eosinophils and other inflammatory cells (fig. 10-54). They measure approximately 500 μm in diameter, and have a cuticle ranging from 5 to 7 μm in thickness (965). A glandular esophagus and ribbon-like, large, unpaired excretory glands are often seen in cross

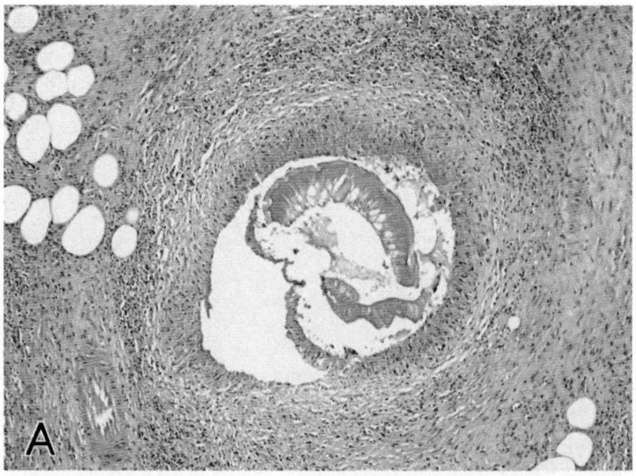

Figure 10-54

ANISAKIDOSIS

A: *Anisakis,* seen in cross section, lies within a granuloma in the perigastric soft tissue.

B: Higher-power view of the worm cut in cross section.

C: The adjacent tissues contain an intense eosinophilic infiltrate. (Courtesy of Dr. John Hart, Chicago, IL.)

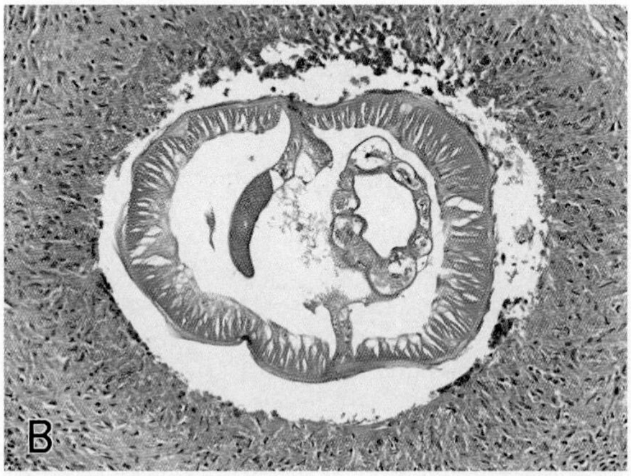

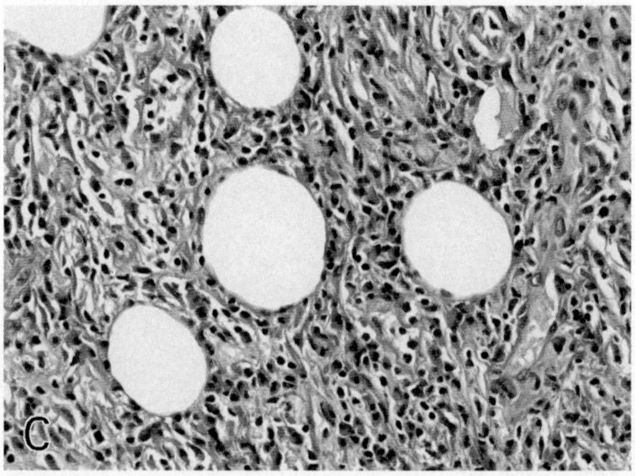

sections of the organism. The organisms also have Y-shaped lateral cords (965,975).

The lymph nodes demonstrate sinus histiocytosis and eosinophilic infiltration without granuloma formation (990). Eosinophilic granulomas may form around a track containing sections of the nematode larvae (975).

Special Techniques. Anisakidosis is diagnosed by radioallergoabsorbent tests, ELISA, or immunofluorescent antibody assays. The diagnosis is also made when worms are seen on endoscopic examination in acute infections.

Differential Diagnosis. Anisakidosis clinically mimics gastric cancer, gastric ulcers, Crohn's disease, appendicitis, ileus, and peritonitis (984,985). It morphologically resembles other roundworm infections. The anisakid larvae morphologically resemble *Ascarid* larvae. *Ascarid* larvae are smaller in diameter and possess bilateral alae that are absent in anisakid larvae. Anisakid larvae have a polymyarian type of musculature with prominent Y-shaped lateral cords. The Y-shaped gastrointestinal lumen of the organism contains numerous tall columnar cells, which are usually prominently featured in cross sections. Reproductive organs appear immature or absent.

Treatment and Prognosis. In Japan, endoscopy is widely used for diagnosis, especially for gastric infections. Surgical resection of the inflamed intestine is the only definitive treatment for intestinal anisakidosis; there are no effective antihelminthic drugs currently in use.

Enterobius Vermicularis Infections

Demography. *Enterobiasis* is a ubiquitous infection, occurring more often in temperate and colder climates. The pinworm, *Enterobius vermicularis,* infects approximately 200 million people worldwide, but is most common in young schoolchildren. It is also prevalent in individuals living in overcrowded conditions and in male homosexuals (996). Four methods of transmission exist: 1) direct infection from the anal canal and perianal regions by fingernail contamination (autoinfection) and soiled night clothes; 2) exposure to viable eggs on soiled bed linen and other contaminated environmental objects; 3) contamination by dust containing embryonated eggs (from bed clothes, pajamas, toys, furniture, and animal fur); and 4) retroinfection, i.e., after hatching on the anal mucosa, larvae migrate into the sigmoid colon and cecum (996).

Etiology. The adult worms are small, yellow-white, and lancet shaped; typically, they inhabit the cecum, the appendix, and adjacent areas of the ileum and ascending colon, although immature worms have occasionally been seen in the rectosigmoid. Females measure 8 to 13 mm in length and the infrequently seen males measure 2 to 5 mm in length. The gravid female migrates through the anal canal at night, deposits approximately 10,000 eggs on the perianal skin and then dies. The eggs typically measure 55 x 25 µm and have a characteristic convexity on one side and flattening on the other. They are infective and fully mature within several hours after being laid and are able to survive for up to 15 days outside the body. They can be found under fingernails and on skin, clothing, sheets, doorknobs, and other objects. After the egg is ingested by a host, the larva emerges in the small intestine and migrates distally to the cecum. In less than a month, newly developed gravid females again discharge ova in the perianal region. The life cycle of the organism is summarized in figure 10-55.

Clinical Features. The predominant symptom of patients with enterobiasis is anal pruritus, thought to possibly be an allergic reaction to the worms or their eggs. In children, these symptoms often lead to irritability, restlessness, and insomnia. A severe scratching response to the pruritus may lead to local bleeding, secondary pyogenic infection, and lichenoid changes. Continued scratching causes local excoriation and weeping of the skin surfaces. Most patients, however, remain asymptomatic. In female children, the worms may lay eggs on the vulva, producing vulvar itching and vulvovaginitis. In very rare cases in girls, adult worms migrate into the cervix, uterus, fallopian tubes, ovaries, or peritoneum (997–1000). In the latter case, abdominal pain may be present. In rare circumstances, the worms

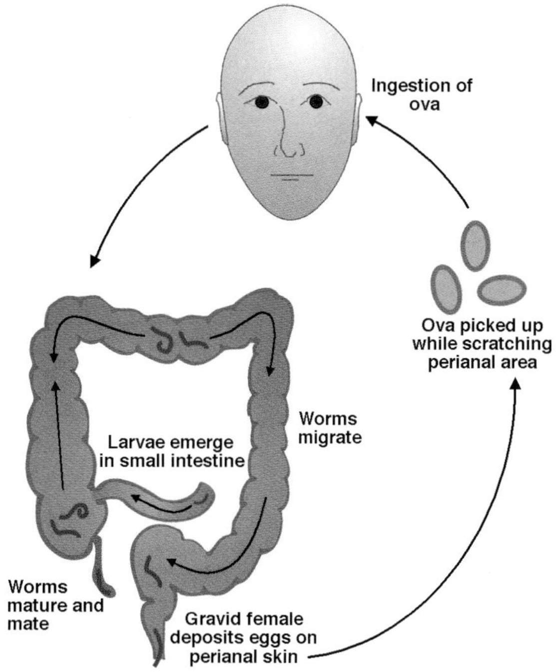

Figure 10-55

DIAGRAM OF THE LIFE CYCLE OF *ENTEROBIUS*

penetrate the intestines, leading to peritoneal signs, and penetrating worms may form granulomas in the anal canal (995,1003).

Gross Findings. *Enterobius* infections are generally mild, and produce no grossly visible lesions. Severe infections, however, may lead to superficial ulceration of the colonic mucosa. Occasionally, adult worms are visible on the surface of the perianal skin.

Microscopic Findings. Specific identification of adult worms in tissue sections depends on demonstrating a pair of cuticular crests, typical eggs in the uterus of the parasite, and the characteristic narrow meromyarian (a type of musculature that consists of two or three muscle layers per quarter section divided by four cords).

Worms are most frequently found in the lumen of the appendix where they fail to elicit an inflammatory response, except for mild mucosal eosinophilia (fig. 10-56) (1002). Severe infections cause pathologic lesions in the colon, cecum, appendix, and lower ileum. The usual manifestations include superficial ulceration, petechial hemorrhages, and sometimes mucosal or submucosal abscesses (993,1002). The

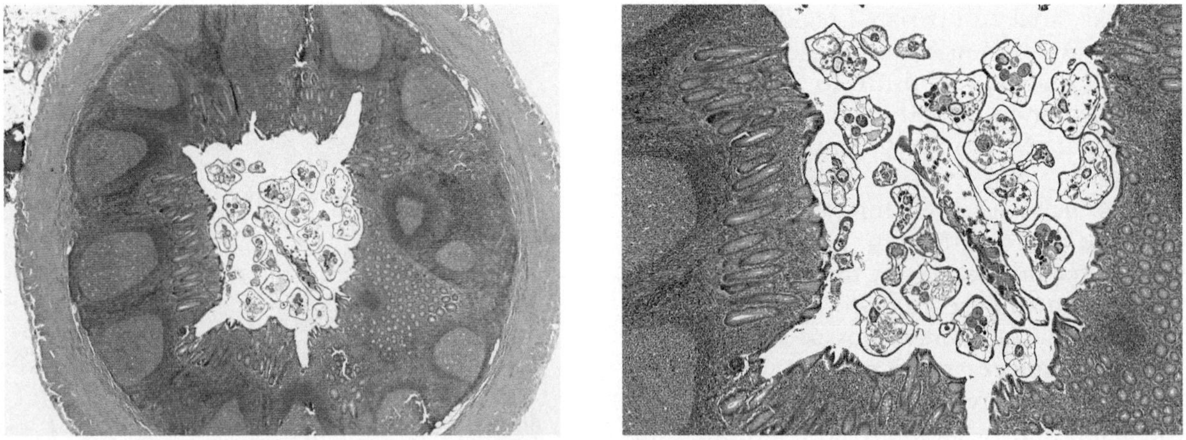

Figure 10-56

ENTEROBIUS VERMICULARIS

Left: Cross sections of numerous *E. vermicularis* organisms in the appendiceal lumen of a child.

Right: Higher-power view shows worms without any associated reaction in the adjacent appendiceal mucosa. (Both figures courtesy of the Division of Gastrointestinal Pathology, Armed Forces Institute of Pathology, Washington, DC.)

parasite only rarely invades the mucosa, but when it does, granulomas form. A rim of granulation tissue, enclosed by a fibrous capsule, surrounds an eosinophilic center. Eosinophils, lymphocytes, giant cells, and Charcot-Leyden crystals infiltrate the granulomas. The granulomas eventually fibrose and hyalinize, and may form obstructive masses when located in the appendix. Rarely, *Enterobius* is a cause of eosinophilic colitis (1001). In some cases, the adult worms migrate into the peritoneum and omentum, where they induce a foreign body inflammatory reaction.

Special Techniques. Conventional stool examination for ova frequently misses the diagnosis. The best method of demonstrating the eggs is to apply clear cellophane tape to the perineum and then place it sticky side down on a microscope slide under low power, examining it for the eggs. The optimum time for applying the tape is early in the morning before the patient has bathed or defecated or when the child is awakened by itching. Three cellophane tapes are sufficient for diagnosis in over 90 percent of cases.

Treatment and Prognosis. Asymptomatic patients do not need treatment. If patients are taught appropriate hygiene to eliminate the risk of autoinfection, the infection becomes self-limited. Symptomatic patients are treated with pyrantel pamoate given as a single dose of 11 mg/kg to a maximum of 1 g (994) or a single dose of 100 mg of mebendazole given orally. Family members of the affected individual should be treated as well since it is likely that they also harbor the organism.

Prevention. Personal cleanliness is the most effective means of prevention. Hands should be frequently washed and the fingernails should be cut short. Infected children should sleep alone and wear tight-fitting pajamas that discourage direct finger contact with the perianal region.

Trichuris Infections

Demography. *Trichuriasis,* caused by the whipworm, *Trichuris trichiura*, is most common in warm, moist, tropical and subtropical regions, but it also occurs in temperate areas. It is estimated to infect over 1 billion persons worldwide (1005a), including 114 million preschool age children and 233 million children ages 5 to 14 years (1005). In the United States, *Trichuris* is found in rural communities of the South. Humans are the principal host for the organism, although it may also infect pigs, lemurs, and monkeys (1007,1012). Another species of *Trichuris*, *T. vulpis*, infects dogs, and has been reported in humans as well (1009). Humans acquire trichuriasis by ingesting embryonated eggs from contaminated hands, soil, food, and water.

Etiology. *T. trichiura* worms are found in the large intestine with their anterior ends deeply

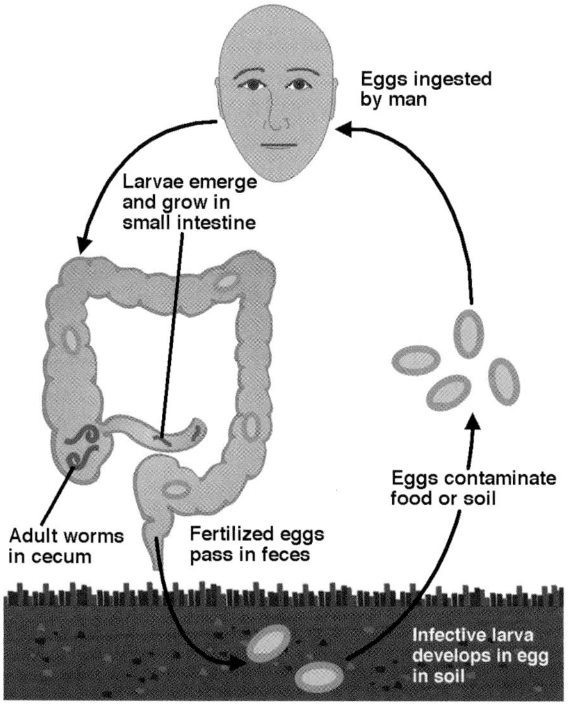

Figure 10-57

DIAGRAM OF THE LIFE CYCLE OF *TRICHURIS*

embedded in the mucosa. The males measure 3.0 to 4.5 cm in length and have a coiled posterior end. The females are 3.5 to 5.0 cm and possess a blunt posterior end. Usually the worms are found in the cecum, with their slender whip-like anterior portion buried in the mucosa. In severe infections, they can be found throughout the large intestine and occasionally in the appendix and terminal ileum. The bile-stained eggs measure 50 to 54 x 22 to 23 µm and have a characteristic bipolar barrel shape with a three-layer shell. The eggs must incubate at least 3 weeks in soil under the proper conditions before the infective larvae emerge (1011). *Trichuris* eggs are sensitive to desiccation and a combination of heat and low humidity is detrimental to their survival. Exposure to sunlight kills them.

The life cycle of *Trichuris* is shown in figure 10-57. After ingestion, eggs pass through the stomach and hatch in the small intestine, where the larvae embed themselves in the intestinal villi. They temporarily penetrate the crypts of Lieberkuhn where they feed and develop further. Gradually, the immature worms make their way to the cecum. They then migrate to the large intestine where they mature into adults in about 30 to 90 days. The slender heads embed themselves into the crypts. Here, the adults mate and the females eventually produce 3,000 to 7,000 eggs daily. In severe infections, worms may be found in sites other than the cecum including the wall of the appendix, terminal ileum, and rectum (1011).

Clinical Features. The severity and consequences of *Trichuris* infection vary widely, depending on the parasite burden, site of infection, and state of the host including age, general health, iron reserves, and history of previous exposure to the organism (1006,1010). Patients with mild infection remain asymptomatic. Moderate infection results in diarrhea, abdominal pain, nausea and vomiting. Severe infections may result in *Trichuris dysentery syndrome*, a condition associated with mucus and bloody diarrhea, tenesmus, abdominal pain, nausea, vomiting, anorexia, dehydration, and weight loss. Rectal prolapse commonly accompanies severe infections. In addition, volvulus or intussusception may occur. Large aggregates of worms can obstruct the appendiceal lumen and cause appendicitis. Peripheral eosinophilia is common.

Gross Findings. The worms burrow into the walls of the small intestine, producing eosinophilic granulomatous lesions that are associated with edema, and thickening and induration of the bowel wall. In cases of rectal prolapse or in patients undergoing endoscopic examination, the worms can be visualized directly (fig. 10-58). Endoscopy also demonstrates the presence of the inflammatory changes.

Microscopic Findings. In many cases, the parasites only elicit minor histologic changes (1008). In some patients, however, the whipworm produces a small inflammatory reaction at the site of its attachment to the colonic mucosa. This may be associated with superficial mucosal erosions and colitis (1004). Acute inflammatory lesions contain neutrophils and eosinophils; more advanced lesions form granulomas with central necrosis and a peripheral zone of macrophages, multinucleated giant cells, and other inflammatory cells.

Differential Diagnosis. The infected bowel appears edematous and diffusely thickened,

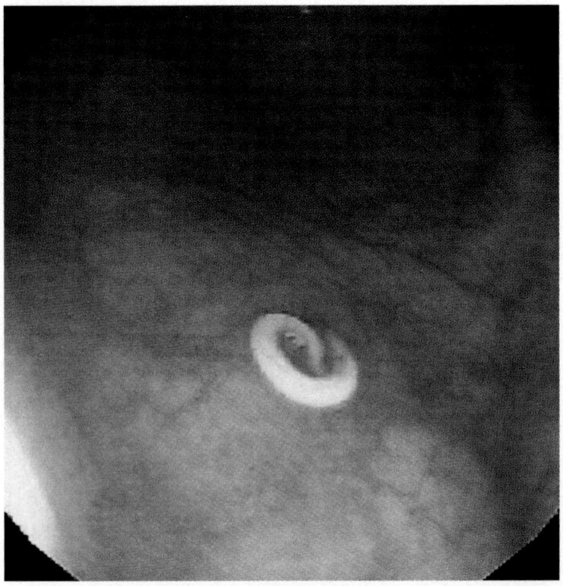

Figure 10-58

TRICHURIS TRICHIURA

The size and appearance of this worm suggest whipworm infection. (Fig. 4-43 from Emory TS, Carpenter HA, Gostout CJ, Sobin LH. Atlas of gastrointestinal endoscopy & endoscopic biopsies. Washington D.C.: Armed Forces Institute of Pathology; 2000:301.)

grossly resembling Crohn's disease. The differential diagnosis also includes other helminth infections.

Treatment and Prognosis. Patients are treated with 100 mg of mebendazole given two times a day for 3 days. The cure rate is approximately 80 percent with this treatment and in those who are not completely cured, there is a marked reduction in worm burden (1013). Albendazole is also effective (1011).

Strongyloides Infections

Demography. *Strongyloidiasis* is estimated to affect from 30 to 100 million people worldwide (1019,1022). The disease is caused by two species of *Strongyloides*, *S. stercoralis* and *S. fuelleborni*. The most common species, *S. stercoralis*, occurs worldwide, but is more common in tropical and subtropical areas. In the United States, it is endemic in Kentucky and eastern Tennessee (1014, 1028,1038); endemic areas are also present in central and southern Europe (1033). *S. fuelleborni* occurs sporadically in Africa and Papua New Guinea (1019,1020,1026).

Disseminated hyperinfection affects individuals with compromised T-cell immunity associated with steroid use, neoplasms, malnutrition, aging, or AIDS. Outbreaks occur in mental institutions and certain urban areas. The disease may also be venereally transmitted (1032).

Etiology. *Strongyloides* is a small nematode measuring 2.0 x 2.0 x 0.4 mm that exists as both a free-living organism and as a tissue parasite within the mucosa of the duodenum or upper jejunum. Strongyloidiasis occurs in one of three major ways (fig. 10-59). In the direct development cycle, rhabditiform larvae that are present in feces develop in the soil into infective filariform larvae that then infect man by penetrating the skin. In the indirect developmental cycle, the rhabditiform larvae undergo several molts in the soil and subsequently mature into free-living adult organisms. Under favorable environmental conditions, this cycle is self-perpetuating. In the autoinfection cycle, rhabditiform larvae convert into infective filariform larvae within the host intestine or on the perianal skin and invade the host directly. This particularly occurs in well-established infections.

The rhabditiform larvae (200 to 300 µm in length) are found in soil contaminated by human feces, where they go through four stages to become male (0.7 mm in length) and female (1 to 2 mm in length) adults. If the climatic conditions are unfavorable, these larvae change directly into filariform or strongyloid larvae, measuring approximately 400 µm in length. They cannot survive for more than a few weeks in the external environment but they can continue development in man. The filariform larvae penetrate the skin where they enter blood vessels and travel to the lung. In the lung, they pass through the alveolar spaces. The adolescent worms migrate into the bronchi, trachea, larynx, and esophagus, where they are swallowed. They mature into adults in the intestine, usually in the duodenum and jejunum. After having fertilized the females, the males are rapidly expelled with the feces while the females penetrate the intestinal mucosa. Here, they deposit up to 30 eggs a day that develop into rhabditiform larvae. The rhabditiform larvae burrow out of the mucosa, into the intestinal lumen, and are excreted with the feces. Alternatively, the rhabditiform larvae may transform into

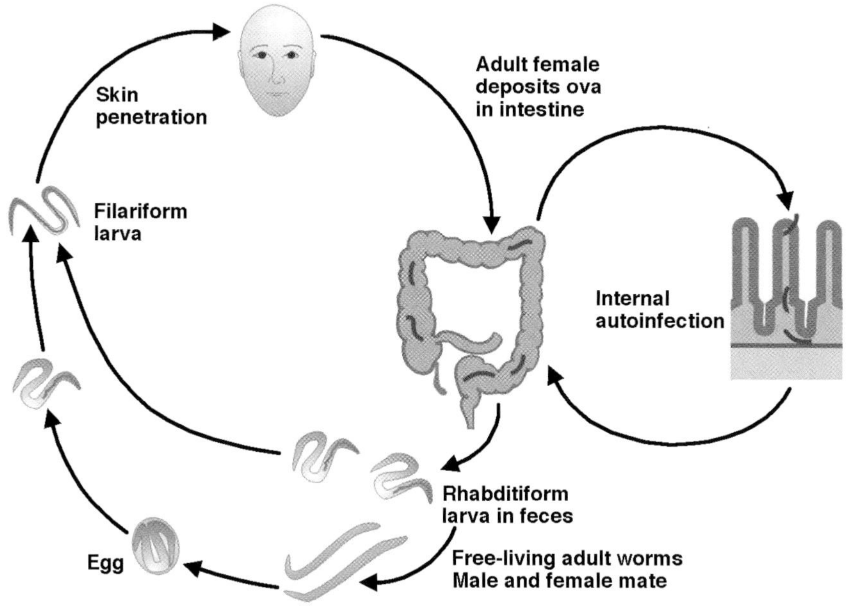

Figure 10-59

DIAGRAM OF THE LIFE CYCLE OF *STRONGYLOIDES*

filariform larvae within 24 hours and then reinvade the host either through the intestinal mucosa (internal autoinfestation) or through the perianal skin (external autoinfestation).

Pathophysiology. The adult form typically lives in the small bowel but autoinfection can affect the large bowel, especially when infestation is heavy. Chronic infection results from the host's inability to eliminate the adult worms from the small bowel, to prevent colonic reinfection by filariform larvae, and to destroy larvae that are in transit back to the intestine. The pathogenesis of strongyloidiasis is related to the host-parasite relationship. Cellular immunity plays an important role in keeping the parasite under control. When cellular immunity is disrupted, the parasite can multiply internally and disseminate.

Clinical Features. The clinical symptoms of *Strongyloides* infection are variable, ranging from asymptomatic cases to severe, debilitating disease. Four basic clinical syndromes occur: acute strongyloidiasis, chronic strongyloidiasis, hyperinfection, and disseminated disease. In acute disease, the earliest manifestation is a pruritic erythematous rash at the site of filariform larval penetration. Some patients develop urticarial lesions. Migration of the larvae through the pulmonary alveoli may result in cough. Tracheal irritation simulating bronchitis also occurs. Gastrointestinal symptoms begin approximately 2 weeks after the initial infection and include diarrhea, abdominal discomfort, bloating, and anorexia (1014,1020,1026).

Chronic strongyloidiasis is usually asymptomatic. Some patients, however, may exhibit intermittent gastrointestinal symptoms such as vomiting, diarrhea, constipation, and borborygmus. Pruritus ani, urticaria, and rash are also common (1031). Recurrent asthma and nephrotic syndrome have been reported (1027,1029,1034,1037,1039).

Hyperinfection is a term that describes a syndrome of accelerated autoinfection that commonly, though not always, is the result of a change in immune status. Patients who were previously asymptomatic may develop gastrointestinal or pulmonary symptoms. Symptomatic patients may experience an exacerbation of their symptoms. Larvae are increased in number, but dissemination beyond the gastrointestinal or respiratory tract does not occur. In such severe infections, patients may experience upper and lower intestinal bleeding, jejunal perforation, ileus, and bowel obstruction (1016,1018,1023, 1030,1036). Malabsorption also occurs. Some patients may develop protein-losing enteropathy leading to hypoalbuminemia, peripheral edema, and ascites (1021,1024).

Extraintestinal manifestations occur in disseminated disease, and include pneumonia, sepsis, meningitis, and brain abscess. Marked peripheral eosinophilia is common but can be absent in patients with overwhelming infections.

Figure 10-60

STRONGYLOIDIASIS

Adult female worms lie within the crypts of the small intestine. (Courtesy of the Division of Gastrointestinal Pathology, Armed Forces Institute of Pathology, Washington, DC.)

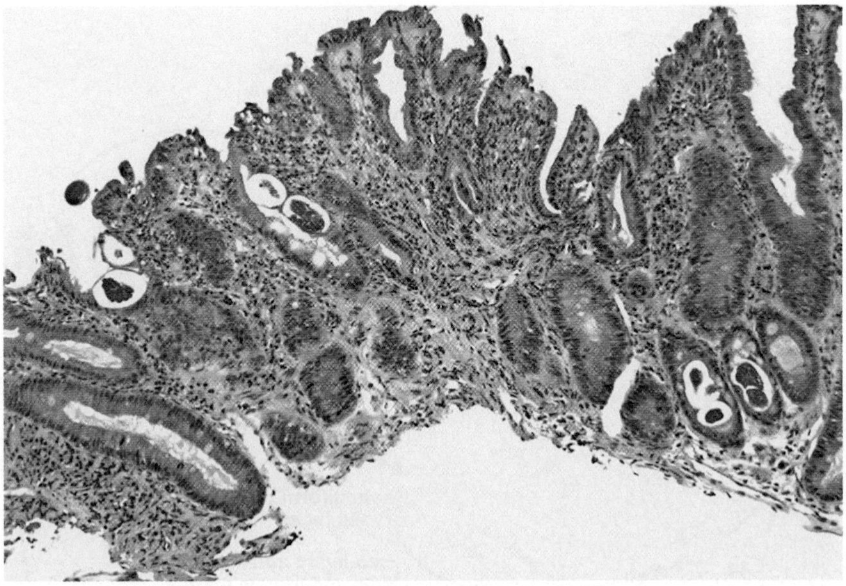

Gross Findings. Most filariform larvae lie within the intestinal lymphatics, and they concentrate in the mesenteric and retroperitoneal lymph nodes. The intestines acquire a dusky red-purple color and a granular mucosa. In patients with well-developed enteritis, the bowel appears grossly thickened, with flattened mucosal folds due to the presence of submucosal edema. Hemorrhagic and ragged mucosal surfaces are covered by friable, greenish tan pseudomembranes. Sigmoidoscopy and colonoscopy may help establish the diagnosis. Erythema, ulcerations, hemorrhage, and rarely, polyps are present along with aphthoid erosions (1015,1035).

Microscopic Findings. Rhabditiform larvae are usually identified in the crypts and the submucosa of the duodenum. They measure 400 μm in length and 20 to 25 μm in width, and are characterized by a short buccal cavity, bulbar esophagus, and longer intestine. Adult female worms may also be seen in the crypts (fig. 10-60). The mucosa may become edematous and usually contains cellular infiltrates composed of numerous eosinophils and mononuclear cells (fig. 10-61). Reactions around the worms may be seen in the lamina propria. Necrotizing granulomas may also be present. In severe cases, mucosal atrophy, villous flattening, and, in long-standing infections, fibrosis with ulceration may be present. Most acute lesions affect the small intestine but similar changes are also seen in the stomach and colon.

In immunocompromised patients, there may be edema, hyperemia, and scattered ulcerations of the bowel. Granulomas are less well developed and Langerhans giant cells are rare. In severe disease, there may be diffuse ulceration of the large bowel with edema and hemorrhage; gravid female worms may be seen nestled in the mucosa as low in the gastrointestinal tract as the colon. The appendix is a frequent site of larval penetration but appendicitis is rare.

Special Techniques. The parasitologic diagnosis of strongyloidiasis requires the detection of *S. stercoralis* larvae or adults in feces, sputum, or duodenal aspirates. It may be necessary to examine several specimens due to the low number of larvae present. In 10 to 30 percent of patients, sampling of duodenal contents by the string test or endoscopic duodenal aspiration may be needed to demonstrate the organism. A clinical diagnosis is suggested by the presence of eosinophilia and a history of travel to an endemic area. In disseminated disease, parasites may be found in unusual sites including sputum, bronchoalveolar lavage fluid, cerebrospinal fluid, ascites fluid, or urine.

Serologic tests or Western blot analysis also detects the disease. Serologic tests for *Strongyloides* are particularly helpful, since extensive stool microscopy fails to detect the disease in a significant number of patients (1031).

Differential Diagnosis. The rhabditiform larvae of *S. stercoralis* must be differentiated from

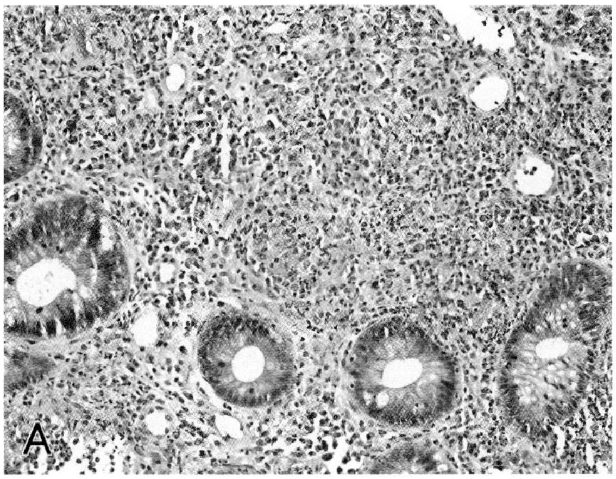

Figure 10-61

STRONGYLOIDIASIS

A: The lamina propria of the colonic mucosa has a dense infiltrate composed of lymphocytes, plasma cells, and numerous eosinophils. A somewhat ill-defined granuloma is also present.

B: Higher-power view shows a granuloma with a surrounding intense eosinophilic infiltrate.

C: A *Strongyloides* larva is present within the lamina propria. The organism is surrounded by numerous eosinophils.

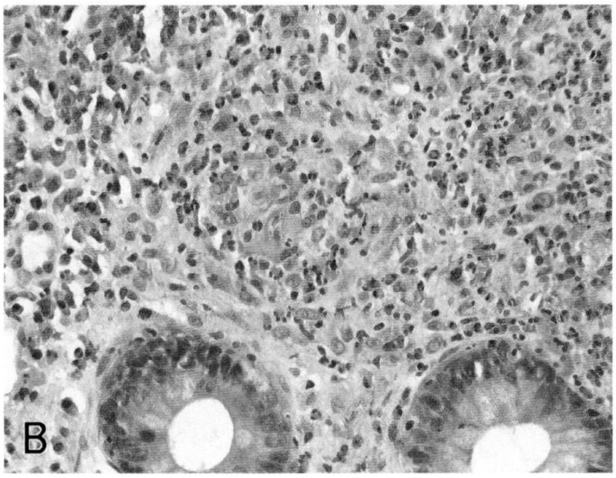

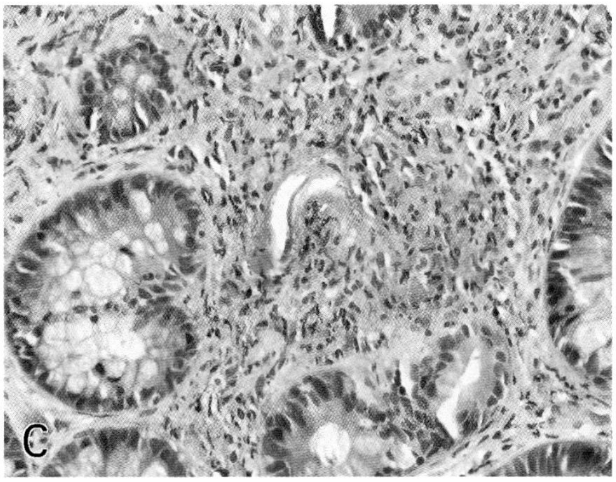

those of hookworm and other nematodes. They can be distinguished by noting either the short buccal cavity and large genital primordium of the rhabditiform larvae of *S. stercoralis* or the long buccal cavity of hookworm larvae. The filariform larvae of *S. stercoralis* have a notch in the tail that differentiates them from hookworms and other larvae.

Eosinophilic gastroenteritis is a disorder often in the differential diagnosis of patients with strongyloidiasis. Eosinophilic enteritis shows mild villous blunting with increased numbers of eosinophils and mononuclear cells in the lamina propria and epithelium. Parasites, however, are absent. Crohn's disease also shows mucosal eosinophils but there are usually signs of more extensive damage, including the presence of ulcers and strictures, as well as occasional granulomas. Crohn's disease often concentrates in the distal ileum and colon, while intestinal strongyloidiasis most often involves the duodenum and jejunum.

Treatment and Prognosis. Because there is a risk of disseminated disease, strongyloidiasis should be treated (1020,1026). Immunocompetent patients with uncomplicated infections are treated with thiabendazole, 20 mg/kg orally twice a day for 2 days (1020,1040). This treatment can be repeated, since it is only effective in approximately two thirds of patients. Retreatment is often necessary. Side effects of thiabendazole include nausea, vomiting, malaise, dizziness, and headache. Albendazole and ivermectin are alternative choices (1013a,1026). Ivermectin is recommended for the treatment of patients with disseminated disease (1017). Sometimes, antibiotics are given to treat concomitant bacterial infections. Even with treatment, disseminated disease frequently results in patient death. Mortality rates due to hyperinfection or disseminated disease are as high as 87 percent (1025).

Angiostrongylus Infections

Demography. *Angiostrongylus* is a nematode that is prevalent in Central and South America from Mexico to Argentina. The disease predominantly affects children, usually boys; most cases occur during the rainy season (1043,1047,1049). Humans appear to be accidental hosts to the organism, and the mode by which the infection is acquired is unknown (1045).

Etiology. *Angiostrongylus* (*Parastrongylus*) (1054) *costaricensis* is a metastrongyloid intestinal nematode found primarily in snails and veronicellid slugs, the obligatory intermediate hosts, and in rodents, the definitive hosts (1049). Man is an accidental host. It is thought that human infections occur when persons ingest vegetables contaminated with third-stage larvae from infected slugs (1045,1049). The time interval from the possible date of ingestion to onset of symptoms is 14 days to several months, or even years (1051,1052,1055).

In rodents, larvae penetrate the gastrointestinal wall and mature in lymphatics and lymph nodes to migrate through the vasculature of the ileocecal region. Adult worms are found in cecal and mesenteric arteries of the definitive hosts and other rodent species. Fertilized eggs embolize to the capillary endothelium where they penetrate and occupy the subendothelium in the submucosal regions. The eggs embryonate and first-stage larvae hatch from the eggs, migrate through the mucosa, and pass into the lumen to be excreted into the feces. In humans, however, the eggs degenerate in the intestinal wall, inciting a granulomatous reaction. Snails and veronicellid slugs, the obligatory intermediate hosts, ingest the larvae in rodent feces. The ingested first-stage larvae develop in the digestive tract of the mollusk into second- and third-stage larvae, which are infectious to certain rodents, monkeys, and humans.

Clinical Features. Angiostrongyliasis causes a highly symptomatic eosinophilic gastroenteritis involving the terminal ileum, cecum, appendix, and ascending colon (1050,1056). The clinical presentation often mimics acute appendicitis or other intra-abdominal emergency lesions and as a result, surgery is performed. Right lower quadrant pain and fever are the main symptoms but nausea, vomiting, diarrhea, or constipation also occur. A palpable mass may be present. Perforation, obstruction, or gastrointestinal bleeding may result (1043,1044,1047,1052).

On physical examination, the abdomen is usually tender in the right lower quadrant, and signs of peritonitis may be elicited. Rectal examination can be painful. Patients exhibit peripheral leukocytosis and eosinophilia. Occasionally patients are ill for months with relapsing episodes of abdominal pain (1044).

Gross Findings. Pathologic changes are usually seen in the cecum, appendix, and terminal ileum. Yellow granulomas in the subserosa, associated with edema and rigidity of the intestinal wall, are common findings. The appendix is often inflamed and may be perforated. Patients may present with gangrenous ischemic enterocolitis or ileitis, sometimes with perforation (1056). In such cases, the intestinal wall appears thickened. Multiple confluent ulcers, some of which perforate, can be observed, particularly in the terminal ileum.

Microscopic Findings. *A. costaricensis* causes an intense, eosinophilic, necrotizing arteritis associated with thrombosis, which leads to severe ischemic necrosis and infarction (1044, 1046). An intense eosinophilic inflammatory infiltrate involves the entire thickness of the intestinal wall. Perforation may occur (1056). Dead organisms may be found in the wall. The worms are characterized morphologically by a thin (2- to 3-μm) keratin cuticle, a lack of lateral cords, and intestines lined by cuboidal to low columnar cells. The worms typically lie within arterial lumens (1056). Eggs are ovoid, usually lying within the submucosa, and possess thin, pale, eosinophilic shells. Eosinophilic granulomas may surround eggs and larvae.

Special Techniques. Larvae and eggs are not found in the stool. In some cases, serologic tests are available.

Differential Diagnosis. The differential diagnosis includes *Trichuris trichiura*, another organism that often lies in the cecum. *Trichuris* adult worms embed within crypts, and are not seen within vascular structures. Gastrointestinal schistosomiasis may also affect this region. Adult *Schistosoma* organisms, however, are typically found in the venous system, not in the arteries. Like *Angiostrongylus*, *Schistosoma* ova may produce granulomas that progress to fibrosis. Anisakid larvae may be similar in size to the adults of *A. costaricensis,* but are distinguished by their thick multilayered cuticles, large Y-shaped lateral cords, and intestines lined by tall columnar cells (1042). Finally, angiostrongyliasis may mimic Crohn's disease (1046).

Treatment and Prognosis. The treatment of *A. costaricensis* infections is often surgical. In some cases, surgery is performed because the patient presents with what clinically appears to be appendicitis. No drug is currently available for the treatment of abdominal angiostrongyliasis. Although vermicidal agents do exist, there is significant concern about the possibility of inducing greater harm to the patient if worms die in their intravascular location (1041,1048,1053). The case-fatality rate among symptomatic patients ranges from 1.8 to 7.4 percent (1044,1047).

Capillaria Philippinensis Infections

Demography. Persons infected with *Capillaria philippinensis* often live in the Philippines and Thailand, where it is common to eat raw freshwater fish. It is also reported in Japan, Korea, Taiwan, Iran, Egypt, the United Arab Emirates, and India (1059,1062,1064–1067). Approximately 2,000 cases have been described. The parasites typically inhabit the mucosa of the small intestine, with the jejunum being the most heavily infiltrated site.

Etiology. *C. philippinensis* is a tiny nematode closely related to *Trichuris* and *Trichinella* species. A fish-bird cycle plays a role in the infection. Male worms measure 1.5 to 3.0 mm in length and females measure 2.5 to 5.0 mm in length. *C. philippinensis* has a long stichosome, which consists of stichocytes surrounding the esophageal tube, with a thin anterior end. The posterior portion of the worm is wider and contains intestines and reproductive organs. Females range in length from 2.5 to 5.3 mm. The vulva is at the end of the stichosome and the uterus may contain thick-shelled bioperculated eggs with a mucoid coat, thin-shelled eggs with a mucoid coat, or embryos. The organism is diagnosed by finding the characteristic ova. The barrel-shaped eggs have flattened bipolar plugs and fully developed larvae. The eggs of *C. philippinensis* average 36 x 19 to 45 x 21 µm, and they resemble those of *Trichuris trichiura.*

Eggs passed in the feces reach the water by indiscriminate defecation in or near water or in fields from which feces are washed into water bodies by torrential tropical rains. The eggs embryonate in water in 5 to 10 days and hatch after ingestion by small freshwater fish. The larvae emerge and grow into infective forms in 3 weeks. When the fish is eaten raw, *C. philippinensis* larvae mature into adult males and females in 12 to 14 days in the small intestine. After mating, the females produce larvae and they in turn mature and the second generation of females produce eggs that pass in the feces. Autoinfection continues by means of a few larviparous female worms that are always present, resulting in hyperinfection.

Clinical Features. *Capillaria* causes diarrhea and malabsorption (1061,1062). Disease onset is acute, with severe malabsorption and 35 percent mortality. Initially, patients present with borborygmus, with or without abdominal pain. Weeks or a month later, patients develop voluminous watery stools passed 5 to 10 times/day, malaise, anorexia, nausea, and vomiting (1057, 1058,1060,1063). There is widespread malabsorption. Patients exhibit hypokalemia, hypocalcemia, hypoproteinemia, and protein-losing enteropathy. The disease progresses over months and the patients exhibit muscle wasting, weakness, hypotension, cardiac abnormalities, abdominal distension, tenderness, edema, anasarca, or hyporeflexia. Patients may die of extreme malnutrition, dehydration, or secondary bacterial infections. The period between symptom onset and death is usually 2 to 3 months.

Gross Findings. The worms inhabit both the large and small intestines, although they are primarily located in the jejunum. Grossly, the small intestine appears thickened, indurated, and hyperemic, and contains large amounts of fluid. Thousands of adult worms, larvae, and ova are seen within the jejunum and the upper portion of the ileum; occasionally, they are seen in the duodenum, and less frequently, in the stomach, esophagus, and colon. Patients with severe infections have many worms embedded in the small bowel mucosa. Barium examinations show diffuse involvement of the small bowel with loss of the normal mucosal pattern, narrowing of the lumen, and separation of the bowel loops.

Microscopic Findings. The worms enter the crypts which subsequently become atrophic. The villi appear flattened, mucosal glands are denuded, and the lamina propria becomes infiltrated with plasma cells, lymphocytes, macrophages, neutrophils, and eosinophils. Histologically, parasites are seen in the intestinal lumen, within the crypts of Lieberkuhn, and in the lamina propria.

Special Techniques. The diagnosis is made by identification of *C. philippinensis* eggs, larvae, or adults in the feces. The parasite is also found in aspirates or biopsies of the duodenum and jejunum. Repeat stool examinations may be required. The eggs are 36 to 45 x 21 µm, have a characteristic shape, bipolar plugs, and a mucoid coat. They must be differentiated from the eggs of *T. trichiura*.

Treatment and Prognosis. In severe cases, treatment consists of electrolyte replacement and antidiarrheal medications. The antihelminthics thiabendazole, mebendazole, or albendazole eliminate the organism. Parasites disappear from the stools in 3 to 4 days and most patients are asymptomatic after a week. Long-term treatment with effective antihelminthics is required because of the worms' ability to multiply in the host. Relapses result from incomplete treatment.

Tapeworm Infections

Definition. Tapeworms are ribbon-shaped, segmented, hermaphroditic, cestode worms that inhabit the intestinal tract of many species. *Taeniasis* is an infection caused by adult tapeworms belonging to the family Taeniidae, particularly *Taenia solium* (pork tapeworm) and *T. saginata* (beef tapeworm). These worms lack a digestive tract and absorb their food through their integument. The worm's body is divided into three regions: scolex or head, neck, and strobila, which consists of immature, mature, and gravid proglottids or segments. *Cysticercosis* is the term used to denote infections by the larval stage of *T. solium* or *T. saginata*.

Demography. Taeniasis has a worldwide distribution. Most cases of cysticercosis result from fecal contamination of food and water, related to poor hygiene and poverty. Therefore cysticercosis is most commonly seen in lower socioeconomic classes in Latin America, Eastern Europe, India, Pakistan, Indonesia, and China. The incidence of this disorder has increased with migration of infected individuals (1074). Infections of *T. solium* are problems in Mexico and other Latin American countries, parts of Europe, China, India, and Africa. They are rare in the United States. *T. saginata* infection is highly prevalent in parts of Europe, Africa, and Asia, and is occasionally reported in the United States.

Infections are associated with eating raw pork and beef. Steak tartare (raw ground beef) is a favorite dish in Europe and America, as is raw pork in Southeast Asia. In Taiwan, *T. saginata* infections are also acquired by eating wild boar and some strains of domestic pig.

Diphyllobothrium latum and other *Diphyllobothrium* species are fish tapeworms that are acquired by humans through consumption of raw fish. Diphyllobothriasis occurs worldwide, and is commonly reported in Russia and parts of Japan (1069). Commonly implicated fish include salmon, whitefish, rainbow trout, pike, perch, turbot, and ruff (1073).

Hymenolepis nana, the dwarf tapeworm, and *H. diminuta*, the rat tapeworm, parasitize both rodents and humans, and insects serve as their intermediate host. *H. nana* has a cosmopolitan distribution but is more common in warm climates (1068). It is the most common autochthonously acquired tapeworm infection in the United States. Most infections occur in the southern states, and are more common in children and institutionalized patients. The infection spreads by an oral-fecal route. Feces of infected children and rats are the usual reservoirs. In some countries, 25 percent of people in rural populations have *H. nana* infection, presumably due to drinking of contaminated water. *H. nana* is unique in that this parasite can be transmitted directly by the egg or by ingestion of fleas or beetles infected with larval cysticercoids.

Etiology. Species that commonly infect humans in the West include the beef tapeworm, *T. saginata;* the pork tapeworm, *T. solium*; and the fish tapeworm, *D. latum*. Adult *T. saginata*, *T. solium*, and *D. latum* are among the largest parasites to infect humans. *T. saginata* measures 1 to 4 meters in length whereas *T. solium* measures 2 to 4 meters. *T. saginata* may have 1,000 to 2,000 proglottids but *T. solium* has less than 1,000. The number of uterine branches in the gravid proglottids differs in the two worms, with those of *T. saginata* being more than12 and those of *T. solium* being less than12. The scolex of a *T. solium* worm has a rostellum armed with rows of hooklets. The rostellum is lacking in *T. saginata* but the scolex of both has four suckers. The two species of *Taenia* produce eggs indistinguishable from one another. The eggs are round, measure 30 to 40 µm in diameter, and have a thick, radially striated shell containing an embryo with six hooklets. The eggs are passed individually in feces or in gravid proglottids that detach from the strobilae and pass from the host. When ingested by intermediate hosts, the eggs hatch and hexacanth embryos or oncospheres migrate to the muscles of the animal. These larvae subsequently develop into fluid-filled, translucent cysts with an invaginated scolex, termed cysticerci. When humans eat the infected beef or pork, raw or uncooked, the cysticercus ruptures in the small intestine and the scolex everts and attaches to the mucosa. The parasites reach sexual maturity and egg production begins in 10 to 12 weeks. These parasites may live in the intestines for as long as 20 years.

D. latum is the largest cestode to infect humans, measuring 2 to 15 meters in length and a maximum of 20 mm in width. The scolex or bothrium is 2 x 1 mm and has dorsal and ventral sucking grooves that serve to attach the worm to the intestinal wall. The strobila has 4,000 proglottids, each with gravid proglottids having male and female sex organs and uteri filled with eggs. The uterine pore is midventral and discharges eggs continuously. Eggs passed in the feces reach cool, fresh water and mature in 10 to 14 days into a ciliated hexacanth larva called a coracidium. The coracidium leaves the egg through the opened operculum and swims freely in the water until ingested by the first intermediate host, a crustacean species, the copepod. It develops into a procercoid larva in the body cavity of the copepod. The infected copepod is then eaten by a fish, the second intermediate host. The procercoid larva migrates from the fish intestines to the muscles and develops into a plerocercoid larva, or sparganum. When the fish is eaten raw by the final host, the plerocercoid larva develops into an adult in the intestine in 3 to 5 weeks and produces large numbers of eggs. The worms are known to live in humans for 10 years or more.

H. nana is the smallest tapeworm infecting man, measuring 1 to 4 cm in length and 1 mm in width. Its scolex has four suckers and an armed rostellum. Approximately 200 proglottids are present which are characterized by their three globular testes. The eggs are oval or spherical and measure 30 to 40 µm in diameter. When the eggs of *H. nana* are ingested by a final host, the oncospheres are released in the small intestine where they burrow into the villi and develop into cysticercoids in 4 days. In about 2 weeks, the larvae reenter the intestinal lumen and attach to the intestinal wall where they become adult worms within the next 2 weeks. Some eggs released by the adult worms hatch in the intestine resulting in autoinfection.

Pathophysiology. All tapeworms are parasitic. They spend their adult lives in the small intestinal lumen of the host. Mucosal attachment occurs via suction cups or grooves located on the head or scolex. The various species of tapeworms are distinguished by counting the number of teeth or cutting plates on the buccal cavity. Behind the scolex is a short neck, from which proglottids develop to form the chain-like strobila of the worm. As each proglottid becomes gravid, eggs are released. Adult worms produce up to 20,000 eggs/day, which disseminate into the environment via stool. Once stuck to the mucosa, the worms suck blood from it. The amount of blood lost varies with the parasite species. Since the worms lack a gastrointestinal tract, adults absorb predigested food across the tegumental surface of each segment. Elimination of *Hymenolepis,* for instance, involves actions by mast cells and hyperplastic goblet cells, with histamine and mucus each playing defensive roles (1072). The goblet cell hyperplasia requires an intact immune system, particularly T cells. Increased mucus from hyperplastic goblet cells entraps the worms, restricting their attachment and expediting their expulsion by peristalsis.

Clinical Features. Usually only one tapeworm is present in the intestine but occasionally two or more are found. Most infected individuals remain asymptomatic and are unaware of the infection until spontaneous passage of proglottids occurs through the anus or in the feces. The most common symptom is intense perianal itching. Abdominal pain, nausea, anorexia or increased appetite, weight loss, headache, and constipation or diarrhea may be present. Abdominal pain and nausea are usually more common in the morning and are relieved by eating breakfast. Allergic manifestations include urticaria, pruritus, or other skin conditions; eosinophilia; and elevated IgE levels. The worms also cause intestinal, appendiceal, biliary, or pancreatic obstruction. *T. solium* may survive 25 years and *T. saginata* 10 years. Therefore, symptomatic patients may have a protracted clinical course.

The major clinical manifestations associated with diphyllobothriasis are diarrhea and pernicious anemia (1070). The parasite splits the vitamin B12 intrinsic factor complex, thereby preventing vitamin B12 absorption by the host.

Most patients with *H. nana* infection remain asymptomatic or have only mild symptoms. Severe infections cause headaches, dizziness, diarrhea, abdominal distress, restlessness, and sometimes convulsions. The clinical manifestations are probably the result of local irritation and absorption of toxic byproducts produced by the parasite.

Gross Findings. Sometimes the worm is found in the intestinal lumen. It measures meters in length. *T. saginata* can be detected on X-ray films of the small bowel as a long, translucent filling defect (1071). Most patients with *D. latum* infection have the parasites in the jejunum. More than one worm can be detected.

Microscopic Findings. The pathologic features of the intestines in taeniasis are rarely described. Much more commonly described are the features of cysticercosis. The adult worms apparently do not seriously damage the gastrointestinal tract except for some superficial damage to the lining mucosa at the site of parasitic attachment (1068). Attachment of the scolex, especially that of *T. solium*, may cause local irritation. The infections cause crypt hyperplasia and a significant increase in the number of endocrine cells. Developing *H. nana* cysticercoids damage villi and large numbers invading the tissue are responsible for enteritis.

Special Techniques. Diagnosing tapeworm infection requires identification of the proglottids or eggs in the stool. The eggs of the various *Taenia* species resemble one another and are thus not diagnostic of a species. Therefore, the gravid segments or the scolex must be examined for characteristic morphologic features. The finding of white, often motile, 1- to 2-cm proglottids passing out of the anus also confirms the diagnosis. Eggs are present in feces and can be detected microscopically, either directly or after concentration of fecal samples. Perianal specimens on cellophane tape swabs may reveal the eggs.

Treatment and Prognosis. The drug of choice for the treatment of *Taenia* infection is praziquantel given after a light meal. *T. saginata* may also be treated with niclosamide, which can result in complete relief of abdominal symptoms within a short period of time (1071). Diphyllobothriasis is treated with antihelminthic agents. This causes a disappearance of the diarrhea and the pernicious anemia. The stool should be examined for the scolex. If the scolex is not removed, the strobila can regenerate and the parasite may become reestablished.

Trematode Infections

Demography. Several species of trematodes infect humans including those belonging to the genera *Fasciolopsis* and *Heterophyes*. *Fasciolopsis* species infect both humans and pigs, and occur most commonly in parts of India and Southeast Asia. Feces from the host reach water bodies containing planorbid snails and freshwater plants. Among these plants are water chestnuts, water bamboo, water lily, water hyacinth, and watercress, and any can be the source of infection if uncooked.

A number of tiny trematodes of the genus *Heterophyes* infect humans but the most common is *H. heterophyes*. Another important heterophyid is *Metagonimus yokogawai*. Most heterophyid infections occur in the Far East except for *H. heterophyes,* which also occurs in the Middle East, the Mediterranean, and parts of Africa. *M. yokogawai* is also reported in Asia.

Etiology. *Fasciolopsis* species are indigenous to China, Taiwan, Laos, Thailand, Bangladesh, and India, and most infections occur in these areas. *F. buski* is the largest intestinal fluke. It measures 20 to 75 mm x 8 to 20 mm and has an oral and ventral sucker. There are two intestinal ceca, two branched testes that occupy most of the body, a central ovary, and a coiled uterus. Eggs pass from the organism into the feces and must reach the water where a ciliated larva, a miracidium, develops in 3 to 7 weeks. The larva emerges and swims in the water seeking a specific snail. A sporocyst develops in the snail and releases rediae, which produce daughter rediae that escape and leave the snail. The cercariae encyst on aquatic plants where they develop into metacercaria. If these aquatic plants are eaten raw, then the metacercaria excyst in the small intestine, attaching to the mucosa, and develop into adults within 3 months. In the intestines, the worms may live for 6 months or more.

Heterophyids are tiny worms measuring 1 to 2 mm in length. They have oral and ventral suckers; tegumentary spines surround the oral sucker. The eggs are small, measuring 27 to 30 x 15 to 17 μm, operculated, ovoid, and yellowish brown. The eggs contain a miracidium which, when laid, hatches after being eaten by the snail intermediate host. Development in the snail is similar to that of other trematodes. The cercaria encyst in fresh water fish. When the fish is eaten raw or undercooked, the metacercariae are digested from the fish tissue and excyst. Tiny parasites develop into adults in the small intestine in 1 to 2 weeks.

Clinical Features. The presence of large numbers of worms causes morbidity, including inflammation, bleeding, ulceration, and excessive mucus secretion, as well as obstruction or abdominal distension, hunger pains, increased appetite, and diarrhea. Absorption of parasitic secretions may cause generalized edema, ascites, nausea, vomiting, cachexia, and leukocytosis with eosinophilia. When death occurs in patients with massive infections, it is usually attributed to toxemia.

Pathologic Findings. In heterophyiasis, worms in the intestine and upper ileum cause mild inflammation and necrosis. When heavy infection is present, chronic diarrhea, upper abdominal pain, anorexia, nausea, vomiting, and abdominal tenderness, similar to peptic ulcer symptoms, can be present. These tiny eggs may be carried into the lymphatics or venules and disseminate to widely dispersed ectopic sites.

Special Techniques. The diagnosis is confirmed by finding eggs in the feces. Fasciolopsis eggs are large, measuring 130 to 140 x 80 to 85 μm, thin-shelled, and operculated.

Treatment and Prognosis. The drug of choice is praziquantel. Niclosamide is also used.

REFERENCES

Introduction

1. Centers for Disease Control and Prevention. Foodborne Diseases Active Surveillance Network, 1996. MMWR Morb Mortal Wkly Rep 1997;46:258–61.
2. Guerrant RL. Why America must care about tropical medicine: threats to global health and security from tropical infectious diseases. Am J Trop Med Hyg 1998;59:3–16.
3. Herikstadt H, Vergia D, Hadler J, et al. Population-based estimate of the burden of diarrheal illnesses: FoodNet 1996-1997, 1st International Conference on Emerging Infectious Diseases (Atlanta), March 1998.
4. LeClere FB, Moss AJ, Everhart JE, Roth HP. Prevalence of major digestive disorders and bowel symptoms, 1989. Adv Data 1992;212:1–15.
5. Mead PS, Slutsker L, Dietz V, et al. Food-related illness and death in the United States. Emerg Infect Dis 1999;5:607–25.
6. World Health Organization. The world health report 1996: fighting disease, fostering development. Report of the Director-General. Geneva: World Health Organization, 1996.

Escherichia Coli Infections

7. Abaas S, Franklin A, Kuhn I, Orskov F, Orskov I. Cytotoxin activity on vero cells among *Escherichia coli* strains associated with diarrhea in cats. Am J Vet Res 1989;50:1294–6.
8. Abdul-Raouf UM, Beuchat LR, Ammar MS. Survival and growth of *Escherichia coli* O157:H7 on salad vegetables. Appl Environ Microbiol 1993;59:1999–2006.
9. Baldwin TJ, Knutton S, Sellers L, Hernandez HA, Aitken A, Williams PH. Enteroaggregative *Escherichia coli* strains secrete a heat-labile toxin antigenically related to *E. coli* hemolysin. Infect Immun 1992;60:2092–5.
10. Bell BP, Griffin PM, Lozano P, Christie DL, Kobayashi JM, Tarr PI. Predictors of hemolytic uremic syndrome in children during a large outbreak of *Escherichia coli* O157:H7 infections. Pediatrics 1997;100:E12.

11. Belongia EA, Osterholm MT, Soler JT, Ammend DA, Braun JE, MacDonald KL. Transmission of *Escherichia coli* O157:H7 infection in Minnesota day-care facilities. JAMA 1993;269:883–8.
12. Bhan MK, Raj P, Levine MM, et al. Enteroaggregative *Escherichia coli* associated with persistent diarrhea in a cohort of rural children in India. J Infect Dis 1989;159:1061–4.
13. Brandt JR, Fouser LS, Watkins SL, et al. *Escherichia coli* O157:H7-associated hemolytic-uremic syndrome after ingestion of contaminated hamburgers. J Pediatr 1994:125;519–26.
14. Brewster DH, Brown MI, Robertson D, Houghton GL, Binson J, Sharp JC. An outbreak of *Escherichia coli* O157 associated with a children's paddling pool. Epidemiol Infect 1994;112:441–7.
15. Buteau C, Proulx F, Chaibou M, et al. Leukocytosis in children with *Escherichia coli* O157:H7 enteritis developing the hemolytic-uremic syndrome. Pediatr Infect Dis J 2000;19:642–7.
16. Camara LM, Carbonare SB, Scaletsky IC, da Silva ML, Carneiro-Sampaio MM. Inhibition of enteropathogenic *Escherichia coli* (EPEC) adhesion to HeLa cells by human colostrum. Detection of specific IgA related to EPEC outer-membrane proteins. Int Arch Allergy Immunol 1994;103:307–10.
17. Cartwright RY. Travellers' diarrhoea. Br Med Bull 1993;49:348–62.
18. Clarke SC. Diarrhoeagenic *Escherichia coli*—an emerging problem? Diagn Microbiol Infect Dis 2001;41:93–8.
19. Consensus conference statement: *Escherichia coli* O157:H7 infections—an emerging national health crisis, July 11-13, 1994. Gastroenterology 1995;108:1923–4.
20. Cravioto A, Tello A, Navarro A, et al. Association of *Escherichia coli* Hep-2 adherence patterns with type and duration of diarrhoea. Lancet 1991;337:262–4.
21. Czeczulin JR, Balepur S, Hicks S, et al. Aggregative adherence fimbria II, a second fimbrial antigen mediating aggregative adherence in enteroaggregative *Escherichia coli*. Infect Immun 1997;65:4135–45.
22. Doyle MP, Schoeni JL. Isolation of *Escherichia coli* O157:H7 from retail fresh meats and poultry. Appl Environ Microbiol 1987;53:2394–6.
23. Doyle MP, Schoeni JL. Survival and growth characteristics of *Escherichia coli* associated with hemorrhagic colitis. Appl Environ Microbiol 1984;48:855–6.
24. Dundas S, Todd WT, Stewart AI, Murdoch PS, Chaudhuri AK, Hutchinson SJ. The central Scotland *Escherichia coli* O157:H7 outbreak: risk factors for the hemolytic uremic syndrome and death among hospitalized patients. Clin Infect Dis 2001;33:923–31.
25. Durrer P, Zbinden R, Fleisch F, et al. Intestinal infection due to enteroaggregative *Escherichia coli* among human immunodeficiency virus–infected persons. J Infect Dis 2000;182:1540–54.
26. Easton L. *Escherichia coli* O157: occurrence, transmission and laboratory detection. Br J Biomed Sci 1997;54:57–64.
27. Echeverria P, Sethabutr O, Serichantalergs O, Lexomboon U, Tamura K. *Shigella* and enteroinvasive *Escherichia coli* in households of children with dysentery in Bangkok. J Infect Dis 1992;165:144–7.
28. Elder RO, Keen JE, Siragusa GR, Barkocy-Gallagher GA, Koohmaraie M, Laegreid WW. Correlation of enterohemorrhagic *Escherichia coli* O157 prevalence in feces, hides, and carcasses of beef cattle during processing. Proc Natl Acad Sci USA 2000;97:2999–3003.
29. Elliott SJ, Nataro JP. Enteroaggregative and diffusely adherent *Escherichia coli*. Revue Med Microbiol 1995;6:196–206.
30. Elliott SJ, Wainwright LA, McDaniel TK, et al. The complete sequence of the locus of enterocyte effacement (LEE) from enteropathogenic *Escherichia coli* E2348/69. Mol Microbiol 1998;28:1–4.
31. Eslava C, Navarro–Garcia F, Czeczulin JR, Henderson IR, Cravioto A, Nataro JP. Pet, an autotransporter enterotoxin from enteroaggregative *Escherichia coli*. Infect Immun 1998;66:3155–63.
32. Friedrich AW, Bielaszewska M, Zhang WL, et al. *Escherichia coli* harboring Shiga toxin 2 gene variants: frequency and association with clinical symptoms. J Infect Dis 2002;185:74–84.
33. Gascon J, Vargas M, Quinto L, Corachan M, Jimenez de Anta MT, Vila J. Enteroaggregative *Escherichia coli* strains as a cause of traveler's diarrhea: a case-control study. J Infect Dis 1998;177:1409–12.
34. Giron JA, Ho AS, Schoolnik GK. An inducible bundle-forming pilus of enteropathogenic *Escherichia coli*. Science 1991;254:713–4.
35. Griffin PM, Ostroff SM, Tauxe RV, et al. Illnesses associated with *Escherichia coli* O157:H7 infections. A broad clinical spectrum. Ann Int Med 1988:109;705–12.
36. Griffin PM, Tauxe RV. The epidemiology of infections caused by *Escherichia coli* O157:H7, other enterohemorrhagic *E. coli*, and the associated hemolytic uremic syndrome. Epidemiol Rev 1991;13:60–98.
37. Guerrant RL, Van Gilder T, Steiner TS, et al. Practice guidelines for the management of infectious diarrhea. Clin Infect Dis 2001;32:331–50.

38. Haider K, Faruque SM, Shahid NS, et al. Enteroaggregative *Escherichia coli* infection in Bangladeshi children: clinical and microbiological features. J Diarrhoeal Dis Res 1991;9: 318–22.
39. Hart CA, Batt RM, Saunders JR. Diarrhoea caused by *Escherichia coli*. Ann Trop Paediatr 1993;13:121–31.
40. Huppertz HI, Rutkowski S, Aleksie S, Karch H. Acute and chronic diarrhoea and abdominal colic associated with enteroaggregative *Escherichia coli* in young children living in Western Europe. Lancet 1997;349:1660–2.
41. Ikeda K, Ida O, Kimoto K, Takatorige T, Nakanishi N, Tatara K. Predictors for the development of haemolytic uraemic syndrome with *Escherichia coli* O157:H7 infections: with focus on the day of illness. Epidemiol Infect 2000;124:343–9.
42. Ina K, Kusugami K, Ohta M. Bacterial hemorrhagic enterocolitis. J Gastroenterol 2003;38: 111–20.
43. Kaper J. EPEC delivers the goods. Trends Microbiol 1998:6;169–72.
44. Karmali MA, Arbus G, Petric M, et al. Hospital-acquired *Escherichia coli* O157:H7 associated haemolytic uraemic syndrome in a nurse (letter). Lancet 1988;i:526.
45. Karmali MA, Petric M, Lim C, Fleming PC, Arbus GS, Lior H. The association between idiopathic hemolytic uremic syndrome and infection by verotoxin-producing *Escherichia coli*. J Infect Dis 1985;151:775–82.
46. Kawamura N, Yamazaki T, Tamai H. Risk factors for the development of *Escherichia coli* O157:H7 associated with hemolytic uremic syndrome. Pediatr Int 1999;41:218–22.
47. Keene WE, Sazie E, Kok J, et al. An outbreak of *Escherichia coli* O157:H7 infections traced to jerky made from deer meat. JAMA 1997:277; 1229–31.
48. Knutton S, Shaw R, Phillips AD, et al. Phenotypic and genetic analysis of diarrhea-associated *Escherichia coli* isolated from children in the United Kingdom. J Pediatr Gastroenterol Nutr 2001;33:32–40.
49. Kravitz GR, Smith K, Wagstrom L. Colonic necrosis and perforation secondary to *Escherichia coli* O157:H7 gastroenteritis in an adult patient without hemolytic uremic syndrome. Clin Infect Dis 2002;35:E103–5.
50. Law D, Chart H. Enteroaggregative *Escherichia coli*. J Appl Microbiol 1998;84:685–97.
51. Ludwig K, Sarkim V, Bitzan M, et al. Shiga toxin–producing *Escherichia coli* infection and antibodies against Stx2 and Stx1 in household contacts of children with enteropathic hemolytic-uremic syndrome. J Clin Microbiol 2002;40:1773–82.
52. Mattila L, Siitonen A, Kyronseppa H, et al. Seasonal variation in etiology of travelers' diarrhea. Finnish-Moroccan Study Group. J Infect Dis 1992;165:385–8.
53. McNamara BP, Koutsouris A, O'Connell CB, Nougayrede JP, Donnenberg MS, Hecht G. Translocated EspF protein from enteropathogenic *Escherichia coli* disrupts host intestinal barrier function. J Clin Invest 2001;107:621–9.
54. Mezoff AG, Giannella RA, Eade MN, Cohen MB. *Escherichia-coli* enterotoxin (STa) binds to receptors, stimulates guanyl cyclase, and impairs absorption in rat colon. Gastroenterology 1992; 102:816–22.
55. Moon HW, Whipp SC, Argenzio RA, Levine MM, Giannella RA. Attaching and effacing activities of rabbit and human enteropathogenic *Escherichia coli* in pig and rabbit intestines. Infection Immun 1983;41:1340–51.
56. Morgan GM, Newman C, Palmer SR, et al. First recognized community outbreak of haemorrhagic colitis due to verotoxin-producing *Escherichia coli* O157:H7 in the UK. Epidemiol Infect 1988;101:83–91.
57. Nataro JP, Kaper JB. Diarrheagenic *Escherichia coli*. Clin Microbiol Rev 1998;11:142–201.
58. Ochoa TJ, Cleary TG. Epidemiology and spectrum of disease of *Escherichia coli* O157. Curr Opin Infect Dis 2003;16:259–63.
59. Okeke IN, Nataro JP. Enteroaggregative *Escherichia coli*. Lancet Infect Dis 2001;1:304–13.
60. O'Loughlin E, Robins-Browne RM. Effect of Shiga toxins on eukaryotic cells. Microb Infect 2001;3:493–507.
61. Ostroff SM, Kobayashi JM, Lewis JH. Infections with *Escherichia coli* O157:H7 in Washington State. The first year of statewide disease surveillance. JAMA 1989:262;355–9.
62. Paul M, Tsukamoto T, Ghosh AR, et al. The significance of enteroaggregative *Escherichia coli* in the etiology of hospitalized diarrhoea in Calcutta, India and the demonstration of a new honey-combed pattern of aggregative adherence. FEMS Microbiol Lett 1994;117:319–25.
63. Pickering LK, Obrig TG, Stapleton FB. Hemolytic-uremic syndrome and enterohemorrhagic *Escherichia coli*. Pediatr Infect Dis J 1994;13: 459–76.
64. Presterl E, Nadrchal R, Wolf D, Rotter M, Hirschl AM. Enteroaggregative and enterotoxigenic *Escherichia coli* among isolates from patients with diarrhea in Austria. Eur J Clin Microbiol Infect Dis 1999;18:209–12.
65. Remis RS, MacDonald KL, Riley LW, et al. Sporadic cases of hemorrhagic colitis associated with *Escherichia coli* O157:H7—clinical, epidemiologic and bacteriologic features. Ann Intern Med 1984;101:624–6.

66. Richardson SE, Karmali MA, Becker LE, Smith CR. The histopathology of the hemolytic uremic syndrome associated with verocytotoxin-producing *Escherichia coli* infections. Hum Pathol 1988;19:1102–8.
67. Riley LW. The epidemiologic, clinical and microbiologic features of hemorrhagic colitis. Ann Rev Microbiol 1987;41:383–407.
68. Riley LW, Remis RS, Helgerson SD, et al. Hemorrhagic colitis associated with a rare *Escherichia coli* serotype. N Engl J Med 1983;308:681–5.
69. Robins-Browne RM, Hartland EL. *Escherichia coli* as a cause of diarrhea. Adv Pediatr Gastroenterol Hepatol 2002;17:467–75.
70. Rothbaum R, McAdams AJ, Giannella R, Partin JC. A clinicopathologic study of enterocyte-adherent *Escherichia coli*: a cause of protracted diarrhea in infants. Gastroenterology 1982;83:441–54.
71. Ryan CA, Tauxe RV, Hosek GW, et al. *Escherichia coli* O157:H7 diarrhoea in a nursing home: clinical, epidemiological and pathological findings. J Infect Dis 1986:154;631–8.
72. Sasagawa C, Buysse JM, Watanabe H. The large virulence plasmid of *Shigella*. Curr Top Microbiol Immunol 1992;180:21–44.
73. Siegler RL. Management of hemolytic-uremic syndrome. J Pediatr 1988;112:1014–9.
74. Steiner TS, Lima AA, Nataro JP, Guerrant RL. Enteroaggregative *Escherichia coli* produce intestinal inflammation and growth impairment and cause interleukin-8 release from intestinal epithelial cells. J Infect Dis 1998;177:88–96.
75. Strockbine NA, Marques LR, Newland JW, et al. Two toxin-converting phages from *Escherichia coli* O157:H7 strain 933 encode antigenically distinct toxins with similar biologic activities. Infect Immun 1986;53:135–40.
76. Su C, Brandt LJ. *Escherichia coli* 0157:H7 infection in humans. Ann Intern Med 1995;123:698–714.
77. Tarr PI, Neill MA, Clausen CR, Newland JW, Neill RJ, Moseley SL. Genotypic variation in pathogenic *Escherichia coli* O157:H7 isolated from patients in Washington, 1984-1987. J Infect Dis 1989;159:344–7.
78. Taylor DN, Echeverria P. Etiology and epidemiology of travelers' diarrhea in Asia. Rev Infect Dis 1986;8:S136–41.
79. Ulshen MH, Rollo JL. Pathogenesis of *Escherichia coli* gastroenteritis in man: another mechanism. N Engl J Med 1980;302:99–101.
80. Wong CS, Jelacic S, Habeeb RL, Watkins SL, Tarr PI. The risk of the hemolytic–uremic syndrome after antibiotic treatment of *Escherichia coli* O157:H7 infections. N Engl J Med 2000;342:1930–6.
81. Wray C, Randall LP, McLaren IM, Woodward MJ. Verocytotoxic *Escherichia coli* from animals, their incidence and detection. In: Karmali MA, Goglio AG, eds. Recent advances in verocytotoxin-producing *Escherichia coli* infections. Amsterdam: Elsevier Science; 1994:69–72.

Salmonella Infections

82. Alpuche-Aranda CM, Berthiaume EP, Mock B, Swanson JA, Miller SI. Spacious phagosome formation within mouse macrophages correlates with *Salmonella* serotype pathogenicity and host susceptibility. Infect Immun 1995;63:4456–62.
83. Bhutta ZA. Impact of age and drug resistance on mortality in typhoid fever. Arch Dis Child 1996;75:214–7.
84. Blaser MJ, Feldman RA. *Salmonella* bacteremia: reports to the Centers for Disease Control. J Infect Dis 1981;143:743–6.
85. Buchwald DS, Blaser MJ. A review of human salmonellosis. Part II: duration of excretion following infection with nontyphi *Salmonella*. Rev Infect Dis 1984;6:345–6.
86. Buck JJ, Nicholls SW. *Salmonella arizonae* enterocolitis acquired by an infant from a pet snake. J Pediatr Gastroenterol Nutr 1997;25:248–9.
87. Butler T, Islam A, Kabir I, Jones PK. Patterns of morbidity and mortality in typhoid fever dependent on age and gender: a review of 522 hospitalized patients with diarrhea. Rev Infect Dis 1991;13:85–90.
88. Cao XT, Kneen R, Nguyen TA, Truong DL, White NJ, Parry CM. A comparative study of ofloxacin and cefixime for treatment of typhoid fever in children. Pediatr Infect Dis J 1999;18:245–8.
89. Carter PB, Collins FM. The route of enteric infection in normal mice. J Exp Med. 1974;139:1189–203.
90. Cartwright KA, Evans BG. Salmon as a food–poisoning vehicle—two successive *Salmonella* outbreaks. Epidemiol Infect 1988;101:249–57.
91. Centers for Disease Control and Prevention. Multistate outbreak of *Salmonella poona* infections—United States and Canada, 1991. MMWR Morb Mortal Wkly Rep 1991;40:549–52.
92. Centers for Disease Control and Prevention. Reptile-associated salmonellosis—selected states, 1996-1998. JAMA 1999;282:2293.
93. Centers for Disease Control and Prevention. Salmonellosis associated with chicks and ducklings—Michigan and Missouri, spring 1999. MMWR Morb Mortal Wkly Rep 2000;49:297–9.

94. Chen LM, Kaniga K, Galan JE. *Salmonella* spp. are cytotoxic for cultured macrophages. Mol Microbiol 1996;21:1101–5.
95. Chinh NT, Parry CM, Ly NT, et al. A randomized controlled comparison of azithromycin and ofloxacin for treatment of multidrug–resistant and nalidixic acid-resistant enteric fever. Antimicrob Agents Chemother 2000;44: 1855–9.
96. Cody SH, Abbott SL, Marfin AA, et al. Two outbreaks of multidrug-resistant *Salmonella* serotype typhimurium DT104 infections linked to raw-milk cheese in Northern California. JAMA 1999;281:1805–10.
97. Cohen ML, Tauxe RV. Drug-resistant *Salmonella* in the United States: an epidemiologic perspective. Science 1986;234:964–9.
98. Collazo CM, Galan JE. The invasion-associated type III secretion system of *Salmonella typhimurium* directs the translocation of the Sip proteins into the host cell. Mol Microbiol 1997;24: 747–56.
99. Collins MA, Peh WC, Evans NS. Aphthous ulcers in *Salmonella* colitis. AJR Am J Roentgenol 1992;158:918.
100. Eggleston FC, Santoshi B, Singh CM. Typhoid perforation of the bowel: experiences in 78 cases. Ann Surg 1979;190:31–5.
101. Fields PI, Swanson RV, Haidaris CG, Heffron F. Mutants of *Salmonella typhimurium* that cannot survive within the macrophage are avirulent. Proc Natl Acad Sci USA 1986;83:5189–93.
102. Frost AJ, Bland AP, Wallis TS. The early dynamic response of the calf ileal epithelium to *Salmonella typhimurium*. Vet Pathol 1997;34: 369–86.
103. Galyov EE, Wood MW, Posqvist R, et al. A secreted effector protein of *Salmonella dublin* is translocated into eukaryotic cells and mediates inflammation and fluid secretion in infected ileal mucosa. Mol Microbiol 1997;25:903–12.
104. Girgis NI, Butler T, Frenck RW, et al. Azithromycin versus ciprofloxacin for treatment of uncomplicated typhoid fever in a randomized trial in Egypt that includes patients with multidrug resistance. Antimicrob Agents Chemother 1999;43:1441–4.
105. Glynn MK, Bopp C, Dewitt W, Dabney P, Mokhtar M, Angulo FJ. Emergence of multidrug-resistant *Salmonella enterica* serotype typhimurium DT104 infections in the United States. N Engl J Med 1998;338:1333–8.
106. Gotuzzo E, Carrillo C. Quinolones in typhoid fever. Infect Dis Clin Pract 1994;3:345–51.
107. Hardt WD, Chen LM, Schuebel KE, Bustelo XR, Galan JE. *S. typhimurium* encodes an activator of Rho GTPases that induces membrane ruffling and nuclear responses in host cells. Cell 1998;93:815–26.
108. Hensel M. *Salmonella* pathogenicity island 2. Mol Microbiol 2000;36:1015–23.
109. Hoffman SL, Punjabi NH, Kumala S, et al. Reduction of mortality in chloramphenicol-treated severe typhoid fever by high-dose dexamethasone. N Engl J Med 1984;310:82–8.
110. Hohmann EL. Nontyphoidal salmonellosis. Clin Infect Dis 2001;32:263–9.
111. Hueck CJ. Type III protein secretion systems in bacterial pathogens of animals and plants. Microbiol Mol Biol Rev 1998;62:379–433.
112. Kraus MD, Amatya B, Kimula Y. Histopathology of typhoid enteritis: morphologic and immunophenotypic findings. Mod Pathol 1999;12:949–55.
113. Lan RT, Reeves PR. Gene transfer is a major factor in bacterial evolution. Mol Biol Evol 1996; 13:47–55.
114. Libby SJ, Goebel W, Ludwig N, et al. A cytolysin encoded by *Salmonella* is required for survival within macrophages. Proc Natl Acad Sci USA 1994;91:489–97.
115. Maguire TM, Wensel RH, Malcolm N, Jewell L, Thomson AB. Massive gastrointestinal hemorrhage cecal ulcers and *Salmonella* colitis. J Clin Gastroenterol 1985;7:249–50.
116. Mandal BK. *Salmonella typhi* and other salmonellas. Gut 1994;35:726–8.
116a. Mattila L, Siitonen A, Kyronseppa H, et al. Seasonal variation in etiology of travelers' diarrhea. Finnish-Moroccan Study Group. J Infect Dis 1992;165:385–8.
117. McGovern VJ, Slavutin LK. Pathology of *Salmonella* colitis. Am J Surg Pathol 1979;3:483–90.
117a. Mead PS, Slutsker L, Dietz V, et al. Food-related illness and death in the United States. Emerg Infect Dis 1999;5:607–25.
118. Miller SI, Mekalanos JJ. Constitutive expression of the RhoP regulon attenuates *Salmonella* virulence and survival within macrophages. J Bacteriol 1990;172:2485–90.
119. Moffet HL. Common infections in ambulatory patients. Ann Intern Med 1978;89:743–5.
120. Nelson JD, Kusmiesz H, Jackson LH, Woodman E. Treatment of *Salmonella* gastroenteritis with ampicillin, amoxicillin or placebo. Pediatrics 1980;65:1125–30.
121. Norris FA, Wilson MP, Wallis TS, Galyov EE, Majerus PW. SopB, a protein required for virulence of *Salmonella dublin*, is an inositol phosphate phosphatase. Proc Natl Acad Sci USA 1998;95:14057–9.
122. Ochman H, Lawrence JG. Phylogenetics and the amelioration of bacterial genomes. In: Neidhardt FC, Curtiss R, eds. Escherictina coli and salmonella: cellular and molecular biology. Washington DC: ASM Press; 1996:2627–37.

123. Ochman H, Wilson AC. Evolution in bacteria: evidence for a universal substitution rate in cellular genomes. J Mol Evol 1987;26:74–86.
124. Parry CM, Hein TT, Dougan G, White NJ, Farrar JJ. Medical progress: typhoid fever. N Engl J Med 2002;347:1770–82.
125. Punjabi NH, Hoffman SL, Edman DC, et al. Treatment of severe typhoid fever in children with high dose dexamethasone. Pediatr Infect Dis J 1988;7:598–600.
126. Quiroga T, Goycoolea M, Tagle R, Gonzalez F, Rodriguez L, Villarroel L. Diagnosis of typhoid fever by two serologic methods: enzyme-linked immunosorbent assay of antilipopolysaccharide of *Salmonella typhi* antibodies and Widal test. Diagn Microbiol Infect Dis 1992;15:651–6.
127. Rampling A. *Salmonella enteritidis* five years on. Lancet 1993;342:317–8.
128. Rodrigue DC, Tauxe RV, Rowe B. International increase in *Salmonella enteritidis*: a new pandemic? Epidemiol Infect 1990;105:21–7.
129. Rogerson SJ, Spooner VJ, Smith TA, Richens J. Hydrocortisone in chloramphenicol-treated severe typhoid fever in Papua New Guinea. Trans R Soc Trop Med Hyg 1991;85:113–6.
130. Schutze GE, Schutze SE, Kirby RS. Extraintestinal salmonellosis in a children's hospital. Pediatr Infect Dis J 1997;16:482–5.
131. Smith JH. Typhoid fever. In: Binford CH, Connor DH, eds. Pathology of tropical and extraordinary diseases. Washington, DC: Armed Forces Institute of Pathology; 1976:123–9.
132. Stevens A, Joseph C, Bruce J, et al. A large outbreak of *Salmonella enteritidis* phage type 4 associated with eggs from overseas. Epidemiol Infect 1989;103:425–33.
133. Stuart BM, Pullen RL. Typhoid: clinical analysis of three hundred and sixty cases. Arch Intern Med 1946;78:629–61.
134. Takeuchi A. Electron microscope studies of experimental *Salmonella* infection. I. Penetration into the intestinal epithelium by *Salmonella typhimurium*. Am J Pathol 1967;50:109–36.
135. White NJ, Parry CM. The treatment of typhoid fever. Curr Opin Infect Dis 1996;9:298–302.
136. Wood MW, Jones MA, Watson PR, et al. SopE, a secreted protein of *Salmonella dublin*, is translocated into the target eukaryotic cell via a sip-dependent mechanism and promotes bacterial entry. Mol Microbiol 1996;22:327–38.

Shigella Infections

137. Anand BS, Malhorta V, Bhattacharya SK, et al. Rectal histology in acute bacillary dysentery. Gastroenterology 1986;90:654–60.
138. Bennish ML, Azad AK, Yousefzadeh D. Intestinal obstruction during shigellosis: incidence, clinical features, risk factors, and outcome. Gastroenterology 1991;101:626–34.
139. Butler T, Dunn D, Dahms B, Islam M. Causes of death and the histopathologic findings in fatal shigellosis. Pediatr Infect Dis J 1989;8:767–72.
139a. Guerrant RL, Van Gilder T, Steiner TS, et al. Practice guidelines for the management of infectious diarrhea. Clin Infect Dis 2001;32:331–50.
140. Islam MM, Azad AK, Bardhan PK, Raqib R, Islam D. Pathology of shigellosis and its complications. Histopathology 1994;24:65–71.
141. Kavaliotis J, Karyda S, Konstantoula T, Kansouzidou A, Tsagaropoulou H. Shigellosis of childhood in northern Greece: epidemiological, clinical and laboratory data of hospitalized patients during the period 1971-96. Scand J Infect Dis 2000;32:207–11.
142. Khuroo MS, Mahajan R, Zargar SA, et al. The colon in shigellosis: serial colonoscopic appearances in *Shigella dysenteriae* I. Endoscopy 1990;22:35–8.
143. Lee LA, Ostroff SM, McGee HB, et al. An outbreak of shigellosis at an outdoor music festival. Am J Epidemiol 1991;133:608–15.
144. Lindberg AA, Pal T. Strategies for development of potential candidate *Shigella* vaccines. Vaccine 1993;11:168–79.
145. Mathan MM, Mathan VI. Morphology of rectal mucosa of patients with shigellosis. Rev Infect Dis 1991;13:S314–8.
146. Maurelli AT, Sansonetti PJ. Genetic determinants of *Shigella* pathogenicity. Annu Rev Microbiol 1988;42:127–50.
147. Morduchowicz G, Huminer D, Siegman-Igra Y, Drucker M, Block CS, Pitlik SD. *Shigella* bacteremia in adults. A report of five cases and review of the literature. Arch Intern Med 1987;147:2034–7.
148. Perdomo OJ, Cavaillon JM, Huerre M, et al. Acute inflammation causes epithelial invasion and mucosal destruction in experimental shigellosis. J Exp Med 1994;180:1307–19.
149. Reeve G, Martin DL, Pappas J, Thompson RE, Greene KD. An outbreak of shigellosis associated with the consumption of raw oysters. N Engl J Med 1989;321:224–7.
150. Sachdev HPS, Chadha V, Malhotra V, Verghese A, Puri RK. Rectal histopathology in endemic *Shigella* and *Salmonella* diarrhea. J Pediatr Gastroenterol Nutr 1993;16:33–8.
151. Sansonetti PJ. Molecular and cellular mechanisms of invasion of the intestinal barrier by enteric pathogens. The paradigm of *Shigella*. Folia Microbiol 1998;43:239–46.
152. Sansonetti PJ, Arondel J, Cavaillon JM, Huerre M. Role of interleukin-1 in the pathogenesis of experimental shigellosis. J Clin Invest 1995;96:884–92.

153. Sansonetti PJ, Clerc P, Maurelli T, Mounier J. Multiplication of *Shigella flexneri* within HeLa cells: lysis of the phagocytic vacuole and plasmid-mediated contact hemolysis. Infect Immun 1986;51:461–9.
154. Sansonetti PJ, Phalipon A. M cells as ports of entry for enteroinvasive pathogens: mechanisms of interaction, consequences for the disease process. Immunology 1999;11:193–203.
155. Speelman P, Kabir I, Islam M. Distribution and spread of colonic lesions in shigellosis: a colonoscopic study. J Infect Dis 1984;150:899–903.
156. van Pelt W, de Wit MA, Wannet WJ, Ligtvoet EJ, Widdowson MA, van Duynhoven YT. Laboratory surveillance of bacterial gastroenteric pathogens in the Netherlands, 1991-2001. Epidemiol Infect 2003;130:431–41.
157. Van Nhieu GT, Sansonetti PJ. Mechanism of *Shigella* entry into epithelial cells. Curr Opin Microbiol 1999;2:51–5.
158. Yoshida S, Sasakawa C. Exploiting host microtubule dynamics: a new aspect of bacterial invasion. Trends Microbiol 2003;11:139–43.
159. Zychlinsky A, Fitting C, Cavaillon JM, Sansonetti PJ. Interleukin 1 is released by murine macrophages during apoptosis induced by *Shigella flexneri*. J Clin Invest 1994;94:1328–32.
160. Zychlinsky A, Perdomo JJ, Sansonetti PJ. Molecular and cellular mechanisms of tissue invasion by *Shigella flexneri*. Ann N Y Acad Sci 1994;730:197–208.
161. Zychlinsky A, Prevost MC, Sansonetti PJ. *Shigella flexneri* induces apoptosis in infected macrophages. Nature 1992;358:167–9.

Staphylococcal Infections

162. Bautista L, Gaya P, Medina M, Nunez M. A quantitative study of enterotoxin production by sheep milk staphylococci. Appl Environ Microbiol 1988;54:566–9.
163. Bone FJ, Bogie D, Morgan-Jones SC. Staphylococcal food poisoning from sheep milk cheese. Epidemiol Infect 1989;103:449–58.
164. Haeghebaert S, Le Querrec F, Gallay A, et al. Les toxi-infections alimentaires collective en France, en 1999 et 2000. Bull Epidemiol Hebdo 2002;23:105–9.
165. Ikejima T, Okusawa S, Ghezzi P, van der Meer JW, Dinarello CA. Interleukin–1 induces tumor necrosis factor (TNF) in human peripheral blood mononuclear cells in vitro and a circulating TNF-like activity in rabbits. J Infect Dis 1990;162:215–23.
166. Khambaty FM, Bennet RW, Shah DB. Application of pulse-field gel electrophoresis to the epidemiological characterization of *Staphylococcus intermedius* implicated in a food-related outbreak. Epidemiol Infect 1994;113:75–80.
167. Le Loir Y, Baron F, Gautier M. *Staphylococcus aureus* and food poisoning. Genet Mol Res 2003;2:63–76.
168. Marrack P, Kappler J. The staphylococcal enterotoxins and their relatives. Science 1990;248:705–11.
169. McCormick JK, Yarwood JM, Schlievert PM. Toxic shock syndrome and bacterial superantigens: an update. Annu Rev Microbiol 2001;55: 77–104.

***Campylobacter* Infections**

170. Allos BM. *Campylobacter jejuni* infections: update on emerging issues and trends. Clin Infect Dis 2001;32:1201–6.
171. Allos BM, Blaser MJ. *Campylobacter jejuni* and the expanding spectrum of related infections. Clin Infect Dis 1995;20:1092–9.
172. Blaser MJ, Reller LB. *Campylobacter* enteritis. N Engl J Med 1981;305:1444–52.
173. Blaser MJ, Waldman RJ, Barrett T, Erlandson AL. Outbreaks of *Campylobacter* enteritis in two extended families. Evidence for person to person transmission. J Pediatrics 1981;98:254–7.
174. Blaser MJ, Wells JG, Feldman RA, Pollard RA, Allen JR. *Campylobacter* enteritis in the United States. A multicenter study. Ann Intern Med 1983;98:360–5.
175. Colgan T, Lambert JR, Newman A, Luk SC. *Campylobacter jejuni* enterocolitis. Arch Pathol Lab Med 1980;104:571–4.
176. Dworkin B, Wormser GP, Abdoo RA, Cabello F, Aguero ME, Sivak SL. Persistence of multiply antibiotic-resistant *Campylobacter jejuni* in a patient with the acquired immune deficiency syndrome. Am J Med 1986;80:965–70.
177. Fauchere JL, Kervella M, Rosenau A, Mohanna K, Veron M. Adhesion to HeLa cells of *Campylobacter jejuni* and *C. coli* outer membrane components. Res Microbiol 1989;140:379–92.
178. Fauchere JL, Veron M, Lellouch-Tubiana A, Pfister A. Experimental infection of gnotobiotic mice with *Campylobacter jejuni*: colonization of intestine and spread to lymphoid and reticuloendothelial organs. J Med Microbiol 1985;20:215–24.
179. Field LH, Headley VL, Underwood JL, Payne SM, Berry LJ. The chicken embryo as a model for *Campylobacter* invasion: comparative virulence of human isolates of *Campylobacter jejuni* and *Campylobacter coli*. Infect Immun 1986;54:118–25.
180. Friedman CR, Neimann J, Wegener HC, Tauxe RV. Epidemiology of *Campylobacter jejuni* infections in the United States and other industrialized nations. In: Nachamkin I, Blaser MJ, eds. *Campylobacter*, 2nd ed. Washington, DC: ASM press; 2000:121–38.

181. Kapperud G, Lassen J, Ostroff SM, Aasen S. Clinical features of sporadic *Campylobacter* infections in Norway. Scand J Infect Dis 1992;24: 741–9.
182. Larvol L, Zeitoun E, Barge J, Valverde A, Delaroque I, Soule JC. Colectasie avec perforation colique compliquant une ilèo–colite a *Campylobacter jejuni*. Gastroenterol Clin Biol 1994;18: 281–4.
183. Lastovica AJ, Skirrow MB. Clinical significance of *Campylobacter* and related species other than *Campylobacter jejuni* and *C. coli*. In: Nachamkin I, Blaser MJ, eds. *Campylobacter*, 2nd ed. Washington, DC: ASM Press; 2000:139–53.
184. Laughon BE, Vernon AA, Druckman DA, et al. Recovery of *Campylobacter* species from homosexual men. J Infect Dis 1988;158:464–7.
185. Lindblom GB, Kaijser B, Sjogren E. Enterotoxin production and serogroups of *Campylobacter jejuni* and *Campylobacter coli* from patients with diarrhea and from healthy laying hens. J Clin Microbiol 1989;27:1272–6.
185a. Mead PS, Slutsker L, Dietz V, et al. Food-related illness and death in the United States. Emerg Infect Dis 1999;5:607–25.
186. Minet J, Grosbois B, Megraud F. *Campylobacter hyointestinalis*: an opportunistic enteropathogen? J Clin Microbiol 1988;26:2659–60.
187. Park CE, Sanders GW. Occurrence of thermotolerant campylobacters in fresh vegetables sold at farmers' outdoor markets and supermarkets. Can J Microbiol 1992;38:313–6.
188. Park SF. The physiology of *Campylobacter* species and its relevance to their role as foodborne pathogens. Int J Food Microbiol 2002;74:177–88.
189. Penner JL. The genus *Campylobacter*: a decade of progress. Clin Microbiol Rev 1988;1:157–72.
190. Perlman DM, Ampel NM, Schifman RB, et al. Persistent *Campylobacter jejuni* infections in patients infected with human immunodeficiency virus (HIV). Ann Intern Med 1988;108: 540–6.
191. Pickett CL. *Campylobacter* toxins and their role in pathogenesis. In: Nachamkin I, Blaser MJ, eds. *Campylobacter*, 2nd ed. Washington, DC: ASM Press; 2000:179–90.
192. Pickett CL, Pesci EC, Cottle DL, Russell G, Erdem AN, Zeytin H. Prevalence of cytolethal distending toxin production in *Campylobacter jejuni* and relatedness of *Campylobacter* sp *cdtB* gene. Infect Immun 1996;64:2070–8.
193. Price AB, Jewkes J, Sanderson PJ. Acute diarrhea: *Campylobacter* colitis and the role of rectal biopsy. J Clin Pathol 1979;32:990–7.
194. Purdy D, Buswell CM, Hodgson AE, McAlpine K, Henderson I, Leach SA. Characterisation of cytolethal distending toxin (CDT) mutants of *Campylobacter jejuni*. J Med Microbiol 2000; 49:473–9.
195. Rautelin H, Koota K, von Essen R, Jahkola M, Siitonen A, Kosunen TU. Waterborne *Campylobacter jejuni* epidemic in a Finnish hospital for rheumatic diseases. Scand J Infect Dis 1990; 22:321–6.
196. Riley LW, Finch MJ. Results of the first year of national surveillance of *Campylobacter* infections in the United States. J Infect Dis 1985; 151:956–9.
197. Slutsker LA, Ries AA, Greene KD, Wells JG, Hutwagner L, Griffin PM. *Escherichia coli* O157:H7 diarrhea in the United States: clinical and epidemiological features. Ann Intern Med 1997;126:505–13.
198. Svedhem A, Kaijser B. Isolation of *Campylobacter jejuni* from domestic animals and pets: probable origin of human infection. J Infect 1981;3:37–40.
199. Totten PA, Fennel CL, Tenover FC, et al. *Campylobacter cinaedi* (sp. nov.) and *Campylobacter fennelliae* (sp. nov.): two new *Campylobacter* species associated with enteric disease in homosexual men. J Infect Dis 1985;151:131–9.
200. Whitehouse CA, Balbo PB, Pesci EC, Cottle DL, Mirabito PM, Pickett CL. *Campylobacter jejuni* cytolethal distending toxin causes a G2-phase cell cycle block. Infect Immun 1998;66:1934–40.
201. Yuki N, Yoshino H, Sato S, Miyatake T. Acute axonal polyneuropathy associated with anti-GM1 antibodies following *Campylobacter* enteritis. Neurology 1990;40:1900–2.

Clostridium Difficile Infections

202. Aktories K, Just I. Monoglucosylation of low-molecular-mass GTP-binding Rho proteins by clostridial cytotoxins. Trends Cell Biol 1995;5: 441–3.
203. Ariano RE, Zhanel GG, Harding GK. The role of anion-exchange resins in the treatment of antibiotic-associated pseudomembranous colitis. Can Med Assoc J 1990;142:1049–51.
204. Bartlett JG. Protein-losing enteropathy associated with *Clostridium difficile* infection. Lancet 1989;1:1353–5.
205. Chaves-Olarte E, Weidmann M, Eichel-Streiber C, Thelestam M. Toxins A and B from *Clostridium difficile* differ with respect to enzymatic potencies, cellular substrate specificities, and surface binding to cultured cells. J Clin Invest 1997;100:1734–41.
206. Cone JB, Wetzel W. Toxic megacolon secondary to pseudomembranous colitis. Dis Colon Rectum 1982;25:478–82.

207. Coyne JD, Dervan PA, Haboubi NY. Involvement of the appendix in pseudomembranous colitis. J Clin Pathol 1997;50:70–1.
208. D'Souza AL, Rajkumar C, Cooke J, Bulpitt CJ. Probiotics in prevention of antibiotic associated diarrhoea: meta-analysis. BMJ 2002;324:1341–5.
209. Emoto M, Kawarabayashi T, Hachisuga MD, Eguchi F, Shirakawa K. *Clostridium difficile* colitis associated with cisplatin-based chemotherapy in ovarian cancer patients. Gynecol Oncol 1996;61:369–72.
210. Fiorentini C, Fabbri A, Falzano L, et al. *Clostridium difficile* toxin B induces apoptosis in intestinal cultured cells. Infect Immunol 1998;6:2660–5.
211. Fiorentini C, Malorni W, Paradisi S, Giuliano M, Mastrantonio P, Donelli G. Interaction of *Clostridium difficile* toxin A with cultured cells: cytoskeletal changes and nuclear polarization. Infect Immun 1990;58:2329–36.
212. Gerding DN, Johnson S, Peterson LR, Mulligan ME, Silva J. *Clostridium difficile*–associated diarrhea and colitis. Infect Control Hosp Epidemiol 1995;16:459–77.
213. Groschel DH. *Clostridium difficile* infection. Crit Rev Clin Lab Sci 1996;33:203–45.
214. Jacobs A, Barnard K, Fishel R, Gradon JD. Extracolonic manifestations of *Clostridium difficile* infections: presentation of 2 cases and review of the literature. Medicine 2001;80:88–101.
215. Kader HA, Picolli DA, Jawad AF, McGowan KL, Maller ES. Single toxin detection is inadequate to diagnose *Clostridium difficile* diarrhea in pediatric patients. Gastroenterology 1998;115: 1329–34.
216. Mahida YR, Hyde SM, Gray T, Borriello SP. Effect of *Clostridium difficile* toxin A on human epithelial cells: induction of interleukin 8 production and apoptosis after cell detachment. Gut 1996;38:337–47.
217. McFarland LV, Surawicz CM, Stamm WE. Risk factors for *Clostridium difficile* carriage and *C. difficile*-associated diarrhea in a cohort of hospitalized patients. J Infect Dis 1990;162:678–84.
218. Reinke CM, Messick CR. Update on *Clostridium difficile*-induced colitis, Part I. Am J Hosp Pharm 1994;51:1771–81.
219. Schiffman R. Signet-ring cells associated with pseudomembranous colitis. Am J Surg Pathol 1996;20:599–602.
220. Schnett S, Antonioli A, Goldman H. Massive mural edema in severe pseudomembranous colitis. Arch Pathol Lab Med 1983:107;211–3.
221. Sidhu JS, Liu D. Signet-ring cells associated with pseudomembranous colitis. Am J Surg Pathol 2001;25:542–3.
222. Thelestam M, Chaves-Olarte E. Cytotoxic effects of the *Clostridium difficile* toxins. Curr Topics Microbiol Immunol 2000;250:85–96.
223. Viscidi R, Wsilley S, Bartlett JG. Isolation rates and toxigenic potential of *Clostridium difficile* isolates from various patient populations. Gastroenterology 1981;81:5–9.
224. Wilcox MH. *Clostridium difficile* infection and pseudomembranous colitis. Best Pract Res Clin Gastroenterol 2003;17:475–93.

Clostridium Septicum Infections

225. Bretzke ML, Bubrick MP, Hitchcock CR. Diffuse spreading *Clostridium septicum* infection, malignant disease and immune suppression. Surg Gynecol Obstet 1988;166:197–9.
226. Hopkins DG, Kushner JP. Clostridial species in the pathogenesis of enterocolitis in patients with neutropenia. Am J Hematol 1983;14:289–95.
227. Katlic MR, Derkac WM, Coleman WS. *Clostridium septicum* infection and malignancy. Ann Surg 1981;193:361–4.
228. Koransky JR, Stargel MD, Dowell VR Jr. *Clostridium septicum* bacteremia: its clinical significance. Am J Med 1979;66:63–6.
229. Kornbluth AA, Danzig JB, Bernstein LH. *Clostridium septicum* infection and associated malignancy: report of 2 cases and review of the literature. Medicine 1989;68:30–7.
230. Pelletier JP, Plumbley JA, Rouse EA, Cina SJ. The role of *Clostridium septicum* in paraneoplastic sepsis. Arch Pathol Lab Med 2000;124: 353–6.
231. Steinberg D, Gold J, Brodin A. Necrotizing enterocolitis in leukemia. Arch Intern Med 1973;131:538–44.
232. Wade DS, Nava HR, Douglass HO. Neutropenic enterocolitis. Clinical diagnosis and treatment. Cancer 1992;69:17–23.
233. Williams N, Scott AD. Neutropenic colitis: a continuing surgical challenge. Br J Surg 1997;84:1200–5.

Clostridium Perfringens and *Clostridium Welchii* Infections

234. Borriello SP, Larson HE, Welch AR, Barclay F, Stringer MF, Bartholomew BA. Enterotoxigenic *Clostridium perfringens*: a possible cause of antibiotic-associated diarrhoea. Lancet 1984;1: 305–7.
235. Brett MM, Rodhouse JC, Donovan TK, Tebbutt GM, Hutchinson DN. Detection of *Clostridium perfringens* and its enterotoxin in cases of sporadic diarrhoea. J Clin Pathol 1992;45:609–11.
236. Brynestad S, Granum PE. *Clostridium perfringens* and foodborne infections. Int J Food Microbiol 2002;74:195–202.
237. Canard B, Saint-Joanis B, Daube G, et al. Genomic diversity and organization of virulence genes in the pathogenic anaerobe *Clostridium perfringens*. Mol Microbiol 1992;6:1421–9.

238. Farrant JM, Traill Z, Conlon C, et al. Pigbel-like syndrome in a vegetarian in Oxford. Gut 1996;39:336–7.
239. Granum PE. *Clostridium perfringens* toxins involved in food poisoning. Int J Food Microbiol 1990;10:101–12.
240. Gui L, Subramony C, Fratkin J, Hughson MD. Fatal enteritis necroticans (pigbel) in a diabetic adult. Mod Pathol 2002;15:66–70.
241. Hardy SP, Parekh N, Denmead M, Granum PE. Cationic currents induced by *Clostridium perfringens* type A enterotoxin in human intestinal CaCo-2 cells. J Med Microbiol 1999;48: 235–43.
242. Hatheway CL. Toxigenic clostridia. Clin Microbiol Rev 1990;3:68–98.
243. Jolivet-Reynaud C, Popoff MR, Vinit MA, et al. Enteropathogenicity of *Clostridium perfringens* beta-toxin and other clostridial toxins. Zb Bacteriol Microbiol Hyg Suppl 1986;15:145–51.
244. Katayama SL, Dupuy B, Daube G, China B, Cole ST. Genome mapping of *Clostridium perfringens* strains with I-*Ceu* 1 shows many virulence genes to be plasmid-borne. Mol Gen Genet 1996;251:720–6.
245. Larson HE, Borrielo SP. Infectious diarrhea due to *Clostridium perfringens*. J Infect Dis 1988;157: 390–1.
246. Lawrence GW. The pathogenesis of enteritis necroticans. In: Rood JI, McClane BA, Songer JG, Titball RW, eds. The clostridia: molecular biology and pathogenesis. London: Academic Press; 1997:197–207.
247. Lawrence GW, Lehmann D, Anian G, et al. Impact of active immunization against enteritis necroticans in Papua New Guinea. Lancet 1990:336;1165–7.
248. Mpamugo O, Donovan T, Brett MM. Enterotoxigenic *Clostridium perfringens* as a cause of sporadic case of diarrhoea. J Med Microbiol 1995;43:442–5.
249. Murrell TG. Pigbel in Papua, New Guinea: an ancient disease rediscovered. Int J Epidemiol 1983;12:211–4.
250. Murrell TG, Walker PD. The pigbel story of Papua New Guinea. Trans R Soc Trop Med Hyg 1991;85:119–22.
251. Petit L, Gibert M, Popoff MR. *Clostridium perfringens*: toxinotype and genotype. Trends Microbiol 1999;7:104–10.
252. Petrillo TM, Beck-Sague CM, Songer JG, et al. Enteritis necroticans (pigbel) in a diabetic child. N Engl J Med 2000;342:1250–3.
253. Rood JI. Virulence genes of *Clostridium perfringens*. Annu Rev Microbiol 1998;52:333–60.
254. Samuel SC, Hancock P, Leigh DA. An investigation into *Clostridium perfringens* enterotoxin-associated diarrhea. J Hosp Infect 1991;18:219–30.
255. Severin WPJ, de la Fuente AA, Stringer MF. *Clostridium perfringens* type C causing necrotizing enteritis. J Clin Pathol 1984;37:942–4.
256. Singh G, Narang V, Malik AK, Khanna SK. Segmental enteritis: "enteritis necroticans." A clinicopathologic study. J Clin Gastroenterol 1996; 22:6–10.
257. Songer JG. Clostridial enteric diseases of domestic animals. Clin Microbiol Rev 1996;9:216–34.
258. Sterne M, Warrack GH. The types of *Clostridium perfringens*. J Pathol Bacteriol 1964;88:279–83.
259. Wada A, Masuda Y, Fukayama M, et al. Nosocomial diarrhoea in the elderly due to enterotoxigenic *Clostridium perfringens*. Microbiol Immunol 1996;40:767–71.
260. Watson DA, Andrew JH, Banting S, Mackay JR, Stillwell RG, Merrett M. Pig-bel but no pig: enteritis necroticans acquired in Australia. Med J Aust 1991;155:47–50.

Vibrio **Infections**

261. Black RE, Merson MH, Rahman AS. A two-year study of bacterial, viral and parasitic agents associated with diarrhea in rural Bangladesh. J Infect Dis 1980;142:660–4.
262. Blake PA, Allegra DT, Snyder JD, et al. Cholera: a possible endemic focus in the United States. N Engl J Med 1980;302:305–9.
263. Blake PA, Merson MH, Weaver RE, Hollis DG, Heublein PC. Disease caused by a marine *Vibrio*: clinical characteristics and epidemiology. N Engl J Med 1979;300:1–5.
264. Carnahan AM, Harding J, Watsky D, Hansman S. Identification of *Vibrio hollisae* associated with severe gastroenteritis after consumption of raw oysters. J Clin Microbiol 1994;32:1805–6.
265. Faruque SM, Albert MJ, Mekalanos JJ. Epidemiology, genetics and ecology of toxigenic *Vibrio cholerae*. Microbiol Mol Biol Rev 1998;62:1301–14.
266. Faruque SM, Nair GB. Molecular ecology of toxigenic *Vibrio cholerae*. Microbiol Immunol 2002;46:59–66.
267. Gangarosa EG, Beisel WR, Benyajati C, et al. The nature of the gastrointestinal lesion in Asiatic cholera and its relation to pathogenesis: a biopsy study. Am J Trop Med Hyg 1960;9:125–35.
268. Klontz KC, Lieb S, Schreiber M, Janowski HT, Baldy LM, Gunn RA. Syndromes of *Vibrio vulnificus* infections. Clinical and epidemiologic features in Florida cases, 1981-1987. Ann Intern Med 1988;109:318–23.
269. Lee SH, Hava DL, Waldor MK, Camilli A. Regulation and temporal expression patterns of *Vibrio cholerae* virulence genes during infection. Cell 1999;99:625–34.

270. Lencer WI. Microbes and microbial toxins: paradigms for microbial-mucosal interactions. *V. cholera*: invasion of the intestinal epithelial barrier by a stably folded protein toxin. Am J Physiol Gastrointest Liver Physiol 2001;280: G781–6.
271. Pavia AT, Campbell JF, Blake PA, Smith JD, McKinley TW, Martin DL. Cholera from raw oysters shipped interstate. JAMA 1987;258: 2374.
272. Ryan ET, Calderwood SB. Cholera vaccines. Clin Infect Dis 2000;31:561–5.
273. Ryan ET, Dhar U, Khan WA, et al. Mortality, morbidity, and microbiology of endemic cholera among hospitalized patients in Dhaka, Bangladesh. Am J Trop Med Hyg 2000;63:12–20.
274. Shandera WX, Hafkin B, Martin DL, et al. Persistence of cholera in the United States. Am J Trop Med Hyg 1983;32:812–7.
275. Sommers HM. Infectious diarrhea. In: Youmans GP, Sommers HM, Patterson PY, eds. Biological and clinical basis of infectious disease, 2nd ed. Philadelphia: WB Saunders; 1980:525.
276. Waldor MK, Mekalanos JJ. Lysogenic conversion by a filamentous phage encoding cholera toxin. Science 1996;272:1910–4.

Aeromonas Infections

277. Abdullah AI, Hart CA, Winstanley C. Molecular characterization and distribution of virulence-associated genes amongst *Aeromonas* isolates from Libya. J Appl Microbiol 2003;95:1001–7.
278. Agger WA, McCormick JD, Gurwith MJ. Clinical and microbiological features of *Aeromonas hydrophila*-associated diarrhea. J Clin Microbiol 1985;21:909–13.
279. Albert MJ, Ansaruzzaman M, Talukder KA, et al. Prevalence of enterotoxin genes in *Aeromonas* spp. isolated from children with diarrhea, healthy controls, and the environment. J Clin Microbiol 2000;38:3785–90.
280. Altwegg M, Martinetti Lucchini G, Luthy-Hottenstein J, Rohrbach M. *Aeromonas*-associated gastroenteritis after consumption of contaminated shrimp. Eur J Clin Microbiol Infect Dis 1991;10:44–5.
281. Altwegg M, Steigerwalt AG, Altwegg-Bissig J, Luthy-Hottenstein J, Brenner DJ. Biochemical identification of *Aeromonas* genospecies isolated from humans. J Clin Microbiol 1990;28: 258–64.
282. Barer MR, Millership SE, Tabaqchali S. Relationship of toxin production to species in the genus *Aeromonas*. J Med Microbiol 1986;22:303–9.
283. Borrell N, Figueras M, Guarro J. Phenotypic identification of *Aeromonas* genomospecies from clinical and environmental sources. Can J Microbiol 1998;44:103–8.
284. Chakraborty T, Montenegro MA, Sanyal SC, Helmuth R, Bulling E, Timmis KN. Cloning of enterotoxin gene from *Aeromonas hydrophila* provides conclusive evidence of production of a cytoxic enterotoxin. Infect Immun 1984;46:435–41.
285. de la Morena ML, Van R, Singh K, Brian M, Murray ME, Pickering LK. Diarrhea associated with *Aeromonas* species in children in day care centers. J Infect Dis 1993;168:215–8.
286. Echeverria P, Blocklow NR, Sanford IB, Cukor GG. Traveler's diarrhea among American Peace Corps volunteers in rural Thailand. J Infect Dis 1981;143:767–71.
287. Gonzalez-Serrano CJ, Santos JA, Garcia-Lopez ML, Otero A. Virulence markers in *Aeromonas hydrophila* and *Aeromonas veronii* biovar *sobria* isolates from freshwater fish and from a diarrhoea case. J Appl Microbiol 2002;93:414–9.
288. Goodwin CS, Harper WE, Stewart JK, Gracey M, Burke V, Robinson J. Enterotoxigenic *Aeromonas hydrophila* and diarrhea in adults. Med J Aust 1983;1:25–6.
289. Hanninen ML, Siitonen A. Distribution of *Aeromonas* phenospecies and genospecies among strains from water, foods or from clinical samples. Epidemiol Infect 1995;115:39–50.
290. Havelaar AH, Schets FM, van Silfhout A, Jansen WH, Wieten G, van der Kooj D. Typing of *Aeromonas* strains from patients with diarrhoea and from drinking water. J Appl Bacteriol 1992;72:435–44.
291. Holmberg SD, Farmer JJ. *Aeromonas hydrophila* and *Plesiomonas shigelloides* as causes of intestinal infections. *Rev Infect Dis* 1984;6:633–9.
292. Joseph SW, Carnahan AM, Brayton PR, et al. *Aeromonas jandaei* and *Aeromonas veronii* dual infection of a human wound following aquatic exposure. J Clin Microbiol 1991;29:565–9.
293. Kirov SM. The public health significance of *Aeromonas* spp. in foods. Int J Food Microbiol 1993;20:179–98.
294. Kirov SM, O'Donovan LA, Sanderson K. Functional characterization of type IV pili expressed on diarrhea-associated isolates of *Aeromonas* species. Infect Immun 1999;67:5447–54.
295. Kuhn I, Albert MJ, Ansaruzzaman M, et al. Characterization of *Aeromonas* spp. isolated from humans with diarrhea, from healthy controls, and from surface water in Bangladesh. J Clin Microbiol 1997;35:369–73.
296. Kuijper EJ, Bol P, Peeters MF, Steigerwalt R, Zanen HC, Brenner DJ. Clinical and epidemiologic aspects of members of *Aeromonas* DNA hybridization groups isolated from human feces. J Clin Microbiol 1989;27:1531–7.

297. Millership SE, Barer MR, Tabaqchali S. Toxin production by *Aeromonas* spp. from different sources. J Med Microbiol 1986;22:311–4.
298. Moyer NP, Martinetti G, Luthy-Hottenstein J, Altwegg M. Value of rRNA gene restriction patterns of *Aeromonas* spp. for epidemiological investigations. Curr Microbiol 1992;24:15–21.
299. Namdari H, Bottone EJ. Cytotoxin and enterotoxin production as factors delineating enteropathogenicity of *Aeromonas caviae*. J Clin Microbiology 1990;28:1796–8.
300. Pazzaglia G, Escalante JR, Sack RB, Rocca C, Benavides V. Transient intestinal colonization by multiple phenotypes of *Aeromonas* species during the first week of life. J Clin Microbiol 1990;28:1842–6.
301. Taylor DN, Echeverria P, Blaser MJ, et al. Polymicrobial aetiology of traveler's diarrhea. Lancet 1985;1:381–3.
302. Teka T, Faruque SG, Hossain MI, Fuchs GJ. Aeromonas-associated diarrhea in Bangladeshi children: clinical and epidemiological characteristics. Ann Trop Pediatr 1999;19:15–20.
303. Thorney JP, Shaw JG, Gryllos IA, Eley A. Virulence properties of clinically significant *Aeromonas* species: evidence of pathogenicity. Rev Med Microbiol 1997;8:61–72.
304. Turnbull PC, Lee JV, Miliotis MD, et al. Enterotoxin production in relation to taxonomic grouping and source of isolation of *Aeromonas* species. J Clin Microbiol 1984;19:175–80.

Plesiomonas Infections

305. Abbott SL, Kokka RP, Janda JM. Laboratory investigation on the low pathogenic potential of *Plesiomonas shigelloides*. J Clin Microbiol 1991;29:148–53.
306. Bai Y, Dai YC, Li JD, et al. Acute diarrhea during army field exercise in southern China. World J Gastroenterol 2004;10:127–31.
307. Baratela KC, Saridakis HO, Gaziri LC, Pelayo JS. Effects of medium composition, calcium, iron and oxygen on haemolysin production by *Plesiomonas shigelloides* isolated from water. J Appl Microbiol 2001;90:482–7.
308. Falcon R, Carbonell GV, Figueredo PM, et al. Intracellular vacuolation induced by culture filtrates of *Plesiomonas shigelloides* isolated from environmental sources. J Appl Microbiol 2003; 95:273–8.
309. Holmberg SD, Wachsmuth IK, Hickman-Brenner FW, Blake PA. *Plesiomonas* enteric infections in the United States. Ann Intern Med 1986;105:690–4.
310. Rautelin H, Sivonen A, Kuikka A, Renkonen OV, Valtonen V, Kosunen TU. Enteric *Plesiomonas shigelloides* infections in Finnish patients. Scand J Inf Dis 1995;27:495–8.
311. Sears CL, Kaper JB. Enteric bacterial toxins: mechanisms of action and linkage to intestinal secretion. Microbiol Rev 1996;60:167–215.
312. Shigematsu M, Kaufmann ME, Charlett A, Niho Y, Pitt TL. An epidemiological study of *Plesiomonas shigelloides* diarrhoea among Japanese travelers. Epidemiol Infect 2000;125:523–30.
313. Tseng HK, Liu CP, Li WC, Su SC, Lee CM. Characteristics of *Plesiomonas shigelloides* infection in Taiwan. J Microbiol Immunol Inf 2002;35:47–52.
314. Wong TY, Tsui HY, So MK, et al. *Plesiomonas shigelloides* infection in Hong Kong: retrospective study of 167 laboratory confirmed cases. Hong Kong Med J 2000;6:375–80.

Yersinia Infections

315. Black RE, Jackson RJ, Tsai T, et al. Epidemic *Yersinia enterocolitica* infection due to contaminated chocolate milk. N Engl J Med 1978;298:76–9.
316. Cornelis G, Laroche Y, Balligand G, Sory MP, Wauters G. *Yersinia enterocolitica*, a primary model for bacterial invasiveness. Rev Infect Dis 1987;9:64–87.
317. Cornelis GR. The *Yersinia* deadly kiss. J Bacteriol 1998;180:5495–504.
318. Cornelis GR. *Yersinia* pathogenicity factors. Curr Top Microbiol Immunol 1994;192:243–63.
319. Cover TL, Aber RC. *Yersinia enterocolitica*. N Engl J Med 1989;321:16–24.
320. De Boer E. Isolation of *Yersinia enterocolitica* from foods. Contrib Microbiol Immunol 1995; 13:71–3.
321. Delorme J, Laverdier M, Martineau B, Lafleur L. Yersiniosis in children. Can Med Assoc J 1974;110:281–4.
322. El-Maraghi NR, Mair NS. The histopathology of enteric infection with *Yersinia pseudotuberculosis*. Am J Clin Pathol 1979;71:631–9.
323. Foberg U, Fryden A, Kihlstrom E, Persson K, Weiland O. *Yersinia enterocolitica* septicemia: clinical and microbiological aspects. Scand J Infect Dis 1986;18:269–79.
324. Fredriksson-Ahomaa M, Korte T, Korkeala H. Contamination of carcasses, offals and the environment with *yad*A-positive *Yersinia enterocolitica* in a pig slaughterhouse. J Food Prot 2000;63:31–5.
325. Fredriksson-Ahomaa M, Lyhs U, Korte T, Korkeala H. Prevalence of pathogenic *Yersinia enterocolitica* in food samples at retail level in Finland. Arch Lebensmittelhyg 2001;52:66–8.
326. Fukushima H, Gomyoda M, Kaneko S. Mice and moles inhabiting mountainous areas of Shimane peninsula as sources of infection with *Yersinia pseudotuberculosis*. J Clin Microbiol 1990;28:2448–55.

327. Gemski P, Lazere JR, Casey T. Plasmid associated with pathogenicity and calcium dependency of *Yersinia enterocolitica*. Infect Immun 1980;27:682–5.
328. Gleason TH, Patterson SD. The pathology of *Yersinia enterocolitica* ileocolitis. Am J Surg Pathol 1982;6:347–55.
328a. Guerrant RL, Van Gilder T, Steiner TS, et al. Practice guidelines for the management of infectious diarrhea. Clin Infect Dis 2001;32:331–50.
329. Kapperud G, Namork E, Skurnik M, Nesbakken T. Plasmid-mediated surface fibrillae of *Yersinia enterocolitica*: relationship to the outer membrane protein YOP1 and possible importance for pathogenesis. Infect Immun 1987;55:2247–54.
330. Keet EE. *Yersinia enterocolitica* septicemia. Source of infection and incubation period identified. NY State J Med 1974;74:2226–30.
331. Lamps LW, Madhusudhan KT, Greenson JK, et al. The role of *Yersinia enterocolitica* and *Yersinia pseudotuberculosis* in granulomatous appendicitis. A histologic and molecular study. Am J Surg Pathol 2001:25;508–15.
332. Merilahti-Palo R, Lahesmaa R, Granfors K, Gripenberg-Lerche C, Toivanen P. Risk of *Yersinia* infection among butchers. Scand J Infect Dis 1991;23:55–61.
333. Miller VL, Falkow S. Evidence for two genetic loci in *Yersinia enterocolitica* that can promote invasion of epithelial cells. Infect Immun 1988;56:1242–8.
334. Miller VL, Farmer JJ 3rd, Hill WE, Falkow S. The *ail* locus is found uniquely in *Yersinia enterocolitica* serotypes commonly associated with disease. Infect Immun 1989;57:121–31.
335. O'Loughlin EV, Humphreys G, Dunn I, et al. Clinical, morphological, and biochemical alterations in acute intestinal yersiniosis. Pediatr Res 1986;20:602–8.
336. Portnoy DA, Moseley SL, Falkow S. Characterization of plasmids and plasmid-associated determinants of *Yersinia enterocolitica* pathogenesis. Infect Immun 1981;31:775–82.
337. Rabinovitz M, Stremple JF, Wells KE, Stone BG. *Yersinia enterocolitica*: infection complicated by intestinal perforation. Arch Intern Med 1987; 147:1662–3.
338. Revell PA, Miller VL. *Yersinia* virulence: more than a plasmid. FEMS Microbiol Lett 2001;205: 159–64.
339. Schiemann DA. Association of *Yersinia enterocolitica* with the manufacture of cheese and occurrence in pasteurized milk. Appl Environ Microbiol 1978;36:274–7.
340. Shayegani M, Stone WB, DeForge I, Root T, Parsons LM, Maupin P. *Yersinia enterocolitica* and related species isolated from wildlife in New York State. Appl Environ Microbiol 1986;52: 420–4.
341. Simmonds SD, Noble MA, Freeman HJ. Gastrointestinal features of culture-positive *Yersinia enterocolitica* infection. Gastroenterology 1987;92:112–7.
342. Stenhouse MA, Milnew LV. *Yersinia enterocolitica:* a hazard in blood transfusion. Transfusion 1982;22:396–8.
343. Tauxe RV, Wauters G, Goossens V, VanNoyen R. *Yersinia enterocolitica* infections and pork: the missing link. Lancet 1987;1:1129–32.
344. Une T. Studies on the pathogenicity of *Yersinia enterocolitica*. II. Interaction with cultured cells in vitro. Microbiol Immunol 1977;21:365–77.
345. Vantrappen G, Ponette E, Geboes K, Bertrand P. *Yersinia enteritis* and enterocolitis: gastroenterological aspects. Gastroenterology 1977; 72:220–7.

Mycobacterium Tuberculosis Infections

346. Barker LP, George KM, Falkow S, Small PL. Differential trafficking of live and dead *Mycobacterium marinum* organisms in macrophages. Infect Immun 1997;65:1497–504.
347. Clemens DL. Characterization of the *Mycobacterium tuberculosis* phagosome. Trends Microbiol 1996;4:113–8.
348. Findlay JM. Medical management of gastrointestinal tuberculosis. J R Soc Med 1982;75:583–4.
349. Gilinsky NH, Marks IN, Kottler RE, Price SK. Abdominal tuberculosis. A 10 year review. S Afr Med J 1983;64:849–57.
350. Hulnick DH, Megibow AJ, Naidich DP, Hilton S, Cho KC, Balthazar EJ. Abdominal tuberculosis: CT evaluation. Radiology 1985;157:199–204.
351. Jayanthi V, Probert CS, Sher KS, Wicks AC, Mayberry JF. The renaissance of abdominal tuberculosis. Dig Dis 1993;11:36–44.
352. Louie E, Rice LB, Holzman RS. Tuberculosis in non-Haitian patients with acquired immunodeficiency syndrome. Chest 1986;90:542–5.
353. Marshall JB. Tuberculosis of the gastrointestinal tract and peritoneum. Am J Gastroenterology 1993;88:989–99.
354. Murray CJ, Lopez AD, eds. The global burden of disease. Global burden of disease and injury series, Vol 1. Cambridge: Harvard University Press; 1996:349–50.
355. Ramakrishnan L, Federspiel NA, Falkow S. Granuloma-specific expression of *Mycobacterium* virulence proteins from the glycine-rich PE-PGRS family. Science 2000;288:1436–9.
356. Rosengart TK, Coppa GF. Abdominal mycobacterial infections in immunocompromised patients. Am J Surg 1990;159:125–30.

357. Schlesinger LS, Bellinger-Kawahara CG, Payne NR, Horwitz MA. Phagocytosis of *Mycobacterium tuberculosis* is mediated by human monocyte complement receptors and complement component C3. J Immunol 1990;144:2771–80.
358. Schorey JS, Carroll MC, Brown EJ. A macrophage invasion mechanism of pathogenic mycobacteria. Science 1997;277:1091–3.
359. Terblanche J. Fistula in ano: a 5 year survey at Groote Schuur Hospital and a review of the literature. S Afr Med J 1964;38:403–8.
360. Venable GS, Rana PS. Colonic tuberculosis. Postgrad Med J 1979;55:276–8.
361. Wales JM, Mumtaz H, MacLeod WM. Gastrointestinal tuberculosis. Br J Chest Dis 1976; 70:39–57.

Neisseria Gonorrhoeae Infections

362. Catterall RD. Anorectal gonorrhoea. Proc R Soc Med 1962;55:871–3.
363. Haines KA, Yeh L, Blake MS, Cristello P, Korchak H, Weissmann G. Protein I, a translocatable ion channel from *Neisseria gonorrhoeae* selectively inhibits exocytosis from human neutrophils without inhibiting O2-generation. J Biol Chem 1988;263:945–51.
364. McMillan A, McNeillage G, Gilmour HM, Lee FD. Histology of rectal gonorrhoea in men, with a note on anorectal infection with *Neisseria meningitidis*. J Clin Pathol 1983:36;511–4.
365. Siegel RM, Schubert CJ, Myers PA, Shapiro RA. The prevalence of sexually transmitted diseases in children and adolescents evaluated for sexual abuse in Cincinnati: rationale for limited STD testing in prepubertal girls. Pediatrics 1995;96: 1090–4.
366. Surawicz CM, Goodell SE, Quinn TC, et al. Spectrum of rectal biopsy abnormalities in homosexual men with intestinal symptoms. Gastroenterology 1986;91:651–9.

Treponemal Infections

367. Centers for Disease Control and Prevention. Primary and secondary syphilis—United States, 1997. MMWR Morb Mortal Wkly Rep 1998;47: 493–7.
368. Jones BV, Lichtenstein JE. Gastric syphilis: radiologic findings. AJR Am J Roentgenol 1993; 160:59–61.
369. Long BW, Johnson JH, Wetzel W, Flowers RH 3rd, Haick A. Gastric syphilis: endoscopic and histological features mimicking lymphoma. Am J Gastroenterology 1995;90:1504–7.

Granuloma Inguinale (Donovanosis)

370. Bozbora A, Erbil Y, Berber E, Ozarmagan S, Ozarmagan G. Surgical treatment of granuloma inguinale. Br J Dermatol 1998;138:1079–81.
371. Carter JS, Bowden FJ, Bastian I, Myers GM, Sriprakash KS, Kemp DJ. Phylogenetic evidence for reclassification of *Calymmatobacterium granulomatis* as *Klebsiella granulomatis* comb nov. Int J Syst Bacteriol 1999;49:1695–700.
372. Coovadia YM, Steinberg JL, Kharsany A. Granuloma inguinale (donovanosis) of the oral cavity: a case report. S Afr Med J 1985;68:815–7.
373. Hart G. Donovanosis. Clin Infect Dis 1997;25: 24–32.
374. Lal S, Nicholas C. Epidemiological and clinical features in 165 cases of granuloma inguinale. Br J Vener Dis 1970;46:461–3.
375. O'Farrell N. Donovanosis. Sex Transm Infect 2002;78:452–7.
376. Ramachander M, Jayalakshmi S, Pankaja P. A study of donovanosis in Guntur. Ind J Dermatol Venereol Leprol 1967;33:237–41.
377. Ramanan C, Sarma PS, Ghorpade A, Das M. Treatment of donovanosis with norfloxacin. Int J Dermatol 1990;29:298–9.

Chancroid

378. Albritton WL. Biology of *Haemophilus ducreyi*. Microbiol Rev 1989;53:377–89.
379. Brentjens RJ, Ketterer M, Apicella MA, Spinola SM. Fine tangled pili expressed by *Haemophilus ducreyi* are a novel class of pili. J Bacteriol 1996;178:808–16.
380. Campagnari AA, Wild LM, Griffiths GE, Karalus RJ, Wirth MA, Spinola SM. Role of lipooligosaccharides in experimental dermal lesions caused by *Haemophilus ducreyi*. Infect Immun 1991;59:2601–8.
381. Chui L, Maclean I, Marusyk R. Development of the polymerase chain reaction for diagnosis of chancroid. J Clin Microbiol 1993;31:659–64.
382. Dicarlo RP, Armentor BS, Mertin DH. Chancroid epidemiology in New Orleans men. J Infect Dis 1995;172:446–52.
383. Fung JC. Chancroid (*Haemophilus ducreyi*). In: Sun T, ed. Sexually related infectious diseases: clinical and laboratory aspects. Philadelphia: Field and Wood; 1986:15.
384. Hobbs MM, San Mateo LR, Orndorff PE, Almond G, Kawula TH. Swine model of *Haemophilus ducreyi* infection. Infect Immun 1995;63: 3094–100.
385. Jonasson JA. *Haemophilus ducreyi*. Int J STD AIDS 1993;4:317–21.
386. Lewis DA. Chancroid: clinical manifestations, diagnosis, and management. Sex Transm Infect 2003;79:68–71.

387. Lewis DA. Chancroid: from clinical practice to basic science. AIDS Patient Care STDs 2000; 14:19–36.
388. Marckmann P, Hojbjerg T, von Eyben FE, Christensen I. Imported pedal chancroid: case report. Genitourin Med 1989;65:126–7.
389. Mertz KJ, Trees D, Levine WC, et al. Etiology of genital ulcers and prevalence of human immunodeficiency virus co-infection in 10 US citizens. J Infect Dis 1998;78:1795–8.
390. Mertz KJ, Weiss JB, Webb RM, et al. An investigation of genital ulcers in Jackson, Mississippi, with use of a multiplex polymerase chain reaction assay: high prevalence of chancroid and human immunodeficiency virus infection. J Inf Dis 1998;178:1060–6.
391. Mohammed KN. Inguinal bubo: problems in diagnosis. Singapore Med J 1992;33:600–2.
392. Nsanze H, Fast MV, D'Costa LJ, Tukei P, Curran J, Ronald A. Genital ulcers in Kenya: clinical and laboratory study. Br J Vener Dis 1981;57: 378–81.
393. Nsanze H, Plummer FA, Maggwa AB, et al. Comparison of media for the primary isolation of *Haemophilus ducreyi*. Sex Transm Dis 1984; 11:6–9.
394. Orle KA, Gates CA, Martin DH, Body BA, Weiss JB. Simultaneous PCR detection of *Haemophilus ducreyi, Treponema pallidum,* and herpes simplex virus type 1 and 2 from genital ulcers. J Clin Microbiol 1996;34:49–54.
395. Purven M, Falsen E, Lagergard T. Cytotoxin production in 100 strains of *Haemophilus ducreyi* from different geographic locations. FEMS Microbiol Lett 1995;129:221–4.
396. Schmid GP, Sanders LL, Blount JH, Alexander ER. Chancroid in the United States. Reestablishment of an old disease. JAMA 1987;258: 3265–8.
397. Seghal VN, Shyam Prasad AL. Chancroid or chancroidal ulcer. Dermatologica 1985;170: 136–41.
398. Seghal VN, Srivastava G. Chancroid: contemporary appraisal. Int J Dermatol 2003;42:182–90.
399. Totten PA, Norn DV, Stamm WE. Characterization of the hemolytic activity of *Haemophilus ducreyi*. Infect Immun 1995;63:4409–16.
400. West B, Wilson SM, Changalucha J, et al. Simplified PCR for detection of *Haemophilus ducreyi* and diagnosis of chancroid. J Clin Microbiol 1995;33:787–90.

Actinomyces Infections

401. Brown JR. Human actinomycosis: a study of 181 subjects. Hum Pathol 1973:4;319–30.
402. Cintron JR, Del Pino A, Duarte B, Wood D. Abdominal actinomycosis. Dis Colon Rectum 1996;39:105–8.
403. Cowgill R, Quan SH. Colonic actinomycosis mimicking carcinoma. Dis Colon Rectum 1978;22:45–6.
404. Ferrari TC, Couto CA, Murta-Oliveira C, Conceicao SA, Silva RG. Actinomycosis of the colon: a rare form of presentation. Scand J Gastroenterol 2000;35:108–9.
405. Koren R, Dekel Y, Ramadan E, Veltman V, Dreznik Z. Periappendiceal actinomycosis mimicking malignancy: report of a case. Pathol Res Pract 2002;198:441–3.
406. Sechas M, Christeas N, Balaroutsos C, Demertzis A, Skalkeas G. Actinomycosis of the colon: report of two cases. Dis Colon Rectum 1972;15:366–9.

Tropheryma Infections

407. Adams M, Rhyner PA, Day J, DeArmond S, Smuckler E. Whipple's disease confined to the central nervous system. Ann Neurol 1987;21: 104–8.
408. Bai JC, Mota AH, Maurino E, et al. Class I and class II HLA antigens in a homogenous Argentinian population with Whipple's disease: lack of association with HLA-B27. Am J Gastroenterol 1991;86:992–4.
409. Bai JC, Sen L, Diez R, et al. Impaired monocyte function in patients successfully treated for Whipple's disease. Acta Gastroenterol Latinoam 1996;26:85–9.
410. Dobbins WO 3rd, Ruffin JM. A light and electron microscopic study of bacterial invasion in Whipple's disease. Am J Pathol 1967;51:225–42.
411. Dutly F, Altwegg M. Whipple's disease and "*Tropheryma whippelii*." Clin Microbiol Rev 2001;14:561–83.
412. Dutly F, Hinrikson HP, Seidel T, Morgenegg S, Altwegg M, Bauerfeind P. *Tropheryma whippelii* DNA in saliva of patients without Whipple's disease. Infection 2000;28:219–22.
413. Dykmann DD, Cuccherini BA, Fuss IJ, Blum LW, Woodward JE, Strober W. Whipple's disease in a father-daughter pair. Dig Dis Sci 1999;44:2542–4.
414. Ectors N, Geboes K, De Vos R, et al. Whipple's disease: a histological, immunocytochemical and electron microscopic study of the immune response in the small intestinal mucosa. Histopathology 1992;21:1–12.
415. Ectors N, Geboes K, Rutgeerts P, et al. RFD7-RFD9 coexpression by macrophages points to T cell-macrophage interaction deficiency in Whipple's disease. Gastroenterology 1992;106:A676.

416. Ehrbar HU, Bauerfeind P, Dutly F, Koelz HR, Altwagg M. PCR-positive tests for *Tropheryma whippelii* in patients without Whipple's disease. Lancet 1999;353:2214.
417. Fenollar F, Lepidi H, Raoult D. Whipple's endocarditis: review of the literature and comparisons with Q fever, *Bartonella* infection, and blood culture–positive endocarditis. Clin Infect Dis 2001;33:1309–16.
418. Feurle GE, Dorken B, Lenhard V. HLA-B27 and defects in the T-cell system in Whipple's disease. Eur J Clin Invest 1979;9:385–9.
419. Feurle GE, Marth T. An evaluation of antimicrobial treatment for Whipple's disease: tetracycline versus trimethoprim-sulfamethoxazole. Dig Dis Sci 1994;39:1642–8.
420. Fleming JL, Wiesner RH, Shorter RC. Whipple's disease: clinical, biochemical, and histopathological features and assessment of treatment in 29 patients. Mayo Clin Proc 1988;63:539–51.
421. Geboes K, Ectors N, Heidbuchel H, Rutgeerts P, Desmet V, Vantrappen G. Whipple's disease: the value of upper gastrointestinal endoscopy for the diagnosis and follow-up. Acta Gastroenterol Belg 1992;55:209–19.
422. Geissdorfer W, Wittmann I, Seitz G, et al. A case of aortic valve disease associated with *Tropheryma whippelii* infection in the absence of other signs of Whipple's disease. Infection 2001;29:44–7.
423. Groll A, Valberg LS, Simon JB, Eidinger D, Wilson B, Forsdyke DR. Immunological defects in Whipple's disease. Gastroenterology 1972;63: 943–50.
424. Gross JB, Wollaeger EE, Sauer WG, et al. Whipple's disease: report of four cases, including two brothers, with observation on pathologic physiology, diagnosis and treatment. Gastroenterology 1959;36:65–93.
425. Gross M, Jung C, Zoller WG. Detection of *Tropheryma whippelii* (Whipple's disease) in faeces. Ital J Gastroenterol Hepatol 1999;31:70–2.
426. Gruner U, Goesch P, Donner A, Peters U. Morbus Whipple und Non–Hodgkin–Lymphom. Z Gastroenterol 2001;39:305–9.
427. Keinath RD, Merrell DE, Vlietstra R, Dobbins WO 3rd. Antibiotic treatment and relapse in Whipple's disease. Gastroenterology 1985;88: 1867–73.
428. Lukacs G, Dobi S, Szabo M. A case of Whipple's disease with repeated operations for ileus and complete cure. Acta Hepatogastroenterol 1978;25:238–42.
429. Maiwald M, Meier-Willersen HJ, Hartmann M, von Herbay A. Detection of *Tropheryma whippelii* DNA in a patient with AIDS. J Clin Microbiol 1995;33:1354–6.
430. Maiwald M, Schuhmacher F, Ditton HJ, von Herbay A. Environmental occurrence of the Whipple's disease bacterium (*Tropheryma whippelii*). Appl Environ Microbiol 1999;64:760–2.
431. Maiwald M, von Herbay A, Persing DH, et al. *Tropheryma whippelii* DNA is rare in the intestinal mucosa of patients without other evidence of Whipple's disease. Ann Intern Med 2001; 134:115–9.
432. Marth T. The diagnosis and treatment of Whipple's disease. Curr Allergy Asthma Rep 2001;1:566–71.
433. Marth T, Kleen N, Stallmach A, et al. Dysregulated peripheral and mucosal Th1/Th2 response in Whipple's disease. Gastroenterology 2002;123:1468–77.
434. Marth T, Neurath M, Cuccherini BA, Strober W. Defects of monocyte interleukin-12 production and humoral immunity in Whipple's disease. Gastroenterology 1997;113:442–8.
435. Marth T, Raoult D. Whipple's disease. Lancet 2003;361:239–46.
436. Marth T, Strober W. Whipple's disease. Semin Gastrointest Dis 1996;7:41–8.
437. Meier-Willersen HJ, Maiwald M, von Herbay A. Whipple's disease associated with opportunistic infections. Dtsch Med Wochenschr 1993;118:854–60.
438. Miksche LW, Blumcke S, Fritsche D, Kuchemann K, Schuler HW, Grozinger KH. Whipple's disease: etiopathogenesis, treatment, diagnosis and clinical course. Case report and review of the world literature. Acta Hepatogastroenterol 1974;21:307–26.
439. Muller N, Schneider T, Zeitz M, Marth T. Whipple's disease: new aspects in pathogenesis and diagnosis. Acta Endoscopica 2001;31:243–53.
440. Olivieri I, Brandi G, Padula A, et al. Lack of association with spondyloarthritis and HLA-B27 in Italian patients with Whipple's disease. J Rheumatol 2001;28:1294–7.
441. Puite RH, Tesluk H. Whipple's disease. Am J Med 1955;19:383–400.
442. Raoult D. A febrile, blood culture negative endocarditis. Ann Intern Med 1999;131:144–6.
443. Raoult D, Birg ML, La Scola B, et al. Cultivation of the bacillus of Whipple's disease. N Engl J Med 2000;342:620–5.
444. Schneider T, Salamon-Looijen M, von Herbay A, et al. Whipple's disease with aortic regurgitation requiring aortic valve replacement. Infection 1998;26:178–180.
445. Suzer T, Demirkan N, Tahta K, Coskun E, Cetin B. Whipple's disease confined to the central nervous system: case report and review of the literature. Scand J Infect Dis 1999;31:411–4.

446. von Herbay A, Ditton HJ, Schumacher F, Maiwald M. Whipple's disease: staging and monitoring by cytology and polymerase chain reaction analysis of cerebrospinal fluid. Gastroenterology 1997;113:434–41.

Chlamydia Infections

447. de la Monte SM, Hutchins GM. Follicular proctocolitis and neuromatous hyperplasia with lymphogranuloma venereum. Hum Pathol 1985;16:1025–32.
448. Mabey D, Peeling RW. Lymphogranuloma venereum. Sex Transm Infect 2002;78:90–2.
449. Quinn TC, Goodell SE, Mkrtichian E, et al. *Chlamydia trachomatis* proctitis. N Engl J Med 1981;305:195–200.
450. Scieux C, Barnes R, Bianchi A, Casin I, Morel P, Perol Y. Lymphogranuloma venereum: 27 cases in Paris. J Infect Dis 1989;160:662–8.

Anthrax

451. Alizad A, Ayoub EM, Makki N. Intestinal anthrax in a two-year-old child. Pediatr Infect Dis J 1995;14:394–5.
452. Bhat P, Mohan DN, Srinivasa H. Intestinal anthrax with bacteriological investigations. J Infect Dis 1985;152:1357–8.
453. Dixon TC, Meselson M, Guillemin J, Hanna PC. Anthrax. N Engl J Med 1999;341:815–26.
454. Dutz W, Kohout E. Anthrax. Pathol Annu 1971;6:209–48.
455. Dutz W, Kohout-Dutz E. Anthrax. Int J Dermatol 1981;20:203–6.
456. Kunanusont C, Limpakarnjanarat K, Foy HM. Outbreak of anthrax in Thailand. Ann Trop Med Parasitol 1990;84:507–12.
457. Leppla SH. The anthrax toxin complex. In: Alouf J, Freer JH, eds. Source book of bacterial protein toxins. London: Academic Press; 1991: 277–302.
458. Meselson M, Guillemin J, Hugh-Jones M, et al. The Sverdlovsk anthrax outbreak of 1979. Science 1994;266:1202–8.
459. Ross JM. The pathogenesis of anthrax following the administration of spores by the respiratory route. J Pathol Bacteriol 1957;73:485–94.
460. Sekhar PC, Singh RS, Sridhar MS, Bhaskar XJ, Rao YS. Outbreak of human anthrax in Ramabhadrapuram village of Chittor district in Andhra Pradesh. Indian J Med Res 1990;91: 448–52.
461. Watson A, Keir D. Information of which to base assessments of risk from environments contaminated with anthrax spores. Epidemiol Infect 1994;113:479–90.

Listeria Infections

462. Altekruse SF, Cohen ML, Swerdlow DL. Emerging foodborne diseases. Emerg Infect Dis 1997; 3:285–93.
463. Aureli P, Fiorucci GC, Caroli D, et al. An outbreak of febrile gastroenteritis associated with corn contaminated with *Listeria monocytogenes*. N Engl J Med 2000;342:1236–41.
464. Centers for Disease Control and Prevention. Multistate outbreak of listeriosis–United States, 2000. MMWR Morb Mortal Wkly Rep 2000;49: 1129–30.
465. Cossart P. Actin-based motility of pathogens: the Arp2/3 complex is a central player. Cell Microbiol 2000;2:195–205.
466. Cossart P, Lecuit M. Interactions of *Listeria monocytogenes* with mammalian cells during entry and actin-based movement: bacterial factors, cellular ligands and signaling. EMBO J 1998;17:3797–806.
467. Dalton CB, Austin CC, Sobel J, et al. An outbreak of gastroenteritis and fever due to *Listeria monocytogenes* in milk. N Engl J Med 1997; 336:100–5.
468. Decatur AL, Portnoy DA. A PEST-like sequence in listeriolysin O essential for *Listeria monocytogenes* pathogenicity. Science 2000;290:992–5.
469. Dramsi S, Biswas I, Maguin E, Braun L, Mastroeni P, Cossart P. Entry of *Listeria monocytogenes* into hepatocytes requires expression of In1B, a surface protein of the internalin multigene family. Mol Microbiol 1995;16:251–61.
470. Eckmann L, Kagnoff MF, Fierer J. Intestinal epithelial cells as watchdogs for the natural immune system. Trends Microbiol 1995;3:118–20.
471. Farber JM, Peterkin PI. *Listeria monocytogenes*, a food-borne pathogen. Microbiol Rev 1991;55:476–511.
472. Frye DM, Zweig R, Sturgeon J, et al. An outbreak of febrile gastroenteritis associated with delicatessen meat contaminated with *Listeria monocytogenes*. Clin Infect Dis 2002;35:943–9.
473. Gaillard JL, Berche P, Frehel C, Gouin E, Cossart P. Entry of *L. monocytogenes* into cells is mediated by internalin, a repeat protein reminiscent of surface antigens from Gram-positive cocci. Cell 1991;65:1127–41.
474. Gill P. Is listeriosis often a foodborne illness? J Infect 1988;17:1–5.
475. Goulet V, Rocourt J, Rebiere I, et al. Listeriosis outbreak associated with the consumption of rillettes in France in 1993. J Infect Dis 1998;177: 155–60.
476. Hof H, Nichterlein T, Kretschmar M. Management of listeriosis. Clin Microbiol Rev 1997;10: 345–57.

477. Janda JM, Abbott SL. Unusual foodborne pathogens: *Listeria monocytogenes*, *Aeromonas*, *Plesiomonas*, and *Edwardsiella* species. Clin Lab Med 1999;19:553–82.
477a. Mead PS, Slutsker L, Dietz V, et al. Food-related illness and death in the United States. Emerg Infect Dis 1999;5:607–25.
478. Mengaud J, Ohayon H, Gounon P, Mege RM, Cossart P. E-cadherin is the receptor for internalin, a surface protein for entry of *Listeria monocytogenes* into epithelial cells. Cell 1996; 84:923–32.
479. Miller JK, Burns J. Histopathology of *Listeria monocytogenes* after oral feeding in mice. Appl Microbiol 1970;19:772–5.
480. Nichterlein T, Kretschmar M, Hof H. Fecal shedding of *Listeria monocytogenes* during murine listeriosis after intravenous infection. Z Bakteriol 1994;281:192–5.
481. Okamoto M, Nakane A, Minagawa T. Host resistance to an intragastric infection with *Listeria monocytogenes* in mice depends on cellular immunity and intestinal bacterial flora. Infect Immun 1994;62:3080–5.
482. Rorvik LM, Aase B, Alvestad T, Caugant DA. Molecular epidemiological survey of *Listeria monocytogenes* in seafoods and seafood-processing plants. Appl Environ Microbiol 2000;66: 4779–84.
483. Salamina G, Dalle Donne E, Niccolini A, et al. A foodborne outbreak of gastroenteritis involving *Listeria monocytogenes*. Epidemiol Infect 1993;117:429–36.
484. Schuchat A, Deaver KA, Wenger JD, et al. Role of foods in sporadic listeriosis. I. Case-control study of dietary risk. JAMA 1992;267:2041–5.
485. Schwartz B, Hexter D, Broome CV, et al. Investigation of an outbreak of listeriosis: new hypotheses for the etiology of epidemic *Listeria monocytogenes* infections. J Infect Dis 1989;159:680–5.
486. Shen Y, Naujokas M, Park M, Ireton K. In1B–dependent internalization of *Listeria* is mediated by the Met receptor tyrosine kinase. Cell 2000;103:501–10.

Tropical Sprue

487. Baker SJ, Mathan VI. Syndrome of tropical sprue in South India. Am J Clin Nutr 1968;21:984–93.
488. Klipstein FA. Recent advances in tropical malabsorption. Scand J Gastroenterol Suppl 1970;6:93–114.
489. Klipstein FA, Falaiye JM. Tropical sprue in expatriates from the tropics living in the continental United States. Medicine 1969;48:475–91.
490. Klipstein F, Baker SJ. Regarding the definition of tropical sprue. Gastroenterology 1970;58: 717–21.
491. Maldonado N, Horta E, Guerra R, Perez-Santiago E. Poorly absorbed sulfonamides in the treatment of tropical sprue. Gastroenterology 1969;57:559–68.
492. O'Brien W. Tropical sprue: a review. J R Soc Med 1979;72:916–20.
493. Tomkins A. Tropical malabsorption: recent concepts in pathogenesis and nutritional significance. Clin Sci 1981;60:131–7.

Bacterial Overgrowth Syndromes

494. Attar A, Flourie B, Rambaud JC, Franchisseur C, Ruszniewski P, Bouhnik Y. Antibiotic efficacy in small intestinal bacterial overgrowth–related chronic diarrhea: a crossover randomized trial. Gastroenterology 1999;117:794–7.
495. Gianella RA, Rout WR, Toskes PP. Jejunal brush border injury and impaired sugar and amino acid uptake in the blind loop syndrome. Gastroenterology 1974;67:965–74.
496. Gianella RA, Toskes PP. Gastrointestinal bleeding and iron absorption in the experimental blind loop syndrome. Am J Clin Nutr 1976;29: 754–7.
497. Justus PG, Fernandez A, Martin JL, King CE, Toskes PP, Mathias JR. Altered myoelectric activity in the experimental blind loop syndrome. J Clin Invest 1983;72:1064–71.
498. King CE, Toskes PP. Protein-losing enteropathy in the human and experimental rat blind loop syndrome. Gastroenterology 1981;80:504–9.
499. Saltzman JR, Russell RM. Nutritional consequences of intestinal bacterial overgrowth. Comp Ther 1994;20:523–30.
500. Singh VV, Toskes PP. Small bowel bacterial overgrowth: presentation, diagnosis and treatment. Curr Gastroenterol Rep 2003;5:365–72.
501. Wanitschke R, Ammon HV. Effects of dihydroxy bile acids and hydroxyl fatty acids on the absorption of oleic acid in the human jejunum. J Clin Invest 1978;61:178–86.
502. Welkos SA, Toskes PP, Baer H. Importance of anaerobic bacteria in the cobalamin malabsorption of experimental rat blind loop syndrome. Gastroenterology 1981;80:313–20.

***Candida* Infections**

503. Alexander JA, Brouillette DE, Chien MC, et al. Infectious esophagitis following liver and renal transplantation. Dig Dis Sci 1988;33:1121–6.
504. Clotet B, Grifol M, Parra O, et al. Asymptomatic esophageal candidiasis in the acquired-immunodeficiency-syndrome-related complex. Ann Intern Med 1986;105:145.
505. Cormack BP, Ghori N, Falkow S. An adhesin of the yeast pathogen *Candida glabrata* mediating adherence to human epithelial cells. Science 1999;285:578–82.

506. DeMuri GP, Hostetter MK. Evidence for a b1 integrin-like fibronectin receptor in *Candida tropicalis*. J Infect Dis 1996;174:127–32.
507. Eras P, Goldstein MJ, Sherlock P. Candida infection of the gastrointestinal tract. Medicine 1972;51:367–79.
508. Gaissert HA, Breuer CK, Weissburg A, Mermel L. Surgical management of necrotizing *Candida* esophagitis. Ann Thor Surg 1999;67:231–3.
509. Gozalbo D, Gil-Navarro I, Asorin I, Renau-Piqueras J, Martinez J, Gil ML. The cell wall-associated glyceraldehyde-3-phosphate dehydrogenase of *Candida albicans* is also a fibronectin and laminin binding protein. Infect Immun 1998;66:2052–9.
510. Haynes K. Virulence in Candida species. Trends Microbiol 2001;9:591–6.
511. Hughes WT. Systemic candidiasis: a study of 109 fatal cases. Pediatr Infect Dis 1982;1:11–8.
512. Kennedy MJ. Adhesion and association mechanisms of *Candida albicans*. Curr Top Med Mycol 1988;2:73–169.
513. Kennedy MJ. Regulation of *Candida albicans* populations in the gastrointestinal tract: mechanisms and significance in GI and systemic candidiasis. Curr Top Med Mycol 1989;3: 315–402.
514. Monod M, Capoccia S, Lechenne B, Zaugg C, Holdom M, Jousson O. Secreted proteases from pathogenic fungi. Int J Med Microbiol 2002; 292:405–19.
515. Santoni G, Gismondi A, Liu JH, et al. *Candida albicans* expresses a fibronectin receptor antigenically related to alpha 5 beta 1 integrin. Microbiology 1994;140:2971–9.
516. Spreghini E, Gismondi A, Piccoli M, Santoni G. Evidence for alphavbeta3 and alphavbeta5 integrin-like vitronectin (VN) receptors in *Candida albicans* and their involvement in yeast cell adhesion to VN. J Infect Dis 1999;180:156–66.
517. Tavitian A, Raufman JP, Rosenthal LE. Oral candidiasis as a marker for esophageal candidiasis in acquired immunodeficiency syndrome. Ann Intern Med 1986;104:54–5.
518. Villanueva A, Gotuzzo E, Arathoon EG, et al. A randomized double-blind study of caspofungin versus fluconazole for the treatment of esophageal candidiasis. Am J Med 2002;113:294–9.

Histoplasma Infections

519. Batanghari JW, Deepe GS Jr, Cera ED, Goldman WE. *Histoplasma* acquisition of calcium and expression of CBP1 during intracellular parasitism. Mol Microbiol 1998;27:531–9.
520. Batanghari JW, Goldman WE. Calcium dependence and binding in cultures of *Histoplasma capsulatum*. Infect Immun 1997;65:5257–61.
521. Bialek R, Feucht A, Aepinus C, et al. Evaluation of two nested PCR assays for detection of *Histoplasma capsulatum* DNA in human tissue. J Clin Microbiol 2002;40:1644–7.
522. Brett MT, Kwan JTC, Bending MR. Cecal perforation in a renal transplant patient with disseminated histoplasmosis. J Clin Pathol 1988; 41:992–5.
523. Bullock WE, Wright SD. Role of adherence-promoting receptors, CR3, LFA-1, and p150,95, in binding of *Histoplasma capsulatum* by human macrophages. J Exp Biol 1987;165:195–210.
524. Byrd TF, Horwitz MA. Interferon gamma-activated human monocytes downregulate transferrin receptors and inhibit the intracellular multiplication of *Legionella pneumophila* by limiting the availability of iron. J Clin Invest 1989;83: 1457–65.
525. Eissenberg LG, Goldman WE, Schlesinger PH. *Histoplasma capsulatum* modulates the acidification of phagolysosomes. J Exp Med 1993;177: 1605–11.
526. Garcia RA, Jagirdar J. Colonic histoplasmosis in acquired immunodeficiency syndrome mimicking carcinoma. Ann Diagn Pathol 2003;7: 14–9.
527. Goodwin RA, Loyd JE, Des Prez RM. Histoplasmosis in the normal host. Medicine 1981;60:1–33.
528. Holzberg M, Artis WM. Hydroxamate siderophore production by opportunistic and systemic fungal pathogens. Infect Immun 1983;40:1134–9.
529. Howard DH, Rafie R, Tiwari A, Faull KF. Hydroxamate siderophores of *Histoplasma capsulatum*. Infect Immun 2000;68:2338–43.
530. Jain S, Koirala J, Castro-Pavia F. Isolated gastrointestinal histoplasmosis: case report and review of the literature. South Med J 2004;97: 172–4.
531. Lamps LW, Molina CP, West AB, Haggitt RC, Scott MA. The pathologic spectrum of gastrointestinal and hepatic histoplasmosis. Am J Clin Pathol 2000;113:64–72.
532. Long KH, Gomez FJ, Morris RE, Newman SL. Identification of heat shock protein 60 as the ligand on *Histoplasma capsulatum* that mediates binding to CD18 receptors on human macrophages. J Immunol 2003;170:487–94.
533. Martagon-Villamil J, Shrestha N, Sholtis M, et al. Identification of *Histoplasma capsulatum* from culture extracts by real-time PCR. J Clin Microbiol 2003;41:1295–8.
534. Newman SL, Gootee L, Morris R, Bullock WE. Digestion of *Histoplasma capsulatum* yeasts by human macrophages. J Immunol 1992;149: 574–80.

535. Retallack DM, Woods JP. Molecular epidemiology, pathogenesis, and genetics of the dimorphic fungus *Histoplasma capsulatum*. Microbes Infect 1999;1:817–25.
536. Rickerts V, Bialek R, Tintelnot K, Jacobi V, Just-Nubling G. Rapid PCR-based diagnosis of disseminated histoplasmosis in an AIDS patient. Eur J Clin Microbiol Infect Dis 2002;21:821–3.
537. Schafer MP, Dean GE. Cloning and sequence analysis of an H^+-ATPase-encoding gene from the human dimorphic pathogen *Histoplasma capsulatum*. Gene 1993;136:295–300.
538. Strasser JE, Newman SL, Ciraolo GM, Morris RE, Howell ML, Dean GE. Regulation of the macrophage vacuolar ATPase and phagosome–lysosome fusion by Histoplasma capsulatum. J Immunol 1999;162:6148–54.
539. Timmerman MM, Woods JP. Ferric reduction is a potential iron acquisition mechanism for *Histoplasma capsulatum*. Infect Immun 1999;67:6403–8.
540. Timmerman MM, Woods JP. Potential role for extracellular glutathione-dependent ferric reductase in utilization of environmental and host ferric compounds by *Histoplasma capsulatum*. Infect Immun 2001;69:7671–8.
541. Wheat J, MaWhinney S, Hafner R, et al. Treatment of histoplasmosis with fluconazole in patients with acquired immunodeficiency syndrome. Am J Med 1997;103:223–32.
542. Wheat J, Sarosi G, McKinsey D, et al. Practice guidelines for the management of patients with histoplasmosis. Clin Infect Dis 2000;30:688–95.
543. Wheat LJ, Slama TG, Zeckel ML. Histoplasmosis in the acquired immunodeficiency syndrome. Am J Med 1985;78:203–10.
544. Wolf JE, Abegg AL, Travis SJ, Kobayashi GS, Little JR. Effects of *Histoplasma capsulatum* on murine macrophage functions: inhibition of macrophage priming, oxidative burst and antifungal activities. Infect Immun 1989;57:513–9.
545. Woods JP. *Histoplasma capsulatum*: molecular genetics, pathogenesis, and responsiveness to its environment. Fungal Genet Biol 2002;35:81–97.
546. Woods JP. Knocking on the right door and making a comfortable home: *Histoplasma capsulatum* intracellular pathogenesis. Curr Opin Microbiol 2003;6:327–31.
547. Woods JP, Heinecke EL, Luecke JW, et al. Pathogenesis of *Histoplasma capsulatum*. Semin Respir Infect 2001;16:91–101.
548. Zancope-Oliveira RM, Reiss E, Lott TJ, Mayer LW, Deepe GS Jr. Molecular cloning, characterization and expression of the M antigen of *Histoplasma capsulatum*. Infect Immun 1999;67:1047–53.
549. Zarabi CM, Thomas R, Adesokan A. Diagnosis of systemic histoplasmosis in patients with AIDS. South Med J 1992;85:1171–5.

Aspergillus Infections

550. Choi JH, Yoo JH, Chung IJ, et al. Esophageal aspergillosis after bone marrow transplant. Bone Marrow Transplant 1997;19:293–4.
551. Denning DW, Stevens DA. Antifungal and surgical treatment of invasive aspergillosis: review of 2,121 published cases. Rev Infect Dis 1990;12:1147–201.
552. Francis P, Walsh TJ. Approaches to management of fungal infections in cancer patients. Part 2. Oncology 1992;6:133–48.
553. Groll AH. Itraconazole—perspectives for the management of invasive aspergillosis. Mycoses 2002;45(Suppl 3):48–55.
554. Hori A, Kami M, Kishi Y, Machida U, Matsumura T, Kashima T. Clinical significance of extra-pulmonary involvement of invasive aspergillosis: a retrospective autopsy-based study of 107 patients. J Hosp Infect 2002;50:175–82.
555. Kinder RB, Jourdan MH. Disseminated aspergillosis and bleeding colonic ulcers in renal transplant patient. J R Soc Med 1985;78:338–9.
556. Obrecht WF, Richter JE, Olympio GA, Gelfand DW. Tracheoesophageal fistula: a serious complication of infectious esophagitis. Gastroenterology 1984;87:1174–9.
557. Peterson PK, McGlave P, Ramsey NK, et al. A prospective study of infectious disease following bone marrow transplantation: emergence of *Aspergillus* and cytomegalovirus as the major causes of mortality. Infect Control 1983:4:81–9.
558. Sanders DL, Pfeiffer RB, Hashimoto LA, Subramony C, Chen F. Pseudomembranous gastritis: a complication of Aspergillus infection. Am Surg 2003;69:536–8.
559. Saral R. *Candida* and *Aspergillus* infections in immunocompromised patients: an overview. Rev Infect Dis 1991;13:487–92.
560. Wolford JL, McDonald GB. A problem-oriented approach to intestinal and liver disease after marrow transplantation. J Clin Gastroenterol 1988;10:419–33.
561. Yong S, Attal H, Chejfec G. Pseudomembranous gastritis: a novel complication of Aspergillus infection in a patient with a bone marrow transplant and graft versus host disease. Arch Pathol Lab Med 2000;124:619–24.

Blastomyces Infections

562. Bradsher RW. Blastomycosis—Systemic fungal infections: diagnosis and treatment I. Infect Dis Clin North Am 1988;2:877–98.
563. Saag MS, Dismukes WE. Treatment of histoplasmosis and blastomycosis. Chest 1988;98:848–51.

Paracoccidioides Infections

564. Restrepo A, Gomez I, Robledo J, Patino MM, Cano LE. Itraconazole in the treatment of paracoccidioidomycosis: a preliminary report. Rev Infect Dis 1987;9:51–6.
565. Restrepo A, Robledo M, Giraldo R, et al. The gamut of paracoccidioidomycosis. Am J Med 1976;61:33–42.
566. Rocha N, Suguiama EH, Maia D, Costa H, Coelho KI, Franco M. Intestinal malakoplakia associated with paracoccidiodomycosis: a new association. Histopathology 1997;30:79–83.

Zygomycosis

567. Neame P, Rayner D. Mucormycosis: a report on 22 cases. Medicine 1986;65:113–23.
568. Rinaldi MG. Zygomycosis—systemic fungal infections: diagnosis and treatment II. Infect Dis Clin North Am 1989;3:19–41.

Cryptococcus Infections

569. Bonacini M, Nussbaum J, Ahluwalia C. Gastrointestinal, hepatic, and pancreatic involvement with Cryptococcus neoformans in AIDS. J Clin Gastroenterol 1990;12:295–7.
570. Daly JS, Porter KA, Chong FK, Robillard RJ. Disseminated, nonmeningeal gastrointestinal cryptococcal infection in an HIV-negative patient. Am J Gastroenterol 1990;85:1421–4.
571. Unat EK, Pars B, Kosyak JP. A case of cryptococcosis of the colon. Br Med J 1960;2:1501–2.
572. Vandepitte J. Clinical aspects of cryptococcoses in patients with AIDS. In: Vanden-Bossche H, ed. Mycoses in AIDS patients. New York: Plenum Press; 1989:115–22.
573. Washington K, Gottfried MR, Wilson ML. Gastrointestinal cryptococcosis. Mod Pathol 1991;4:707–11.

Coccidioides Infections

574. Centers for Disease Control and Prevention. Coccidioidomycosis—Arizona, 1990-1995. MMWR Morb Mortal Wkly Rep 1996;45:1069–73.
575. Chowfin A, Tight R. Female genital coccidioidomycosis (FGC), Addison's disease and sigmoid loop abscess due to *Coccidioides immitis*; case report and review of the literature on FGC. Mycopathologia 1999;145:121–6.
576. Cuen KTK. Coccidioidal peritonitis. Am J Clin Pathol 1983;80:514–6.
577. Drutz DJ, Catanzaro A. Coccidioidomycosis Part II. Am Rev Respir Dis 1978;117:727–71.
578. Harris RE. Coccidioidomycosis complicating pregnancy. Obstet Gynecol 1966;24:401.
579. Weisman IM, Moreno AJ, Parker AL, Sippo WC, Liles WJ. Gastrointestinal dissemination of coccidioidomycosis. Am J Gastroenterol 1986;81:589–93.

Rotavirus and Rotavirus-Like Particle Infections

580. Anderson EJ, Weber SG. Rotavirus infection in adults. Lancet Infect Dis 2004;4:91–9.
581. Arias CF, Isa P, Guerrero CA, et al. Molecular biology of rotavirus cell entry. Arch Med Res 2002;33:356–61.
582. Bolivar R, Conklin RH, Vollet JJ, et al. Rotavirus in travelers' diarrhea: study of an adult student population in Mexico. J Infect Dis 1978;137:324–7.
583. Centers for Disease Control and Prevention. Foodborne outbreak of a group A rotavirus gastroenteritis among college students, Washington, DC—March 2000. MMWR Morb Mortal Wkly Rep 2000;49:1131–3.
584. Cox MJ, Medley GF. Serological survey of anti-group A rotavirus IgM in UK adults. Epidemiol Infect 2003;131:719–26.
585. Cubit WD, Holzel H. An outbreak of rotavirus infection in a long-stay ward of a geriatric hospital. J Clin Pathol 1980;33:306–8.
586. Davidson GP, Barnes GL. Structural and functional abnormalities of the small intestine in infants and young children with rotavirus enteritis. Acta Paediatr Scand 1979;68:181–6.
587. del Refugio Gonzalez-Losa M, Polanco-Marin GG, Manzano-Cabrera L, Puerto-Solis M. Acute gastroenteritis associated with rotavirus in adults. Arch Med Res 2001;32:164–7.
588. De Wit MA, Koopmans MP, Kortbeek LM, van Leeuwen NJ, Vinje I, van Duynhoven YT. Etiology of gastroenteritis in sentinel general practices in the Netherlands. Clin Infect Dis 2001;33:280–8.
589. De Zoysa I, Feachem R. Interventions for the control of diarrhoeal diseases among young children: rotavirus and cholera immunization. Bull World Health Org 1985;63:569–83.
590. Dickman KG, Hempson SJ, Anderson J, et al. Rotavirus alters paracellular permeability and energy metabolism in Caco-2 cells. Am J Physiol Gastrointest Liver Physiol 2000;279:G757–66.
591. Echeverria P, Blacklow NR, Cukor GG, Vibulbandhitkit S, Changchawalit S, Boonthai P. Rotavirus as a cause of severe gastroenteritis in adults. J Clin Microbiol 1983;18:663–7.
592. Flewett TH, Bryden AS, Davies H, Woode GN, Bridger JC, Derrick JM. Relationship between viruses from acute gastroenteritis of children and newborn calves. Lancet 1974;2:61–3.
593. Glass RI, Kilgore PE, Holman RC, et al. The epidemiology of rotavirus diarrhea in the United States: surveillance and estimate of disease burden. J Infect Dis 1996;174:S5–11.

594. Grimood K, Abbott GD, Fergusson DM, Jennings LC, Allan JM. Spread of rotavirus within families: a community based study. BMJ 1983;287:575–7.
595. Grimwood K, Lund JC, Coulson BS, Hudson IL, Bishop RF, Barnes GL. Comparison of serum and mucosal antibody responses following severe acute rotavirus gastroenteritis in young children. J Clin Microbiol 1988;26:732–8.
596. Guarino A, Canani RB, Russo S, et al. Oral immunoglobulins for treatment of acute rotaviral gastroenteritis. Pediatrics 1994;93:12–6.
597. Halaihel N, Lievin V, Alvarado F, Vasseur M. Rotavirus infection impairs intestinal brush-border membrane Na(+)-solute cotransport activities in young rabbits. Am J Physiol Gastrointestin Liver Physiol 2000;279:G587–96.
598. Halvorsrud J, Orstavik I. An epidemic of rotavirus-associated gastroenteritis in a nursing home for the elderly. Scand J Infect Dis 1980;12:161–4.
599. Holmes IH, Rich B, Bishop R, Davidson G. Infantile enteritis: morphogenesis and morphology. J Virol 1975;16:937–43.
600. Hopkins RS, Gaspard GB, Williams FP, Karlin RJ, Cukor G, Blacklow NR. A community waterborne gastroenteritis outbreak: evidence for rotavirus as the agent. Am J Public Health 1984;74:263–5.
601. Horie Y, Nakagomi O, Koshimura Y, et al. Diarrhea induction by rotavirus NSP4 in the homologous mouse model system. Virology 1999;262:398–407.
602. Iturriza-Gomara M, Green J, Brown DW, Ramsay M, Desselberger U, Gray JJ. Molecular epidemiology of human group A rotavirus infections in the United Kingdom between 1995 and 1998. J Clin Microbiol 2000;38:4394–401.
603. Jewkes J, Larson HE, Price AB, Sanderson PJ, Davies HA. Aetiology of acute diarrhoea in adults. Gut 1981;22:388–92.
604. Johansen K, Stintzing G, Magnusson KE, et al. Intestinal permeability assessed with polyethylene glycols in children with diarrhea due to rotavirus and common bacterial pathogens in a developing community. J Pediatr Gastroenterol Nutr 1989;9:307–13.
605. Kanfer EJ, Abrahamson G, Taylor J, Coleman JC, Samson DM. Severe rotavirus-associated diarrhoea following bone marrow transplantation: treatment with oral immunoglobulin. Bone Marrow Transplant 1994;14:651–2.
606. Kapikian AZ. Viral gastroenteritis. JAMA 1993;269:627–30.
607. Kapikian AZ, Kim HW, Wyatt RG, et al. Human reovirus-like agent as the major pathogen associated with "winter" gastroenteritis in hospitalized infants and young children. N Engl J Med 1976;294:965–72.
608. Kapikian AZ, Wyatt RG, Levine MM, et al. Oral administration of human rotavirus to volunteers: induction of illness and correlates of resistance. J Infect Dis 1983;147:95–106.
609. Keljo DJ, MacLeod RJ, Perdue MH, Butler DG, Hamilton JR. D-glucose transport in piglet jejunal brush-border membranes: insights from a disease model. Am J Physiol 1985;249:G751–60.
610. Keswick BH, Blacklow NR, Cukor GC, DuPont HL, Vollet JL. Norwalk virus and rotavirus in travellers' diarrhoea in Mexico. Lancet 1982;1:109–10.
611. Koopman JS, Monto AS. The Tecumseh study. XV: rotavirus infection and pathogenicity. Am J Epidemiol 1989;130:750–9.
612. Loosli J, Gyr K, Stalder H, et al. Etiology of acute infectious diarrhea in a highly industrialized area of Switzerland. Gastroenterology 1985;88:75–9.
613. Losonsky GA, Johnson JP, Winkelstein JA, Yolken RH. Oral administration of human serum immunoglobulin in immunodeficient patients with viral gastroenteritis: a pharmacokinetic and functional analysis. J Clin Invest 1985;76:2362–7.
614. Lundgren O, Peregrin AT, Persson K, Kordasti S, Uhnoo I, Svensson L. Role of the enteric nervous system in fluid and electrolyte secretion of rotavirus diarrhea. Science 2000;287:491–5.
615. MacLeod RJ, Hamilton JR. Absence of a cAMP-mediated antiabsorptive effect in an undifferentiated jejunal epithelium. Am J Physiol 1987;252:G776–82.
616. Nakagima H, Nakagomi T, Kamisawa T, et al. Winter seasonality and rotavirus diarrhoea in adults. Lancet 2001;357:1950.
617. Obert G, Peiffer I, Servin AL. Rotavirus-induced structural and functional alterations in tight junctions of polarized intestinal Caco–2 cell monolayers. J Virol 2000;74:4645–51.
618. Oyofo BA, Subekti D, Tjaniadi P, et al. Enteropathogens associated with acute diarrhea in community and hospital patients in Jakarta, Indonesia. FEMS Immunol Med Microbiol 2002;34:139–46.
619. Steffen R, Collard F, Tornieporth N, et al. Epidemiology, etiology and impact of traveler's diarrhea in Jamaica. JAMA 1999;281:811–7.
620. Svenungsson B, Lagergren A, Ekwall E, et al. Enteropathogens in adult patients with diarrhea and healthy control subjects: a 1-year prospective study in a Swedish clinic for infectious diseases. Clin Infect Dis 2000;30:770–8.
621. Tucker AW, Haddix AC, Bresee JS, Holman RC, Parashar UD, Glass RI. Cost-effectiveness analysis of a rotavirus immunization program for the United States. JAMA 1998;279:1371–6.

622. Velazques FR, Matson DO, Calva JJ, et al. Rotavirus infections in infants as protection against subsequent infections. N Engl J Med 1996;335:1022–8.
623. Vollet JJ, Ericsson CD, Gibson G, et al. Human rotavirus in an adult population with travelers' diarrhea and its relationship to the location of food consumption. J Med Virol 1979; 4:81–7.
624. Ward RL, Bernstein DI, Shukla R, et al. Effects of antibody to rotavirus on protection of adults challenged with a human rotavirus. J Infect Dis 1989;159:79–88.
625. Ward RL, Bernstein DI, Shukla R, et al. Protection of adults rechallenged with a human rotavirus. J Infect Dis 1990;161:440–5.
626. Ward RL, Bernstein DI, Young EC, Sherwood JR, Knowlton DR, Schiff GM. Human rotavirus studies in volunteers: determination of infectious dose and serological response to infection. J Infect Dis 1986;154:871–80.
627. Wenman WM, Hinde D, Feltham S, Gurwith M. Rotavirus infection in adults. Results of a prospective family study. N Engl J Med 1979;301:303–6.
628. Wilde J, Yolken R, Willoughby R, Eiden J. Improved detection of rotavirus shedding by polymerase chain reaction. Lancet 1991;337:323–6.
629. Yolken RH, Wilde J. Assays for detecting human rotavirus. In: Kapikian AZ, ed. Viral infections of the gastrointestinal tract, 2nd ed. New York: M Dekker; 1994:251–78.

Norwalk and Norwalk-Like Virus Infections

630. Becker KM, Moe CL, Southwick KL, MacCormack JN. Transmission of Norwalk virus during a football game. N Engl J Med 2000;343: 1223–7.
631. Berg DE, Kohn MA, Farley TA, McFarland LM. Multi-state outbreaks of acute gastroenteritis traced to fecal-contaminated oysters harvested in Louisiana. J Infect Dis 2000;181(suppl 2):S381–6.
632. Blacklow NR, Greenberg HB. Viral gastroenteritis. N Engl J Med 1991;325:252–64.
633. Bresee JS, Widdowson MA, Monroe SS, Glass RI. Foodborne viral gastroenteritis: challenges and opportunities. Clin Infect Dis 2002;35:748–53.
634. Centers for Disease Control and Prevention. Norwalk-like viruses: public health consequences and outbreak management. MMWR Morb Mort Wkly Rep 2001;50:1–18.
635. Centers for Disease Control and Prevention. Norwalk-like viral gastroenteritis in U.S. army trainees—Texas, 1998. MMWR Morb Mort Wkly Rep 1999;48:225–7.
636. Centers for Disease Control and Prevention. Outbreak of acute gastroenteritis associated with Norwalk-like viruses among British military personnel—Afghanistan, May 2002. MMWR Morb Mort Wkly Rep 2002;51:477–9.
637. Chatterjee NK, Moore DW, Monroe SS, et al. Molecular epidemiology of outbreaks of viral gastroenteritis in New York State, 1998–1999. Clin Infect Dis 2004;38(suppl 3):S303–10.
638. Daniels NA, Bergmire-Sweat DA, Schwab KJ, et al. A foodborne outbreak of gastroenteritis associated with Norwalk-like viruses: first molecular traceback to deli sandwiches contaminated during preparation. J Infect Dis 2000;181: 1467–70.
639. Dowell SF, Groves C, Kirkland KB, et al. A multistate outbreak of oyster-associated gastroenteritis: implications for interstate tracing of contaminated shellfish. J Infect Dis 1995;171: 1497–503.
640. Fankhauser RL, Noel JS, Monroe SS, Ando TA, Glass RI. Molecular epidemiology of "Norwalk-like viruses" in outbreaks of gastroenteritis in the United States. J Infect Dis 1998;178:1571–8.
641. Gotz H, Ekdahl K, Lindback J, de Jong B, Hedlund KO, Giesecke J. Clinical spectrum and transmission characteristics of infection with Norwalk-like virus: findings from a large community outbreak in Sweden. Clin Infect Dis 2001;33:622–8.
642. Ho MS, Glass RI, Monroe SS, et al. Viral gastroenteritis aboard a cruise ship. Lancet 1989;2:961–5.
643. Marks PJ, Vipond IB, Carlisle D, Deakin D, Fey RE, Caul EO. Evidence for airborne transmission of Norwalk-like virus (NLV) in a hotel restaurant. Epidemiol Infect 2000;124:481–7.
644. Mounts AW, Ando T, Koopmans M, Bresee JS, Noel J, Glass RI. Cold weather seasonality of gastroenteritis associated with Norwalk-like viruses. J Infect Dis 2000;181(suppl 2):S284–7.
645. Rockx B, de Wit M, Vennema H, et al. Natural history of human *Calicivirus* infection: a prospective cohort study. Clin Infect Dis 2002;35: 246–53.
646. Sawyer LA, Murphy JJ, Kaplan JE, et al. 25- to 30-nm virus particle associated with a hospital outbreak of acute gastroenteritis with evidence for airborne transmission. Am J Epidemiol 1988;127:1261–71.
647. Schreiber DS, Blacklow NR, Trier JS. The mucosal lesion of the proximal small intestine in acute infectious nonbacterial gastroenteritis. N Engl J Med 1973;288:1318–23.

648. Shieh YS, Monroe SS, Fankhauser RL, Langlois GW, Burkhardt W III, Baric RS. Detection of Norwalk-like virus in shellfish implicated in illness. J Infect Dis 2000;181(suppl 2):S360–6.
649. Vinje J, Koopmans MP. Molecular detection and epidemiology of small round structured viruses in outbreaks of gastroenteritis in the Netherlands. J Infect Dis 1996;174:610–5.

Sapporo and Sapporo-Like Virus Infections

650. Chiba S, Nakata S, Numata-Kinoshita K, Honma S. Sapporo virus: history and recent findings. J Infect Dis 2000;181(suppl 2):S303–8.
650a. Rockx B, de Wit M, Vennema H, et al. Natural history of human *Calicivirus* infection: a prospective cohort study. Clin Infect Dis 2002;35: 246–53.

Enteric Adenovirus Infections

651. Baldwin A, Kingman H, Darville M, et al. Outcome and clinical course of 100 patients with adenovirus infection following bone marrow transplantation. Bone Marrow Transplant 2000; 26:1333–8.
652. Baskin GB, Soike KF. Adenovirus enteritis in SIV-infected Rhesus monkeys. J Infect Dis 1989;160: 905–7.
653. Bates PR, Bailey AS, Wood DJ, et al. Comparative epidemiology of rotavirus, subgenus-F (types 40 and 41) adenovirus, and astrovirus gastroenteritis in children. J Med Virol 1993;39:224–8.
654. Bhisitkul DM, Todd KM, Listernick R. Adenovirus infection and childhood intussusception. Am J Dis Child 1992;146:1331–3.
654a. Blacklow NR, Greenberg HB. Viral gastroenteritis. N Engl J Med 1991;325:252–64.
655. Brandt CD, Rodriguez WJ, Kim HW, et al. Rapid presumptive recognition of diarrhea-associated adenoviruses. J Clin Microbiol 1984;20:1008–9.
656. Gonzalez GG, Pujol FH, Liprandi F, Deibis L, Ludert JE. Prevalence of enteric viruses in human immunodeficiency virus seropositive patients in Venezuela. J Med Virol 1998;55:288–92.
657. Guarner J, de Leon-Bojorge B, Lopez-Corella E, et al. Intestinal intussusception associated with adenovirus infection in Mexican children. Am J Clin Pathol 2003;120:845–50.
658. Hsu HY, Kao CL, Huang LM, et al. Viral etiology of intussusception in Taiwanese childhood. Pediatr Infect Dis J 1998;17:893–8.
659. Janoff EN, Orenstein JM, Manischewitz JF, Smith PD. Adenovirus colitis in the acquired immunodeficiency syndrome. Gastroenterology 1991;100:976–9.
660. Landry ML, Fong CK, Neddermann K, Solomon L, Hsiung GD. Disseminated adenovirus infection in an immunocompromised host: pitfalls in diagnosis. Am J Med 1987;83:555–9.
661. Lin HC, Kao CL, Lu CY, et al. Enteric adenovirus infection in children in Taipei. J Microbiol Immunol Infect 2000;33:176–80.
662. Orenstein JM, Dieterich DT. The histopathology of 103 consecutive colonoscopy biopsies from 82 symptomatic patients with acquired immunodeficiency syndrome: original and look-back diagnoses. Arch Pathol Lab Med 2001;125:1042–6.
663. Retter M, Middleton PJ, Tam JS, et al. Enteric adenoviruses: detection, replication, and significance. J Clin Microbiol 1979;10:574–8.
664. Sabin CA, Clewley GS, Deayton JR, et al. Shorter survival of HIV-positive patients with diarrhoea who excrete adenovirus from the GI tract. J Med Virol 1999;58:280–5.
665. Saderi H, Roustai MH, Sabahi F, Sadeghizadeh M, Owlia P, de Jong JC. Incidence of enteric adenovirus gastroenteritis in Iranian children. J Clin Virol 2002;24:1–5.
666. Thomas PD, Pollok RC, Gazzard BG. Enteric viral infections as a cause of diarrhoea in the acquired immunodeficiency syndrome. HIV Med 1999;1:19–24.
667. Waters V, Ford-Jones EL, Petric M, et al. Etiology of community-acquired pediatric viral diarrhea: a prospective longitudinal study in hospitals, emergency departments, pediatric practices and child care centers during the winter rotavirus outbreak 1997 to 1998. Pediatr Infect Dis J 2000;19:843–8.
668. Yan Z, Nguyen S, Poles M, Melamed J, Scholes JV. Adenovirus colitis in human immunodeficiency virus infection. An underdiagnosed entity. Am J Surg Pathol 1998;22:1101–6.
669. Yolken RH, Bishop CA, Townsend TR, et al. Infectious gastroenteritis in bone-marrow transplant recipients. N Engl J Med 1982;306: 1010–2.

Astrovirus Infections

670. Abad FX, Villena C, Guix S, Caballero S, Pinto RM, Bosch A. Potential role of fomites in the vehicular transmission of human astroviruses. Appl Environ Microbiol 2001;67:3904–7.
671. Cubit WD, Mitchell DK, Carter MJ, Willcocks MM, Holzel H. Application of electromicroscopy, enzyme immunoassay, and RT-PCR to monitor an outbreak of astrovirus type 1 in a paediatric bone marrow transplant unit. J Med Virol 1999;57:313–21.
672. Dennehy PH, Nelson SM, Spangenberger S, Noel JS, Monroe SS, Glass RI. A prospective case-control study of the role of astrovirus in acute diarrhea among hospitalized young children. J Infect Dis 2001;184:10–5.

673. Esahli H, Breback K, Bennet R, Ehrnst A, Eriksson M, Hedlund KO. Astroviruses as a cause of nosocomial outbreaks of infant diarrhea. Pediatr Infect Dis J 1991;10:511–5.
674. Ford-Jones EL, Mindorff CM, Gold R, Petric M. The incidence of viral-associated diarrhea after admission to a pediatric hospital. Am J Epidemiol 1990;131:711–8.
675. Gaggero A, O'Ryan M, Noel JS, et al. Prevalence of astrovirus infection among Chilean children with acute gastroenteritis. J Clin Microbiol 1998;36:3691–3.
676. Gray JJ, Wreghitt TG, Cubitt WD, Elliot PR. An outbreak of gastroenteritis in a home for the elderly associated with astrovirus type 1 and human calicivirus. J Med Virol 1987;23:377–81.
677. Grohmann GS, Glass RI, Pereira HG, et al. Enteric viruses and diarrhea in HIV-infected patients. N Engl J Med 1993;329:14–20.
678. Jonassen TO, Kjeldsberg E, Grinde B. Detection of human astrovirus serotype-1 by the polymerase chain reaction. J Virol Methods 1993; 44: 83–8.
679. Kurtz JB, Lee TW, Craig JW, Reed SE. Astrovirus infection in volunteers. J Med Virol 1979;3: 221–30.
680. Mitchell DK, Matson DO, Jiang X, et al. Molecular epidemiology of childhood astrovirus infection in child care centers. J infect Dis 1999;180:514–7.
681. Oishi I, Yamazaki K, Kimoto T, Minekawa Y, Nishimura H, Kitaura T. A large outbreak of acute gastroenteritis associated with astrovirus among students and teachers in Osaka Japan. J Infect Dis 1994;170:439–43.
682. Oseto M, Yamshita Y, Yoshida K, et al. Serotypes of astrovirus isolated from children in sporadic gastroenteritis cases in Ehime Prefecture 1981-1997. Jpn J Infect Dis 1999;52:134–5.
683. Pang XL, Vesikari T. Human astrovirus–associated gastroenteritis in children under 2 years of age followed prospectively during a rotavirus vaccine trial. Acta Paediatr 1999;88:532–6.
684. Pinto RM, Abad FX, Gajardo R, Bosch A. Detection of infectious astroviruses in water. Appl Environ Microbiol 1996;62:1811–3.
685. Pinto RM, Villena C, Le Guyader FS, et al. Astrovirus detection in wastewater samples. Water Sci Technol 2001;12:73–6.
686. Qiao H, Nilsson M, Abreu ER, et al. Viral diarrhea in children in Beijing, China. J Med Virol 1999;57:390–6.
687. Shastri S, Doane AM, Gonzales J, Upadhyayula U, Bass DM. Prevalence of astroviruses in a children's hospital. J Clin Microbiol 1998;36: 2571–4.
688. Walter JE, Mitchell DK. Role of astroviruses in childhood diarrhea. Curr Opin Pediatr 2000;12: 275–9.

Herpesvirus Infections

689. Adler M, Goldman M, Liesnard C, Hardy N, Van Gossum A, Engelholm L. Diffuse herpes simplex virus colitis in a kidney transplant recipient successfully treated with acyclovir. Transplantation 1987;43:919–21.
690. Bacon TH, Levin MJ, Leary JJ, Sarisky RT, Sutton D. Herpes simplex virus resistance to acyclovir and penciclovir after two decades of antiviral therapy. Clin Microbiol Rev 2003;16:114–28.
691. Boulton AJ, Slater DN, Hancock BW. Herpes virus colitis: a new cause of diarrhoea in a patient with Hodgkin's disease. Gut 1982;23:47–9.
692. Buss DH, Scharyj M. Herpesvirus infection of the esophagus and other visceral organs in adults. Incidence and clinical significance. Am J Med 1979;66:457–62.
693. Colemont LJ, Pen JH, Pelckmans PA, Degryse HR, Pattyn SR, Van Maercke YM. Herpes simplex virus type I colitis: an unusual cause of diarrhea. Am J Gastroenterol 1990;85:1182–5.
694. Corey L. Herpesviruses. In: Sherris J, ed. Medical microbiology, 2nd ed. New York: Elsevier; 1990:559–75.
695. Daley AJ, Craven P, Holland AJ, Jones CA, Badawi N, Isaacs D. Herpes simplex virus colitis in a neonate. Pediatr Infect Dis J 2002;21: 887–8.
696. Delis S, Kato T, Ruiz P, Mittal N, Babinski L, Tzakis A. Herpes simplex colitis in a child with combined liver and small bowel transplant. Pediatr Transplantation 2001;5:374–7.
697. Deshmukh M, Shah R, McCallum RW. Experience with herpes esophagitis in otherwise healthy patients. Am J Gastroenterol 1984;79: 173–6.
698. el-Serag HB, Zwas FR, Cirillo NW, Eisen RN. Fulminant herpes colitis in a patient with Crohn's disease. J Clin Gastroenterol 1996;22: 220–3.
699. Galbraith JC, Shafran SD. Herpes simplex esophagitis in the immunocompetent patient: report of four cases and review. Clin Infect Dis 1992;14:894–901.
700. Goodgame RW. Viral infections of the gastrointestinal tract. Curr Gastroenterol Rep 1999;1: 292–300.
701. Kingreen D, Nitsche A, Beyer J, Siegert W. Herpes simplex infection of the jejunum occurring in the early post-transplantation period. Bone Marrow Transplant 1997;20:989–91.
702. Kurahara K, Aoyagi K, Nakamura S, et al. Treatment of herpes simplex esophagitis in an immunocompetent patient with intravenous acyclovir: a case report and review of the literature. Am J Gastroenterol 1998;93:2239–40.

703. Naik HR, Chandrasekar PH. Herpes simplex virus (HSV) colitis in a bone marrow transplant recipient. Bone Marrow Transplant 1996;17:85–6.
704. Nash G, Ross JS. Herpetic esophagitis. A common cause of esophageal ulceration. Hum Pathol 1974;5:339–45.
705. Pazin GJ. Herpes simplex esophagitis after trigeminal nerve surgery. Gastroenterology 1978;74:741–3.
706. Ramanathan J, Rammouni M, Baran J, Khatib R. Herpes simplex virus esophagitis in the immunocompetent host: an overview. Am J Gastroenterol 2000;95:2171–6.
707. Rattner HM, Cooper DJ, Zaman MB. Severe bleeding from herpes esophagitis. Am J Gastroenterol 1985;80:523–5.
708. Reyes M, Shaik NS, Graber JM, et al. Acyclovir-resistant genital herpes among persons attending sexually transmitted disease and human immunodeficiency virus clinics. Arch Intern Med 2003;163:76–80.
709. Rompalo AM, Mertz GJ, Davis LG, et al. A double-blind study of oral acyclovir for the treatment of first episode herpes simplex virus proctitis in homosexual men. JAMA 1988;259: 2879–81.
710. Shortsleeve MJ, Levine MS. Herpes esophagitis in otherwise healthy patients: clinical and radiographic findings. Radiology 1992;182: 859–61.
711. Yuhan R, Orsay C, DelPino A, et al. Anorectal disease in HIV-infected patients. Dis Colon Rectum 1998;41:1367–70.

Varicella Zoster Virus Infections

711a. Corey L. Herpesviruses. In: Sherris J, ed. Medical microbiology, 2nd ed. New York: Elsevier; 1990:559–75.
712. Debinski HS, Kamm MA, Talbot IC, Khan G, Kangro HO, Jeffries DJ. DNA viruses in the pathogenesis of sporadic chronic idiopathic intestinal pseudo–obstruction. Gut 1997;41:100–6.
713. Feldman S. Varicella zoster infections of the fetus, neonate and immuno-compromised child. Adv Pediatr Infect Dis 1986;1:99–115.
713a. Goodgame RW. Viral infections of the gastrointestinal tract. Curr Gastroenterol Rep 1999;1: 292–300.
714. Hong JJ, Elgart ML. Gastrointestinal complications of dermatomal herpes zoster successfully treated with famciclovir and lactulose. J Am Acad Dermatol 1998;38:279–80.
715. Luber AD, Flaherty JF Jr. Famciclovir for treatment of herpesvirus infections. Ann Pharmacother 1996;30:978–85.
716. Patel PA, Yoonessi S, O'Malley J, Freeman A, Gershon A, Ogra PL. Cell-mediated immunity to varicella-zoster virus infection in subjects with lymphoma or leukemia. J Pediatrics 1979; 94:223–30.
717. Pui JC, Furth EE, Minda J, Montone KT. Demonstration of varicella-zoster virus infection in the muscularis propria and myenteric plexi of the colon in an HIV-positive patient with herpes zoster and small bowel pseudo-obstruction (Ogilvie's syndrome). Am J Gastroenterol 2001; 96:1627–30.
718. Sherman RA, Silva J Jr, Gandour-Edwards R. Fatal varicella in an adult: case report and review of the gastrointestinal complications of chickenpox. Rev Infect Dis 1991;13:424–7.

Cytomegalovirus Infections

719. Aqel NM, Tanner P, Drury A, Francis ND, Henry K. Cytomegalovirus gastritis with perforation and gastrocolic fistula formation. Histopathology 1991;18:165–8.
719a. Corey L. Herpesviruses. In: Sherris J, ed. Medical microbiology, 2nd ed. New York: Elsevier; 1990:559–75.
720. DeRiso AJ, Kemeny MM, Torres RA, Oliver JM. Multiple jejunal perforations secondary to cytomegalovirus in a patient with acquired immune deficiency syndrome: case report and review. Dig Dis Sci 1989;34:623–9.
721. Frager DH, Frager JD, Wolf EL, et al. Cytomegalovirus colitis in acquired immune deficiency syndrome. Gastrointest Radiol 1986;11:241–6.
722. Grefte A, Blom N, van der Giessen M, van Son W, The TH. Ultrastructural analysis of circulating cytomegalic cells in patients with active cytomegalovirus infection: evidence for virus production and endothelial origin. J Infect Dis 1993;168:1110–8.
723. Ho M. Epidemiology of cytomegalovirus infections. Rev Infect Dis 1990;12:S701–10.
724. Huang ES, Roche JK. Cytomegalovirus DNA and adenocarcinomas of the colon: evidence for latent viral infection. Lancet 1978;1:957–60.
725. Kyriazis AP, Mitra SK. Multiple cytomegalovirus-related intestinal perforations in patients with acquired immunodeficiency syndrome. Arch Pathol Lab Med 1992;116:495–9.
726. McDonald GB, Sharma P, Hackman RC, Meyers JD, Thomas ED. Esophageal infections in immunosuppressed patients after marrow transplantation. Gastroenterology 1985;88:1111–7.
727. Merigan TC, Resta S. Cytomegalovirus: where have we been and where are we going? Rev Infect Dis 1990;12:S693–700.
728. Myerson D, Hackman RC, Nelson JA, Ward DC, McDougall JK. Widespread presence of histologically occult cytomegalovirus. Hum Pathol 1984;15:430–9.

729. Occena RO, Taylor SF, Robinson CC, Sokol RJ. Association of cytomegalovirus with Menetrier's disease in childhood: report of two new cases with a review of literature. J Pediatr Gastroenterol Nutr 1993;17:217–24.
730. Orloff JJ, Saito R, Lasky S, Dave H. Toxic megacolon in cytomegalovirus colitis. Am J Gastroenterol 1989;84:794–7.
731. Page MJ, Dreese JC, Poritz LS, Koltun WA. Cytomegalovirus enteritis: a highly lethal condition requiring early detection and intervention. Dis Col Rectum 1998;41:619–23.
732. Rene E, Marche C, Chevalier T, et al. Cytomegalovirus colitis in patients with acquired immunodeficiency syndrome. Dig Dis Sci 1988; 33:741–50.
733. Schneiderman DJ, Cello JP, Laing FC. Papillary stenosis and sclerosing cholangitis in the acquired immunodeficiency syndrome. Ann Intern Med 1987;106:546–9.
734. Tatum ET, Sun PC, Cohn DL. Cytomegalovirus vasculitis and colon perforation in a patient with the acquired immunodeficiency syndrome. Pathology 1989;21:235–8.
735. Weber JN, Thom W, Barrison I, et al. Cytomegalovirus colitis and oesophageal ulceration in the context of AIDS: clinical manifestations and preliminary report of treatment with foscarnet. Gut 1987;28:482–7.

Human Papilloma Virus Infections

736. Broker TR. Structure and genetic expression of papillomaviruses. Obstet Gynecol Clin North Am 1987;4:329–48.
737. Frazer IH, Medley G, Crapper RM, Brown TC, Mackay IR. Association between anorectal dysplasia, human papillomavirus and human immunodeficiency virus infection in homosexual men. Lancet 1986;2:657–60.
738. Gross G, Ikenberg H, Gissman L, Hagedorn M. Papillomavirus of the anogenital region: correlation between histology, clinical picture, and virus type: proposal of a new nomenclature. J Invest Dermatol 1985;85:147–52.
739. Hill SA, Coghill SB. Human papillomavirus in squamous carcinoma of anus. Lancet 1986:2; 1333.
740. Moore GE, Norton LW, Meiselbaugh DM. Condyloma. A new epidemic. Arch Surg 1978;113: 630–1.
741. Noffsinger A, Witte D, Fenoglio–Preiser CM. The relationship of human papillomaviruses to anorectal neoplasia. Cancer 1992;70:1276–87.
742. Noffsinger AE, Hui YZ, Yochman L, Miller MA, Hurtubise P, Fenoglio-Preiser CM. The relationship of human papillomavirus to ploidy and proliferation in anal carcinomas. Cancer 1995; 75:958–67.
743. Palefsky J. Human papillomavirus infection among HIV-infected individuals: implications for development of malignant tumors. Hematol Oncol Clin North Am 1991;5:357–70.
744. Prasad CJ, Sheets E, Selig AM. The binucleate squamous cell: histologic spectrum and relationship to low-grade squamous intraepithelial lesions. Mod Pathol 1993;6:313–7.
745. Stone KM. Epidemiologic aspects of genital HPV infection. Clin Obstet Gynecol 1989;32: 112–6.
746. Syrjanen KJ. Epidemiology of human papillomavirus infections and their association with genital squamous cell cancer. APMIS 1989;97: 957–70.
747. Taichman LB, LaPorta RF. The expression of papillomaviruses in epithelial cells. In: Salzman NP, Howley PM, eds. The papovaviridae. New York: Plenum Press; 1987:109.
748. Wells M, Griffiths S, Lewis F, Bird CC. Demonstration of the human papillomavirus types in paraffin processed tissue from human anogenital lesions by in-situ hybridization. J Pathol 1987;152:77–82.
749. Zachow KR, Ostrow RS, Bender M, et al. Detection of human papillomavirus DNA in anogenital neoplasia. Nature 1982;300:771–3.

Giardia Infections

750. Ali SA, Hill DR. *Giardia intestinalis*. Curr Opin Infect Dis 2003;16:453–60.
751. Anonymous. Nitazoxanide (Alinia)—a new anti-protozoal agent. Med Lett Drug Ther 2003;45:29–31.
752. Bauer B, Engelbrecht S, Bakker-Grunwald T, Scholze H. Functional identification of alpha 1-giardin as an annexin of *Giardia lamblia*. FEMS Microbiol Lett 1999;173:147–53.
753. Char S, Cevallos AM, Yamson P, Sullivan PB, Neale G, Farthing MJ. Impaired IgA response to *Giardia* heat shock antigen in children with persistent diarrhoea and giardiasis. Gut 1993;34:38–40.
754. Cruz A, Sousa MI, Azeredo Z, et al. Isolation, excystation and axenization of *Giardia lamblia* isolates: in vitro susceptibility to metronidazole and albendazole. J Antimicrob Chemother 2003;51:1017–20.
755. D'Anchino M, Orlando D, De Feudis L. *Giardia lamblia* infections become clinically evident by eliciting symptoms of irritable bowel syndrome. J Infect 2002;45:169–72.
756. Di Prisco MC, Hagel I, Lynch NR, et al. Association between giardiasis and allergy. Ann Allergy Asthma Immunol 1998;81:261–5.

757. Dutta AK, Phadke MA, Bagade AC, et al. A randomized multicenter study to compare the safety and efficacy of albendazole and metronidazole in the treatment of giardiasis in children. Indian J Pediatr 1994;61:689–93.
758. Esfandiari A, Swartz J, Teklehaimanot S. Clustering of giardiasis among AIDS patients in Los Angeles County. Cell Mol Biol 1997:43:1077–83.
759. Farthing MJ. The molecular pathogenesis of giardiasis. J Pediatr Gastroenterol Nutr 1997;24: 79–88.
760. Farthing MJ, Varon SR, Keusch GT. Mammalian bile promotes growth of *Giardia lamblia* in axenic culture. Trans R Soc Trop Med Hyg 1983;77:467–9.
761. Garcia LS, Shimizu RY. Evaluation of nine immunoassay kits (enzyme immunoassay and direct fluorescence) for detection of *Giardia lamblia* and *Cryptosporidium parvum* in human fecal specimens. J Clin Microbiol 1997;35:1526–9.
762. Garcia LS, Shimizu RY, Novak S, Carroll M, Chan F. Commercial assay for detection of *Giardia lamblia* and *Cryptosporidium parvum* antigens in human fecal specimens by rapid solid–phase qualitative immunochromatography. J Clin Microbiol 2003;41:209–12.
763. Gardner TB, Hill DR. Treatment of giardiasis. Clin Microbiol Rev 2001;14:114–28.
764. Geldreich EE. Drinking water microbiology—new directions toward water quality enhancement. Int J Food Microbiol 1989;9:295–312.
765. Ghosh S, Debnath A, Sil A, De S, Chattopadhyay DJ, Das P. PCR detection of *Giardia lamblia* in stool: targeting intergenic spacer region of multicopy rRNA gene. Mol Cell Probes 2000;14:181–9.
766. Jimenez JC, Uzcanga G, Zambrano A, Di Prisco MC, Lynch NR. Identification and partial characterization of excretory/secretory products with proteolytic activity in *Giardia intestinalis*. J Parasitol 2000;86:859–62.
767. Johnston SP, Ballard MM, Beach MJ, Causer L, Wilkins PP. Evaluation of three commercial assays for detection of *Giardia* and *Cryptosporidium* organisms in fecal specimens. J Clin Microbiol 2003;41:623–6.
768. Kramer MH, Herwaldt BL, Craun GF, Calderon RL, Juranek DD. Surveillance for waterborne-disease outbreaks—United States, 1993-1994. MMWR Morb Mortal Rep1996;45(SS1):1–33.
769. Lane S, Lloyd D. Current trends in research into the waterborne parasite *Giardia*. Crit Rev Microbiol 2002;28:123–47.
770. Letts M, Davidson D, Lalonde F. Synovitis secondary to giardiasis in children. Am J Orthop 1998;27:451–4.
771. Levy DA, Bens MS, Craun GF, Calderon RL, Herwaldt BL. Surveillance for waterborne-disease outbreaks—United States, 1995-1996. MMWR Morb Mortal Wkly Rep 1998;47:6–7.
772. Markell E, Krotoski W. Markell and Vogel's medical parasitology. Philadelphia: WB Saunders; 1989.
773. Meyers JD, Kuharic HA, Holmes KK. *Giardia lamblia* infection in homosexual men. Br J Vener Dis 1977;53:54–5.
774. Moorehead WP, Guasparini R, Donovan CR, Mathias RG, Gottle R, Baytalan G. Giardiasis outbreak from a chlorinated community water supply. Can J Public Health 1990;81:358–62.
775. Olson ME, Ceri H, Morck DW. *Giardia* vaccination. Parasitol Today 2000;16:213–7.
776. Ortega YR, Adam RD. *Giardia*: overview and update. Clin Infect Dis 1997;25:545–50.
777. Osterholm MT, Forfang JC, Ristinen TL, et al. An outbreak of foodborne giardiasis. N Engl J Med 1981;304:24–8.
778. Ozbilgin A, Ertan P, Yereli K, et al. Giardiasis treatment in Turkish children with a single dose of ornidazole. Scand J Infect Dis 2002;34:918–20.
779. Petersen LR, Cartter ML, Hadler JL. A foodborne outbreak of *Giardia lamblia*. J Infect Dis 1988;157:846–8.
780. Pickering LK, Woodward WE, DuPont HL, Sullivan P. Occurrence of *Giardia lamblia* in children in day care centers. J Pediatr 1984;104: 522–6.
781. Porter JD, Ragazzoni HP, Buchanon JD, Waskin HA, Juranek DD, Parkin W. *Giardia* transmission in a swimming pool. Am J Public Health 1988;78:659–62.
782. Rauch AM, Van R, Bartlett AV, Pickering LK. Longitudinal study of *Giardia lamblia* in a day care center population. Pediatr Infect Dis J 1990;9:186–9.
783. Roberts-Thomson IC, Mitchell GF, Anders RF, et al. Genetic studies in human and murine giardiasis. Gut 1980;21:397–401.
784. Sacky ME, Weigel MM, Armijos RX. Predictors and nutritional consequences of intestinal parasitic infections in rural Ecuadorian children. J Trop Pediatr 2003;49:17–23.
785. Scott KG, Logan MR, Klammer GM, Teoh DA, Buret AG. Jejunal brush border microvillus alterations in *Giardia muris*-infected mice: role of T lymphocytes and interleukin-6. Infect Immun 2000;68:3412–8.
786. Steiner TS, Thielman NM, Guerrant RL. Protozoal agents: what are the dangers for the public water supply? Annu Rev Med 1997;48:329–40.

787. Teoh DA, Kamieniecki D, Pang G, Buret AG. *Giardia lamblia* rearranges F-actin and alpha-actinin in human colonic and duodenal monolayers and reduces transepithelial electric resistance. J Parasitol 2000;86:800–6.
788. Zimmerman SK, Needham CA. Comparison of conventional stool concentration and preserved-smear methods with Merifluor *Cryptosporidium/Giardia* Direct Immunofluorescence Assay and ProSpecT *Giardia* EZ Microplate Assay for detection of *Giardia lamblia*. J Clin Microbiol 1995;33:1942–3.

Amoeba Infections

789. Clark CG. *Entamoeba dispar*, an organism reborn. Trans R Soc Trop Med Hyg 1998;92:361–4.
790. De Meester F, Shaw E, Scholze H, Stolarsky T, Mirelman D. Specific labeling of cysteine proteinases in pathogenic and nonpathogenic *Entamoeba histolytica*. Infect Immun 1990;58: 1396–401.
791. Diamond LS, Clark CG. A redescription of *Entamoeba histolytica* Schaudinn, 1903 (Emended Walker, 1911) separating it from *Entamoeba dispar* Brumpt, 1925. J Eukaryot Microbiol 1993;40:340–4.
792. Espinosa-Catellano M, Martinez-Palomo A. Pathogenesis of intestinal amebiasis: from molecules to disease. Clin Microbiol Rev 2000;13: 318–31.
793. Gilman R, Islam M, Paschi S, Goleburn J, Ahmad F. Comparison of conventional and immunofluorescent techniques for the detection of *Entamoeba histolytica* in rectal biopsies. Gastroenterology 1980;78:435–9.
793a. Guerrant RL, Van Gilder T, Steiner TS, et al. Practice guidelines for the management of infectious diarrhea. Clin Infect Dis 2001;32:331–50.
794. Kretschmer R, Collado ML, Pacheco MG, et al. Inhibition of human monocyte locomotion by products of axenically grown *E. histolytica*. Parasite Immunol 1985;7:527–43.
795. Krogstad DJ. Isozyme patterns and pathogenicity in amebic infection. N Engl J Med 1986;315: 390–1.
796. Martinez-Palomo A, Espinosa-Cantellano M. Amoebiasis: new understanding and new goals. Parasitol Today 1998;14:1–3.
797. Muller FW, Franz A, Werries E. Secretory hydrolases of *E. histolytica*. J Protozool 1988;35: 291–5.
798. Okhuysen PC. Traveler's diarrhea due to intestinal protozoa. Clin Infect Dis 2001;33:110–4.
799. Ostoa-Saloma P, Cabrera N, Becker I, Perez–Montfort R. Proteinases of *Entamoeba histolytica* associated with different subcellular fractions. Mol Biochem Parasitol 1989;32:133–44.
800. Patterson M, Healy GR, Shabot JM. Serologic testing for amoebiasis. Gastroenterology 1980;78:136–41.
801. Perez-Montfort R, Ostoa-Saloma P, Velazquez-Medina L, Montfort I, Becker I. Catalytic classes of proteinases of *Entamoeba histolytica*. Mol Biochem Parasitol 1987;26:87–98.
802. Petri WA, Chapman MD, Snodgrass T, Mann BJ, Broman J, Ravdin JI. Subunit structure of the galactose and N-acetyl-D-galactosamine–inhibitable adherence lectin of *Entamoeba histolytica*. J Biol Chem 1989;264:3007–12.
803. Prathap K, Gilman R. The histopathology of acute intestinal amebiasis. Am J Pathol 1970;60:229–39.
804. Saffer LD, Petri WA Jr. Role of the galactose lectin of *Entamoeba histolytica* in adherence-dependent killing of mammalian cells. Infect Immun 1991;59:4681–3.
805. Samuelson J, Acuna-Soto R, Reed S, Biagi F, Wirth D. DNA hybridization probe for clinical diagnosis of *Entamoeba histolytica*. J Clin Microbiol 1989;27:671–6.
806. Sargeaunt PG. Zymodemes of *Entamoeba histolytica*. In: Ravdin JI, ed. Amebiasis: human infection by *Entamoeba histolytica*. New York: John Wiley & Sons; 1988:370–7.
807. Spice WM, Ackers JP. The effects of *Entamoeba histolytica* lysates on human colonic mucins. J Eukaryot Microbiol 1998;45:24S–7S.
808. Tannich E, Scholze H, Nickel R, Horstmann RD. Homologous cysteine proteases of pathogenic and nonpathogenic *Entamoeba histolytica*. Differences in structure and expression. J Biol Chem 1991;266:4798–803.
809. Trissl D. Glycosidases of *E. histolytica*. Z Parasitenkd 1983;69:291–8.

Balantidium Infections

810. Castro J, Vazquez-Iglesias JL, Arnal-Monreal F. Dysentery caused by *Balantidium coli*: report of two cases. Endoscopy 1983;15:272–4.
811. Esteban JG, Aguirre C, Angles R, Ash LR, Mas-Coma S. Balantidiasis in Aymara children from the northern Bolivian Altiplano. Am J Trop Med Hyg 1998;59:922–7.
812. Gendrel D, Treluyer JM, Richard-Lenoble D. Parasitic diarrhea in normal and malnourished children. Fundam Clin Pharmacol 2003;17: 189–97.
813. Juckett G. Intestinal protozoa. Am Fam Physician 1996;53:2507–16.
814. Kaur R, Rawat D, Kakkar M, Uppal B, Sharma VK. Intestinal parasites in children with diarrhea in Delhi, India. Southeast Asian J Trop Med Public Health 2002;33:725–9.

815. Swartzwelder JC. Balantidiasis. Am J Dig Dis 1950;17:173–9.
816. Urbina D, Arzuza O, Young G, Parra E, Castro R, Puello M. Rotavirus type A and other enteric pathogens in stool samples from children with acute diarrhea on the Colombian northern coast. Int Microbiol 2003;6:27–32.
817. Walzer PD, Judson FN, Murphy KB, Healy GR, English DK, Schultz MG. Balantidiasis outbreak in Truk. Am J Trop Med Hyg 1973;22:33–41.

Cryptosporidium Infections

818. Blanshard C, Jackson SM, Shanson DC, Francis N, Gazzard BG. Cryptosporidiosis in HIV-seropositive patients. Q J Med 1992;85:813–23.
819. Chen XM, Gores GJ, Paya CV, LaRusso NF. *Cryptosporidium parvum* induces apoptosis in biliary epithelia by a Fas/Fas ligand-dependent mechanism. Am J Physiol 1999;277:G599–608.
820. Chen XM, Keithly JS, Paya CV, LaRusso NF. Current concepts: cryptosporidiosis. N Engl J Med 2002;346:1723–31.
821. Chen XM, LaRusso NF. Mechanisms of attachment and internalization of *Cryptosporidium parvum* to biliary and intestinal epithelial cells. Gastroenterology 2000;118:368–79.
822. Chen XM, Levine SA, Splinter PL, et al. *Cryptosporidium parvum* activates nuclear factor kappa B in biliary epithelia preventing biliary cell apoptosis. Gastroenterology 2001;120:1774–83.
823. Chen XM, Levine SA, Tietz P, et al. *Cryptosporidium parvum* is cytopathic for cultured human biliary epithelia via an apoptotic mechanism. Hepatology 1998;28:906–13.
824. Clavel A, Arnal AC, Sanchez EC, et al. Respiratory cryptosporidiosis: case series and review of the literature. Infection 1996;24:341–6.
825. Current WL, Reese NC, Ernst JV, Bailey WS, Heyman MB, Weinstein WN. Human cryptosporidiosis in immunocompetent and immunodeficient persons: studies of an outbreak and experimental transmission. N Engl J Med 1983;308:1252–7.
826. Duombo O, Rossignol JF, Pichard E, et al. Nitazoxanide in the treatment of cryptosporidial diarrhea and other intestinal parasitic infections associated with acquired immunodeficiency syndrome in tropical Africa. Am J Trop Med Hyg 1997;56:637–9.
827. Elwin K, Chalmers RM, Roberts R, Guy EC, Casemore DP. Modification of a rapid method for the identification of gene-specific polymorphisms in *Cryptosporidium parvum* and its application to clinical and epidemiological investigations. Appl Environ Microbiol 2001;67:5581–4.
828. Forney JR, DeWald DB, Yang S, Speer CA, Healey MC. A role for host phosphoinositide 3-kinase and cytoskeletal remodeling during *Cryptosporidium parvum* infection. Infect Immun 1999;67:844–52.
829. Godwin TA. Cryptosporidiosis in the acquired immunodeficiency syndrome: a study of 15 autopsy cases. Hum Pathol 1991;22:1215–24.
830. Goodgame R, Genta R, White A, Chappell C. Intensity of infection in AIDS-associated cryptosporidiosis. J Infect Dis 1993;167:704–9.
831. Goodgame RW, Kimball K, Ou CN, et al. Intestinal function and injury in acquired immunodeficiency syndrome-related cryptosporidiosis. Gastroenterology 1995;108:1075–82.
832. Guerrant RL. Cryptosporidiosis: an emerging, highly infectious threat. Emerg Infect Dis 1997;3:51–7.
833. Higgins JA, Fayer R, Trout JM, et al. Real-time PCR for the detection of *Cryptosporidium parvum*. J Microbiol Methods 2001;47:323–37.
834. Iturriaga R, Zhang S, Sonek GJ, Stibbs H. Detection of respiratory enzyme activity in *Giardia* cysts and *Cryptosporidium* oocysts using redox dyes and immunofluorescence techniques. J Microbiol Methods 2001;46:19–28.
835. Jokipii L, Jokipii AM. Timing of symptoms and oocyst excretion in human cryptosporidiosis. N Engl J Med 1986;315:1643–7.
836. Kazlow PG, Shah K, Benkov KJ, Dische R, LeLeiko NS. Esophageal cryptosporidiosis in a child with acquired immune deficiency syndrome. Gastroenterology 1986;91:1301–3.
837. Kosek M, Alcantara C, Lima AA, Guerrant RL. Cryptosporidiosis: an update. Lancet Infect Dis 2001;1:262–9.
838. Laurent F, Eckmann L, Savidge TC, et al. *Cryptosporidium parvum* infection of human intestinal epithelial cells induces polarized secretions of C-X-C chemokines. Infect Immun 1997;65:5067–73.
839. Lopez-Velez R, Tarazona R, Garcia Camacho A, et al. Intestinal and extraintestinal cryptosporidiosis in AIDS patients. Eur J Clin Microbiol Infect Dis 1995;14:677–81.
840. MacKenzie WR, Hoxie NJ, Proctor ME, et al. A massive outbreak in Milwaukee of *Cryptosporidium* infection transmitted through the public water supply. N Engl J Med 1994;331:161–7.
841. Maillot C, Gargala G, Delaunay A, et al. *Cryptosporidium parvum* infection stimulates the secretion of TGF-beta, IL-8 and RANTES by Caco-2 cell line. Parasitol Res 2000;86:947–9.
842. Mallon M, MacLeod A, Wastling J, Smith H, Reilly B, Tait A. Population structures and the role of genetic exchange in the zoonotic pathogen *Cryptosporidium parvum*. J Mol Evol 2003;56:407–17.

843. Manabe YC, Clark DP, Moore RD, et al. Cryptosporidiosis in patients with AIDS: correlates of disease and survival. Clin Infect Dis 1998;27: 536–42.
844. McLauchlin J, Amar C, Pedraza-Diaz S, Nichols GL. Molecular epidemiological analysis of *Cryptosporidium* spp. in the United Kingdom: results of genotyping *Cryptosporidium* spp. in 1,705 fecal samples from humans and 105 fecal samples from livestock animals. J Clin Microbiol 2000;38:3984–90.
845. Meinhardt PL, Casemore DP, Miller KB. Epidemiologic aspects of human cryptosporidiosis and the role of waterborne transmission. Epidemiol Rev 1996;18:118–36.
846. Morgan U, Weber R, Xiao L, et al. Molecular characterization of *Cryptosporidium* isolates obtained from human immunodeficiency virus-infected individuals living in Switzerland, Kenya, and the United States. J Clin Microbiol 2000;38:1180–3.
847. O'Donoghue PJ. *Cryptosporidium* and cryptosporidiosis in man and animals. Int J Parasitol 1995;25:139–95.
848. Pieniazek NJ, Bornay-Llinares FJ, Slemenda SB, et al. New *Cryptosporidium* genotypes in HIV-infected persons. Emerg Infect Dis 1999;5:444–9.
849. Rossi P, Rivasi F, Codeluppi M, et al. Gastric involvement in AIDS associated with cryptosporidiosis. Gut 1998;43:476–7.
850. Rossignol JF, Hidalgo H, Feregrino M, et al. A double-'blind' placebo-controlled study of nitazoxanide in the treatment of cryptosporidial diarrhea in AIDS patients in Mexico. Trans R Soc Trop Med Hyg 1998;92:663–6.
851. Smith NH, Cron S, Valdez LM, Chappell CL, White AC Jr. Combination drug therapy for cryptosporidiosis in AIDS. J Infect Dis 1998;178:900–3.
852. Stehr-Green JK, McCaig L, Remsen HM, Rains CS, Fox M, Juranek DD. Shedding of oocysts in immunocompetent individuals infected with *Cryptosporidium*. Am J Trop Med Hyg 1987;36:338–42.
853. Tangermann RH, Gordon S, Wiesner P, Kreckman L. An outbreak of cryptosporidiosis in a day-care center in Georgia. Am J Epidemiol 1991;133:471–6.
854. Tzipori S, Ward H. Cryptosporidiosis: biology, pathogenesis and disease. Microbes Infect 2002;4:1047–58.
855. Tzipori S, Widmer G. The biology of *Cryptosporidium*. Contrib Microbiol 2000;6:1–32.
856. Ventura G, Cauda R, Larocca LM, Riccioni ME, Tumbarello M, Lucia MB. Gastric cryptosporidiosis complicating HIV infection: case report and review of the literature. Eur J Gastroenterol Hepatol 1997;9:307–10.
857. Xiao L, Bern C, Limor J, et al. Identification of 5 types of *Cryptosporidium* parasites in children in Lima, Peru. J Infect Dis 2001;183:492–7.

Cyclospora Infections

858. Caceres VM, Ball RT, Somerfeldt SA, et al. A foodborne outbreak of cyclosporiasis caused by imported raspberries. J Fam Pract 1998;47:231–4.
859. Centers for Disease Control and Prevention. Outbreak of diarrhoeal illness associated with cyanobacteria (blue-green algae)-like bodies—Chicago and Nepal, 1989 and 1990. MMWR Morb Mort Wkly Rep 1991;40:325–7.
860. Connor BA, Shlim DR, Scholes JV, Rayburn JL, Reidy J, Rajah R. Pathologic changes in the small bowel in nine patients with diarrhoea associated with a coccidia-like body. Ann Int Med 1993;119:377–82.
861. Eberhard ML, Ortega YR, Hanes DE, et al. Attempts to establish experimental *Cyclospora cayetanensis* infection in laboratory animals. J Parasitol 2000;86:577–82.
862. Eberhard ML, Pieniazek NJ, Arrowood MJ. Laboratory diagnosis of *Cyclospora* infections. Arch Pathol Lab Med 1997;121:792–7.
863. Fleming CA, Caron D, Gunn JE, Barry MA. A foodborne outbreak of *Cyclospora cayetanensis* at a wedding: clinical features and risk factors for illness. Arch Intern Med 1998;158:1121–5.
864. Herwaldt BL. *Cyclospora cayetanensis*: a review, focusing on the outbreaks of cyclosporiasis in the 1990s. Clin Infect Dis 2000;31:1040–57.
865. Ho AY, Lopez AS, Eberhart MG, et al. Outbreak of cyclosporiasis associated with imported raspberries, Philadelphia, Pennsylvania, 2000. Emerg Infect Dis 2002;8:783–8.
866. Hoge CW, Shlim DR, Echeverria P. Cyanobacterium-like *Cyclospora* species. N Engl J Med 1993;329:1504–5.
867. Hoge CW, Shlim DR, Ghimire M, et al. Placebo-controlled trial of co-trimoxazole for *Cyclospora* infections among travellers and foreign residents in Nepal. Lancet 1995;345:691–3.
868. Hoge CW, Shlim DR, Rajah R, et al. Epidemiology of diarrhoeal illness associated with coccidian-like organism among travellers and foreign residents in Nepal. Lancet 1993;341:1175–9.
869. Negm AY. Identification of *Cyclospora cayetanensis* in stool using different stains. J Egypt Soc Parasitol 1998;28:429–36.
870. Ortega YR, Nagle R, Gilman RH, et al. Pathologic and clinical findings in patients with cyclosporiasis and a description of intracellular parasite life-cycle stages. J Infect Dis 1997;176:1584–9.

871. Pollok RC, Bendall RP, Moody AH, Chiodini PL, Churchill DR. Travellers' diarrhoea associated with cyanobacterium-like bodies. Lancet 1992;340:556–7.
872. Relman DA, Schmidt TM, Gajadhar A, et al. Molecular phylogenetic analysis of *Cyclospora*, the human intestinal pathogen, suggests that it is closely related to *Eimeria* species. J Infect Dis 1996;173:440–5.
873. Richardson RF Jr, Remler BF, Katirji B, Murad MH. Guillain-Barre syndrome after *Cyclospora* infection. Muscle Nerve 1998;21:669–71.
874. Sifuentes-Osornio J, Porras-Cortes, Bendall RP, Morales-Villareal F, Reyes-Teran G, Ruiz-Palacios GM. *Cyclospora cayetanensis* infection in patients with and without AIDS: biliary disease as another clinical manifestation. Clin Infect Dis 1995;21:1092–7.
875. Sterling CR, Ortega YR. *Cyclospora*: an enigma worth unraveling. Emerg Infect Dis 1999;5:48–53.
876. Wurtz R. *Cyclospora*: a newly identified intestinal pathogen of humans. Clin Infect Dis 1994;18:620–3.

Leishmania Infections

877. Alvar J, Canavate C, Gutierrez-Solar B, et al. Leishmania and human immunodeficiency virus coinfection: the first 10 years. Clin Microbiol Rev 1997;10:298–319.
878. Berman JD. Human leishmaniasis: clinical, diagnostic, and chemotherapeutic developments in the last 10 years. Clin Infect Dis 1997;24: 684–703.
879. Cascio A, Calattini S, Colomba C, et al. Polymerase chain reaction in the diagnosis and prognosis of Mediterranean visceral leishmaniasis in immunocompetent children. Pediatrics 2002;109:E27.
880. Cerf BJ, Jones TC, Badaro R, Sampaio D, Teixeira R, Johnson WD. Malnutrition as a risk factor for severe visceral leishmaniasis. J infect Dis 1987;156:1030–3.
881. Croft SL, Coombs GH. Leishmaniasis—current chemotherapy and recent advances in the search for novel drugs. Trends Parasitol 2003; 19:502–8.
882. Desjeux P. Leishmaniasis. Public health aspects and control. Clin Dermatol 1996;14:417–23.
883. Guerin PJ, Olliaro P, Sundar S, et al. Visceral leishmaniasis: current status of control, diagnosis, and treatment, and a proposed research and development agenda. Lancet Infect Dis 2002;2:494–501.
884. Laguna F, Adrados M, Alvar J, et al. Visceral leishmaniasis in patients infected with the human immunodeficiency virus. Eur J Clin Microbiol Infect Dis 1997;16:898–903.
885. Laguna F, Garcia-Samaniego J, Soriano V, et al. Gastrointestinal leishmaniasis in human immunodeficiency virus-infected patients: report of five cases and review. Clin Infect Dis 1994;19: 48–53.
886. Laguna F, Lopez-Velez R, Pulido F, et al. Treatment of visceral leishmaniasis in HIV-infected patients: a randomized trial comparing meglumine antimonate with amphotericin B. AIDS 1999;13:1063–9.
887. Murray HW. Clinical and experimental advances in treatment of visceral leishmaniasis. Antimicrob Agents Chemother 2001;45:2185–97.
888. Russo R, Nigro LC, Minniti S, et al. Visceral leishmaniasis in HIV infected patients: treatment with high dose liposomal amphotericin B (AmBisome). J Infect Dis 1996;32:133–7.
889. Salotra P, Sreenivas G, Pogue GP, et al. Development of a species-specific PCR assay for detection of *Leishmania donovani* in clinical samples from patients with kala-azar and post-kala-azar dermal leishmaniasis. J Clin Microbiol 2001;39:849–54.
890. Sendino A, Barbado FJ, Mostaza JM, Fernandez-Martin J, Larrauri J, Vazquez-Rodriguez JJ. Visceral leishmaniasis with malabsorption syndrome in a patient with acquired immunodeficiency syndrome. Am J Med 1990;89:673–5.
891. Solano JG, Sanchez CS, Romero SM, et al. Visceral leishmaniasis of atypical location in immunodepressed patients. A report of two cases. Int J Surg Pathol 1996;3:241–3.
892. World Health Organization. Intestinal protozoan and helminthic infections. Report of a WHO Scientific Group. WHO Tech Rep Ser 666. Geneva: World Health Organization; 1981.

Chagas' Disease

893. Brener Z. Immunity of *Trypanosoma cruzi*. Adv Parasitol 1980;18:247–92.
894. Chamond N, Coatnoan N, Minoprio P. Immunotherapy of *Trypanosoma cruzi* infections. Curr Drug Targets Immune Endocr Metabol Disord 2002;2:247–54.
895. Dias JC. Acute Chagas' disease. Mem Inst Oswaldo Cruz 1984;79:85–92.
896. Goin JC, Sterin-Borda L, Bilder CR, et al. Functional implications of circulating muscarinic cholinergic receptor autoantibodies in chagasic patient with achalasia. Gastroenterology 1999;117:798–805.
897. Kirchhoff LV. American trypanosomiasis (Chagas' disease). Gastroenterol Clin North Am 1996;25:517–33.

898. Koberle F. Chagas' disease and Chagas' syndromes: the pathology of American trypanosomiasis. Adv Parasitol 1968;6:63–116.
899. Tarleton RL, Sun J, Zhang L, Postan M. Depletion of T-cell subpopulations results in exacerbation of myocarditis and parasitism in experimental Chagas' disease. Infect Immun 1994;62:1820–9.

Blastocystis Infections

900. al-Tawil YS, Gilger MA, Gopalakrishna GS, Langston C, Bommer KE. Invasive *Blastocystis hominis* infection in a child. Arch Pediatr Adolesc Med 1994;148:882–5.
901. Chen TL, Chan CC, Chen SP, et al. Clinical characteristics and endoscopic findings associated with *Blastocystis hominis* in healthy adults. Am J Trop Med Hyg 2003;69:213–6.
902. Cirioni O, Giacometti A, Drenaggi D, Ancarani F, Scalise G. Prevalence and clinical relevance of *Blastocystis hominis* in diverse patient cohorts. Eur J Epidemiol 1999;15:389–93.
903. Doyle PW, Helgason MM, Mathias RG, Proctor EM. Epidemiology and pathogenicity of *Blastocystis hominis*. J Clin Microbiol 1990;28:116–21.
904. El Masry NA, Bassily S, Farid Z, Aziz AG. Potential clinical significance of *Blastocystis hominis* in Egypt. Trans R Soc Trop Med Hyg 1990;84:695.
905. Horiki N, Maruyama M, Fujita Y, Yonekura T, Minato S, Kaneda Y. Epidemiologic survey of *Blastocystis hominis* infection in Japan. Am J Trop Med Hyg 1997;56:370–4.
906. Jelinek T, Peyerl G, Loscher T, von Sonnenburg F, Nothdurft HD. The role of *Blastocystis hominis* as a possible intestinal pathogen in travellers. J Infect 1997;35:63–6.
907. Lee MG, Rawlins SC, Didier M, DeCeulaer K. Infective arthritis due to *Blastocystis hominis*. Ann Rheum Dis 1990;49:192–3.
908. Nigro L, Larocca L, Massarelli L, et al. A placebo-controlled treatment trial of *Blastocystis hominis* infection with metronidazole. J Travel Med 2003;10:128–30.
909. Nimri LF. Evidence of an epidemic of *Blastocystis hominis* infections in preschool children in northern Jordan. J Clin Microbiol 1993;31:2706–8.
910. Nimri L, Batchoun R. Intestinal colonization of symptomatic and asymptomatic schoolchildren with *Blastocystis hominis*. J Clin Microbiol 1994;32:2865–6.
911. Ok UZ, Girginkardesler N, Balcioglu C, Ertan P, Pirildar T, Kilimcioglu AA. Effect of trimethoprim-sulfamethoxazole in *Blastocystis hominis* infection. Am J Gastroenterol 1999;94:3245–7.
912. Sheehan DJ, Raucher BG, McKitrick JC. Association of *Blastocystis hominis* with signs and symptoms of human disease. J Clin Microbiol 1986;24:548–50.
913. Stenzel DJ, Boreham PFL. *Blastocystis hominis* revisited. Clin Microbiol Rev 1996;9:563–84.
914. Taamasri P, Leelayoova S, Rangsin R, Naaglor T, Ketupanya A, Mungthin M. Prevalence of *Blastocystis hominis* carriage in Thai army personnel based in Chonburi, Thailand. Military Med 2002;167:643–6.
915. Tan KSW, Singh M, Yap EH. Recent advances in *Blastocystis hominis* research: hot spots in terra incognita. Int J Parasitol 2002;32:789–804.
916. Telalbasic S, Pikula ZP, Kapidzic M. *Blastocystis hominis* may be a potential cause of intestinal disease. Scand J Infect Dis 1991;23:389–90.
917. van Saanen-Ciurea M, El Achachi HE. *Blastocystis hominis*: culture and morphological study. Experientia 1985;41:546.
918. Windsor JJ, Macfarlane L, Hughes-Thapa G, Jones SK, Whiteside TM. Incidence of Blastocystis hominis in faecal samples submitted for routine microbiological analysis. Br J Biomed Sci 2002;59:154–7.
919. Zaki M, Daoud AS, Pugh RN, Al-Ali G, Al-Mutairi G, Al-Saleh Q. Clinical report of *Blastocystis hominis* infection in children. J Trop Med Hyg 1991;94:118–22.
920. Zierdt CH. *Blastocystis hominis*—past and future. Clin Microbiol Rev 1991;4:61–79.
921. Zierdt CH, Rude WS, Bull BS. Protozoan characteristics of *Blastocystis hominis*. Am J Clin Pathol 1967;48:495–501.
922. Zierdt CH, Tna H. Endosymbiosis in *Blastocystis hominis*. Parasitology 1976;39:422–30.
923. Zuckerman MJ, Ho H, Hooper L, Anderson B, Polly SM. Frequency of recovery of *Blastocystis hominis* in clinical practice. J Clin Gastroenterol 1990;12:525–32.
924. Zuckerman MJ, Watts MT, Ho H, Meriano FV. *Blastocystis hominis* infection and intestinal injury. Am J Med Sci 1994;308:96–101.

Ascaris Infections

925. Albonico M, Crompton DW, Savioli L. Control strategies for human intestinal nematode infections. Adv Parasitol 1999;42:278–341.
926. Albonico M, Smith PG, Hall AS, Chwaya HM, Alawi KS, Savioli L. A randomized controlled trial comparing mebendazole and albendazole against *Ascaris*, *Trichuris* and hookworm infections. Trans R Soc Trop Med Hyg 1994;88:585–9.
927. Anderson RM. The population dynamics and epidemiology of intestinal nematode infections. Trans R Soc Trop Med Hyg 1986;80:686–96.

928. Chai JY, Cho SY, Lee SH, Seo BS. Reduction in the incidence of biliary and other surgical complications of ascariasis according to the decrease of its national egg prevalence in Korea. Korean J Parasitol 1991;29:101–11.
929. Chu WG, Chen PM, Huang CC, Hsu CT. Neonatal ascariasis. J Pediatr 1972;81:783–5.
930. Chrungoo RK, Hangloo VK, Faroqui MM, Khan M. Surgical manifestations and management of ascariasis in Kashmir. J Indian Med Assoc 1992;90:171–4.
931. Crompton DW, Savioli L. Intestinal parasitic infections and urbanization. Bull World Health Organ 1993;71:1–7.
932. Khuroo MS, Zargar SA, Mahajan R. Hepatobiliary and pancreatic ascariasis in India. Lancet 1990;335:1503–6.
933. O'Lorcain P, Holland CV. The public health importance of *Ascaris lumbricoides*. Parasitology 2000;121:S51–71.
934. Pawlowski ZS, Arfaa F. Ascariasis. In: Warren KS, Mahmoud AA, eds. Tropical and geographic medicine. New York: McGraw-Hill; 1984:347.
935. Quinnell RJ. Genetics of susceptibility to human helminth infection. Int J Parasitol 2003;33:1219–31.
936. Rahman WA. Comparative trials using albendazole and mebendazole in the treatment of soil-transmitted helminths in schoolchildren on Penanag, Malaysia. Southeast Asian J Trop Med Public Health 1996;27:765–7.
937. Sinniah B. Daily egg production of *Ascaris lumbricoides*: the distribution of eggs in the faeces and the variability of egg counts. Parasitology 1982;84:167–75.
938. Sinniah B, Chew PI, Subramaniam K. A comparative trial of albendazole, mebendazole, pyrantel pamoate and oxantel pyrantel pamoate against soil transmitted helminthiases in school children. Trop Biomedicine 1990;7:129–34.
939. Storey GW, Phillips RA. The survival of parasite eggs throughout the soil profile. Parasitology 1985;91:585–90.
940. Thein–Hlaing. Ascariasis and childhood malnutrition. Parasitology 1993;107:S125–36.
941. Thein-Hlaing, Myat-Lay-Kyin, Hlaing-Mya, Maung-Maung. Role of ascariasis in surgical abdominal emergencies in the Rangoon Children's Hospital Burma. Ann Trop Paediatr 1990;10:53–60.

Hookworm Infections

942. Croese JA, Loukas A, Opdebeeck J, Fairley S, Prociv P. Human enteric infection with canine hookworms. Ann Intern Med 1994;120:369–74.
943. Crompton DW. How much human helminthiasis is there in the world? J Parasitol 1999;85:397–403.
944. Dowd AJ, Dalton JP, Loukas AC, Prociv P, Brindley PJ. Secretion of cysteine proteinase activity by the zoonotic hookworm *Ancylostoma caninum*. Am J Trop Med Hyg 1994;51:341–7.
945. Hotez P, Capello M, Hawdon J, Beckers C, Sakanari J. Hyaluronidases of the gastrointestinal invasive nematodes *Ancylostoma caninum* and *Anisakis simplex*: possible functions in the pathogenesis of human zoonoses. J Infect Dis 1994;170:918–26.
946. Loukas A, Prociv P. Immune responses in hookworm infections. Clin Microbiol Rev 2001;14:689–703.
947. Palmer ED. Course of egg output over a 15 year period in a case of experimentally induced necatoriasis americanus, in the absence of hyperinfection. Am J Trop Med Hyg 1955;4:756–7.
948. Prociv P, Croese J. Human enteric infection with *Ancylostoma caninum*: hookworms reappraised in the light of a new zoonosis. Acta Trop 1996;62:23–44.
949. Walker NI, Croese J, Clouston AD, Parry M, Loukas A, Prociv P. Eosinophilic enteritis in northeastern Australia. Pathology, association with *Ancylostoma caninum*, and implications. Am J Surg Pathol 1995;19:328–37.

Schistosoma Infections

950. Bethlem EP, Schettino G, Carvalho CR. Pulmonary schistosomiasis. Curr Opin Pulm Med 1997;3:361–5.
951. Chen MG. Relative distribution of *Schistosoma japonicum* eggs in the intestine of man: a subject of inconsistency. Acta Trop 1991;48:163–71.
952. Chen MC, Chang PY, Chuang CY, et al. Colorectal cancer and schistosomiasis. Lancet 1981;1:971–3.
953. Chitsulo L, Engels D, Montresor A, Savioli L. The global status of schistosomiasis and its control. Acta Trop 2000;77:41–51.
954. Cooke GS, Lalvani A, Gleeson FV, Conlon CP. Acute pulmonary schistosomiasis in travelers returning from Lake Malawi, sub-Saharan Africa. Clin Infect Dis 1999;29:836–9.
955. Doherty JF, Moody AH, Wright SG. Katayama fever: an acute manifestation of schistosomiasis. BMJ 1996;313:1071–2.
956. Garcia LS, Shimizu RY, Plamer JC. Algorithms for detection and identification of parasites. In: Murray PR, ed. Manual of clinical microbiology, 7th ed. Washington, DC: American Society for Microbiology Press; 1999:1336–54.

957. Hussein A, Medany S, Abou el Magd AM, Sherif SM, Williams CB. Multiple endoscopic polypectomies for schistosomal polyposis of the colon. Lancet 1983;1:673–4.
958. Ismail M, Botros S, Metwally A, et al. Resistance to praziquantel: direct evidence from *Schistosoma mansoni* isolated from Egyptian villagers. Am J Trop Med Hyg 1999;60:932–5.
959. Nebel OT, el-Masry NA, Castell DO, Farid Z, Fornes MF, Sparks HA. Schistosomal disease of the colon: a reversible form of polyposis. Gastroenterology 1974;67:939–43.
960. Patz J, Graczyk T, Geller N, Vittor A. Effects of environmental change on emerging parasitic diseases. Int J Parasitol 2000;30:1395–405.
961. Ross AG, Bartley PB, Sleigh AC, et al. Current concepts: schistosomiasis. N Engl J Med 2002; 346:1212–20.
962. van der Werf MJ, de Vlas SJ, Brooker S, et al. Quantification of clinical morbidity associated with schistosome infection in sub-Saharan Africa. Acta Trop 2003;86:125–39.
963. William S, Botros S, Ismail M, Farghally A, Day TA, Bennett JL. Praziquantel-induced tegumental damage in vitro is diminished in schistosomes derived from praziquantel-resistant infections. Parasitology 2001;122:63–6.

Anisakis Infections

964. Audicana T, Fernandez de Corres L, Munoz D, Fernandez E, Navarro JA, del Pozo MD. Recurrent anaphylaxis caused by *Anisakis simplex* parasitizing fish. J Allergy Clin Immunol 1995; 96:558–60.
965. Couture C, Measures L, Gagnon J, Desbiens C. Human intestinal anisakiosis due to consumption of raw salmon. Am J Surg Pathol 2003;27: 1167–72.
966. Deardorff TL, Kayes SG, Fukumura T. Human anisakiasis transmitted by marine food products. Hawaii Med J 1991;50:9–16.
967. Gardiner MA. Survival of *Anisakis* in cold smoked salmon. Can Institute Food Sci Tech J 1990;23:143–4.
968. Hauck AK. Occurrence and survival of the larval nematode *Anisakis* sp. in the flesh of fresh, frozen, brined and smoked Pacific herring, *Clupea harengus pallasi*. J Parasitol 1977;63:515–9.
969. Hays R, Measures LN, Huot J. Euphausiids as intermediate hosts of *Anisakis simplex* in the St. Lawrence estuary. Can J Zool 1998;76:1126–35.
970. Hays R, Measures LN, Huot J. Capelin (*Mallotus villosus*) and herring (*Clupea harengus*) as paratenic hosts of *Anisakis simplex*, a parasite of beluga (*Delphinapterus leucas*) in the St. Lawrence estuary. Can J Zool 1998;76:1411–7.
971. Ishikura H, Kikuchi K, Nagasawa K, et al. Anisakidae and anisakidosis. In: Sun T, ed. Progress in clinical parasitology. New York: Springer Verlag; 1992:43–102.
972. Kagei N, Orikasa H, Hori E, et al. A case of hepatic anisakiasis with a literal survey for extragastrointestinal anisakiasis. Jpn J Parasitol 1995;44:346–51.
973. Kakizoe S, Kakizoe H, Kakizoe K, et al. Endoscopic findings and clinical manifestation of gastric anisakiasis. Am J Gastroenterol 1995;90:761–3.
974. Kasuya S, Hamano H, Izumi S. Mackerel-induced urticaria and *Anisakis*. Lancet 1990;335: 665.
975. Kim HJ, Park C, Cho SY. A case of extra gastrointestinal anisakiasis involving a mesocolic lymph node. Korean J Parasitol 1997;35:63–6.
976. Kliks MM. Anisakiasis in the western United States: four new case reports from California. Am J Trop Med Hyg 1983;323:526–32.
977. Lewis R, Shore JH. Anisakiasis in the United Kingdom. Lancet 1985;2:1019.
978. Lucas SB, Cruse JP, Lewis AA. Anisakiasis in the United Kingdom. Lancet 1985;2:843–4.
979. Margolis L, Arthur JR. Synopsis of the parasites of fishes of Canada. Bull Fisheries Research Board Can 1979;199:269.
980. McDonald TE, Margolis L. Synopsis of the parasites of fishes of Canada. Supplement (1978-1993). Can Special Publ Fisheries Aquatic Sci 1995;122:265.
981. Moreno-Ancillo A, Caballero MT, Cabanas R, et al. Allergic reactions to *Anisakis simplex* parasitizing seafood. Ann Allergy Asthma Immunol 1997;79:246–50.
982. Myers B. Anisakine nematodes in fresh commercial fish from waters along the Washington, Oregon and California coasts. J Food Prot 1979;42:380–4.
983. Oshima T. *Anisakis* and anisakiasis in Japan and adjacent areas. In: Morishita K, Komiya Y, Matsubayashi H, eds. Progress of medical parasitology in Japan. Tokyo: Tokyo Meguro Parasitological Museum; 1972:201–393.
984. Oshima T, Kliks MM. Effects of marine mammal parasites on human health. Inter J Parasitol 1986;17:415–21.
985. Pampiglione S, Rivasi F, Criscuolo M, et al. Human anisakiasis in Italy: a report of eleven new cases. Pathol Res Pract 2002;198:429–34.
986. Sakanari JA, Loinaz HM, Deardorff TL, Raybourne RB, McKerrow JH, Frierson JG. Intestinal anisakiasis: a case diagnosed by morphologic and immunologic methods. Am J Clin Pathol 1988;90:107–13.

987. Sakanari JA, McKerrow JH. Anisakiasis. Clin Microbiol Rev 1989;2:278–84.
988. Smith JW. Ascaridoid nematodes and pathology of the alimentary tract and its associated organs in vertebrates, including man: a literature review. Helminthological Abstr 1999;68: 49–96.
989. Sugimachi K, Inokuchi K, Odiwa, Fujino T, Ishii Y. Acute gastric anisakiasis: analysis of 178 cases. JAMA 1985;253:1012–3.
990. Tunon T, Zozaya E, Tabar AI, Dorronsoro ML, Gomez B, Valenti C. Eosinophilic enteritis due to Anisakis: a call for pathologists' attention. Int J Surg Pathol 1997;5:69–76.
991. Whitaker DJ. A parasite survey of juvenile chum salmon (*Oncorhynchus keta*) from the Nanaimo River. Can J Zool 1985;63:2875–7.
992. Yasuma J. Studies on the in vitro axenic development of *Anisakis* larvae (I). Jpn J Parasitol 1965;16:723–8.

Enterobius Vermicularis Infections

993. Beattie RM, Walker-Smith JA, Domizio P. Ileal and colonic ulceration due to enterobiasis. J Pediatr Gastroenterol Nutr 1995;21:232–4.
994. Bumbalo TS, Fugazotto DJ, Wyczalek JV. Treatment of enterobiasis with pyrantel pamoate. Am J Trop Med Hyg 1969;18:50–2.
995. Chandrasoma PT, Mendis KN. *Enterobius vermicularis* in ectopic sites. Am J Trop Med Hyg 1977;26:644–9.
996. Cook GC. Enterobius vermicularis infection. Gut 1994;35:1159–62.
997. Das DK, Pathan SK, Hira PR, Madda JP, Hasaniah WF, Juma TH. Pelvic abscess from *Enterobius vermicularis*. Report of a case with cytologic detection of eggs and worms. Acta Cytol 2001;45:425–9.
998. Dundas KC, Calder AA, Alyusuf R. *Enterobius vermicularis* threadworm infestation of paraovarian tissue in a woman who has had a hysterectomy. Br J Obstet Gynaecol 1999;106:605–7.
999. Erhan Y, Zekioglu O, Ozdemir N, Sen S. Unilateral salpingitis due to *Enterobius vermicularis*. Int J Gynecol Pathol 2000;19:188–9.
1000. Hong ST, Choi MH, Chai JY, Kim YT, Kim MK, Kim KR. A case of ovarian enterobiasis. Korean J Parasitol 2002;40:149–51.
1001. Liu LX, Chi J, Upton MP, Ash LR. Eosinophilic colitis associated with larvae of the pinworm *Enterobius vermicularis*. Lancet 1995;346:410–2.
1002. Sinniah B, Leopairut J, Neafie RC, Connor DH, Voge M. Enterobiasis: a histopathological study of 259 patients. Ann Trop Med Parasitol 1991;85:625–35.
1003. Vafai M, Mohit P. Granuloma of the anal canal due to *Enterobius vermicularis*. Report of a case. Dis Colon Rectum 1983;26:349–50.

Trichuris Infections

1004. Bundy DA. Epidemiological aspects of *Trichuris* and trichuriasis in Caribbean communities. Trans R Soc Trop Med Hyg 1986;80:706–18.
1005. Chan MS. The global burden of intestinal nematode infections—fifty years on. Parasitol Today 1997;13:438–43.
1005a. Crompton DW. How much human helminthiasis is there in the world? J Parasitol 1999; 85:397–403.
1006. Gilman RH, Chong YH, Davis C, Greenberg HK, Virik HK, Dixon HB. The adverse consequences of heavy *Trichuris* infection. Trans R Soc Trop Med Hyg 1983;77:432–8.
1007. Horii Y, Usui M. Experimental transmission of *Trichuris* ova from monkeys to man. Trans R Soc Trop Med Hyg 1985;79:423.
1008. MacDonald TT, Choy MY, Spencer J, et al. Histopathology and immunohistochemistry of the caecum in children with *Trichuris* dysentery syndrome. J Clin Pathol 1991;44:194–9.
1009. Mirdha BR, Singh YG, Samantray JC, Mishra B. *Trichuris vulpis* infection in slum children. Ind J Gastroenterol 1988;17:154.
1010. Pawlowski ZS. Trichuriasis. In: Warren KS, Mahmoud AA, eds. Tropical and geographic medicine. New York: McGraw Hill; 1984:380–5.
1011. Stephenson LS, Holland CV, Cooper ES. The public health significance of *Trichuris trichiura*. Parasitology 2000;121:S73–95.
1012. Wolfe MS. *Oxyuris*, *Trichostongylus* and *Trichuris*. Clin Gastroenterol 1978;7:211–7.
1013. Wolfe MS, Wershing JM. Mebendazole: treatment of trichuriasis and ascariasis in Bahamian children. JAMA 1974;240:1408–11.

Strongyloides Infections

1013a. Albonico M, Smith PG, Hall AS, Chwaya HM, Alawi KS, Savioli L. A randomized controlled trial comparing mebendazole and albendazole against *Ascaris*, *Trichuris* and hookworm infections. Trans R Soc Trop Med Hyg 1994;88:585–9.
1014. Berk SL, Verghese A, Alvarez S, Hall K, Smith B. Clinical and epidemiologic features of strongyloidiasis. A prospective study in rural Tennessee. Arch Intern Med 1987;147:1257–61.
1015. Carp NZ, Nejman JH, Kelly JJ. Strongyloidiasis: an unusual cause of colonic pseudopolyposis and gastrointestinal bleeding. Surg Endosc 1987;1:175–7.

1016. Chaudhuri B, Nanos S, Soco JN, McGrew EA. Disseminated *Strongyloides stercoralis* infestation detected by sputum cytology. Acta Cytol 1980;24:360–2.
1017. Daubenton JD, Buys HA, Hartley PS. Disseminated strongyloidiasis in a child with lymphoblastic lymphoma. J Pediatr Hematol Oncol 1998;20:260–3.
1018. Dees A, Batenburg PL, Umar HM, Menon RS, Verweij J. *Strongyloides stercoralis* associated with a bleeding gastric ulcer. Gut 1990;31:1414–5.
1019. Genta RM. Global prevalence of strongyloidiasis: critical review with epidemiologic insights into the prevention of disseminated disease. Rev Infect Dis 1989;11:755–67.
1020. Grove DI. Human strongyloidiasis. Adv Parasitol 1996;38:251–309.
1021. Ho PL, Luk WK, Chan AC, Yuen KY. Two cases of fatal strongyloidiasis in Hong Kong. Pathology 1997;29:324–6.
1022. Jorgensen T, Montresor A, Savioli L. Effectively controlling strongyloidiasis. Parasitol Today 1996;12:164.
1023. Kennedy S, Campbell RM, Lawrence JE, Nichol GM, Rao DM. A case of severe *Strongyloides stercoralis* infection with jejunal perforation in an Australian ex-prisoner-of-war. Med J Aust 1989;150:92–3.
1024. Liepman M. Disseminated *Strongyloides stercoralis*. A complication of immunosuppression. JAMA 1975;231:387–8.
1025. Link K, Orenstein R. Bacterial complications of strongyloidiasis: *Streptococcus bovis* meningitis. South Med J 1999;92:728–31.
1026. Liu LX, Weller PF. Strongyloidiasis and other intestinal nematode infections. Infect Dis Clin North Am 1993;7:655–82.
1027. McNeely D, Inouye T, Tam PY, Ripley D. Acute respiratory failure due to strongyloidiasis in polymyositis. J Rheumatol 1980;7:745–50.
1028. Milder JE, Walzer PD, Kilgore G, Rutherford I, Klein M. Clinical features of *Strongyloides stercoralis* infection in an endemic area of the United States. Gastroenterology 1981;80:1481–8.
1029. Mori S, Konishi T, Matsuoka K, et al. Strongyloidiasis associated with nephrotic syndrome. Intern Med 1998;37:606–10.
1030. Newton RC, Limpuangthip P, Greenberg S, Gam A, Neva FA. *Strongyloides stercoralis* hyperinfection in a carrier of HTLV-1 virus with evidence of selective immunosuppression. Am J Med 1992;92:202–8.
1031. Pelletier LL Jr, Baker CB, Gam AA, Nutman TB, Neva FA. Diagnosis and evaluation of treatment of chronic strongyloidiasis in ex-prisoners of war. J Infect Dis 1988;157:573–6.
1032. Phillips SC, Mildvan D, William DC, Gelb AM, White MC. Sexual transmission of enteric protozoa and helminths in a venereal-disease-clinic population. N Engl J Med 1981;305:603–6.
1033. Scaglia M, Brustia R, Gatti S, et al. Autochthonous strongyloidiasis in Italy: an epidemiological and clinical review of 150 cases. Bull Soc Pathol Exot Filiales 1984;77:328–32.
1034. Sen P, Gil C, Estrellas B, Middleton JR. Corticosteroid induced asthma: a manifestation of limited hyperinfection syndrome due to *Strongyloides stercoralis*. South Med J 1995;88:923–7.
1035. Stoopack PM, Raufman JP. Aphthoid ulceration of the colon in strongyloidiasis. Am J Gastroenterol 1991;86:639–42.
1036. Thomas MC, Costello SA. Disseminated strongyloidiasis arising from a single dose of dexamethasone before stereotactic radiosurgery. Int J Clin Pract 1998;52:520–1.
1037. Tullis TC. Bronchial asthma associated with intestinal parasites. N Engl J Med 1970;282:370–2.
1038. Walzer PD, Milder JE, Banwell JG, Kilgore G, Klein M, Parker R. Epidemiologic features of *Strongyloides stercoralis* infection in an endemic area of the United States. Am J Trop Med Hyg 1982;31:313–9.
1039. Wong TY, Szeto CC, Lai FF, Mak CK, Li PK. Nephrotic syndrome in strongyloidiasis: remission after eradication with antihelminthic agents. Nephron 1998;79:333–6.
1040. Zaha O, Hirata T, Kinjo F, Saito A. Strongyloidiasis—progress in diagnosis and treatment. Intern Med 2000;39:695–700.

Angiostrongylus Infections

1041. Ambu S, Mak JW, Ng CS. Efficacy of ivermectin against *Parastrongylus malaysiensis* infection in rats. J Helminthol 1992;66:293–6.
1042. Ash LR. Human anisakiasis misdiagnosed as abdominal angiostrongyliasis. Clin Infect Dis 1993;16:332–4.
1043. Duarte Z, Morera P, Vuong PN. Abdominal angiostrongyliasis in Nicaragua: a clinico-pathological study on a series of 12 cases reports. Ann Parasitol Hum Comp 1991;66:259–62.
1044. Graeff-Teixeira C, Camillo-Coura L, Lenzi HL. Histopathological criteria for the diagnosis of abdominal angiostrongyliasis. Parasitol Res 1991;77:606–11.
1045. Kramer MH, Greer GJ, Quinonez JF, et al. First reported outbreak of abdominal angiostrongyliasis. Clin Infect Dis 1998;26:365–72.

1046. Liacouras CA, Bell LM, Aljabi MC, Piccoli DA. *Angiostrongylus costaricensis* enterocolitis mimics Crohn's disease. J Pediatr Gastroenterol Nutr 1993;16:203–7.
1047. Loria-Cortes R, Lobo-Sanahuja JF. Clinical abdominal angiostrongylosis: a study of 116 children with intestinal eosinophilic granuloma caused by *Angiostrongylus costaricensis*. Am J Trop Med Hyg 1980;29:538–44.
1048. Mentz MB, Graeff-Teixeira C. Drug trials for treatment of human angiostrongyliasis. Rev Inst Med Trop S Paulo 2003;45:179–84.
1049. Morera P. Life history and redescription of *Angiostrongylus costaricensis* Morera and Cespedes, 1971. Am J Trop Med Hyg 1973;22:613–21.
1050. Morera P, Perez F, Mora F, Castro L. Visceral larva migrans-like syndrome caused by *Angiostrongylus costaricensis*. Am J Trop Med Hyg 1982;30:67–70.
1051. Neafie RC, Marty AM. Unusual infections in humans. Clin Microbiol Rev 1993;6:34–56.
1052. Silvera CT, Ghali VS, Roven S, Heimann J, Gelb A. Angiostrongyliasis: a rare cause of gastrointestinal hemorrhage. Am J Gastroenterol 1989;84:329–32.
1053. Terada M, Rodriguez BO, Dharejo AM, Ishii AI, Sano M. Studies on chemotherapy of various parasitic helminths (XXVI): comparative in vitro effects of various antihelmintics on the motility of *Angiostrongylus costaricensis* and *A. cantonensis*. Jpn J Parasitol 1986;35:365–7.
1054. Ubelaker JE. Systematics of species referred to the genus *Angiostrongylus*. J Parasitol 1986;72: 237–44.
1055. Vazquez JJ, Boils PL, Sola JJ, et al. Angiostrongyliasis in a European patient: a rare cause of gangrenous ischemic enterocolitis. Gastroenterology 1993;105:1544–9.
1056. Wu SS, French SW, Turner JA. Eosinophilic ileitis with perforation caused by *Angiostrongylus (Parastrongylus) costaricensis*. A case study and review. Arch Pathol Lab Med 1997;121:989–91.

Capillaria Philippinensis Infections

1057. Ahmad L, El-Dib N, El-Boraey Y, Ibrahim M. *Capillaria philippinensis*: an emerging parasite causing severe diarrhea in Egypt. J Egypt Soc Parasitol 1999;29:483–93.
1058. Belizario YY, de Leon WU, Esparar DJ, Galang JM, Fantone J, Verdadero C. Compostela Valley: a new endemic focus for *Capillaria philippinensis*. Southeast Asian J Trop Med Public Health 2000;31:478–81.
1059. Chen CY, Hsieh WC, Lin JT, Liu MC. Intestinal capillariasis: report of a case. J Formosan Med Assoc 1989;88:617–20.
1060. Chunlertrith K, Mairiang P, Sukeepaisarnjaroen W. Intestinal capillariasis: a cause of chronic diarrhea and hypoalbuminemia. Southeast Asian J Trop Med Public Health 1992;23:433–6.
1061. Cross JH. Intestinal capillariasis. Parasitol Today 1990;6:26–8.
1062. Cross JH. Intestinal capillariasis. Clin Microbiol Rev 1992;5:120–9.
1063. El-Dib N, Doss W. Intestinal capillariasis in Egypt: a case report. J Egypt Soc Parasit 2002; 32:145–54.
1064. Kang G, Mathan M, Ramakrishna BS, Mathai E, Sarada V. Human intestinal capillariasis: first report from India. Trans R Soc Trop Med Hyg 1994;88:204.
1065. Khalifa RM, Sakla AA, Hassan AA. *Capillaria philippinensis*—a human intestinal nematode newly introduced to upper Egypt. Helminthologia 2000;37:23–7.
1066. Lee SH, Hong ST, Chai JY, et al. A case of intestinal capillariasis in the Republic of Korea. Am J Trop Med Hyg 1993;48:542–6.
1067. Youssef G, Mikhail EM, Mansour NS. Intestinal capillariasis in Egypt: a case report. Am J Trop Med Hyg 1989;40:195–6.

Tapeworm Infections

1068. Castillo M. Intestinal taeniasis. In: Marcial-Rojas RA, ed. Pathology of protozoal and helminthic diseases. Baltimore: Williams & Wilkins; 1971:618.
1069. Dick TA, Nelson PA, Choudhury A. Diphyllobothriasis: update on human cases, foci, patterns and sources of human infections and future considerations. Southeast Asian J Trop Med Public Health 2001;32(suppl 2):59–76.
1070. Jones T. Cestodes. Clin Gastroenterol 1978;7: 105–28.
1071. Matuchansky C, Lenormand Y. *Taenia saginata*. N Engl J Med 1999;341:1737.
1072. McKay DM, Halton DW, McCaigue MD, Johnston CF, Fairweather I, Shaw C. *Hymenolepis diminuta*: intestinal goblet cell response to infection in male C57 mice. Exp Parasitol 1990;71:9–20.
1073. Munoz J. Foodborne diseases: seafood. Pediatr Infect Dis J 1999;18:910–1.
1074. Nash TE, Neva FA. Recent advances in the diagnosis and treatment of cerebral cysticercosis. N Engl J Med 1984;331:1491–6.

11 GASTROINTESTINAL DISEASES IN IMMUNOCOMPROMISED PATIENTS

Gastrointestinal diseases are extremely common in the growing population of immunocompromised and immunosuppressed patients, including those with human immunodeficiency virus (HIV) infection and those who have undergone solid organ or bone marrow transplantation. Symptoms of gastrointestinal origin in this group of patients occur as a result of opportunistic infection, drug-induced injury, or as a direct result of the process that initially led to the immune dysfunction.

HUMAN IMMUNODEFICIENCY VIRUS INFECTION

Definition. *Acquired immunodeficiency syndrome* (AIDS) results from infection with HIV. It is associated with a number of defining abnormalities (Table 11-1).

Demography. More than 30 million people are infected with HIV-1 worldwide. The major risk groups for developing AIDS vary with geographic locale. In Africa and Asia, the major risk group is sexually active heterosexuals; women are more often infected than men (17,45). In the United States, over 70 percent of cases affect homosexual or bisexual men; another 15 percent develop in intravenous drug users. Other high-risk groups include prostitutes, hemophiliacs, children born to HIV-positive mothers, patients transfused with HIV infected blood or blood products, and heterosexual contacts of any of the above groups (50). HIV-infected mothers pass the virus transplacentally, through the birth canal at the time of delivery, or through breast milk. AIDS especially affects Hispanics and African-Americans (15). The AIDS patient population in the United States is disproportionately male, black, and poor (9). In 1994, 18 percent of patients in the United States were women. Sexual transmission is now the dominant route by which women become infected (20). HIV is also endemic in Central Africa and Haiti. Substantial declines have occurred in AIDS incidence and related deaths in recent years (15), probably due to an increased awareness in at-risk populations and the introduction of antiretroviral therapies.

Table 11-1

DEFINITION OF ACQUIRED IMMUNODEFICIENCY SYNDROME (AIDS)

Any patient with one or more of the following reliably diagnosed diseases in the absence of a known cause of immunodeficiency; laboratory evidence regarding human immunodeficiency virus (HIV) infection either positive or not available:
Candidiasis of esophagus, trachea, bronchi, or lungs
Cryptococcosis, extrapulmonary
Cryptosporidiosis with diarrhea persisting more than 1 month
Cytomegalovirus disease, extranodal, in patient >1 month of age
Herpes simplex virus infection with ulceration persisting >1 month
Kaposi's sarcoma in patient <60 years of age
Lymphoma, brain (primary), in patient <60 years of age
Lymphoid interstitial pneumonia or pulmonary lymphoid hyperplasia in child <13 years of age
Mycobacterium avium-intracellulare or *M. kansasii* disease, disseminated
Pneumocystosis
Progressive multifocal leukoencephalopathy
Any patient with one or more of the following reliably diagnosed diseases plus laboratory evidence of HIV infection:
Bacterial infections, multiple or recurrent, in child <13 years of age
Coccidioidomycosis, disseminated
HIV encephalopathy
Histoplasmosis, disseminated
Isosporiasis with diarrhea persisting more than 1 month
Kaposi's sarcoma at any age
Lymphoma, brain (primary), at any age
Other non-Hodgkin's lymphomas of certain types
Mycobacteriosis caused by mycobacteria other than *M. tuberculosis*, disseminated
Tuberculosis, extrapulmonary
Salmonella (nontyphoid) septicemia, recurrent
HIV wasting syndrome

Since 1996, profound changes have taken place in the epidemiology, clinical presentation, complications, and management of HIV infection. Primarily, these changes are the result of the introduction of highly active antiretroviral

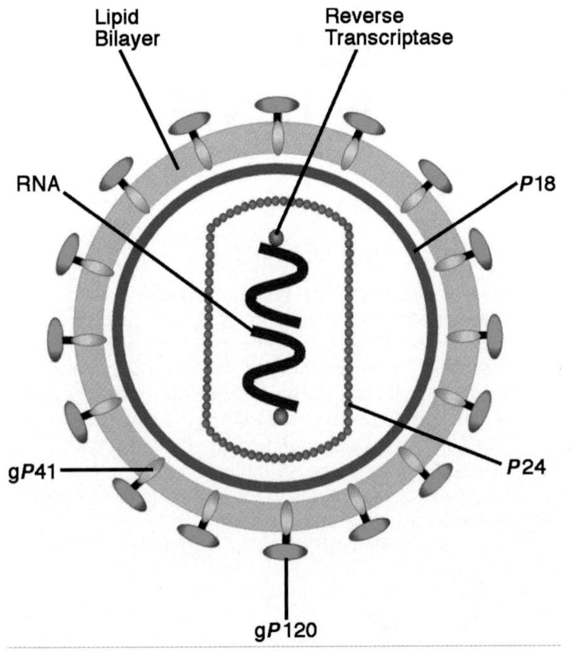

Figure 11-1

SCHEMATIC DIAGRAM OF THE HUMAN IMMUNODEFICIENCY VIRUS (HIV) VIRION

The envelope proteins (GP120 and GP41) and nuclear capsid proteins (P24 and P18) are identified. The diploid RNA genome contains reverse transcriptase and an RNA-dependent DNA polymerase.

treatment (HAART). Gastrointestinal and hepatobiliary complications were universally recognized during the course of HIV infection; however, in the era of HAART, these complications have dramatically decreased. Monkemuller et al. (36) showed a substantial reduction in the number of opportunistic infections associated with HIV infection in a group of patients on HAART. Although substantially effective in suppressing opportunistic infections, the antiretroviral medications are associated with gastrointestinal side effects in up to 10 percent of cases (8). Currently, drug-induced side effects and nonopportunistic diseases are among the most common causes of gastrointestinal symptoms in HIV-positive patients (11,36).

Etiology. Two HIV types exist: HIV-1 and HIV-2. Both viruses belong to the lentivirus family of nononcogenic retroviruses. HIV-1 is the predominant virus in the United States, Europe, and eastern Africa; HIV-2 infection predominates in parts of western Africa. Fewer AIDS cases develop in HIV-2–infected than in HIV-1–infected populations. Viral transmission is similar for both viruses, except that perinatal transmission occurs less frequently with HIV-2 infections. HIV-2 also has a longer latency period before AIDS appears, the course is less aggressive, and the mortality rate is lower than for those with HIV-1 infection. HIV-2–infected patients typically have a lower viral load and higher CD4 counts than HIV-1–infected individuals.

HIV easily mutates, leading to the emergence of new viral strains that can resist immune attack or drug therapy or alter the clinical or histopathologic features of the disease. The number of active replicating viruses is proportional to the number of CD4-positive lymphocytes.

The HIV virion measures approximately 100 nm in diameter and contains a dense cylindrical core (fig. 11-1). Its life cycle is shown in figure 11-2. The virion contains two single RNA strands, structural proteins, and the enzymes required for viral replication. The HIV genome is diagramed in figure 11-3. HIV genes encode core proteins (GAG), reverse transcriptase, protease, an endonuclease (Pol), and envelope glycoproteins (Env). At least five other genes exert regulatory functions that may affect viral pathogenicity including: *vif, tat3, rev, nef*, and *vpr* (Table 11-2). The viruses use the enzyme reverse transcriptase to transcribe viral RNA into proviral DNA in host cells. The proviral DNA resides in the cells during viral latency. The lipid envelope surrounding the viral core is derived from the host cell surface as the virions bud from the infected cell. As a result, this lipid envelope contains host membrane protein remnants as well as the viral envelope glycoprotein gp120 and the transmembrane protein gp41, two proteins involved in viral attachment and entry into host cells (fig. 11-2) (29).

The CD4 protein and its co-receptor, CXCR4, and possibly CD26 on helper T-cell surfaces, serve as high affinity receptors for the viral envelope gp120, mediating rapid, firm cellular attachments. T-cell trophic viruses requiring CXCR4 for entry are termed X4 viruses (4).

Some HIV strains (named R5 viruses to reflect their co-receptor requirement) bind to macrophages via the beta-chemokine receptor CCR5 (1,39,51). Genetic polymorphisms in the chemokine receptor genes that mediate HIV

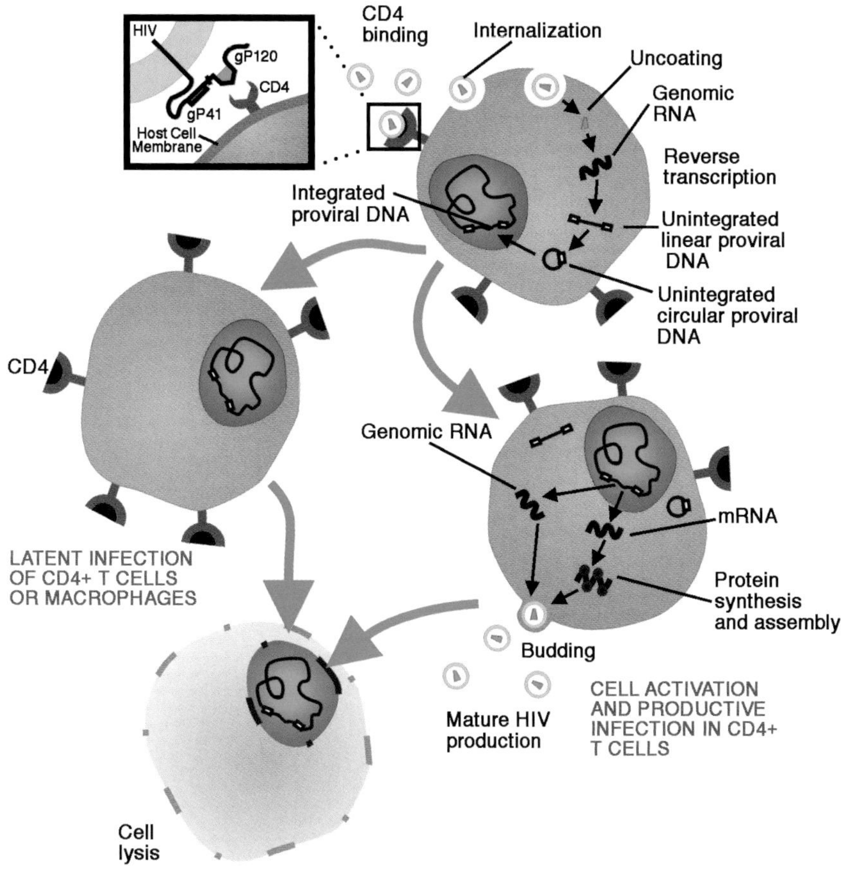

Figure 11-2

HIV LIFE CYCLE

Following the interaction of gP120 with the CD4 membrane receptor, gP41-mediated membrane fusion occurs, leading to viral entry into the cell. Reverse transcription of the viral RNA results in the production of double-stranded DNA from the virus. The viral integrase promotes insertion of the viral DNA duplex into the host genome. The first mRNA produced corresponds to the multiply spliced variants of viral DNA encoding the tat, rev, and nef regulatory proteins. Subsequently, viral structural proteins are produced, allowing the assembly of viral particles. Free HIV-1 virions are then released by viral budding from the host cell membranes, which may then reinitiate the retroviral life cycle.

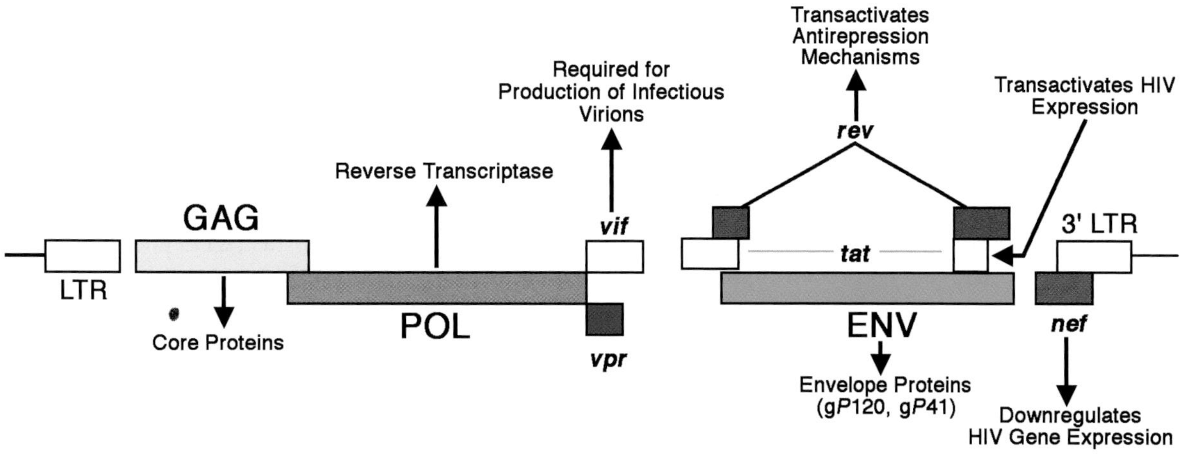

Figure 11-3

HIV GENOME

Each of the genes of HIV-1 are depicted, as are their primary functions. The 5' and 3' long terminal repeats (LTRs) contain regulatory sequences recognized by various host transcription factors. The positions of the tat and rev RNA response elements and the nef response element are also shown.

Table 11-2
HIV-ENCODED PROTEINS

Envelope	Envelope surface (SU) protein
Gag	Capsid (CA) structural protein; matrix (MA) protein—myristoylated: role in budding; nucleocapsid (NC) protein: helps in reverse transcription
gP4	Required for fusion and entry into host cell
gP120	Involved in chemokine receptor binding
Integrase (IN)	Viral cDNA integration
Nef	Removes CD4 surface expression or infected cells by accelerating endocytosis; enhances infectivity of cell free virus
Polymerase (Pol)	Reverse transcriptase (RT); RNase H—inside core
Protease (PR)	Post-translational processing of viral proteins
Rev	Involved in RNA splicing and RNA nuclear-cytoplasmic transport; regulation of viral mRNA expression
Tat	Promotes viral transcription
Tev	Tat/rev activities
Vif	Transports virions to cell nucleus; stabilizes virion DNA intermediates; increases virus infectivity and cell-cell transmission
Vpr	Allows transport of viral RNA into the nucleus of nondividing cells and upregulates viral gene expression; induces G2 arrest in dividing cells
Vpu	Membrane spanning protein that binds CD4 in the endoplasmic reticulum and targets it for proteolysis, downregulating its expression; enhances virion release from infected cells; helps in virion release
Vpx	Helps in infectivity

disease progression affect disease expression (37). Cells with absent or reduced *CCR5* expression or *CCR5* mutation have a reduced sensitivity to HIV infection (31,42), and these cells are resistant to HIV infection even in the face of a high risk of infection (31).

Pathophysiology. The most common mode of HIV-1 infection is sexual transmission through the anogenital mucosa. Monocytes, macrophages, dendritic cells, and CD4-positive T lymphocytes are the primary viral targets (29). The virus is initially acquired via one of the following: rectal mucosal tears, M cells overlying lymphoid follicles, direct infection of the rectal epithelium, or infection of lamina propria dendritic cells subjacent to the anorectal epithelium (48).

HIV-1 adhering to the luminal membranes of rectal M cells are endocytosed and delivered to intraepithelial lymphocytes, macrophages, and the mononuclear cells of the lymphoid follicles (2). The infected cells fuse with CD4-positive lymphocytes and spread into deeper tissues. Within 2 days of the initial infection, viruses can be detected in draining internal iliac lymph nodes. Shortly thereafter, systemic dissemination occurs. HIV can be cultured from the plasma 1 to 2 weeks after infection (38).

The gastrointestinal mucosa serves as an important reservoir for HIV, with lamina propria macrophages frequently harboring the virus (2, 30). The gastrointestinal epithelium and lamina propria are also a rich source of CD4-positive T cells. These cells are also abundant in the regional lymph nodes. The intestinal mucosa becomes profoundly and selectively depleted of CD4-positive cells within days of the infection, even before similar changes occur in peripheral lymphoid tissues. In contrast, CD8-positive T cells increase early in the infection and then display increased levels of activation antigens and abnormal major histocompatibility class (MHC)-restricted HIV-specific and -nonspecific cytotoxic abilities. A specific increase in apoptotic CD8-positive T cells eventually leads to their depletion (30). This change, sometimes referred to as the *CD8 lymphocytosis syndrome*, predominantly affects black males who have MHC human leukocyte antigen (HLA) DR5; it is associated with a favorable host response (24). A nearly complete absence of CD4-positive intraepithelial lymphocytes and decreased CD11-positive intraepithelial lymphocytes characterizes the intestinal mucosa of severely ill AIDS patients (22)

Host factors also play a major role in the pathogenesis of HIV-related disease. A complex network of endogenous cytokines provides a delicate balance between HIV induction and suppression. The β-chemokines RANTES, MIP-1α, and MIP-1β act as suppressors of macrophage-trophic HIV strains (19) and elevated β-chemokine expression levels probably help control HIV load and replication in individuals who do not progress to AIDS (1,49).

Clinical Features. Acute HIV-1 infection is a transient, symptomatic illness associated with high viral titers and a robust immunologic antiviral response (27). Signs and symptoms of acute HIV-1 infection occur within days to weeks of the initial viral exposure. In the several days or weeks after the infection is acquired, 30 to70 percent of patients experience an acute viral syndrome that includes the first gastrointestinal symptoms. The most common systemic signs and symptoms are fever, fatigue, a maculopapular rash, headache, lymphadenopathy, pharyngitis, myalgia, arthralgia, aseptic meningitis, retroorbital pain, weight loss, depression, gastrointestinal distress, night sweats, and oral or genital ulcers. The acute illness coincides with a small decline in the number of CD4-positive cells. Later, the CD4-positive cell count decreases further, the CD8-positive cell count increases, and the CD4 to CD8 ratio becomes inverted. The acute illness lasts for a few days to more than 10 weeks, but averages less than 14 days (46). Since the early signs and symptoms are nonspecific, acute HIV-1 infection is frequently confused with other viral illnesses. Initial laboratory studies may show lymphopenia and thrombocytopenia but atypical lymphocytes are infrequent (18). Standard serologic tests only become positive 3 to 4 weeks after the initial infection (10). Severe and prolonged symptoms correlate with rapid disease progression (3).

After the initial infection, there is rapid viremia resulting in widespread viral dissemination, seeding of lymphoid organs (14), and entrapment by follicular dendritic cells (25). Individuals with the highest viral loads have the highest rates of disease progression (33).

AIDS develops after a long latent period, averaging 7 to 10 years following the initial infection. During the latency period, the immune system remains relatively intact, preventing most secondary infections, but viral replication actively continues in lymphoid tissues (47). A CD4 count less than 500/mL heralds the development of clinical AIDS. A drop to less than 200/mL defines AIDS and indicates a high probability of developing AIDS-related infections, neoplasms, and death.

Diarrhea affects 30 to 50 percent of North American and European and 90 percent of African HIV-infected patients (17,26). AIDS patients who present with diarrhea have a greater degree of immunosuppression than those without diarrhea, predisposing the gut to the infections that contribute to morbidity and death. Diarrhea occurred in up to 90 percent of patients in the pre-HAART era. More recent data suggest that diarrhea is still a frequent complaint, but is more commonly attributable to drug-induced injury or non-HIV–related pathologic processes. Diarrhea in HIV-infected patients, therefore, results from the presence of: 1) enteric pathogenic infections; 2) complications of the drugs used to treat the HIV infection; 3) the presence of "AIDS enteropathy" or "AIDS gastropathy"; 4) AIDS-related motility disturbances; and 5) tumor development. Often it is impossible to attribute any AIDS-associated gastrointestinal sign or symptom to a specific underlying cause, since patients usually have numerous gastrointestinal pathologies (Table 11-3). The coccidian parasites *Cryptosporidium parvum, Isospora belli,* and *Cyclospora,* and the microsporidia account for at least 50 percent of cases of persistent diarrhea in the industrialized and developing world, with major contributions from *Mycobacterium avium* complex and other bacteria, as well as cytomegalovirus (CMV) infection (23).

The gastrointestinal manifestations of HIV change according to the stage of the infection. Early and intermediate gastrointestinal manifestations include diarrhea without detectable pathogens (*AIDS enteropathy*) and low-grade bacterial overgrowth. Well-established infections, particularly parasitic and viral infections, characterize late-stage disease. Severe recurrent systemic or gastrointestinal parasitic, viral, fungal,

Table 11-3

GASTROINTESTINAL LESIONS IN PATIENTS WITH AIDS

Infections	Parasites	HIV enteropathy
Bacteria	*Entamoeba histolytica*	HIV ganglioneuritis
Spirochetosis	*Giardia lamblia*	Motility problems
Salmonella typhimurium	*Cyclospora* species	Idiopathic esophageal ulcers
Shigella species	*Enterobius vermicularis*	Tumors
Mycobacterium tuberculosis	*Cryptosporidium*	Anal condylomas
Mycobacterium avium-intracellulare	*Toxoplasma*	Kaposi's sarcoma
Escherichia coli	*Taenia saginata*	Smooth muscle tumors
Campylobacter species	*Isospora belli*	Lymphomas
Aeromonas hydrophilia	Microsporidia group	Various carcinomas
Neisseria gonorrheae	Leishmaniasis	Traumatic lesions
Lymphogranuloma venereum	*Strongyloides*	Drug effects
Syphilis	*Blastocystis hominis*	Nutritional deficiencies
Chlamydial infections	Fungi	Lymphoid change
Viruses	*Candida*	Depletions
Epstein-Barr virus (EBV)	*Histoplasma*	Hyperproliferation
Cytomegalovirus (CMV)	*Blastocystis hominis*	
Herpes simplex virus (HSV)	*Pneumocystis carinii*	
Human immunodeficiency virus (HIV)	*Aspergillus fumigatus*	
Human papilloma virus (HPV)	*Cryptococcus neoformans*	
? Rotavirus		
? Adenovirus		

and protozoal infections, along with the development of neoplasms and other HIV-associated pathologies, often result in a fatal outcome.

Esophageal symptoms like dysphagia and odynophagia were reported to occur in up to one third of AIDS patients before HAART was available. Opportunistic infections, particularly *Candida* infections, are a frequent cause of esophageal symptoms. Infections with viral organisms like herpes simplex virus (HSV) and CMV are infrequent. The incidence of HIV-unrelated causes of esophageal symptoms such as gastroesophageal reflux disease and pill-induced esophagitis is rising (36). Severe odynophagia is more likely to be associated with idiopathic ulcerative esophagitis or possibly a neoplasm.

Abdominal pain in AIDS patients may or may not be related to HIV infection. Abdominal pain is more severe, however, when associated with the consequences of HIV infection (40). The pain is variable in character; it ranges from the dull, aching pain of infectious enteritis to the acute, severe pain of perforation and pancreatitis.

Depending upon the etiology, diarrhea can be transient or chronic. It may be associated with blood in stool, tenesmus, malabsorption, and other gastrointestinal complaints. Gastrointestinal bleeding is an uncommon clinical feature of AIDS, affecting less than 1 percent of the patient population (41). Studies have found that upper gastrointestinal bleeding is most commonly associated with non-HIV–related causes like peptic ulcer (5). The most common cause of lower gastrointestinal bleeding in HIV-positive patients is CMV colitis (6,16).

Anorectal signs and symptoms seen in HIV-infected patients include perirectal abscesses, anal fistulas, infectious proctitis, and idiopathic ulcerations. Human papilloma virus (HPV)-associated squamous lesions are also common in these patients.

Infants born with HIV infections tend to be small for their gestational age and display various abnormalities, including diarrhea, failure to thrive, and weight loss. Some manifestations become life threatening (7,47) due to the presence of opportunistic infections, increased gastrointestinal permeability (32), lymphoproliferative diseases, and cancer. In children with AIDS, infections are more severe, often relapse, and are harder to eradicate than in adults. Children, especially those in the developing world, are prone to develop diarrhea.

Endoscopic procedures on AIDS patients with gastrointestinal symptomatology should determine whether the gut is directly affected by the AIDS virus (e.g., AIDS enteropathy) or whether a complication related to the immunosuppressed state is present. The latter includes opportunistic infections or the development of neoplasias (e.g., Kaposi's sarcoma, lymphoproliferative disorders). The endoscopist relies on the pathologist to utilize specialized staining techniques to determine this. In addition, sufficient tissue should be obtained to allow histologic, immunologic, viral, and even mycologic analyses. Communication between the endoscopist and specialized laboratories is important as the clinician may not always be aware of how specimens are best transported to obtain optimal results.

Special Techniques. In the past, the best predictor of AIDS onset was the percentage or absolute number of circulating CD4-positive T cells. Currently, viral quantification in plasma is a better predictor of progression to AIDS and death. Measurements of viral burden also currently form the basis for decisions concerning initiation and modification of antiviral therapies. Still, the CD4 cell count monitors the immune system and is a useful guide for decisions concerning prophylaxis for opportunistic infections. In addition, the CD4 count helps predict the type of infection that may be responsible for a given patient's symptoms. A CD4 count greater than 200/mL suggests common bacteria as possible infectious agents. In patients with CD4 counts above 200/mL, nonopportunistic pathogens should be considered in the differential diagnosis. When CD4 counts are lower than 100/mL, fungi, mycobacteria, CMV, and unusual protozoa should be considered as possible causative agents.

Three techniques are currently available for viral load testing: reverse transcriptase polymerase chain reaction (RT-PCR), nucleic acid sequence–based amplification, and branched chain DNA (bDNA) analysis. Viral load testing should be obtained prior to initiation of antiretroviral therapy, 3 to 4 weeks after initiating or changing therapy, and periodically, perhaps on the same schedule as CD4 counts, i.e., every 3 to 4 months.

In general, patients with viral loads of more than 5,000 copies/mL of plasma should be started on treatment. The goal of therapy is to decrease the HIV RNA level to an undetectable amount or to have at least a decrease of 1.0 log in the viral load. Failure of therapy and the need to change therapy is signaled by an HIV RNA increase of 0.5 log or greater.

Treatment and Prognosis. In recent years, significant advances have been made in the prevention and treatment of opportunistic infections, including *Pneumocystis carinii* pneumonia, CMV retinitis, disseminated *Mycobacterium avium* complex infection, and mucosal candidiasis, due to use of intensive, highly active antiretroviral therapies (39). Mortality overall in AIDS patients has declined in excess of 80 percent since the introduction of HAART (34,35).

A recent panel of experts recommended immediate therapy be considered for persons with acute HIV infections (12,13). Early treatment restores the virus-specific cellular immune responses required to control early viremia (44) so that the extent of viral dissemination is limited, the damage to the immune system is restricted, antigen-presenting cells are protected, and the chance of disease progression is reduced. There are drawbacks to the institution of such therapy, however, and recent trends are leaning toward more conservative treatment with HAART. Recent recommendations are that HAART be instituted at a time when CD4 counts suggest an immediate risk of progression to AIDS, or in patients at risk of dying (12,43). Risks of early therapy include the adverse effects of these drugs on the quality of the patient's life as well as potential serious side effects that may result from drug toxicity. In addition, the duration of the beneficial effects of HAART is currently unknown (34). Previously treated patients are known to experience a poorer response to the reinstitution of HAART, perhaps as a result of acquisition of some degree of drug resistance (28,34).

Five classes of drugs have been approved for the treatment of HIV infection: 1) nucleoside reverse transcriptase inhibitors, 2) nucleotide reverse transcriptase inhibitors, 3) non-nucleoside reverse transcriptase inhibitors, 4) protease inhibitors, and 5) fusion inhibitors. In addition, various new anti-HIV drugs are under clinical or preclinical development (21). Updates for treatment guidelines are available from the World Wide Web site of the HIV/AIDS Treatment

Information Service (ATIS) at http://www.hivatis.org.

HIV Enteropathy

Definition. *HIV enteropathy*, in its broadest sense, refers to gastrointestinal damage resulting from an HIV infection. A more specific definition of HIV enteropathy is the presence of chronic (more than 1 month's duration) diarrhea, malabsorption, and wasting without evidence of an enteric infection after complete evaluation (55). Synonyms include *AIDS enteropathy* and *AIDS enterocolitis*.

Etiology. Multiple enteric pathogenic bacteria cause diarrhea in AIDS patients including *Campylobacter jejuni* or *C. fetus*, *Clostridium difficile*, *Enterobacter aerogenes*, *Salmonella*, *Shigella flexneri*, *Klebsiella*, and other Gram-negative bacilli. The most common etiologic agent detected in the large bowel of AIDS patients is CMV followed by *Mycobacterium avium*. Patients may also have fungal or parasitic infections (Table 11-3). The degree of inflammation seen in AIDS enteropathy correlates with mucosal levels of p24 antigen and clinical symptoms, supporting an etiologic role for HIV.

Pathophysiology. Proposed explanations for HIV-associated enteropathy include any or all of the following: 1) the presence of an occult enteric infection (56); 2) the direct effect of the virus on the gastrointestinal epithelium; 3) the indirect effects of a localized immunologic dysfunction; 4) an immune-mediated enterocolitis; 5) a drug-induced change; or 6) an effect of some nutritional deficiency. Arguments in favor of a direct HIV-related viral cytopathic effect include the identification of the virus in epithelial cells by in situ hybridization or Southern blot analysis and the absence of other pathogens.

Clinical Features. Diarrhea often develops before full-blown AIDS develops, sometimes only occurring during the clinically latent period. Patients may develop steatorrhea and low lactase activity secondary to epithelial damage. Vitamin B12 deficiency and abnormalities of xylose absorption also occur. Overt bleeding, in the absence of coexisting anal disease, is unusual.

Gross Findings. The colonoscopic mucosal pattern shows diffuse abnormalities consisting of contact bleeding, edema, superficial ulcerations, exudates, and loss of the normal vascular pattern. The features are nonspecific and the diagnosis is by exclusion of other pathologies, especially opportunistic infections.

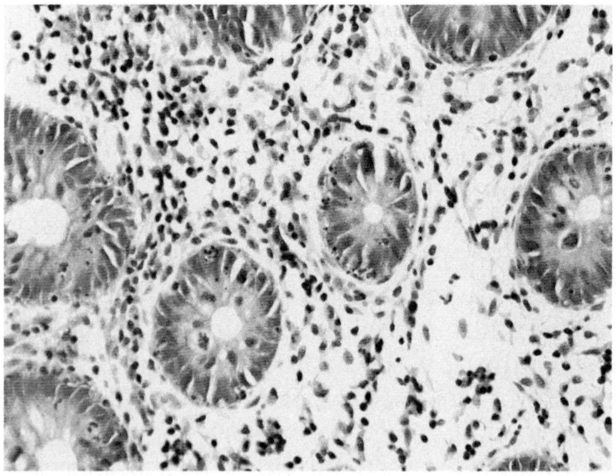

Figure 11-4

HIV ENTEROPATHY

Numerous apoptotic bodies lie in the bases of the crypts. The histologic changes are similar to those seen in graft versus host disease (see figs. 11-23, 11-24).

Microscopic Findings. The intestinal inflammation is often nonspecific in AIDS-associated enteropathy (fig. 11-4). It consists of degranulating eosinophils, activated lymphocytes, and plasma cells with increased numbers of intraepithelial and lamina propria T lymphocytes (52). Early in the disease, the lymphocyte density is normal but lymphoid depletion develops in patients with full-blown AIDS. In this latter phase, macrophage and eosinophilic infiltrates are prominent and apoptosis is common. In end-stage disease, opportunistic infections are present together with eosinophilia, neutrophilia, apoptosis, and tissue injury.

Either the mucosal T-cell alterations in AIDS or the direct viral infection of the enterocytes may alter the mucosal architecture and produce an enteropathy or colopathy. This is characterized by a decreased villus to crypt ratio secondary to villous atrophy and crypt hyperplasia (56). The epithelial mitotic index varies with respect to disease duration and severity; it increases early and then decreases.

Histologically, the intestinal mucosa exhibits nonspecific apoptosis, edema, enlarged nuclei, increased numbers of mononuclear cells in the lamina propria, and intraepithelial

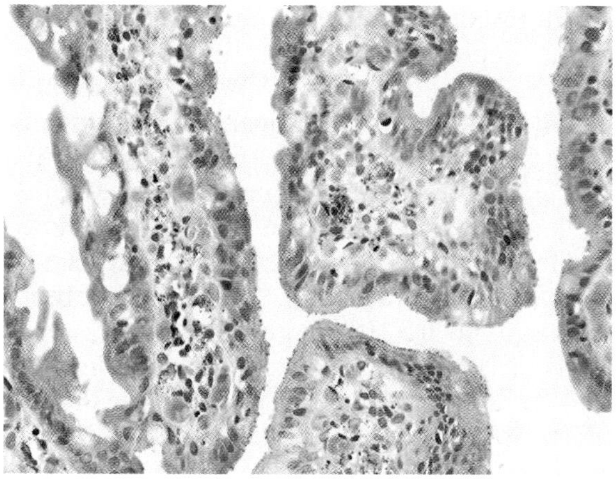

Figure 11-5

DUODENAL IRON PIGMENT DEPOSITION IN A PATIENT WITH ACQUIRED IMMUNODEFICIENCY SYNDROME (AIDS)

Blue-stained iron pigment granules are in the lamina propria of the villus tips. The patient also has cryptosporidiosis, seen here as blue dots on the villus surface (iron-stained section).

lymphocytosis. Aphthous ulcers may be present. The apoptotic changes seen in AIDS resemble the apoptosis in grade I graft versus host disease. As the disease evolves, cell loss results in a population of functionally immature enterocytes incapable of absorbing nutrients due to the immaturity of their brush border enzymes. The changes resemble those seen in celiac disease (see chapter 12).

Another change that affects the small intestinal mucosa of AIDS patients more often than non-AIDS patients is pseudomelanosis. The reason for this is unclear. It appears as areas of spotty brownish or blackish pigmentation in the duodenal mucosa that can be seen at the time of endoscopy; it is maximal in the second portion of the duodenum. Most patients have received oral iron supplements. Histologically, iron pigment is seen in the villus tips (fig. 11-5).

Colonic biopsies show a more or less normal architecture with nonspecific inflammatory changes and a mixed cell infiltrate, including intraepithelial lymphocytosis, focal crypt epithelial cell apoptosis, endothelial tubuloreticular bodies, lymphocytes, and monocytes (53). Other changes include crypt atrophy coexisting with regenerative crypts. This presumably represents the end stage of the epithelial apoptosis that causes the crypts to appear to vanish from the mucosa. The crypts superficially resemble dilated lymphatics. Closer examination discloses that the cystic spaces in the lamina propria are lined by variably flattened epithelium; often, the lumens contain apoptotic cells.

Vascular calcification with intimal fibrosis, fragmentation of the internal elastic lamina, and fibrosis of the media with luminal narrowing, changes designated as *AIDS arteriopathy*, develop in the small to medium-sized systemic arteries, including those in the gastrointestinal tract and within the mesocolon. This may lead to secondary ischemic changes and mucosal ulceration.

Small collections of foamy histiocytes may superficially suggest the presence of *Mycobacterium avium* complex or Whipple's disease but these are negative for microorganisms. These lesions are relatively common in the colon and probably represent a nonspecific response to mucosal damage from many etiologies. In our experience, it is always wise to stain biopsies containing these collections for the presence of mycobacteria and fungi, especially if the collections are large and prominent.

Another change that may affect the intestines is a nonspecific motility disorder. This may be the result of the drug therapy causing muscle fiber atrophy or due to the presence of CMV within enteric ganglia.

Special Techniques. In tissue sections, HIV is detected by in situ hybridization in both the crypt cells and in the stromal cells of the lamina propria (54).

Differential Diagnosis. The changes of AIDS enteropathy may resemble microscopic colitis, celiac disease, or graft versus host disease. The clinical setting, results of HIV testing, and tissue transglutaminase status serve to distinguish among these possibilities.

Treatment. In the absence of the identification of a specific treatable pathogen or disease process by stool studies or endoscopic examination with biopsy of the upper and lower digestive tracts, consideration of a trial of antimicrobial therapy (e.g., ciprofloxacin, metronidazole) may be reasonable in the hope of treating an elusive infection or the presence of bacterial overgrowth. Nutritional, fluid, and electrolyte support is important, and the clinician may have to employ parenteral means in order to replace ongoing losses. Luminal agents (fiber preparations, cholestyramine) may add bulk to the stool. Antimotility agents (loperamide, diphenoxylate with atropine, codeine, paregoric, morphine, tincture of opium) may be necessary for support. Octreotide may be effective in some patients, but its use is controversial and should not be employed indefinitely if no response is achieved in a few weeks.

HIV-ASSOCIATED DISEASES IN SPECIFIC GASTROINTESTINAL LOCATIONS

Esophageal Disease

Demography. The majority of AIDS patients with esophageal erosions or ulcers have no known etiologic agent or have viral or fungal infection. Esophageal candidiasis occurs so commonly that it is an AIDS-defining lesion.

Etiology. AIDS patients often present with esophageal disease due to 1) infection (*Candida*, CMV, HSV, Epstein-Barr virus [EBV], *Mycobacterium avium*, *Cryptosporidium*, *Pneumocystis*, *Leishmania*); 2) the development of a tumor (papilloma, Kaposi's sarcoma, lymphomas); 3) idiopathic ulcers; 4) ordinary gastroesophageal reflux disease; 5) pill-induced esophagitis; and 6) strictures secondary to healed inflammatory disease.

Clinical Features. The clinical symptoms of esophageal disease include dysphagia and severe odynophagia. Ulcers develop in the first month or so following the HIV infection, complicating a mononucleosis-like febrile illness. Progressive weight loss results from the presence of multiple hypopharyngeal and esophageal ulcers. The ulcers often become quite large, sometimes developing into "giant esophageal ulcers." These can progress to a life-threatening size, eroding vessels, limiting oral nutrition, and leading to secondary pulmonary problems, including fistula formation. Healing predisposes to stricture development, especially if gastroesophageal reflux is also present. The majority of esophageal problems encountered are readily treatable on an ambulatory basis.

Gross Findings. Gross findings include areas of whitish exudates, plaques, erosions, and ulcers ranging in size from aphthous ulcers to giant esophageal ulcers. Most patients with *Candida* have plaques. Strictures may be present.

Microscopic Findings. The histologic features of the esophagus depend on the etiology of the lesions. In the absence of endoscopic lesions, biopsies rarely yield significant histologic findings. The most common infections are CMV and HSV when ulcers are present and *Candida* if plaques are present. The viruses are identified by the presence of characteristic inclusions. Prospective evaluation of the number of biopsies required for the diagnosis of viral esophagitis in HIV patients discloses that at least 10 may be required. Three biopsies are usually sufficient to diagnose CMV infection (59). Esophageal *M. avium* complex usually represents an extension of mediastinal nodal infection, so that the organisms may only be present deep in the esophageal wall and not in the mucosa. This implies that one needs to examine deep biopsies if the clinical question is "rule out mycobacteria." Esophageal biopsy specimens should first be examined with hematoxylin and eosin (H&E). Silver and acid-fast stains should be performed if a fungal or mycobacterial infection is suspected but not seen with H&E stains.

In the absence of a specific infection, the esophagus exhibits variable inflammatory reactions, erosions, and ulcers. Alternatively, there may only be focal edema coexisting with rare apoptotic cells. Large numbers of apoptotic bodies can be seen in the cells immediately adjacent to idiopathic esophageal ulcers, contrasting with the lack of apoptotic bodies in esophageal ulcers with known etiologies. This feature is thought to be a manifestation of the HIV infection. The submucosa may become densely infiltrated with neutrophils, and a few mononuclear cells extend to the level of the muscularis propria (60). Many patients have ordinary gastroesophageal reflux disease and all of its complications (see chapter 3).

Special Studies. Infections are evaluated by culture, special stains, immunohistochemical studies, in situ hybridization, and polymerase chain reaction (PCR). The decision to use these modalities depends on the clinical implications of the diagnosis. For example, every effort must be made to exclude an opportunistic infection when a diagnosis of an idiopathic esophageal ulcer is being entertained. If three levels of H&E-stained sections fail to document the infection, special stains should be used to rule out the presence of the organism if the clinicians plan to aggressively treat the infection. In this situation, the pathology request form typically states "rule out. . ." We rarely use any in situ or PCR reactions to diagnose viral infections.

Treatment. Idiopathic esophageal and aphthous ulcers respond well to corticosteroids, with symptomatic response generally occurring within several days. Thalidomide (which reduces tumor necrosis factor) is also useful in this situation. Resolution of severe ulcerative disease may result in stricture formation and the development of dysphagia. Endoscopic dilatation is the strategy of choice in this case. Patients with tracheoesophageal fistulas often experience dramatic relief from their intractable cough following placement of an esophageal stent. Gastroesophageal reflux is treated along conventional lines by means of acid suppressive therapy. One needs to be cognizant of the potential for severe drug interactions if prokinetic agents are used.

Gastric Disease

Etiology. In AIDS patients, infectious gastritis, other than that related to *Helicobacter pylori*, usually results from bacterial, viral, and protozoal infections; of these, CMV is the most common. *H. pylori* infections may be particularly virulent in AIDS patients. The AIDS-associated viruses and the inflammation associated with it causes mucosal damage.

Some patients develop *AIDS gastropathy*, a disorder characterized by a reduction in parietal cell mass, and gastric acid and pepsinogen secretion, and an increase in mucus secretion (60). The disease is mediated by the presence of antiparietal cell antibodies. Hypochlorhydria results in high bacterial counts in the stomach and predisposes the patient to intestinal bacterial infections. Kaposi's sarcoma and lymphoma represent the most prevalent gastric malignancies seen in AIDS patients. AIDS patients also develop suppurative gastritis.

Clinical Features. Abdominal pain is common and usually secondary to gastritis, ulcer, or gastric outlet obstruction. Other signs and symptoms include dyspepsia, bloating, and rarely, upper gastrointestinal bleeding.

Gross Findings. Gross findings include red inflamed mucosa due to gastritis, ulcer, or mass lesion secondary to lymphoma or Kaposi's sarcoma. Cryptosporidial (58) and syphilitic infections of the antral mucosa cause isolated antral narrowing.

Microscopic Findings. CMV viral inclusions are frequently seen in the gastric epithelium. *H. pylori* gastritis is more severe in AIDS patients. Phlegmonous gastritis shows marked acute inflammation, vascular thrombosis, necrosis, and hemorrhage. The histologic features of AIDS gastropathy are similar to those of chronic atrophic gastritis described in chapter 4.

Kaposi's sarcoma is predominantly submucosal and can be missed on endoscopic biopsy. Highly vascularized nodules composed of elongated spindle cells with narrow thin blood vessels are characteristic. Pink acellular globules are admixed with the spindle cells. Gastric B-cell lymphoma is the second most common neoplasm seen in AIDS patients. Low-grade lymphoma of mucosa-associated lymphoid tissue (MALT) type, follicular center cell lymphoma, and diffuse large B-cell lymphoma have been described.

Treatment. Treatment is targeted against the offending agent.

Anorectal Disease

Demography. Anorectal disease is very common in AIDS patients. Traumatic injury, infection, condylomas, and anal squamous cell neoplasia are the most common lesions.

Etiology. The anorectal lesions found in active homosexuals result from opportunistic infections (HSV, HPV, syphilis, *Chlamydia*, CMV, scabies, molluscum contagiosum), tumors (lymphoma, squamous cell carcinoma, Kaposi's sarcoma), and trauma. Ulcerative disease of the anorectum may be due to trauma, *Chlamydia*, HSV, syphilis, benign fissures, idiopathic AIDS-related ulceration, and malignancies. Trauma from the use of rectal instruments and the insertion of foreign bodies can cause significant mucosal inflammation and sphincter damage, predisposing to fecal incontinence.

Clinical Features. Pain may be due to HSV proctitis, which often involves the sacral root. Constant discomfort may be due to an abscess or neoplasm. Pain on defecation is usually due to a fissure or ulceration. Lacerations, abrasions, and perforations leading to exsanguinating hemorrhage occur, especially if foreign bodies are inserted into the rectum when the patient is under the influence of illicit psychoactive drugs or excessive alcohol consumption.

Herpetic ulceration is probably the most common anal AIDS infection, whereas *Neisseria gonorrhoeae* probably represents the most common infective cause of acute and chronic proctitis in this population. Masses may be due to tumor, condylomata, or even mucosal prolapse. *Chlamydia trachomatis*/lymphogranuloma venereum may mimic Crohn's disease and is a cause of chronic stricturing fistulas and painful proctitis. AIDS-related idiopathic anal ulceration occurs more proximally than benign fissures.

Rectal lymphoma may mimic an anal fissure or present as a mass lesion. Kaposi's sarcoma presents as submucosal raised purple lesions. The patient often has difficulty tolerating the anorectal examination because of the pain (57), and topical and even general anesthesia may be necessary to completely examine this area.

Gross Findings. Findings include diffuse hemorrhage, anal fissures, ulcers, fistula-in-ano, perianal abscesses, and condyloma acuminata. Lymphogranuloma venereum produces strictures and proctitis and may be difficult to distinguish from idiopathic inflammatory bowel disease (for further discussion, see chapter 10).

Microscopic Findings. The usual anorectal abnormality is acute inflammation, a feature seen more often in patients with pathogens than in those without pathogens. Chronic inflammation suggests the presence of an infection. When the mucosa is examined, an extremely florid proctitis is present. The inflammation may extend high into the rectum. Deep perirectal ulcers or abscesses develop, and they may contain large numbers of bacteria. Prominent lymphoid aggregates are often present. Gram stains demonstrate numerous cocci. Syphilitic chancres mimic fissures, fistulas, or malignant tumors. There is increased apoptosis. Parasitic infections are common.

Treatment. Anal fissures may be treated with high fiber diet and topical antiinflammatory agents, including nitrates. Sphincterotomy should be avoided as it may precipitate incontinence. Perianal suppuration must be drained and cultured to include acid-fast organisms. Anorectal HSV and CMV are treated with standard therapies as for disease elsewhere. Treatment of syphilitic proctitis consists of intramuscular benzathine penicillin while rectal gonorrhea, with or without proctitis, usually responds to a single dose of ceftriaxone intramuscularly followed by a 10-day course of doxycycline. It is recommended that these patients be reevaluated after 3 months as recurrence of infection is common.

BACTERIAL INFECTIONS IN IMMUNOCOMPROMISED PATIENTS

Mycobacterium Avium Complex

Demography. *Mycobacterium avium* and *Mycobacterium intracellulare* (collectively referred to as *Mycobacterium avium* complex) are ubiquitous organisms, isolated worldwide from soil, dust, fresh water, ocean water, animal feed, poultry, and animals commonly used as meat (67,77). In non-AIDS patients, *Mycobacterium avium* complex (MAC) is characteristically restricted to the lung. Disseminated infection is almost exclusively seen in AIDS patients, although the incidence of colonization and infection has declined in the era of HAART (65). The frequency of disseminated MAC infection among AIDS patients is not influenced by patient sex or the route of infection (67). Hispanics are less likely to acquire the infection than non-Hispanic whites or blacks. Persons acquire the infection through environmental exposure to organisms in aerosols, water, food, and soil (68,74–76). The frequency of the infection declines with age. The major risk factor for infection is the level of immune dysfunction, as reflected by the CD4-positive cell count. Between 76 and 90 percent of MAC infections develop late in the course of AIDS when other AIDS-defining diagnoses have already developed and CD4 counts measure less than 60/mm^3 (67).

Pathophysiology. Disseminated MAC usually results from primary infection. Asymptomatic colonization of the respiratory or gastrointestinal tract often precedes disseminated disease. The organisms bind to the apical surface of enterocytes, and are internalized via a mechanism that involves rearrangement of the cytoskeleton of the affected cell (63). Growth of the organism within epithelial cells results in expression of an invasive phenotype (73). Significant differences in virulence exist among different strains (72).

Clinical Features. In AIDS patients, the gastrointestinal tract is involved twice as frequently as the lungs (78). At the time of autopsy, up to two thirds of AIDS patients with MAC infection have gastrointestinal involvement (69). All gastrointestinal segments become infected but the most dramatic changes occur in the small bowel, particularly the duodenum. Occasionally, MAC causes discrete esophageal ulcers, but this is uncommon. Rarely, localized infections develop (66).

Patients typically present with nausea, chronic diarrhea, abdominal pain, malabsorption, fever, sweats, chills, weight loss, lymphadenopathy, hepatosplenomegaly, and pancytopenia. Peripancreatic and porta hepatis lymph node involvement may obstruct the bile duct, causing jaundice. Lymphoid hyperplasia in Peyer patches and lymph nodes predisposes to intestinal intussusception.

Rising cholestatic liver enzymes in the absence of dilated bile ducts on imaging suggests hepatic infection, drug effect, or sclerosing cholangitis. Patients with hepatic MAC involvement often have easily palpable hepatomegaly. Multiorgan involvement invariably occurs and the diagnosis may be made relatively noninvasively from culture of blood, stool, urine, or sputum, or bone marrow examination. Occasionally, liver biopsy may be necessary.

Gross Findings. Endoscopically, MAC may appear as yellow-white nodules. The duodenum and small bowel are often involved. The colonic mucosa may be edematous and erythematous. Involvement may be patchy and asymptomatic. Ulceration may occur, and may be complicated by fistulization, hemorrhage, and perforation. Occasionally, the mucosa appears endoscopically normal and the disorder is diagnosed by random biopsies taken during the workup of unremitting diarrhea. Regional lymph nodes typically enlarge, grossly resembling lymphoma until the nodes are cut and examined in cross section. These enlarged nodes are often visible on computerized tomography (CT) scans.

Microscopic Findings. Mycobacteria are beaded rods measuring 4 to 6 µm in length and less than 1 µm in diameter. These acid-fast bacilli are not distinguishable by their shape or size from other mycobacteria, including *Mycobacterium tuberculosis*. However, their intracellular location and the presence of large numbers of intracellular organisms sometimes arranged in stacks are distinctive (fig. 11-6). In patients with extensive disease the infiltrates are easily recognized in H&E-stained sections using low-power microscopy (fig. 11-7). A diffuse histiocytic infiltrate fills the lamina propria, pushing apart the crypts and causing mucosal atrophy with villous blunting and distortion. The severity of the infection determines both the number of intracellular organisms and the number of infected histiocytic cells. Focal disease is harder to detect and may require the use of special stains. Duodenal biopsies or brushings often contain the organism.

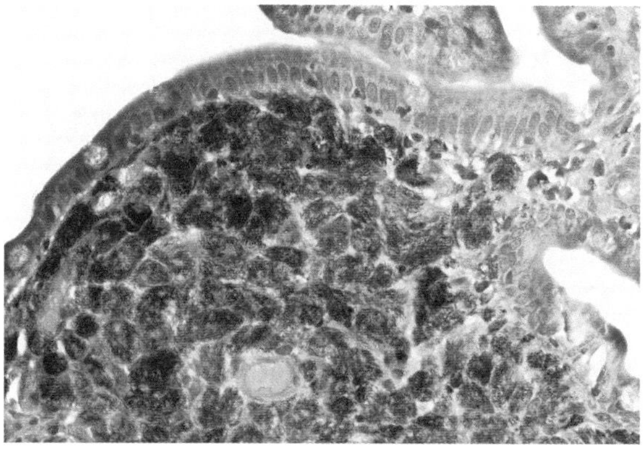

Figure 11-6

ACID-FAST STAIN IN A PATIENT WITH DISSEMINATED *MYCOBACTERIUM AVIUM* COMPLEX (MAC) INFECTION

Thousands of organisms pack the cytoplasm of the histiocytes within the lamina propria.

Lymphocytes, plasma cells, and neutrophils are sparse, if present at all. Occasionally, there are poorly circumscribed, noncaseating, epithelioid granulomas containing lymphocytes and rare multinucleated giant cells. These granulomas are less well formed than the granulomas typical of *M. tuberculosis* infection and they lack necrosis. Villous blunting accompanies the infiltrate in the lamina propria, leading to malabsorption. Gastric and large intestinal infiltrates tend to be less prominent than those in the small intestine. Rarely, mycobacteria-containing macrophages are seen in all of the bowel layers. Small bowel and regional lymph nodes are commonly massively infiltrated in

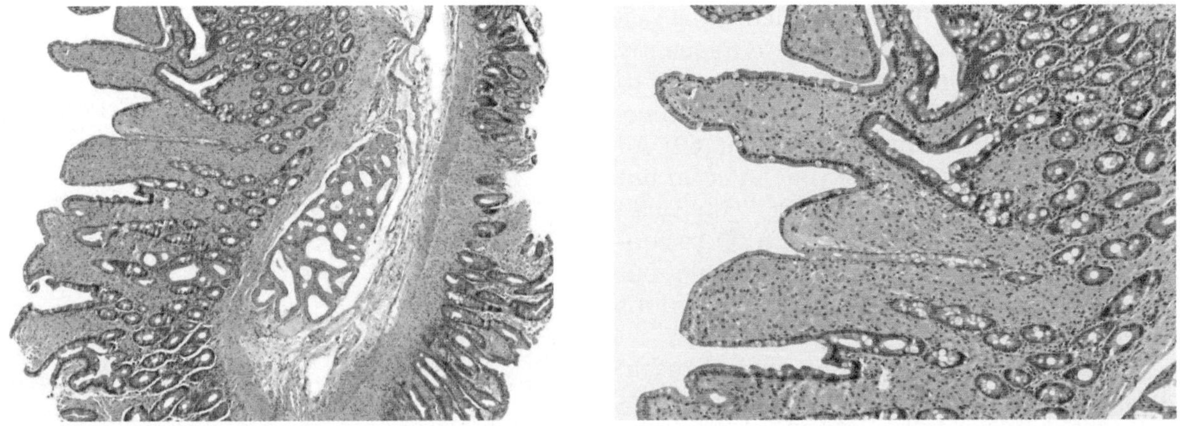

Figure 11-7

MAC INFECTION

Left: Low-power view of a duodenal biopsy specimen from a patient with disseminated MAC infection. The lamina propria contains a dense infiltrate of eosinophilic histiocytes. This infiltrate distorts the normal architecture of the duodenum, separating the crypts and blunting the villi.

Right: Higher-power view of the dense histiocyte collection. No granulomas are formed.

disseminated disease but single, scattered, infected histiocytes may also be seen.

Special Techniques. The diagnosis of gastrointestinal MAC infection is best made by endoscopic biopsy. Fecal smear is less sensitive than culture. Mycobacterial cultures require 1 to 2 weeks for organism growth, contrasting with light microscopic interpretation of biopsy sections, which requires 1 to 2 days. The organism can also be identified by the use of DNA probes applied to primary cultures. The most commonly used test is the Gen-Probe culture confirmation test, which uses hybridization probes complementary to ribosomal mycobacterial RNA (62). PCR analysis also identifies the organism. Culture, which takes from a few weeks to several months, is helpful in establishing drug sensitivity.

Differential Diagnosis. MAC histologically resembles both Whipple's disease and severe *Histoplasma* infection because all three infections cause periodic acid–Schiff (PAS)-positive macrophages to accumulate in the lamina propria. The PAS-positive globules seen in Whipple's disease are larger than the positively staining MAC bacteria. Additionally, MAC are acid-fast while the Whipple's bacilli are not. *Histoplasma* are larger organisms and are easily identified using the Grocott methenamine silver stain. The organism responsible for classic tuberculosis histologically resembles *M. avium*. It is important to distinguish between the two species since the treatment for *M. tuberculosis* differs from that for *M. avium*. Features that favor a diagnosis of MAC include diffuse histiocytic aggregates containing large numbers of bacteria in the lamina propria, without granulomas or caseation.

Treatment and Prognosis. Prophylactic treatment is recommended for the prevention of disseminated MAC in AIDS patients with CD4 counts under 200/mm^3 (71). Prophylactic therapy with rifabutin, clarithromycin, and azithromycin is effective and synergistic effects can be expected when they are administered together unless the organisms have become resistant to the drugs (70). Two quadruple drug regimens provide benefits to patients with disseminated disease. The first regimen includes amikacin plus ciprofloxacin, ethambutol, and rifampin (64); the second regimen includes isoniazid, ethambutol, ansamycin, and clofazimine (61). Mycobacterial therapy with clarithromycin can significantly reduce the bacteremia and improve the quality of life and the rate of survival in patients with disseminated MAC. More than 12 weeks' therapy is required to decrease bacterial load and to improve symptoms. Lifelong suppressive therapy is often required to prevent relapse.

Mycobacterium Tuberculosis Infections

Demography. *Tuberculosis* occurred so commonly in HIV-infected patients that it became an AIDS-defining illness in 1987 (80). Although extrapulmonary tuberculosis is still common in AIDS patients, luminal gastrointestinal tract involvement remains infrequent (82). Tuberculosis may be diagnosed before or after the AIDS diagnosis. Patients with both diagnoses tend to be Haitian, black (other than Haitian), or Hispanic. AIDS patients with tuberculosis are younger (median age at diagnosis of tuberculosis, 34 years compared with 44 years) and are more likely to be male than patients without AIDS.

Pathophysiology. In immunocompetent individuals, macrophages ingest the bacterium, and process and present mycobacterial antigens to host T cells. Lymphokines secreted by CD4 cells, the cell population that becomes selectively depleted in AIDS patients, enhance macrophage capacity to ingest and kill the bacteria. In AIDS patients, however, the CD4 depletion makes them very susceptible to tuberculosis. Patients acquire the infection through reactivation of latent tuberculosis or by developing a primary infection. Reactivation of latent tuberculosis occurs secondary to defective T cell and/or macrophage function (79).

Clinical Features. Newly acquired tuberculous infections in HIV-infected patients progress rapidly to disseminated active disease (81). AIDS patients are more likely to have extrapulmonary tuberculosis and a nonreactive tuberculin skin test than are non-AIDS patients (80). Gastrointestinal infections result from swallowing the organisms. Abdominal mycobacterial infections affect the intestine, peritoneum, liver, psoas muscles, and stomach. The pattern of bowel involvement parallels the distribution of lymphoid tissue so that the ileocecal and rectal areas are most commonly infected. The infection is generally segmental, contrasting with the more diffuse involvement seen with MAC infections. Typical symptoms include weight loss, fatigue, abdominal pain, and fever. Diarrhea and hematochezia occur less commonly. Laboratory findings include anemia and abnormal liver function tests. Acid-fast stains of stool smears may be positive. The pathologic features resemble those seen in patients without AIDS (see chapter 10).

Spirochetosis

Definition. *Intestinal spirochetosis* is an overgrowth of spirochetes or an infestation of the intestinal epithelium by spirochetes. The diagnosis requires a biopsy.

Demography. Spirochetosis is common in homosexual men, including those without evidence of immunodeficiency. The infection was present in 53.7 percent of rectal biopsy specimens from homosexual men attending a sexually transmitted disease clinic (88). Spirochetosis also affects a small percentage of healthy heterosexual individuals.

Etiology. A heterogeneous group of phenotypically and genotypically distinct, nontreponemal, weakly beta-hemolytic, intestinal spirochetes cause diarrheal disease in humans. Patients with symptomatic disease usually have *Serpulini jonessii* infection, whereas asymptomatic persons are more likely to have *Brachyspira alborgia* infection (87). *Serpulini pilosicoli* may also be etiologically responsible for the infection (83,88).

Clinical Features. Spirochetes colonizing the intestines may be true pathogens or they may be enteric commensals that become opportunistic pathogens when the local environment is altered by changes such as chronic stasis. The bacteria can cause various gastrointestinal disturbances, including chronic diarrhea, rectal bleeding, constipation, purulent discharge, and abdominal and perianal pain (84). Some have suggested that the clinical symptoms result from an immune reaction elicited by the penetration of the spirochetes into the mucosa rather than from the bacteria themselves (84).

Gross Findings. Spirochetosis does not usually produce any gross or endoscopic lesion. The diagnosis is made by careful examination of biopsy specimens.

Microscopic Findings. The colonic epithelium and lamina propria usually appear normal, but the surface epithelium has a dense, blue luminal fringe measuring 2 to 3 µm in thickness (fig. 11-8) due to the presence of hundreds of adherent spirochetes. The organisms stain strongly with PAS and Warthin-Starry stains and weakly with Alcian blue (fig. 11-9). They also stain with Giemsa, Fontana-Masson, and Dieterle silver stains. The rare patients with endoscopic evidence of colitis may have ulcers,

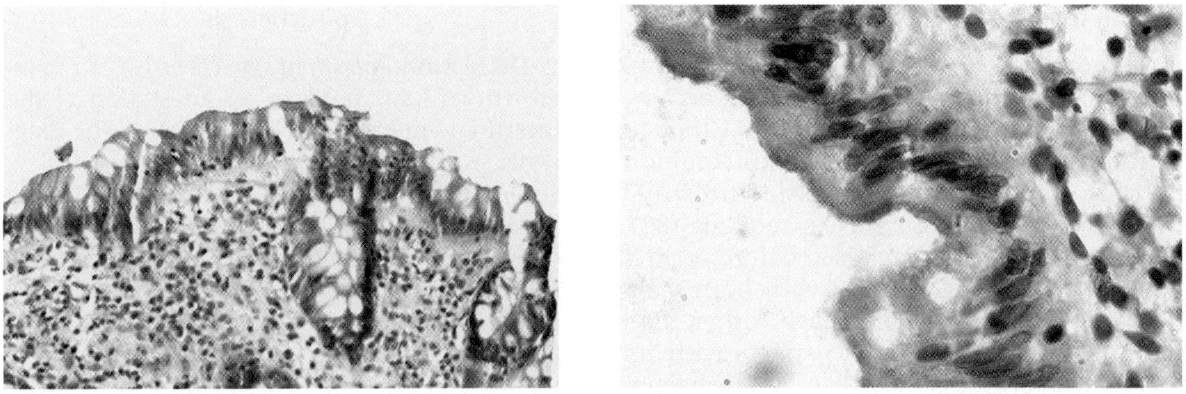

Figure 11-8

INTESTINAL SPIROCHETOSIS

Left: Low-power photomicrograph shows relatively well-preserved colonic mucosal architecture. There is no significant increase in inflammation within the lamina propria. A faint bluish fringe covers the luminal surface of the epithelial cells.

Right: High-power view of numerous adherent organisms aligned on the mucosal surface.

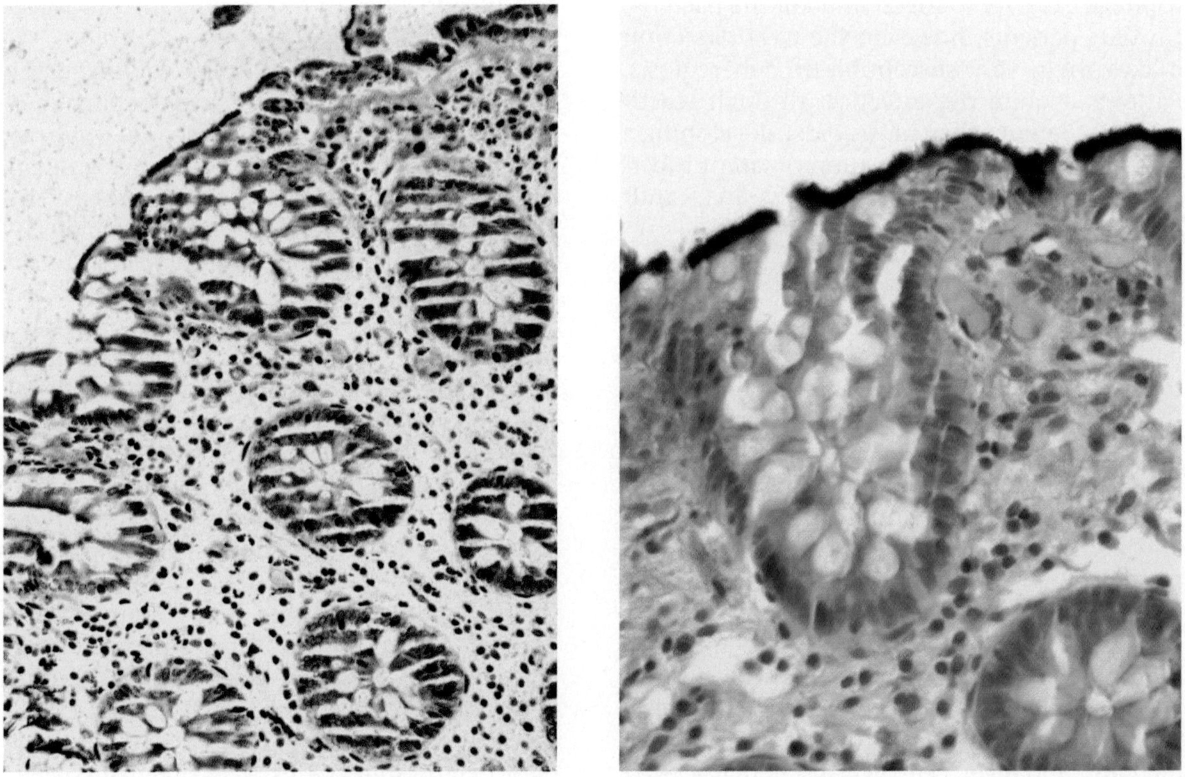

Figure 11-9

SPIROCHETOSIS

Left: The Warthin-Starry stain highlights the organisms attached to the surface of the epithelial cells.

Right: An immunohistochemical stain for spirochetes (*Treponema pallidum*) also confirms the presence of the organisms.

extensive superficial cell necrosis, and acute inflammation of the mucosa and lamina propria. Bacteria can extend down into the crypts, causing a conspicuous inflammatory response consisting of macrophages in the underlying lamina propria (85,86).

Special Studies. Ultrastructural examination discloses the presence of numerous thin, spiral-shaped microorganisms attached to the epithelial surface, situated between and parallel to the microvilli or parallel to the epithelial surface. Intestinal spirochetes are differentiated by the number and arrangement of periplasmic flagella, and the number of more axial filaments linearly inserted somewhat subterminally at each end. *B. alborgia* have four flagella (85); *S. pilosicoli* have 8 to 12 periplasmic flagella per cell.

Treatment and Prognosis. In some patients, treatment results in an improvement in symptoms; in others, therapy fails to induce any changes. The organism can be eradicated with metronidazole, but symptoms often persist, raising questions as to the relevance of the organism with respect to symptom generation.

VIRAL INFECTIONS IN IMMUNOCOMPROMISED PATIENTS

Cytomegalovirus Infections

Demography. *Enteric CMV infections* are a well-recognized problem in immunodeficient patients and CMV is the most common viral pathogen identified in autopsied AIDS patients. The presence of colonic or distal ileal CMV infection usually signifies the presence of disseminated disease. The frequency of CMV colitis among AIDS patients is about 13 percent (97); however, recent data suggest that the incidence of CMV reactivation in the AIDS population is decreasing in the era of HAART (98,100). CMV infection is also common in transplant patients and in those with primary immunodeficiencies. CMV may additionally infect patients with inflammatory bowel disease who are on immunosuppressive or chronic steroid therapy. Most cases of CMV infection in immunocompromised patients probably represent reactivation of latent infection. Approximately 1 to 2 percent of newborns, 10 to 40 percent of children, and 50 to 90 percent of adults in the general population are seropositive for CMV (89,92).

Pathophysiology. Immunocompromised individuals with decreased CD4 lymphocyte counts (below 100/mL) tend to develop CMV viremia, endothelial infections, endotheliolitis, submucosal ischemia, and secondary ulceration (94,95). CMV-associated vasculitis in the gastrointestinal tract is especially well documented in the AIDS population, where it preferentially involves the colon in up to 67 percent of CMV-infected patients. The affected vessels, including arteries and veins, undergo segmental necrosis, perivascular hemorrhage, and thrombosis, predisposing to secondary ischemia. CMV also predisposes to bacterial or fungal infection by compromising mucosal barrier integrity.

Clinical Features. Adults typically acquire CMV infection prior to alterations in their immune status (91). In contrast, children acquire primary CMV infection either at the same time or after they become immunocompromised (96). CMV-infected HIV-positive individuals exhibit two major types of problems: those related to the CMV infection and those related to the HIV infection. Some postulate that CMV acts as a cofactor in the pathogenesis of AIDS. Indeed, HIV-infected infants who acquire CMV infection in the first 18 months of life have a significantly higher rate of disease progression and central nervous system involvement than those infected by HIV alone (96). In infants, the CMV infection appears to progress more rapidly than the HIV infection, and more than half of the infants born with CMV infection have an AIDS-defining condition or die by 18 months of age.

CMV infections occur throughout the gastrointestinal tract, from the esophagus to the anus (96), often showing the most serious complications in the large bowel. The symptoms generally depend on the location and severity of the infection and the immune status of the patient. The most common presentation is abdominal pain associated with chronic diarrhea. Other common manifestations include odynophagia, dysphagia, dyspepsia, nausea, vomiting, malabsorption, weight loss, gastrointestinal bleeding, protein-losing enteropathy, severe wasting, colitis, ulcers, perforation, peritonitis, obstruction from the formation of inflammatory masses, and appendicitis. Abdominal pain may be marked and rebound tenderness is often present, indicating full-thickness involvement of the bowel wall.

The clinical presentation of CMV esophagitis differs from other viral and fungal infections in that symptom onset occurs gradually. Painful, difficult swallowing and retrosternal pain occur less commonly than in herpetic esophagitis, although odynophagia is almost uniformly present.

Gross Findings. CMV can involve the entire alimentary tract, usually producing multiple mucosal erosions and ulcers.

Esophagus. Most typically, CMV esophagitis affects the mid to distal esophagus as superficial erosions with geographic, serpiginous, nonraised borders. These vary in number, size, and appearance. Because of their lack of endoscopic uniformity, they are easily confused with other ulcerating esophageal conditions. Most ulcers measure less than 1 cm in greatest diameter but giant ulcers are seen in 28 percent of patients. Endoscopically, there is diffuse erosive disease, deep linear ulcers, mucosal friability, erythema, and sometimes pseudotumoral masses. As the infection progresses, ulcers extend from 10 to 15 cm in length. Complications include strictures, bacterial infection, and bronchoesophageal fistulas (90). Patients become rapidly nutritionally depleted as dysphagia and odynophagia complicate their wasting disease. Biopsies must be taken in order to determine the cause of the ulcer.

Stomach. Gastric CMV usually produces an endoscopic appearance of nonspecific gastritis. Other gastric manifestations include thickened and edematous mucosal folds, erosions, and ulcers. Mucosal biopsy is necessary to establish the diagnosis. Gastroparesis with recurrent vomiting may occur as a complication.

Intestines. Although any region of the gastrointestinal tract may be involved, the colon is most commonly affected. CMV colitis reveals a spectrum of nonspecific changes, including ulcers, granularity, thumbprinting, a coarse mucosal pattern, edematous folds, and nodular defects often corresponding to pseudomembranes. CT scans may show a focally or diffusely thickened colonic wall, a finding that correlates with histologic evidence of submucosal inflammation.

The cecum and right colon are more commonly infected than the distal colon; the rectum and sigmoid colon may also be involved. The endoscopic appearance of CMV colitis is highly variable, ranging from normal to diffuse erythema with submucosal hemorrhages, to erosions and discreet deep ulceration (fig. 11-10). Superinfections may be superimposed and toxic megacolon may occur, leading to perforation and peritonitis. Colectomy may be necessary and should not be withheld in situations of medically intractable disease. A CMV endotheliolitis may result in ischemia with resultant complicating thromboses.

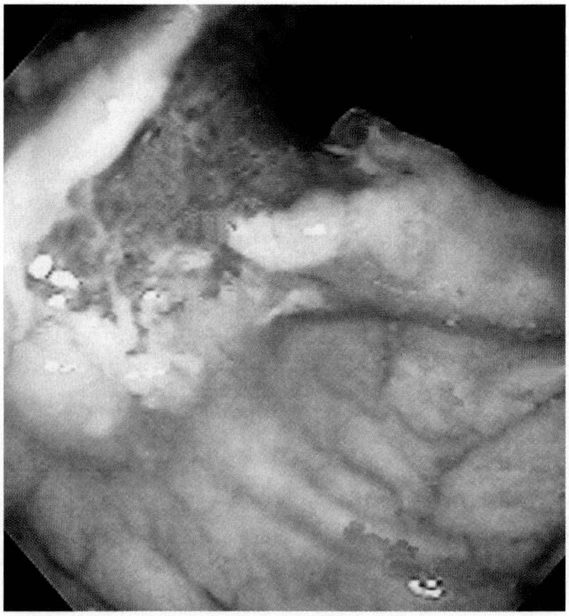

Figure 11-10

ENDOSCOPIC APPEARANCE OF CYTOMEGALOVIRUS (CMV) COLITIS

A large ulcer is present in the colon.

Microscopic Findings. The histologic diagnosis of CMV in fixed tissues usually requires finding characteristic intranuclear or cytoplasmic inclusions. Sampling error leads to a lack of sensitivity of the histologic examination, but when the virus is identified, histology has a high degree of specificity. CMV infects epithelium, endothelium, smooth muscle cells, fibroblasts, histiocytes, and ganglion cells. CMV-infected cells appear enlarged (cytomegalic) and they often contain eosinophilic intranuclear inclusions surrounded by a halo and granular basophilic cytoplasm (fig. 11-11). Nuclear and cytoplasmic inclusions often coexist. Atypical inclusions may appear as irregular smudgy cells with basophilic nuclear enlargement and elongated eosinophilic cytoplasm or cells containing small granular cytoplasmic inclusions. Deep biopsies may be necessary to detect stromal disease.

The intensity of the inflammation and necrosis generated by CMV infection varies widely. The pathologic changes range from a relatively bland lesion to extensive acute and chronic inflammation with widespread necrosis and gastrointestinal perforation. The accompanying inflammatory infiltrate consists of lymphocytes, histiocytes, plasma cells, and polymorphonuclear leukocytes. The number of inclusions generally parallels the severity of the inflammation, although occasional cases show numerous inclusions in the absence of significant inflammation. Tissues examined from the base of CMV-induced ulcers show acute inflammation and granulation tissue.

CMV may be difficult to demonstrate histologically. If CMV is suspected, numerous biopsies should be taken in order not to miss the cytomegalic or inclusion-bearing cells. Goodgame et al. (95) obtained 8 to 10 biopsy specimens from mucosal erosions and ulcers in AIDS patients known to have CMV infection and found that often only one revealed cytomegalic inclusion-bearing cells. Diagnostic cytologic brushings exhibit characteristic cytomegaly, marginated chromatin, large basophilic intranuclear inclusions surrounded by a clear halo, and granular eosinophilic intracytoplasmic inclusions.

Esophagus. The esophageal squamous epithelium virtually never becomes infected by CMV. Rather, the virus affects the stromal cells underlying ulcers (fig. 11-12). CMV inclusions may sometimes be seen in the epithelial cells of the esophageal submucosal glands (fig. 11-13). Coexisting *Candida* or HSV infection may complicate the histologic features. Perivascular macrophage aggregates in the granulation tissue and exudates of esophageal ulcers can be found in CMV esophagitis. These lesions do not usually contain viral inclusions and immunostains must be used to demonstrate the virus.

Stomach. There are two major patterns of gastric involvement. One pattern consists of abundant CMV cytoplasmic and nuclear inclusion-bearing cells in the gastric glands (fig. 11-14) and stromal cells, including macrophages, endothelial cells, and smooth muscle cells. The second

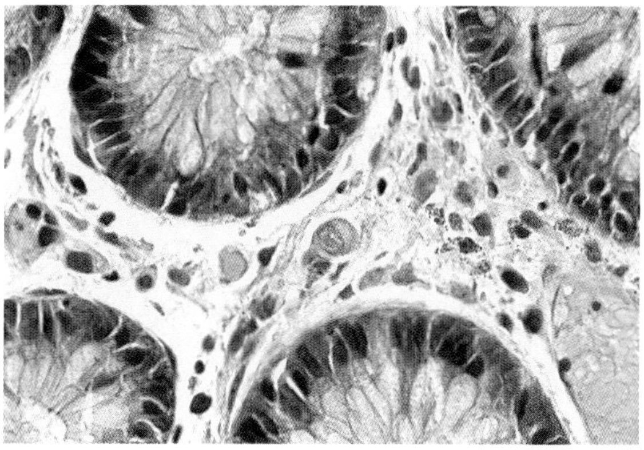

Figure 11-11

CMV COLITIS

A characteristic CMV inclusion-bearing cell lies in the lamina propria (center). The cell is large, and contains a slightly eosinophilic nuclear inclusion surrounded by a clear halo.

pattern occurs with less severe disease and the infection is very subtle. One may have to search for a long time to find characteristic inclusions. The lamina propria in either pattern may appear normocellular, hypercellular, or hypocellular.

Intestines. Intestinal lesions also vary in their severity. Inclusion-bearing stromal (fig. 11-15) or epithelial cells are associated with variable degrees of inflammation. Some intestinal lesions exhibit severe CMV-related occlusive vasculitis. Cytomegalic inclusions occur within endothelial cells of medium-sized arteries and veins, as well as arterioles, venules, and capillaries. The affected endothelial cells appear enlarged, leading to partial or complete vascular occlusion with occasional thrombus formation. A leukocytoclastic vasculitis and lymphoplasmacytic perivascular infiltrate develops, leading to lost vascular integrity with complete or segmental necrosis, ischemia, intestinal ulceration, and perforation. The vasculitis may be associated with exuberant fibroblastic reactions that are especially prominent in ulcer bases (99). Small blood vessels with endothelial cells containing cytomegalic inclusions lie among the fibroblasts. The surrounding tissues show ischemic changes.

Special Techniques. The diagnosis of gastrointestinal CMV infection is best established by demonstrating viral cytopathic effects in tissue specimens. Alternatively, immunohistochemical techniques can be used to detect viral

Figure 11-12

CMV ESOPHAGITIS

A: Low-power photomicrograph of a large esophageal ulcer from a patient with a previous history of radiation therapy for lung carcinoma. The biopsy shows reactive-appearing squamous epithelium and a fibrin thrombus in an underlying vessel. The presence of such fibrin thrombi should raise the possibility of CMV infection because of the tendency of the virus to infect endothelial cells.

B: An enlarged endothelial cell highly suspicious for CMV infection is in another vessel.

C: Higher-power view shows a more typical CMV inclusion–containing cell within the stromal tissue.

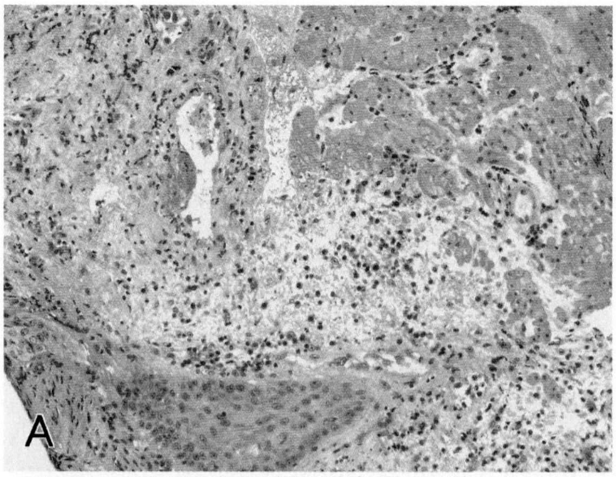

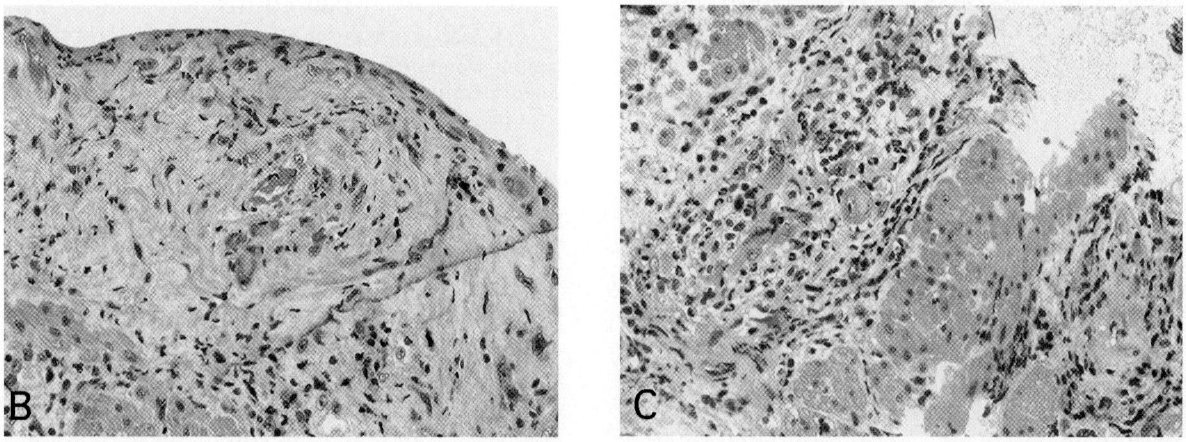

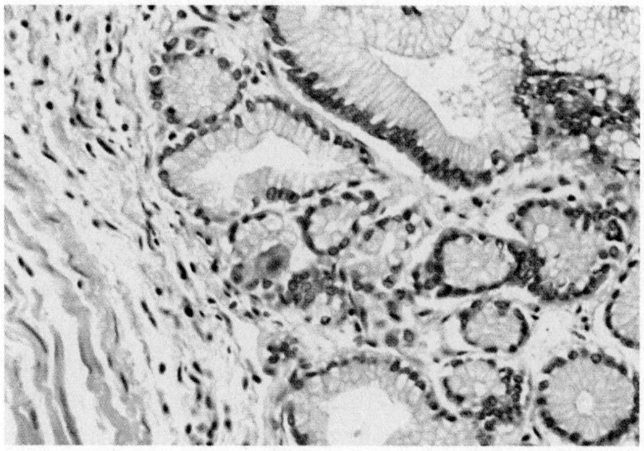

Figure 11-13

CMV INCLUSION

Esophageal submucosal gland contains an epithelial cell with a typical CMV inclusion.

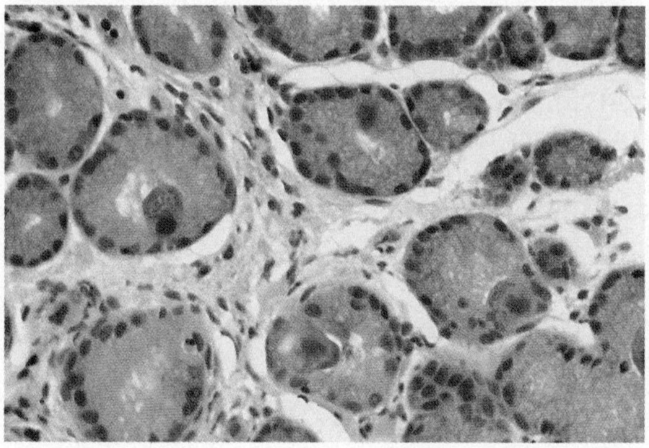

Figure 11-14

CMV GASTRITIS IN AN AIDS PATIENT

Numerous inclusions are within the cells lining the gastric glands.

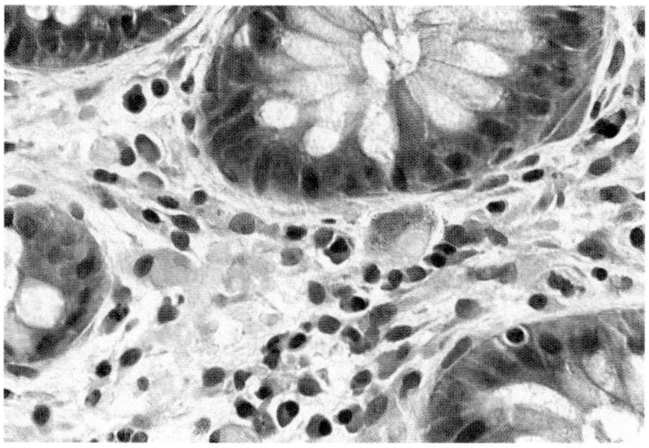

Figure 11-15

CMV COLITIS

An inclusion-bearing cell lies in the lamina propria.

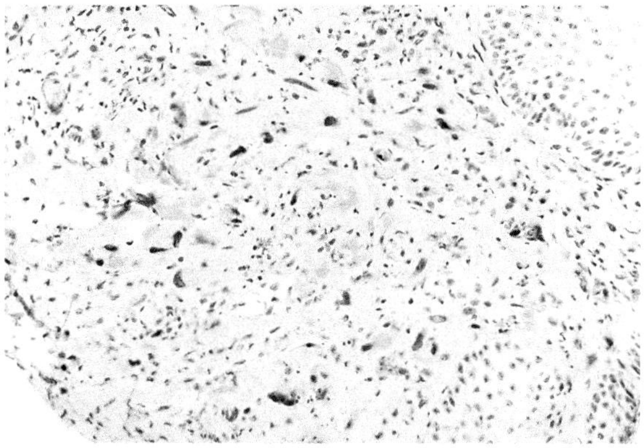

Figure 11-16

IN SITU HYBRIDIZATION FOR CMV

Numerous brown-staining nuclei are present in cells within the base of an esophageal ulcer. This staining indicates the presence of CMV viral DNA in the affected cells.

antigens in fixed tissue sections or cytologic preparations (fig. 11-16). The virus may also be detected using various DNA detection systems, including in situ hybridization, dot blot hybridization, or PCR on DNA extracted from paraffin sections of small biopsies. CMV may be detected by direct viral isolation from clinical specimens via conventional tissue culture or rapid shell viral culture systems, or by serologic methods used to detect CMV-specific immunoglobulin (Ig)G antibodies. Cultures for CMV are usually positive when inclusions are present, but they are less sensitive and specific than histopathologic identification (94).

Differential Diagnosis. In the esophagus, the clinical differential diagnosis includes HSV, varicella-zoster virus, and *Candida* infections. In the stomach, the infection may produce pseudotumors that mimic neoplasia. Colonic CMV infections mimic numerous other pathologic processes, especially idiopathic inflammatory bowel disease or ischemia. Violaceous CMV lesions may resemble Kaposi's sarcoma, while white-yellow plaques and nodules suggest ischemia or pseudomembranous colitis.

Treatment and Prognosis. CMV infection can independently contribute to AIDS-related morbidity and mortality and can be an independent predictor of death (93). Treatment with foscarnet, acyclovir, or ganciclovir reverses many of the disease manifestations. Most patients respond to intravenous ganciclovir, using a 2- to 3-week induction period. Partial responders may benefit from a repeat course or switching therapy to foscarnet. Cidofovir is the newest agent that has similar efficacy rates as ganciclovir but has the advantage of having a longer half-life. Each antiviral agent has unique toxicities, but in general, remission may be achieved in up to 90 percent of patients. The role of maintenance therapy is currently being studied. Many CMV patients have other co-morbidities that adversely impact long-term survival. Relapse is common when therapy is discontinued and most patients require lifelong maintenance therapy.

Herpes Simplex Virus Infections

Demography. Predisposing factors to *HSV infection* in immunocompromised patients include nasogastric intubation, steroid therapy, and anticancer therapies (102).

Pathophysiology. In immunosuppressed patients, HSV infections are either a primary infection or result from reactivation of latent infection when CD4-positive cells fall below 50/mm^3 (101). AIDS patients may have esophagitis due to either HSV type I or type II. In contrast, non-HIV and immunocompetent patients are most commonly infected with HSV type I.

Clinical Features. Most immunocompromised patients develop herpetic esophagitis. Proctocolitis and severe perianal ulceration with a prominent mucopurulent discharge occur, but are much less common. Odynophagia and chest pain affect the majority of patients with esophageal disease. Pain and tenesmus

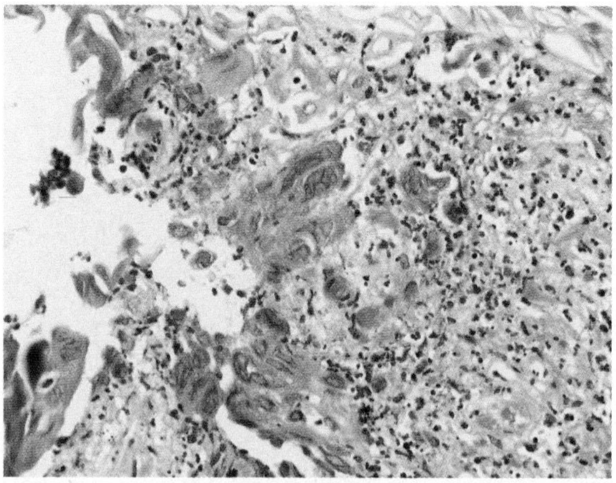

Figure 11-17

HERPES ESOPHAGITIS

This biopsy taken from the edge of an esophageal ulcer shows numerous herpes simplex virus (HSV)–infected squamous epithelial cells. The nuclear inclusions are glassy in appearance, and the chromatin is marginated to the periphery of the nucleus. Numerous giant cells have multiple, molded nuclei that contain typical inclusions.

predominate in large intestinal disease. Sacral nerve involvement is accompanied by urinary bladder problems.

Gross Findings. Esophageal involvement develops in approximately 90 percent of patients with visceral HSV infection. The middle and distal thirds of the esophagus are the most commonly affected areas. Mucosal involvement begins as bullous lesions with central umbilicated areas and a pale yellow peripheral rim. Rupture gives rise to a multiple, sharply defined, punched-out, linear ulcers with elevated margins and a hemorrhagic base. The ulcers may develop an overlying pseudomembrane. The intervening mucosa often appears normal unless the patients have concomitant *Candida* or CMV infection. Large areas of denuded mucosa develop in severe disease. Herpetic ulcers usually stop at the gastroesophageal junction. Hemorrhage, stenosis, and fistulas may occur. The presence of preexisting damage by other causes like gastroesophageal reflux or drug-induced injury may obscure the classic pathologic features of the viral infection.

Microscopic Findings. HSV predominantly infects squamous epithelium. It causes erosions that coalesce to produce ulcers surrounded by dense inflammatory exudates. Herpetic esophagitis is usually easy to recognize if a biopsy is taken at the edge of the herpetic ulcer. Multinucleated giant cells contain characteristically molded nuclei and Cowdry type A intranuclear inclusions (fig. 11-17). The diagnosis rests on identifying the characteristic epithelial viral inclusions. This may be difficult in AIDS patients, in the absence of clear inclusions or multinucleated giant cells. Instead, only large mononuclear cell aggregates containing convoluted nuclei lying adjacent to the infected epithelium may be seen. The presence of macrophage aggregates highly suggests the diagnosis. Occasionally, there is histologic evidence of herpetic infection in the ducts and acini of the submucosal glands beneath the ulcer.

Special Techniques. Immunohistochemistry or in situ hybridization may be required to either confirm the nature of an inclusion that is found or even to detect the presence of the virus in the absence of characteristic inclusions. Viral culture not only increases the diagnostic yield on the tissues, but also distinguishes between viral infections with overlapping histologic and cytologic features.

Differential Diagnosis. The differential diagnosis of HSV includes other viral or fungal infections, particularly in the esophagus. It also includes idiopathic esophageal ulcers or disease related to reflux esophagitis. In the large intestine, the differential diagnosis usually involves other infectious diseases. The appropriate diagnosis can be established by finding characteristic inclusions or with the use of special stains or genetic probes.

Treatment. Acyclovir is the treatment of choice, administered orally for 2 to 3 weeks or intravenously for 7 days. Long-term treatment may be necessary for recurrences. Foscarnet may also be used but resistance is common following repeated viral exposure.

Other Viral Infections

A number of other viruses including *Norwalk virus*, *astrovirus*, and *picornavirus* (103) have been identified in both symptomatic and asymptomatic AIDS patients. Their overall contribution to diarrheal disease is small (104).

Adenovirus infection, although uncommon, can be overlooked due to the subtle associated morphologic changes. Adenovirus affects the stomach, small intestine, and colon (107,110). Occasional cases of hemorrhagic colitis due to adenovirus infection have been described (106). The adenovirus-infected epithelial cells appear amphophilic because of the presence of intranuclear inclusions that vary in shape and size (see chapter 10). These intranuclear inclusions are often overlooked or are mistaken for those of CMV (108). Adenovirus is usually seen only in mucosal cells, especially goblet cells, sparing cells of the lamina propria, such as endothelial cells and smooth muscle cells, which are frequent targets of CMV. The virus can be detected by in situ hybridization, electron microscopy, or culture of inflamed colonic tissue (105,109).

FUNGAL INFECTIONS IN IMMUNOCOMPROMISED PATIENTS

Candida Infections

Demography. The most common opportunistic disease in HIV-infected individuals is *Candida esophagitis*, a disease that represents an AIDS-defining illness. *Candida* infection affects up to 90 percent of AIDS patients (113). Patients with low CD4 counts and a low CD4 to CD8 ratio are most likely to develop candidiasis. Disease prevalence varies considerably among various high-risk groups, and is particularly high among blacks (80 percent) (113). *Candida* gastritis and enteritis are less common than esophageal disease, presumably because neutrophil function usually remains intact in AIDS patients, thereby effectively preventing widespread fungal dissemination.

Oral thrush often predicts concurrent esophageal involvement, with a positive and negative predictive value of 90 and 82 percent, respectively (114).

Candidiasis also affects patients on antibiotics, hemodialysis, and chemotherapy; transplant patients; and immunocompetent patients with serious postoperative complications, cancer, severely debilitating diseases, penetrating abdominal trauma, or with indwelling vascular access devices.

Etiology. Although most cases of *Candida* esophagitis result from *Candida albicans* organisms, other fungi, such as *C. tropicalis* and *C. glabrata* also cause disease. The pathophysiology of *Candida* infection is discussed in more detail in chapter 10.

Clinical Features. Upper gastrointestinal symptoms include abdominal pain, upper gastrointestinal bleeding, or refractory nausea and vomiting. Dysphagia and odynophagia cause significant discomfort and represent a major cause of weight loss in infected patients. The infection is associated with weakness, fatigue, and a diminished quality of life; patients may also remain asymptomatic.

The clinical presentation of intestinal candidiasis consists of watery, sometimes explosive diarrhea, occasional cramps, mild diffuse abdominal tenderness, and weight loss. *Candida* colitis consists of multiple, variably sized ulcers with heaped-up edges and necrotic bases distributed throughout the colon, grossly resembling CMV infections (112).

Gross Findings. The endoscopic appearance of esophageal candidiasis is characteristic and consists of multiple creamy yellow plaques, often in a longitudinal arrangement. Plaques may also be diffuse. Mucosal friability and erosive disease underlie the plaque. Esophageal candidiasis may involve the entire esophagus; more often it remains localized to the distal region. With increasing severity, scattered mucosal plaques coalesce, resulting in circumferential disease and luminal impingement. Complications such as strictures and fistulas may develop.

Microscopic Findings. The diagnosis is usually made by demonstrating the organism in smears, cytologic preparations, or biopsies. Some believe that brushings are preferable to biopsies to confirm a diagnosis that is frequently endoscopically obvious (111). Microscopically, characteristic budding yeasts and pseudohyphae, associated with varying degrees of inflammation, are seen (fig. 11-18). The grossly visible plaques consist of desquamated, superficial, hyperplastic, and hyperkeratotic squamous epithelium; inflammatory cells; fungi; and bacteria. Surface colonization typically consists of yeast on intact mucosal surfaces or confined to the necrotic tissue. It is rare to see fungus invade underlying tissues. If invasion is present, however, it is important to transmit this information to the clinician. Penetration of hyphal-like elements into the underlying tissues characterizes invasive disease.

Treatment and Prognosis. Given the high frequency of *Candida* esophagitis in patients with

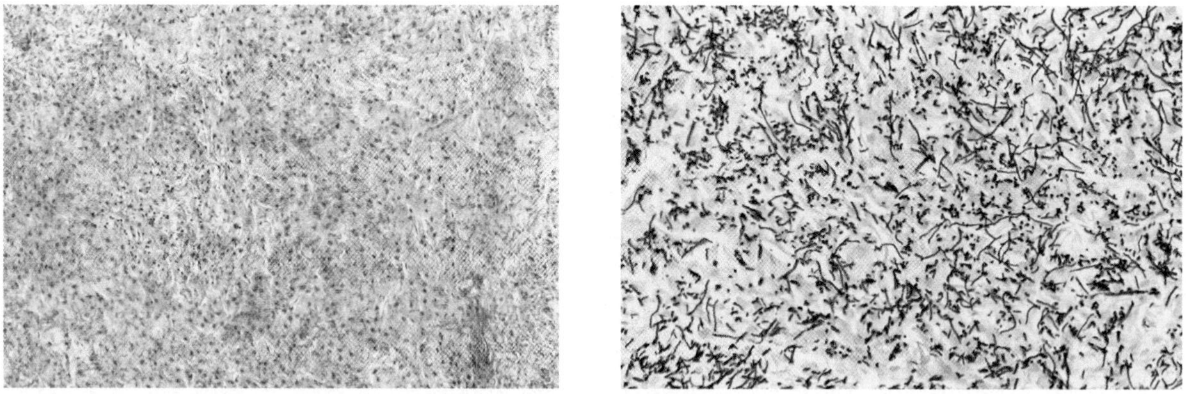

Figure 11-18

CANDIDA ESOPHAGITIS

Left: Hematoxylin and eosin (H&E)-stained section of an esophageal biopsy demonstrates keratin, desquamated squamous epithelial cells, and admixed fungal organisms.

Right: The yeast and pseudohyphal forms are easily seen on a Grocott methenamine silver–stained section.

AIDS, the current recommendation is to treat new-onset esophageal symptoms empirically with oral fluconazole for 2 weeks. Fluconazole taken prophylactically reduces the frequency of esophageal candidiasis, especially in those with 50 or fewer CD4-positive lymphocytes/mm^3. The drug does not reduce overall mortality.

Histoplasmosis

In advanced HIV disease, a CD4 count below 200/mm^3 predisposes patients to disseminated histoplasmosis. Histoplasmosis is discussed further in chapter 10.

Other Fungal Infections

Fungal infection due to *Penicillium marneffei* has been reported as a cause of colitis and chronic diarrhea in AIDS patients in Southeast Asia (115). *Coccidioidomycosis* and *cryptococcal infection* of the gut are rare and usually occur in the context of systemic disease. These organisms more frequently involve the liver than the luminal gastrointestinal tract.

DISSEMINATED *PNEUMOCYSTIS CARINII* INFECTION

Demography. Disseminated *Pneumocystis carinii* infection affects AIDS patients.

Clinical Features. Disseminated infections involve the lungs, stomach, jejunum, ileum, mesoappendix, abdominal lymph nodes, diaphragm, pancreas, and thyroid gland (116,117).

Gross Findings. Small intestinal changes consist of large patches of necrosis affecting the serosal side of the bowel wall. The corresponding mucosal surface appears normal. Mesenteric lymph nodes are enlarged, with areas of soft caseous necrosis.

Microscopic Findings. There is widespread mucosal destruction by foamy histiocytes containing organisms similar to those seen in the pulmonary alveoli. The lesions appear eosinophilic and acellular on stained slides. Numerous *P. carinii* cysts are evident within histiocytes in Giemsa- or Grocott-stained sections. The enlarged, lymphoid-depleted mesenteric lymph nodes show paracortical angiomatous transformation and contain necrotic areas surrounded by eosinophilic material. The eosinophilic material consists of masses of *P. carinii* trophozoites and cysts. Vacuolated macrophages, foreign body giant cells, small numbers of neutrophils, and fibroblastic proliferations surround the necrotic foci.

Differential Diagnosis. The differential diagnosis includes all lesions associated with diffuse histiocytic lamina propria infiltrates.

Treatment. The recommended treatment for extrapulmonary infection is intravenous trimethoprim-sulfamethoxazole or pentamidine.

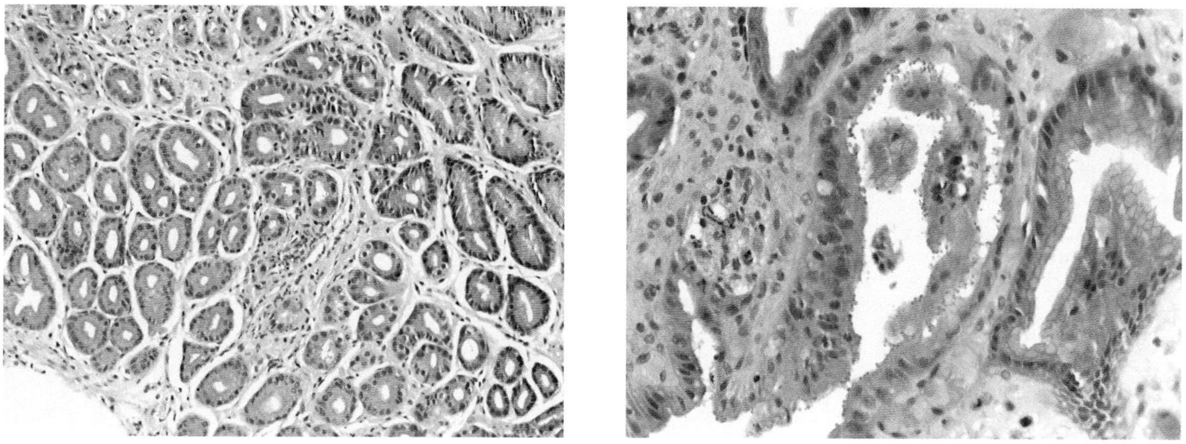

Figure 11-19

GASTRIC *CRYPTOSPORIDIUM* INFECTION

Left: The lamina propria of the stomach shows patchy acute inflammation.
Right: High-power microscopy delineates numerous bluish organisms adhering to the apical surface of the epithelial cells.

PARASITIC INFECTIONS IN IMMUNOCOMPROMISED PATIENTS

Cryptosporidium Infections

Demography. *Cryptosporidium parvum*, a coccidial organism, causes diarrhea in 3 to 11 percent of AIDS patients in the United States and in 40 to 55 percent of AIDS patients in developing countries (122a). It is the most frequently encountered protozoan parasite among AIDS patients. HIV-positive patients with self-limited infections have significantly higher CD4 counts than patients with persistent infections (123, 124). The latter frequently have CD4 counts measuring less than 100 cells/mm^3, usually even less than 50 cells/mm^3. *Cryptosporidium* also infects immunocompetent patients, and is discussed in detail in chapter 10.

Clinical Features. The clinical features of cryptosporidiosis in immunocompromised patients differ depending on where the organisms are located. Patients with infection in the proximal small intestine typically have mild diarrhea that progresses to voluminous, debilitating, watery diarrhea associated with dehydration, malabsorption, and profound weight loss. Secondary malabsorption often occurs and is related to decreased absorptive surface area in heavily infested individuals. The chronic, relentless diarrhea lasts for months and is accompanied by vomiting, anorexia, cramps, and abdominal pain.

Since AIDS patients with CD4 counts under 180/mm^3 cannot clear the organism, the infection often persists throughout the patient's life, manifesting as chronic illness with exacerbations and remissions. Gastroduodenal involvement may produce partial gastric outlet obstruction. Patients with only a colonic infection tend to have less severe symptoms. Patients with CD4 counts over 180/mm^3 often experience spontaneous resolution within a few weeks.

Gross Findings. Radiologically, the mucosal folds in the proximal small intestine are thickened and blunted, and occasionally, the gastric antrum is thick and contracted (121). Endoscopically, the mucosa is generally well preserved and the diagnosis is made by examination of the biopsy specimen.

Microscopic Findings. Cryptosporidia involve the esophagus, stomach, bile ducts, and intestines. The sensitivity of endoscopic mucosal biopsy in detecting the organism varies by anatomic location as follows: stomach, 11 percent; duodenum, 53 percent; terminal ileum, 91 percent; and colon, 60 percent (127). The presence of gastroesophageal infection usually reflects concomitant intestinal involvement.

The diagnosis of cryptosporidial infection requires close scrutiny of all epithelial surfaces, including those in the lumens of intestinal or gastric glands for the presence of the characteristic organisms (fig. 11-19). The latter appear as

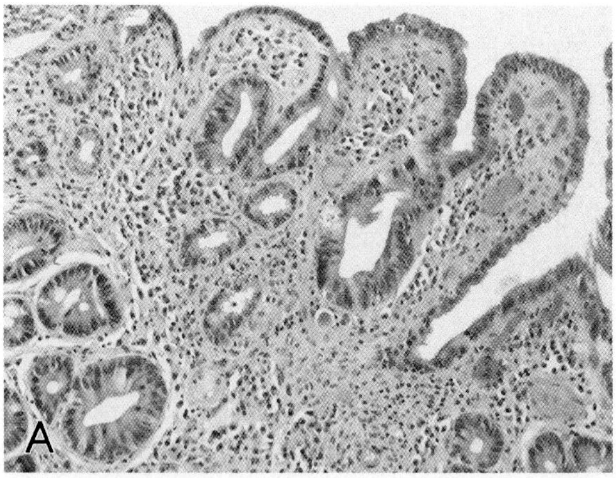

Figure 11-20

SMALL INTESTINAL CRYPTOSPORIDIOSIS

A: Low-power view shows mild villous blunting. The epithelium appears regenerative.

B: The inflammation is acute and chronic.

C: The apical surfaces of many epithelial cells are covered with round, faintly bluish-staining *Cryptosporidium* organisms.

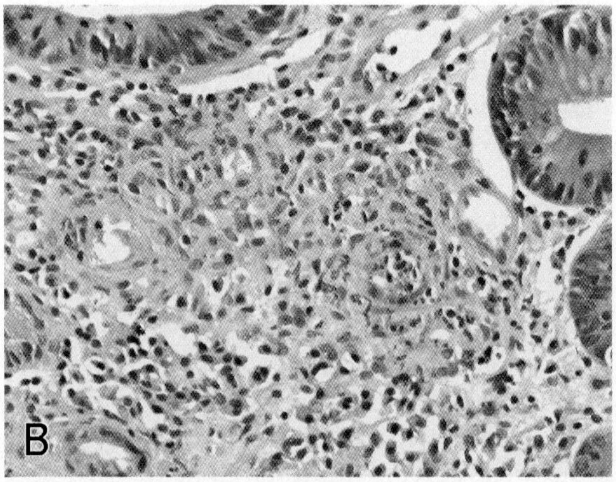

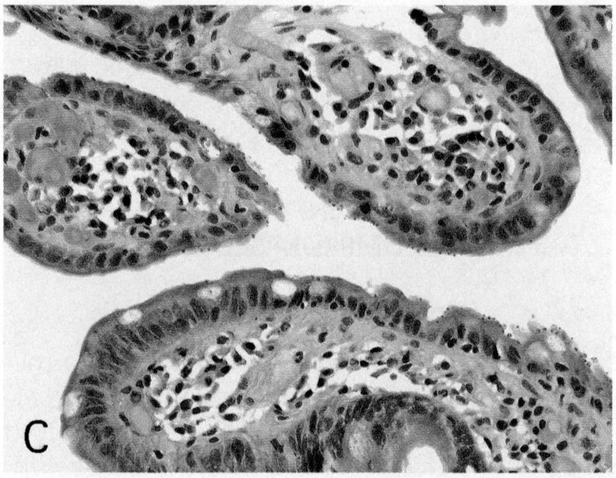

clusters of spherical or oval bluish bodies, measuring 2 to 4 µm in diameter, attached to the epithelial surfaces (fig. 11-20). In the esophagus, the organisms are attached to the superficial squamous mucosa and the luminal borders of the submucosal glands and ducts. All stages of cryptosporidia can be found at all levels of the gastrointestinal tract.

Low intensity infections have a normal histology, whereas high intensity infections show severe inflammation and varying degrees of villous atrophy (including complete villous flattening with crypt hyperplasia) (122) and mild to moderate chronic inflammatory cell infiltrates (fig. 11-20). Focal cryptitis, crypt abscesses, gland dilatation, and crypt rupture also occur. There may be associated intraepithelial lymphocytosis. Eosinophils and prominent neutrophilic infiltrates may be present. Since cryptosporidiosis is commonly associated with other bowel pathogens, the intensity of the inflammation reflects the entire spectrum of organisms that are present.

In tissue sections, cryptosporidia stain deep blue with H&E, Giemsa, and Gram stains; positively with PAS stains; and negatively with the Gomori methenamine silver (GMS) stain. A fluorescein-labeled IgG monoclonal antibody to the wall of cryptosporidial oocysts is very sensitive (126) and can detect small numbers of organisms in tissue sections or gastrointestinal brushings.

Special Techniques. The diagnosis of cryptosporidiosis is most reliably made by detection of oocysts in stool specimens. The 5-µm acid-fast oocysts are found in concentrated fresh stool specimens examined by modified Ziehl-Neelsen, Kinyoun, auramine-phenol, or safranin-methylene blue staining methods (118–120). Individual stool samples are insensitive for diagnosis, since only 53 percent demonstrate the organism; in contrast, when multiple stool samples are evaluated from a patient, 73 percent of patients demonstrate *C. parvum* in at least one stool sample. Immunofluorescent detection methods have greater sensitivity and specificity than conventional staining methods (120). Enzyme immunoassay kits allow simple, rapid, and less subjective ways of detecting cryptosporidia in fecal samples submitted to busy diagnostic laboratories (125).

Differential Diagnosis. Cryptosporidia can be easily overlooked or mistaken for mucus droplets or cellular debris. They can be differentiated from mucin by the Giemsa stain combined with the Alcian blue, neutral red, or mucicarmine stain. Cryptosporidia are mucicarmine negative. *Cyclospora cayetanensis* produces an unsporulated oocyst that occurs in feces and resembles *Cryptosporidium*. The oocyst of *Cyclospora* is larger, however, typically measuring 8 to 10 µm in diameter. Ultrastructurally, *Cyclospora* organisms develop within a vacuole at the luminal end of the enterocyte cytoplasm rather than in the brush border, as is seen with *Cryptosporidium*. The features of *Cyclospora* infection are discussed in detail in chapter 10.

Treatment. To date, there is no effective therapy for cryptosporidiosis. The agent that has shown most efficacy is paromomycin, an oral aminoglycoside (128). Some have reported resolution of cryptosporidial infections with spiramycin (123a), bovine colostrum (127), somatostatin (119), zidovudine, and other agents. Although not pathogen specific, the most effective therapy for cryptosporidiosis in HIV-positive patients is HAART. Correction of the dehydration and electrolyte imbalance may require hospitalization for intravenous replacement. Most patients are able to continue with a good quality of life on conventional antidiarrheal agents.

Isospora Belli Infections

Demography. Most *Isospora belli* infections affect patients in tropical and subtropical countries, particularly in Africa and South America. They account for diarrhea in 15 percent of AIDS patients in Haiti and 0.2 percent in the United States. The organism spreads by ingestion of contaminated food or water or via homosexual transmission.

Etiology. *I. belli* infections follow the ingestion of infective sporulated oocysts. These excyst in the proximal small intestine, releasing eight sporozoites that invade epithelial cells where they become trophozoites. Although the organism preferentially infects the small bowel, it can spread to the stomach, esophagus, biliary tree, and large intestine; only rarely does it disseminate to extraintestinal lymph nodes (131), liver, or spleen.

The life cycle involves a sexual (gametocytes) and asexual (trophozoites) phase. During the schizogonous (asexual) phase, each trophozoite divides into numerous merozoites which, when released from parasitized cells, invade other epithelial cells. Each merozoite may then pass through one or more repetitive cycles of asexual division or proceed to the sexual phase by maturing into macrogametes (female) and microgametes (male). Zygotes, resulting from the fertilization of the gametes, mature into oocysts. These are released into the bowel lumen, passing into stool where they undergo sporulation. Released trophozoites parasitize downstream enterocytes, reinitiating the reproductive cycle. All stages of both asexual (trophozoite, schizont, and merozoite) and sexual (macrogametocyte) phases of the parasitic life cycle occur within the epithelial cytoplasm, always enclosed within a parasitophorous vacuole. The nonsporulated (immature) oocytes excreted in stool mature into infective mature oocysts within 48 to 72 hours. They can also remain dormant for long periods of time. *Isospora* organisms do not sporulate until they are passed from the host and are exposed to oxygen and temperatures below body temperature.

Clinical Features. The symptoms produced by *Isospora* resemble those seen in cryptosporidial infections but the distinction between the two infections is important, since *Isospora* infections are easily treated by appropriate antibiotic therapy. The infection usually remains confined to the small intestine. The immunocompetent host presents with watery diarrhea lasting 3 to 5 weeks (130,132); diarrhea in AIDS patients may last for months. Patients experience weight loss, severe colicky abdominal pain, anorexia, malaise, nausea, vomiting, steatorrhea, and wasting. About 50 percent of patients develop peripheral eosinophilia. Fat malabsorption, vitamin B12 deficiency, and lactose intolerance can occur.

Microscopic Findings. *Isospora* organisms lie within small intestinal villous enterocytes, or less commonly, in the colonic mucosa. They cause moderate mucosal villous atrophy, crypt hyperplasia, and lamina propria inflammation by lymphocytes, plasma cells, polymorphonuclear leukocytes, and eosinophils. Eosinophils may be so prominent that a diagnosis of eosinophilic enteritis is suggested. The flattened mucosa may show clubbed tips, marked dilatation of the vascular spaces, and excessive lamina propria collagen deposits. The epithelium generally appears well preserved except for focal vacuolization. Close epithelial examination usually discloses intracellular organisms in different stages of the sexual and asexual life cycles.

The organisms are difficult to see on routine H&E-stained sections, but Giemsa staining highlights them. The organisms stain faintly with H&E, dark blue with Giemsa or H&E plus Alcian blue, and red with PAS stains. The large schizont stage is best seen in over-stained Giemsa preparations.

As parasitized cells are destroyed, the adjacent cells remain intact and appear normal. Occasional extracellular merozoites may be seen in the intestinal lumen and in the lamina propria near or within lymphatic vessels. Rare schizonts are present in the lamina propria and the submucosa. Mesenteric lymph nodes may also become involved. The merozoite has a banana shape and is seen at all levels in the enterocyte cytoplasm. The central nucleus, large nucleolus, perinuclear halo, and location within a thick parasitophorous (PAS-negative) vacuole give the merozoite a characteristic appearance. Free merozoites and gametocytes are more difficult to detect than intracellular organisms.

Special Techniques. Patients with isosporiasis intermittently shed oocysts, so that multiple stool specimens should be examined to increase the likelihood of detecting the organism. The oocysts are concentrated from fresh stool samples by sucrose flotation and highlighted by the Kinyoun acid-fast stain. Fecal specimens are best examined after 1 to 2 days at room temperature, allowing oocysts to mature.

Ultrastructurally, unizoite tissue cysts occur with a single organism in a parasitophorous vacuole. The zoite lies within a multilayered wall. The middle of the parasite has a well-defined nucleus and the posterior part contains a crystalloid body.

Differential Diagnosis. The differential diagnosis includes cryptosporidiosis, but the *Isospora* oocyst is considerably larger (25 to 30 µm in length) than *Cryptosporidium* (4 to 5 µm), with a thin wall enveloping two large sporoblasts or a single large zygote (an immature oocyst) when shed in the feces. The oocyst of *Cyclospora,* also in the differential diagnosis, measures 8 to 10 µm in length.

Treatment. The most effective antimicrobial agents for *I. belli* are trimethoprim-sulfamethoxazole and ciprofloxacin. The infection recurs in as many as 50 percent of patients, however, requiring repeated and sometimes long-term suppressive therapy (129). Pyrimethamine has also been recommended.

Microsporidium Infections

Demography. *Microsporidia* have an extensive host range, including most invertebrates and all classes of vertebrates. Most animals acquire the infection through ingestion. Microsporidia are primarily waterborne, but foodborne disease also occurs. Microsporidiosis predominantly, but not exclusively, affects severely immunodepressed persons with AIDS. In fact, *Microsporidium* species has emerged as one of the most common intestinal infections in persons with AIDS, varying from 15 to 39 percent (141,143, 148,157,159). Patients with microsporidial infections are usually homosexual with a history of foreign travel or residence in tropical regions. The prevalence of *Enterocytozoon bieneusi* infection ranges from 10 to 50 percent in AIDS patients with unexplained diarrhea and no other known pathogens (134,147,152). The organism infects both adults and children. Infected individuals tend to have profound immunosuppression with less than 100 CD4-positive cells/mL.

Etiology. Microsporidia constitute a separate phylum of ubiquitous, spore-forming, obligate intracellular protozoans that cause a wide range of diseases, including enteritis. They are ancient, intracellular, eukaryotic spore-forming protozoans that lack mitochondria. Distinctive features of the phylum Microspora include: 1) a lack of mitochondria; 2) a merogonic and sporogonic life cycle that gives rise to generations of sporoblasts which become mature spores; and 3) spores with a coiled polar filament; the number of coils is unique to each species (134). Many microsporidial species infect humans, predominantly AIDS patients, including *Enterocytozoon* *bieneusi, Enterocytozoon, Nosema, Pleistophora, Microsporidium bieneusi,* and the encephalitozoons, *Encephalitozoon hellem, E. cuniculi,* and *E. intestinalis,* formerly *Septata intestinalis* (153,154). Of these genera, only *Enterocytozoon* and *Encephalitozoon intestinalis* infect the gut. *E. bieneusi* is the most frequently identified microsporidian. Three distinct genotypic forms of *E. bieneusi* infect humans. *E. intestinalis* probably only accounts for 10 to 20 percent of cases of intestinal microsporidiosis (139) and is the second most prevalent microsporidian infection reported in AIDS patients (138).

Two phases of the life cycle of *E. bieneusi* are identified ultrastructurally: 1) a proliferative phase (merogony) and 2) a spore-forming phase (sporogony). During the proliferative phase, the organisms appear as small, electron-lucent, round objects containing 1 to 6 nuclei. The spore-forming phase begins with the presence of stacks of electron-dense discs that later aggregate end-to-end to form the curved profiles of polar tubes. The nuclei continue to divide, resulting in larger organisms with up to 12 nuclei surrounded by several coils of the polar tube. These large multinucleated forms break up into sporoblasts (immature spores) that then develop into mature spores. The mature spores are very electron dense, have a single nucleus, and possess an exceptional tubular extrusion apparatus for injecting spore contents, termed "sporoplasm," into host cells. The extrusion apparatus consists of several coils of polar tube, an anchoring tube, and a polarplast. Each spore also contains a posterior polar vacuole, and a polar filament with 5 to 7 overlapping coils of the polar tubules, which appear in cross section as a series of doublets.

Spores are infective when released in the feces. Intracellularly, spores differentiate into trophozoites that undergo asexual multiplication to form merozoites. The merozoites invade new host cells and certain types develop into male and female microgametes. Fertilization produces oocysts that are either excreted or produce sporozoites in situ to repeat the cycle.

E. intestinalis has a life cycle with four stages: meront, sporont, sporoblast, and spore. Like *E. bieneusi,* the spores contain a polar tube that injects membrane-bound sporoplasm into uninfected host cells. The earliest stage, the meront, is an ovoid, uninucleate organism measuring 2.7 x 1.5 μm that replicates by binary fission. The nuclear division sometimes outstrips cytoplasmic division, leading to binucleate and tetranucleate forms. As a result, organisms aggregate within a vacuole in the host cell cytoplasm. The second stage, the sporont, divides by binary fission, each producing two or four sporoblasts (135). Sporoblasts are uninucleate organisms that develop a polar tube and as these mature, these organelles become more conspicuous. Transformation to the final or fourth stage of the spore is marked by the development of a thick coat. The spores measure approximately 2.0 x 1.2 μm and contain a single nucleus and a polar tube, as well as some other organelles. They infect target cells by sticking to the cell membrane by means of the anterior attachment organ and injecting sporoblasts into the host cell via the polar tube. This is followed by merogony.

Clinical Features. Clinically, microsporidiosis in HIV patients is indistinguishable from cryptosporidiosis, although the symptoms are usually milder in the former. The diverse clinical manifestations of microsporidiosis include intestinal, biliary, pulmonary, ocular, muscular, and renal disease, depending on the infecting organism (143,151). *E. bieneusi* tends to remain localized to the gastrointestinal tract, spreading from the small intestine to contiguous intraluminal structures such as the biliary tract, the colon, the pancreatic duct, and the upper respiratory tract (149). *E. hellem* and *E. intestinalis* behave more like classic mammalian microsporidia. *E. cuniculi, E. hellem,* and *E. intestinalis* not only spread contiguously, but infect macrophages and disseminate from their points of entry to the respiratory tract and other organs (150).

Primary *E. bieneusi* infections preferentially involve the proximal small intestine. The cardinal feature is persistent diarrhea with increased fecal volumes of up to several liters/24 hours. The chronic diarrhea (lasting up to 30 months) causes severe wasting (134) and fluid and electrolyte imbalance.

E. intestinalis causes similar gastrointestinal disease but it is also associated with systemic disease (134). The initial symptoms usually localize to the gastrointestinal tract, but the organisms disseminate to bronchi, renal tubules, and nasal epithelium (151), leading to renal failure and rhinosinusitis (142).

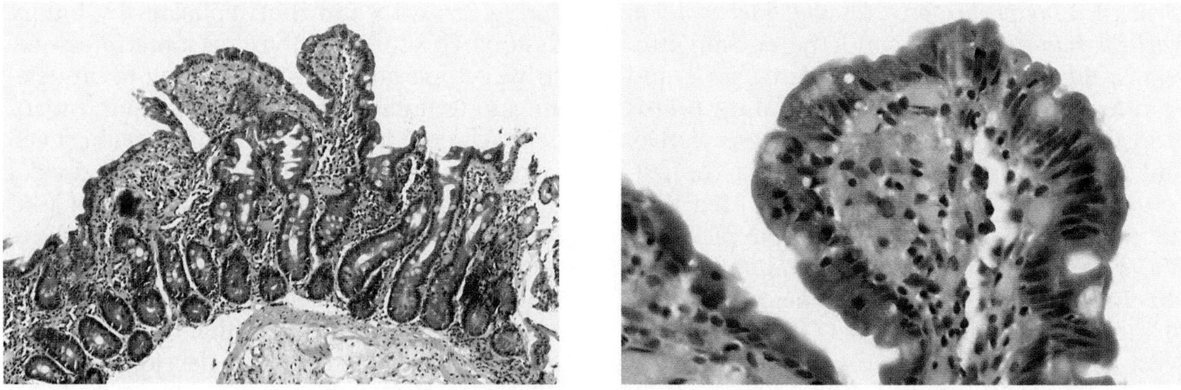

Figure 11-21

MICROSPORIDIOSIS

Left: Low-power view of a duodenal biopsy specimen from an AIDS patient with microsporidiosis. The normal villous architecture is distorted, and the crypts appear hyperplastic.

Right: Higher-power view of the duodenal epithelium shows minimal changes on a routine H&E-stained section.

Gross Findings. Endoscopically, patients with microsporidial infections usually lack discrete ulcers or masses, but the villi often appear abnormal under the dissecting microscope. Exceptionally, the infection may cause severe ulcerating disease, and even lead to perforation (155).

Microscopic Findings. *E. bieneusi* occurs throughout the length of the small intestine. *E. intestinalis* infects both the small and large intestines (139,151). Microsporidial infections can be diagnosed by identifying spores in the stool, by small bowel biopsy, by microscopy of intestinal aspirates, and by examination of touch preparations of mucosal brushings (158). The intracellular organisms have a pale blue cytoplasm and irregularly shaped, supranuclear eosinophilic nuclei that indent the nucleus in Giemsa-stained preparations (153,154). The lack of contrast between the organisms and host cell cytoplasm makes it difficult to appreciate their presence. Stool examination for microsporidial spores using the modified chromophobe stain is the simplest method, and perhaps the most sensitive method, for diagnosing the intestinal infection (154).

The histopathologic features of intestinal microsporidiosis parallel the parasite burden and consist of a spectrum of degenerative changes. Characteristically, the parasitic burden and histopathologic changes of *E. bieneusi* affect the villus tip; *E. intestinalis* may also infect the deeper crypt. Typically, there is a focal distribution of the parasite in the lining epithelium of the duodenal mucosa, although massive infestations also occur (fig. 11-21). The most typical changes include villous atrophy, crypt hyperplasia, enterocyte pleomorphism, and intraepithelial lymphocytosis. Neutrophils are not typically present. Increased numbers of macrophages or plasma cells are present in the lamina propria. The enterocytes become increasingly abnormal as the villi shorten and become broader and more irregular. Infected cells have irregular hyperchromatic nuclei, vacuolated cytoplasm, and irregular outlines. The tips of the villi appear progressively more disorganized, with aggregates of crowded cells that pile up, degenerate, and become necrotic. In heavier infections, disorganized aggregates of crowded, irregularly shaped, degenerating necrotic cells that often contain organisms and spores affect the villus tips, which eventually slough into the lumen. Since the organisms are more frequently found in degenerating cells than in intact ones, it is useful to examine the detached and degenerating surface epithelium as well as intact tissue fragments. Individual enterocytes may contain multiple stages of the *E. intestinalis* life cycle (154).

The clustered, dark, refractile, oval spores measure approximately 0.7 to 1.0 µm in width and 1.0 to 1.6 µm in length, and are less frequent than the parasite. They lie in a supranuclear location, and are surrounded by an inner unit

Table 11-4

COMPARISON OF MICROSPORIDIA

Organism	Polar Tubes	Appearance in Enterocytes	Infection	Size (Diameter)	Treatment
E. bieneusi	Double coil	Organism free in cell cytoplasm	Restricted to gut; only infects epithelium	1-2 µm	No specifically effective treatment
E. intestinalis	Single coil	Organism encased in parasitophorous vesicles	Disseminates widely; infects epithelium, fibroblasts, macrophages, endothelial cells	1.2-2.5 µm	Albendazole

membrane, an electron-lucent endospore, and a thin electron-dense exospore. Spores are often seen in degenerating enterocytes.

Microsporidia are often missed, even on careful examination, and even by experienced pathologists, because of their small size, intracellular location, and poor staining with usual tissue stains. Therefore, visualization of the parasite is best accomplished by staining methods that enhance the contrast between the very small microsporidial spores and other cellular contents and background debris. Stains that are helpful in this regard include acid-fast, Giemsa, Brown-Hopp, PAS, and methenamine silver stains. Spores are more easily seen as refractile objects when the microscope condenser is lowered or removed.

Schwarz (154) recommends identification of the microsporidia to the level of the genus, since *Encephalitozoon* has the propensity to disseminate, whereas *Enterocytozoon* does not. Furthermore, they each exhibit different drug sensitivities (Table 11-4) (139,151).

Special Techniques. Microsporidia can be identified to the level of species by electron microscopy, indirect immunofluorescence (133), and Western blot and genetic analyses. The best way to classify microsporidia, however, is by ultrastructural examination. The diagnosis is based on the ultrastructural features of the spores in the proliferative forms, the method of division, and the nature of the host cell-parasite interface. *E. bieneusi* is uniquely characterized by its development up through late sporogony as large, multinucleated plasmodia that maintain intimate contact with the cell cytoplasm (145). Development of polar filaments or tubules from discs derived from clear cleft-like structures also represent a unique feature (fig. 11-22) (146).

Evaluation of urinary sediment may aid in the diagnosis of disseminated *E. intestinalis*. The use of fluorescent stains is a sensitive and rapid method for detecting microsporidia spores in stool and intestinal fluid, biopsy imprints, tissue specimens, and archival material (137). *Encephalitozoon* organisms may also be diagnosed using an antibody for a panspecific antiexosporum (140). The immunologically based assays may be fraught with serologic cross reactivity between microsporidian species (139). PCR evaluation of stool provides a powerful tool for the specific diagnosis in epidemiologic investigations of enteric microsporidial infections. A 12/65 base-pair fragment of the small subunit ribosomal RNA (*RRS*) gene can be amplified in patients infected with *E. bieneusi*. A 930 base-pair fragment of the *RRS* gene can be amplified from patients infected with *E. intestinalis* (144). The organism may also be identified by in situ hybridization (156).

Treatment. Effective therapy for microsporidia has not been fully defined. Symptomatic improvement has been shown with metronidazole and atovaquone. Albendazole is effective for *E. intestinalis* but not for *E. bieneusi* (139). Like cryptosporidiosis, institution of HAART in HIV-infected individuals may result in resolution of diarrhea and loss of the pathogen from stool and small bowel biopsies (136). Left untreated, small bowel infection can lead to perforation and peritonitis (155). Octreotide can control the diarrhea.

Toxoplasmosis

Demography. *Toxoplasma gondii* most frequently affects patients with AIDS, although those who have lymphomas, have received transplants, or have chronic inflammatory

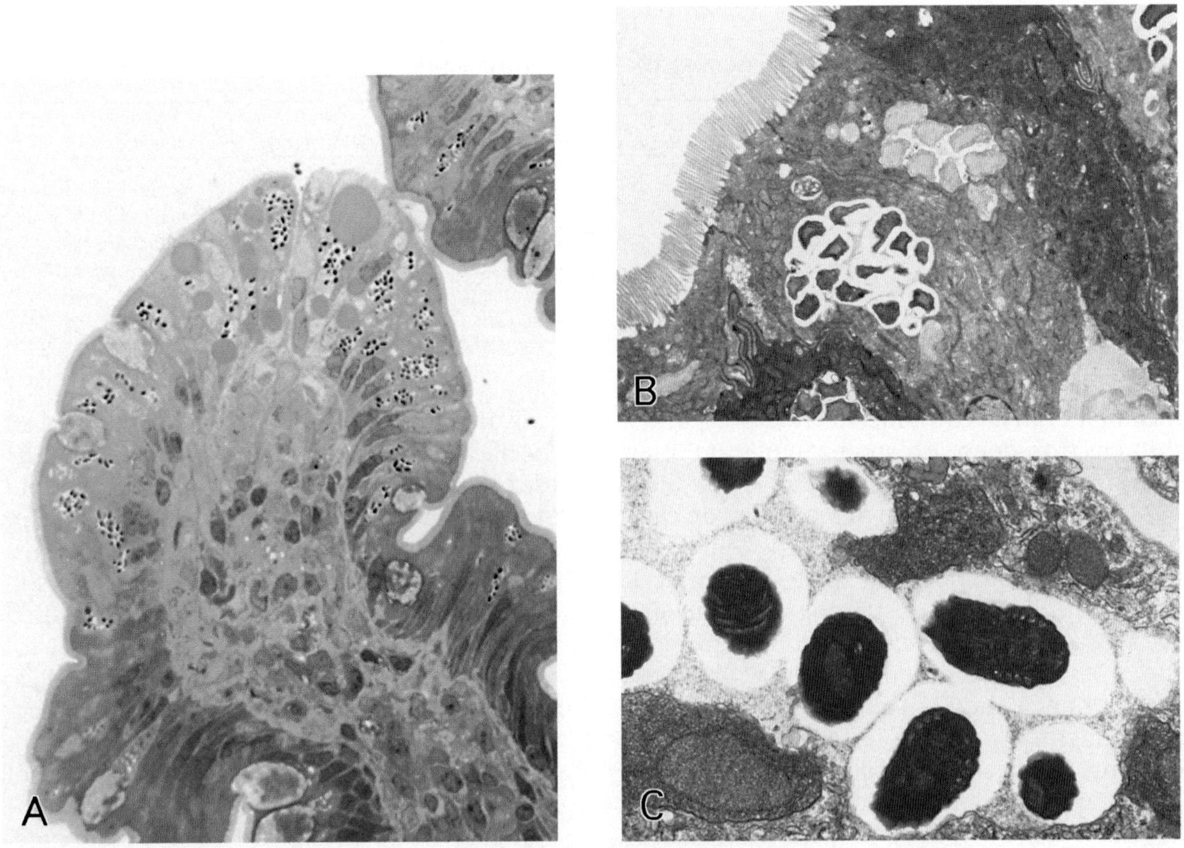

Figure 11-22

MICROSPORIDIOSIS

A: Thick epon-embedded, toluidine blue–stained section of the biopsy shown in figure 11-21. Numerous dark-staining microorganisms lie within the supranuclear cytoplasm of many of the enterocytes.

B: Transmission electron micrograph shows the organisms more clearly within the enterocyte cytoplasm.

C: A typical coiled polar filament is identifiable in some of the organisms, a diagnostic feature of microsporidia.

diseases of the connective tissues are also affected by this pathogen.

Pathophysiology. *T. gondii* is an obligate, intracellular coccidian protozoan that frequently infects birds and mammals, including humans. Infection is usually asymptomatic in normal human hosts, but in immunodeficient individuals frequently results in symptomatic ocular, central nervous system, or pulmonary disease. Gastrointestinal manifestations of toxoplasmosis occur but are infrequent.

T. gondii most commonly infects cats, the host in which they undergo the sexual reproductive phase of their life cycle. Oocysts are formed in the intestinal mucosa and passed into the environment in the feces. Human infection occurs as a result of ingestion of infective oocysts from contaminated soil or undercooked meat from infected animals. Oocysts excyst in the duodenum, releasing sporozoites that invade the intestinal tissues. Within the tissues, *T. gondii* exists in two forms. Tachyzoites infect many different cell types. They multiply within infected cells, eventually destroying them. Bradyzoites arise as the host begins to develop an immune reaction to the infection. This *T. gondii* form preferentially infects muscle and nervous tissue. The cysts containing bradyzoites may remain in the host in a latent state, only to be reactivated at a later time when the host's immune system becomes impaired.

Clinical Features. Most immunocompetent persons with acute *Toxoplasma* infection are asymptomatic. Occasionally, acute infection may produce a transient flu-like illness. In immunocompromised patients, toxoplasmosis may represent a life-threatening illness primarily as a result of its central nervous system effects.

Gastrointestinal toxoplasmosis is rare, and occurs in the setting of disseminated infection where it occurs in 6 to 20 percent of patients (162–164). Any or all gastrointestinal sites may be involved. Patients most commonly complain of abdominal pain, but diarrhea, nausea, vomiting, and anorexia may also occur (160,161). Ascites may be present.

Gross Findings. Endoscopically, ulcers or thickened gastric folds may be seen in association with gastrointestinal toxoplasmosis. Thickening of the gastric wall and antral narrowing may be seen radiographically (161).

Microscopic Findings. The microscopic features of toxoplasmosis in the gastrointestinal tract are a result of the variable acute and chronic inflammation. The diagnosis is established by the identification of bradyzoites, tachyzoites, or cysts in the tissues.

Special Studies. Bradyzoites in cysts are PAS positive. In addition, organisms may be identified with the use of immunohistochemistry or PCR (161).

Other Parasites

AIDS patients develop a number of other parasitic infections. Among the more common are *giardiasis* and *amebiasis*. In addition, *Strongyloides* infections occur in some immunocompromised patients. These are discussed in chapter 10.

GRAFT VERSUS HOST DISEASE

Definition. *Graft versus host disease* (GVHD) is an immunologic disorder that may result in severe gastrointestinal damage. GVHD most commonly follows bone marrow or organ transplantation, and represents the response of immunocompetent donor cells to the histocompatibility antigens of the recipient. Less commonly, it complicates maternal-fetal cell transfer in immunodeficient children (178) or transfusion of nonirradiated cells and blood products (165,170).

Demography. The incidence of GVHD in bone marrow transplant patients ranges from less than 10 percent to more than 80 percent, depending on the degree of incompatibility, the number of T cells in the graft, the patient age, and the nature of the immunosuppressive regimen the patient has undergone. GVHD may occur even in fully matched MHC donors and recipients due to incompatibilities in minor histocompatibility antigens (172,176,192). The incidence of GVHD is possibly higher in African-Americans than in other individuals (171).

Etiology. The basic requirements for GVHD to occur include the following: 1) the graft must contain immunocompetent cells; 2) the host must be sufficiently genetically different from the graft to be perceived as antigenically foreign; and 3) the host must be unable to reject the graft. These conditions allow engrafted cells to react to the host through immunologically mediated processes (166).

The principal target organs of GVHD are skin, gastrointestinal tract, biliary tree, bone marrow, and lymphoid tissues. These organs have high cell turnover rates and may continually express differentiation antigens, resulting in increased immune surveillance (188). Alternatively, cells in these organs may harbor latent viruses that could act as targets for donor immune surveillance.

Pathophysiology. CD8-, CD3- and TiA1-positive cytotoxic T cells mediate epithelial cell death in GVHD (167,193). CD8 cells recognize class II MHC-restricted antigens which produce the lymphokines that lead to the development of the enteropathy associated with GVHD (175,180). Apoptosis may occur through the Fas/Fas ligand pathway (183).

Clinical Features. Acute GVHD occurs within days (7 to 100) in recipients who are not HLA matched or in patients without any prophylaxis. Rarely, acute GVHD occurs later than 100 days post-transplant (175). The typical clinical presentation of acute GVHD includes rash, nausea, anorexia, profuse watery diarrhea, intestinal hemorrhage, crampy abdominal pain, abdominal tenderness, paralytic ileus, malabsorption, and jaundice. The intestine and stomach are involved in most patients; colonic involvement is less frequent (168,190,191,194). Esophageal GVHD may also be seen (181,182,184).

Chronic GVHD is less common than acute GVHD and occurs more than 100 days following transplantation, either as an extension of acute GVHD or following a quiescent disease-free interval. Fifteen to 40 percent of long-term transplantation survivors have chronic GVHD

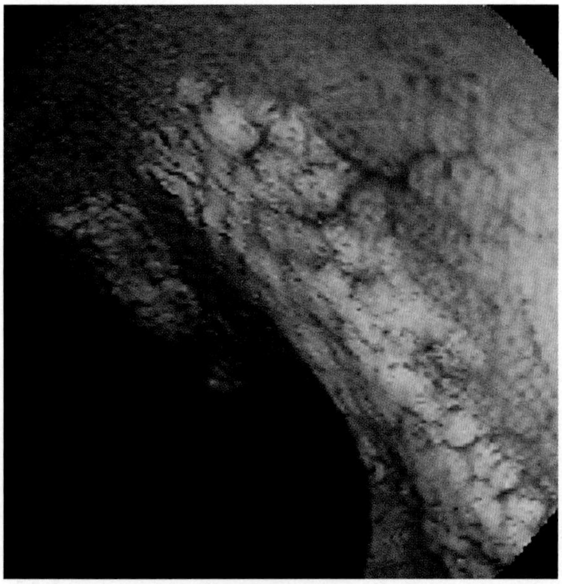

Figure 11-23

GRAFT VERSUS HOST DISEASE

There are atypical white plaques. The honeycomb mucosal pit pattern is accentuated, suggesting mucosal edema. (Fig. 4-123 from Emory TS, Carpenter HA, Gostout CJ, Sobin LH. Atlas of gastrointestinal endoscopy & endoscopic biopsies. Washington DC: Armed Forces Institute of Pathology; 2009:332.)

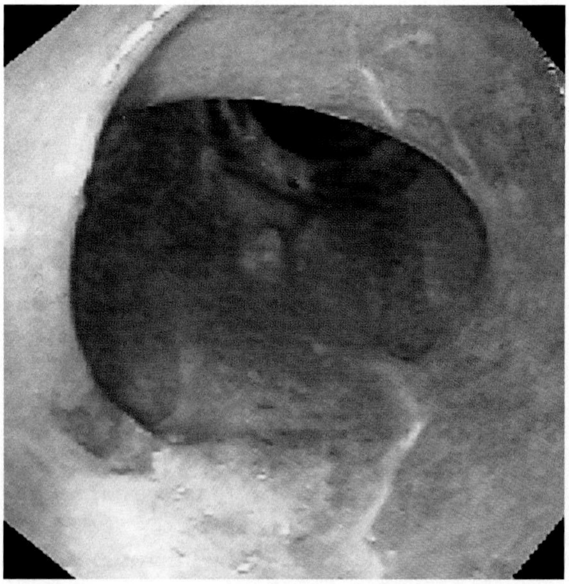

Figure 11-24

GRAFT VERSUS HOST DISEASE

There is ulceration with mucosal sloughing in the terminal ileum. (Fig. 4-124 from Emory TS, Carpenter HA, Gostout CJ, Sobin LH. Atlas of gastrointestinal endoscopy & endoscopic biopsies. Washington DC: Armed Forces Institute of Pathology; 2009:333.)

Table 11-5

HISTOLOGIC GRADING OF GRAFT VERSUS HOST DISEASE

Grade	Histology
1	Mild necrosis of individual crypts
2	Crypt abscesses and crypt cell flattening
3	Dropout of many crypts
4	Flat mucosa

(177). It may result from long-living lymphocytes of donor origin that have become sensitized to unknown antigens, probably minor histocompatibility antigens of the host (177). Symptoms of chronic GVHD are nonspecific and include diarrhea, nausea, vomiting, and in some cases, complete gastrointestinal intolerance necessitating total parenteral nutrition (186).

Gross Findings. Endoscopic findings in patients with GVHD are variable, ranging from normal to severely inflamed, with erythema, ulceration, and exudates (figs. 11-23, 11-24). The degree to which the endoscopic appearance correlates with a histologic diagnosis of GVHD varies from study to study (169,173,187).

Microscopic Findings. Mucosal biopsy provides a sensitive test for detecting GVHD in the gastrointestinal tract. The biopsy should not be taken during the first 3 weeks of immunosuppressive therapy because all patients show some degree of inflammation in the immediate post-transplant period. The lesions of acute GVHD range from necrosis of individual crypt cells to total mucosal loss (Table 11-5). Apoptotic bodies are the sine qua non of the diagnosis. Apoptotic bodies collect at the crypt bases in the intestine, and in the neck region of the gastric glands (fig. 11-25). As a result, the base of the glands may appear dilated and may contain apoptotic debris (194).

As the lesions evolve, an entire crypt may drop out, creating single crypt loss. The mucosal architecture is progressively lost with increasing ulceration, mucosal denudation, and submucosal edema (fig. 11-26). The epithelium may appear degenerated and cuboidal. In some

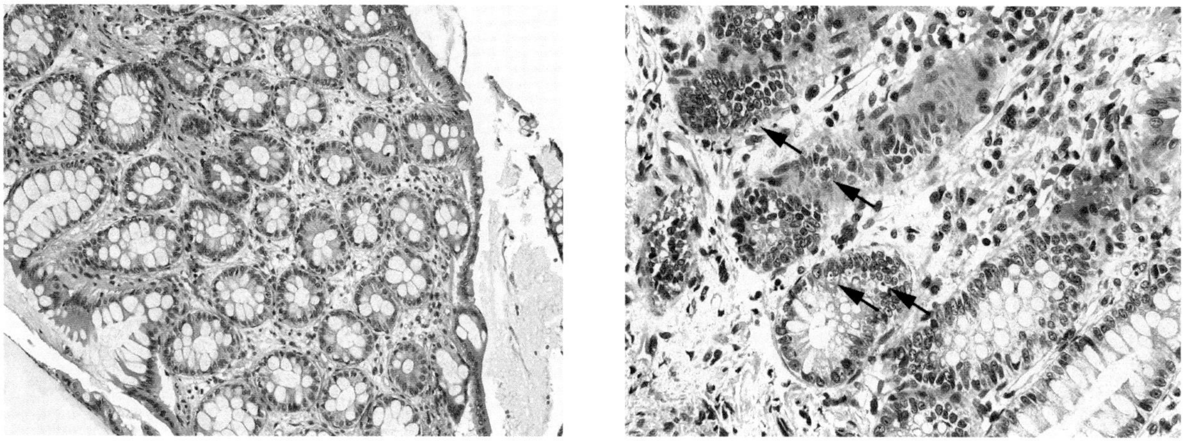

Figure 11-25

GRAFT VERSUS HOST DISEASE

Left: Low-power photograph of the colonic mucosa from a patient with early graft versus host disease (GVHD). The mucosal architecture is normal, and there is no evidence of inflammation.

Right: On high power, scattered apoptotic bodies are within the colonic glands (arrows).

cases, the epithelium appears as a flattened monolayer. Ulcer healing leads to fibrosis and stricture formation.

In chronic GVHD, there is segmental lamina propria fibrosis and submucosal fibrosis extending to the serosa. These lesions occur throughout the entire length of the gastrointestinal tract, from the esophagus to the colon.

Occasional patients pass ropey, tan material resembling strands of sloughed mucosal tissue, known as mucosal casts, per rectum. The composition of the material is rarely clear-cut. It usually contains fibrin, neutrophils, cellular debris, bacteria, or fungi, and very little identifiable tissue (189). The presence of free intestinal epithelium may be confirmed by immunostaining for cytokeratin (189).

Differential Diagnosis. Changes similar to those found in GVHD sometimes occur in immunosuppressed or immunodeficient patients, without a history of transplant or transfusion. Patients have various associated diseases including lymphoma, leukemia, combined immune deficiency, or severe T-cell deficiency. The signs and symptoms resemble those developing following bone marrow transplantation but they occur more rapidly and tend to be associated with a higher fatality rate. A novel T-lymphocyte population has been identified in combined immunodeficiency associated with features of GVHD (195). Some patients have other autoimmune diseases. This entity probably overlaps with autoimmune enteropathy.

Histologic features similar to those of GVHD may be a result of drug injury. Mycophenolate mofetil, a drug used to reduce acute graft rejection in solid organ transplant patients, may produce such a pattern of injury (fig. 11-27) (179,185).

It is important to rule out the possibility of CMV infection in patients suspected of GVHD since this virus commonly infects immunocompromised patients, and has histologic features similar to GVHD (179,190,194).

Treatment and Prognosis. The treatment for patients with both acute and chronic GVHD is increased immunosuppression. Despite improvements in immunosuppressive regimens, some patients are refractory to therapy. Patients with chronic intestinal GVHD usually have multisystem or multiorgan involvement. Complete recovery occurs in slightly more than half of patients. Mortality is approximately 18 percent (186). Extracorporeal photopheresis is a novel therapeutic intervention that may be efficacious in some patients refractory to increased immunosuppressive therapy (174). Clinical responses to this treatment have been reported in patients with both skin and visceral GVHD.

Figure 11-26

GRAFT VERSUS HOST DISEASE

This patient had more severe disease than the patient in figure 11-23.

A: Low-power view of the colonic mucosa demonstrates areas of glandular loss.

B: There is mild architectural change and the lamina propria contains an increased number of inflammatory cells. Scattered crypt abscesses are present.

C: Higher-power view shows apoptotic colonic epithelial cells (arrows). The crypts are infiltrated by neutrophils.

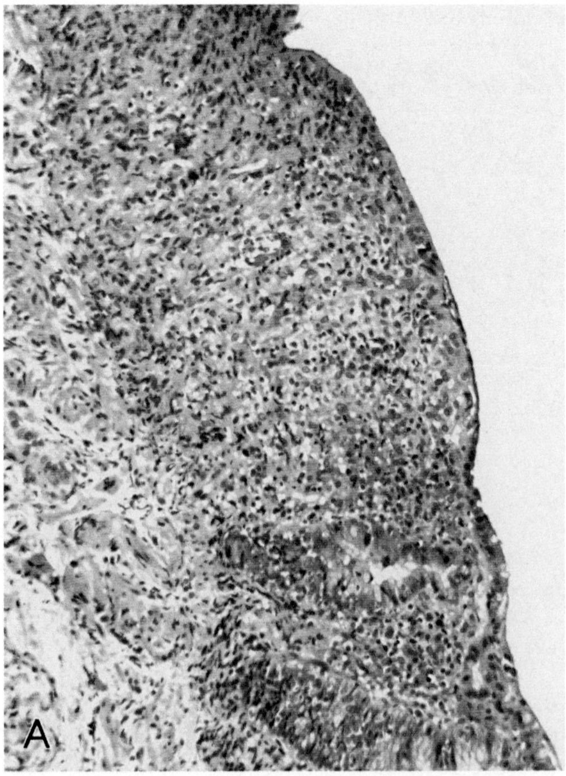

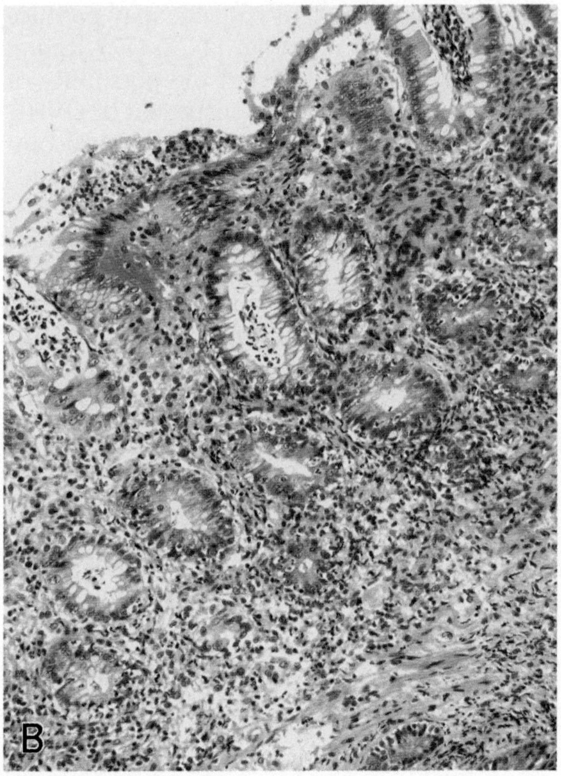

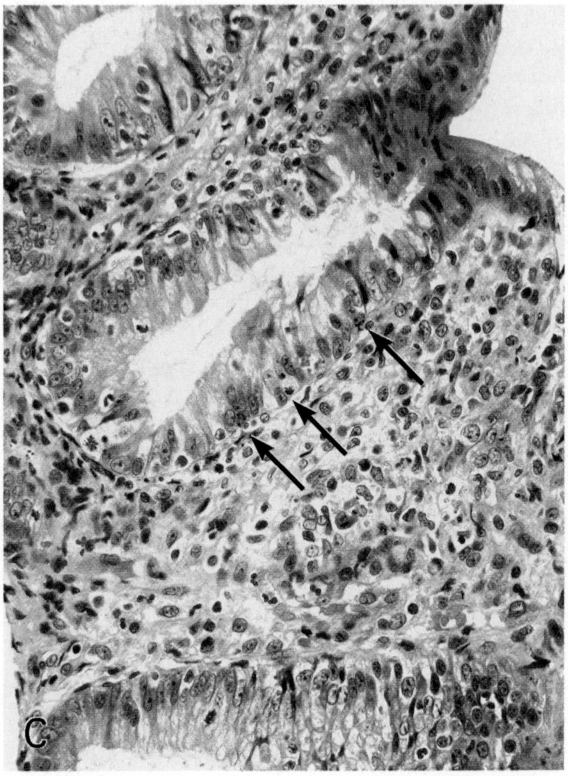

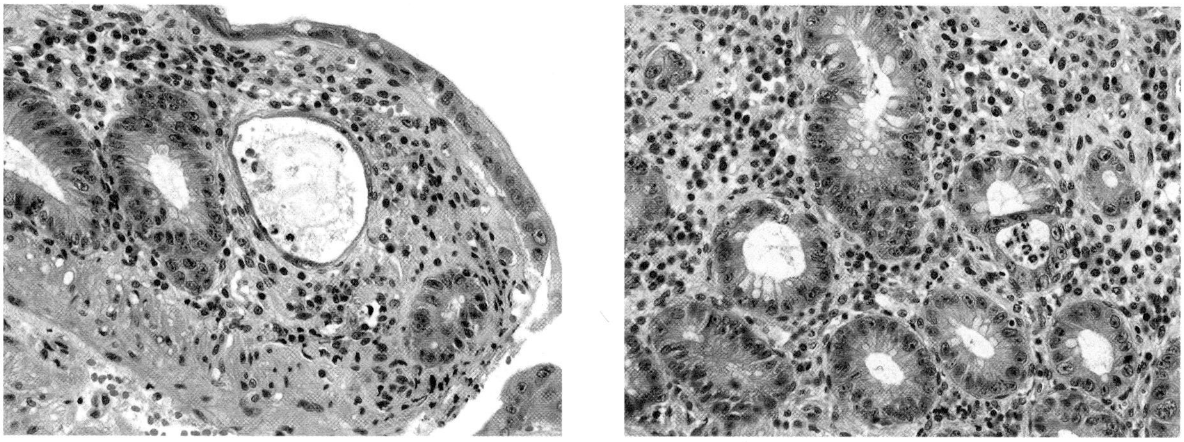

Figure 11-27

MYCOPHENOLATE MOFETIL COLONIC INJURY

Left: Individual crypts appear to be dropping out of the mucosa. The center crypt contains apoptotic and inflammatory debris. The epithelium is flattened.

Right: Cryptitis with a crypt abscess.

REFERENCES

Human Immunodeficiency Virus Infections

1. Alkhatib G, Combadiere C, Broder CC, et al. CC CKR5: A RANTES, MIP1-alpha, MIP 1-beta receptor as a fusion cofactor for macrophage-tropic HIV-1. Science 1996;272:1955–8.
2. Amerongen HM, Weltzin R, Farnet CM, Michetti P, Haseltine WA, Neutra MR. Transepithelial transport of HIV-1 by intestinal M cells: a mechanism for transmission of AIDS. J Acquir Immune Defic Syndr 1991;4:760–5.
3. Balslev E, Thomsen KH, Weisman K. Histopathology of acute human immunodeficiency virus exanthema. J Clin Pathol 1990;43:201–2.
4. Berger EA, Doms RW, Fenyo EM, et al. A new classification for HIV-1. Nature 1998;391:240.
5. Bini EJ, Micale PL, Weinshel EH. Risk factors for rebleeding and mortality from acute upper gastrointestinal hemorrhage in human immunodeficiency virus infection. Am J Gastroenterol 1999;94:358–63.
6. Bini EJ, Weinshel EH, Falkenstein DB. Risk factors for recurrent bleeding and mortality in human immunodeficiency virus infected patients with acute lower GI hemorrhage. Gastrointest Endosc 1999;49:748–53.
7. Blanche S, Tardieu M, Duliege A, et al. Longitudinal study of 94 symptomatic infants with perinatally acquired human immunodeficiency virus infection. Evidence for bimodal expression of clinical and biological symptoms. Am J Dis Child 1990;144:1210–5.
8. Bonfanti P, Valsecchi L, Parazzini F, et al. Incidence of adverse reactions in HIV patients treated with protease inhibitors: a cohort study. J Acquir Immune Defic Syndr 2000;23:236–45.
9. Bozette SA, Berry SH, Duan N, et al. The care of HIV-infected adults in the United States. N Engl J Med 1998;339:1897–904.
10. Busch MP, Lee LL, Satten GA, et al. Time course of detection of viral and serologic markers preceding human immunodeficiency virus type 1 seroconversion: implications for screening of blood and tissue donors. Transfusion 1995;35:91–7.
11. Call SA, Heudebert G, Saag M, Wilcox CM. The changing etiology of chronic diarrhea in HIV-infected patients with CD4 cell counts less than 200 cells/mm^3. Am J Gastroenterol 2000;95:3142–6.
12. Carpenter CC, Fischl MA, Hammer SM, et al. Antiretroviral therapy of HIV in 1996: recommendations of an international panel. JAMA 1996;276:146–54.
13. Carpenter CC, Fischl MA, Hammer SM, et al. Antiretroviral therapy for HIV infection in 1997: updated recommendations of the International AIDS Society—USA panel. JAMA 1997;277:1962–9.

14. Cavert W, Notermans DW, Staskus K, et al. Kinetics of response in lymphoid tissues to antiretroviral therapy of HIV-1 infection. Science 1997;276:960–4.
15. Center for Disease Control. Update: Trends in AIDS incidence, deaths, and prevalence—United States, 1996. JAMA 1997;277:874–5.
16. Chalasani N, Wilcox CM. Etiology and outcome of lower gastrointestinal bleeding in patients with AIDS. Am J Gastroenterol 1998;93:175–8.
17. Chin J. Current and future dimensions of the HIV/AIDS pandemic in women and children. Lancet 1990;336:221–4.
18. Clark SJ, Shaw GM. The acute retroviral syndrome and pathogenesis of HIV-1 infection. Semin Immunol 1993;5:149–55.
19. Cocchi F, De Vico AL, Garzino-Demo A, Arya SK, Gallo RC, Lusso P. Identification of RANTES, MIP-1 alpha, and MIP-1 beta as the major HIV suppressor factors produced by CD8+ T cells. Science 1995;270:1811–5.
20. Cu-Urvin S, Flanigan TP, Rich JD, Mileno MD, Mayer KH, Carpenter CC. Human immunodeficiency virus infection and acquired immunodeficiency syndrome among North American women. Am J Med 1996;101:316–22.
21. De Clerq E. Antivirals and antiviral strategies. Nature Rev Microbiol 2004;2:704–720.
22. Ellakany S, Whiteside TL, Schade RR, van Thiel DH. Analysis of intestinal lymphocyte subpopulations in patients with AIDS and AIDS-related complex. Am J Clin Pathol 1987;87:356–64.
23. Farthing MJG, Kelly MP, Veitch AM. Recently recognised microbial enteropathies and HIV infection. J Antimicrob Chemother 1996;37:61–70.
24. Gillin JS, Shike M, Alcock N, et al. Malabsorption and mucosal abnormalities of the small intestine in the acquired immunodeficiency syndrome. Ann Intern Med 1985;102:619–22.
25. Heath SL, Tew TG, Tew JG, Szakal AK, Burton GF. Follicular dendritic cells and human immunodeficiency virus infectivity. Nature 1995;377: 740–4.
26. Janoff EN, Smith PD. Perspectives on gastrointestinal infections in AIDS. Gastroenterol Clin North Am 1988;17:451–63.
27. Kahn JO, Walker BD. Acute human immunodeficiency virus type I infection. N Engl J Med 1998;339:33–9.
28. Ledergerber B, Egger M, Opravil M, et al. Clinical progression and virological failure on highly active retroviral therapy in HIV-1 patients: a prospective cohort study. Lancet 1999;353:863–8.
29. Levy JA. Infection by human immunodeficiency virus—CD4 is not enough. N Engl J Med 1996;335:1528–30.
30. Lewis DE, Tang DS, Adu-Oppong A, Schober W, Ridgers JR. Anergy and apoptosis in CD8+ T cells from HIV-infected persons. J Immunol 1994;153:412–20.
31. Liu R, Paxton WA, Choe S, et al. Homozygous defect in HIV-1 coreceptor accounts for resistance for some multiply-exposed individuals to HIV-infection. Cell 1996;86:367–77.
32. McLoughlin LC, Nord KS, Joshi VV, Oleske JM, Connor EM. Severe gastrointestinal involvement in children with acquired immunodeficiency syndrome. J Pediatr Gastroenterol Nutr 1987;6:517–24.
33. Mellors JW, Rinaldo CR Jr, Gupta P, White RM, Todd JA. Prognosis in HIV-1 infection predicted by the quantity of virus in plasma. Science 1996;272:1167–70.
34. Mocraft A, Lundgren JD. Starting highly active antiretroviral therapy: why, when and response to HAART. J Antimicrob Chemother 2004;54: 10–3.
35. Mocraft A, Vella S, Benfield TL, et al. Changing patterns of mortality across Europe in patients infected with HIV-1. Lancet 1998;352:1725–30.
36. Monkemuller KE, Wilcox CM. Investigation of diarrhea in AIDS. Can J Gastroenterol 2000;14: 933–40.
37. Mummidi S, Ahuja SS, Gonzalez E, et al. Genealogy of the CCR5 locus and chemokine system gene variants associated with altered rates of HIV-1 disease progression. Nat Med 1998; 4:786–801.
38. Niu MT, Stein DS, Schnittman SM. Primary human immunodeficiency virus type 1 infection: review of pathogenesis and early treatment intervention in humans and animal retrovirus infections. J Infect Dis 1993;168:1490–501.
39. Palella FJ Jr, Delaney KM, Moorman AC, et al. Declining morbidity and mortality among patients with advanced human immunodeficiency virus infection. N Engl J Med 1998;338:853–60.
40. Parente F, Cernuschi M, Antinori S, et al. Severe abdominal pain in patients with AIDS: frequency, clinical aspects, causes, and outcome. Scand J Gastroenterol 1994;29:511–5.
41. Parente F, Cernuschi M, Valsecchi L, et al. Acute upper gastrointestinal bleeding in patients with AIDS: a relatively uncommon condition associated with reduced survival. Gut 1991;32:987–90.
42. Paxton WA, Martin SR, Tse D, et al. Relative resistance to HIV-1 infection of CD4 lymphocytes from persons who remain uninfected despite multiple high-risk sexual exposure. Nat Med 1996;2:2412–7.
43. Phillips AN, Lepri AC, Lampe F, Johnsn M, Sabin CA. When should antiretroviral therapy be started for HIV invedtion? Interpreting the evidence from observational studies. AIDS 2003;17: 1863-1869.
44. Rosenberg ES, Billingsley JM, Caliendo AM, et al. Vigorous HIV-1 specific CD4+ T cell responses associated with control of viremia. Science 1997;278:1447-50.

45. Rwandan HIV Seroprevalence Study Group. Nationwide community-based serological survey of HIV-1 and other human retrovirus infections in a central African country. Lancet 1989;1:941–3.
46. Schacker T, Collier AC, Hughes J, Shea T, Corey L. Clinical and epidemiological features of primary HIV infection. Ann Intern Med 1996;125: 257–64.
47. Scott GB, Buck BE, Leterman JG, Bloom FL, Parks WP. Acquired immunodeficiency syndrome in infants. N Engl J Med 1984;310:76–81.
48. Sneller MC, Strober W. M cells and host defense. J Infect Dis 1986;154:737–41.
49. Weiss RA. HIV receptors and the pathogenesis of AIDS. Science 1996;272:1885–6.
50. World Health Organization and Centers for Disease Control: Statistics from the World Health Organization and the Centers for Disease Control. AIDS 1990;4:605–10.
51. Zaitseva M, Blauvelt A, Lee S, et al. Expression and function of CCR5 and CXCR4 on human Langerhans cells and macrophages: implications for HIV primary infection. Nat Med 1997;3: 1369–75.

HIV Enteropathy

52. Ferreira RC, Forsyth LE, Richman PI, Wells C, Spencer J, MacDonald TT. Changes in the rate of crypt epithelial cell proliferation and mucosal morphology induced by a T-cell-mediated response in human small intestine. Gastroenterology 1990;98:1255–63.
53. Hing MC, Goldschmidt C, Mathijs JM, Cunningham AL, Cooper DA. Chronic colitis associated with human immunodeficiency virus infection. Med J Aust 1992;156:683–7.
54. Nelson JA, Wiley CA, Reynolds-Kohler CA, Reese CE, Margaretten W, Levy JA. Human immunodeficiency virus detected in bowel epithelium from patients with gastrointestinal symptoms. Lancet 1988;1:259–62.
55. Simon D, Brandt LJ. Diarrhea in patients with the acquired immunodeficiency syndrome. Gastroenterology 1993;105:1238–42.
56. Ullrich R, Zeitz M, Heise W, et al. Mucosal atrophy is associated with loss of activated T cells in the duodenal mucosa of human immunodeficiency virus (HIV)-infected patients. Digestion 1990;46:302–7.

Disease in Specific Gastrointestinal Locations

57. Denis BJ, May T, Bigard MA, Canton P. Anal and perianal diseases in symptomatic HIV infection: a prospective study in 190 patients. Gastroenterol Clin Biol 1992;16:148–54.
58. Moskovitz BL, Stanton TL, Kusmierek JJ. Spiramycin therapy for cryptosporidial diarrhea in immunocompromised patients. J Antimicrob Chemother 1988;22:189–91.
59. Wilcox CM, Straub RF, Schwartz DA. Prospective evaluation of biopsy number for the diagnosis of viral esophagitis in patients with HIV infection and esophageal ulcer. Gastrointest Endosc 1996;44:587–93.
60. Wilcox CM, Zaki SR, Coffield LM, Greer PW, Schwartz DA. Evaluation of idiopathic esophageal ulceration for human immunodeficiency virus. Mod Pathol 1996;8:568–72.

Mycobacterium Avium Complex

61. Agins BD, Berman DS, Spiechandler D, el-Sadr W, Simberkoff MS, Rahal JJ. Effect of combined therapy with ansamycin, clofazimine, ethambutol and isoniazid for *Mycobacterium avium* infection in patients with AIDS. J Infect Dis 1989;159:784–7.
62. Body BA, Warren NG, Spicer A, Henderson D, Chery M. Use of Gen-Probe and BACTEC for rapid isolation and identification of mycobacteria. Am J Clin Pathol 1990;93:415–20.
63. Burmudez LE, Parker A, Goodman JR. Growth within macrophages increases the efficiency of *Mycobacterium avium* in invading other macrophages by a complement receptor independent pathway. Infect Immun 1997;65:1916–25.
64. Chiu J, Nussbaum J, Bozzette S, et al. Treatment of disseminated *Mycobacterium avium* complex infection in AIDS with amikacin, ethambutol, rifampin, and ciprofloxacin. Ann Intern Med 1990;113:358–61.
65. Gadelha A, Accacio N, Grinzstejn B, et al. Low incidence of colonization and no cases of disseminated *Mycobacterium avium* complex infection (DMAC) in Brazilian AIDS patients in the HAART era. Braz J Infect Dis 2002;6:252–7.
66. Gray JR, Rabeneck L. Atypical mycobacterial infection of the gastrointestinal tract in AIDS patients. Am J Gastroenterol 1989;84:1521–4.
67. Horsburgh CR Jr. *Mycobacterium avium* complex infection in the acquired immunodeficiency syndrome. N Engl J Med 1991;324:1332–8.
68. Horsburgh CR Jr, Chin DP, Yajko DM, et al. Environmental risk factors for acquisition of *Mycobacterium avium* complex in persons with human immunodeficiency virus infection. J Infect Dis 1994;170:362–7.
69. Klatt EC, Jensen DF, Meyer PR. Pathology of *Mycobacterium avium-intracellulare* infection in acquired immunodeficiency syndrome. Hum Pathol 1987;18:709–14.
70. Mizutani S. Nontuberculous mycobacteroides: the present status and in the future. Infection with human immunodeficiency virus (HIV) and nontuberculous mycobacteriosis. Kekkaku 1998;73:87–92.

71. Nightingale SD, Cameron DW, Gordin FM, et al. Two controlled trials of rifabutin prophylaxis against *Mycobacterium avium* complex infection in AIDS. N Engl J Med 1993;329:828–33.
72. Okhusu K, Bermudez LE, Nash KA, MacGregor RR, Inderlied CB. Differential virulence of *Mycobacterium avium* strains isolated from HIV-infected patients with disseminated *M. avium* complex disease. J Infect Dis 2004;190:1347–54.
73. Sangari FJ, Goodman J, Bermudez LE. *Mycobacterium avium* enters intestinal epithelial cells through the apical membrane, but not by the basolateral surface, activated small GTPase Rho and, once within epithelial cells, expresses an invasive phenotype. Cell Microbiol 2000;2:561–8.
74. von Reyn CF, Arbeit RD, Horsburgh CR, et al. Sources of disseminated *Mycobacterium avium* infection in AIDS. J Infect 2002;44:166–70.
75. von Reyn CF, Arbeit RD, Tosteson AN, et al. The international epidemiology of disseminated *Mycobacterium avium* complex infection in AIDS. AIDS 1996;10:1025–32.
76. von Reyn CF, Maslow JN, Barber TW, Falkinham JO, Arbeit RD. Persistant colonization of potable water as a source of *Mycobacterium avium* infection in patients with AIDS. Lancet 1994;343:1137–41.
77. von Reyn CF, Waddell RD, Eaton T, et al. Isolation of *Mycobacterium avium* complex from water in the United States, Finland, Zaire, and Kenya. J Clin Microbiol 1993;31:3227–30.
78. Wallace JM, Hannah JB. *Mycobacterium avium* complex infection in patients with the acquired immunodeficiency syndrome. A clinicopathologic study. Chest 1988;93:926–32.

Mycobacterium Tuberculosis Infections

79. Bender BS, Davidson BL, Kline R, Brown C, Quinn TC. Role of the mononuclear phagocyte system in the immunopathogenesis of human immunodeficiency virus infection and the acquired immunodeficiency syndrome. Rev Infect Dis 1988;10:1142–54.
80. Centers for Disease Control. Tuberculosis outbreak among HIV-infected persons. JAMA 1991;15:2058–61.
81. Daley CL, Small PM, Schechter GF, et al. An outbreak of tuberculosis with accelerated progression among persons infected with the human immunodeficiency virus. N Engl J Med 1992;326:231–5.
82. Monkemuller KE, Wilcox CM. Diagnosis and treatment of colonic disease in AIDS. Gastrointest Endosc Clin North Am 1998;8:889–911.

Spirochetosis

83. Duhamel GE, Trott DJ, Muniappa N, et al. Canine intestinal spirochetes consist of *Serpulina pilosicoli* and a newly identified group provisionally designed "*Serpulina canis*" sp nov. J Clin Microbiol 1998;36:2264–70.
84. Gebbers JO, Ferguson DJ, Mason C, Kelly P, Jewell DP. *Spirochaetosis* of the human rectum associated with an intraepithelial mast cell and IgE plasma cell response. Gut 1987;28:588–93.
85. Guccion JG, Benator DA, Zeller J, Termanini B, Saini N. Intestinal spirochetosis and acquired immunodeficiency syndrome: ultrastructural studies of two cases. Ultrastruc Pathol 1995;19:15–22.
86. Kostman JR, Patel M, Catalano E, Camacho J, Hoffpauir J, DiNubile MJ. Invasive colitis and hepatitis due to previously uncharacterized spirochetes in patients with advanced human immunodeficiency virus infection. Clin Infect Dis 1995;21:1159–65.
87. Lee FD, Kraszewski A, Gordon J, Howie JG, McSeveney D, Harland WA. Intestinal spirochetosis. Gut 1971;12:126–33.
88. Trivett-Moore NL, Gilbert GL, Law CL, Trott DJ, Hampson DJ. Isolation of *Serpulina pilosicoli* from rectal biopsy specimens showing evidence of intestinal spirochetosis. J Clin Microbiol 1998;36:261–5.

Cytomegalovirus Infections

89. Alford CA, Stagno S, Pass RF, Britt WJ. Congenital and perinatal cytomegalovirus infections. Rev Infect Dis 1990;12(Suppl 7):S745–53.
90. Chalasani N, Parker KM, Wilcox CM. Bronchoesophageal fistula as a complication of cytomegalovirus esophagitis in AIDS. Endoscopy 1997;29:S28–9.
91. Collier AC, Meyers JD, Corey L, Murphy VL, Roberts PL, Handsfield HH. Cytomegalovirus infection in homosexual men: relationship to sexual practices, antibody to human immunodeficiency virus, and cell-mediated immunity. Am J Med 1987;82:593–601.
92. Fowler KB, Stagno S, Pass RF. Maternal age and congenital cytomegalovirus infection: screening of two diverse newborn populations, 1980-1990. J Infect Dis 1993;168:552–6.
93. Gallant JE, Moore RD, Richman DD, Keruly J, Chaisson RE. Incidence and natural history of cytomegalovirus disease in patients with advanced human immunodeficiency virus disease treated with zidovudine. The Zidovudine Epidemiology Study Group. J Infect Dis 1992;166:1223–7.
94. Goodgame RW. Gastrointestinal cytomegalovirus disease. Ann Intern Med 1993;119:924–35.
95. Goodgame RW, Genta RM, Estrada R, Demmler G, Buffone G. Frequency of positive tests for cytomegalovirus in AIDS patients: endoscopic lesions compared with normal mucosa. Am J Gastroenterol 1993;88:338–43.
96. Kovacs A, Schluchter M, Easley K, et al. Cytomegalovirus infection and HIV-1 disease progression in infants born to HIV-1-infected women. N Engl J Med 1999;341:77–84.

97. Mentec H, Leport C, Leport J, Marche C, Harzic M, Vilde JL. Cytomegalovirus colitis in HIV-1-infected patients: a prospective research in 55 patients. AIDS 1994;8:461–7.
98. Pallela FP Jr, Delaney KM, Moorman AC, et al. Declining morbidity and mortality among patients with advanced human immunodeficiency virus infection. N Engl J Med 1998;338: 853–60.
99. Shintaku M, Inoue N, Sasaki M, Izuno Y, Ueda Y, Ikehara S. Cytomegalovirus vasculitis accompanied by an exuberant fibroblastic reaction in the intestine of an AIDS patient. Acta Pathol Jpn 1991;41:900–4.
100. Springer KL, Weinberg A. Cytomegalovirus infection in the era of HAART: fewer reactivations and more immunity. J Antimicrob Chemother 2004;54:582–6.

Herpes Simplex Virus Infections

101. Bagdades EK, Pillay D, Squire SB, O'Neil C, Johnson MA, Griffiths PD. Relationship between herpes simplex virus ulceration and CD4+ cell counts in patients with HIV infection. AIDS 1992;6:1317–20.
102. Genereau T, Lortholary O, Bouchaud O, et al. Herpes simplex esophagitis in patients with AIDS: report of 34 cases. The Cooperative Study Group on Herpetic Esophagitis in HIV Infection. Clin Infect Dis 1996;22:926–31.

Other Viral Infections

103. Gonzalez GG, Pujol FH, Liprandi F, Deibis L, Ludert JE. Prevalence of enteric viruses in human immunodeficiency virus seropositive patients in Venezuela. J Med Virol 1998;55:288–92.
104. Grohmann GS, Glass RI, Pereira HG, et al. Enteric viruses and diarrhea in HIV-infected patients. Enteric Opportunistic Infections Working Group. N Engl J Med 1993;329:14–20.
105. Janoff EN, Orenstein JM, Manischewitz JF, Smith PD. Adenovirus colitis in the acquired immunodeficiency syndrome. Gastroenterology 1991;100:976–9.
106. Khoo SH, Bailey AS, de Jong JC, Mandal BK. Adenovirus infections in human immunodeficiency virus-positive patients: clinical features and molecular epidemiology. J Infect Dis 1995;172:629–37.
107. Maddox A, Francis N, Moss J, Blanshard C, Gazzard B. Adenovirus infection in the large bowel in HIV positive patients. J Clin Pathol 1992;45:684–8.
108. Parkin J, Tums S, Roberts A, et al. "Cytomegalovirus" colitis: can it be caused by adenovirus? III International Conference on AIDS, Abstracts, no volume editor, University Publishing Group, Frederick MD, Conference date: June 1-5, 1987, Washington DC.
109. Smith PD, Lane HC, Gill VJ, et al. Intestinal infection in patients with acquired immunodeficiency syndrome (AIDS). Etiology and response to therapy. Ann Intern Med 1988;108:328–33.
110. Yi ES, Powell HC. Adenovirus infection of the duodenum in an AIDS patient: an ultrastructural study. Ultrastructural Pathol 1994;18:549–51.

Candida Infections

111. Bonacini M, Laine L, Gal AA, Lee MH, Martin SE, Strigle S. Prospective evaluation of blind brushing of the esophagus for *Candida* esophagitis in patients with human immunodeficiency virus infection. Am J Gastroenterol 1990;85:385–9.
112. Jayagopal S, Cervia JS. Colitis due to *Candida albicans* in a patient with AIDS. Clin Infect Dis 1992;15:555.
113. Malebranche R, Arnoux E, Guerin JM, et al. Acquired immunodeficiency syndrome with severe gastrointestinal manifestations in Haiti. Lancet 1983;2:873–8.
114. Wilcox CM, Straub RF, Clark WS. Prospective evaluation of oropharyngeal findings in human immunodeficiency virus-infected patients with esophageal ulceration. Am J Gastroenterol 1995;90:1938–41.

Other Fungal Infections

115. Wei SC, Hung CC, Chen MY, Wang CY, Chuang CY, Wong JM. Endoscopy in acquired immunodeficiency syndrome patients with diarrhea and negative stool studies. Gastrointest Endosc 2000;51:427–32.

Disseminated *Pneumocystis carinii* Infections

116. Carter TR, Cooper PH, Petri, WA Jr, Kim CK, Walzer PD, Guerrant RL. *Pneumocystis carinii* infection of the small intestine in a patient with acquired immune deficiency syndrome. Am J Clin Pathol 1988;89:679–83.
117. Matsuda S, Urata Y, Shiota T, et al. Disseminated infection of *Pneumocystis carinii* in a patient with the acquired immunodeficiency syndrome. Virchows Arch A Cell Pathol 1989;414: 523–7.

Cryptosporidium Infections

118. Angus KW, Campbell I, Gray EW, Sherwood D. Staining of faecal yeasts and *Cryptosporidium* oocysts. Vet Rec 1981;108:173.
119. Cook DJ, Kelton JG, Stainsz AM, Collins SM. Somatostatin treatment for cryptosporidial diarrhea in a patient with the acquired immunodeficiency syndrome (AIDS). Ann Intern Med 1988;108:708–9.

120. Garcia LS, Brewer TC, Bruckner DA. Incidence of *Cryptosporidium* in all patients submitting stool specimens for ova and parasite examination: monoclonal antibody IFA method. Diagn Microbiol Infect Dis 1988;11:25–7.
121. Garone MA, Winston BJ, Lewis JH. Cryptosporidiosis of the stomach. Am J Gastroenterol 1986;81:465–70.
122. Goodgame RW, Kimball K, Ou CN, et al. Intestinal function and injury in acquired immunodeficiency syndrome-related cryptosporidiosis. Gastroenterology 1995;108:1075–82.
122a. Malebranche R, Arnoux E, Guerin JM, et al. Acquired immunodeficiency syndrome with severe gastrointestinal manifestations in Haiti. Lancet 1983;2:873–8.
123. Manabe YC, Clark DP, Moore RD, et al. Cryptosporidiosis in patients with AIDS: correlates of disease and survival. Clin Infect Dis 1998;27: 536–42.
123a. Moskovitz BL, Stanton TL, Kusmierek JJ. Spiramycin therapy for cryptosporidial diarrhea in immunocompromised patients. J Antimicrob Chemother 1988;22:189–91.
124. Pozio E, Rezza G, Boschini A, et al. Clinical cryptosporidiosis and human immunodeficiency virus (HIV)-induced immunosuppression: findings from a longitudinal study of HIV-positive and HIV-negative former injection drug users. J Infect Dis 1997;176:969–75.
125. Siddons CA, Chapman PA, Rush BA. Evaluation of an enzyme immunoassay kit for detecting cryptosporidium in faeces and environmental samples. J Clin Path 1992;45:479–82.
126. Sterling CR, Arrowood MJ. Detection of cryptosporidium sp. infections using a direct immunofluorescence assay. Pediatr Infect Dis 1986;5:S139–42.
127. Ungar BL, Ward DJ, Fayer R, Quinn CA. Cessation of *Cryptosporidium*-associated diarrhea in an acquired immunodeficiency syndrome patient after treatment with hyperimmune bovine colostrum. Gastroenterology 1990;98:486–9.
128. White AC Jr, Chappell CL, Hayat CS, Kimball KT, Flanigan TP, Goodgame RW. Paromomycin for cryptosporidiosis in AIDS: a prospective, double-blind trial. J Infect Dis 1994;170: 419–24.

Isospora Belli Infections

129. DeHovitz JA, Pape JW, Boncy M, Johnson WD Jr. Clinical manifestations and therapy of *Isospora belli* infection in patients with the acquired immunodeficiency syndrome. N Engl J Med 1986;315:87–90.
130. Ma P, Kaufman D. *Isospora belli* diarrheal infection in homosexual men. AIDS Res 1984;1: 327–38.
131. Michiels JF, Hofman P, Bernard E, et al. Intestinal and extraintestinal *Isospora belli* infection in an AIDS patient. Path Res Pract 1994; 190:1089–93.
132. Restrepo C, Macher AM, Radany EH. Disseminated extraintestinal isosporiasis in a patient with acquired immune deficiency syndrome. Am J Clin Pathol 1987;87:536–42.

Microsporidium Infections

133. Aldras AM, Orenstein JM, Kotler, Shadduck JA, Didier ES. Detection of microsporidia by indirect immunofluorescence antibody test using polyclonal and monoclonal antibodies. J Clin Microbiol 1994;32:608–12.
134. Bryan RT, Cali A, Owen RL, Spencer HC. Microsporidia: opportunistic pathogens in patients with AIDS. Prog Clin Parasitol 1991;2:1–26.
135. Canning EU, Hollister WS. The Microsporidia of Vertebrates. New York: Academic Press; 1986.
136. Carr A, Marriott D, Field A, Vasak E, Cooper DA. Treatment of HIV-1-associated microsporidiosis and cryptosporidiosis with combination antiretroviral therapy. Lancet 1998;351:256–61.
137. Conteas CN, Sowerby T, Berlin GW, et al. Fluorescence techniques for diagnosing intestinal microsporidiosis in stool, enteric fluid, and biopsy specimens from acquired immunodeficiency syndrome patients with chronic diarrhea. Arch Pathol Lab Med 1996;120:847–53.
138. Croppo GP, Croppo GP, Moura H, et al. Ultrastructure, immunofluorescence, western blot, and PCR analysis of eight isolates of *Encephalitozoon (Septata) intestinalis* established in culture from sputum and urine samples and duodenal aspirates of five patients with AIDS. J Clin Microbiol 1998;36:1201–8.
139. Dore GJ, Marriott DJ, Hing MC, Harkness JL, Fields AS. Disseminated microsporidiosis due to *Septata intestinalis* in nine patients infected with the human immunodeficiency virus: response to therapy with albendazole. Clin Infect Dis 1995;21:70–6.
140. Enriquez FJ, Ditrich O, Palting JD, Smith K. Simple diagnosis of *Encephalitozoon* sp. microsporidial infections by using a panspecific antiexospore monoclonal antibody. J Clin Microbiol 1997;35:724–9.
141. Gumbo T, Sarbah S, Gangaidzo IT, et al. Intestinal parasites in patients with diarrhea and human immunodeficiency virus infection in Zimbabwe. AIDS 1999;13:819–21.
142. Gunnarsson G, Hurlbut D, DeGirolami PC, Federman M, Wanke C. Multiorgan microsporidiosis: report of five cases and review. Clin Infect Dis 1995;21:37–44.
143. Kotler DP, Orenstein JM. Prevalence of intestinal microsporidiosis in HIV-infected individuals referred for gastroenterologic evaluation. Am J Gastroenterol 1994;89:1998–2002.

144. Ligoury O, David F, Sarfati C, et al. Diagnosis of infections caused by *Enterocytozoon bieneusi* and *Encephalitozoon intestinalis* using polymerase chain reaction in stool specimens. AIDS 1997;11:723–6.
145. Lumb R, Swift J, James C, Papanaoum K, Mukherjee T. Identification of the microsporidian parasite, *Enterocytozoon bieneusi* in faecal samples and intestinal biopsies from an AIDS patient. Int J Parasitol 1993;23:793–801.
146. Michiels JF, Hofman P, Saint Paul C, Loubière R. Pathological features of intestinal microsporidiosis in HIV positive patients: a report of 13 new cases. Path Res Pract 1993;189:377–83.
147. Molina JM, Sarfati C, Beauvais B, et al. Intestinal microsporidiosis in human immunodeficiency virus-infected patients with chronic unexplained diarrhea: prevalence and clinical and biological features. J Infect Dis 1993;167: 217–21.
148. Navin TR, Weber R, Vugia DJ, et al. Declining CD4+ T-lymphocyte counts are associated with increased risk of enteric parasitosis and chronic diarrhea: results of a 3-year longitudinal study. J Acquir Immune Defic Syndr Hum Retrovirol 1999;20:154–9.
149. Orenstein JM. Intestinal microsporidiosis. Adv Anat Pathol 1996;3:46–58.
150. Orenstein JM, Dietrich DT, Lew EA, Kotler DP. Albendazole as a treatment for intestinal and disseminated microsporidiosis due to *Septata intestinalis* in AIDS patients: a report of four patients. AIDS 1993;7:S40–2.
151. Orenstein JM, Tenner M, Cali A, Kotler DP. A microsporidian previously undescribed in humans, infecting enterocytes and macrophages, and associated with diarrhea in an acquired immunodeficiency syndrome patient. Hum Pathol 1992;23:722–8.
152. Rabeneck L, Genta RM, Gyorkey F, Clarridge JE, Gyorkey P, Foote LW. Observations on the pathological spectrum and clinical course of microsporidiosis in men infected with the human immunodeficiency virus: follow-up study. Clin Infect Dis 1995;20:1229–35.
153. Schwartz DA, Bryan RT, Hewan-Lowe KO, et al. Disseminated microsporidiosis (*Encephalitozoon hellem*) and acquired immunodeficiency syndrome: autopsy evidence for respiratory acquisition. Arch Pathol Lab Med 1992;116:660–8.
154. Schwartz DA, Sobottka I, Leitch GJ, Cali A, Visvesvara GS. Pathology of microsporidiosis: emerging parasitic infections in patients with acquired immunodeficiency syndrome. Arch Pathol Lab Med 1996;120:173–88.
155. Soule JB, Halverson AL, Becker RB, Pistole MC, Orenstein JM. A patient with acquired immunodeficiency syndrome and untreated *Encephalitozoon (Septata) intestinalis* microsporidiosis leading to small bowel perforation. Response to albendazole. Arch Pathol Lab Med 1997;121: 880–7.
156. Velasquez JN, Carnevale S, Labbe JH, Chertcoff A, Cabrera MG, Oelemann W. In situ hybridization: a molecular approach for the diagnosis of the microsporidian parasite *Enterocytozoon bieneusi*. Hum Pathol 1999;30:54–8.
157. Wanachiwanawin D, Manatsathit S, Lertlaituan P, Thakerngpol K, Suwanagool P. Intestinal microsporidiosis in HIV infected patients with chronic diarrhea in Thailand. Southeast Asian J Trop Med Public Health 1998;29:767–71.
158. Weber R, Bryan RT, Owen RL, Wilcox CM, Gorelkin L, Visvesvara GS. Improved light-microscopic detection of microsporidia spores in stool and duodenal aspirates. The Enteric Opportunistic Infections Working Group. N Engl J Med 1992;326:161–6.
159. Weber R, Ledergerber B, Zbinden R, et al. Enteric infections and diarrhea in human immunodeficiency virus-infected persons: prospective community-based cohort study. Swiss HIV Cohort Study. Arch Intern Med 1999;159: 1473–80.

Toxoplasmosis

160. Alpert L, Miller M, Alpert E, Satin R, Lamoureux E, Trudel L. Gastric toxoplasmosis in acquired immunodeficiency syndrome: antemortem diagnosis with histopathologic characterization. Gastroenterology 1996;110:258–64.
161. Ganji M, Tan A, Maitar MI, Weldon-Linne CM, Weisenberg E, Rhone DP. Gastric toxoplasmosis in a patient with acquired immunodeficiency syndrome. A case report and review of the literature. Arch Pathol Lab Med 2003;127: 732–4.
162. Garcia LW, Hemphill RB, Marasco WA, Ciano PS. Acquired immunodeficiency syndrome with disseminated toxoplasmosis presenting as an acute pulmonary and gastrointestinal illness. Arch Pathol Lab Med 1991;115:459–63.
163. Gleason TH, Hamlin WB. Disseminated toxoplasmosis in the compromised host: a report of five cases. Arch Intern Med 1974;134:1059–62.
164. Jautzke G, Sell M, Thalmann U, et al. Extracerebral toxoplasmosis in AIDS. Histological and immunohistological findings based on 80 autopsy cases. Pathol Res Pract 1993;189:428–36.

Graft Versus Host Disease

165. Anderson KC, Weinstein HJ. Transfusion-associated graft-versus-host disease. N Engl J Med 1990;323:315–21.

166. Billingham RE. The biopsy of graft-versus-host reactions. Harvey Lect 1966-1067;62:21–78.
167. Burdick JF, Vogelsang GB, Smith WJ, et al. Severe graft-versus-host disease in a liver-transplant recipient. N Engl J Med 1988;318:689–91.
168. Cox GJ, Matsui SM, Lo RS, et al. Etiology and outcome of diarrhea after marrow transplantation: a prospective study. Gastroenterology 1994;107:1398–407.
169. Cruz-Correa M, Poonawala A, Abraham SC, et al. Endoscopic findings predict the histologic diagnosis of gastrointestinal graft-versus-host disease. Endoscopy 2002;34:808–13.
170. Dinsmore RE, Straus DJ, Pollack MS, et al. Fatal graft-v-host disease following blood transfusion in Hodgkin's disease documented by HLA typing. Blood 1980;55:831–4.
171. Easaw S, Lake D, Beer M, Seiter K, Feldman EJ, Ahmed T. Graft-versus-host disease. Possible higher risk for African American patients. Cancer 1996;78:1492–7.
172. Falkenburg JH, van de Corput L, Marijt EW, Willemze R. Minor histocompatibility antigens in human stem cell transplantation. Exp Hematol 2003;31:743–51.
173. Forbes GM, Rule SA, Herrmann RP, et al. A prospective study of screening upper gastrointestinal (GI) endoscopy prior to and after bone marrow transplantation (BMT). Aust N Z J Med 1995;25:32–6.
174. Foss FM, Gorgun G, Miller KB. Extracorporeal photopheresis in chronic graft-versus-host disease. Bone Marrow Transplant 2002;29:719–25.
175. Glucksburg H, Storb R, Fefar A, et al. Clinical manifestations of graft-versus-host disease in human recipients of marrow from HLA-matched sibling donors. Transplantation 1984;18:295–304.
176. Goulet O, Revillon Y, Jan D, et al. Small-bowel transplantation in children. Transplant Proc 1990;22:2499–500.
177. Graze PR, Gale RP. Chronic graft-versus-host disease: a syndrome of disordered immunity. Am J Med 1979;66:611–20.
178. Grogan TM, Odom RB, Burgess JH. Graft-vs-host reaction. Arch Dermatol 1977;113:806–12.
179. Gulbuhce HE, Brown CA, Wick M, Segall M, Jessurun J. Graft-versus-host disease after solid organ transplant. Am J Clin Pathol 2003;119: 568–73.
180. Mason DW, Dallman M, Barclay AN. Graft-versus-host disease induces expression of Ia antigen in rat epidermal cells and gut epithelium. Nature 1981;293:150–1.
181. McDonald GB, Sullivan KM, Schuffler MD, Shulman HM, Thomas ED. Esophageal abnormalities in chronic graft-versus-host disease in humans. Gastroenterology 1981;80:914–21.
182. Minocha A, Mandanas RA, Kida M, Jazzar A. Bullous esophagitis due to chronic graft-versus-host disease. Am J Gastroenterol 1997;92:529–30.
183. Nagata S. Apoptosis by death factor. Cell 1997; 88:355–65.
184. Otero Lopez-Cubero S, Sale GE, McDonald GB. Acute graft-versus-host disease of the esophagus. Endoscopy 1997;29:S35–6.
185. Papadimitriou JC, Cangro CB, Lustberg A, et al. Histologic features of mycophenolate mofetil-related colitis: a graft-versus-host disease-like pattern. Int J Surg Pathol 2003;11:295–302.
186. Patey-Mariaud de Serre N, Reijasse D, Verkarre V, et al. Chronic intestinal graft-versus-host disease: clinical, histological and immunohistochemical analysis of 17 children. Bone Marrow Transplant 2002;29:223–30.
187. Ponec RJ, Hackman RC, McDonald GB. Endoscopic and histologic diagnosis of intestinal graft-versus-host disease after marrow transplantation. Gastrointest Endosc 1999;49:612–21.
188. Sale GE, Shulman HM, Galluci BD, Thomas ED. Young rete ridge keratinocytes are preferred targets in cutaneous graft-versus-host disease in man. Am J Pathol 1985;118:278–87.
189. Silva MR, Henne K, Sale GE. Positive identification of enterocytes by keratin antibody staining of sloughed intestinal tissue in severe GVHD. Bone Marrow Transplant 1993;12:35–6.
190. Snover DC. Mucosal damage simulating acute graft-versus-host reaction in cytomegalovirus colitis. Transplantation 1985;39:669–70.
191. Snover DC, Weisdorf SA, Vercelloti GM, Rank B, Hutton S, McGlave P. A histopathologic study of gastric and small intestinal graft-versus-host disease following allogeneic bone marrow transplantation. Hum Pathol 1985;16:387–92.
192. Storb R. Marrow transplantation: the Seattle experience. Tokai J Exp Clin Med 1985;10:75–83.
193. Takata M. Immunohistochemical identification of perforin-positive cytotoxic lymphocytes in graft-versus-host disease. Am J Clin Pathol 1995;103:324–9.
194. Washington K, Bentley R, Green A, Olson J, Treem WR, Krigman HR. Gastric graft-versus-host disease: a blinded histologic study. Am J Surg Pathol 1997;21:1037–46.
195. Wirt DP, Brooks EG, Vaidya S, Klimpel GR, Waldmann TA, Goldblum RM. Novel T-lymphocyte population in combined immunodeficiency with features of graft-vs-host disease. N Engl J Med 1989;321:370–4.

12 MALABSORPTION SYNDROMES

INTRODUCTION

Malabsorption syndromes result from the deficient uptake of various types of nutrients, so that there are insufficient nutrients and calories available to maintain normal homeostasis. Although *malabsorption* and *maldigestion* are related in terms of clinical presentation and complications, pathophysiologically they are different. Maldigestion results from defective intraluminal hydrolysis of nutrients, while malabsorption occurs secondarily to defective mucosal nutrient uptake following digestion. In addition, intestinal motility, solubilization of nutrients, and various exocrine and endocrine hormones are involved in normal absorption.

Demography

Malabsorption syndromes affect people of all ages. Age incidence depends upon the underlying etiology. Celiac disease, the most common cause of malabsorption in developed countries, is detected at almost any age. Congenital enzyme deficiencies present as malabsorption in children. In elderly patients, chronic intestinal ischemia, congestive heart failure, and bacterial overgrowth are common causes of malabsorption. The prevalence of a particular type of malabsorption syndrome may also vary in different ethnic groups. For example, celiac disease is the most common cause of malabsorption in Western Europe and the United States while infectious diseases, lactase deficiency, and nutritional deficiencies are the usual causes of malabsorption in the developing world.

Etiopathogenesis

Malabsorption syndromes occur by one of three broad categories of pathogenetic mechanisms. These categories form the basis of the laboratory approach used to make a specific diagnosis.

The first category is that of premucosal disease. Defective digestion and absorption result from pancreatic or other systemic diseases and reduced local bile salt concentration. The second, and most common group of disorders that a surgical pathologist is likely to face, is that of mucosal diseases. Mucosal defects are due to anatomic or biochemical alterations in the epithelium, the presence of microorganisms, or inflammatory or infiltrative processes affecting the lamina propria. The third group of disorders is the postmucosal diseases. Malabsorption occurs because of lymphatic obstruction, vascular disease, or congestive cardiac failure. Table 12-1 summarizes the various causes of malabsorption.

Because clinically diagnosed malabsorption may be due to diverse causative factors, it is essential that the pathologist be supplied with sufficient clinical information, including results of laboratory or serologic tests, before any attempt to arrive at a specific diagnosis is undertaken. The presence of a normal small intestinal biopsy does not exclude many conditions leading to malabsorption (Tables 12-2, 12-3). Table 12-4 lists the information that should be provided to the pathologist interpreting small bowel biopsies for malabsorption.

Choice of Specimen

Small intestinal biopsies can be obtained by either a suction capsule or by forceps after endoscopic visualization. The suction capsule method requires radiographic guidance and is more expensive than the more commonly used forceps biopsy. Studies have shown no significant difference in diagnostic yield between these two techniques (2). Focal or patchy lesions can be visualized and then biopsied by the endoscopic method (1,3). This technique also permits visualization of the gastrointestinal tract, and radiation exposure associated with suction biopsy is avoided. Capsule biopsies are still preferred to endoscopic biopsies by some gastroenterologists when a diagnosis is being sought in a child younger than 2 years of age.

Either the duodenum or the jejunum is an appropriate site for biopsy. Most endoscopic

Table 12-1

CAUSES OF MALABSORPTION

Inadequate Digestion
Postgastrectomy steatorrhea
Deficient activation of pancreatic lipase
Chronic pancreatitis
Pancreatic carcinoma
Cystic fibrosis
Pancreatic resection
Reduced intestinal bile salt concentration (with impaired micelle formation)
Abnormalities in Bile Production and Metabolism
Parenchymal liver disease
Extrahepatic biliary obstruction
Interrupted enterohepatic circulation of bile salts
Inadequate Absorptive Surface Secondary to Surgical Procedures
Blind loop syndrome
Ileal resection
Drugs
Neomycin
Calcium carbonate
Cholestyramine
Colchicine
Lymphatic Obstruction
Intestinal lymphangiectasia
Whipple's disease
Lymphoma
Inflammatory or Infiltrative Disorders
Crohn's disease
Infectious enteritis
Tropical sprue
Eosinophilic enteritis
Celiac disease
Collagenous sprue
Radiation enteritis
Amyloidosis
Scleroderma
Mastocytosis
Biochemical or Genetic Abnormalities
Disaccharidase deficiency
Hypogammaglobulinemia
Abetalipoproteinemia
Hartnup's disease
Cystinuria
Monosaccharide malabsorption
Endocrine and Metabolic Disorders
Diabetes mellitus
Hypoparathyroidism
Adrenal insufficiency
Hyperthyroidism
Zollinger-Ellison syndrome
Carcinoid syndrome
Cardiovascular Disorders
Constrictive pericarditis
Congestive heart failure
Mesenteric vascular insufficiency
Vasculitis

Table 12-2

CAUSES OF MALABSORPTION WITH NORMAL-APPEARING PROXIMAL JEJUNAL BIOPSIES

Dermatosis other than dermatitis herpetiformis
Pancreatitis
Alcoholism
Cirrhosis
Hepatitis
Iron deficiency anemia
Ulcerative colitis
Postgastrectomy without bacterial overgrowth
Malignancy outside the gastrointestinal tract
Cholera
Biliary obstruction

forceps biopsies are procured from the duodenum. The biopsy should be procured no more proximal than the second part of the duodenum to avoid artifacts due to prominent Brunner glands or the nonspecific duodenitis commonly seen in the bulb and proximal duodenum.

There are no definite established guidelines regarding the number of biopsy fragments that should be taken. In general, three to four fragments, procured preferably by jumbo forceps, should be sufficient for diagnosis. Biopsies may also be procured with the use of the more routinely used smaller forceps; in this case, the number of biopsies taken should be increased to four to six.

In many cases, prior communication between the gastroenterologist and pathologist is necessary to decide whether a portion of the specimen is to be kept for enzyme or other biochemical studies, electron microscopy, or microbiologic examination. The clinical history and endoscopic findings should be provided on the surgical pathology requisition slip.

Handling the Specimen

A nonfragmented, well-oriented biopsy specimen aids in establishing an accurate diagnosis. Biopsies of 3 to 4 mm in thickness preferably procured by a jumbo forceps give reproducible results. Immediate orientation by the gastroenterologist is best, but is impractical in regular clinical practice. The optimal method of orienting the specimen is to put the base of

Table 12-3

MALABSORPTION WITH NORMAL VILLI BUT OTHER DIAGNOSTIC FEATURES

Disease	Specific Histologic Features
Abetalipoproteinemia	Vacuolated enterocytes containing lipids involving upper two thirds of the villi; acanthocytes
Crohn's disease	Noncaseating granulomas; transmural inflammation
X-linked immunodeficiency	Absent lamina propria plasma cells
Lipid storage disease	Vacuolated ganglion cells, capillaries, and macrophages
Amyloidosis	Congo red–positive material in muscularis and blood vessels
Chronic granulomatous disease	Pigmented vacuolated macrophages in lamina propria
Melanosis	Brown pigmented macrophages in lamina propria
Systemic mastocytosis	Mast cell infiltrates in lamina propria
Hemochromatosis	Iron deposits in epithelium and macrophages
Mycobacterium avium complex	PAS[a]-positive diastase-resistant macrophages containing acid-fast organisms

[a]PAS = periodic acid–Schiff.

Table 12-4

CLINICAL INFORMATION REQUIRED FOR INTERPRETATION OF SMALL BOWEL BIOPSIES FOR MALABSORPTION

Patient age
Patient sex
Ethnicity
Country of domicile
Travel history
Reason for the biopsy
Drug use
History of associated diseases
Acquired immunodeficiency syndrome
Neoplasias
Infections
Metabolic diseases
Immune deficiencies
Prior surgery

the mucosa on filter paper and float it upside down in a bottle of fixative. This technique allows the villi in the specimen to float freely, minimizing artifactual distortion of the mucosal architecture. Appropriate orientation can also be achieved by scanning under a dissecting microscope. An initial impression of the villous architecture can also be obtained by this method. Its applicability in clinical practice, however, is limited. In most institutions, adequate orientation is achieved by asking an experienced histotechnologist to embed the biopsies on edge.

Although Bouin, Hollande, and B5 fixatives yield little shrinkage artifact and give optical nuclear detail, most pathology departments use neutral buffered formalin as the fixative. Adequate fixation for histology and superior preservation of DNA for ancillary studies are possible with formalin fixation. Formalin is also inexpensive and easy to discard.

There is a lack of consensus among pathologists regarding the number of slides and levels that should be prepared and examined histologically. Examination of multiple sections and levels increases the likelihood of finding patchy changes and well-oriented villi.

Histologic Approach to Biopsies Obtained for Malabsorption

A systemic approach for the evaluation of each compartment of the small intestinal mucosa and submucosa is necessary in order to identify a pattern of injury and to determine a possible cause of the patient's symptoms.

Assessment of Villi. An adequate small intestinal biopsy should have a row of at least four well-oriented villi in the section (fig. 12-1). Obliquely sectioned villi are the most common source of diagnostic misinterpretation. Such poorly oriented villi look broad and flat and have a multilayered epithelial lining (fig. 12-2).

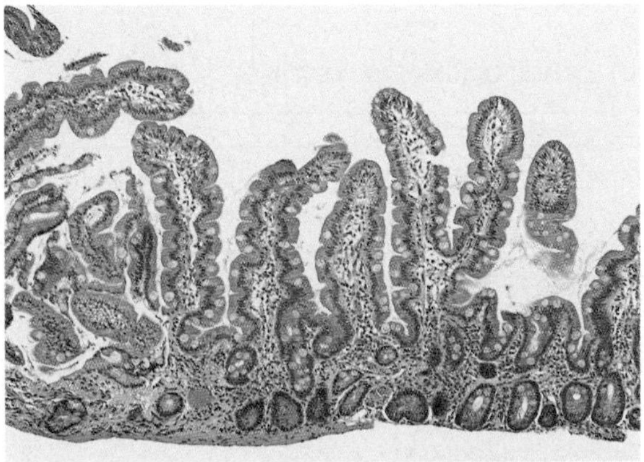

Figure 12-1

NORMAL VILLOUS ARCHITECTURE

Normal villous architecture is best assessed in areas where at least four adjacent, well-oriented villi are identifiable. In this section, the villi are three to four times the length of the intestinal crypts.

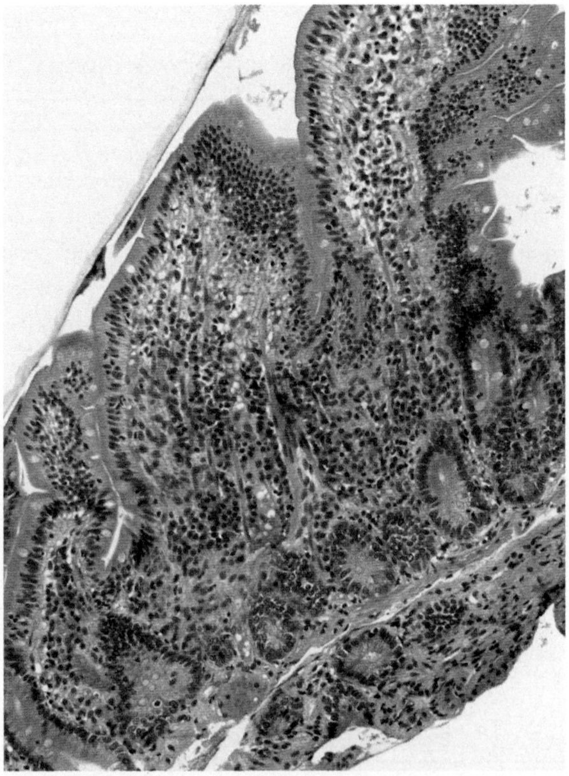

Figure 12-2

ARTIFACTUAL CHANGES MAKING VILLUS ASSESSMENT DIFFICULT

Oblique sectioning and poor orientation of small intestinal biopsies make interpretation of the architecture difficult. In this section, the specimen was oriented upside down on a piece of filter paper, making the villi appear blunted. In addition, the biopsy is tangentially sectioned making the epithelial layer appear stratified.

Villi may appear atrophied, normal, or hypertrophied in patients presenting with malabsorption. The latter is rare. Villi should be assessed by their normal relationship with the small intestinal crypt. In adults overall, the villous height is approximately three or more times the depth of the crypts, whereas in children this ratio is typically 2 to 1. Villous height is also lower in elderly patients. The duodenal crypt/villus ratio is 3–1 to 7–1, whereas the ileal crypt/villus ratio is 4 to 1. Villi overlying lymphoid aggregates are often stubby or absent, and therefore, should not be evaluated in these areas. Causes of villous atrophy are listed in Table 12-5. Villous atrophy occurs in three different patterns.

Villous Atrophy and Crypt Hyperplasia. This is the usual type of injury pattern observed, and is typical of celiac disease as well as many other disorders. The villous enterocytes are the target of the injury. The villus to crypt ratio is decreased and crypts show elongation and a marked increase in mitotic activity (fig. 12-3). A system for grading the degree of villous atrophy is shown in Table 12-6. Such grading helps assess the severity of damage. Evaluation of the degree of villous atrophy present in a biopsy is also necessary to apply the Marsh classification in celiac disease (see below).

Villous Atrophy with Crypt Hypoplasia. In this pattern of injury, the crypt is the site of damage. The crypt to villus ratio is minimally altered. This pattern is seen in advanced celiac disease, cytotoxic drug-induced injury, and vitamin B12 and folic acid deficiencies.

Villous Hyperplasia. This unusual pattern is seen following intestinal resection or with glucagonoma. The length of the villi and depth of the crypts are both increased, resulting in minimal alteration of the villus to crypt ratio.

Other changes, including villous expansion due to lamina propria alterations, erosion, metaplasia, and the presence of microorganisms, should be evaluated in all small intestinal biopsies taken for malabsorption.

Enterocyte Changes. The appearance of the brush border, size and shape of the cells, intracytoplasmic and nuclear alterations, and regenerative activity should be evaluated.

Table 12-5

CAUSES OF VILLOUS ATROPHY

Sprue Syndromes
- Celiac Sprue
- Refractory sprue
- Collagenous sprue
- Mesenteric lymph node cavitation syndrome
- Other protein injury (soy, milk)

Infectious Causes
- Gastroenteritis
- Parasitic infections (*Giardia* most common)
- Mycobacterial infections
- Fungal infections (histoplasmosis most common)
- Viral infections (cytomegalovirus most common)
- Tropical sprue
- Whipple's disease
- Bacterial overgrowth

Immunologic Disorders
- IgA deficiency
- Common variable immunodeficiency
- X-linked agammaglobulinemia
- Acquired immunodeficiency syndrome (AIDS)
- Autoimmune enteropathy

Nutritional Deficiency Disorders
- Kwashiorkor
- Zinc deficiency
- Vitamin B12 and folic acid deficiencies

Others
- Crohn's disease
- Graft versus host disease
- Immunoproliferative disorders (lymphoma, macroglobulinemia)
- Intestinal lymphangiectasia
- Zollinger-Ellison syndrome
- Microvillous inclusion disease
- Radiation enteropathy
- Eosinophilic gastroenteritis
- Chronic ischemia

Table 12-6

GRADES OF VILLOUS ATROPHY

Mild
- Most villi appear branched, broadened, or fused; some remain normal
- Surface epithelium appears abnormal
  - loss of polarity
  - increased intraepithelial lymphocytes
- Increased mitoses outside the normal proliferative compartment
- Increased acute and chronic inflammatory cells in lamina propria

Moderate (partial villous atrophy)
- Villi broadened and shortened
- Cuboidal surface epithelium
- Large numbers of intraepithelial lymphocytes
- Increased mononuclear cells in the lamina propria

Severe (subtotal or total villous atrophy)
- Villi almost or completely absent
- Marked mononuclear cell infiltrates

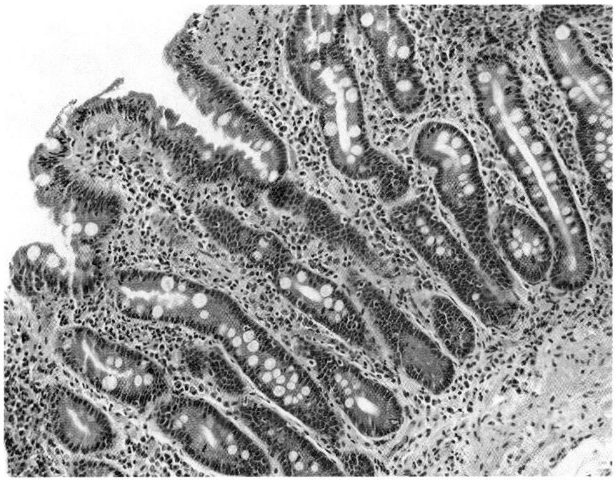

Figure 12-3

VILLOUS ATROPHY AND CRYPT HYPERPLASIA

The mucosal surface of this duodenal biopsy specimen is nearly flat, and the crypts are markedly elongated.

Enterocyte changes can be nonspecific, but may indicate a specific etiology in certain cases.

Nonspecific injury often results in an attenuated or absent brush border. The enterocytes lose their normal columnar shape and become more cuboidal. The cytoplasm becomes amphophilic to basophilic with vacuolization and the nuclei are irregular in size and shape. The regenerating enterocytes show tufting, and mitoses are present higher in the crypt than normal (fig. 12-4).

Specific changes include the presence of intracytoplasmic accumulations, for example, iron in hemochromatosis; characteristic vacuolization of the enterocytes in abetalipoproteinemia; or microvillous inclusion disease. Viral inclusions and parasites are also seen (see chapter 10). Macrocytosis is often seen in vitamin B12 or folic acid deficiency or following treatment with chemotherapeutic agents. Increased apoptosis is seen in autoimmune enteropathy and graft versus host disease (see chapters 11 and 14).

Intraepithelial lymphocytosis is seen most frequently in association with celiac disease. The causes of intraepithelial lymphocytosis are listed in Table 12-7.

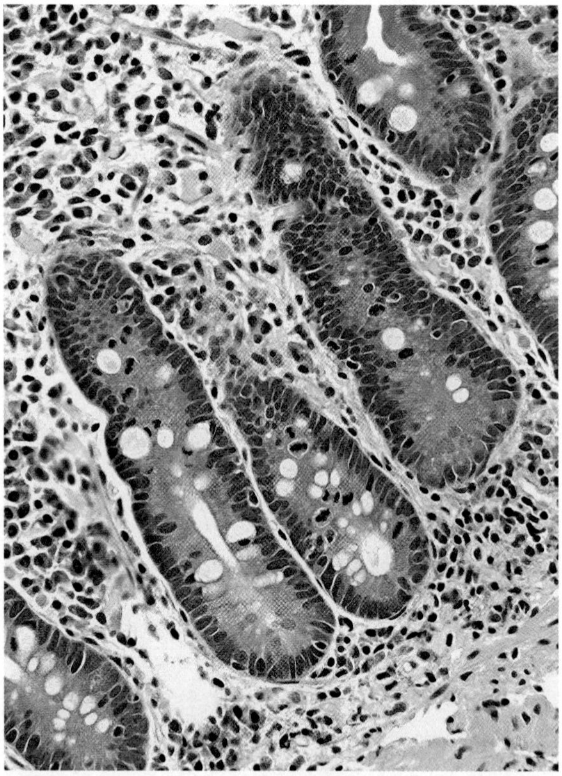

Figure 12-4

CELIAC DISEASE

The intestinal crypts in this biopsy from a patient with celiac disease are hyperplastic. Numerous mitoses extend upward into the superficial portion of the crypts.

Crypt Changes. Crypts may show hyperplasia or hypoplasia as described previously. Although not specific, increased numbers of Paneth and endocrine cells are commonly seen in celiac disease. Paneth cell abnormalities are also seen in acrodermatitis enteropathica (3).

Lamina Propria Changes. The character of any lamina propria inflammatory infiltrate may help to determine the etiology of the patient's malabsorption. It is important to note that a mild degree of lymphoplasmacytosis is normal in duodenal biopsies. A marked increase in chronic inflammatory cells is seen in many conditions including celiac disease, peptic duodenitis, drug injury, infection, and nonspecific chronic duodenitis. Acute inflammation suggests etiologies such as peptic duodenitis, drug-induced injury, and Crohn's disease. Crypt abscesses indicate acute enteritis or Crohn's disease. The presence of large numbers of eosinophils suggests allergic injury, parasitic infection, or eosinophilic gastroenteritis. Mast cells are increased in mastocytosis, allergic disorders, and Crohn's disease.

Table 12-7

CAUSES OF INTRAEPITHELIAL LYMPHOCYTOSIS

Celiac disease
Relatives of patients with celiac disease
Autoimmune enteropathy
Systemic autoimmune disorders like systemic lupus erythematosus, rheumatoid arthritis
Nonsteroidal antiinflammatory medications
Crohn's disease
Infections
Lymphocytic colitis and enterocolitis

Inflammatory infiltrates that are predominantly histiocytic in nature may be seen in infections such as *Mycobacterium avium* complex infection, histoplasmosis, and Whipple's disease. In addition, various storage diseases may present with diffuse lamina propria histiocytic collections.

It is also important to determine which cell types are not present in the biopsy. For example, an absence of plasma cells is a strong indicator of immunodeficiency disease, particularly common variable immunodeficiency. A decreased number of chronic inflammatory cells is seen in patients who are on steroids or who have other types of immunodeficiency.

Lymphatic dilatation is seen with lymphangiectasia or lymphatic outflow obstruction. Blood vessels are primarily affected in ischemic diseases, radiation injury, amyloid deposition, and thromboembolic disorders. The lamina propria may also show deposition of material as occurs in amyloidosis, macroglobulinemia, melanosis, and hemochromatosis. The conditions leading to mucosal deposits are listed in Table 12-8.

Submucosal Changes. The submucosa may not be present in some biopsy specimens. If present, blood vessels, lymphatics, inflammation, Brunner gland hyperplasia, and metaplastic changes should be evaluated. If available, the submucosal plexus should be evaluated for ganglion cell changes. It is not uncommon to find ganglion cells in the muscularis mucosae or

Table 12-8

CAUSES OF INTESTINAL MUCOSAL DEPOSITS

Amyloid light chains
Macroglobulins
Collagenous sprue and collagenous enterocolitis
Infantile systemic hyalinosis
Lipid proteinosis
Melanosis
Pseudomelanosis
Xanthomas
Muciphages
Storage diseases
Tangier disease
Fabry's disease
Tay-Sachs and other gangliosidoses
Niemann-Pick disease
Wolman's disease
Cystinosis
Mucopolysaccharidoses

lower mucosa of the small intestine. These should not be interpreted as representing neuronal dysplasia (see chapter 17).

CELIAC DISEASE

Definition: *Celiac disease* is a malabsorptive disorder in which the small intestinal mucosa of sensitive individuals is injured as a result of ingestion of gluten-containing foods. Synonyms include *celiac sprue* and *gluten-sensitive enteropathy*.

Epidemiology. Celiac disease is the most common cause of malabsorption in Western populations. The disease prevalence in most of Europe is estimated at approximately 1/1,000, but is up to 10-fold higher in many Western European countries (8,9,31,40,47,48,52,54). Recent estimates of the disease prevalence suggest that worldwide as many as 1/266 people are affected (18). Celiac disease is rarely seen in Japanese, Chinese, and African individuals. The disorder affects women more commonly than men.

Celiac disease appears to have a strong genetic component, demonstrating a higher incidence in siblings than in the general population (43,53). There is 70 percent concordance for celiac disease in identical twins (23). About 10 percent of first-degree relatives of celiac patients also have the disease (29,45), although a significant proportion (about 50 percent) remain asymptomatic and are said to have latent celiac disease (29,45).

Pathophysiology. The complex etiology of celiac disease results from the interaction of environmental agents, genetic predisposition, and immunologic factors to produce intestinal injury (fig. 12-5).

Gluten and Other Prolamines. Celiac disease has been recognized as an autoimmune enteropathy triggered by ingestion of wheat gluten (gliadins), barley (hordeins), rye (secalins), and possibly oats (avenins). Gluten is found in grains such as wheat and buckwheat, as well as in many processed foods such as gravies, sausage, beer, ale, bread, and bread products.

Gluten can be separated electrophoretically into four major fractions: alpha, beta, gamma, and omega gliadins (6). Gliadins are prolamines with a high content of proline and glutamic acid. All four types appear to be toxic, although alpha-gliadin has the most pathogenic properties (11). Toxic gliadins contain pro-ser-gln-gln and gln-gln-gln-pro amino acid sequences. These sequences are absent from nontoxic peptides (15,59). A recent study demonstrated that a 33-mer peptide generated by digestion of alpha-gliadin with intestinal enzymes in vivo and in vitro is a highly stimulatory antigen for CD4-positive T cells (56). This peptide is resistant to further digestion by intestinal brush border enzymes and is a highly specific substrate for deamidation by tissue transglutaminase. This 33-mer peptide is not present in cereal proteins that do not cause celiac disease.

A possible pathogenetic role of enteric pathogens has been suggested in the etiology of celiac disease. This hypothesis was supported by a study in which analysis of alpha-gliadin demonstrated an amino acid region that was homologous to the 54-kDa E1b protein coat of adenovirus (32). In addition, patients with celiac disease have been reported to have a significantly higher prevalence of past adenovirus 12 infection than control subjects (5).

Celiac disease demonstrates the strongest association of any illness with a specific class II human leukocyte antigen (HLA) molecule (28, 41,42,60,61). The disorder is triggered by an environmental insult (gluten consumption),

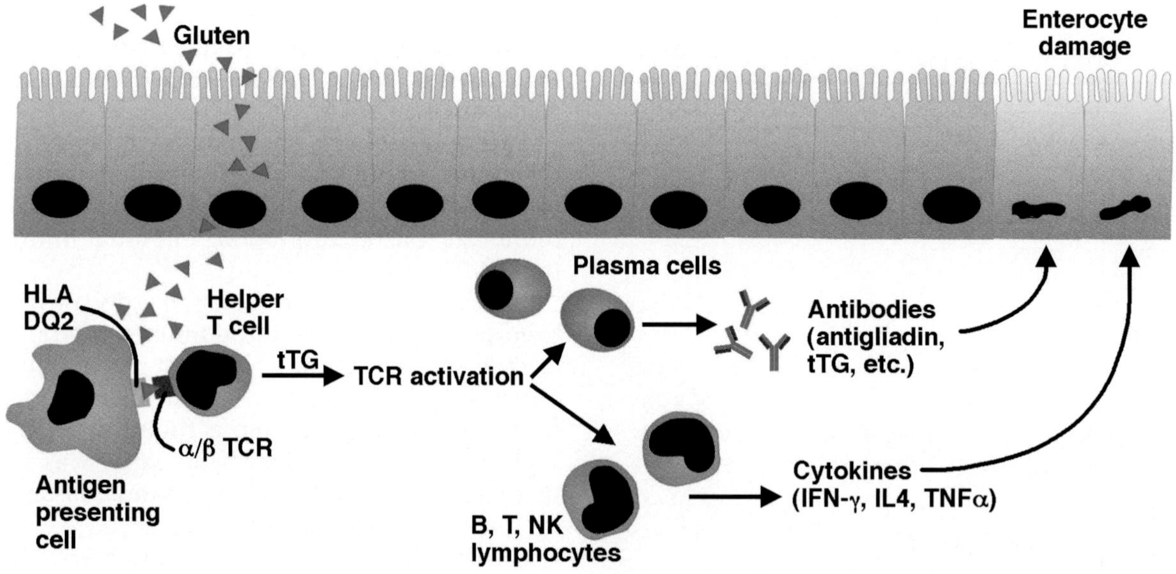

Figure 12-5

PATHOPHYSIOLOGY OF CELIAC DISEASE

Dietary gluten is absorbed from the intestinal lumen and enters the lamina propria of the small intestine. Gliadin is presented, in conjunction with HLA-DQ2 or DQ8 cell surface antigens on antigen-presenting cells, to T lymphocytes expressing the α/β T-cell receptor (TCR). Tissue transglutaminase deamidates the gliadin, generating negatively charged glutamic acid residues from neutral glutamines on the gliadin molecule. These negatively charged glutamate residues interact with positions 4, 6, and 7 in the antigen-binding groove of the human leukocyte antigen (HLA) molecule, eliciting an enhanced T-cell response to the antigen. Activated T lymphocytes then activate other lymphocytes, resulting in the production of cytokines and immunoglobulins that damage enterocytes.

and the HLA haplotype acts as a classic immune response gene that operates at either the T cell or antigen-presenting cell level to favor gliadin-specific responses (41,60,61). The primary HLA association in the majority of patients is with DQ2 (61); fewer patients are of haplotype DQ8. An increased risk for celiac disease also exists among individuals who are DR3-DQ2 homozygous and DR3-DQ2/DR7-DQ2 heterozygous (40).

In addition to the HLA linkage, celiac disease has been linked to several other chromosomal regions. Linkage to 2q33, an area of regulation for T-lymphocyte activation, has been seen in a Finnish family (27). Linkage to other regions on other chromosomes has additionally been reported (22,35,48,51,65,70), but linkage to 5p31-33 is the most consistently identified (22,37,48).

Gluten-reactive T cells can be isolated from small intestinal biopsies of celiac patients but not from nonceliac controls. These T cells are CD4 positive and express the α/β T-cell receptor (TCR). A number of distinct T-cell epitopes within gluten exist. Lamina propria antigen-presenting cells that express HLA-DQ2 or -DQ8, present gliadin peptides bound to their α/β heterodimer antigen-presenting grooves to sensitized T lymphocytes that express the α/β TCR. These lymphocytes then activate B lymphocytes to produce immunoglobulins, and stimulate other T cells to produce cytokines including interferon (IFN)-γ, interleukin (IL)4, IL5, IL6, IL10, tumor necrosis factor (TNF)-γ, and transforming growth factor (TGF)-β (fig. 12-5).

Tissue Transglutaminase (tTG) and Other Autoantigens. tTG is expressed in many different tissues, and is found both extracellularly and intracellularly. tTG is expressed just beneath the epithelium in the gut wall. Calcium-dependent tTG catalyzes selective cross-linking or deamidation of protein-bound glutamine residues. Deamidation of the glutamine residues of gliadin by tTG prepares the gliadin molecule to bind with HLA-DQ molecules (46,66). In addition, tTG can cross-link glutamine residues of peptides to lysine residues in other proteins, including tTG itself. This may result in the formation of gluten-tTG complexes. These complexes may permit gluten-reactive T cells to stimulate tTG-specific B cells by a mechanism of intramolecular help, thereby explaining the occurrence of gluten-dependent tTG autoantibodies, a characteristic feature of active celiac disease. Furthermore, tTG-catalyzed cross-linking and consequent haptenization of gluten with extracellular matrix proteins allow for storage and extended availability of gluten in the mucosa. tTG is necessary for activation of TGF-β which is involved in the differentiation of intestinal epithelium (54), regulates immunoglobulin (Ig)A expression (14), and modulates immune responses. In addition, antibodies to tTG in patients with celiac disease interfere with fibroblast-induced differentiation of epithelial cells, possibly by inhibiting the cross-linking activity of tTG.

Cell-Mediated and Antibody-Mediated Immune Responses. Gluten ingestion in untreated patients with celiac disease induces nonproliferative activation of CD4-positive T α/β receptor-positive cells in the lamina propria. This is accompanied by proliferative activation of intraepithelial lymphocytes (α/β- and γ/δ-positive T cells) in the epithelial compartment.

Activated CD4-positive T cells activate B lymphocytes and plasma cells to produce autoantibodies. These T cells also stimulate other T lymphocytes to secrete cytokines, most notably IFN-γ, but also IL4, IL5, IL6, IL10, TNF-γ and TGF-β. These cytokines not only damage the enterocytes, but also induce expression of aberrant HLA class II cell surface antigens on the luminal surface of enterocytes. This facilitates additional direct antigen presentation by these cells to the sensitized lymphocytes. Cytokines produced by DQ2-restricted T cells are of Th1 type and are dominated by the secretion of IFN-γ. Cytokines produced by DQ8-restricted T cells have a Th0 profile. Increased γ/δ T cells in the epithelium and lamina propria of the small intestine have also been observed in celiac patients, and these cells persist even after gluten withdrawal. These cells may play a protective role through activation of a nonspecific immune response that helps to lessen the antigen-specific immune response.

Celiac disease characteristically results in the accumulation of IgA-, IgM-, and IgG-producing plasma cells within the mucosa (7,69). These antibodies are directed against gliadin, transglutaminase, endomysium, reticulin, and enterocyte actin. The exact physiologic role of these antibodies is still unclear.

Recent evidence suggests that gliadin or its metabolites may directly injure the intestinal mucosa. Up-regulation of mucosal HLA-DR and intercellular adhesion molecule within 2 hours of in vitro exposure to gliadin suggests an early effect that may not be immune mediated (49). This early effect is followed by activation of CD4-, CD25-positive T cells, producing the immunologic injury.

Associated Diseases. Table 12-9 shows the wide variety of systemic diseases that are associated with celiac disease. Dermatitis herpetiformis and celiac disease are both associated with IgA-mediated epithelial injury. Initially, dermatitis herpetiformis was considered a skin disease that occurred often concomitantly with celiac disease, but currently it is believed that dermatitis herpetiformis is a cutaneous manifestation of celiac disease, affecting approximately 25 percent of patients. tTG, the autoantigen for

Table 12-9

CONDITIONS ASSOCIATED WITH CELIAC DISEASE

Common Associations
Developmental delay
Short stature
Dermatitis herpetiformis
Vasculitis
Arthritis
Autoimmune hepatitis
Polyglandular autoimmune syndrome
Autoimmune thyroid disease
Insulin-dependent diabetes
IgA nephropathy
Lymphoma
Carcinoma
Uncommon or Rare Associations
Ulcerative colitis
Sarcoidosis
Primary biliary cirrhosis
Pericarditis
Cystic fibrosis
Epilepsy
Facial anomalies
Hypoparathyroidism
Bronchiolitis
Interstitial pulmonary fibrosis
Alopecia areata
Alpha-1-antitrypsin deficiency

antiendomysial antibody, is also the autoantigen in dermatitis herpetiformis (34). Restriction of patients to a gluten-free diet is essential in the treatment of both conditions.

Another IgA-mediated autoimmune disease associated with celiac disease is IgA nephropathy. Patients with IgA nephropathy carry a risk of contracting celiac disease; however, there is no increase in celiac-type HLA-DQ in IgA nephropathy patients. It has been hypothesized that the increased intestinal permeability in IgA nephropathy may predispose genetically susceptible patients to celiac disease.

Many hepatobiliary diseases occur in association with celiac disease, including asymptomatic elevations of liver enzymes, nonspecific hepatitis, nonalcoholic fatty liver disease, and autoimmune and cholestatic liver disease. Increased levels of alanine aminotransferase, aspartate aminotransferase, and/or alkaline phosphatase are seen in up to 47 percent of celiac disease patients (4). Two main mechanisms underlying the development of the liver damage have been proposed: 1) celiac disease may result in increased intestinal permeability to toxins and antigens injurious to the liver and 2) chronic intestinal mucosal inflammation may represent a primary trigger.

Other associated autoimmune disorders include insulin-dependent diabetes, autoimmune thyroid disease, Addison's disease, Sjögren's syndrome, alopecia areata, and rheumatoid arthritis. Approximately 5 percent of insulin-dependent diabetics have associated celiac disease, and one third of insulin-dependent diabetics with DQ2 have celiac disease (58,63). It is possible that chronic autoimmune stimulation of lymphocytes in the intestine predisposes to increased formation of other autoantibodies.

Another important association is with trisomy 21 (Down's syndrome) (57). The prevalence of celiac disease is 20 times that of the general population in patients with Down's syndrome (57).

There is a well-established relationship between celiac disease and lymphocytic colitis and lymphocytic gastritis (figs. 12-6, 12-7). Rectal gluten challenge in patients with celiac disease induces a mild proctitis characterized by lymphocytosis of the rectal lamina propria (38). Patients with celiac disease and microscopic colitis share certain predisposing HLA-DQ genes; however, these are not exactly related conditions. The intraepithelial lymphocytes in lymphocytic colitis are predominantly CD8-positive unlike those of celiac disease. In addition, epithelial abnormalities and increased mononuclear inflammation are more prevalent in patients with lymphocytic colitis. The watery diarrhea that is characteristic of lymphocytic colitis often does not respond to a gluten-free diet.

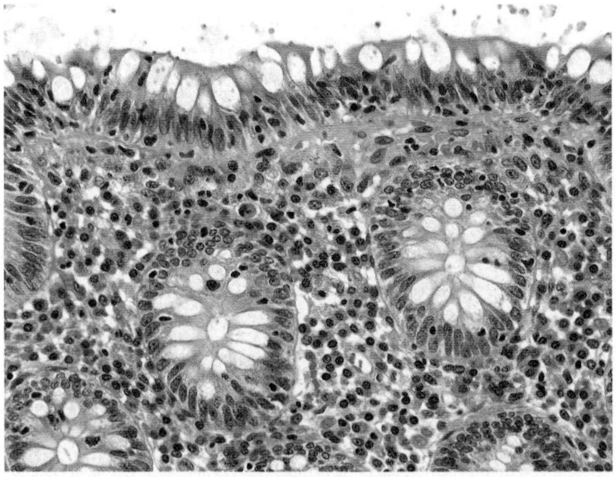

Figure 12-6

LYMPHOCYTIC COLITIS

The lamina propria of the colon contains an increased number of lymphocytes and plasma cells. Numerous intraepithelial lymphocytes are also present. The normal mucosal architecture is preserved.

Clinical Features. The clinical spectrum of celiac disease is diverse and includes the following forms. *Typical celiac disease* is fully expressed gluten-sensitive enteropathy associated with the classic features of malabsorption. The full expression includes positive serology for endomysial and tTG antibodies and a diagnostic biopsy. This form of the disease usually affects younger patients.

In *atypical celiac disease*, fully expressed gluten-sensitive enteropathy is associated with atypical manifestations including short stature, anemia, and infertility.

Patients with *latent celiac disease* have normal small bowel villous architecture on biopsy, but villous atrophy develops later on. Two variants have been described. The first includes patients diagnosed in childhood and who recovered completely with gluten-free diet. The

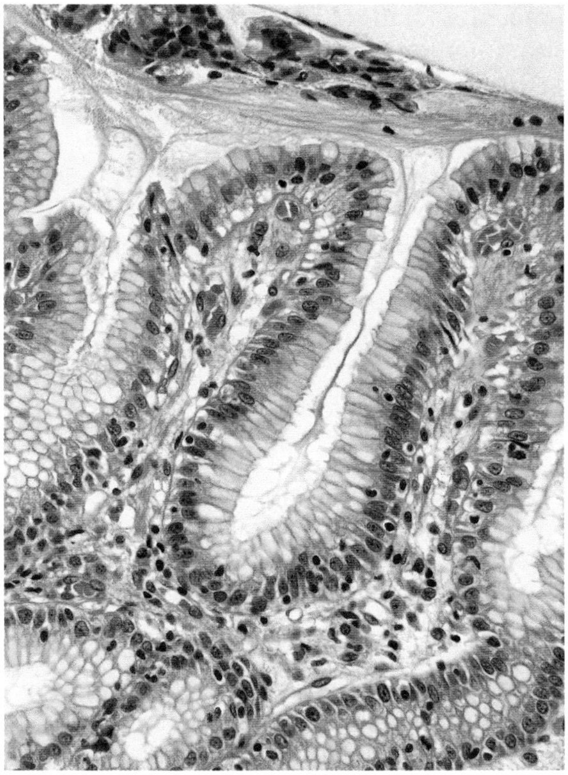

Figure 12-7

LYMPHOCYTIC GASTRITIS ASSOCIATED WITH CELIAC DISEASE

The gastric glands contain numerous intraepithelial lymphocytes. Lymphocytes are somewhat increased in number in the lamina propria.

disease then remains latent in these individuals even after normal diet is adopted. In the second variant, a normal mucosa was present on early biopsies while the patient was consuming gluten, but more typical features of celiac disease develop later.

Those with *potential celiac disease* never had biopsy changes but have characteristic immunologic abnormalities. HLA-DQ2 is more frequent in these patients and they frequently have a first-degree relative affected by the disease.

Asymptomatic patients with positive serologic autoantibodies and diagnostic biopsy have *silent celiac disease*. Patients with *refractory celiac disease* have severe, symptomatic, intestinal atrophy that does not respond to at least 6 months of a strict gluten-free diet.

The clinical presentation of any given patient with celiac disease depends on the severity of the damage and their age at presentation. The classic presentation is that of steatorrhea with abdominal cramps and vomiting. In infants, the symptoms begin after weaning, when cereals are first introduced into the diet. Signs of nutritional deficiency, such as anemia, occur next in frequency in children. Other manifestations include failure to thrive, short stature, muscle wasting, hypotonia, abdominal distension, and watery diarrhea. Atypical modes of presentation include neurologic manifestations, osteopenia, and primary presentation with associated conditions like dermatitis herpetiformis without gastrointestinal manifestations. The most common neurologic finding is ataxia, followed by epilepsy, cerebral calcification, cerebral white-matter lesions on magnetic resonance imaging (MRI), myelopathy, peripheral neuropathy, and myopathy (25,68).

Celiac disease in adults is most often diagnosed in the third and fourth decades of life, but may develop at any age. Approximately 20 percent of cases are diagnosed in individuals over the age of 60 (26). Women are more frequently affected than men and are generally diagnosed at a younger age. Many adult patients present with diarrhea, but as many as 50 percent do not (17,39). Since the introduction of highly sensitive autoantibody tests, the number of patients presenting with classic features of celiac disease has decreased. In fact, iron deficiency anemia, formerly regarded as an atypical presenting sign, is now the most common presentation of adult patients (17). Iron deficiency is primarily due to iron malabsorption. Gastrointestinal bleeding does occur occasionally, and may represent an indicator of disease complicated by ulcerative jejunoileitis or malignancy.

Other extraintestinal features of the disease include vague abdominal pain, bone disease, abnormal peripheral blood smear findings, infertility (both male and female), amenorrhea, recurrent abortion or low birth weight babies, hypoglycemia, peripheral neuropathy, ataxia, and seizures (13,16,23,67). Up to 8 percent of patients are detected by mucosal changes on duodenal endoscopy performed for other conditions like gastroesophageal reflux disease or gastritis (23); 7 to 15 percent are detected through serum antibody tests performed because of a family history of celiac disease.

Table 12-10

EXTRAINTESTINAL SYMPTOMS OF CELIAC DISEASE

Deficiency	Manifestations
Iron	Hemorrhage, hemolysis, microcytic anemia
Vitamin B12	Macrocytic anemia
Calcium	Osteomalacia, bone pain, compression fractures
Vitamin D	Osteomalacia, compression fractures
Vitamin A	Night blindness, follicular hyperkeratosis of the skin
Vitamin B	Neuropathies
Pituitary, adrenal, and parathyroid hormones	Endocrine gland hypofunction

Physical examination shows changes that are attributable to malabsorption and deficiency of minerals, vitamins, and other essential nutrients (Table 12-10). The clinical presentation often reflects the degree of malabsorption present.

Serologic Testing. In the last decade, the application of serologic testing for autoantibodies has changed the clinical evaluation of patients with malabsorption syndromes. Tests for IgA endomysial and IgA tTG antibodies are based on the target antigen tTG. IgA antigliadin antibody (AGA) and IgG AGA evaluations are based on the target antigen gliadin (44). Antireticulin and antismooth muscle actin antibodies are additional autoantibodies that may be seen in celiac patients, but are not generally evaluated in routine clinical practice.

IgA Endomysial Antibodies. Endomysial antibodies bind to the connective tissue surrounding smooth muscle cells (10,44). In the laboratory, IgA endomysial antibodies are usually detected by indirect immunofluorescence examination of sections of human umbilical cord (69). The test is reported as either positive or negative. The IgA endomysial antibody test has a sensitivity of 85 to 90 percent and a specificity of 97 to 100 percent (10,20,44). Antibody levels decrease when the patient is placed on a gluten-free diet, and may become undetectable in treated patients (33). The sensitivity of this test is lower in children younger than 2 years of age.

IgA tTG Antibodies. IgA tTG antibodies are detected by an automated enzyme-linked immunosorbent test. This test is less expensive and easier to perform than the test used to detect IgA endomysial antibodies. The test for IgA tTG has a sensitivity of 95 to 98 percent and a specificity of 94 to 95 percent (17,62). Like endomysial antibody tests, sensitivity is lower in children younger than 2 to 3 years.

IgA and IgG Antigliadin Antibodies. The IgA antigliadin assay has a sensitivity of 75 to 90 percent and a specificity of 82 to 95 percent. The IgG antigliadin assay has a sensitivity of 69 to 85 percent and a sensitivity of 73 to 90 percent (17). Most reports suggest that tests for antigliadin antibodies are more sensitive than endomysial antibody studies in infants and children younger than 2 to 3 years. High antigliadin antibody levels, however, have been reported in some normal individuals (64).

Assays for IgA endomysial and IgA tTG antibodies are used interchangeably as first-line tests for the diagnosis of celiac disease. In patients with IgA deficiency, IgG tTG testing is recommended as the first-line serologic test. Antibody levels decrease during treatment with a gluten-free diet and are useful in assessing dietary compliance. An IgA antigliadin antibody test is the most commonly used marker to monitor response to a gluten-free diet. A normal baseline value is reached within 3 to 6 months of dietary restriction. Currently, experience with IgA tTG antibodies in assessing dietary response is limited.

Other Laboratory Tests. Biochemical tests performed in the evaluation of celiac disease patients include serum iron, folate, albumin, calcium, and potassium levels. Liver function studies should be tested since serum transaminases are elevated in up to 40 percent of patients with untreated celiac disease (4).

Peripheral blood smears show features of iron deficiency anemia in the form of hypochromic microcytic anemia with low mean cell volume (MCV), mean cell hemoglobin (MCH), and mean cell hemoglobin concentration (MCHC). Many target cells, siderocytes, Heinz bodies, and Howell-Jolly bodies are seen in patients with splenic atrophy. Patients with folic acid or vitamin B12 (unusual) deficiency have macrocytosis and ovalocytosis with hypersegmented neutrophils on peripheral blood smears.

Microscopic stool examination to detect steatorrhea as a screening test for malabsorption

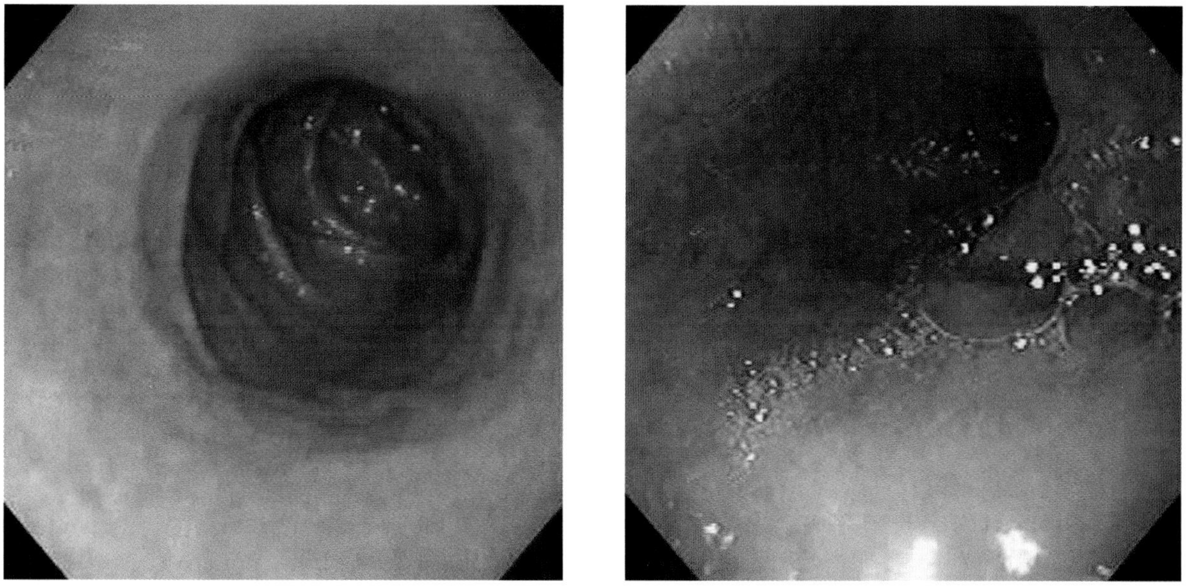

Figure 12-8

ENDOSCOPIC FINDINGS IN CELIAC DISEASE

Left: The duodenal folds have the scalloped appearance typical of celiac disease.
Right: In this view, the mucosa appears atrophic with a mosaic-like appearance.

is useful in the early stages of patient evaluation. Quantitative estimation of stool fat content is necessary to document steatorrhea. This and the D-xylose absorption test, however, do not provide a specific diagnosis and are not part of the routine workup of celiac patients.

Endoscopic Findings. Endoscopic examination with biopsy is considered the gold standard for the diagnosis of celiac disease. Celiac disease can be patchy in its early stages and targeted biopsy of affected areas is necessary. Endoscopic findings include loss of villi, a mosaic pattern affecting the mucosa, scalloping of the duodenal folds, micronodularity, and visible vascularity (fig. 12-8). The endoscopic findings, however, are not specific for celiac disease, as similar changes are seen in patients with eosinophilic gastroenteritis, giardiasis, tropical sprue, and other diseases (55). A biopsy is necessary to define the presence and extent of injury. The severity of the changes seen on biopsy appears to correlate well with the endoscopic findings.

Radiologic Findings. Small bowel barium studies may be normal in early celiac disease. In well-developed cases, intestinal dilatation and an abnormal mucosal pattern with obliteration of mucosal folds, flocculation, and segmentation are seen. Patients with mild to moderate disease show involvement of the proximal small intestine. In severe cases, the distal small intestine may be affected. Barium studies can exclude other causes of malabsorption such as Crohn's disease or bacterial overgrowth. They are primarily used, however, to exclude complications of celiac disease including lymphoma and carcinoma. Abdominal computerized tomography (CT) may be useful in documenting the presence of hyposplenism, ascites, lymphadenopathy, and mesenteric lymph node cavitation.

Microscopic Findings. Small intestinal biopsy is not only the gold standard for diagnosing celiac disease, but is essential in excluding other causes of malabsorption, assessing the severity of the damage, and identifying life-threatening complications of the disease. Histologic changes are seen in villi, crypts, enterocytes, and lamina propria.

Intraepithelial Lymphocytosis. The hallmark of celiac disease is intraepithelial lymphocytosis (fig. 12-9), which may be seen in the absence of villous atrophy (fig. 12-10). Intraepithelial lymphocyte counts should be performed on 3- to 4-μm, well-oriented sections. Normal small bowel epithelium contains up to 20 lymphocytes/100

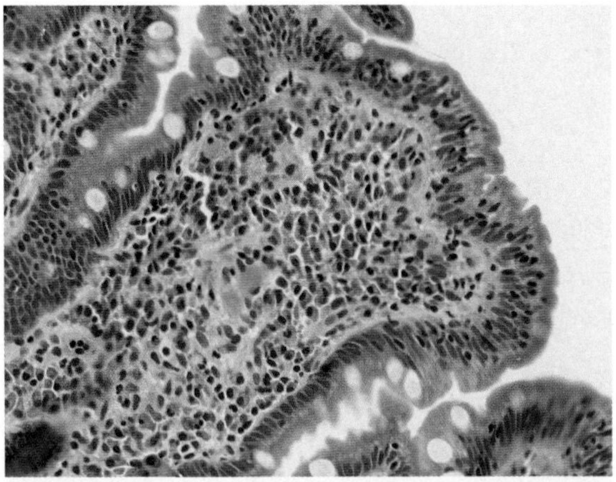

Figure 12-9

INTRAEPITHELIAL LYMPHOCYTES IN CELIAC DISEASE

Intraepithelial lymphocytes are markedly increased in number in celiac disease, as shown here. Lymphocytes in the surface epithelium in this case number more that 30/100 enterocytes, and are concentrated at the tips of the villi.

enterocytes on hematoxylin and eosin (H&E)-stained sections (19). Slightly greater numbers of lymphocytes may be observed in immunostained sections. Higher numbers of lymphocytes are also seen overlying lymphoid follicles and lymphoid aggregates. As a result, intraepithelial lymphocytes should not be counted in these areas. According to the modified Marsh classification for the diagnosis of celiac disease (Table 12-11), a significant increase in intraepithelial lymphocytes is defined as more than 40 lymphocytes/100 surface or upper crypt enterocytes. In addition, some authors report that the clustering of lymphocytes (greater than 12) in the epithelium at the tips of the villi and extending evenly along the sides of the villus, is strongly indicative of celiac disease (21). Others have observed a significant increase in villus tip lymphocytes in early celiac disease compared to controls, but did not find any difference in

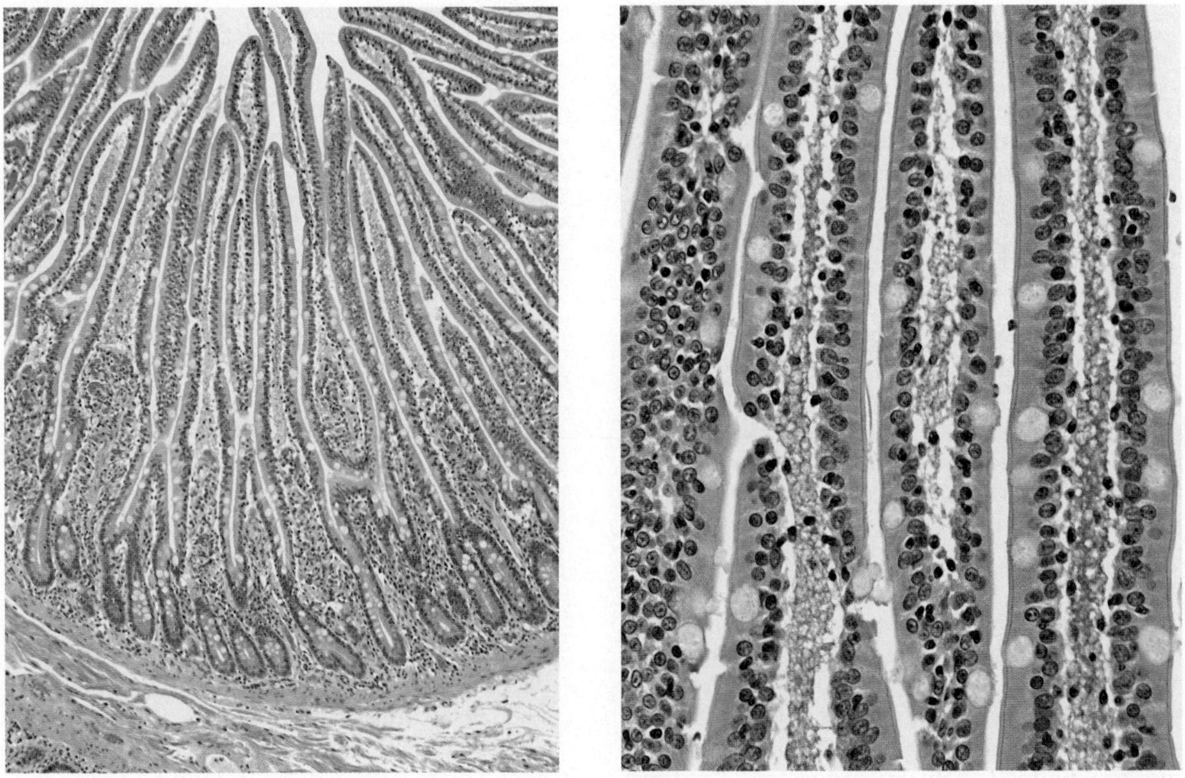

Figure 12-10

LYMPHOCYTIC ENTERITIS

Left: Low-power view shows an essentially normal villous architecture in the small intestine.

Right: On higher power, a prominent increase in intraepithelial lymphocytes is seen despite the normal appearance of the mucosal architecture.

distribution of intraepithelial lymphocytes between controls and patients with early celiac disease (30). Intraepithelial lymphocytosis is not specifically diagnostic for celiac disease, but may also seen in a number of other conditions (see Table 12-6).

Enterocyte Changes. Enterocytes show nonspecific changes in celiac disease including attenuation of the brush border, a cuboidal appearance, supranuclear cytoplasmic vacuolation, cytoplasmic basophilia, loss of polarity, and loss of basal nuclear orientation (fig. 12-11). Surface erosion is uncommon, but can be seen in severe cases.

Villous Atrophy. Villous atrophy in celiac disease is due to increased enterocyte destruction by immune-mediated injury. Villous atrophy is variable in degree, with complete atrophy only present in severe cases (fig. 12-12). Villous atrophy is nonspecific, and can be seen in other conditions as well (see Table 12-5).

Crypt Hyperplasia. Crypt hyperplasia and elongation accompany the villous atrophy (fig. 12-13). The proliferative zone of the crypt is expanded and there is an increase in enterocyte mitotic activity. The enterocytes at the bases of the crypts appear regenerative and goblet cells are decreased in number.

Lamina Propria Changes. Edema, vascular congestion, and a variable degree of inflammatory cell infiltration of the lamina propria are seen in celiac disease patients. The inflammatory infiltrate consists predominantly of lymphocytes and

Table 12-11

MODIFIED MARSH CLASSIFICATION OF CELIAC DISEASE

Marsh Type	IEL[a]	Crypts	Villi
Type 0	<40	Normal	Normal
Type 1	>40	Normal	Normal
Type 2	>40	Hypertrophic	Normal
Type 3a	>40	Hypertrophic	Mild atrophy
Type 3b	>40	Hypertrophic	Marked atrophy
Type 3c	>40	Hypertrophic	Absent

[a]IEL = Intraepithelial lymphocytes/100 enterocytes.

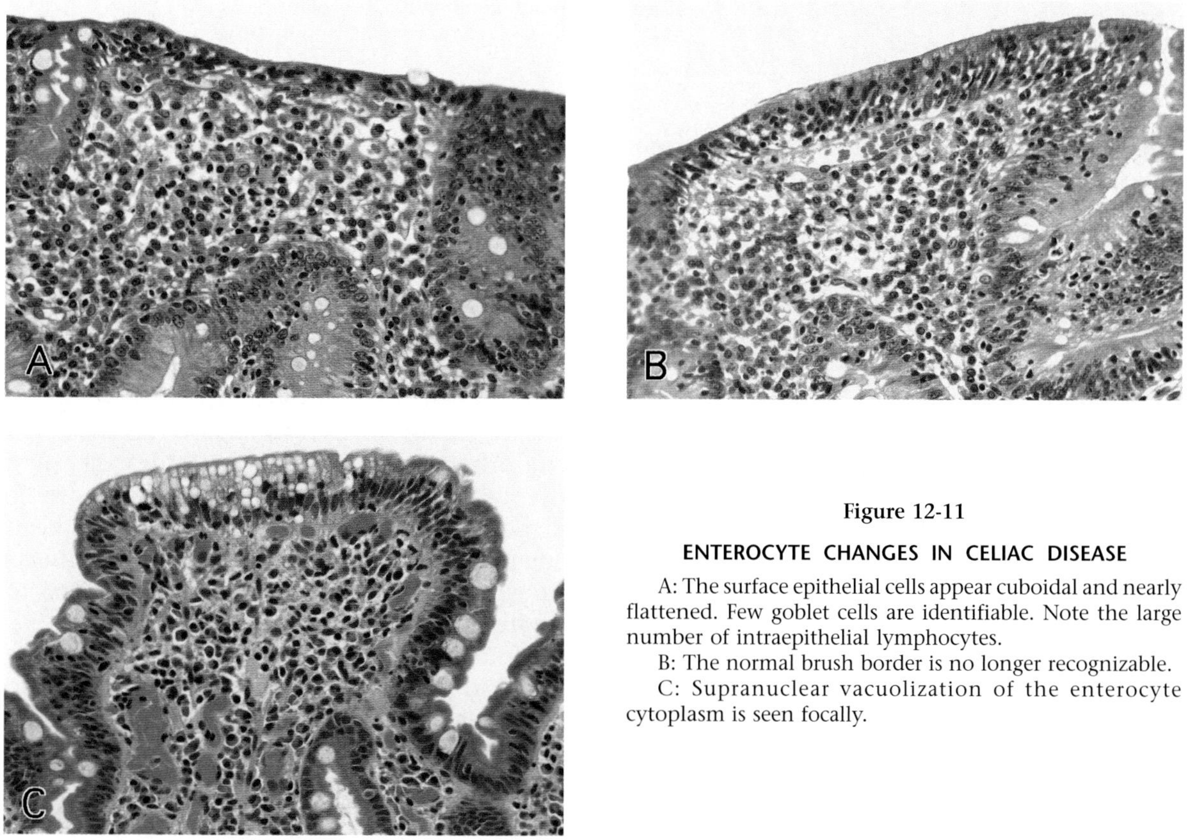

Figure 12-11

ENTEROCYTE CHANGES IN CELIAC DISEASE

A: The surface epithelial cells appear cuboidal and nearly flattened. Few goblet cells are identifiable. Note the large number of intraepithelial lymphocytes.

B: The normal brush border is no longer recognizable.

C: Supranuclear vacuolization of the enterocyte cytoplasm is seen focally.

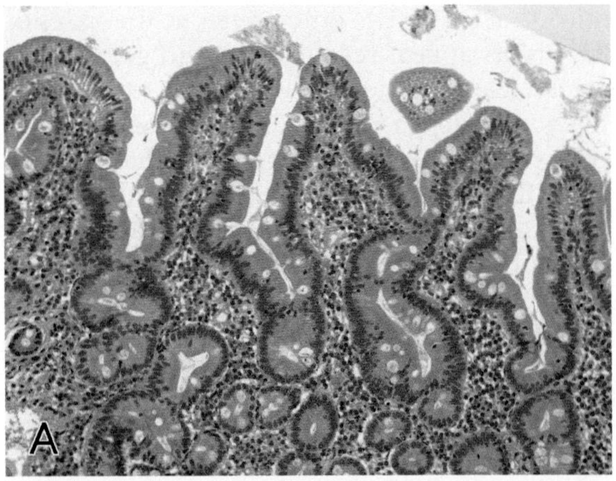

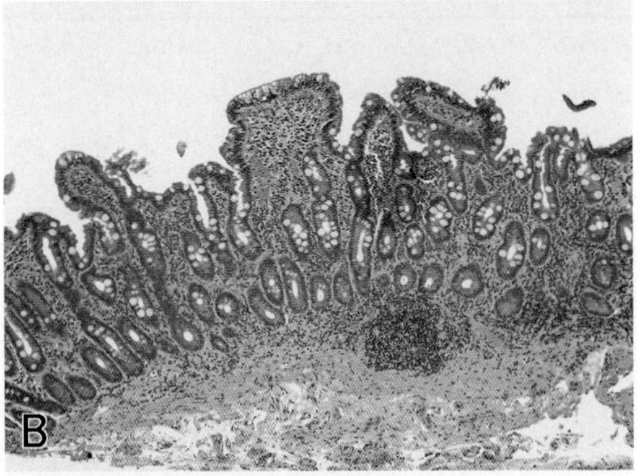

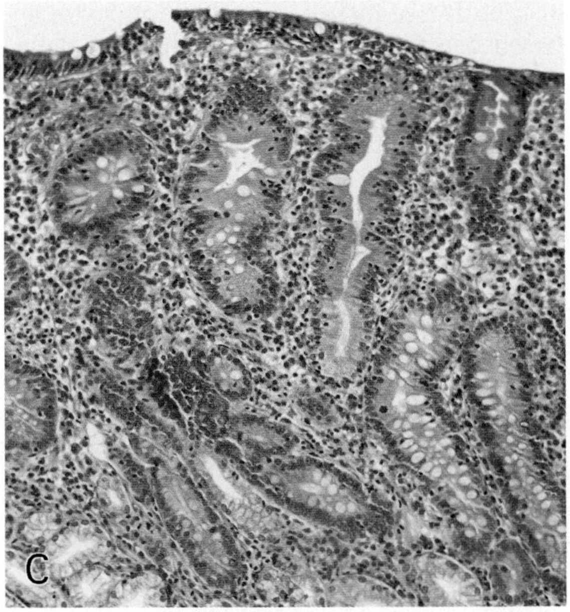

Figure 12-12

VARIABLE VILLOUS ATROPHY IN CELIAC DISEASE

A: This biopsy shows a mildly altered villous architecture. Many villi are still identifiable.

B: Biopsy from another patient with celiac disease shows more prominent villous blunting.

C: Complete villous atrophy is seen in another patient.

plasma cells, although eosinophils, and sometimes, neutrophils are also seen (fig. 12-14). The presence of cryptitis and crypt abscesses is very unusual in patients with celiac disease, and points to another etiology such as infection or Crohn's disease. IgA-, IgG-, and IgM-producing cells are increased 2- to 6-fold, with IgA-producing cells predominating. As a result, patients with IgA deficiency and celiac disease show a lower intensity of chronic inflammatory infiltration in the lamina propria. Immunophenotypically, lamina propria T lymphocytes in celiac patients are CD4-positive and intraepithelial T lymphocytes are CD8-positive, a distribution that is similar to that seen in normal mucosa.

As previously mentioned, the histologic changes of celiac disease are often patchy in distribution. As a result, multiple biopsy specimens from endoscopically normal and abnormal areas should be examined in order to establish the diagnosis. The histologic changes are most pronounced in the second and third parts of the duodenum. The microscopic features become less severe and patchier in the distal small bowel, particularly in the ileum.

The severity of the histologic changes does not correlate well with the clinical signs and symptoms. The extent of the small intestinal disease, however, does correlate with the clinical severity the disease. Celiac patients with severe villous atrophy can be asymptomatic provided that the length of involved small bowel is short. On the other hand, minimal histologic changes involving a longer segment of intestine can be associated with clinical symptoms. It has been suggested that in clinically severe disease, a longer length of small intestine is exposed to higher concentrations of dietary gluten.

Histologic Response to Gluten-Free Diet. Table 12-12 shows the chronology of the clinical and histologic responses to a gluten-free diet. Partial villous atrophy is seen in more than 50 percent of patients on a gluten-free diet. The degree of intraepithelial lymphocytosis, however, does

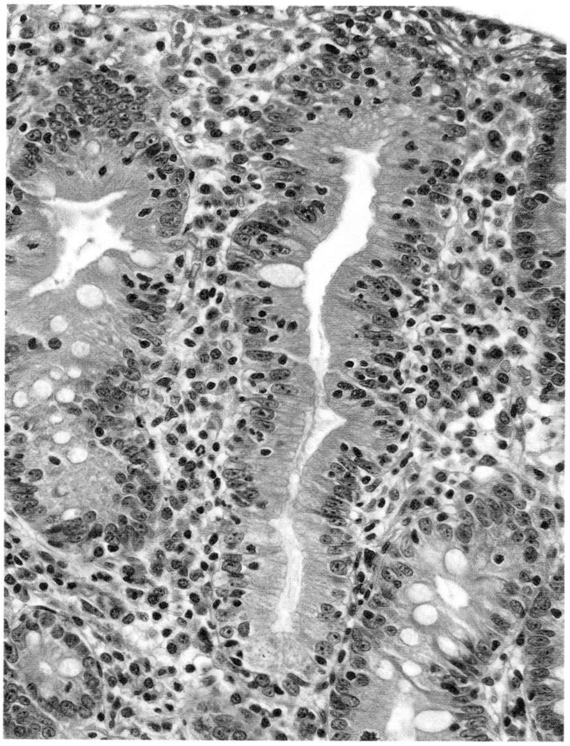

Figure 12-13

CRYPT HYPERPLASIA IN CELIAC DISEASE

The crypt is markedly elongated and villi were completely absent from the mucosal surface. The number of intraepithelial lymphocytes is increased.

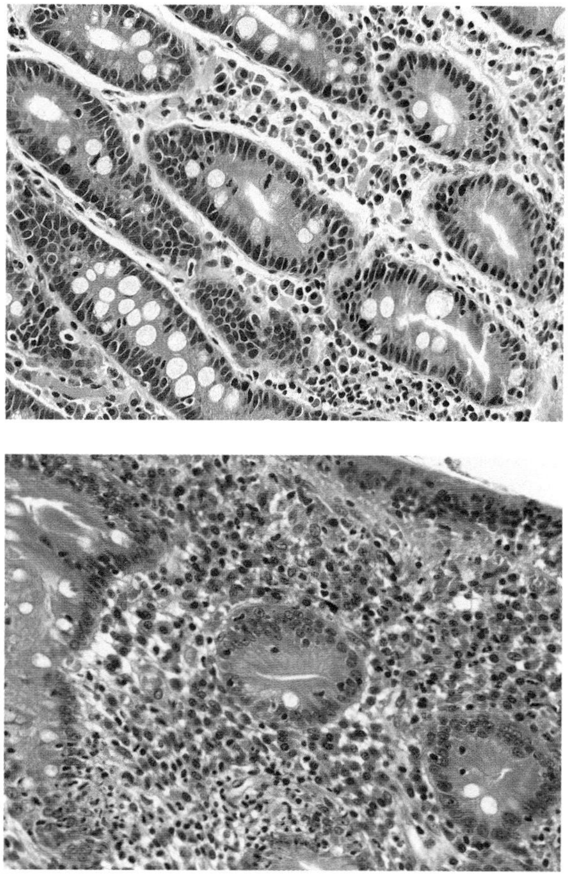

Figure 12-14

CELIAC DISEASE

Top: The lamina propria contains a mixed inflammatory infiltrate composed of lymphocytes, numerous plasma cells, and variable numbers of eosinophils.

Bottom: Neutrophils are present in some cases, as seen here.

decrease with gluten restriction, and is probably a more specific indicator of dietary response than is villous atrophy. The resolution of abnormal histologic changes occurs distal to proximal in the small intestine. Therefore, it may take more than 6 months of gluten restriction before histologic improvement is seen in the duodenum. In some patients, histologic improvement may take as long as 2 years (24).

Treatment and Prognosis. Removal of gluten from the diet is essential for the treatment of patients with celiac disease, and generally is required lifelong. Symptomatic response to the institution of a gluten-free diet is often rapid, with many patients responding within 48 hours (50); in others, weeks or even months may be required before clinical remission is achieved. In addition to a gluten-free diet, patients with severe celiac disease may require supplemental therapy to correct nutritional deficiencies related to malabsorption.

The prognosis is excellent for those patients who are diagnosed early, and adhere strictly to the gluten-free diet. Late diagnosis or noncompliance with dietary restrictions may result in malnutrition and debilitation. In general, both treated adult and pediatric patients have life expectancies similar to those of the general population (12,36).

COMPLICATIONS AND RELATED DISORDERS OF CELIAC DISEASE

Refractory Sprue

Definition. *Refractory sprue* is defined as symptomatic, severe villous atrophy that does not respond to a strict gluten-free diet for at

Table 12-12

DIETARY RESPONSE IN CELIAC DISEASE

Normal Diet
Malabsorption
Flat small intestinal biopsy (absent or severely blunted villi) with:
Damaged surface epithelium
Numerous intraepithelial lymphocytes
Chronic inflammation in lamina propria
Crypt hyperplasia
Short-Term Gluten-Free Diet (1 Week to 3 Months)
Early onset of clinical improvement
Within days, evidence of diminished surface epithelial damage
Reduced number of intraepithelial lymphocytes
Reduced chronic inflammation
Mild to moderate villous atrophy
Gluten-Free Diet >3 Months
Villi gradually become normal
No crypt hyperplasia
Decreased mitoses
Chronic inflammation diminished
Gluten Challenge
Early increase in intraepithelial lymphocytes
Eventual return of all other histologic abnormalities
Malabsorption returns

least 6 months. Since refractory sprue is a diagnosis of exclusion, the possibilities of inadvertent gluten ingestion and other causes of villous atrophy including disaccharidase deficiency, protein enteropathy, and bacterial overgrowth should be ruled out.

Etiology. Recent evidence suggests that refractory sprue may represent a manifestation of an aberrant clonal intraepithelial lymphocyte-mediated neoplastic process. Cellier et al. (71) demonstrated that intraepithelial lymphocytes in patients with refractory sprue represent a monoclonal population that lacks CD8, a marker found in normal intraepithelial lymphocytes. These histologically undetected monoclonal T cells may be designated *cryptic intestinal T-cell lymphoma* (72). The lymphocyte-induced injury leads to intestinal ulceration and lymph node cavitation in some patients. In some, but not all, the condition progresses to full-blown lymphoma.

Treatment. At present, patients with suspected refractory sprue are given a trial of glucocorticoids. In steroid-unresponsive cases, a search for clonal *TCR* gene rearrangements and immunostains for CD8 are advised.

Collagenous Sprue

Definition. *Collagenous sprue* is diagnosed histologically and is characterized by the development of a subepithelial collagen band thicker than 10 µm.

Demography. Collagenous sprue typically affects patients with a long history of celiac disease, but has been regarded by some as a distinct entity.

Clinical Features. The typical clinical history is of a patient with celiac disease who initially responded to a gluten-free diet, but subsequently became refractory to treatment.

Microscopic Findings. The small bowel biopsy shows a variable degree of villous atrophy and other features typical of celiac disease. In addition, a prominent subepithelial collagen band is present (fig. 12-15). This thickened collagen table can be highlighted with the use of a trichrome stain.

Treatment and Prognosis. Although patients with collagenous sprue should be given a trial of a gluten-free diet, the prognosis is poor and many patients develop other complications such as ulcerative jejunoileitis and lymphoma (73).

Ulcerative Jejunoileitis

Definition. *Ulcerative jejunoileitis* is an uncommon, but serious complication of celiac disease, characterized by multiple, chronic small intestinal ulcers. Although this entity has been regarded by many as synonymous with lymphoma, ulcerative jejunoileitis without any evidence of lymphoma has been documented in a few cases (75).

Clinical Features. The ulcers affect adults, generally after many years of malabsorption. Patients typically present with worsening of their malabsorption symptoms, abdominal pain, and complications including obstruction, perforation, and hemorrhage (74). Patients are often diagnosed late in the course of the disease (74). Radiographic studies, and in some cases laparotomy, are required to establish the diagnosis. Intestinal perforation and peritonitis may develop.

Pathologic Findings. The linear and shallow ulcers have a transverse orientation and little surrounding fibrosis, but are morphologically

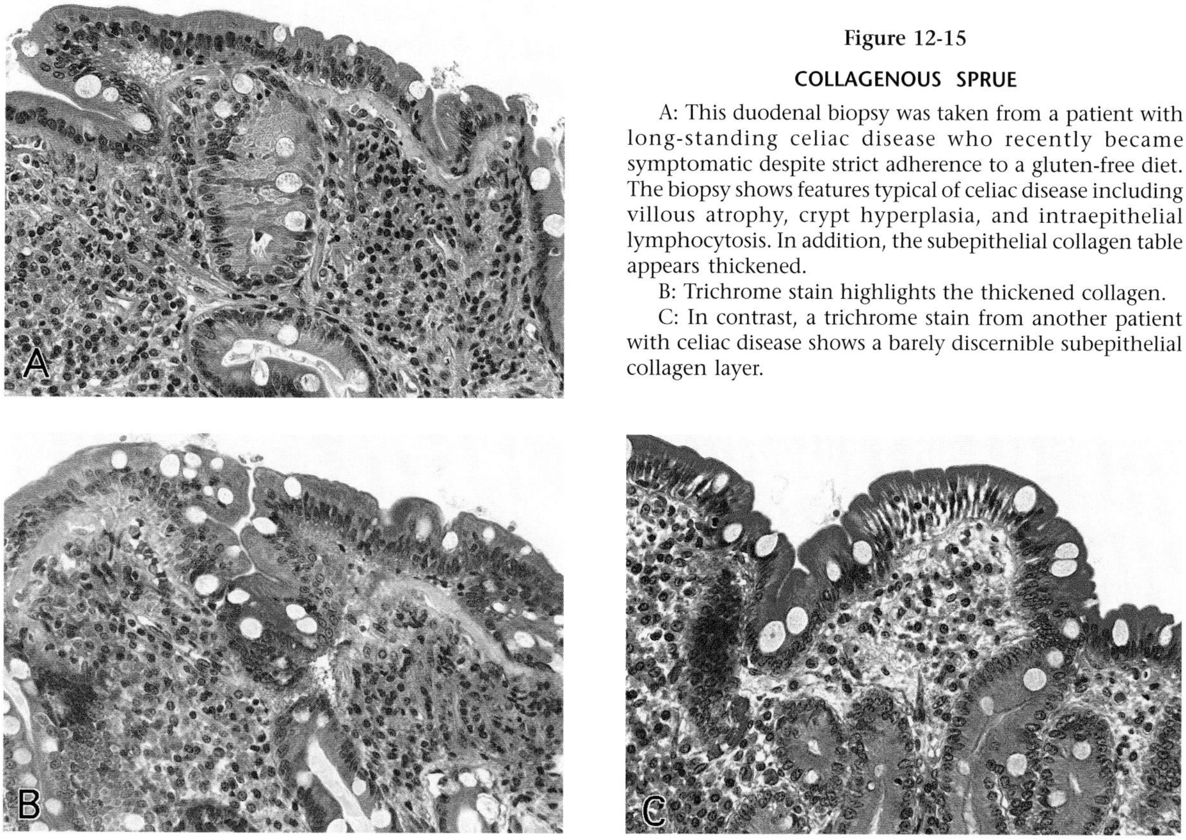

Figure 12-15

COLLAGENOUS SPRUE

A: This duodenal biopsy was taken from a patient with long-standing celiac disease who recently became symptomatic despite strict adherence to a gluten-free diet. The biopsy shows features typical of celiac disease including villous atrophy, crypt hyperplasia, and intraepithelial lymphocytosis. In addition, the subepithelial collagen table appears thickened.

B: Trichrome stain highlights the thickened collagen.

C: In contrast, a trichrome stain from another patient with celiac disease shows a barely discernible subepithelial collagen layer.

nonspecific, usually multiple, and predominantly jejunal in location (fig. 12-16). Histologically, the bases of the ulcers consist of purulent exudate overlying granulation tissue and fibrosis. The inflammation extends into the submucosa or even the muscle. The serosa may appear edematous and inflamed.

Treatment and Prognosis. Surgical excision is the most effective therapy. Some patients respond to glucocorticoids and azathioprine. Diffuse or multifocal enteropathy-associated T-cell lymphoma develops in the majority of untreated patients.

Enteropathy-Associated T-Cell Lymphoma

Definition. *Enteropathy-associated T-cell lymphoma* (EATL) is a T-cell lymphoma that occurs in the setting of celiac disease. It is a life-threatening complication that occurs in a small percentage of patients.

Demography. A variable incidence in EATL has been reported, ranging from 3 to 15 percent. Lymphoma usually occurs late in the

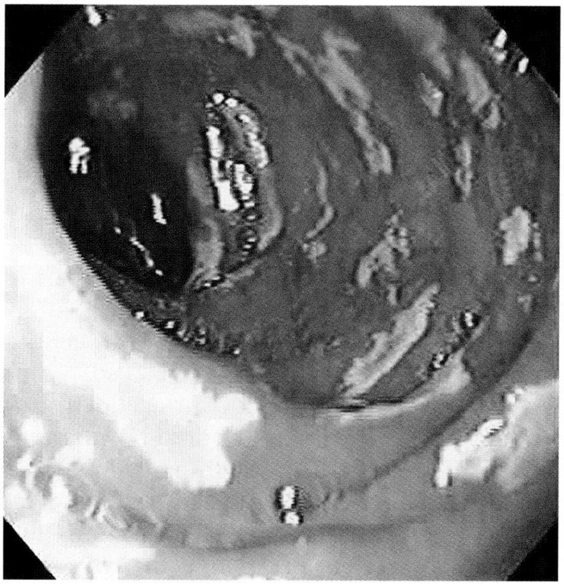

Figure 12-16

ULCERATIVE JEJUNOILEITIS

Endoscopic view demonstrates the presence of numerous ulcers within the small intestine.

course of celiac disease, frequently 20 to 30 years after the original onset of the disease. As a result, it is seen in an older age group, with the majority of patients more than 50 years of age.

Clinical Features. The clinical features of EATL are similar to those of refractory sprue and ulcerative jejunoileitis. Radiographic studies may show a mass lesion. The overall prognosis is extremely poor, with a 5-year survival rate of approximately 10 percent.

Other Malignancies

Small bowel adenocarcinoma is the most common nonlymphomatous malignant neoplasm seen in celiac patients. Patients may also develop nodal lymphomas and carcinomas in other gastrointestinal sites, the oropharynx, or breast.

INFECTIONS CAUSING MALABSORPTION

Bacterial Overgrowth

Bacterial overgrowth occurs following intestinal resection, gastrectomy, or in patients with diverticulosis or stasis due to disorders affecting intestinal motility. Bacterial overgrowth leads to malabsorption due to increased deconjugation and dehydroxylation of bile salts, rendering them unavailable for absorption of fat. In addition, unconjugated bile salts and bacterial proteases damage the brush border, decreasing absorption. Bacteria also compete for nutrients. The diagnosis is established by an appropriate clinical history and radiologic examination. Biopsy has no role in this diagnosis, other than to exclude other causes of malabsorption.

Other Infections

Multiple protozoal organisms may infect the small intestine and result in malabsorption. Common organisms include intracellular protozoa such as *Isospora* and microsporidia and extracellular organisms such as *Giardia* and *Cryptosporidium*. Whipple's disease, tropical sprue, viral gastroenteritis, and bacterial infections also cause malabsorption. Infections with such organisms reduce the absorptive capacity of the small intestine as a result of their invasion of the epithelium or by the damage they cause to the brush border. Infections leading to malabsorption are discussed in detail in chapters 10 and 11.

Malabsorption in Acquired Immunodeficiency Syndrome

Opportunistic bacterial, fungal, or protozoal infections; impaired oral intake; acquired immunodeficiency syndrome (AIDS)-associated motility disorders; drug-induced injury; and malignancy affecting the small intestine are all causes of malabsorption in human immunodeficiency virus (HIV)-positive patients. HIV/AIDS is discussed in detail in chapter 11.

POSTOPERATIVE MALABSORPTION SYNDROMES

Extensive Small Bowel Resection

The severity and type of malabsorption that occurs following small bowel resection depend upon the length and portion of small intestine resected. Jejunal resection leads to water and nutrient malabsorption. Ileal resection leads to malabsorption of vitamin B12 and disruption of bile acid–mediated absorptive processes. When the ileocecal valve is compromised loss of neurohumoral mechanisms, slow intestinal transit time, and bacterial overgrowth contribute to the malabsorption.

The symptoms are worst in the immediate postoperative period. Later, intestinal adaptation in the form of hypertrophy and hyperplasia of the remaining intestine occurs. This increases absorption of some nutrients and symptoms improve to a certain extent. Careful pathologic examination of the resected bowel segment is necessary to exclude an additional etiology of malabsorption.

Gastric Surgery

Rapid transit through the stomach, hypoacidity leading to bacterial overgrowth, and dilution of pancreatic enzymes by rapid emptying of gastric liquid are some of the mechanisms causing malabsorption following gastric surgery. Unlike small bowel resection, the malabsorption is mild and not specific to any nutrients.

SYSTEMIC DISEASES CAUSING MALABSORPTION

Systemic Mastocytosis

Definition. *Systemic mastocytosis* is a clonal proliferation of mast cells, which accumulate in skin, bones, lymph nodes, and parenchymal organs.

Demography. Mastocytosis in children is generally limited to skin manifestations (84). Adult-onset mastocytosis is usually a systemic disease that results from a clonal proliferation of mast cell precursors.

Etiology. Systemic mastocytosis is associated with activating mutations in the *c-kit* gene within mast cell progenitor cells. The protein product of *c-kit* is a receptor tyrosine kinase that is activated when bound by stem cell factor, the major mast cell growth and differentiation factor (76,78,84). Gastrointestinal symptoms occur as a result of the release of active mediators from the proliferating mast cells or from infiltration of tissues by these neoplastic cells.

Clinical Features. Eighty percent of patients present with dermatologic findings, usually urticaria pigmentosa (87). Typical symptoms include pruritus, flushing, tachycardia, asthma, and headache, all thought to result from the release of histamine from the proliferating mast cells (80,81). Fifty to 80 percent of patients have gastrointestinal symptoms, including peptic ulcers, malabsorption, steatorrhea, nausea, vomiting, copious watery diarrhea, and abdominal pain (80–82). These features are also thought to be due to effects of histamine and prostaglandins on the intestinal and gastric epithelia (77,79–81,85). Symptoms are often induced by alcohol consumption (80). The hyperhistaminemia produces gastric hypersecretion (77, 83). Gastric acid levels correlate with the degree of histaminemia and with the presence of acid peptic disease, including peptic duodenitis (77,83). The release of mediators from mast cells results in increased intestinal permeability and altered smooth muscle function (88). Malabsorption may also be related in part to mucosal infiltration by mast cells.

Endoscopic and Radiologic Findings. Endoscopically, urticaria-like lesions are seen in the gastrointestinal tract. Radiographically, "bulls-eye" lesions resembling metastases, edema, thickened folds, and a nodular mucosal pattern may be present (86). Small intestinal involvement may be suggested radiographically by the presence of small nodular filling defects, particularly in the duodenum.

Microscopic Findings. Histologic changes include mucosal villous atrophy, marked submucosal edema, and clumps of mast cell infiltrates in the lamina propria (fig. 12-17). Large numbers of mast cells infiltrate the lamina propria, muscularis mucosae, and submucosa, with aggregates of mast cells within the gland lumens and evidence of glandular destruction. Eosinophils may also be seen. Immunohistochemical stains for tryptase or CD117 highlight the presence of the mast cells (fig. 12-17).

Diabetes Mellitus

Diabetes mellitus can cause malabsorption by several different mechanisms. There is a known association between insulin-dependent diabetes and celiac disease. Diabetics may also have abnormalities in pancreatic exocrine secretion and develop bacterial overgrowth leading to malabsorption. Steatorrhea occurring in the absence of these conditions in diabetic patients may be attributed to rapid intestinal transit.

Endocrine Abnormalities

Hypothyroidism is associated with celiac disease and partial villous atrophy. Malabsorption associated with hypothyroidism is characterized by the failure of multiple endocrine organs due to autoimmune damage (autoimmune polyglandular syndrome type 1). *Hyperthyroidism* can cause malabsorption by altering intestinal secretion and altering intestinal transit time. Other endocrinopathies that may result in malabsorption include *Addison's disease* and *hypoparathyroidism*.

Collagen Vascular Diseases

Collagen vascular diseases, particularly *scleroderma*, cause malabsorption as a result of their effects on gastrointestinal motility. In patients with scleroderma or other connective tissue diseases, the muscularis propria may undergo atrophy and fibrous replacement, resulting in a predisposition to bacterial overgrowth (fig. 12-18). Associated vasculitis may also contribute to impaired nutrient absorption.

IMMUNOLOGIC DISORDERS

Selective IgA Deficiency

Definition. *Selective IgA deficiency* is a condition in which the major mucosal immunoglobulin, IgA, is not produced.

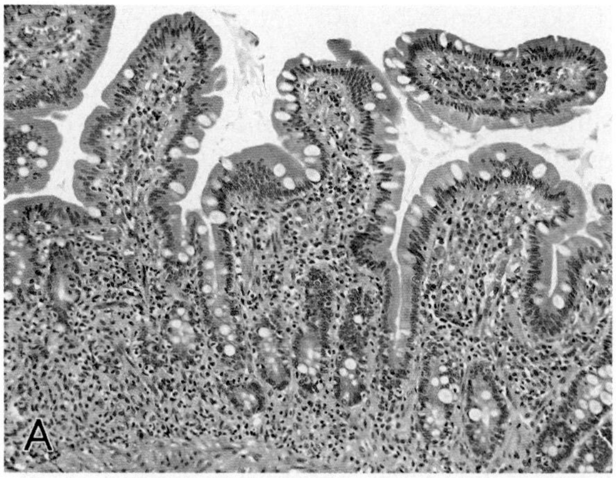

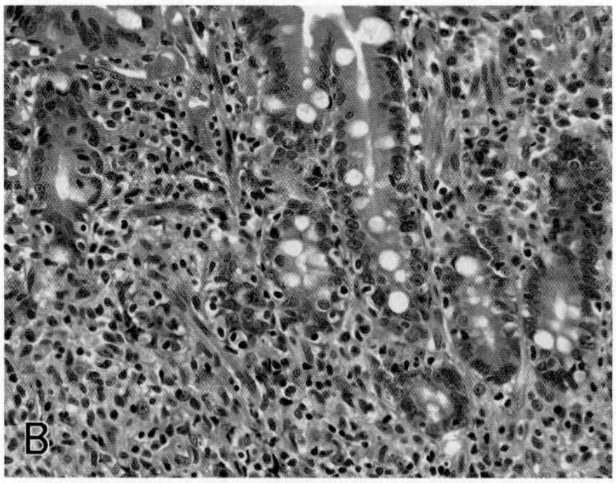

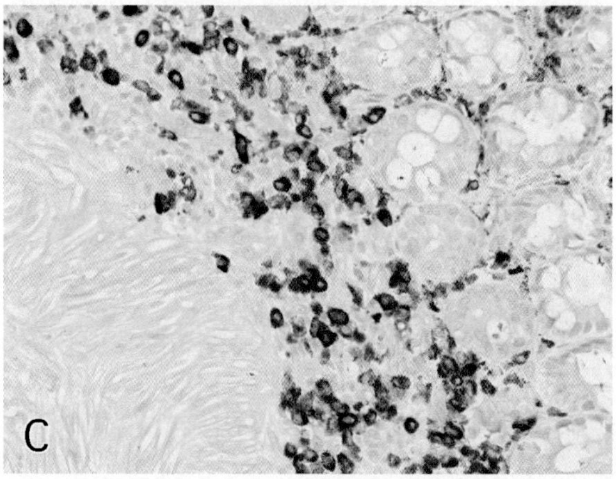

Figure 12-17

SYSTEMIC MASTOCYTOSIS

A: Low-power photomicrograph demonstrates mild villous blunting in a patient with systemic mastocytosis.

B: The lamina propria contains numerous infiltrating cells including eosinophils and mast cells. Mast cells also appear to be infiltrating the glandular epithelium.

C: An immunostain for mast cell tryptase highlights the mast cell infiltrate.

Demography. Selective IgA deficiency is the most common immunodeficiency in Caucasians, occurring in about 1/600 individuals in the general population (95,97). The incidence varies, however, depending on the population being studied. Published figures range from 1/400 in Finland to 1/1,500 in Japan (91). IgA deficiency is 10 to 15 times more common in patients with celiac disease than in the general population.

Etiology. In most cases, the cause of the immunoglobulin deficiency is unknown. The disease may be congenital or induced by viral infections, leukopenia, and drugs (89,92,94,96,98, 100–102). Unusual cases result from deletion of an *IgA* gene on chromosome 14 (100). Selective IgA deficiency is associated with extended HLA haplotypes that include either a C4A null allele (C4AQ0), 21-hydroxylase gene deletions in the HLA class III region, or rare class IIIC gene haplotypes (98), especially in Caucasians. These haplotypes are rare in blacks and Asians. The presence of suppressor cells specific for IgA synthesis causes the abnormalities (89).

Most patients have defective B-cell maturation with abnormal terminal differentiation of membrane IgA-positive B cells into IgA-secreting plasma cells. A smaller percentage of individuals have a defect in the immune regulation of a putative suppressor T cell that selectively inhibits IgA production.

Clinical Features. Many patients with selective IgA deficiency lack clinical abnormalities due to a compensatory increase in IgM (90). Other patients, especially if deficient in IgG subclasses, present with diarrhea, malabsorption, autoimmune disease (93,99,103), or bacterial infections, including gastrointestinal, sinus, and respiratory infections. Patients with IgA deficiency also frequently have antibodies directed against cow's milk and ruminant serum proteins, immunoglobulins, thyroglobulin, and collagen. Selective IgA deficiency leads to depletion of

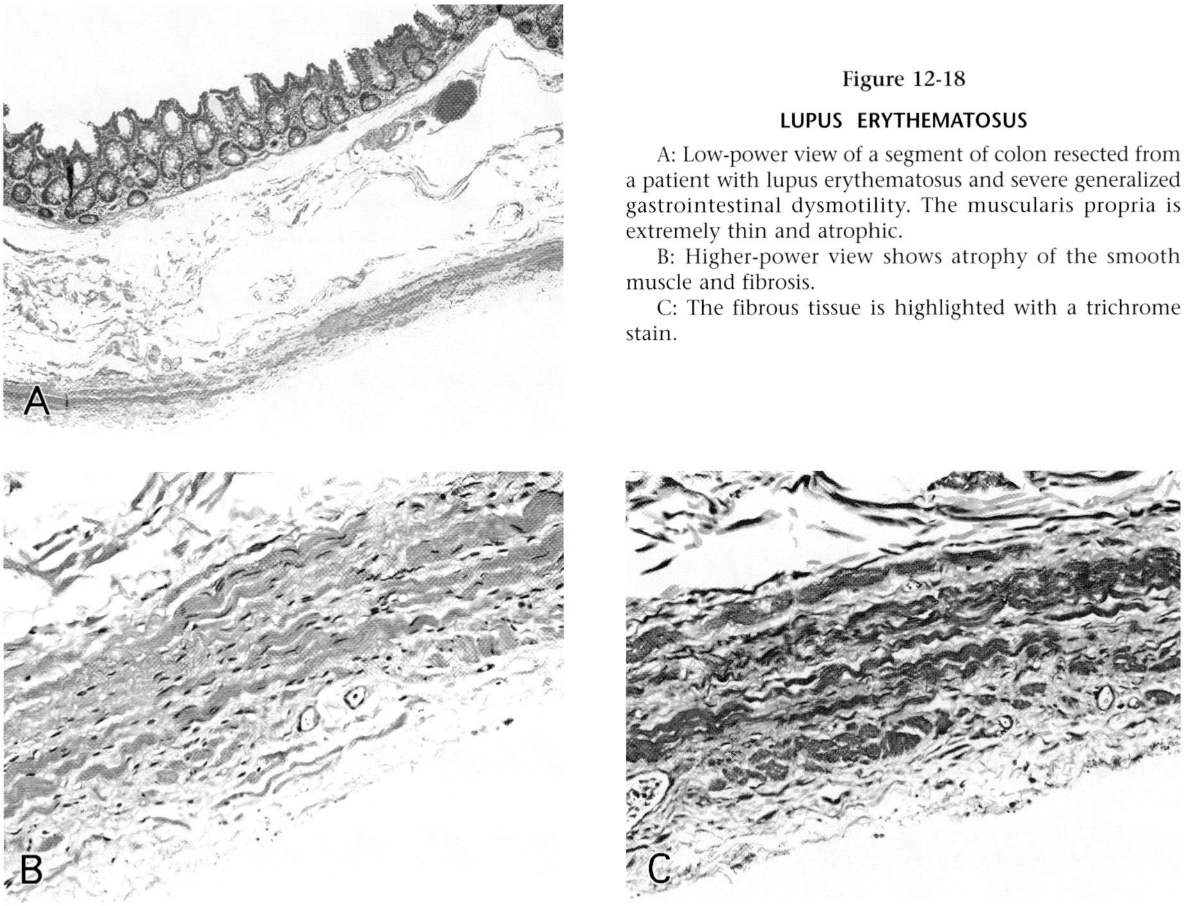

Figure 12-18

LUPUS ERYTHEMATOSUS

A: Low-power view of a segment of colon resected from a patient with lupus erythematosus and severe generalized gastrointestinal dysmotility. The muscularis propria is extremely thin and atrophic.

B: Higher-power view shows atrophy of the smooth muscle and fibrosis.

C: The fibrous tissue is highlighted with a trichrome stain.

IgA-producing plasma cells in the lamina propria. Serum IgA levels are low to undetectable.

Pathologic Findings. Biopsies in IgA-deficient patients may appear completely normal with a seemingly full complement of lymphocytes and plasma cells in the lamina propria, especially in adults. In some patients, slightly decreased numbers of lymphocytes and plasma cells are seen. Immunohistochemical analysis for immunoglobulins demonstrates that the lamina propria plasma cells produce IgM and IgG, but not IgA. Patients may also have evidence of coexisting celiac disease or bacterial infection. Rarely, patients with a selective IgA deficiency present with a completely flat mucosa in the absence of bacterial overgrowth or *Giardia* infection.

Common Variable Immunodeficiency

Definition. *Common variable immunodeficiency* (CVID) represents a heterogeneous group of immunologic diseases characterized by low levels of immunoglobulins and an inability to mount an antibody response to antigens. Synonyms include *acquired hypogammaglobulinemia*, *adult-onset hypogammaglobulinemia*, and *dysgammaglobulinemia*

Demography. CVID is the second most common primary immunodeficiency, following isolated IgA deficiency. It affects 6 to 12/1 million live births (105,111,117). The disorder is almost equally distributed between the sexes. The disease is usually sporadic, but familial clustering associated with an autosomal dominant mode of transmission occurs in 20 percent of patients (122).

Etiology. The major defect in CVID is a failure of B-cell differentiation, with impaired secretion of immunoglobulins, but it is not clear whether this is due to a primary B-cell defect or abnormalities in T cells. B cells in CVID are immature, and show impaired upregulation of markers of activation (104,112,115). In some patients, a defect in *IgV* gene somatic hypermutation is

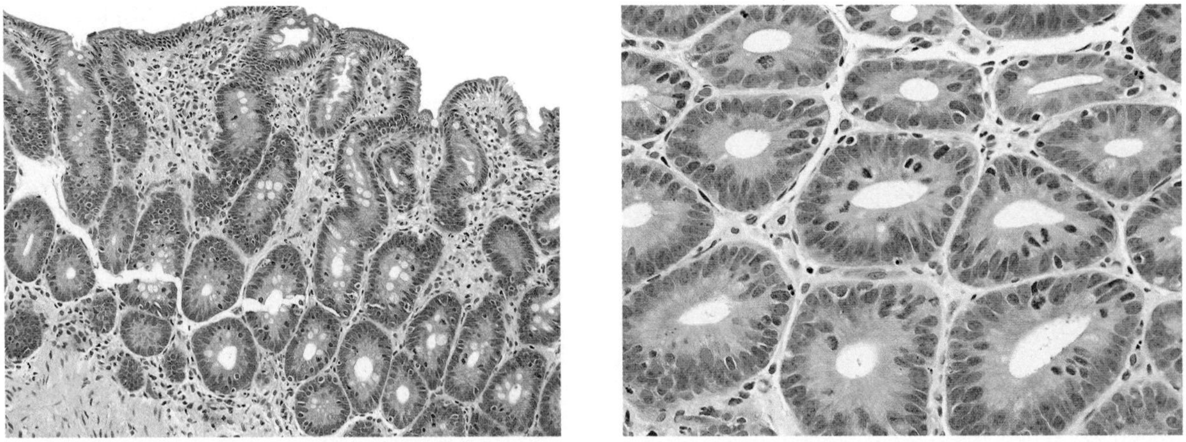

Figure 12-19

COMMON VARIABLE IMMUNODEFICIENCY

Left: At low power, the biopsy features of common variable immunodefiency (CVID) appear quite similar to those of celiac disease. There is prominent blunting of the villi and crypt hyperplasia.

Right: Higher-power view shows numerous mitoses in the hyperplastic crypts. (Courtesy of Dr. John Hart, Chicago, IL.)

present, an abnormality that results in the production of immunoglobulins with reduced or absent affinity for antigens (120). In addition to B-cell abnormalities, CVID patients also show abnormalities in T cell function. CVID patients exhibit decreased T-cell proliferation and activation, defective antigen-driven response, and reduced production of cytokines (113,118,123).

Since some cases of CVID appear to be familial, an active search for the responsible genetic abnormality has been sought. Haplotype analysis and linkage studies indicate that the HLA-DQ/DR locus is the major site of involvement (119). An association between CVID and homozygosity for genes encoding HLA class II molecules, especially HLA-DQ, has been reported (109). In some patients, there is an association with the TNF-α +488 A allele (121). In one recent study, 4 of 32 patients with adult-onset CVID demonstrated a homozygous deletion of the *ICOS* gene, an inducible co-stimulator found on activated T cells (114).

Clinical Features. Chronic and recurrent sinopulmonary infections are the hallmark of the disease (106,124,125). Approximately 60 percent of patients with CVID develop diarrhea (126). Twenty to 30 percent of patients have mild to moderate malabsorption frequently due to small intestinal infection with *Giardia*. The CVID-associated enteropathy may be accompanied by a deficiency in jejunal brush border enzymes (108). Achlorhydria, due to the presence of chronic atrophic gastritis, is seen in 33 to 50 percent of patients (116). Patients develop a pernicious anemia-like syndrome with intrinsic factor deficiency, gastric atrophy, loss of parietal cells, and low vitamin B12 levels. Lactose and gluten intolerance may result from mucosal inflammation and increased mucosal permeability.

Pathologic Findings. Histologically, variable degrees of villous atrophy are seen, and in some cases, the histologic picture closely resembles that seen in celiac disease (fig. 12-19). In contrast to celiac disease, however, a marked intraepithelial lymphocytosis is not present. In addition, the lamina propria in CVID appears variably cellular, with a distinct absence of plasma cells (fig. 12-20). Other inflammatory cells, including eosinophils and neutrophils, may be present. Infection, particularly with *Giardia*, should be ruled out microscopically in all patients.

Treatment and Prognosis. The mainstay of therapy for patients with CVID is replacement of immunoglobulins. As a result, patients receive immunoglobulin intravenously every 3 to 4 weeks. Some patients report side effects from therapy such as fatigue, malaise, vomiting, chills, and fever. Rarely, anaphylactic reactions occur. In some patients with impaired T-cell function, long-term treatment with IL-2 has been administered (110).

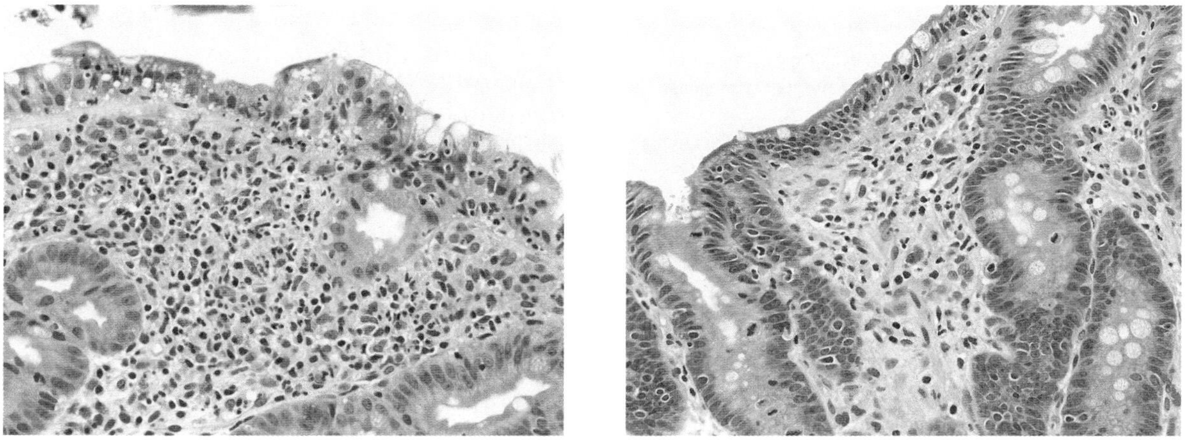

Figure 12-20

COMMON VARIABLE IMMUNODEFICIENCY

Left: The lamina propria appears hypercellular as in celiac disease, but plasma cells are absent from the infiltrate.
Right: The surface epithelium contains scattered neutrophils, but the prominent increase in intraepithelial lymphocytes characteristically seen in celiac disease is not present. (Courtesy of Dr. John Hart, Chicago, IL.)

Overall, the 20-year survival for CVID patients following diagnosis is 64 to 67 percent (107). In comparison, the 20-year survival rate is 92 to 94 percent for individuals in the general population.

Other Immunodeficiency Conditions Leading to Malabsorption

Severe combined immunodeficiency and *chronic granulomatous disease* are other disorders in which malabsorption can occur. Malabsorption is not the primary mode of presentation in patients with these conditions. The basic injury leading to malabsorption is recurrent infection by a variety of microorganisms.

Autoimmune Enteropathy

Autoimmune enteropathy is a rare cause of malabsorption. Antienterocyte antibodies, and in rare cases, antigoblet cell antibodies are present and lead to intestinal injury. Histologically, the disease is similar to celiac disease. Increased apoptotic activity is seen in the enterocytes. This entity is discussed more extensively in chapter 14.

Amyloidosis

Demography. *Primary amyloidosis* involves the gastrointestinal tract and may produce malabsorption, primarily in elderly individuals.

Clinical Features. Diarrhea, steatorrhea, weight loss, and anorexia are the usual symptoms (127). Diarrhea may be mediated by rapid intestinal transit time due to autonomic neuropathy and intestinal myopathy. Malabsorption may occur because the deposition of amyloid is a physical barrier to nutrient absorption. In addition, the motility disorder that occurs in patients with amyloidosis may result in bacterial overgrowth. Symptoms that occur as a result of involvement of other organs may help in establishing the diagnosis.

Microscopic Findings. The small intestinal biopsy shows amyloid deposition around blood vessels, and in the lamina propria, muscle layer, and enteric nerves. The changes may be patchy in distribution. Congo red stains or immunostains for amyloid protein are confirmatory.

LIPID MALABSORPTION

Lipid malabsorption and accumulation of lipids in enterocytes are seen in a number of conditions (Table 12-13).

Abetalipoproteinemia

Definition. *Abetalipoproteinemia* is an autosomal recessive genetic disease characterized by the virtual absence of apolipoprotein (apo)B and apoB-containing lipoproteins in plasma. It is also known as *Bassen-Kornzweig syndrome*.

Demography. Affected patients are usually individuals of Jewish or Mediterranean descent.

Table 12-13

CAUSES OF INTESTINAL LIPID ACCUMULATION

Abetalipoproteinemia
Familial hypobetalipoproteinemia
Diabetes mellitus
Gluten-sensitive enteropathy
Cow's milk enteropathy (and related entities)
Anderson's disease (chylomicron retention disease)
Fasting states
Impaired chylomicron metabolism
Juvenile nutritional megaloblastic anemia
Tropical sprue

Approximately one third of the cases result from consanguineous marriages, and family studies suggest an autosomal recessive mode of inheritance (129). The sex ratio is 1 to 1.

Etiology. In abetalipoproteinemia, chylomicron assembly is defective as a result of mutations in the microsomal triglyceride transfer protein (MTP) (131,132,134–136). MTP is a resident lipid transfer protein within the endoplasmic reticulum of hepatocytes and enterocytes. It is a heterodimer composed of a unique large subunit and a small subunit, protein disulfide isomerase. It catalyzes the transport of a wide variety of neutral lipids and phospholipids in in-vitro assays. The absence of MTP in abetalipoproteinemia occurs secondary to mutations in the gene for the large subunit of the protein. The absence of MTP results in an absence of apoB100 and apoB48 from the plasma, because apoB-containing lipoprotein assembly is disrupted in the liver and intestine.

Clinical Features. At birth, infants with abetalipoproteinemia are asymptomatic. Signs and symptoms begin within months after birth, once a diet rich in lipids has been started. The initial symptoms are diarrhea, bloating, and vomiting. Over time, anemia, weight loss, and failure to thrive occur. Spinocerebellar degeneration, peripheral neuropathy, and retinitis pigmentosa occur as a result of deficiencies in fat-soluble vitamins (vitamin E levels are characteristically extremely low). The gastrointestinal manifestations of the disease often improve with time, in part because affected patients learn to avoid dietary fats.

Acanthocytes are characteristically seen in the peripheral blood. Serum hypolipidemia is present, with reduced cholesterol, triglycerides, low density lipoproteins (LDL), and chylomicrons. Patients have undetectable levels of serum apolipoprotein B.

Endoscopic Findings. Examination of the small intestine demonstrates a "gelee blanche," or "white hoar frost," appearance to the mucosal surface (128,130,133,137). This feature is a reflection of the infiltration of mucosal lipids.

Microscopic Findings. On low-power examination, the villous architecture is minimally abnormal. The diagnostic changes are seen in the enterocytes, which appear pale with vaculated cytoplasm (fig. 12-21). This appearance is due to numerous subnuclear and apical fat microvacuoles within the enterocyte cytoplasm. These cytoplasmic droplets do not stain for mucin, but are positive with oil red-O. The lamina propria may contain macrophages with bizarre inclusions. Acanthocytes may occasionally be seen in the lumens of mucosal capillaries. In contrast to other conditions associated with lipid accumulation, abetalipoproteinemia is not associated with dilation of lacteals or lipid accumulation within the lamina propria.

Treatment and Prognosis. Early diagnosis and treatment are essential to avoid growth retardation and neuroretinal complications in patients with this disease. Many of the gastrointestinal symptoms can be relieved by placing affected patients on lipid-poor diets. Essential fatty acids may be replaced by dietary enrichment, or may be provided parenterally. Lipid-soluble vitamin replacement, particularly of vitamin E, should be undertaken. Interestingly, patients rarely achieve normal plasma alpha-tocopherol levels despite long-term therapy (129).

Familial Hypobetalipoproteinemia

Definition. *Familial hypobetalipoproteinemia,* also known as *homozygous hypobetalipoproteinemia,* is a rare inborn error of metabolism characterized by the inability to synthesize the apoproteins required for the export of lipoproteins from mucosal cells. By definition, patients present with low density lipoprotein (LDL) levels in the lowest fifth percentile (140).

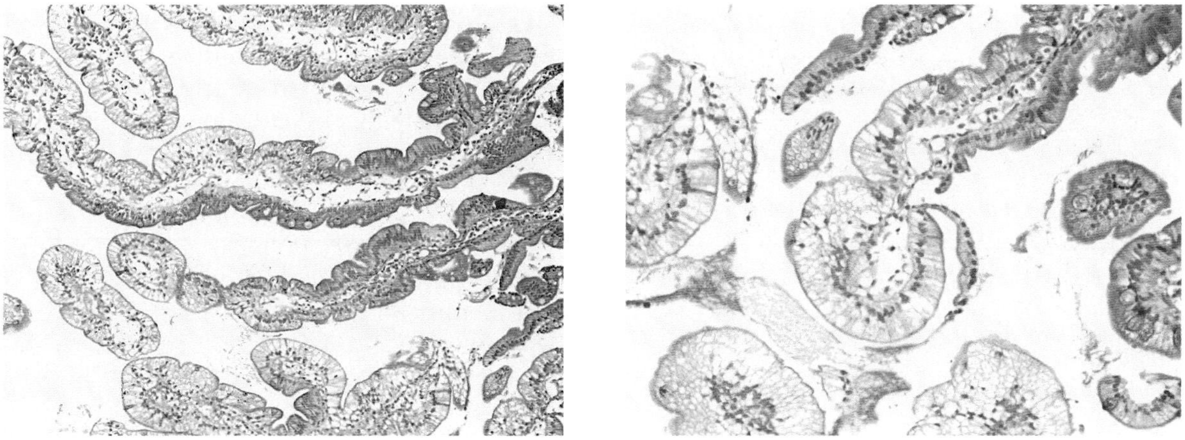

Figure 12-21

ABETALIPOPROTEINEMIA

Left: Low-power view shows the normal villous architecture.
Right: On higher power, the enterocytes are pale staining and vacuolated.

Demography. This autosomal co-dominant disorder is characterized by very low levels of total and LDL cholesterol, triglycerides, and apolipoprotein B. Betalipoprotein levels in heterozygous individuals are about 50 percent of normal; these patients usually remain asymptomatic except for mild fat intolerance. Homozygous individuals suffer the sequelae of intestinal fat malabsorption (138,139). Although typically decreased, the LDL fraction and apoprotein B are present in blood.

Etiology. The disease results from mutations in the *APOB* gene, leading to the formation of prematurely truncated apoB proteins.

Clinical Features. Heterozygotes for familial hypobetalipoproteinemia are usually asymptomatic, but have LDL cholesterol and apoB plasma levels that are 25 to 33 percent that of normal individuals. The clinical features seen in compound heterozygotes or homozygotes are similar to those seen in patients with abetalipoproteinemia.

Treatment and Prognosis. Treatment for homozygous patients includes restriction of fats from the diet.

Anderson's Disease

Definition. *Anderson's disease,* also known as *chylomicron retention disease,* is a rare autosomal recessive disease of intestinal lipid transport in which apoB48 is absent.

Clinical Features. Symptoms begin during the first few months of life and include chronic diarrhea, significant fat malabsorption, and failure to thrive (142). Unlike abetalipoproteinemia, acanthocytosis rarely occurs and neuromuscular manifestations are much less severe. Fasting triglyceride levels are normal but fat-soluble vitamins, especially A and E, are severely decreased. Plasma cholesterol levels are low but do not reach the levels observed in abetalipoproteinemia. ApoB, apoAI, and apoIV are decreased. Immunoperoxidase localization of apoB in fasting biopsy specimens shows normal to elevated staining of the lipid-laden intestinal epithelial cells (142).

Pathologic Findings. Morphologic studies demonstrate that the enterocytes contain large numbers of fat particles (chylomicrons) in the endoplasmic reticulum and the Golgi complex. Thus, the defect appears to be in the translocation of Golgi-derived vesicles to the plasma membrane for excretion. Hence, little or no fat is observed in the intercellular spaces and lacteals (142). The ultrastructural features differ from those seen in abetalipoproteinemia in that chylomicrons and larger lipid vacuoles are seen in the apical enterocyte cytoplasm (141).

Table 12-14

DRUGS AND SUPPLEMENTS ASSOCIATED WITH MALABSORPTION

Acarbose	Octreotide
Alcohol	Olestra
Antacids	Oral contraceptive agents
Anthraquinone laxatives	Orlistat
Biguanides	Paraaminosalicylate
Bisacodyl	Phenolphthalein
Carbamazepine	Phenytoin
Cholestyramine	Phytates
Colchicine	Proton pump inhibitors
Glucocorticoids	Pyrimethamine
Histamine-2 receptor agonists	Sulfonamides
Methotrexate	Tetracycline
Methyldopa	Thiazides
Neomycin	Triamterene

DRUG-INDUCED MALABSORPTION

Many drugs and dietary supplements lead to malabsorption. Some of these are listed in Table 12-14.

MALNUTRITION

Severe nutritional deficiency can produce marked small intestinal abnormalities (150) as is seen in the severe form of childhood malnutrition known as kwashiorkor. Malnutrition of this severity seldom occurs in developed countries, but less severe forms may be recognized after gastric surgery or in patients with chronic diseases. Malnutrition results from a lack of a suitable diet, faulty metabolism, and inadequate absorption of dietary constituents. Since the gastrointestinal mucosa is constantly renewed, it is highly sensitive to protein-calorie malnutrition.

Kwashiorkor

Definition. *Kwashiorkor* is a disease with characteristic clinical findings caused when physiologic stress is superimposed on chronic protein-calorie malnutrition.

Demography. Kwashiorkor is one of the most common pediatric illnesses of underdeveloped areas of the world. It was first reported in Africa, particularly in eastern and southern Africa, but can be seen in many parts of the developing world, mainly in the tropics and subtropics.

Etiology. Kwashiorkor results from severe protein deprivation. Nutrient malabsorption exacerbates the protein-caloric malnutrition, further damaging the gut, impairing immune competence, and increasing the risk of infections. Most organs are adversely affected due to malnutrition or concomitant infections.

Clinical Features. Typical clinical findings include growth retardation, peripheral edema, a protuberant abdomen, intestinal distension, hepatomegaly, and characteristic changes involving the skin and hair. Children with kwashiorkor are typically lethargic and apathetic.

Pathologic Findings. The small intestinal abnormalities are indistinguishable from those of untreated celiac disease. Histologically, the mucosa appears flattened. The crypts are elongated and coiled, but show a lower than normal mitotic index. The crypt changes are not uniformly distributed. The villi may be atrophic in some areas, whereas in others they appear normal or hyperplastic (162). Epithelial cell height decreases and the nuclei are arranged irregularly. Ultrastructurally, the microvilli appear shortened or deformed with branching and fusion. Free ribosomes are markedly reduced. In fatal cases, severe hypoplasia develops along with megaloblastic changes in the enterocytes. Paneth cells are reduced in number. The lamina propria becomes infiltrated with mononuclear cells and the basement membrane thickens (148). The presence of neutrophilic infiltrates suggests a coexisting infection. Affected patients respond to reinstitution of a normal diet with concomitant improvement in the histologic appearance of the intestinal mucosa.

VITAMIN DEFICIENCIES

Vitamin B12 Deficiency

Etiology. The ileum is the primary site of absorption of vitamin B12. Mucosal disease or resection of the terminal ileum leads to *vitamin B12 malabsorption*. Vitamin B12 malabsorption may also be congenital as a result of isolated absence of intrinsic factor secretion, a selective ileal absorptive defect known as *Imerslund syndrome*, or absence of transcobalamin II. More common causes of B12 deficiency include autoimmune gastritis (see chapter 4), caloric malnutrition, eating disorders, the presence of ileal diseases such as Crohn's disease, or complicating chemotherapy.

Normally, vitamin B12 ingested in the food is released by acid digestion in the stomach. The free B12 is preferentially picked up by R protein secreted by the salivary glands. Bound B12 is then transported to the small intestine where proteolysis by trypsin releases it for subsequent binding to intrinsic factor in the distal ileum. The intrinsic factor–B12 complex binds to the brush border of ileal enterocytes and is taken up and transported across the basolateral membrane. Here it is picked up by transcobalamin II for transport to the portal circulation. Defects in vitamin B12 absorption can result from decreased B12 in the diet, failed synthesis of intrinsic factor as in gastritis, decreased acid release of B12, loss of ileal receptors in a host of mucosal diseases, or defective receptors as seen in some immunologic diseases.

Clinical Features. Vitamin B12 deficiency results in megaloblastic anemia, leukopenia, thrombocytopenia, and neurologic changes predominantly involving the posterolateral spinal tracts.

Microscopic Findings. Histologically, the mucosa shows macrocytosis from the deficiency state.

Folate Deficiency

Etiology. Congenital folate malabsorption is rare. Most cases of *folate deficiency* occur because of insufficient dietary intake. Folate is found in wheat flour, beans, nuts, liver, and green, leafy vegetables. It is heat labile, and therefore becomes depleted from many cooked foods. In addition, oral contraceptives, antiepileptic agents, chronic diseases, malabsorption syndromes, alcohol, and smoking all impede folate absorption and metabolism.

Clinical Features. Patients develop megaloblastic anemia secondary to folate deficiency. Patients with eating disorders or malnourished alcoholics with severe nutritional folic acid deficiency who have secondary folate deficiencies have gastrointestinal lesions. These changes reverse following therapy (144,149).

Pathologic Findings. Some patients develop partial villous atrophy. The small intestinal villi appear stunted or club-shaped, and in some areas the mucosa appears flat. The enterocytes may also appear megaloblastic. The brush border appears indistinct and the nuclei of the surface epithelium are rounder than normal. Goblet cells and Paneth cells are normal. Neutrophils and plasma cells may be seen infiltrating the lamina propria.

Vitamin A Deficiency

Vitamin A deficiency affects the mucous membranes, particularly of the respiratory tract (165), but small intestinal abnormalities occur as well. These take the form of crystalline lysosomal inclusions in Paneth cells (157).

Vitamin E Deficiency and Brown Bowel Syndrome

Definition. *Brown bowel* is a rare syndrome characterized by lipofuscin deposition in the smooth muscle cells of the muscularis propria of the intestine, although any part of the gastrointestinal tract may be affected. Vitamin E deficiency is associated with brown bowel syndrome.

Demography. Vitamin E deficiency occurs alone or complicates other diseases. Brown bowel syndrome is endemic in the Thai-Lao ethnic group (159) and is induced in various species of animals by vitamin E deprivation (164).

Etiology. Vitamin E is an antioxidant that serves to scavenge free radicals throughout the body. The lipofuscin pigment deposition that occurs in brown bowel syndrome is the result of oxidative injury to smooth muscle cells.

Clinical Features. Vitamin E deficiency has been associated with both eosinophilic enteritis (154) and brown bowel syndrome. Patients range in age from the 20s to the late 70s, with an average age of 51 years (151). They present with epigastric pain, mild diarrhea, and chronic malabsorption. Brown bowel syndrome occasionally produces intestinal pseudoobstruction, but this is uncommon (147,161). It is not known whether the pigment deposition causes intestinal smooth muscle dysfunction.

Pathologic Findings. Grossly, the outer aspect of the bowel appears variably orange-brown and is often retrospectively described as darker than usual by the surgeon. The segmental or diffuse brownish discoloration can be appreciated from the serosal aspect of the gastrointestinal tract as well as on cut section (151). The disorder more commonly affects the small intestine and the stomach, but it can involve the colon. The

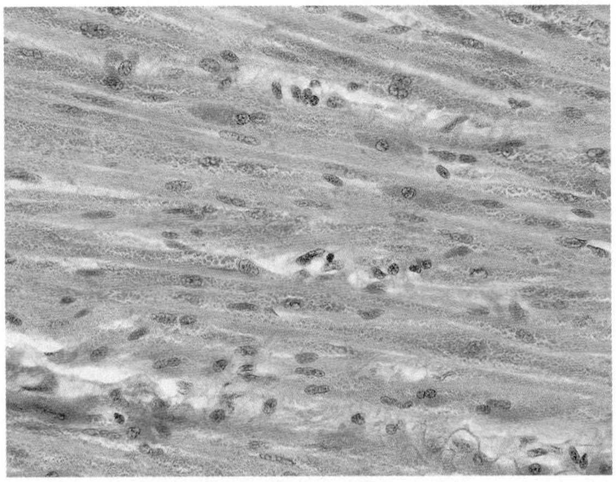

Figure 12-22

BROWN BOWEL SYNDROME

The smooth muscle cells of the muscularis propria contain a coarsely granular, light brown pigment (hematoxylin and eosin [H&E] stain).

esophagus may also be affected. No correlation exists between the degree of pigmentation and the severity of the associated symptoms.

Histologically, the mucosa usually appears normal, although occasionally, the villi appear blunted. There is usually no inflammation or fibrosis present, although eosinophils may populate the submucosa and muscular layer. Coarsely autofluorescent, granular, golden brown lipofuscin fills the smooth muscle cells of the muscularis propria, muscularis mucosae, and vascular walls (fig. 12-22). The pigment appears as round to oval granules, often lying in a perinuclear or central cellular location. The muscularis mucosae contains only minimal amounts of pigment; however, the vascular smooth muscle of the submucosa and subserosa frequently contains abundant pigment granules. The muscle fibers themselves may appear frayed. In advanced cases, large lipofuscin deposits result in considerable smooth muscle cell loss. In areas of minimal involvement, the pigment is barely visible. Macrophages also contain collections of pigment, especially in the muscular layer.

The pigment granules are positive with periodic acid–Schiff (PAS) after diastase digestion and fail to stain for melanin (fig. 12-23). The Fontana-Masson stain is the most sensitive stain for detecting the pigment, especially when the cells contain scant amounts (fig. 12-23).

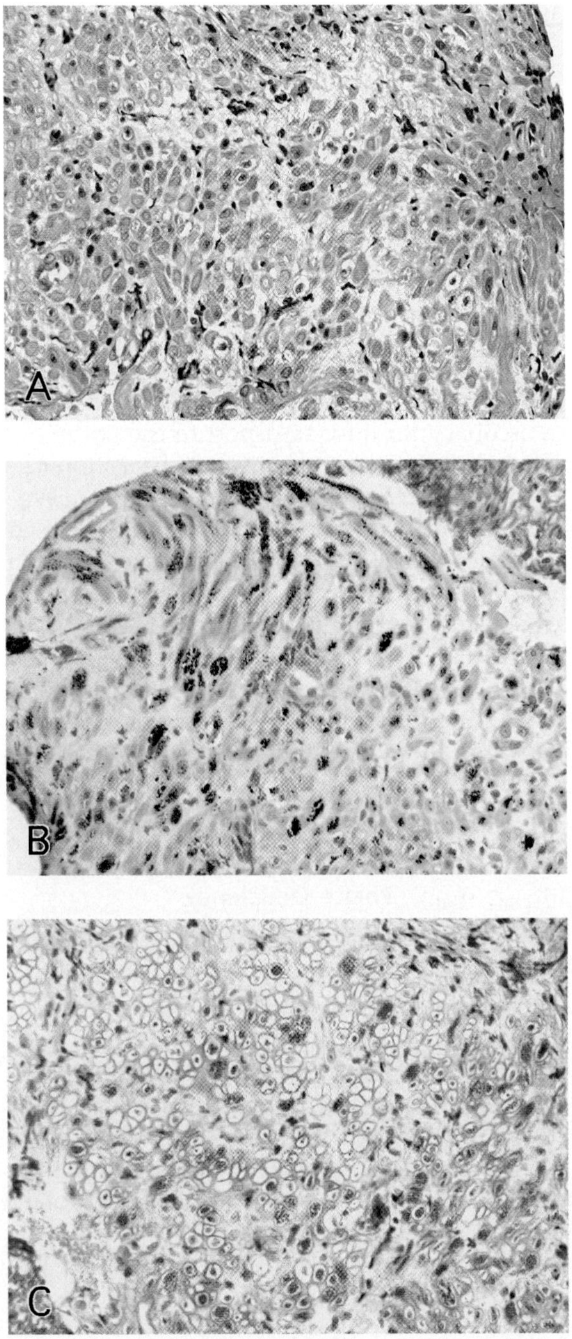

Figure 12-23

BROWN BOWEL INVOLVING THE ESOPHAGUS

A: H&E-stained section from an esophageal ulcer in a patient with severe malnutrition and known vitamin E deficiency. Many of the smooth muscle fibers in the ulcer base contain light brown pigment.

B: Fontana-Masson stain highlights the lipofuscin granules.

C: The lipofuscin also stains with periodic acid–Schiff (PAS).

Zinc Deficiency and Acrodermatitis Enteropathica

Definition. *Acrodermatitis enteropathica* is an autosomal recessive inborn error of metabolism resulting in zinc malabsorption and severe *zinc deficiency*.

Etiology. Zinc is a normal constituent of more than 100 enzymes. As a result, zinc deficiency has an overall detrimental effect on nucleic acid metabolism and protein and amino acid synthesis, eventually leading to growth arrest. Acquired deficiencies result from decreased zinc intake (as in total parenteral nutrition), increased zinc excretion (such as occurs in hepatic cirrhosis, proteinuria, burns, and penicillamine therapy), decreased intestinal absorption (as occurs in malabsorption syndromes, chronic alcoholic pancreatitis, and Crohn's disease), and increased zinc demands (as occurs in growth states, such as pregnancy or in patients with anemia) (143,156,158).

Zinc deficiency is associated with reduced absorption of unsaturated fats and impaired desaturation of linoleic and alpha-linoleic acids or their metabolites.

Clinical Features. The clinical manifestations of zinc deficiency include rash, stomatitis, glossitis, conjunctivitis, alopecia, nail dystrophy, growth retardation, psychologic disturbances, hypogonadism, photophobia, diarrhea, anorexia, impaired wound healing, defective cell-mediated immunity, and recurrent viral, fungal, and bacterial infections (152,153,163). Diarrhea and anorexia occur commonly, especially in infants. Growth retardation, alopecia, weight loss, and recurrent infections are prevalent in toddlers and schoolchildren. The diagnosis is made clinically and by documentation of the zinc deficiency. Zinc levels in serum, urine, and hair are approximately 50 percent of normal. Administration of zinc supplements leads to rapid and complete recovery. Severe cases may be fatal.

Pathologic Findings. Small intestinal biopsies of zinc-deficient individuals demonstrate focal villous shortening with mild crypt hyperplasia and slight infiltration of the lamina propria by mixed inflammatory cells. Electron microscopy of Paneth cells demonstrates the characteristic pleomorphic cytoplasmic inclusion bodies typical of acrodermatitis enteropathica (145,146). The ultrastructural abnormalities disappear after initiation of zinc therapy (145).

Other Mineral Deficiencies

Experimental animals made *selenium deficient* develop eosinophilic enteritis (160). Eosinophilia also complicates *magnesium deficiency* (155). The magnesium deficiency prompts mast cell degranulation and histamine release, causing subsequent tissue eosinophilia.

REFERENCES

Introduction

1. Dickey W, Hughes D. Prevalence of celiac disease and its endoscopic markers among patients having routine upper gastrointestinal endoscopy. Am J Gastroenterol 1999;94:2182–6.
2. Mee AS, Burke M, Vallon AG, Newman J, Cotton PB. Small bowel biopsy for malabsorption: comparison of the diagnostic accuracy of endoscopic forceps and capsule biopsy specimens. Br Med J 1985;291:769–72.
3. Wilson ID, McClain CJ, Erlandsen SL. Ileal Paneth cells and IgA system in rats with severe zinc deficiency: an immunohistochemical and morphological study. Histochemistry 1980;12: 457–71.

Celiac Disease

4. Abdo A, Meddings J, Swain M. Liver abnormalities in celiac disease. Clin Gastroenterol Hepatol 2004;2:107–12.
5. Arato A, Kosnai I, Szonyi L, Toth M. Frequent past exposure to adenovirus 12 in coeliac disease. Acta Paediatr Scand 1991;80:1101–2.
6. Autran JC, Ellen J, Law L, et al. N-terminal amino acid sequencing of prolamins of wheat and related species. Nature 1979;282:527–9.
7. Baklien K, Brandtzaeg P, Fausa O. Immunoglobulins in jejunal mucosa and serum from patients with adult coeliac disease. Scand J Gastroenterol 1977;12:149–59.

8. Catassi C, Ratsch IM, Fabiani E, et al. Coeliac disease in the year 2000: exploring the iceberg. Lancet 1994;343:200–3.
9. Cavell B, Stenhammar L, Ascher H, et al. Increasing incidence of childhood coeliac disease in Sweden. Results of a national study. Acta Paediatr 1992;81:589–92.
10. Chorzelski TP, Beutner EH, Sulej J, et al. IgA anti-endomysium antibody. A new immunological marker of dermatitis herpetiformis and coeliac disease. Br J Dermatol 1984;111:395–402.
11. Ciclitira PJ, Ellis HJ. Investigation of cereal toxicity in coeliac disease. Postgrad Med J 1987;63: 767–75.
12. Collin P, Reunala T, Pukkala E, Laippala P, Keyrilainen O, Pasternack A. Coeliac disease—associated disorders and survival. Gut 1994;35:1215–8.
13. Collin P, Vilska S, Heinonen PK, Hallstrom O, Pikkarainen P. Infertility and coeliac disease. Gut 1996;39:382–4.
14. Cox DA, Maurer T. Transforming growth factor-beta. Clin Immunol Immunopathol 1997; 83:25–30.
15. De Ritis G, Occorsio P, Auricchio S, Gramenzi F, Morisi G, Silano V. Toxicity of wheat flour proteins and protein-derived peptides for in vitro developing intestine from rat fetus. Pediatr Res 1979;13:1255–61.
16. De Santis A, Addolorato G, Romito A, et al. Schizophrenic symptoms and SPECT abnormalities in a coeliac patient: regression after a gluten-free diet. J Intern Med 1997;242:421–3.
17. Farrell RJ, Kelly CP. Celiac sprue. N Engl J Med 2002;346:180–8.
18. Fasano A, Catassi C. Current approaches to diagnosis and treatment of celiac disease: an evolving spectrum. Gastroenterology 2001;120:636–51.
19. Ferguson A, Murray D. Quantitation of intraepithelial lymphocytes in human jejunum. Gut 1971;12:988–94.
20. Ferreira M, Davies SL, Butler M, Scott D, Clark M, Kumar P. Endomysial antibody: is it the best screening test for coeliac disease? Gut 1992;33:1633–7.
21. Goldstein NS, Underhill J. Morphologic features suggestive of gluten sensitivity in architecturally normal duodenal biopsy specimens. Am J Clin Pathol 2001;116:63–71.
22. Greco L, Corazza G, Barbon MC, et al. Genome search in celiac disease. Am J Hum Genet 1998;62:669–72.
23. Green PH, Shane E, Rotterdam H, Forde KA, Grossbard L. Significance of unsuspected celiac disease detected at endoscopy. Gastrointest Endosc 2000;51:60–5.
24. Grefte JM, Bouman JG, Grond J, Jansen W, Kleibeuker JH. Slow and incomplete histological and functional recovery in adult gluten sensitive enteropathy. J Clin Pathol 1988;41:886–91.
25. Hadjivassiliou M, Gibson A, Davies-Jones GA, Lobo AJ, Stephenson TJ, Milford-Ward A. Does cryptic gluten sensitivity play a part in neurological illness? Lancet 1996;347:369–71.
26. Hankey GL, Holmes GK. Coeliac disease in the elderly. Gut 1994;35;65–7.
27. Holopainen P, Naluai AT, Moodie S, et al. Candidate gene region 2q33 in European families with coeliac disease. Tissue Antigens 2004;63:212–22.
28. Howell MD, Austin RK, Kelleher D, Nepom GT, Kagnoff MF. An HLA-D region restriction fragment length polymorphism associated with celiac disease. J Exp Med 1986;164:333–8.
29. Howell MD, Smith JR, Austin RK, et al. An extended HLA-D region haplotype associated with celiac disease. Proc Natl Acad Sci USA 1988;85:222–6.
30. Jarvinen TT, Collin P, Rasmussen M, et al. Villous tip intraepithelial lymphocytes as markers of early-stage coeliac disease. Scand J Gastroenterol 2004;39:428–33.
31. Johnston SD, Watson RG, McMillan SA, Sloan J, Love AH. Coeliac disease detected by screening is not silent—simply unrecognized. Q J Med 1998;91:853–60.
32. Kagnoff MF, Paterson YJ, Kumar PJ, et al. Evidence for the role of a human intestinal adenovirus in the pathogenesis of coeliac disease. Gut 1987;28:995–1001.
33. Kapuscinska A, Zalewski T, Chorzelski TP, et al. Disease specificity and dynamics of changes in IgA class anti-endomysial antibodies in celiac disease. J Pediatr Gastroenterol Nutr 1987;6: 529–34.
34. Karpati S. Dermatitis herpetiformis: close to unraveling a disease. J Dermatol Sci 2004;34:83–90.
35. King AL, Yiannakou JY, Brett PM, et al. A genome-wide family-based linkage search of coeliac disease. Ann Hum Genet 2000;64:497–500.
36. Kolsteren MM, Koopman HM, Schalekamp G, Mearin ML. Health-related quality of life in children with celiac disease. J Pediatr 2001;138:593–5.
37. Liu J, Juo SH, Holopainen P, et al. Genomewide linkage analysis of celiac disease in Finnish families. Am J Hum Genet 2002;70:51–9.
38. Loft DE, Marsh MN, Crowe PT. Rectal gluten challenge and diagnosis of coeliac disease. Lancet 1990;335:1293–5.
39. Logan RF, Tucker G, Rifkind EA, Heading RC, Ferguson A. Changes in clinical features of coeliac disease in adults in Edinburgh and the Lothians 1960-79. Br Med J 1983;286:95–7.

40. Louka AS, Sollid LM. HLA in coeliac disease: unraveling the complex genetics of a complex disorder. Tissue Antigens 2003;61:105–17.
41. Lundin KE, Scott H, Fausa O, Thorsby E, Sollid LM. T cells from the small intestinal mucosa of a DR4, DQ7/DR4, DQ8 celiac disease patient preferentially recognize gliadin when presented by DQ8. Hum Immunol 1994;41:285–91.
42. Lundin KE, Scott H, Hansen T, et al. Gliadin-specific, HLA-DQ(a1*0501, 1*0201) restricted T cells isolated from the small intestinal mucosa of celiac disease patients. J Exp Med 1993;178: 187–96.
43. MacDonald WC, Dobbins WO 3rd, Rubin CE. Studies of the familial nature of celiac sprue using biopsy of the small intestine. N Engl J Med 1965;272:448–56.
44. Maki M. The humoral immune system in coeliac disease. Baillieres Clin Gastroenterol 1995;9:231–49.
45. Marsh MN, Bjarnason I, Shaw J, Ellis A, Baker R, Peters TJ. Studies of intestinal lymphoid tissue. XIV-HLA status, mucosal morphology, permeability and epithelial lymphocyte populations in first degree relatives of patients with coeliac disease. Gut 1990;31:32–6.
46. Molberg O, McAdam SN, Korner R, et al. Tissue transglutaminase selectively modifies gliadin peptides that are recognized by gut-derived T cells in celiac disease. Nature Med 1998;4: 713–7.
47. Mylotte M, Egan-Mitchell B, McCarthy CF, McNicholl B. Coeliac disease in the West of Ireland. Br Med J 1973;3:498–9.
48. Naluai AT, Nilsson S, Gudjonsdottir AH, et al. Genome-wide linkage analysis of Scandinavian affected sib-pairs supports presence of susceptibility loci for celiac disease on chromosomes 5 and 11. Eur J Hum Genet 2001;9:938–44.
49. Oberhuber G, Schwarzenhofer M, Vogelsang H. In vitro model of the pathogenesis of celiac disease. Dig Dis 1998;16:341–4.
50. Pink IJ, Creamer B. Response to a gluten-free diet of patients with the coeliac syndrome. Lancet 1967;1:300–4.
51. Popat S, Bevan S, Braegger CP, et al. Genome screening of coeliac disease. J Med Genet 2002; 39:328–31.
52. Rossipol E. Incidence of coeliac disease in children in Austria. Z Kinderheilkd 1975;119:143–9.
53. Schuppan D. Current concepts of celiac disease pathogenesis. Gastroenterology 2000;119:234–42.
54. Schuppan D, Dieterich W, Riecken EO. Exposing gliadin as a tasty food for lymphocytes. Nature Med 1998;4:666–7.
55. Shah VH, Rotterdam H, Kotler DP, Fasano A, Green PH. All that scallops is not celiac disease. Gastrointest Endosc 2000;51:717–20.
56. Shan L, Molberg O, Parrot I, et al. Structural basis for gluten intolerance in celiac sprue. Science 2002;297:2275–9.
57. Simila S, Kokkonen J. Coexistence of celiac disease and Down syndrome. Am J Ment Retard 1990;95:120–2.
58. Sjoberg K, Eriksson KF, Bredgerg A, Wassmuth R, Eriksson S. Screening for coeliac disease in adult insulin-dependent diabetes mellitus. J Intern Med 1998;243:133–40.
59. Sjostrom H, Friis SU, Noren O, Anthonsen D. Purification and characterisation of antigenic gliadins in coeliac disease. Clin Chim Acta 1992;207:227–37.
60. Sollid LM, Markussen G, Ek J, Gjerde H, Vartdal F, Thorsby E. Evidence for a primary association of celiac disease to a particular HLA-DQ alpha/beta heterodimer. J Exp Med 1989;169:345–50.
61. Sollid LM, Thorsby E. HLA susceptibility genes in celiac disease—genetic mapping and role in pathogenesis. Gastroenterology 1993;105:910–22.
62. Sulkanen S, Halttunen T, Laurila K, et al. Tissue transglutaminase autoantibody enzyme-linked immunosorbent assay in detecting celiac disease. Gastroenterology 1998;115:1322–8.
63. Talal AH, Murray JA, Goeken JA, Sivitz WI. Celiac disease in an adult population with insulin-dependent diabetes mellitus: use of endomysial antibody testing. Am J Gastroenterol 1997;92:1280–4.
64. Uibo O, Uibo R, Kleimola V, Jogi T, Maki M. Serum IgA anti-gliadin antibodies in an adult population sample. High prevalence without celiac disease. Dig Dis Sci 1993;38:2034–7.
65. van Belzen MJ, Vrolijk MM, Meijer JW, et al. A genomewide screen in a four-generation Dutch family with celiac disease: evidence for linkage to chromosomes 6 and 9. Am J Gastroenterol 2004;99:466–71.
66. van de Wal Y, Kooy Y, van Veelen P, et al. Selective deamidation by tissue transglutaminase strongly enhances gliadin-specific T cell reactivity. J Immunol 1998;161:1585–8.
67. Vasquez H, Mazure R, Gonzalez D, et al. Risk of fractures in celiac disease patients: a cross-sectional, case-control study. Am J Gastroenterol 2000;95:183–9.
68. Volta U, De Giorgio R, Petrolini N, et al. Clinical findings and anti-neuronal antibodies in coeliac disease with neurological disorders. Scand J Gastroenterol 2002;37:1276–81.
69. Volta U, Molinaro N, Fratangelo D, Bianchi FB. IgA subclass antibodies to gliadin in serum and intestinal juice of patients with coeliac disease. Clin Exp Immunol 1990;80:192–5.

70. Zhong F, McCombs CC, Olson JM, et al. An autosomal screen for the genes that predispose to celiac disease in the western counties of Ireland. Nat Genet 1996;14:329–33.

Refractory Sprue

71. Cellier C, Delabesse E, Helmer C, et al. Refractory sprue, coeliac disease, and enteropathy-associated T-cell lymphoma. French Coeliac Disease Study Group. Lancet 2000;356:203–8.
72. Murray A, Cuevas EC, Jones DB, Wright DH. Study of the immunohistochemistry and T cell clonality of enteropathy-associated T cell lymphoma. Am J Pathol 1995;146:509–19.

Collagenous Sprue

73. Guller R, Anabitarte M, Mayer M. Collagenous sprue and ulcerative jejuno-ileitis in a patient with gluten-induced enteropathy. Schweiz Med Wochenschr 1986;116:1343–9.

Ulcerative Jejunoileitis

74. Bayless TM, Kapelowitz RF, Shelley WM, Ballinger WF 2nd, Hendrix TR. Intestinal ulceration—a complication of celiac disease. N Engl J Med 1967;276:996–1002.
75. Enns R, Lay T, Bridges R. Use of azathioprine for nongranulomatous ulcerative jejunoileitis. Can J Gastroenterol 1997;11:503–6.

Systemic Mastocytosis

76. Akin C, Metcalfe DD. Systemic mastocytosis. Annu Rev Med 2004;55:419–32.
77. Barriere H, Dreno B, Pecquet C, Le Bodic MF, Bolze JL. Systemic mastocytosis and intestinal malabsorption. Semin Hop Paris 1983;59:2925–31.
78. Carter MC, Metcalfe DD. Paediatric mastocytosis. Arch Dis Child 2002;86:315–9.
79. Cherner JA, Jensen RT, DuBois A, O'Dorisio TM, Gardner JD, Metcalfe DD. Gastrointestinal dysfunction in systemic mastocytosis: a prospective study. Gastroenterology 1988;95:657–67.
80. Fishman RS, Fleming CR, Li CY. Systemic mastocytosis with review of gastrointestinal manifestations. Mayo Clin Proc 1979;54:51–4.
81. Horan RF, Austen KF. Systemic mastocytosis: retrospective review of a decade's clinical exprience at the Brigham and Women's Hospital. J Invest Dermatol 1991;96:5S–13S.
82. Jensen RT. Gastrointestinal abnormalities and involvement in systemic mastocytosis. Hematol Oncol Clin N Am 2000;14:579–623.
83. Keller RT, Roth HP. Hyperchlorhydria and hyperhistaminemia in a patient with systemic mastocytosis. N Engl J Med 1970;301:1449–50.
84. Kettelhut BV, Metcalfe DD. Pediatric mastocytosis. J Invest Dermatol 1991;96:15S–9S.
85. Ouwendijk RJ, Zijlstra FJ, Wilson JH, Bonta IL, Vincent JE, Stolz E. Raised plasma levels of thromboxane B2 in systemic mastocytosis. Eur J Clin Invest 1983;13:227–9.
86. Quinn SF, Shaffer HA, Willard MR, Ross S. Bull's eye lesions: a new gastrointestinal presentation of mastocytosis. Gastrointest Radiol 1984;9:13–5.
87. Soter NA. The skin in mastocytosis. J Invest Dermatol 1991;96:32S–8S.
88. Vermillion DL, Ernst PB, Scicchitano R, Collins SM. Antigen-induced contraction of jejunal smooth muscle in the sensitized rat. Am J Physiol 1988;255:G701–8.

Selective IgA Deficiency

89. Atwater JS, Tomasi TB Jr. Suppressor cells and IgA deficiency. Clin Immunol Immunopathol 1978;9:379–84.
90. Buckley RH. Breakthroughs in the understanding and therapy of primary immunodeficiency. Clin Immunol 1994;41:665–90.
91. Cunningham-Rundles C. Selective IgA deficiency. J Pediatr Gastroenterol Nutr 1988;7:482–4.
92. Farr M, Struthers GR, Scott DG, Bacon PA. Fenclofenac-induced selective IgA deficiency in rheumatoid arthritis. Br J Rheumatol 1985;24: 3679.
93. Hodgson HJ, Jewell DP. Selective IgA deficiency and Crohn's disease: report of two cases. Gut 1977;18:644–6.
94. Leickly FE, Buckley RH. Development of IgA and IgG2 subclass deficiency after sulfasalazine. J Pediatrics 1986;108:481–2.
95. Ropars C, Muller A, Paint N, et al. Large scale detection of IgA deficient blood donors. J Immunol Methods 1982;54:183–9.
96. Savilahti E. Sulphasalazine induced immunodeficiency. Br Med J 1983;287:759.
97. Schaffer FM, Monteiro RC, Volanakis JE, Cooper MD. IgA deficiency. Immunodeficiency 1991;3:15–44.
98. Schaffer FM, Palermos J, Zhu ZB, Barger BO, Cooper MD, Volanakis JE. Individuals with IgA deficiency and common variable immunodeficiency share polymorphisms of major histocompatibility complex class III genes. Proc Natl Acad Sci USA 1989;86:8015–9.
99. Strober W, Sneller M. IgA deficiency. Ann Allergy 1991;66:363–75.
100. van Loghem E, Zegers BJ, Bast EJ, Kater L. Selective deficiency of immunoglobulin A2. J Clin Invest 1983;72:1918–23.

101. van Riel PL, van de Putte LB, Gribnau FW, de Waal RM. IgA deficiency during aurothioglucose treatment. A case report. Scand J Rheumatol 1984;13:334–6.
102. Webster AD. Immune deficiency. In: Booth CC, Neale G, eds. Disorders of the small intestine. London: Blackwell Scientific; 1985:135.
103. Wells JV, Micheali D, Fudenberg HH. Antibodies to human collagen in subjects with selective IgA deficiency. Clin Exp Immunol 1973;13:203–8.

Common Variable Immunodeficiency

104. Agematsu K, Futatani T, Hokibara S, et al. Absence of memory B cells in patients with common variable immunodeficiency. Clin Immunol 2002;103:34–42.
105. Bjorkander J, Bake B, Hanson LA. Primary hypogammaglobulinaemia: impaired lung function and body growth with delayed diagnosis and inadequate treatment. Eur J Respir Dis 1984;65:529–36.
106. Cunningham-Rundles C. Clinical and immunologic analyses of 103 patients with common variable immunodeficiency. J Clin Immunol 1989;9:22–33.
107. Cunningham-Rundles C, Bodian C. Common variable immunodeficiency: clinical and immunological features of 248 patients. Clin Immunol 1999;92:34–48.
108. Dawson J, Bryant MG, Bloom SR, Peters TJ. Jejunal mucosal enzyme activities, regulatory peptides and organelle pathology of the enteropathy of common variable immunodeficiency. Gut 1986;27:273–7.
109. De La Concha EG, Fernandez-Arquero M, Martinez A, et al. HLA class II homozygosity confers susceptibility to common variable immunodeficiency (CVID). Clin Exp Immunol 1999;116:516–20.
110. Di Renzo M, Pasqui AL, Auteri A. Common variable immunodeficiency: a review. Clin Exp Med 2004;3:211–7.
111. Fasth A. Primary immunodeficiency disorders in Sweden: cases among children. J Clin Immunol 1982;2:86–92.
112. Fiorilli M, Crescenzi M, Carbonari M, et al. Phenotypically immature IgG-bearing B cells in patients with hypogammaglobulinemia. J Clin Immunol 1986;6(1):21–5.
113. Funauchi M, Farrant J, Moreno C, Webster AD. Defects in antigen-driven lymphocyte responses in common variable immunodeficiency (CVID) are due to a reduction in the number of antigen-specific CD4+ T cells. Clin Exp Immunol 1995;101:82–8.
114. Grimbacher B, Hutloff A, Schlesier M, et al. Homozygous loss of ICOS is associated with adult-onset common variable immunodeficiency. Nature Immunol 2003;4(3):261–8.
115. Groth C, Drager R, Warnatz K, et al. Impaired up-regulation of CD70 and CD86 in naive (CD27-) B cells from patients with common variable immunodeficiency (CVID). Clin Exp Immunol 2002;129:133–9.
116. Hermans PE, Diaz-Buxo JA, Stobo JD. Idiopathic late-onset immunoglobulin deficiencies. Am J Med 1976;61:221–37.
117. Hosking CS, Roberton DM. Epidemiology and treatment of hypogammaglobulinemia. Birth Defects Orig Artic Ser 1993;19:223–7.
118. Jolles S, Tyrer M, Johnson M, Webster D. Long term recovery of IgG and IgM production during HIV infection in a patient with common variable immunodeficiency (CVID). J Clin Pathol 2001;54:713–5.
119. Kralovicova J, Hammarstrom L, Plebani A, Webster AD, Vorechovsky I. Fine-scale mapping at IGAD1 and genome-wide genetic linkage analysis implicate HLA-DQ/DR as a major susceptibility locus in selective IgA deficiency and common variable immunodeficiency. J Immunol 2003;170:2765–75.
120. Levy Y, Gupta N, Le Deist F, et al. Defect in IgV gene somatic hypermutation in common variable immuno-deficiency syndrome. Proc Nat Acad Sci USA 1998;95:13135–40.
121. Mullighan CG, Fanning GC, Chapel HM, Welsh KI. TNF and lymphotoxin-alpha polymorphisms associated with common variable immunodeficiency: role in the pathogenesis of granulomatous disease. J Immunol 1997;159:6236–41.
122. Nijenhuis T, Klasen I, Weemaes CM, Preijers F, de Vries E, van der Meer JW. Common variable immunodeficiency (CVID) in a family: an autosomal dominant mode of inheritance. Neth J Med 2001;59:134–9.
123. North ME, Webster AD, Farrant J. Defects in proliferative responses of T cells from patients with common variable immunodeficiency on direct activation of protein kinase C. Clin Exp Immunol 1991;85(2):198–201.
124. Sneller MC, Strober W, Eisenstein E, Jaffe JS, Cunningham-Rundles C. NIH conference. New insights into common variable immunodeficiency. Ann Intern Med 1993;118:720–30.
125. Spickett GP. Current perspectives on common variable immunodeficiency (CVID). Clin Exp Allergy 2001;31:536–42.

126. Washington K, Stenzel TT, Buckley RH, Gottfried MR. Gastrointestinal pathology in patients with common variable immunodeficiency and X-linked agammaglobulinemia. Am J Surg Pathol 1996;20:1240–52.

Amyloidosis

127. Gilat T, Spiro HM. Amyloidosis and the gut. Am J Dig Dis 1968;13:619–33.

Abetalipoproteinemia

128. Akamatsu K, Sakaue H, Mizukami Y, Yamaguchi S, Tanaka A, Ohta Y. A case report of abetalipoproteinemia (Bassen-Kornzweig syndrome): the first case in Japan. Jpn J Med 1983;22:231–6.
129. Berriot-Varoqueaux N, Aggerbeck LP, Samson-Bouma ME, Wetterau JR. The role of the microsomal triglyceride transfer protein in abetalipoproteinemia. Annu Rev Nutr 2000;20: 663–97.
130. Delpre G, Kadish U, Glantz I, Avidor I. Endoscopic assessment in abetalipoproteinemia. Endoscopy 1978;10:59–62.
131. Narcisi TM, Shoulders CC, Chester SA, et al. Mutations of the microsomal triglyceride transfer protein gene in abetalipoproteinemia. Am J Hum Genet 1995;57:1298–310.
132. Ohashi K, Ishibashi S, Osuga JI, et al. Novel mutations in the microsomal triglyceride transfer protein gene causing abetalipoproteinemia. J Lipid Res 2000;41:1199–204.
133. Scully RE, Mark EJ, McNeely WF, McNeely BU. Case records of the Massachusetts general hospital. N Engl J Med 1992;327:628–35.
134. Sharp D, Blinderman L, Combs KA, et al. Cloning and gene defects in microsomal triglyceride transfer protein associated with abetalipoproteinemia. Nature 1993;365:65–9.
135. Shoulders CC, Brett DJ, Bayliss JD, et al. Abetalipoproteinemia is caused by defects in the gene encoding the 97 kDa subunit of a microsomal triglyceride transfer protein. Hum Mol Genet 1993;2:2109–16.
136. Wetterau JR, Aggerbeck LP, Bouma ME, et al. Absence of microsomal triglyceride transfer protein in individuals with abetalipoproteinemia. Science 1992;258:999–1001.
137. Willemin B, Coumaros D, Zerbe S, et al. L'abetalipoproteinemie. A propros de deux cas. Gastroenterol Clin Biol 1987;11:704–8.

Familial Hypobetalipoproteinemia

138. Malloy MJ, Kane JP. Hypolipidemia. Med Clin N Am 1982;66:469–84.
139. Malloy MJ, Kane JP, Hardman DA, Hamilton RL, Dalal KB. Normotriglyceridemic abetalipoproteinemia: absence of the B-100 apolipoprotein. J Clin Invest 1981;67:1441–50.
140. Schonfeld G. Familial hypobetalipoproteinemia: a review. J Lipid Res 2003;44:878–83.

Anderson's Disease

141. Boldrini R, Biselli R, Bosman C. Chylomicron retention disease—the role of ultrastructural examination in differential diagnosis. Pathol Res Pract 2001;197:753–7.
142. Bouma ME, Beucler I, Aggerbeck LP, Infante R, Schmitz J. Hypobetalipoproteinemia with accumulation of an apoprotein B-like protein in intestinal cells: immunoenzymatic and biochemical characterization of seven cases of Anderson's disease. J Clin Invest 1986;78:398–410.

Malnutrition

143. Atkinson RL, Dahms WT, Bray GA, Jacob R, Sandstead HH. Plasma zinc and copper in obesity and after intestinal bypass. Ann Intern Med 1978;89:491–3.
144. Bianchi A, Chipman D, Dreskin A, Rosensweig N. Nutritional folic acid deficiency with megaloblastic changes in the small-bowel epithelium. N Engl J Med 1970;282:859–61.
145. Bohane TD, Cutz E, Hamilton JR, Gall DG. Acrodermatitis enteropathica, zinc, and the Paneth cell. A case report with family studies. Gastroenterology 1977;73:587–92.
146. Braun OH, Heilmann K, Rossner JA, Pauli W, Bergmann KE. Acrodermatitis enteropathica zinc deficiency and ultrastructural findings. Eur J Pediatrics 1977;125:153–62.
147. Cluysenaer OJ, van Tongeren JH. Pseudo-obstruction in coeliac sprue. Neth J Med 1987;31:300–4.
148. Cook GC, Lee FD. The jejunum after kwashiorkor. Lancet 1966;2:1263–7.
149. Dawson DW. Partial villous atrophy in nutritional megaloblastic anaemia corrected by folic acid therapy. J Clin Pathol 1971;24:131–5.
150. Duque E, Bolanos O, Lotero H, Mayoral LG. Enteropathy in adult protein malnutrition: light microscopic findings. Am J Clin Nutr 1975;28:901–13.
151. Gallager RL. Intestinal ceroid deposition—"brown bowel syndrome": a light and electron microscopic study. Virchows Arch A Pathol Anat Histol 1980;389:143–51.
152. Golden MH, Harland PS, Golden BE, Jackson AA. Zinc and immunocompetence in protein energy malnutrition. Lancet 1978;1:1226–8.

153. Hambidge KM, Hambidge C, Jacobs M, Baum JD. Low levels of zinc in hair, anorexia, poor growth, and hypogeusia in children. Pediatr Res 1972;6:868–74.
154. Hong CB, Chow CK. Induction of eosinophilic enteritis and eosinophilia in rats by vitamin E and selenium deficiency. Exp Mol Pathol 1988;48:182–92.
155. Hungerford GF. Role of histamine in producing the eosinophilia of magnesium deficiency. Proc Soc Exp Biol Med 1964;115:182–5.
156. Kay RG, Tasman-Jones C, Pybus J, Whiting R, Black H. A syndrome of acute zinc deficiency during parental alimentation in man. Ann Surg 1976;183:331–40.
157. Koch MJ, Biesalski HK, Stofft E, et al. Crystalloid lysozyme inclusions in Paneth cells of vitamin A-deficient rats. Cell Tissue Res 1990;260: 625–8.
158. Navert B, Sandstrum B, Cederblad A. Reduction of the phytate content of bran by leavening in bread and its effect on zinc absorption in man. Br J Nutr 1985;53:47–53.
159. Nye SW, Chittayasothorn K. Ceroid in the gastrointestinal smooth muscle of the Thai-Lao ethnic group. Am J Pathol 1967;51:287–99.
160. Reddy CC, Massaro EJ. Biochemistry of selenium: a brief overview. Fund Appl Toxicol 1983;3:431–6.
161. Ruchti C, Eisele S, Kaufmann M. Fatal intestinal pseudo-obstruction in brown bowel syndrome. Arch Pathol Lab Med 1990;114:76–80.
162. Stanfield JP, Hutt MS, Tunnicliffe R. Intestinal biopsy in kwashiorkor. Lancet 1965;2:802–4.
163. Walravens PA, Krebs NF, Hambidge KM. Linear growth of low income preschool children receiving a zinc supplement. Am J Clin Nutr 1983;38:195–201.
164. Yarrington JT, Wiehair CK. Ultrastructure of gastrointestinal smooth muscle in ducks with a vitamin E-selenium deficiency. J Nutr 1975;105:782–90.
165. Zile MH, Bunge EC, De Luca HF. DNA labeling of the rat epithelial tissues in vitamin A-deficiency. J Nutr 1981;111:777–88.

13 DISEASES OF THE APPENDIX

CONGENITAL ANOMALIES

Congenital anomalies involving the appendix are rare, and include *congenital agenesis* and *complete* or *partial duplication* (4). Appendiceal agenesis has an incidence of 1/100,000 appendices examined at the time of autopsy (3). The agenesis may occur in the presence of a normal cecum or in association with cecal dysgenesis. Appendiceal agenesis also sometimes accompanies ileal atresia (7), thalidomide ingestion (1), or trisomy 18. Patients with trisomy 18 usually display multiple congenital abnormalities involving the gastrointestinal tract as well as other organ systems (3).

Appendiceal duplication is found in 1/12,500 patients treated for appendicitis (4). Three types of appendiceal duplication exist as described by the Cave-Wallbridge classification. Type A consists of incomplete duplication in which both appendices have a common base; type B consists of complete appendiceal duplication in which each appendix arises at a different location; and type C consists of complete duplication of the cecum in which each cecum has an accompanying duplicated appendix (2,6). Triplication of the appendix can also occur (5).

DIVERTICULA

Demography. *Diverticula* affect 2 to 3 percent of histologically examined appendices from surgical and autopsy material (9,11). They can be single or multiple, and are usually asymptomatic and discovered incidentally at the time of surgery for other reasons. Occasionally, however, they become inflamed, leading to symptoms of acute appendicitis. Diverticula affect both sexes equally.

Etiology. Most appendiceal diverticula are acquired (8a). In one series, acquired diverticula were present 10 times more frequently than their congenital counterparts (8). Several factors may play a role in the development of appendiceal diverticula: 1) luminal obstruction with distension of the appendix increases intraluminal pressure and causes mucosal herniation and 2) increased muscular contractions and muscular hypertrophy may lead to increased intraluminal pressure and mucosal herniation. The mucosa herniates through areas of weakness in the appendiceal wall. This occurs in areas where blood vessels pass through the muscularis propria, or in areas weakened or destroyed by previous episodes of inflammation and necrosis.

Patients with mucoceles, regardless of their cause, may develop outpouchings of the appendiceal wall, presumably as the result of the increased pressure of the accumulated mucus in the appendiceal lumen. A similar mechanism may be responsible for the relatively high frequency (14 percent) of appendiceal diverticulosis in patients with cystic fibrosis (10). Thick mucus accumulates in the appendiceal lumen, sometimes massively distending it.

Clinical Features. The symptoms of patients with appendiceal diverticulitis may mimic those of acute appendicitis. Diverticulitis, however, is generally seen in older patients than those with acute appendicitis, and symptom onset may be insidious, occurring over the course of several days or weeks. In addition, some patients complain of previous similar symptoms (12).

Gross Findings. Acquired diverticula are commonly multiple and lie along the mesenteric and antimesenteric borders, usually of the distal third of the appendix. Their size varies from 2 to 5 mm. When multiple, they may give the outer surface of the appendix a beaded appearance. Like their counterparts in the colon, appendiceal diverticula are subject to inflammation or perforation. Fecaliths lying in their lumens predispose to the development of diverticulitis.

Microscopic Findings. Normal-appearing mucosa lines the diverticula (fig. 13-1). The walls contain muscularis mucosae, submucosa, and the longitudinal muscle of the muscularis propria. Acquired diverticula lack the circular muscular coat; congenital diverticula, in contrast, have all of the normal layers of the bowel wall. When a diverticulum becomes inflamed, the inflammation is often localized to it, but it sometimes spreads to involve the appendix proper, producing appendicitis or periappendicitis. When extensive, the inflammation may distort, obliterate, or disrupt the diverticulum.

Histologically, early diverticulitis is characterized by a peridiverticular neutrophilic infiltrate. Later, this infiltrate is replaced by mononuclear cells. When the inflammatory process spreads to the periappendiceal tissues, an abscess may result. Perforation is common in the setting of diverticulitis (8a,11).

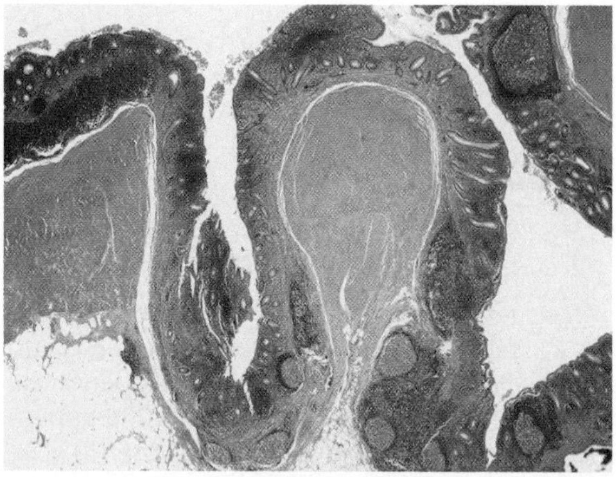

Figure 13-1

APPENDICEAL DIVERTICULOSIS

Low-power view demonstrates several diverticula of the appendix. Each diverticulum is lined by normal-appearing appendiceal mucosa and submucosa, and an attenuated layer of smooth muscle.

INTUSSUSCEPTION

Definition. An *intussusception* results from invagination or telescoping of the distal appendix into the proximal appendix or cecum.

Clinical Features. Appendiceal intussusception is rare, occurring in 0.1 percent of patients undergoing appendectomy (13). It is more common in males, presents in patients of all ages, but is most frequently seen in the first decade of life (14,15). The symptoms often suggest acute appendicitis, although the lesions may also remain asymptomatic. Factors that may predispose to the development of appendiceal intussusception include the presence of a fetal cone-shaped appendix, an unusually thin mesoappendix, and the presence of endometriosis, lymphoid hyperplasia, or appendiceal neoplasms (16–18,20).

Endoscopic Findings. Currently employed endoscopes are unable to enter the appendiceal lumen. The stoma of the appendix opening can be inspected, however, and has the appearance of a diverticulum with characteristic surrounding folds at the convergence of the muscle layers at the apex of the cecum. Occasionally, this stoma may be the site of a polypoid growth, inflammatory change, or other lesions that could be sampled if removed endoscopically. An inverted appendiceal stump or intussusception may assume a polypoid appearance and may confound an unsuspecting endoscopist. Snaring such a lesion with a polypectomy snare could result in perforation and resultant peritonitis.

Pathologic Findings. Intussusception should be suspected when the concentric ring sign is seen on ultrasound, an appearance that probably corresponds to the "coiled spring" radiographic appearance of appendiceal intussusception. In one form of the disease, the distal appendix intussuscepts into the proximal appendix. In other forms, the proximal appendix intussuscepts into the cecoappendicular valvular opening or the whole appendix intussuscepts into the cecum, sometimes presenting as an edematous cecal "polyp" that may be seen endoscopically (19). Biopsy of such "polyps" demonstrates a histologic picture that appears to be the reverse of normal (fig. 13-2). The epithelium lies on the external surface and the submucosa and muscularis propria lie inside the mucosa. The submucosa becomes edematous and the muscularis propria may appear hyperplastic, fibrotic, or as though it has been subjected to traction. The epithelium sometimes appears hyperplastic, inflamed, or eroded, especially if secondary ischemic damage develops. A helpful clue to the diagnosis is the presence of both the circular and longitudinal layers of the muscularis propria with its myenteric plexus in the submucosa of a polypoid lesion. The amount of tissue inversion seen depends on the extent of the intussusception.

Occasionally, the appendix undergoes autoamputation following intussusception or volvulus. The presence of cecal scarring and hemosiderin in the absence of other cecal abnormalities provides clues that the appendix was present at birth.

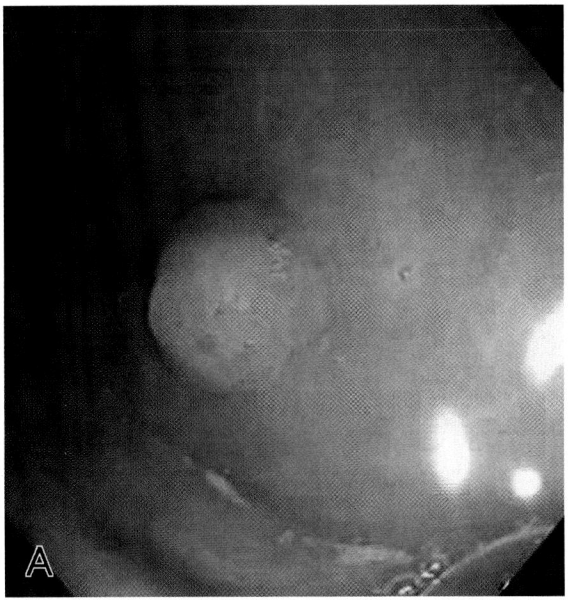

Figure 13-2

INVERTED APPENDIX

A: Endoscopic view of an inverted appendiceal stump. The lesion has a polypoid appearance.

B: Low-power view of a biopsy specimen of a "cecal polyp." The polyp is composed of mucosa, submucosa, and muscularis propria arranged in an "inside out" fashion.

C: Higher-power view shows the mucosa and submucosa of the inverted appendix.

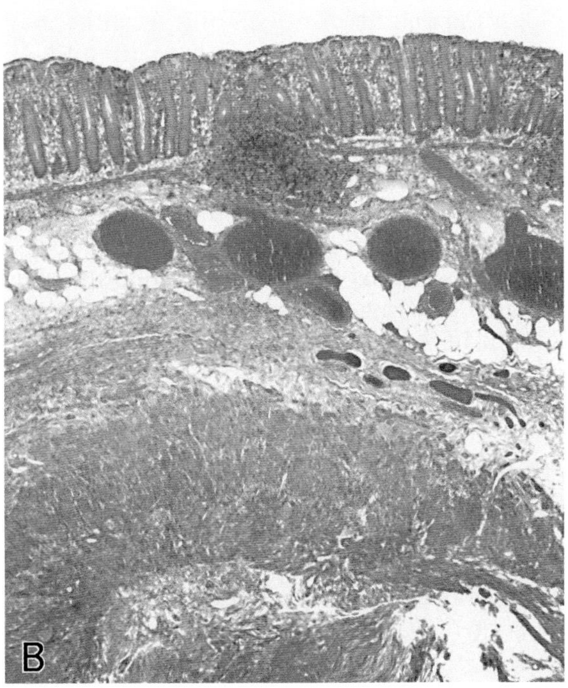

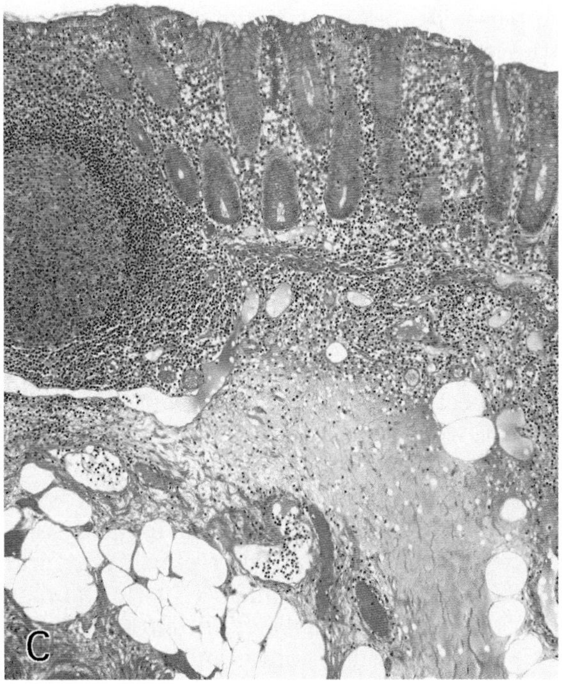

SEPTA

Single or multiple, complete or incomplete *septa* consisting of mucosa and submucosa may divide the appendiceal lumen into compartments. The presence of complete septa predisposes the appendix to appendicitis. Septa occur most often in the second decade of life; there is a clear male predominance (21).

AMYAND HERNIA

The finding of an appendix in an inguinal hernia constitutes an *Amyand hernia*. Acute appendicitis or its complications in inguinal hernias are rare, and a symptomatic appendix lying in an inguinal hernia is not usually suspected preoperatively (22,23).

APPENDICITIS

Demography. *Acute appendicitis* is one of the most common and readily curable inflammatory diseases of the gastrointestinal tract. Seven to 12 percent of the population in the United States will develop appendicitis at some time in their life (42). Acute appendicitis may develop at any age, but the peak incidence is in the second decade of life (25,26,50). Appendicitis affects males more commonly than females, particularly during early childhood (25,26,46,50,57). In addition, there is seasonal variation in the incidence of acute appendicitis (25,26,57), with a peak in the summer months. Appendicitis occurs more commonly in Western than in Eastern countries, although the overall incidence has declined in many regions in recent years (25,27,48,71). This variation in disease incidence is likely attributable to dietary differences between populations (64). Appendicitis develops less frequently in countries where the population consumes a high-fiber diet, as opposed to a higher incidence in populations that consume a low-residue, high-sugar diet (24,27,34,56). Heredity may also play a role in the pathogenesis of the disorder (31,38, 40). Finally, hygiene represents an additional etiologic factor (29,30).

Although appendicitis more commonly affects younger individuals, it also occurs in the elderly. The incidence of appendicitis in the elderly may, in fact, be increasing due to longer life expectancies. When the disease affects the elderly, there is a high mortality and complication rate (35,44,45,52).

Pathophysiology. Acute appendicitis is associated with luminal obstruction in most cases. Secretions accumulate under pressure behind the obstruction and normal peristaltic drainage fails to occur. The increased intraluminal pressure then leads to a compromised blood flow, which in turn leads to ischemic damage. Mucosal damage occurs early, impairing mucosal defenses to infection. Once an infection becomes established, arteriolar occlusion by intravascular thrombi, by pressure from inflammatory edema, or by a fecalith predisposes to the rapid development of gangrene, perforation, and peritonitis. With age, as the appendix becomes progressively fibrotic, it is less likely to distend from partial obstruction.

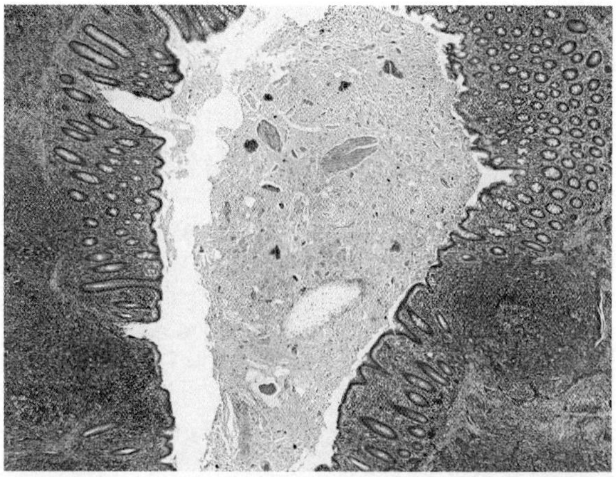

Figure 13-3

FECALITH

Fecal material composed of vegetable material, bacteria, and amorphous debris can be seen in the appendiceal lumen.

Both appendiceal calculi and fecaliths may obstruct the appendiceal lumen (fig. 13-3). Fecaliths are hard, but crushable, fecal material, whereas true calculi are hard, calcified, non-crushable stones. Fecaliths and calculi form when feces and mucus trapped in the appendiceal lumen remain continuously bathed in minerals and become inspissated. The inspissated concretions then serve as a continuous irritant, causing pressure necrosis and ulceration. The fecalith or calculus progressively increases in size until it obstructs the lumen and elevates distal intraluminal pressure. Fecaliths occur more commonly than calculi, but calculi are more likely to lead to perforation and periappendiceal abscess formation (61). The prevalence of calculi ranges from less than 1 to 2 percent (66). Fecaliths are seen in 2 percent of appendices removed incidentally and in 11 percent of patients with appendicitis. Acute appendicitis may also occur secondary to obstruction from passed gallstones or from obstructing aggregates of helminths.

Reactive lymphoid hyperplasia causing partial appendiceal obstruction following some form of antigenic stimulation (infectious, allergic) probably accounts for the high rate of appendicitis in young individuals, as they have more abundant lymphoid tissue than the elderly. When an older patient develops appendicitis, one should suspect, and rule out, appendiceal obstruction due to a neoplasm of the appendix (e.g., carcinoid) or of the cecum (e.g., adenoma or carcinoma).

Organisms Associated with Appendicitis. No single microorganism—bacterial, viral, or parasitic—is regularly associated with appendicitis. In some cases, multiple organisms cause the disease. Organisms enter tissues in which the mucosal barrier is already damaged secondary to obstruction and ischemia. The organisms commonly cultured from patients with acute appendicitis are listed in Table 13-1 (28,32,55,58). The appendix may become involved in patients who have a more generalized bacterial enterocolitis, such as that caused by *Salmonella*, *Shigella*, *Campylobacter*, and *Yersinia* (see below) (36,58).

Clinical Features. Acute appendicitis initially causes periumbilical, colicky pain that later localizes to the right lower quadrant. The pain usually develops over a short period of time, and is often accompanied by nausea, vomiting, or localized jejunal ileus. A mass may be palpable on rectal examination. Fever and leukocytosis develop with the onset of peritoneal inflammatory signs in the right lower quadrant. These classic symptoms often do not occur in elderly patients with acute appendicitis: abdominal pain may be of longer duration and fever may be absent (45,67).

Atypical clinical symptoms of acute appendicitis may be seen when the appendix is situated in an aberrant location or when inflammation spreads to involve adjacent organs. Occasionally patients present with urogenital symptoms including right renal colic, dysuria, frequency, and urinary retention (39).

Complications of appendicitis are relatively common, particularly in very young children or in the elderly. The most common complication is perforation, which can lead to generalized peritonitis, periappendiceal or subdiaphragmatic abscess formation, and serosal pneumatosis. The frequency of perforation in infants is as high as 50 percent, but is less (10 to 20 percent) in individuals aged 10 to 40 years. The frequency of perforation rises to 30 percent in patients 60 years of age, and in those over 75, increases to 50 percent or more (49,62,67).

Suppurative pyelophlebitis is an additional complication. Infected thrombi involve the small vessels of the serosa and medial appendix; these thrombi may extend or embolize to distant sites such as the liver where they establish secondary bacterial infections, cholangitis, and hepatic abscesses. If infective thrombophlebitis occurs, the patient may develop sepsis, shock, and disseminated intravascular coagulopathy. If the inflammation becomes walled off by fibrous connective tissue, then a localized periappendiceal abscess forms. Fistulas may form between the appendix and other structures of the gastrointestinal tract, vagina, or bladder. Other complications include fibrous adhesions, lumbar abscesses, and appendicocutaneous fistulas.

Table 13-1

ORGANISMS ASSOCIATED WITH ACUTE APPENDICITIS
Bacteroides fragilis
Bilophila wadsworthia
Campylobacter jejuni
Eggerthella lenta
Escherichia coli
Fusobacterium nucleatum
Haemophilus influenzae
Klebsiella
Lactobacillus
Peptostreptococcus micros
Pseudomonas
Shigella
Staphylococcus aureus
β-Hemolytic *Streptococcus* group A
Streptococcus milleri
Streptococcus pneumoniae
Streptococcus anginosus
Yersinia enterocolitica

A recurring clinical problem is that many diseases masquerade as acute appendicitis. In the past, the mortality associated with appendiceal perforation was so high that most patients with symptoms suggestive of appendicitis underwent laparotomy and appendectomy (47). This practice continues to some degree even today. As a result, every pathologist will encounter an appendix that was removed with the clinical diagnosis of appendicitis but appears histologically normal. The rate of negative appendectomy in some centers is as high as 20 to 30 percent (33,47). More recent studies in which

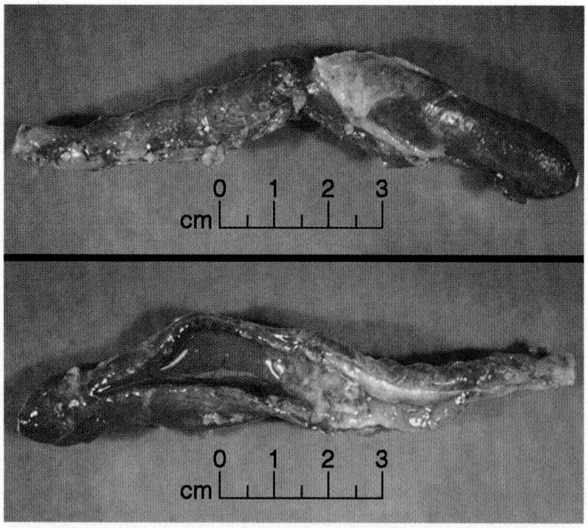

Figure 13-4

ACUTE APPENDICITIS

Top: The serosal surface is erythematous, and a yellowish white inflammatory exudate is present in one area.

Bottom: The mucosa of the opened specimen appears erythematous and ulcerated.

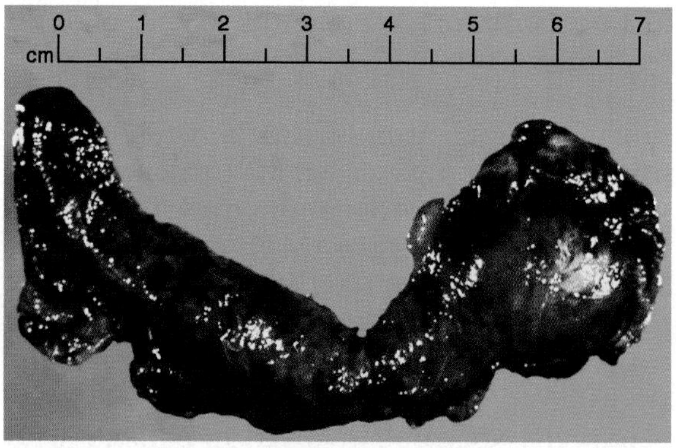

Figure 13-5

ACUTE APPENDICITIS

A more advanced case of acute appendicitis than that seen in figure 13-4 shows a purple-black serosal surface, and an area of inflammatory exudate in the proximal portion of the specimen. (Courtesy of the Division of Gastrointestinal Pathology, Armed Forces Institute of Pathology, Washington, DC.)

active observation of patients with potential acute appendicitis was performed show lower rates of negative appendectomy (47,51).

Endoscopic Findings. Endoscopy plays no role in the diagnosis of acute appendicitis, and is contraindicated when this diagnosis is being entertained.

Gross Findings. Acute appendicitis can be classified as simple, gangrenous, or perforated based on operative and pathologic features. Normally, the appendiceal mucosa appears smooth and light yellow-tan. The serosa is pink-tan, smooth, and glistening. Dilatation and congestion of serosal vessels in acute appendicitis produce localized or generalized hyperemia and constitute the earliest visible external changes. In contrast, an appendix with well-developed acute appendicitis shows marked congestion with a serosal granular fibrinous or purulent coating and vascular engorgement (fig. 13-4). The mesoappendix appears edematous and contiguous structures may become inflamed. Upon opening the appendix, purulent material often exudes from the surface and an impacted fecalith or calculus may be seen in the lumen. The acute inflammatory process can localize to one segment of the organ or the entire appendix may be affected. Extension of the inflammation further reduces the blood flow so that gangrene develops, causing possible rupture. By the time full-blown gangrenous appendicitis develops, the organ appears soft, purplish, and hemorrhagic, sometimes with visible thrombi in the mesoappendix (fig. 13-5).

Microscopic Findings. The gross and microscopic appearance of the appendix often closely correlate with one another (53). The histologic changes seen in acute appendicitis depend on the duration and severity of the disease. They range from minimal inflammation to marked necrosis with complete mural destruction and rupture. In early lesions, neutrophils appear at the base of the crypts adjacent to a small epithelial defect. White blood cells collect in the lamina propria or in the glandular lumens, sometimes forming crypt abscesses (fig. 13-6). Acute inflammatory cells can be easily identified migrating through the vasculature (fig. 13-7). Some appendices contain a prominent eosinophilic infiltrate (fig. 13-8). Submucosal edema and congestion are also often prominent. After the inflammatory process reaches the submucosa, it spreads quickly to involve the remaining appendix. Eventually, the mucosa becomes eroded, the wall becomes necrotic, and vascular thrombosis occurs (fig. 13-9). If the appendix becomes perforated, an intense, nonspecific, serosal inflammatory and fibrous process ensues.

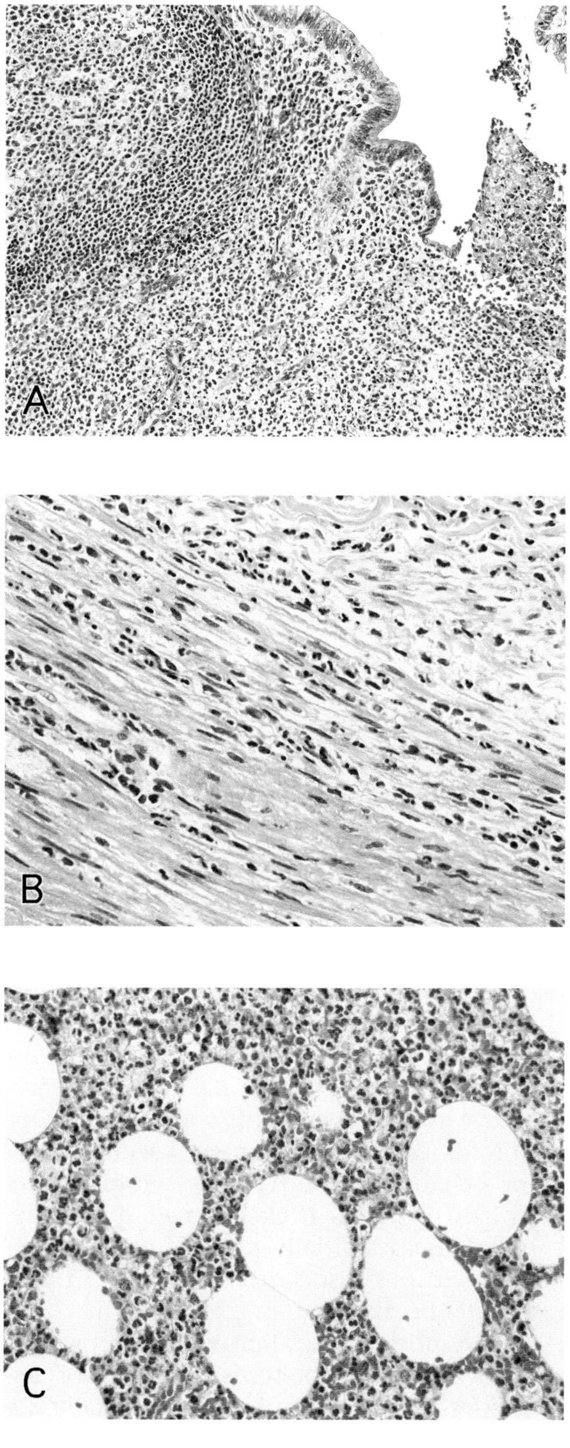

Figure 13-6

ACUTE APPENDICITIS

A: Patchy mucosal erosion and ulceration. The lamina propria contains numerous neutrophils.

B: Neutrophils infiltrate the muscularis propria.

C: Neutrophils are also present in the periappendiceal fat.

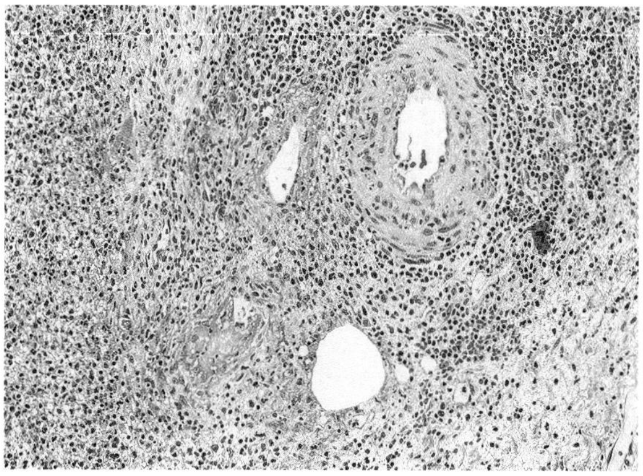

Figure 13-7

ACUTE APPENDICITIS

Neutrophils are migrating through the wall of an artery. An adjacent vein contains a fibrin thrombus.

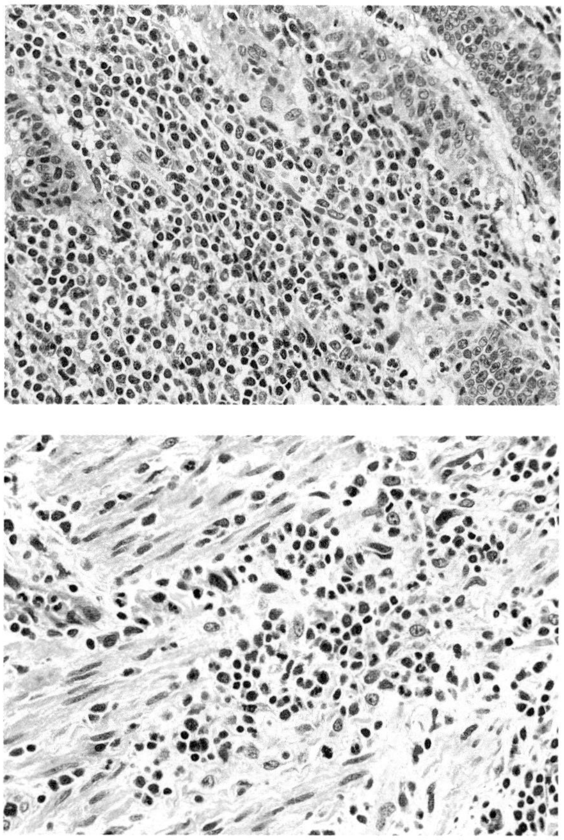

Figure 13-8

ACUTE APPENDICITIS

Top: The mucosal inflammatory infiltrate contains numerous eosinophils.

Bottom: Numerous eosinophils are also seen infiltrating the muscularis propria.

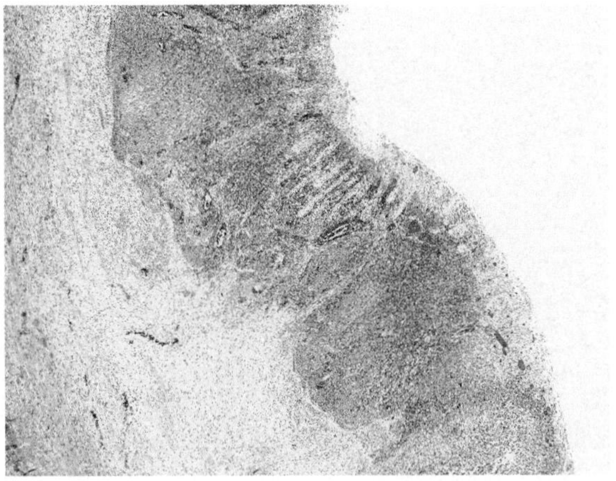

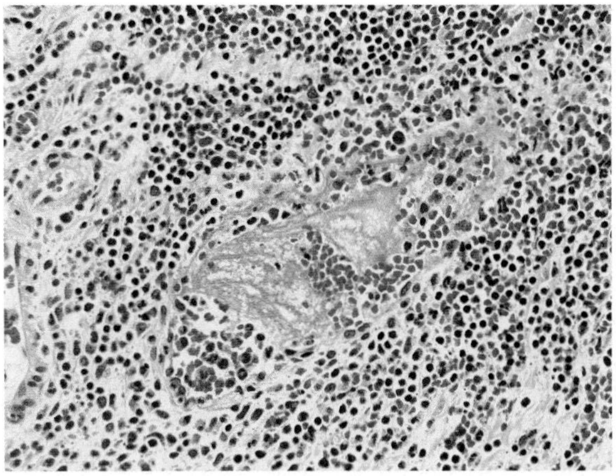

Figure 13-9

ACUTE APPENDICITIS

Left: Low-power view of a specimen from the appendix of a patient with necrotizing appendicitis. There is widespread necrosis of the mucosa and underlying tissues. The histologic changes are reminiscent of ischemic injury.

Right: Fibrin thrombi are in submucosal and mucosal vessels.

Patients who develop acute appendicitis with perforation are often treated with antibiotics, and then, after a period of 6 to 8 weeks, undergo appendectomy. Such appendices frequently demonstrate the presence of granulomatous or xanthogranulomatous inflammation (41). In addition, changes resembling Crohn's disease may sometimes be seen, including transmural lymphoid aggregates, mural fibrosis, distortion of crypt architecture, focal cryptitis, and formation of crypt abscesses. Later signs or symptoms of Crohn's disease do not develop in these patients (41).

Specific Forms of Appendicitis

***Campylobacter* Appendicitis.** Most patients with *Campylobacter* infection are children who present with a clinical picture of appendicitis. The appendix may appear normal, but the mesenteric lymph nodes are usually enlarged and swollen (69). The findings resemble those seen with *Campylobacter* colitis. Histologic features include mucosal infiltration by neutrophils and eosinophils, crypt abscesses, mucosal edema, and histiocytic collections that may resemble granulomas. The curved rods of *Campylobacter* organisms can be identified with the Warthin-Starry stain, electron microscopy, and immunologic stains.

***Yersinia Enterocolitica* Appendicitis.** *Yersinia enterocolitica* is a common cause of granulomatous appendicitis (32,54). The organism produces characteristic irregular granulomas containing a central zone of necrotizing inflammation. The granulomas contain neutrophils and are surrounded by palisading histiocytes and a cuff of lymphocytes (fig. 13-10) (54). Eosinophils may be quite prominent. Grossly, mesenteric lymph nodes appear enlarged, matted, fleshy, and reddish gray with central yellowish microabscesses. The histologic changes often remain limited to the mucosa and submucosa, sparing the muscularis propria and serosa. Transmural inflammation may also be seen, however, making the distinction of *Yersinia* appendicitis from Crohn's appendicitis difficult. Organism-specific polymerase chain reaction (PCR) or serologic tests establish or confirm the correct diagnosis. Crohn's disease initially presenting as appendicitis, without associated ileocecal or other involvement, although rare, does occur.

Tuberculosis Appendicitis. Tuberculous appendicitis usually represents extension of disease from the ileocecal area or occasionally the urogenital tract. In extensive cases, the appendix may become incorporated into a large granulomatous tissue mass that also involves the cecum and mesoappendix. The presence of confluent, nondiscrete, necrotizing granulomas containing acid-fast bacilli confirms the diagnosis. In tuberculosis, the necrosis and fibrosis

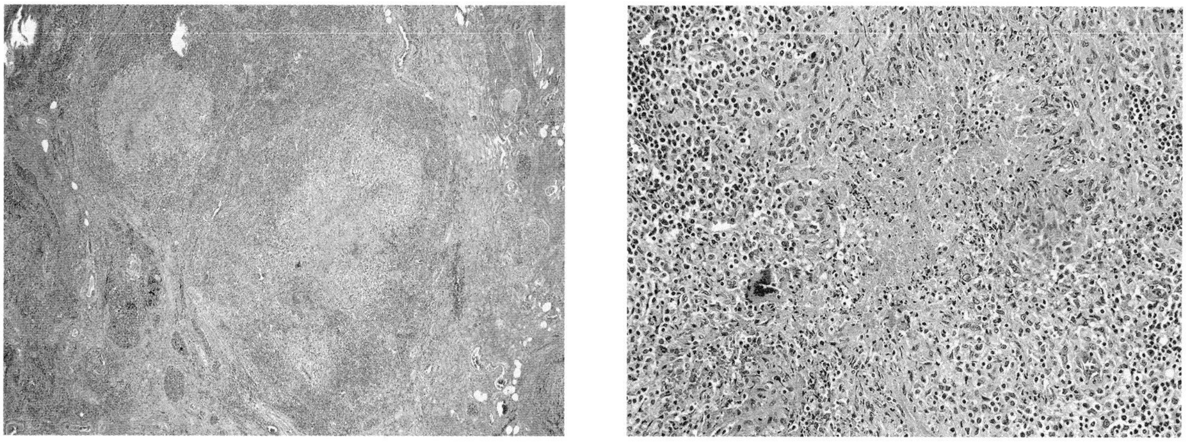

Figure 13-10

YERSINIA APPENDICITIS

Left: Low-power view of the appendiceal wall in a 12-year-old patient with symptoms of acute appendicitis. Two necrotizing granulomas are present.

Right: Higher-power view shows epithelioid histiocytes, giant cells, and central necrosis.

tend to destroy the muscularis propria whereas in Crohn's disease the structure of the muscularis propria is preserved, even though it may contain granulomas. Additionally, Crohn's disease-associated granulomas are almost exclusively non-necrotizing.

Actinomycosis Appendicitis. *Actinomyces israelii* is part of the normal intestinal flora in approximately 5 percent of people. Yet the same organism can become pathogenic, producing chronic suppurative appendicitis. Mycelia are easily identifiable in inflamed areas (43). *Actinomyces israelii* preferentially involves the ileocecal area, sometimes causing formation of a granulomatous mass or multiple sinus tracts that drain through the overlying skin. The fluid draining from the sinuses usually contains characteristic "sulfur granules." A dense fibrous connective tissue mass surrounds the actinomycotic mycelia. It is important to recognize true acute actinomycotic appendicitis when it occurs and treat it because it may spread locally and cause pelvic abscesses. The diagnosis should be suspected in any patient who develops sinus tracts or fistulas following appendectomy.

Viral Appendicitis. The appendix is seldom removed in patients with viral appendicitis because the disease usually remains self-limited. Patients often complain of generalized symptoms associated with viral illness, including fever, headache, pharyngitis, and myalgias. Appendicitis results from viral infections localized to the lymphoid tissue of Peyer patches. As the infected lymphoid follicles enlarge, they temporarily block the outflow of luminal secretions from the appendix, producing characteristic symptoms associated with appendicitis (fig. 13-11).

Patients with viral appendicitis occasionally undergo appendiceal intussusception; therefore, a viral infection should be suspected in patients with appendiceal intussusception without an obvious underlying mechanical basis.

Fungal Appendicitis. Mucormycosis is an acute mycosis that usually develops in immunosuppressed or debilitated patients. The fungi are ubiquitous in nature, growing as saprophytes on fruits and vegetables. They have broad, very rarely septate, haphazardly branched hyphae that characteristically stain deeply with hematoxylin. The irregular branching contrasts with the regular branching seen in *Aspergillus*. *Mucor* has a tendency to invade blood vessels, causing thrombosis and vascular dissemination. Fungi are demonstrable in the appendiceal lumen and invading the underlying tissues. Extensive mucosal necrosis and ulceration result.

Histoplasma capsulatum may be identified in the appendix of individuals living in endemic areas. When present, it produces granulomatous inflammation. South American blastomycosis, cryptococcosis, geotrichosis, and sporotrichosis also affect the appendix.

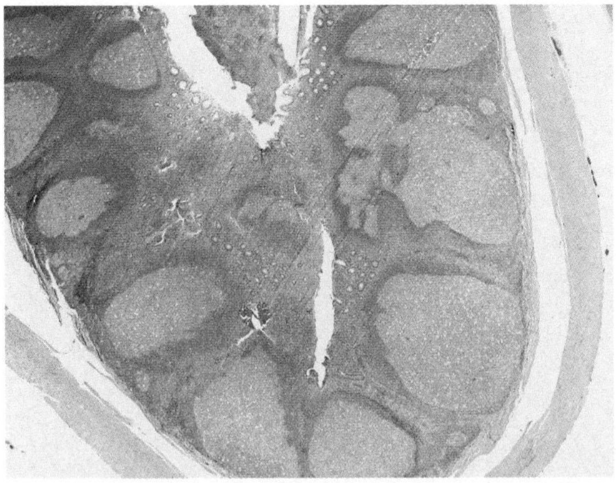

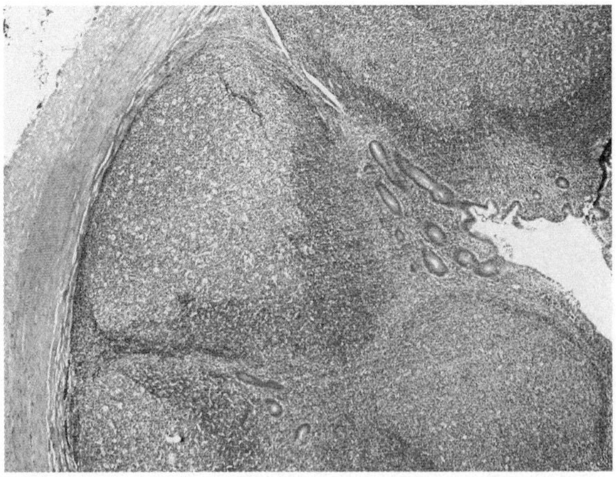

Figure 13-11

REACTIVE LYMPHOID HYPERPLASIA

Left: The patient had symptoms of acute appendicitis. There is massive lymphoid hyperplasia, resulting in marked narrowing of the appendiceal lumen.

Right: Higher-power view of the mucosa overlying the hyperplastic lymphoid follicles. No acute inflammatory infiltrates are present. The changes are likely due to viral infection.

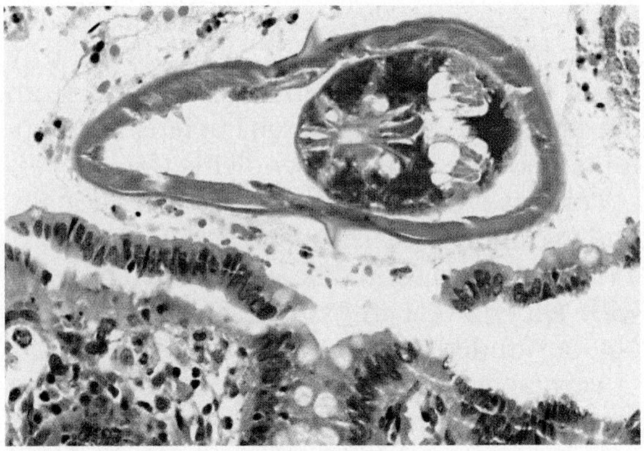

Figure 13-12

ENTEROBIUS VERMICULARIS APPENDICITIS

A cross section of a worm is seen in the lumen of the appendix. The two cuticular crests characteristic of the organism are easily seen.

***Enterobius Vermicularis* Appendicitis.** *Enterobius* has a worldwide distribution, but the organism appears more frequently in temperate and cold climates than in the tropics. *Enterobius vermicularis* is found in approximately 3 to 4 percent of appendix specimens in the United States and European countries (59,70). Infection rates among children in Asian countries are 25 to 75 percent (63). Poor sanitation, crowded habitation, and lack of exposure to sunshine all favor transmission of the infection (37). Children are especially susceptible to the infection. Enterobiasis is more fully discussed in chapter 12.

E. vermicularis, also referred to as pinworm or threadworm, is the causative agent. Adult female worms measure 6 to 12 mm and males, 2 to 5 mm in length. The ova hatch in the duodenum where the larvae molt and become sexually mature. Mating of adults takes place in the cecum, appendix, or, occasionally, the ileum. The males die soon after copulation; females migrate to the perianal and perineal regions to lay eggs. The females die shortly after oviposition. The eggs of *Enterobius* species are highly contagious and highly resistant to commonly used disinfectants.

Adult worms are sometimes found in tissue sections. They are most commonly identified within the lumen of the appendix (fig. 13-12). Usually, they fail to elicit an inflammatory response, except for mild mucosal eosinophilia. Severe infections cause pathologic lesions in the colon, cecum, appendix, and lower ileum, including superficial ulceration, petechial hemorrhages, and sometimes mucosal or submucosal abscesses (59). The parasite only rarely invades the mucosa, but when it does, granulomas form.

***Schistosoma* Appendicitis.** Schistosomiasis, a waterborne trematode infection, represents one of the most widespread parasitic diseases. An estimated 300 million people are affected world-

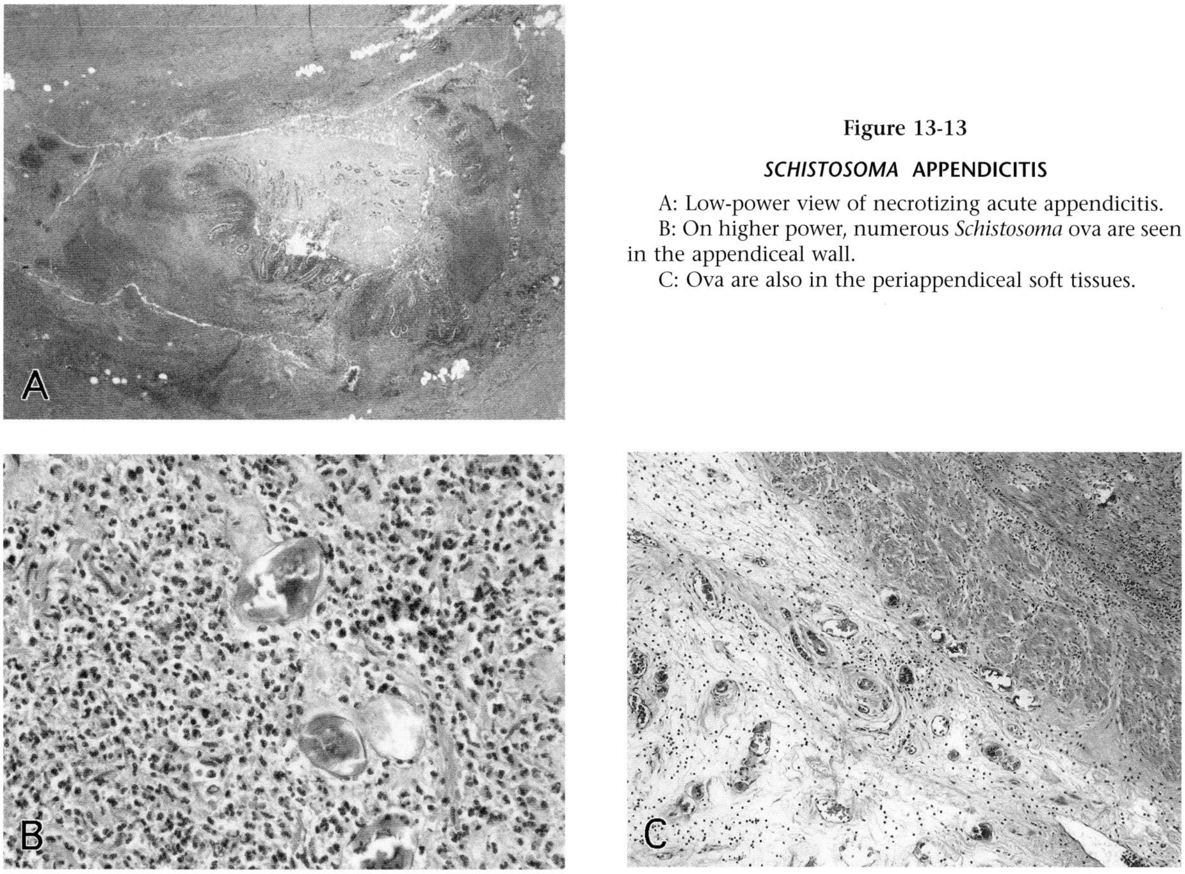

Figure 13-13

***SCHISTOSOMA* APPENDICITIS**

A: Low-power view of necrotizing acute appendicitis.

B: On higher power, numerous *Schistosoma* ova are seen in the appendiceal wall.

C: Ova are also in the periappendiceal soft tissues.

wide (60). In endemic areas, schistosomes are found in 1 to 15 percent of appendiceal resection specimens (62,65). Granulomatous appendicitis develops in younger patients during the early phase of egg laying in the appendix when acute granulomatous inflammation surrounds viable ova (fig. 13-13). Concomitant tissue necrosis, tissue eosinophilia, and neutrophil exudation ensue. Obstructive appendicitis develops in older individuals. It results from fibrosis of the appendiceal wall secondary to a long-standing inflammatory reaction to the *Schistosoma* eggs; these may appear calcified in tissue sections.

Other Parasites Causing Appendicitis. *Ascaris, Fasciola, Amoeba, Balantidium coli, Toxocara* species, *Trichuris, Rictularia, Strongyloides, Taenia,* and *Capillaria hepatica* may all affect the appendix, either alone or in conjunction with infestation of other parts of the intestine. Appendiceal amebiasis shows the typical flask-like ulcers seen elsewhere, a feature that should alert the pathologist to look for typical trophozoites. The histologic findings resemble those seen in the small intestine or colon. Granulomas can form around the eggs of the dead adult or larval forms. Eosinophils may be quite prominent.

PERIAPPENDICITIS

Definition. *Periappendicitis* is an inflammation in the periappendiceal soft tissues.

Clinical Features: A commonly encountered problem when assessing acute appendicitis is the presence of an acute inflammation restricted to the appendiceal serosa. In this situation, it is likely that the patient has inflammatory disease elsewhere in the abdominal cavity or pelvis that has extended to involve the appendiceal serosa. Periappendicitis occurs most commonly in boys below the age of 12 years and in females between the ages of 17 and 21. Primary causes include pelvic inflammatory disease, diverticulitis, inflammatory bowel disease, or inflammation associated with intestinal tumors (Table 13-2). Serious complications develop in a large percentage of patients preoperatively presumed to have acute appendicitis, but who are subsequently found to have periappendicitis. This finding suggests that establishing a diagnosis of periappendicitis has clinical significance and merits further clinical investigation into its cause (72).

Table 13-2

CAUSES OF PERIAPPENDICITIS

Appendicitis in another appendiceal segment
Pelvic inflammatory disease
Ectopic pregnancy
Urologic disease
Inflammatory bowel disease
Colonic neoplasms
Colitis
Colonic diverticular disease
Abdominal aortic aneurysm
Chlamydial infections

Pathologic Findings. The histologic findings reflect the duration of the inflammatory process and its nature. Most commonly, acute inflammation and edema are limited to the serosa and muscularis propria (fig. 13-14). In some cases, there is a prominent fibrinous exudate with little associated inflammation. As the process begins to resolve, fibrous tissue and chronic inflammatory cells replace the acute inflammation and edema, and fibrosing strands penetrate the mesoappendix.

NEUROGENIC APPENDICOPATHY

Definition. *Neurogenic appendicopathy* is a condition in which neural abnormalities within the appendix produce symptoms that mimic acute appendicitis. This condition is also referred to as *neurogenic appendicitis* and *neuroimmune appendicitis*.

Pathologic Findings. The rate of negative appendectomy in patients with symptoms suggestive of acute appendicitis ranges from 10 to 20 percent. Histologic evaluation of such appendices reveals the presence of distinct neuroma-like lesions in from 45 to 57 percent of cases

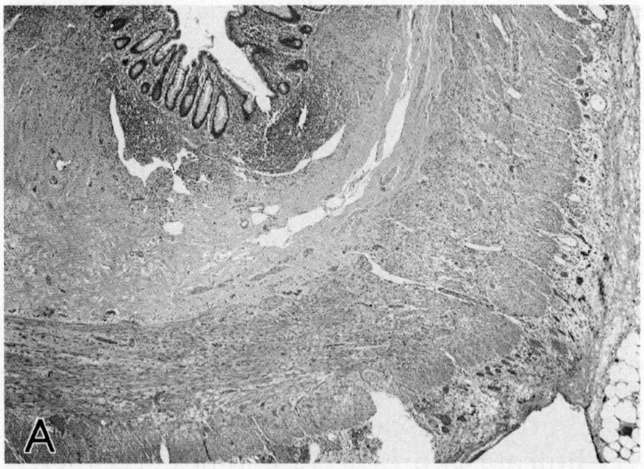

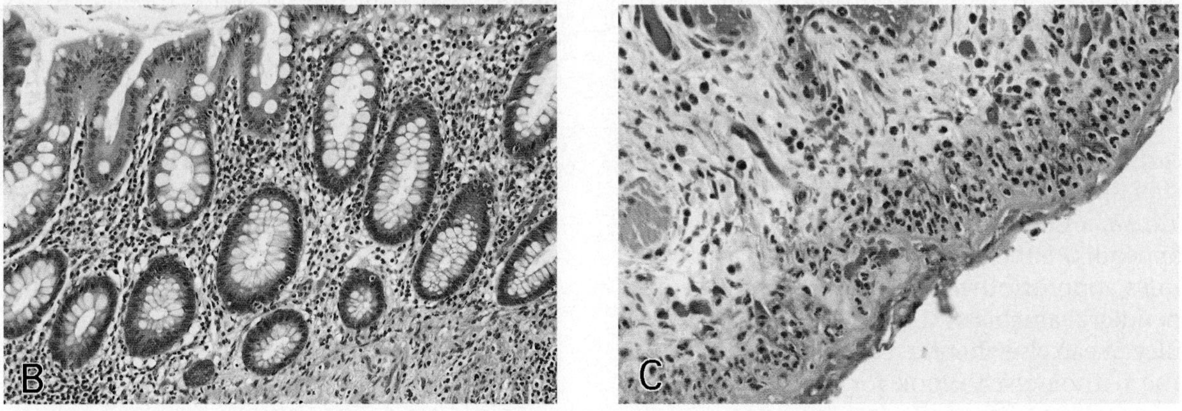

Figure 13-14

PERIAPPENDICITIS

A: The appendix was removed from a patient with a tuboovarian abscess. The subserosa is thickened and contains inflammatory cells. The remainder of the appendix, however, appears normal.

B: Higher-power view of the appendiceal mucosa shows no evidence of inflammation.

C: High-power view shows acute appendiceal serositis.

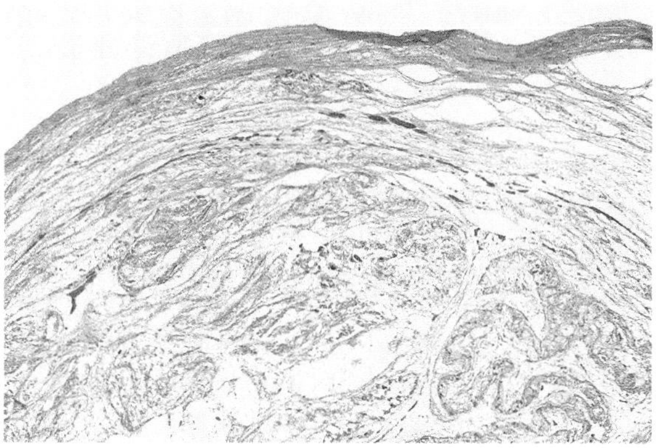
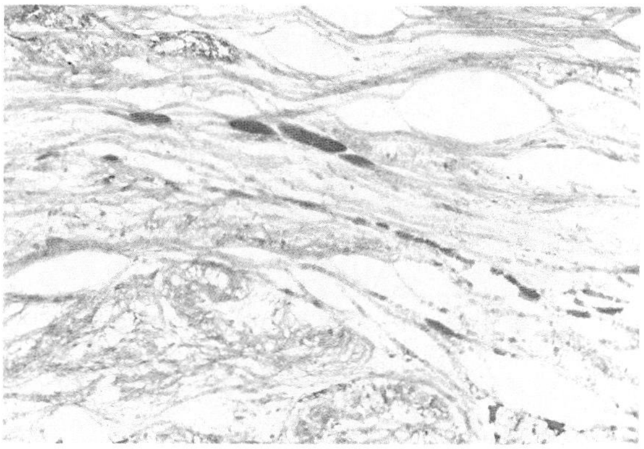

Figure 13-15

MYXOGLOBULOSIS

Left: There is a rounded collection of mucinous material containing rare cells.
Right: Higher-power view of the relatively acellular mucin making up the lesion.

(74,75). These lesions are characterized histologically as collections of pale-staining, spindle-shaped cells located within the lamina propria or in an area of fibrous obliteration. These cellular aggregates stain with S-100 protein. The significance of this finding remains controversial, although one recent study found that appendices demonstrating such neuromatous collections also produced the neurotransmitters substance P and vasoactive intestinal peptide (73). The elaboration of such substances may be associated with the symptoms of abdominal pain that these patients report. Other studies have shown that histologically noninflamed appendices from patients with symptoms of acute appendicitis frequently produce inflammatory cytokines including tumor necrosis factor alpha, interleukin-2, cyclooxygenases 1 and 2, and prostaglandin E2 (76,77).

MYXOGLOBULOSIS

Definition. *Myxoglobulosis* is a variant of appendiceal mucocele characterized by the presence of mucinous, occasionally calcified, pearl-like globules in the lumen of the appendix (fig. 13-15) (78,79). The distinctive features of the globules have given rise to terms such as *"fish-egg"* or *"caviar" appendix*.

Clinical and Pathologic Features. The incidence of myxoglobulosis ranges between 0.35 and 8.0 percent of mucoceles (78,79). The lesions can present clinically as acute appendicitis or may be an incidental finding at the time of laparotomy or autopsy. Perforation is an infrequent complication, with the usual consequence of either peritonitis or pseudomyxoma peritonei. In some perforated appendices, the white globules become walled off by fibrous adhesions in a pericecal collection.

Grossly, the characteristic finding is a group of opaque white globules consisting of calcified amorphous material without an underlying architecture. The factors that lead to the transformation of mucin into the globular masses are unknown. The lesions may form around a mucin or necrotic tissue core that acts as a nidus for the concentric deposition of mucin.

PROGRESSIVE FIBROUS OCCLUSION

Definition. *Progressive fibrous occlusion* refers to a process in which the normal appendiceal lumen is obliterated and replaced by fibrous tissue.

Etiology. Fibrous occlusion (fibrous obliteration) probably occurs as part of the natural aging process. The process starts distally and progresses proximally, eventually resulting in the loss of the normal appendiceal mucosa and Peyer patches. Fibrosis replaces the mucosa and submucosa (fig. 13-16).

Pathologic Findings. Distal fibrous occlusion may be accompanied by neural hyperplasia. The incidence of neural hyperplasia varies geographically, but it is more common in countries with a high incidence of appendicitis. A Western-style diet may induce the hyperplasia, possibly eventually resulting in the formation of carcinoid

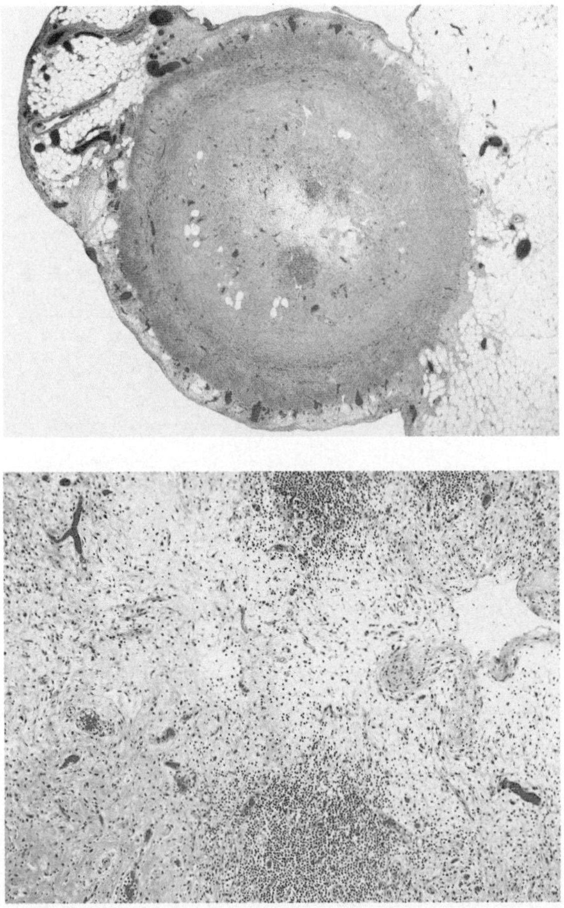

Figure 13-16

FIBROUS OBLITERATION OF THE APPENDIX

Top: Low-power view of a cross section of the distal portion of the appendix. The lumen has been obliterated by a proliferation of loose connective tissue.

Bottom: Higher-power view demonstrates the presence of numerous pale-staining spindled cells admixed with lymphocytes and plasma cells. Several clusters of lymphocytes are present, which represent the remains of the submucosal lymphoid aggregates characteristically seen in the normal appendix.

tumors. The distinction between neural hyperplasia, neuroma, and normal is subjective. When the neural proliferation is associated with fibrosis or when the histologic pattern becomes disorganized, resembling that seen in amputation neuroma, we prefer to designate the proliferation as hyperplasia. Histologically, there are small nodules of Schwann cells with spindled comma-shaped nuclei and scant indistinct cytoplasm. These are aggregated in onionskin-like lamellae in a myxoid stroma, producing a vaguely whorled pattern. These features may be best appreciated using immunostains for neural markers such as S-100 protein, PGP9.5, or Leu-7.

FOREIGN BODIES

Foreign bodies lodged in the appendix may cause localized appendicitis. Fecaliths represent the most common foreign body encountered (80, 80a), accounting for about 44 percent of all foreign objects found in the appendix. Other common foreign materials include barium and parasites. Almost every other type of conceivable foreign body may be present, such as pins, nails, bubble gum, teeth, and seeds.

DRUG EFFECTS

Drugs affect the appendix in a manner similar to that seen in the remainder of the intestines. Chemotherapy severely depletes the normal lymphoid tissues, producing a hypocellular lamina propria and loss of Peyer patches. The epithelial cells may appear necrotic or megaloblastic. Thalidomide is associated with appendiceal agenesis (81,82).

INFLAMMATORY BOWEL DISEASE

Both *ulcerative colitis* and *Crohn's disease* may affect the appendix. The diagnosis of appendiceal ulcerative colitis and Crohn's disease relies on a combination of clinical manifestations, radiologic features, and morphologic findings. When the disease remains isolated to the appendix, as happens in fewer than 5 percent of patients, one must rely on the histologic features alone (83,87,89). The histologic changes resemble those seen in the remainder of the colon.

Crohn's Disease

The appendix is involved in as many as 50 percent of patients with evidence of ileal Crohn's disease (87). Appendiceal disease can also be found synchronously with disease at a considerable distance from the ileocecal region, such as in the rectum or upper small intestine.

Grossly, the appendix appears enlarged, thickened, and sometimes adherent to the terminal ileum or cecum. Mesenteric lymph nodes may be enlarged. A transmural mixed cellular infiltrate, consisting of lymphocytes, plasma cells, neutrophils, and eosinophils, is usually present (fig. 13-17). The prominent transmural inflammation

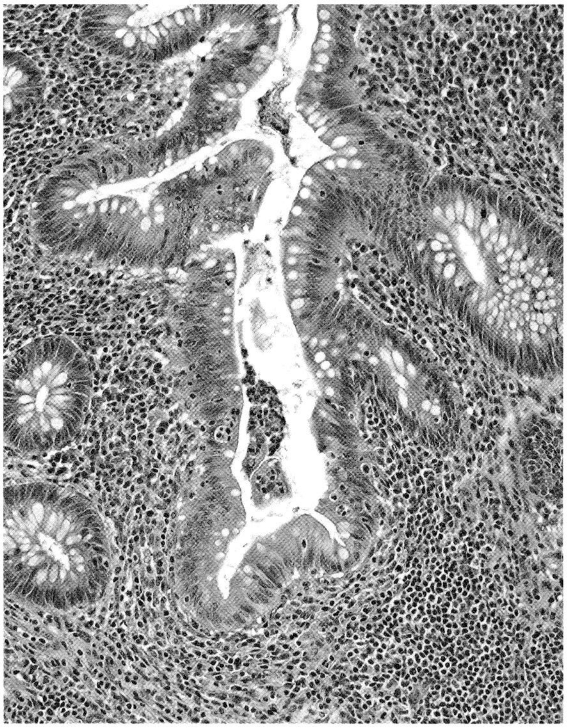

Figure 13-17

CROHN'S DISEASE INVOLVING THE APPENDIX

The appendiceal mucosa shows evidence of distortion of the crypt architecture and active inflammation with the formation of crypt abscesses.

is characterized by fibrosis and giant cell epithelioid granulomas. The deep submucosa and muscularis propria/serosa junction are particularly involved by the disease, although granulomas can be seen anywhere. Granulomas often lie in a paravascular or paralymphatic location. Lymphoid aggregates lie in the thickened serosa and are associated with the granulomas. Hypertrophy of the muscularis propria develops in about half of the cases. Other findings include marked mucosal ulceration, focal crypt inflammation, crypt abscesses, fissures, ulcers, perforation, abscess formation, neural hyperplasia, and sometimes, subserosal fibrosis. An accompanying spectrum of acute inflammation also occurs. Epithelioid granulomas are often seen in the periappendiceal lymph nodes.

The histologic differential diagnosis includes other entities that produce granulomatous appendicitis (fig. 13-18) including tuberculosis; yersiniosis; parasitic, fungal, and actinomycotic infections; and sarcoidosis.

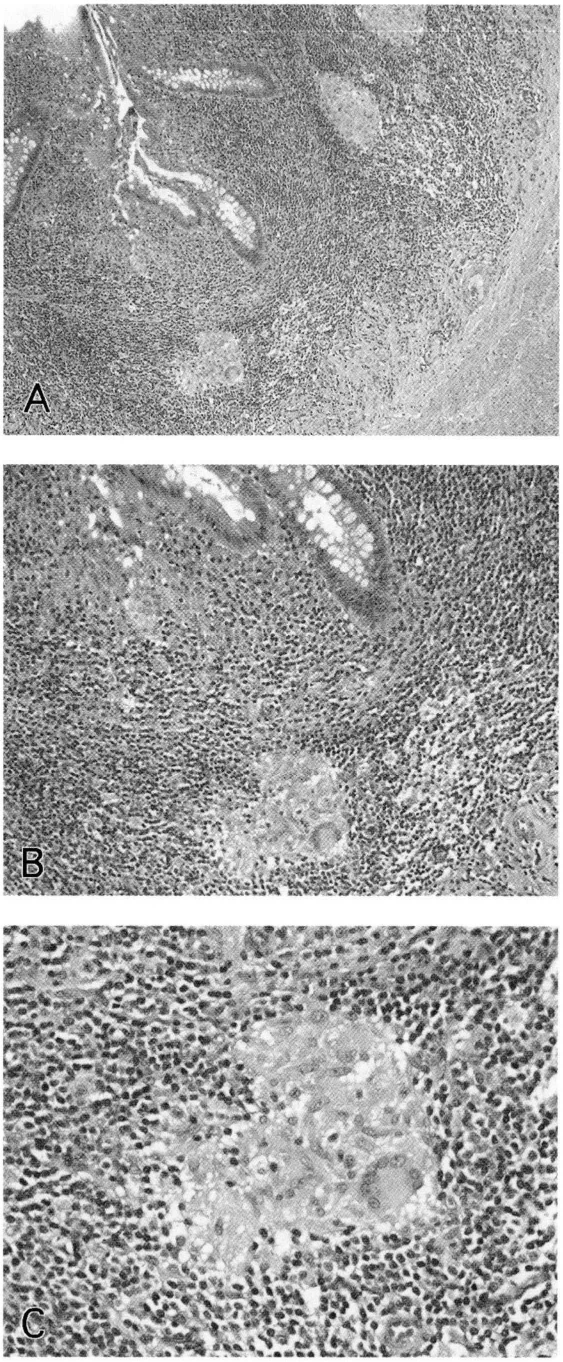

Figure 13-18

GRANULOMATOUS APPENDICITIS IN A PATIENT WITH CROHN'S DISEASE

A: Numerous well-formed, compact, non-necrotizing granulomas are present in the mucosa.

B: The mucosa contains abundant lymphoid tissue, but is not actively inflamed.

C: Higher-power view shows one of the compact sarcoid-like granulomas. A multinucleated giant cell is present.

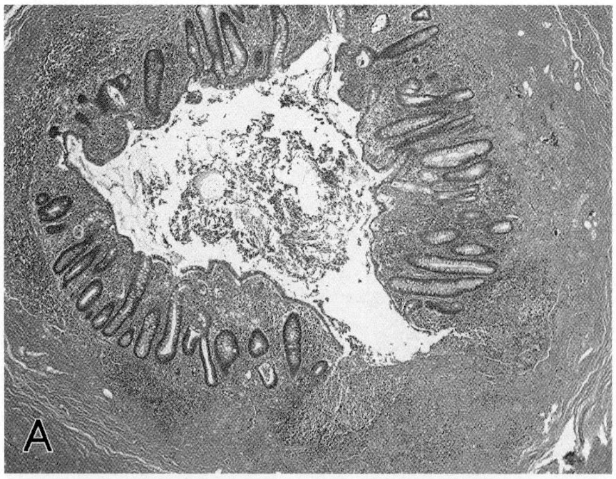

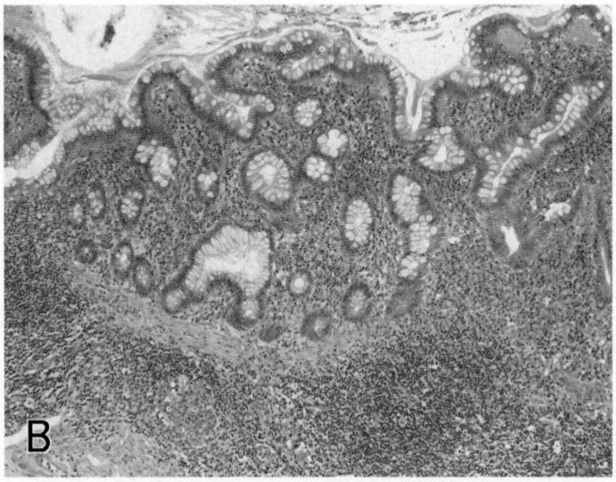

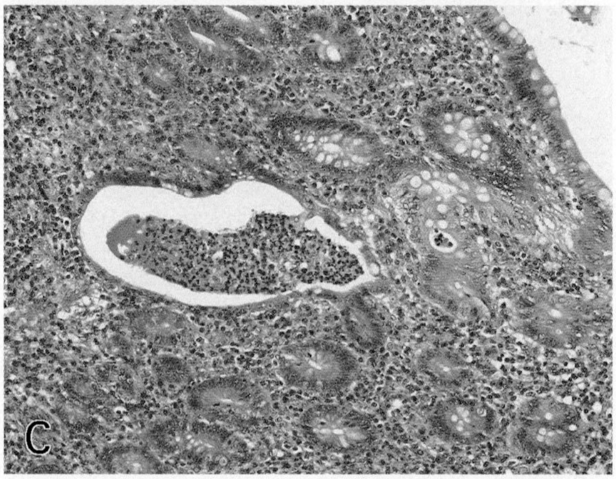

Figure 13-19

ULCERATIVE COLITIS INVOLVING THE APPENDIX

A: Focal ulceration of the appendiceal mucosa.

B: There is architectural distortion of crypts as characterizes inflammatory bowel disease.

C: Higher-power view of the mucosa shows a large crypt abscess and dense chronic inflammation of the lamina propria.

Ulcerative Colitis

Approximately 50 percent of patients with ulcerative colitis have appendiceal involvement (85), usually in continuity with cecal involvement. Isolated appendiceal ulcerative colitis may also be seen in some patients with left sided disease that spares the proximal bowel ("cecal patch") (84–86,88). It may be very difficult to distinguish between acute appendicitis and ulcerative colitis, particularly if the entire clinical history is unknown. The histologic features of ulcerative colitis in the appendix are identical to those in the colon (fig. 13-19).

GYNECOLOGIC ABNORMALITIES AFFECTING THE APPENDIX

Endometriosis

Endometriosis affects approximately 1 percent of appendices (94,95). It can present as appendicitis or appendiceal intussusception (93,96,97). Perforation may also develop (92). Endometriosis usually involves the serosal surface or the muscular layers of the appendix, and only rarely involves the mucosa. Grossly, endometriosis appears as discrete brownish foci, although more often it is an incidental histologic finding that was not appreciated grossly. Both endometrial glands and stroma are associated with variable amounts of fibrosis and hemosiderin deposition.

Endosalpingiosis

Endosalpingiosis, the ectopic location of benign glandular epithelium resembling that lining the normal fallopian tube, often involves the peritoneal surfaces. It can also be encountered on the serosal surface of the bowel, including the appendix (90,91), where it affects either the serosa or the muscularis propria. The distinction of this lesion from endometriosis is relatively straightforward because the endometrial epithelium and stroma, areas of periglandular hemorrhage, and hemosiderin-laden macrophages present in endometriosis are absent in endosalpingiosis. The identification of müllerian types of cells differentiates this lesion from mesonephric remnants and mesothelial inclusion cysts. The absence of goblet cells precludes a gastrointestinal origin.

Decidual Nodules

Decidual nodules may stud the appendiceal serosa (fig. 13-20). The masses of decidual cells may be quite prominent. Histologically they resemble decidua found elsewhere. This change is usually seen in those who are pregnant or are undergoing a postpartum tubal ligation with elective appendectomy.

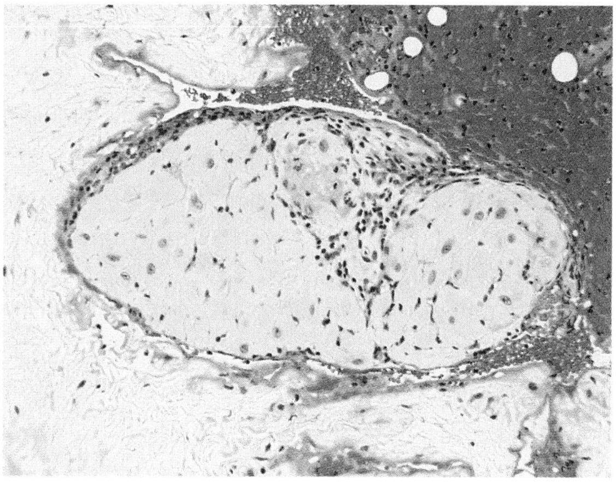

Figure 13-20

DECIDUAL NODULES

A small cluster of decidualized cells is present on the serosa of the appendix. This patient had recently been pregnant.

MUCOCELE

Definition. The term *mucocele* refers to any dilatation of the appendiceal lumen resulting from mucus accumulation, but it does not indicate a specific pathogenic mechanism or underlying histologic diagnosis. Both neoplastic and non-neoplastic lesions can produce a mucocele.

Clinical Features. Non-neoplastic mucoceles occur in middle-aged individuals, and affect both sexes equally. Patients often present with abdominal pain, with or without a palpable mass. The mucocele results from obstruction of the appendiceal lumen.

Pathologic Findings. Progressive accumulation of mucinous debris within the appendix causes cystic dilatation associated with flattening and atrophy of the epithelium (fig. 13-21). The wall of the appendix may be focally fibrotic and contain chronic inflammatory cells. Rupture of a retention mucocele produces localized mucin accumulations that are usually easily resectable. The mucin does not reaccumulate under these circumstances. The epithelium lining a non-neoplastic mucocele may also become hyperplastic, resembling that seen in hyperplastic polyps.

CYSTIC FIBROSIS

The common denominator for the gastrointestinal abnormalities occurring in the setting of cystic fibrosis is abnormal mucus production. In the appendix, increased numbers of hyperdistended goblet cells line the entire length of the crypts. The goblet cells release their abnormal mucin content and the appendix swells and becomes hyperdistended with inspissated eosinophilic secretions (fig. 13-22). Appendicitis results when the lumen is obstructed by the thick secretions. Symptomatic patients often present with appendiceal abscesses at the time of surgery (98,99).

NON-NEOPLASTIC POLYPS

Hyperplastic Polyps

Localized, small hyperplastic polyps arise in the appendix but their incidence is unknown. Histologically, they resemble hyperplastic polyps occurring elsewhere in the large intestine. The glands have serrated lumens lined by benign epithelium demonstrating an orderly progression of cellular maturation. The collagen table appears thickened and cytologic atypia is absent.

Sessile serrated polyps and serrated adenomas also affect the appendix. Differentiation of these lesions from hyperplastic polyps is important because they are associated with an increased risk for the development of adenocarcinoma.

Other Polyps

Both *Peutz-Jeghers* and *juvenile polyps* can affect the appendix as part of a more generalized syndrome. They resemble similar polyps arising elsewhere in the gut.

Figure 13-21

NON-NEOPLASTIC MUCOCELE

A: A dilated appendix is filled with thick mucinous material.

B: Low-power view shows an attenuated appendiceal wall and abundant luminal mucin.

C: The mucosa appears flattened and atrophic. No adenomatous changes are present in this mucocele.

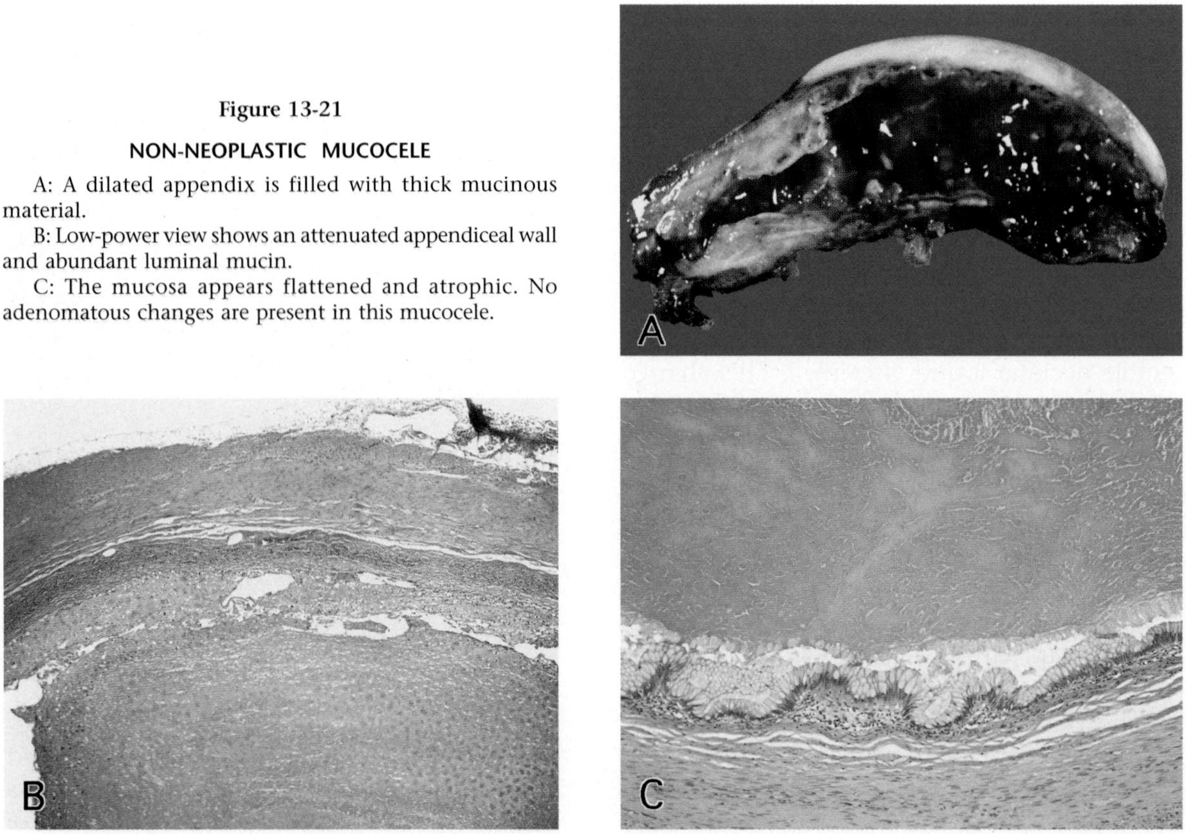

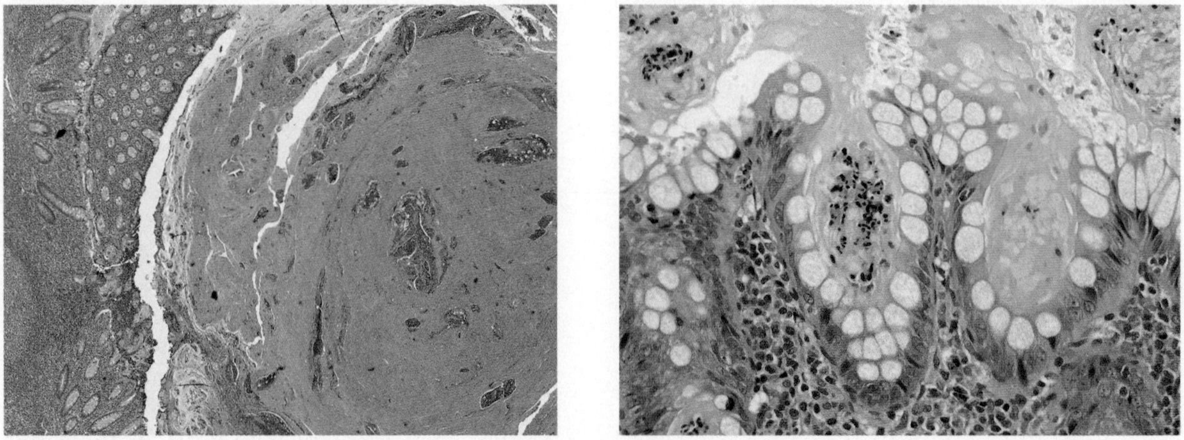

Figure 13-22

CYSTIC FIBROSIS

Left: The appendiceal lumen is filled with dense eosinophilic mucinous secretions.

Right: The epithelium contains numerous hyperdistended goblet cells and dilated crypt lumens.

REFERENCES

Congenital Anomalies

1. Bremner DN, Mooney G. Agenesis of appendix: a further thalidomide anomaly. Lancet 1978;1: 826.
2. Cave AJ. Appendix vermiformis duplex. J Anat 1936;70:283–92.
3. Collins DC. Agenesis of the vermiform appendix. Am J Surg 1951;82:689–96.
4. Collins, DC. A study of 50,000 specimens of the human vermiform appendix. Surg Gynecol Obstet 1955;101:437–55.
5. Tinckler LF. Triple appendix vermiformis—a unique case. Br J Surg 1968;55:79–81.
6. Wallbridge PH. Double appendix. Br J Surg 1962; 50:346–7.
7. Yokose Y, Maruyama H, Tsutsumi M, Uchida K, Shiraiwa K, Konishi Y. Ileal atresia and absence of appendix. Acta Pathol Jpn 1986;36:1403–10.

Diverticula

8. Collins, DC. A study of 50,000 specimens of the human vermiform appendix. Surg Gynecol Obstet 1955;101:437–55.

8a. Esparza AR, Pan CM. Diverticulosis of the appendix. Surgery 1970;67:922–8.

9. Favara BE. Multiple congenital diverticula of the vermiform appendix. Am J Clin Pathol 1968; 49:60–4.
10. George DH. Diverticulosis of the vermiform appendix in patients with cystic fibrosis. Hum Pathol 1987;18:75–9.
11. Lipton S, Estrin J, Glasser I. Diverticular disease of the appendix. Surg Gynecol Obstet 1989;168: 13–6.
12. Phillips BJ, Perry CW. Appendiceal diverticulitis. Mayo Clinic Proc 1999;74:890–2.

Intussusception

13. Collins DC. 71,000 human appendix specimens, a final report summarizing forty years' study. Am J Proctol 1963;14:365–81.
14. Fink VH, Santos AL, Goldberg SL. Intussusception of the appendix. Case reports and review of the literature. Am J Gastroenterol 1964;42: 431–40.
15. Forshall I. Intussusception of the vermiform appendix with a report of seven cases in children. Br J Surg 1953;40:305–12.
16. Ho L, Rosenman LD. Complete invagination of the vermiform appendix with villous adenoma, intussuscepting to the splenic flexure of the colon. Surgery 1975;77:505–6.
17. Lauwers GY, Prendergast NC, Wahl SJ, Bagchi S. Invagination of vermiform appendix. Dig Dis Sci 1993;38:565–8.
18. Nissen ED, Goldstein AI. Intussusception of the appendix associated with endometriosis. Int J Gynecol Obstet 1973;11:184–9.
19. Ozuner G, Davidson P, Church J. Intussusception of the vermiform appendix: preoperative colonoscopic diagnosis of two cases and review of the literature. Int J Colorectal Dis 2000; 15:185–7.
20. Rodriguez MA, Wasdahl WA. Mucinous carcinoid and endometriosis in an inside-out appendix. Am J Gastroenterol 1978;69:199–202.

Septa

21. De La Fuente AA. Septa in the appendix: a previously undescribed condition. Histopathology 1985;9:1329–37.

Amyand Hernia

22. D'Alia C, Lo Schiavo MG, Tonante A, et al. Amyand's hernia: case report and review of the literature. Hernia 2003;7:89–91.
23. Hutchinson R. Amyand's hernia. J R Soc Med 1993;86:104–5.

Appendicitis

24. Adamidis D, Roma-Giaanikou E, Karamolegou K, Tselalidou E, Constantopoulus A. Fiber intake and childhood appendicitis. Int J Food Sci Nutr 2000;51:153–7.
25. Addiss DG, Shaffer N, Fowler BS, Tauxe RV. The epidemiology of appendicitis and appendectomy in the United States. Am J Epidemiol 1990;132:910–25.
26. Al-Omran M, Mamdani MM, McLeod RS. Epidemiologic features of acute appendicitis in Ontario, Canada. Can J Surg 2003;46:263–8.
27. Arnbjornsson E. Acute appendicitis and dietary fiber. Arch Surg 1983;118:868–70.
28. Astagneau P, Goldstein FW, Francoual S, Baviera E, Barthalon M, Acar JF. Appendicitis due to both *Streptococcus pneumoniae* and *Haemophilus influenzae*. Eur J Clin Microbiol Infect Dis 1992;11:559–60.
29. Barker DJ, Morris J. Acute appendicitis, bathrooms, and diet in Britain and Ireland. Br Med J 1988;296:953–5.
30. Barker DJ, Osmond C, Golding J, Wadsworth ME. Acute appendicitis and bathrooms in three samples of British children. Br Med J 1988;296:956–8.

31. Basta M, Morton NE, Mulvihill JJ, Radovanovic Z, Radojicic C, Marinkovic D. Inheritance of acute appendicitis: familial aggregation and evidence of polygenic transmission. Am J Hum Genet 1990;46:377–82.
32. Bennion RS, Thompson JE Jr, Gil J, Schmit PJ. The role of *Yersinia enterocolitica* in appendicitis in the southwestern United States. Am Surg 1991;57:766–8.
33. Blair NP, Bugis SP, Turner LJ, MacLeod MM. Review of the pathologic diagnoses of 2,216 appendectomy specimens. Am J Surg 1993;165: 618–20.
34. Brender JD, Weiss NS, Koepsell TD, Marcuse EK. Fiber intake and childhood appendicitis. Am J Public Health 1985;75:399–400.
35. Campbell KL, De Beaux AC. Non-steroidal anti-inflammatory drugs and appendicitis in patients aged over 50 years. Br J Surg 1992;79:967–8.
36. Chan FT, Stringel G, Mackenzie AM. Isolation of *Campylobacter jejuni* from an appendix. J Clin Microbiol 1983;18:422–4.
37. Cook GC. *Enterobius vermicularis* infection. Gut 1994;35:1159–62.
38. Duffy DL, Martin NG, Matthews JD. Appendectomy in Australian twins. Am J Hum Genet 1990;47:590–92.
39. Gardikis S, Touloupidis S, Dimitriadis G, et al. Urological symptoms of acute appendicitis in childhood and early adolescence. Int Urol Nephrol 2002;34:189–92.
40. Gauderer MW, Crane MM, Green JA, DeCou JM, Abrams RS. Acute appendicitis in children: the importance of family history. J Ped Surg 2001;36:2124–7.
41. Guo G, Greenson JK. Histopathology of interval (delayed) appendectomy specimens: strong association with granulomatous and xanthogranulomatous appendicitis. Am J Surg Pathol 2003;27:1147–51.
42. Hardin D. Acute appendicitis: review and update. Am Fam Physician 1999;60:2027–34.
43. Hickey K, McKenna P, O'Connell PR, Gillan JE. Actinomycosis presenting as appendicitis in pregnancy. Br J Obstet Gynaecol 1993;100:595–6.
44. Horattas MC, Guyton DP, Wu D. A reappraisal of appendicitis in the elderly. Am J Surg 1990; 160:291–3.
45. Hui TT, Major KM, Avital I, Hiatt JR, Margulies DR. Outcome of elderly patients with appendicitis: effect of computed tomography and laparoscopy. Arch Surg 2002;137:995–1000.
46. Janik JS, Firor HV. Pediatric appendicitis: a 20-year study of 1,640 children at Cook County (Illinois) Hospital. Arch Surg 1979;114:717–9.
47. Jones PF. Suspected acute appendicitis: trends in management over 30 years. Br J Surg 2001;88:1570–7.
48. Kang JY, Hoare J, Majeed A, Williamson RC, Maxwell JD. Decline in admission rates for acute appendicitis in England. Br J Surg 2003;90: 1586–92.
49. Koepsell TD, Inui TS, Farewell VT. Factors affecting perforation in acute appendicitis. Surg Gynecol Obstet 1981;153:508–10.
50. Korner H, Sondenaa K, Soreide JA, et al. Incidence of acute nonperforated and perforated appendicitis: age-specific and sex-specific analysis. World J Surg 1997;21:313–7.
51. Kosloske AM, Love CL, Rohrer JE, Goldthorn JF, Lacey SR. The diagnosis of appendicitis in children: outcomes of a strategy based on pediatric surgical evaluation. Pediatrics 2004;113:29–34.
52. Kraemer M, Franke C, Ohmann C, Yang Q. Acute Abdominal Pain Study Group. Acute appendicitis in late adulthood: incidence, presentation, and outcome. Results of a prospective multicenter acute abdominal pain study and review of the literature. Langenbecks Arch Surg 2000;385:470–81.
53. Kraemer M, Ohmann C, Leppert R, Yang Q. Macroscopic assessment of the appendix at diagnostic laparoscopy is reliable. Surg Endosc 2000;14:625–33.
54. Lamps LW, Madhusudhan KT, Greenson JK, et al. The role of *Yersinia enterocolitica* and *Yersinia pseudotuberculosis* in granulomatous appendicitis: a histologic and molecular study. Am J Surg Pathol 2001;25:508–15.
55. Lau WY, Teoh-Chan CH, Fan ST, Yam WC, Lau KF, Wong SH. The bacteriology and septic complication of patients with appendicitis. Ann Surg 1984;200:576–81.
56. Lee JA. The influence of sex and age on appendicitis in children and young adults. Gut 1962;3: 80–4.
57. Luckmann R, Davis P. The epidemiology of acute appendicitis in California: racial, gender, and seasonal variation. Epidemiology 1991;2:323–30.
58. Madden NP, Hart CA. *Streptococcus milleri* in appendicitis in children. J Pediatr Surg 1985;20:6–7.
59. Moreno E. Enterobiasis (oxyuriasis, pinworm infection). In: Marcial-Rojas RA, ed. Pathology of protozoa and helminthic diseases. Baltimore: Williams & Wilkins; 1971:760.
60. Nash TE, Cheever AW, Ottesen EA, Cook JA. Schistosome infections in humans: perspectives and recent findings. NIH Conference. Ann Intern Med 1982;97:740–54.

61. Nitecki S, Karmeli R, Sarr MG. Appendiceal calculi and fecaliths as indications for appendectomy. Surg Gynecol Obstet 1990;171:185–8.
62. Onuigbo WI. Appendiceal schistosomiasis. Method of classifying oviposition and inflammation. Dis Colon Rectum 1985;28:397–8.
63. Pawlowski ZS. Enterobiasis. In: Warren KS, Mahmoud AA, eds. Tropical and geographical medicine. New York: McGraw-Hill; 1984:386.
64. Rode J, Dhillon AP, Hutt MS. Appendicitis revisited: a comparative study of Malawian and English appendices. J Pathol 1987;153:357–63.
65. Satti MB, Tamimi DM, Al Sohaibani MO, Al Quorain A. Appendicular schistosomiasis: a cause of clinical acute appendicitis? J Clin Pathol 1987;40:424–8.
66. Shin MS, Ho KJ. Appendicolith. Significance in acute appendicitis and demonstration by computed tomography. Dig Dis Sci 1985;30:184–7.
67. Storm-Dickerson TL, Horattas MC. What have we learned over the past 20 years about appendicitis in the elderly? Am J Surg 2003;185:198–201.
68. Tovar JA, Trallero EP, Garay J. Appendiceal perforation and shigellosis. Z Kinderchir 1983;38:419.
69. van Spreeuwel JP, Lindeman J, Bax R, Elbers HJ, Sybrandy R, Meijer CJ. *Campylobacter*-associated appendicitis: prevalence and clinicopathologic features. Pathol Annu 1987;22:55–65.
70. Wiebe BM. Appendicitis and *Enterobius vermicularis*. Scand J Gastroenterol 1991;26:336–8.
71. Williams NM, Jackson D, Everson NW, Johnstone JM. Is the incidence of acute appendicitis really falling? Ann R Coll Surg Engl 1998;80:122–4.

Periappendicitis

72. Fink AS, Kosakowski CA, Hiatt JR, Cochran AJ. Periappendicitis is a significant clinical finding. Am J Surg 1990;159:564–8.

Neurogenic Appendicopathy

73. Di Sebastiano P, Fink T, di Mola FF, et al. Neuroimmune appendicitis. Lancet 1999;354:461–6.
74. Franke C, Gerharz CD, Bohner H, et al. Neurogenic appendicopathy: a clinical disease entity? Int J Colorectal Dis 2002;17:185–91.
75. Franke C, Gerharz CD, Bohner H, et al. Neurogenic appendicopathy in children. Eur J Ped Surg 2002;12:28–31.
76. Nemeth L, Reen DJ, O'Briain DS, McDermott M, Puri P. Evidence of an inflammatory pathologic condition in "normal" appendices following emergency appendectomy. Arch Pathol Lab Med 2001;125:759–64.
77. Wang Y, Reen DJ, Puri P. Is a histologically normal appendix following emergency appendicectomy always normal? Lancet 1996:347:1076–9.

Myxoglobulosis

78. Gonzalez JE, Hann SE, Trujillo YP. Myxoglobulosis of the appendix. Am J Surg Pathol 1988; 12:962–6.
79. Lubin J, Berle E. Myxoglobulosis of the appendix. Report of two cases. Arch Pathol 1972;94: 533–6.

Foreign Bodies

80. Balch CM, Silver D. Foreign bodies in the appendix. Report of eight cases and review of the literature. Arch Surg 1971;102:14–20.
80a. Collins, DC. A study of 50,000 specimens of the human vermiform appendix. Surg Gynecol Obstet 1955;101:437–55.

Drug Effects

81. Shand JE, Bremner DN. Agenesis of the vermiform appendix in a thalidomide child. Br J Surg 1977;64:203–4.
82. Smithells RW. Thalidomide, absent appendix, and sweating. Lancet 1978;1:1042.

Inflammatory Bowel Disease

83. Ariel I, Vinograd I, Hershlag A, et al. Crohn's disease isolated to the appendix: truths and fallacies. Hum Pathol 1986;17:1116–21.
84. Davison AM, Dixon MF. The appendix as a 'skip lesion' in ulcerative colitis. Histopathology 1990;16:93–5.
85. Goldblum JR, Appelman HD. Appendiceal involvement in ulcerative colitis. Mod Pathol 1992;5:607–10.
86. Groisman GM, George J, Harpaz N. Ulcerative appendicitis in universal and nonuniversal ulcerative colitis. Mod Pathol 1994;7:322–5.
87. Kahn E, Markowitz J, Daum F. The appendix in inflammatory bowel disease in children. Mod Pathol 1992;5:380–3.
88. Kroft SH, Stryker SJ, Rao MS. Appendiceal involvement as a skip lesion in ulcerative colitis. Mod Pathol 1994;7:912–4.
89. Prieto-Nieto I, Perez-Robledo JP, Hardisson D, Rodriguez-Montes JA, Larrauri-Martinez J, Garcia-Sancho-Martin L. Crohn's disease limited to the appendix. Am J Surg 2001;182:531–3.

Gynecologic Abnormalities

90. Cajigas A, Axiotis CA. Endosalpingiosis of the vermiform appendix. Int J Gynecol Pathol 1990; 9:291–5.

91. McCluggage WG, Clements WD. Endosalpingiosis of the colon and appendix. Histopathology 2001;39:645–6.
92. Nakatani Y, Hara M, Misugi K, Korehisa H. Appendiceal endometriosis in pregnancy. Report of a case with perforation and review of the literature. Acta Pathol Jpn 1987;37:1685–90.
93. Nycum LR, Moss H, Adams JQ, Macri CI. Asymptomatic intussusception of the appendix due to endometriosis. South Med J 1999;92:524–5.
94. Ortiz-Hidalgo C, Cortes-Aguilar D, Ortiz de la Pena J. Endometriosis of the vermiform appendix (EVA) is an uncommon lesion with a frequency < 1% of all cases of pelvic endometriosis. Recent case. World J Surg 1999;23:427.
95. Prystowsky JB, Stryker SJ, Ujiki GT, Poticha SM. Gastrointestinal endometriosis. Incidence and indications for resection. Arch Surg 1988;123:855–8.
96. Sakaguchi N, Ito M, Sano K, Baba T, Koyama M, Hotchi M. Intussusception of the appendix: a report of three cases with different clinical and pathologic features. Pathol Int 1995;45:757–61.
97. Sriram PV, Seitz U, Soehendra N, Schroeder S. Endoscopic appendectomy in a case of appendicular intussusception due to endometriosis, mimicking a cecal polyp. Am J Gastroenterol 2000;95:1594–6.

Cystic Fibrosis

98. Martens M, De Boeck K, Van Der Steen K, Smet M, Eggermont E. A right lower quadrant mass in cystic fibrosis: a diagnostic challenge. Eur J Pediatrics 1992;151:329–31
99. Shields MD, Levison H, Reisman JJ, Durie PR, Canny GI. Appendicitis in cystic fibrosis. Arch Dis Child 1991;66:307–10.

14 MISCELLANEOUS INTESTINAL DISORDERS

EOSINOPHILIC DISEASES

Food Allergy

Demography. Up to 45 percent of the population report adverse reactions to food (1). The incidence appears to be increasing, although this may reflect increased reporting of allergic symptoms by patients and physicians (2). Food sensitivity occurs particularly commonly in infants and young children.

Etiology. Numerous antigens may play a role in the pathogenesis of conditions loosely termed "food allergies," and many conditions are associated with an allergy to food (Table 14-1). Patients with diseases such as eczema and asthma exhibit a clear-cut relationship between exposure to ingested allergens and symptom development. A definitive diagnosis of a food allergy requires the demonstration of an unequivocal clinical reaction after a controlled food challenge and elimination of the symptom complex subsequent to removal of the offending food.

Pathophysiology. The increased susceptibility of infants to food allergic reactions results from their general immunologic immaturity and the overall immaturity of their gastrointestinal tracts (4,5). The majority of allergic reactions to food are immunoglobulin (Ig)E-mediated, mast cell–dependent, immediate hypersensitivity type reactions. The interaction of an antigen with an antibody or immunocyte triggers the allergic reaction. It is mediated by soluble factors from activated neutrophils, mast cells, and macrophages, or by direct membrane interactions between immune cells and antigens on their cell surfaces. Released cytokines and inflammatory mediators act directly on the epithelium, endothelium, or muscle, or indirectly through nerves and mesenchymal cells. The immediate consequences of these mediators include a local change in vascular permeability, stimulation of mucus production, increased muscle contraction, stimulation of pain fibers, recruitment of inflammatory cells, edema of mucosal epithelial villi, increased protein loss from the gut, and increased absorption of foreign antigens. Eosinophils, lymphocytes, and monocytes are attracted to the reaction site where they release additional inflammatory mediators and cytokines. Repeated ingestion of an allergen stimulates mononuclear cells to secrete histamine-releasing factors, some of which interact with IgE molecules bound to basophil and mast cell surfaces (3). If significant mast cell degranulation occurs, mast cell mediators may provoke potentially fatal systemic anaphylaxis.

Clinical Features. The clinical manifestations of food allergy vary widely in location, severity, and time of onset, and correlate with the site and extent of mast cell degranulation. The principal organ systems affected by allergic food reactions are the intestinal tract, skin, and lungs. In some patients, the signs and symptoms of an immediate reaction remain limited to the gastrointestinal tract, with cramping, bloating, nausea, vomiting, diarrhea, growth failure in children, and weight loss in adults. Factors such as the quantity and quality of the food ingested, and the presence of other existing medical conditions, may also influence the clinical features.

Table 14-1

CONDITIONS ASSOCIATED WITH FOOD ALLERGY

Systemic anaphylaxis
Rhinitis
Conjunctivitis
Asthma
Allergic alveolitis
Celiac disease
Cow's milk protein enteropathy
Urticaria
Angioedema
Atopic eczema
Dermatitis herpetiformis

Gross Findings. Affected regions of the gastrointestinal tract may appear grossly unremarkable, or may demonstrate variable degrees of edema.

Microscopic Findings. Biopsies of the small intestine may show partial villous atrophy with vacuolated cytoplasm, particularly at the surface, and prominent eosinophilic infiltrates. Eosinophils may aggregate in the lamina propria or infiltrate into the epithelium. Since these infiltrates are usually focal, multiple biopsies are often required to make the diagnosis.

Cow's Milk Intolerance and Related Disorders

Demography. An adverse reaction to the ingestion of cow's milk is the most common food allergy in young children. It affects 0.1 to 7.5 percent of children in developed countries (6,7).

Etiology. Sensitivity to cow's milk is the most frequent cause of an intolerance reaction, but it also occurs with soy, egg, and wheat ingestion.

Pathophysiology. Reactions to cow's milk proteins are classified clinically as quick onset (symptoms develop within 1 hour of food ingestion) or slow onset (symptoms develop more than 1 hour from food ingestion). Quick-onset allergic reactions are IgE-mediated, and do not result in structural gastrointestinal damage (12). Slow-onset reactions may also be IgE-mediated, or they may be the result of T-cell–mediated immune reactions. Such reactions may result in macrophage influx associated with cytokine release and direct damage to gastrointestinal tissues (12).

Clinical Features. Several clinical syndromes associated with cow's milk allergy have now been defined (Table 14-2). Patients with *cow's milk esophagitis* present with symptoms similar to those of gastroesophageal reflux disease. Infants with *cow's milk enteropathy* or *colitis* generally present at 1 week to 3 months of age with protracted vomiting, malabsorption, diarrhea, and dehydration (10a). Infants with a more insidious symptom onset have diarrhea, protein-losing enteropathy, iron deficiency anemia due to chronic intestinal blood loss, weight loss, and failure to thrive. Fecal examination demonstrates occult blood, neutrophils, and eosinophils. The abnormalities resolve on a cow's milk–free diet and only recur on cow's milk challenge. Important predisposing factors are age less than 3 years, transient IgA immunodeficiency, atopy, and early bottle feeding.

Table 14-2

CLINICAL SYNDROMES ASSOCIATED WITH COW'S MILK INTOLERANCE

Clinical Presentation	Syndrome
Quick onset	Acute cow's milk allergy
Slow onset	Cow's milk esophagitis
	Cow's milk sensitivity enteropathy
	Cow's milk colitis
Varied	Multiple food allergy

Pathologic Findings. Cow's milk esophagitis is characterized by dense infiltration of eosinophils into the esophageal mucosa. The histologic changes are indistinguishable from eosinophilic esophagitis (see chapter 3). In cow's milk enteropathy, the intestinal mucosa typically appears thin, with patchy areas of villous atrophy that produce a pattern resembling celiac disease (8–11). Biopsy specimens reveal flattened villi, edema, a prominent mononuclear cell infiltrate of the epithelium and lamina propria, and an accompanying small number of eosinophils. Intraepithelial lymphocytes are usually fewer than seen in celiac disease.

Treatment and Prognosis. Patients recover following elimination of milk, soy, or other offending antigens from the diet.

Eosinophilic Esophagitis

Eosinophilic esophagitis most likely represents food allergy. This entity is discussed in detail in chapter 3.

Allergic Proctocolitis

Demography. *Allergic proctocolitis* commonly affects infants ranging from a few days to 1 year of age (20).

Etiology. The disorder often results from exposure to cow's milk or soy protein in the formula (13,16–18). It also occurs in infants receiving breast milk (15).

Clinical Features. Affected infants present primarily with acute rectal bleeding, with or without associated diarrhea (14,19,21). Other common manifestations include weight loss, an allergic history, anemia, and peripheral eosinophilia (19,20).

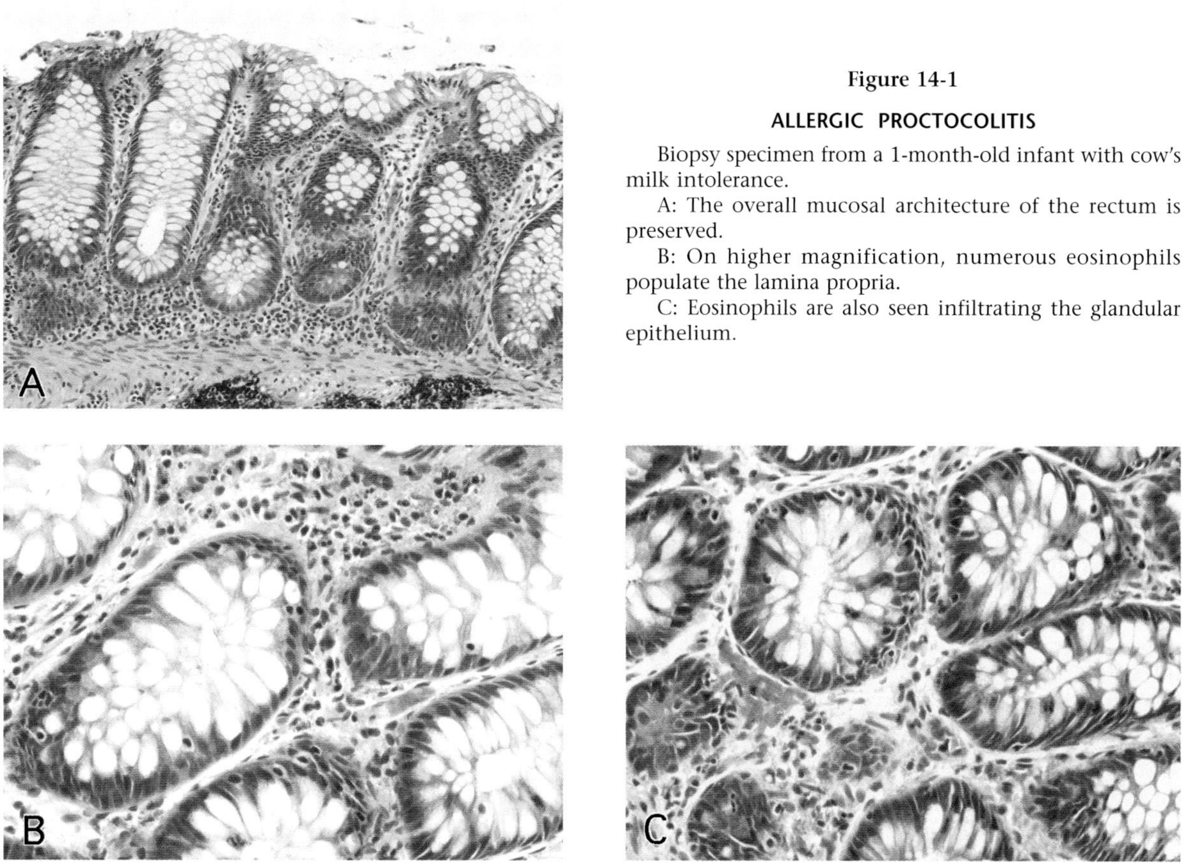

Figure 14-1

ALLERGIC PROCTOCOLITIS

Biopsy specimen from a 1-month-old infant with cow's milk intolerance.

A: The overall mucosal architecture of the rectum is preserved.

B: On higher magnification, numerous eosinophils populate the lamina propria.

C: Eosinophils are also seen infiltrating the glandular epithelium.

Gross Findings. Allergic proctocolitis involves any colonic segment, but the rectosigmoid is preferentially involved. Endoscopic features include focal erythema (19), a friable-appearing mucosa, and increased mucosal nodularity suggestive of lymphoid hyperplasia. Zones of entirely normal mucosa separate abnormal areas. In severe cases, there is decreased mucosal vascularity, multiple superficial aphthous erosions, or frank ulceration covered by a surface exudate.

Microscopic Findings. Increased numbers of eosinophils populate the lamina propria, particularly surface epithelium, crypt epithelium, and the muscularis mucosae (fig. 14-1). Eosinophils are characteristically present in large numbers (over 60 eosinophils per 10 high-power fields in the lamina propria). In addition, numerous intact or degranulated eosinophils may be seen in the deep mucosa and interspersed among muscle fibers of the muscularis mucosae (13,19,20,22). Often, the eosinophilic aggregates are closely associated with lymphoid nodules. The intensity of the eosinophilic infiltrate varies, not only between biopsies at different sites but within individual biopsy specimens. Biopsy specimens appear normal in about 50 percent of patients; in other patients, only one or two biopsies may be abnormal. No significant correlation exists between the number of mucosal eosinophils, patient age, illness duration, endoscopic appearance, and type of inciting allergen.

The overall mucosal architecture is maintained in allergic proctocolitis without histologic features of chronicity, such as distorted, branched, or atrophic crypts; Paneth cell metaplasia; basally located lymphoid aggregates; or diffuse plasmacytosis (fig. 14-1). The eosinophilia is an excellent marker of infantile allergic proctocolitis, but given the focal distribution of the lesion, multiple mucosal biopsy specimens must be obtained, and several levels of each should be examined (13,19,20).

Treatment and Prognosis. Pediatric patients with allergic proctocolitis generally respond promptly to dietary changes.

Eosinophilic Gastroenteritis

Definition. *Eosinophilic gastroenteritis* is a diagnosis applied to a diverse group of diseases seen in patients who share the following: 1) gastrointestinal symptoms; 2) gastrointestinal eosinophilic infiltrates; and 3) no demonstrable cause of the eosinophilia such as parasitic infection or a specific allergic response.

Demography. Eosinophilic gastroenteritis is an uncommon condition, with an estimated frequency of less than 1/100,000 population (32). The disease affects all races and ages, from infancy to adulthood, but the incidence peaks between the 2nd and 6th decades of life. The incidence is slightly higher in males, in a ratio of 3 to 2 (24,29). Approximately 70 percent of patients have a history of allergy, including hay fever, allergic rhinitis, eczema, asthma, drug sensitivities, or elevated IgE levels (30,40,42). Some patients have associated connective tissue diseases, specifically scleroderma, scleroderma variants, polymyositis, and dermatomyositis.

Etiology. Food allergy has been postulated as an etiologic factor in this disease since many patients have food-specific antibodies of the IgE isotype (25). In most cases, however, there is no specific allergen that triggers the disease and some patients have few or no allergic features (40).

Pathophysiology. The mechanism(s) whereby eosinophilic infiltrates cause gastrointestinal dysfunction remains unclear. Eosinophils are attracted to the site of inflammation by eotaxin, a substance produced by epithelial cells (23). In addition, eosinophils produce various cytokines, including transforming growth factor, granulocyte-macrophage colony-stimulating factor, interleukin (IL)3, and IL5 (48). These cytokines are known to be chemotactic for eosinophils, and therefore, contribute to the propagation of the inflammatory response in an autocrine fashion. Eosinophils produce a number of inflammatory mediators that may contribute to tissue damage including leukotrienes, platelet activating factor, major basic protein, eosinophil-derived neurotoxin, eosinophil cationic protein, and eosinophil peroxidase (32); all of these can directly damage gastrointestinal tissues. Major basic protein and eosinophil peroxidase also cause indirect injury by activating mast cells and by releasing histamine and other potentially harmful substances (28,36). Eosinophil-derived neurotoxins damage gastric nerves and muscles, causing gastroparesis and obstruction.

Clinical Features. The clinical manifestations of eosinophilic gastroenteritis correlate with the depth of the eosinophilic infiltration of the bowel wall and its location. A preponderance of eosinophils in a particular portion of the gut wall is the basis for classifying the disease into mucosal, muscular, and serosal subtypes (32). Patients with predominantly mucosal disease experience postprandial nausea, vomiting, abdominal pain, diarrhea, and protein-losing enteropathy (34). The muscular pattern of disease results in thickening and rigidity of the muscularis propria, causing functional gastric outlet obstruction and motility disturbances. Subserosal involvement is associated with higher levels of peripheral eosinophilia and bloating (45). Occasionally, patients present with an acute abdominal emergency such as acute appendicitis or intestinal perforation (27). Rare fatalities have been described (31,47).

Gross Findings. Involvement of gastrointestinal segments measuring up to 50 cm in length produces diffuse bowel thickening (24,46). A variable degree of antral stenosis with mucosal irregularity or gastric pseudopolyposis may be seen in the stomach on barium studies. Endoscopically, the bowel may appear normal or may show nonspecific features such as erythema, friability, erosions, ulcerations, and nodularity (32). Ascites may be present, and is thought to develop when eosinophils infiltrate the serosa or muscularis propria.

Microscopic Findings. Establishing the diagnosis of eosinophilic gastroenteritis by endoscopic biopsy can be problematic (37). In about 10 percent of cases, mucosal biopsies are nondiagnostic, either because of the sampling error inherent in diagnosing a patchy process, or due to mucosal sparing (fig. 14-2). In these instances, the diagnosis is established by multiple biopsies, full-thickness biopsy, or surgical resection. An eosinophil count of greater than 20 cells per high-power field is generally used to define eosinophilic gastroenteritis histologically (33,45,49).

In the stomach, mucosal edema, capillary lymphatic dilatation, and an intense but patchy eosinophilic infiltrate displace and destroy gastric pits and glands. Often, there is a

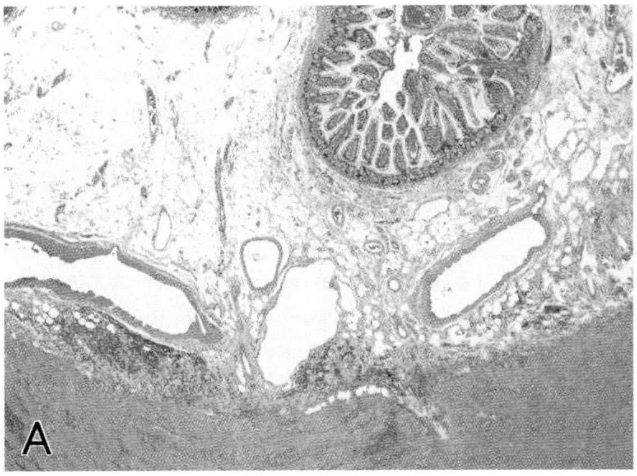

Figure 14-2

EOSINOPHILIC GASTROENTERITIS

A: Low-power view shows prominent submucosal edema in a resected segment of small intestine from a patient with eosinophilic gastroenteritis. Eosinophils infiltrate the muscularis propria and deep submucosa.

B: The mucosal architecture is preserved.

C: Higher-power view shows that the mucosa is spared by the heavy eosinophilic infiltrates. If lesions involve the deeper bowel layers, mucosal biopsy is often nondiagnostic.

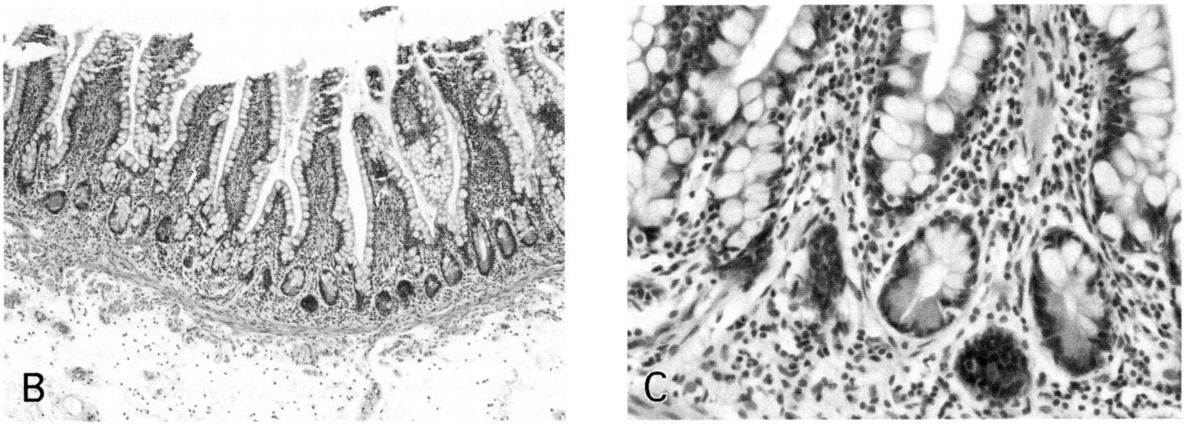

concomitant increase in the number of IgE-secreting plasma cells. Epithelial necrosis and degeneration develop, but frank ulceration rarely occurs. There may be pronounced hypertrophy of the muscularis propria, and the smooth muscle bundles become separated by dense eosinophilic infiltrates. Charcot-Leyden crystals can be found in these areas. In some cases, loose granulomas develop and acute vasculitis affects small arteries. Postinflammatory fibrous strictures sometimes complicate involvement of the muscularis propria.

In the small intestine, localized eosinophilic infiltrates cause crypt hyperplasia, epithelial cell necrosis, and villous atrophy. In a minority of cases (approximately 10 percent), diffuse enteritis develops, with complete villous loss producing an appearance identical to that seen in celiac disease. Submucosal edema is common, and destruction of the wall and fibrosis may occur (fig. 14-2). Contiguous smooth muscle fibers in the muscularis mucosae appear hyperchromatic, enlarged, and irregular, with reactive nuclei separated by eosinophils. The submucosa, muscularis propria, and even the subserosal soft tissue may show some degree of eosinophilic infiltration (fig. 14-3). Sometimes the mesenteric lymph nodes become hyperplastic and infiltrated with eosinophils.

Differential Diagnosis. Eosinophilic gastroenteritis must be distinguished from other disorders associated with eosinophilia. These include parasitic infections, collagen vascular diseases, inflammatory bowel disease, and neoplastic processes including Langerhans cell histiocytosis and lymphoma (Table 14-3).

Treatment and Prognosis. Patients generally respond dramatically to a short course of corticosteroid therapy (33,39,45). Some patients are treated with cromolyn sodium (26,41,49). Other therapies include elimination diets (30) and the use of antihistamines and other drugs used for asthma therapy (ketotifen, montelukast, and suplatast tosilate) (35,38,43,44).

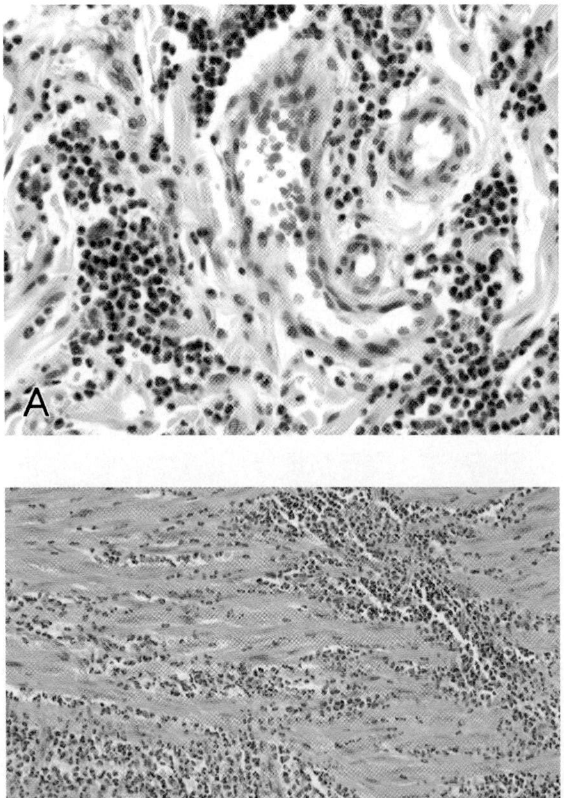

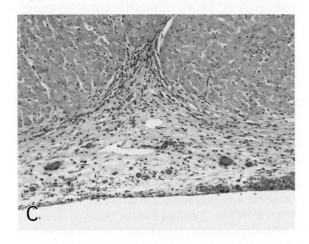

Figure 14-3

EOSINOPHILIC GASTROENTERITIS

A: The submucosal eosinophilic infiltration is intense.

B: Large numbers of eosinophils extend into the muscularis propria.

C: Subserosal collections of eosinophils are present.

Table 14-3

INTESTINAL LESIONS CHARACTERIZED BY EOSINOPHILIA

Parasitic infections
Crohn's disease
Allergic enteritis
Eosinophilic gastroenteritis
Hypereosinophilic syndrome and eosinophilic leukemia
Cow's milk intolerance and related entities
Hyperimmunoglobulinemia E
Gluten-sensitive enteropathy
Peptic duodenitis
Magnesium deficiency
Vitamin E deficiency
Selenium deficiency
Toxic oil syndrome
L-tryptophan-associated myalgia syndrome
Peritoneal dialysis
Inflammatory fibroid polyps
Non-Hodgkin's lymphoma
Hodgkin's disease

INFLAMMATORY FIBROID POLYP

Definition. *Inflammatory fibroid polyp* (IFP) is a pseudotumorous lesion of the gastrointestinal tract. It was first described by Vanek in 1949 (75), and therefore is also known as *Vanek's polyp*.

Demography. IFPs are relatively rare tumors that affect all areas of the gastrointestinal tract (59,62,65). They are most common in the stomach and small intestine (74). Colonic and esophageal IFPs are rare (51,53,56,66,71,73). Most lesions develop in adults, although some occur in children (54,65). The average patient is 63 years old (74).

Etiology. IFPs are postulated to occur as a result of a reactive process (allergic or foreign body reaction). It is likely that the lesion represents a peculiar form of granulation tissue (61,68). Associated lesions include *Helicobacter pylori* infection (69,71), gastric ulcer, adenoma (61), and carcinoma (68).

Clinical Features. Many patients with IFPs are asymptomatic (57). When symptoms do develop, they vary depending on the site of involvement within the gastrointestinal tract and the size of the polyp. Patients with gastric IFPs

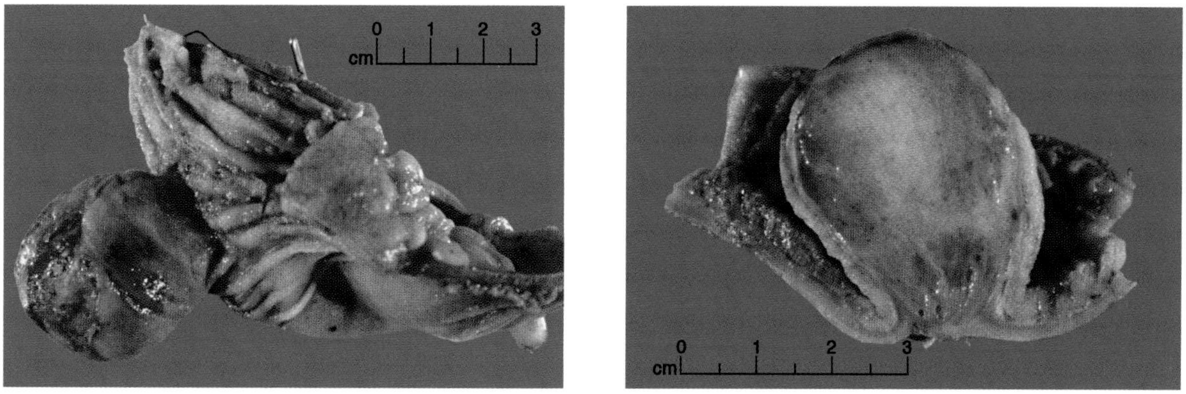

Figure 14-4

INFLAMMATORY FIBROID POLYP

Left: A polypoid mass arises in the small intestine. The mucosa overlying the polyp is, for the most part, intact.

Right: On cut section, the polyp appears to arise in the submucosa. It has a uniform, white-tan cut surface without areas of necrosis or hemorrhage.

present with nausea, vomiting, vague abdominal pain, anemia, or bleeding (57,72). Patients with small intestinal IFPs present with diarrhea, small bowel obstruction, or intussusception (50,52,67,70).

Gross Findings. Grossly, IFPs are sessile or polypoid, solitary or multiple masses ranging in size from less than 1 to 12 cm in diameter (64). Most lesions measure less than 3 cm.

IFPs originate in the submucosa, where they appear as circumscribed, oval to round nodules of firm, gray-tan connective tissue that project into the lumen of the stomach or intestine (fig. 14-4). This gross appearance simulates an ulcerated leiomyoma with its homogeneous white-gray color and firm consistency. Occasionally, IFPs present as nodular thickenings of the wall near an area of ulceration. Small bowel lesions sometimes extend into the muscularis propria and may reach the serosa. The mucosa overlying the polyp may be eroded or ulcerated, although it is frequently intact.

Microscopic Findings. Histologically, IFPs consist of loosely structured fibrous tissue (fig. 14-5). The predominant cell types are spindled fibroblast or myofibroblast-like cells intermingled with inflammatory cells. Whorls of spindle cells surround thin-walled vessels in a concentric or onion-skin–like fashion. Vascularity and cellularity vary from lesion to lesion. The spindle cells appear uniform and contain abundant cytoplasm and pale, spindle-shaped nuclei. Occasional mitotic figures are seen, but these are not usually numerous. Atypical forms are never present. Varying numbers of inflammatory cells infiltrate the lesions. Eosinophils may be seen in large numbers, but not in all cases. Multinucleated giant cells can also be observed. The distinction of the lesion from surrounding tissue becomes blurred and there is no pseudocapsule.

IFPs characteristically demonstrate diffuse immunostaining for vimentin, and focal staining for smooth muscle actin, CD68, CD34, and CD31 (55,58,61,63). The tumors are negative for CD117 (55,61).

Differential Diagnosis. The differential diagnosis includes inflammatory lesions as well as mesenchymal tumors. Eosinophils may be prominent in IFPs (fig. 14-5). As a result, other eosinophil-containing lesions must be considered in the differential diagnosis. Eosinophilic gastroenteritis is distinguished from IFP by the younger age of the patient, by the diffuse infiltration of eosinophils that may involve long bowel segments, and by the presence of peripheral eosinophilia. In addition, eosinophilic gastroenteritis usually does not show a marked proliferation of fibroblasts and blood vessels.

Differentiating IFP from mesenchymal tumors such as leiomyomas and gastrointestinal stromal tumors is usually not difficult since these

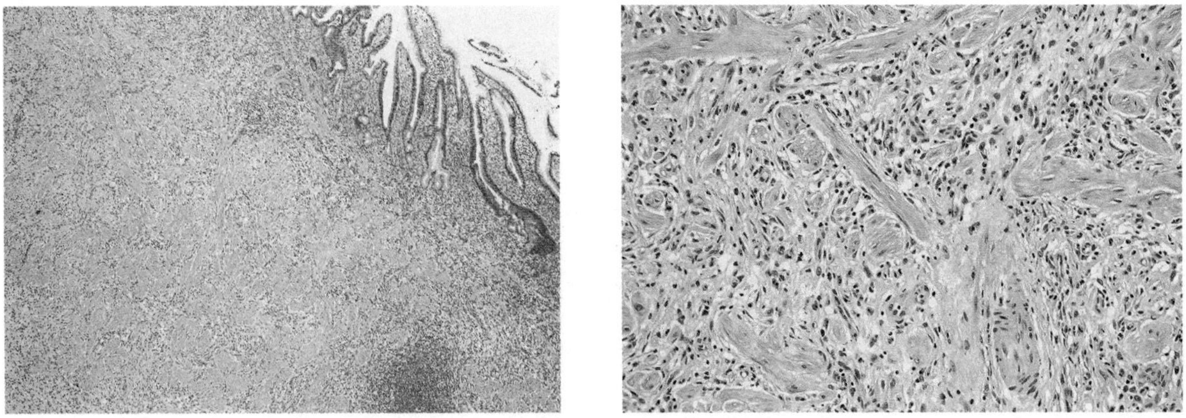

Figure 14-5

INFLAMMATORY FIBROID POLYP

Left: Low-power view of a gastric inflammatory fibroid polyp. The lesion is composed of spindle cells with numerous admixed inflammatory cells. The borders of the polyp are poorly demarcated and difficult to discern from the adjacent submucosal connective tissue and muscle. The overlying mucosa is intact.

Right: On higher power, the tumor is composed of myofibroblast-like spindle cells and numerous inflammatory cells. Eosinophils are particularly prominent.

Table 14-4

GASTROINTESTINAL DISEASES ASSOCIATED WITH GRANULOMAS

Foreign Body Granulomas
Food granulomas
Suture granulomas
Barium granulomas
Talc granulomas
Beryllium granulomas
Infectious Granulomas
Syphilis
Mycobacterial infections
Helicobacter pylori infection
Yersiniosis
Lymphogranuloma venereum
Histoplasmosis
Coccidioidomycosis
Zygomycosis
Blastomycosis
Amebiasis
Prototheca infection
Anisakiasis
Schistosomiasis
Strongyloidiasis
Neoplastic
Associated with carcinoma
Associated with lymphoma
Langerhans cell histiocytosis
Miscellaneous
Crohn's disease
Sarcoidosis
Chronic granulomatous disease of childhood
Allergic granulomatosis and vasculitis
Wegener's granulomatosis
Tumoral amyloidosis
Rheumatoid nodules

lesions almost never contain abundant inflammatory cells. In difficult cases, immunohistochemical staining distinguishes these lesions.

Treatment and Prognosis. IFPs are benign lesions. They may be resected endoscopically or surgically in symptomatic patients.

GRANULOMATOUS AND XANTHOMATOUS DISEASES

Gastrointestinal granulomas form in many disorders (Table 14-4). The etiology of granulomas or histiocytic collections differ depending on whether they are compact or loose, diffuse or localized, contain giant cells or not, and are associated with areas of necrosis or not. Small crypt-associated mucin granulomas complicate infections and other forms of mucosal injury. Vessel-associated histiocytic collections complicate certain infections, especially cytomegalovirus infection. Histiocytic cells surround foreign bodies or the air spaces characteristic of pneumatosis intestinalis. Necrotizing granulomatous inflammation may accompany infection with mycobacteria or fungi (see chapter 10). Small, compact granulomas are seen in Crohn's disease (see chapter 15) and sarcoidosis.

Sarcoidosis

Definition. *Sarcoidosis* is a systemic granulomatous disease that preferentially affects lymph nodes, lungs, and spleen, but also involves many other organs, including, rarely, the gastrointestinal tract.

Demography. Sarcoidosis is a relatively common disease, occurring in 3 to 500 persons/100,000 in Europe (88). In the United States, the disease is seen in 5/100,000 Caucasians and in 40/100,000 African-Americans (105). The disease usually affects the 20- to 40-year-old age group, and in some studies, occurs more commonly in women (98). The incidence of gastrointestinal involvement in these patients is not known.

Etiology. The etiology of sarcoidosis in unknown.

Clinical Features. The gastrointestinal abnormalities that may occur in patients with sarcoidosis include achalasia, gastric ulcer and localized hypertrophic gastropathy, upper gastrointestinal hemorrhage, malabsorption, protein-losing enteropathy, diarrhea, hematochezia, constipation, and abdominal pain (77, 82–84,91,94,95,108). Lymphangiectasia may develop secondarily to lymphatic obstruction from abnormal lymph nodes (101). Small bowel or colonic obstruction has also been reported as a result of stricture formation (78,80,86,87, 109). Rarely, colonic polyps simulating adenomas occur (110).

Pathologic Findings. It is not possible to make a definitive diagnosis of sarcoidosis in the absence of classic disease in the liver or lungs. Histologically, gastrointestinal sarcoidosis consists of compact, bland granulomas that lack necrosis. These may involve both the bowel wall and the regional lymph nodes. If a prominent rim of lymphocytes and plasma cells surrounds the granulomas, a diagnosis of Crohn's disease should be excluded. Areas of necrosis suggest the presence of an infectious process such as tuberculosis or *Yersinia* infection.

Granulomas Associated with Foreign Material

Granulomas develop around foreign material such as talc or sutures. *Suture granulomas* usually contain a central suture surrounded by palisading histiocytes and foreign body giant cells (fig. 14-6). *Talc granulomas* typically contain foreign body type giant cells and can be distinguished from other granulomas by the use of polarizing lenses, which reveal typical birefringent crystals. Starch-based glove powders also produce granulomas recognizable under polarized light by the presence of a distinctive "Maltese cross." Accidental entry of barium into the intestinal wall during radiologic examinations may provoke *barium granulomas*. The histiocytic collections contain birefringent granular material of a pale green color.

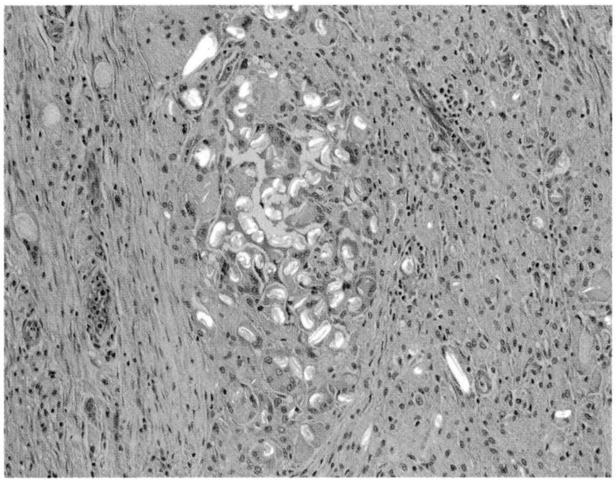

Figure 14-6

SUTURE GRANULOMA

Fragments of old suture material are surrounded by epithelioid histiocytes and giant cells. The suture granuloma was taken from the serosal surface of the colon of a patient who had previous abdominal surgery. The suture fragments are easily seen under polarized light.

Xanthomatosis

Small mucosal histiocytic aggregates are encountered throughout the gastrointestinal tract and are most common in the rectum (fig. 14-7). The lesions are sometimes detected endoscopically as yellowish nodules. The cells comprising these aggregates are muciphages, and presumably represent vestiges of some prior minor mucosal damage. Generalized or localized muciphage collections may complicate motility disorders (107). True *xanthomatosis* consists of accumulations of lipid-laden macrophages that form mural plaques or nodules. Gastrointestinal xanthomatosis occurs in patients with hypercholesterolemia and hypertriglyceridemia (81).

MALAKOPLAKIA

Definition. *Malakoplakia* is a distinctive, rare granulomatous lesion that usually involves the urinary bladder. The colon is the most common site of extraurogenital involvement.

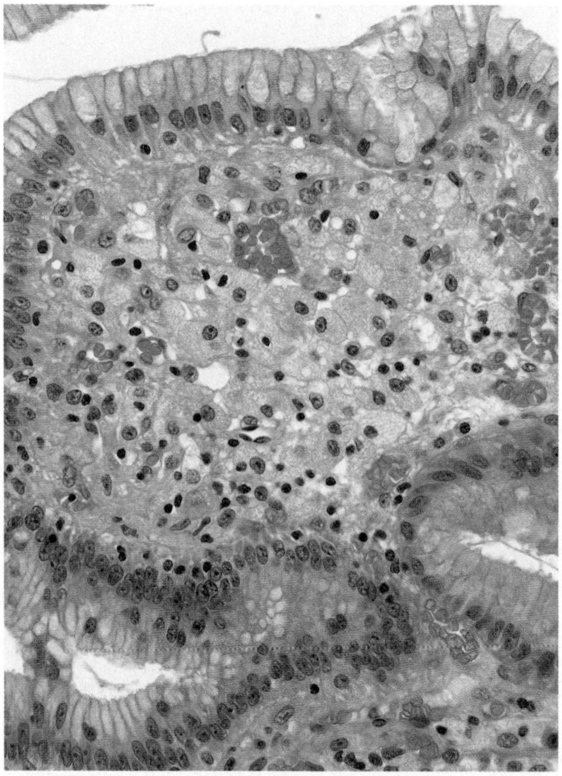

Figure 14-7

XANTHOMA

A collection of foamy histiocytes is present in the superficial mucosa in this gastric biopsy. This lesion appeared as a small yellowish white plaque at the time of endoscopy.

Table 14-5

DISEASES ASSOCIATED WITH COLONIC MALAKOPLAKIA

Inflammatory bowel disease
Neurofibromatosis
Immunodeficiency diseases
Alpha chain disease
Miliary tuberculosis
Tuberculosis
Mycobacterium avium complex infection
Klebsiella infection
Escherichia coli infection
Lymphoreticular diseases
Villous adenoma
Carcinoma

Demography. Patients with colonic malakoplakia range in age from 6 weeks to 88 years. The sex distribution is equal (79,96,100,106).

Etiology. Malakoplakia complicates various diseases (Table 14-5), including infections with *Escherichia coli*, *Klebsiella*, and *Mycobacterium tuberculosis* (93,97).

Pathophysiology. Malakoplakia results from an abnormal macrophage lysosomal response and abnormal microtubule assembly, which lead to defective handling of phagocytosed bacteria. These abnormalities may result from an immunologic defect affecting cellular digestion, absence of the necessary lysosomal enzymes, or decreased levels of cyclic guanosine monophosphate (GMP) (76,90,93,111,112).

Clinical Features. The gastrointestinal tract, particularly the colon, is the dominant site of involvement in most patients. Most patients with colonic malakoplakia have symptoms (102). Adults present with rectal bleeding, diarrhea, and abdominal pain (92). Patients with extensive disease experience intractable diarrhea, bowel obstruction, ulcers, fistulas, and even death. Children present with fever, failure to thrive, bloody diarrhea, and malnutrition (79,93,89,99,103,104).

Gross Findings. Endoscopically, gastrointestinal malakoplakia assumes three gross forms: 1) unifocal lesions, 2) widespread mucosal multinodular lesions, and 3) large mass lesions. Radiographic features vary. Colonic involvement is segmental or diffuse, with the rectosigmoid and cecum being the most commonly affected sites. Early lesions appear soft, flat, and yellowish tan. Later, lesions become raised and tan-gray, with an irregular hyperemic margin and a central depressed area (85). Submucosal lesions secondarily elevate the mucosa into soft yellow-tan plaques or nodules. Often the overlying mucosa appears intact.

Microscopic Findings. Histologic examination of the lesions reveals the presence of numerous histiocytic granular cells with eosinophilic cytoplasm (fig. 14-8). Ultrastructurally, these histiocytes contain giant phagolysosomes containing various forms of mineralized debris and partially digested bacteria (89). The presence of characteristic intracellular and extracellular Michaelis-Gutmann bodies clinches the diagnosis. Michaelis-Gutmann bodies vary in size from 2 to 10 µm and have a round, dense, or

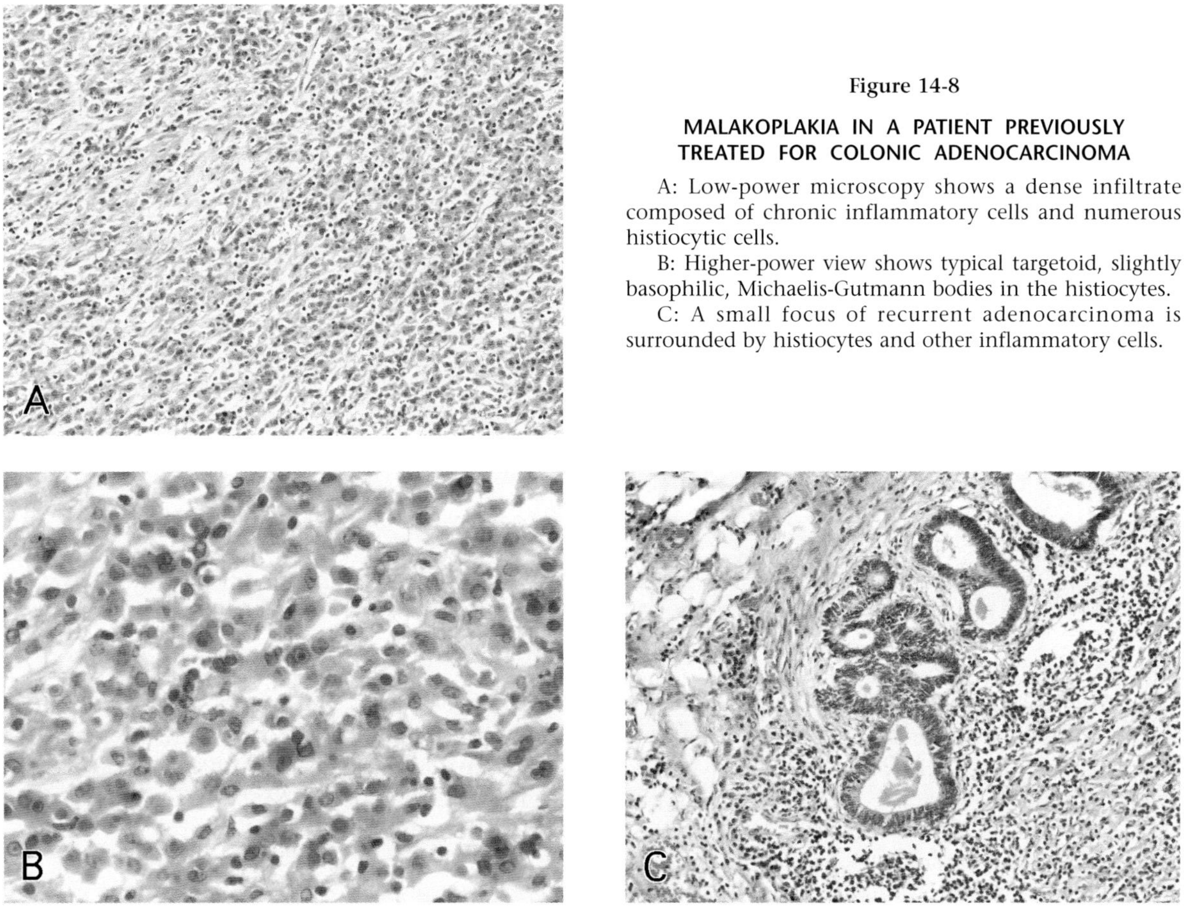

Figure 14-8

MALAKOPLAKIA IN A PATIENT PREVIOUSLY TREATED FOR COLONIC ADENOCARCINOMA

A: Low-power microscopy shows a dense infiltrate composed of chronic inflammatory cells and numerous histiocytic cells.

B: Higher-power view shows typical targetoid, slightly basophilic, Michaelis-Gutmann bodies in the histiocytes.

C: A small focus of recurrent adenocarcinoma is surrounded by histiocytes and other inflammatory cells.

targetoid appearance due to the presence of concentric laminations (fig. 14-8). These stain blue with hematoxylin and are highlighted with the Von Kossa stain for calcium or with iron stains. They also contain lipid and are periodic acid–Schiff (PAS) and Alcian blue positive. Because malakoplakia tends to be associated with both adenomas and carcinomas, the tissues should be carefully evaluated for the presence of these neoplastic conditions (fig. 14-8).

Differential Diagnosis. Malakoplakia superficially resembles several other disorders, including storage diseases, Whipple's disease, *Mycobacterium avium-intracellulare* infection, and fungal infections because of the histiocytic infiltrates, but none of the other disorders contain the pathognomonic Michaelis-Gutmann bodies. Special stains identify the specific infection in fungal or tuberculous lesions.

Treatment and Prognosis. Surgical resection is usually curative in limited disease.

IMMUNE-MEDIATED DISEASES

Autoimmune Enteropathy

Definition. *Autoimmune enteropathy* is a life-threatening disorder of infancy characterized by intractable diarrhea and a constellation of associated autoimmune diseases, including membranous glomerulonephritis, insulin-dependent diabetes, hemolytic or sideroblastic anemia, autoimmune hepatitis, sclerosing cholangitis, and hypothyroidism (120). The disease rarely occurs in adults (114,116,118).

Pathophysiology. Infants with autoimmune enteropathy have circulating systemic antibodies against enterocytes (115). The autoantigen is a 75-kDa protein encoded on chromosome 19p13, and has homology to the tumor suppressor *MCC* gene, and has therefore been named MCC2 (119,121,122). Some patients also have antigoblet cell antibodies.

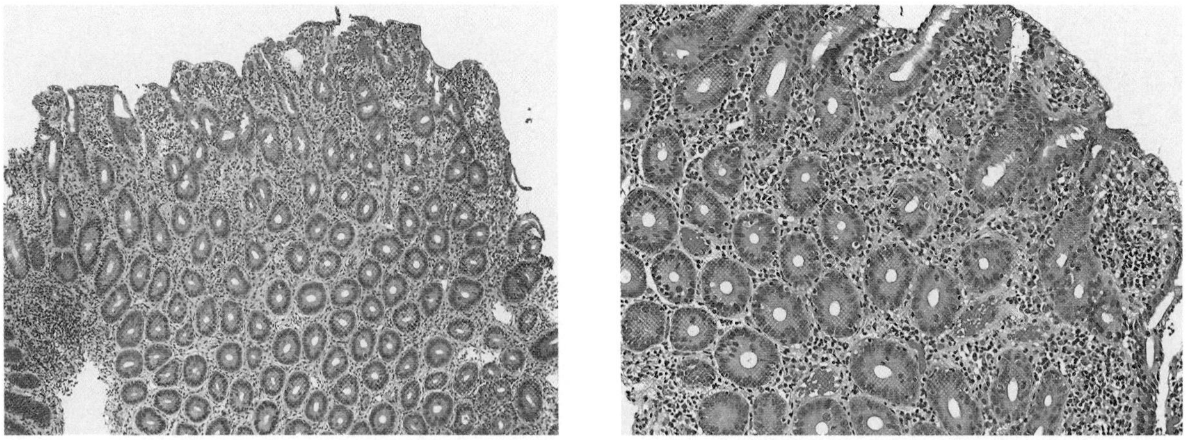

Figure 14-9

AUTOIMMUNE ENTEROPATHY

Left: On low power, a duodenal biopsy shows villous blunting and crypt hyperplasia.

Right: The lamina propria contains a prominent lymphoplasmacytic infiltrate. Intraepithelial lymphocytes are mildly increased in number in some areas, but not to the extent normally seen in celiac disease. Note the absence of goblet cells.

Clinical Features. Affected infants present with unexplained episodes of protracted diarrhea and no response to dietary therapy. The diarrhea usually develops after the first 8 weeks of life (117). The course of the disease is typically severe and is often refractory to treatment, and as a result, may be fatal. Only a subset of patients has an immunodeficiency, even though the etiology is thought to be related to abnormal T-cell or B-cell regulation (123). Some patients demonstrate associated IgA deficiencies and T-cell abnormalities (123). At least 50 percent of patients have antienterocyte antibodies as shown by indirect immunofluorescent microscopy.

Pathologic Findings. The histologic features may be surprisingly subtle and may involve the large and small intestines. The histologic changes may be minimal and patchy. Often, the most consistent feature is a nonspecific increase in lymphocytes involving both the epithelium and the lamina propria. Apoptotic bodies are prominent in the crypts, a finding that mimics graft versus host disease. Small bowel biopsies may show partial or complete villous atrophy, crypt hyperplasia, a mononuclear cell infiltrate of the lamina propria, and increased expression of major histocompatibility complex (MHC) class II antigens (fig. 14-9) (113). Goblet cells may be completely absent from the biopsies in patients with antigoblet cell antibodies.

Treatment and Prognosis. Tacrolimus may be useful in treating autoimmune enteropathy in patients who do not respond to steroids or cyclosporin (113,118). Mycophenolate mofetil may also be effective (124).

Microscopic Colitis

Read et al. (142) introduced the term *microscopic colitis* to describe patients with diarrhea of unknown origin who had a normal barium enema and colonoscopic examination but whose colorectal biopsies showed mucosal inflammation. The histologic features of biopsies taken from many such patients show a distinctive lymphocytic infiltration of the colonic epithelium, and therefore, the term *lymphocytic colitis* has been applied to these cases (133,134). Others show a prominent thickening of the subepithelial collagen table, and therefore, the term *collagenous colitis* has been used to describe these biopsies.

Lymphocytic Colitis

Demography. In Europe, the incidence of *lymphocytic colitis* is 4 to 16 cases/100,000 people/year (125,136,140). Lymphocytic colitis occurs most commonly in middle-aged or elderly patients. The median age at diagnosis is 65 to 70 years, and the female to male ratio ranges from 1.6-5.0 to 1 (125,131,135).

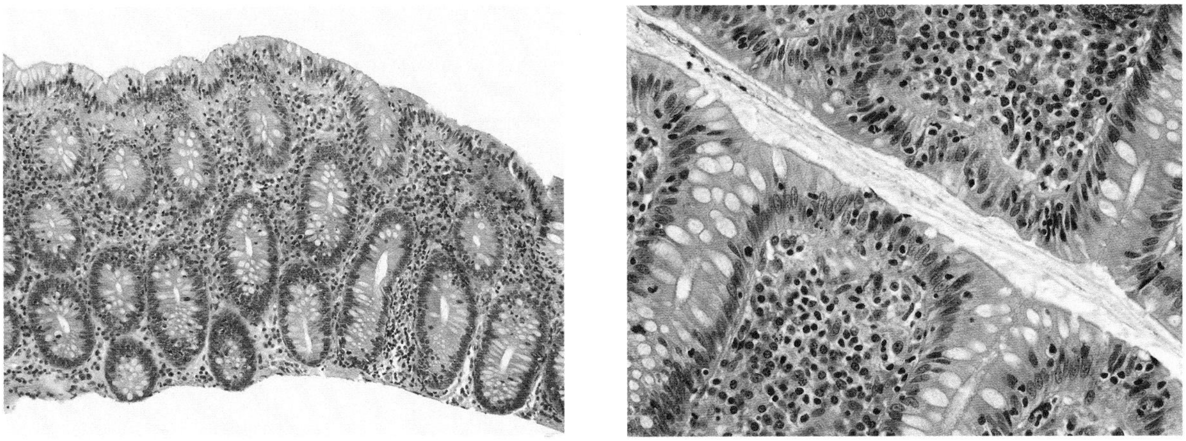

Figure 14-10

LYMPHOCYTIC COLITIS

Left: A biopsy specimen from a patient with chronic watery diarrhea. The overall mucosal architecture is preserved, but the lamina propria contains a dense mononuclear infiltrate.

Right: On higher magnification, the intraepithelial lymphocytosis is apparent in both the crypts and on the mucosal surface.

Pathophysiology. The pathogenesis of lymphocytic colitis is unknown. A number of hypotheses, however, have been proposed. First, the disease shows a female predominance, and therefore, may have an autoimmune or hormonal basis. Autoantibodies, such as antinuclear antibody and rheumatoid factor, are found in up to 50 percent of patients with lymphocytic colitis (133). In addition, patients with lymphocytic colitis commonly have associated autoimmune diseases including thyroid disease, rheumatoid arthritis, celiac disease, and diabetes mellitus (129,130,135,139).

Several milk-associated or waterborne outbreaks of diarrhea endoscopically and histologically similar to lymphocytic colitis have been reported, but to date no associated infectious agent has been identified (128,137,141).

Clinical Features. Patients with lymphocytic colitis present with chronic watery diarrhea that can be intermediate or continuous, ranging in duration from 2 months to 25 years. Related symptoms include mild crampy abdominal pain, moderate weight loss, and an essentially normal physical examination. Nocturnal diarrhea and incontinence may develop. Up to one third of patients with histologic evidence of gluten-sensitive enteropathy (GSE) in the small bowel exhibit lymphocytic colitis and this accounts for the steatorrhea present in some patients (129).

Gross Findings. Endoscopically, the bowel almost invariably appears normal, accounting for the use of the term "microscopic" colitis. When changes are present, they usually involve patchy mucosal erythema, congestion, decreased vascular markings, or mild friability. The relationship of the bowel preparation to the endoscopic changes is not clear.

Microscopic Findings. The most distinctive feature of lymphocytic colitis is the presence of increased intraepithelial lymphocytes, particularly at the luminal surface (fig. 14-10). To be of diagnostic significance, the increase of lymphocytes must average at least 20 lymphocytes/100 epithelial cells (126). This threshold compares with an average of 4 to 5 lymphocytes/100 epithelial cells in the normal colon, inflammatory bowel disease, and infectious colitis (127); a mean of 8.4 in GSE cases without colonic epithelial lymphocytosis; and a mean of 25.0 to 32.4 in patients with lymphocytic colitis without concurrent GSE (fig. 14-10) (143). The lamina propria also contains increased numbers of lymphocytes and eosinophils (fig. 14-10). Occasional neutrophils may be present. Unlike collagenous colitis, the histologic features of lymphocytic colitis are usually uniform throughout the large bowel.

Differential Diagnosis. Increased intraepithelial lymphocytes are common to several diseases (Table 14-6), but when diffusely present

Table 14-6

DISEASES ASSOCIATED WITH INCREASED INTRAEPITHELIAL LYMPHOCYTES

Reflux esophagitis
Lymphocytic gastritis
Gluten-sensitive enteropathy
Tropical sprue
Whipple's disease
Giardiasis
Cryptosporidiosis
Lymphocytic enteritis
Small bowel transplant rejection
Lymphocytic colitis
Crohn's disease
Graft versus host disease
Human immunodeficiency virus (HIV) disease

Table 14-7

COMPARISON OF FEATURES OF LYMPHOCYTIC AND COLLAGENOUS COLITIS

Feature	Collagenous Colitis	Lymphocytic Colitis
Patient age	Middle aged, elderly	Middle aged, elderly
Female to male ratio	up to 20 to 1	1.6-5.0 to 1
Collagen table	Markedly thickened	Not thickened
Intraepithelial lymphocytes	Increased	Markedly increased
Distribution	May be patchy	Diffuse
Autoimmune diseases	Associated	Associated
Gluten-sensitive enteropathy	Not associated	Associated
Changes in small intestine	Occasionally	Occasionally
Changes in stomach	Occasionally	Occasionally

they are more likely to be associated with lymphocytic colitis. Focal lesions, sometimes taking the form of lymphoid aggregates, are more likely to be associated with polyps, diverticula, or Crohn's disease. Table 14-7 compares collagenous colitis and lymphocytic colitis.

Treatment and Prognosis. Few treatment trials have been performed to date on patients with lymphocytic colitis. Antidiarrheal therapy with loperamide hydrochloride or diphenoxylate hydrochloride/atropine is frequently effective, particularly for patients with mild to moderate diarrhea (139). If these agents are not effective, bismuth subsalicylate is beneficial in many patients (132,138,139). Other drugs that have been used with variable success in refractory colitis include sulfasalazine, mesalamine, or corticosteroids (138).

Collagenous Colitis

Definition. The term *collagenous colitis* was introduced in 1976 by Lindstrom (162) to describe a disease in which patients suffered from chronic, watery diarrhea and had accumulations of a collagenous ground substance containing amorphous proteins and immunoglobulins in the subluminal colonic basement membrane, at the lamina propria interface.

Demography. There is a marked female predominance, with the female to male ratio ranging from 6-20 to 1 (149a,164a). The median age at which collagenous colitis presents is 58 to 68 years, but the age range is wide (163). The disorder sometimes affects children (155) and is sometimes familial (157,168). A significant percentage of patients have a history of using nonsteroidal antiinflammatory drugs (NSAIDs) (144,152,166). Other agents such as lansoprazole, ticlopidine, and flutamide have also been suspected, but a definite association has not been proven (146,167,171).

Etiology. The female predominance of collagenous colitis and its association, like lymphocytic colitis, with other autoimmune diseases suggests the possibility of an autoimmune etiology (149a).

Pathophysiology. Surface epithelial damage appears to cause secretory diarrhea, whereas the thickened subepithelial collagen table appears to represent a variable response to the surface damage. The injury in collagenous colitis may result from bile acid malabsorption (165), mast cell infiltration (145,164), and use of NSAIDs (144, 152,166), and possibly, other drugs. The development of clinical symptoms correlates with the thickness of the collagen deposits and the total epithelial surface area involved (150,151).

Clinical Features. Symptoms include watery, nonbloody diarrhea with up to 20 stools per day. The diarrhea can last for months, or even years. Colicky abdominal pain occurs in up to

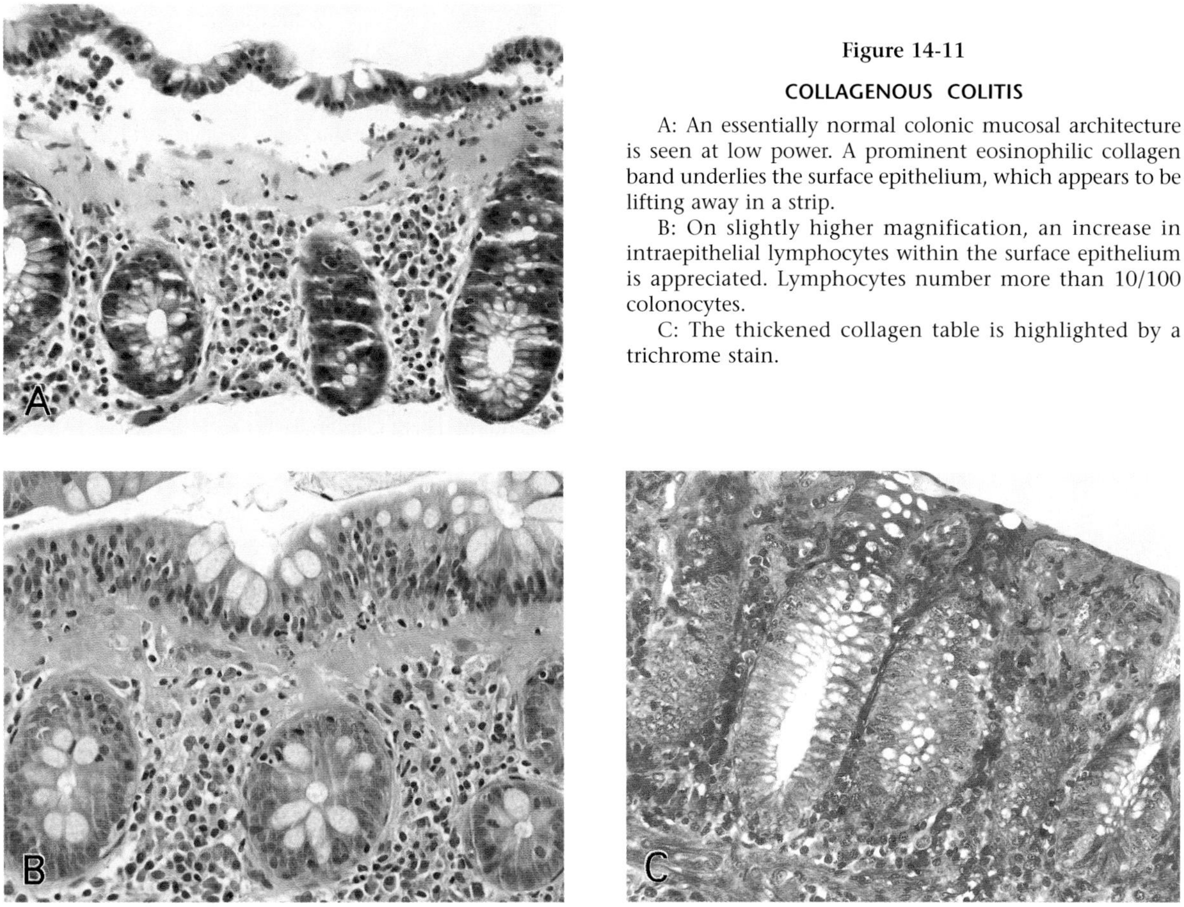

Figure 14-11

COLLAGENOUS COLITIS

A: An essentially normal colonic mucosal architecture is seen at low power. A prominent eosinophilic collagen band underlies the surface epithelium, which appears to be lifting away in a strip.

B: On slightly higher magnification, an increase in intraepithelial lymphocytes within the surface epithelium is appreciated. Lymphocytes number more than 10/100 colonocytes.

C: The thickened collagen table is highlighted by a trichrome stain.

three quarters of patients (149a). Nausea, vomiting, flatulence, urgency, incontinence, and weight loss vary in frequency.

Joint disease, including chronic arthritis, affects some patients (149,153,169). Abnormal thyroid function (149a,156,159), the CRST (calcinosis, Raynaud's phenomenon, sclerodactyly, telangiectasia) syndrome (161), and discoid lupus (148), are also associated with collagenous colitis. Autoantibodies such as antinuclear and antireticulin antibodies or rheumatoid factor are found some patients (154,164a).

Gross Findings. The colon appears grossly and endoscopically normal, although mild erythema is sometimes seen.

Microscopic Findings. The histologic hallmark of collagenous colitis is chronic mucosal inflammation associated with a broad, continuous, hypocellular, eosinophilic, linear, subepithelial fibrous band immediately subjacent to the surface epithelium (fig. 14-11). In collagenous colitis, the subepithelial collagen band measures greater than 10 μm in thickness, and contains entrapped capillaries, red blood cells, and inflammatory cells. There is little, if any, extension of the thickened collagen table around the crypts. The thickened subepithelial layer stains light pink with the PAS and green with the Masson trichrome stain. The changes are most marked in the proximal colon, with the distal portion being spared. The changes are often continuous, but may also exhibit a patchy distribution.

Additional histologic findings include epithelial vacuolization and desquamation, as well as intraepithelial lymphocytosis (fig. 14-11). The intraepithelial lymphocytosis seen in collagenous colitis, however, is not as dramatic as that seen in lymphocytic colitis (147). Focally, the superficial lamina propria contains slightly to moderately increased numbers of lymphocytes, plasma cells, and mast cells admixed with variable numbers of eosinophils and neutrophils

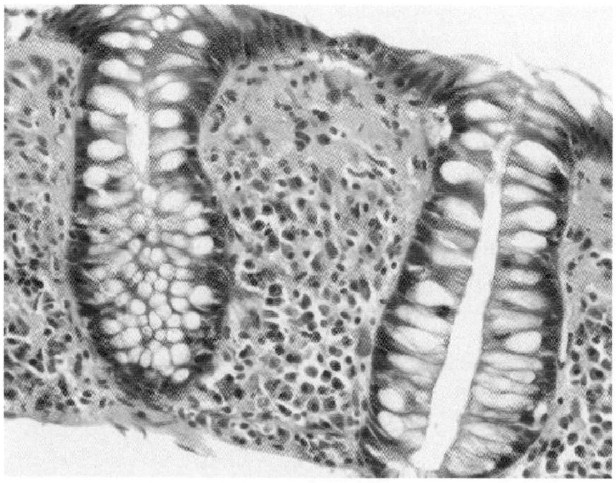

Figure 14-12

COLLAGENOUS COLITIS

Prominent eosinophils and other inflammatory cells are entrapped within the collagen layer, but are also numerous in the lamina propria.

Table 14-8

FEATURES OF DISEASES THAT MIMIC COLLAGENOUS COLITIS ON BIOPSY

Collagenous colitis: Subluminal collagen thickening, intraepithelial lymphocytosis, inflammation in upper mucosa.

Ulcerative colitis: Diffuse continuous process with numerous crypt abscesses, cryptitis, glandular destruction, and signs of chronicity; no subluminal collagen thickening.

Radiation colitis: Mucosal telangiectasia, submucosal vascular changes, atypical fibroblasts, fibrosis.

Infectious colitis: Diffuse lamina propria inflammation, significant neutrophils in lamina propria; usually no subluminal collagen thickening.

Mucosal prolapse syndromes: Glandular distortion, mucosal ulceration, mucosal fibrosis, perpendicular smooth muscle fibers in lamina propria.

Ischemic colitis: Coagulative necrosis, fibrin thrombi, architectural distortion if disease is chronic, mucosal fibrosis, glandular dropout.

Amyloidosis: Perivascular, muscular, or lamina propria eosinophilic deposits; positivity with Congo red stains.

Progressive systemic sclerosis: Fibrosis along all basement membranes, including crypts.

Diverticulosis: Chronic inflammation, thickened basement membranes.

Diversion colitis: Prominent nodular lymphoid hyperplasia, ulceration, acute inflammation, aphthous ulcers, cryptitis.

(fig. 14-12). Eosinophils can be focally prominent. Damaged epithelial cells appear flattened, mucin depleted, vacuolated, and irregularly oriented. Focally, small strips of interglandular surface epithelium lift off their basement membrane and a subepithelial cleft filled with neutrophils and eosinophils forms (fig. 14-12). Despite all of these changes, the crypt epithelium appears relatively normal. Frank ulceration and active inflammation may be signs of NSAID-associated injury (160).

Differential Diagnosis. Subepithelial collagen thickening occurs in various diseases. As a result, the diagnosis of collagenous colitis can only be made in the proper clinical and histologic settings. Tangential sectioning of normal colonic mucosa results in an artifactually thickened basement membrane and such cases can be wrongly interpreted as collagenous colitis. If biopsies lack the characteristic inflammatory pattern, a tangentially cut thick basement membrane should be ignored. The key to a correct diagnosis of collagenous colitis is analyzing the summation of various inflammatory changes plus the subepithelial collagenization.

Other entities in the differential diagnosis are lymphocytic colitis, ulcerative colitis, ischemic colitis, radiation colitis, amyloidosis, progressive systemic sclerosis, acute infectious colitis, colonic carcinoma, hyperplastic polyp, mucosal prolapse syndrome, fecal stream diversion, and diverticular disease. Biopsies with increased subepithelial collagen deposition from patients without characteristic clinical symptoms generally come from the rectum or rectosigmoid. Since collagenous colitis generally affects the proximal colon more severely, the most reliable biopsies for the diagnosis of collagenous colitis come from that region. Features that distinguish the diseases that mimic collagenous colitis are listed in Table 14-8.

Treatment and Prognosis. Spontaneous remissions and relapses are characteristic; occasionally the disease resolves spontaneously (164b). Symptoms may resolve following treatment with bismuth subsalicylate. Refractory patients may respond to treatment with octreotide, methotrexate, cyclosporine, or antibiotics (164a). Fecal stream diversion can induce clinical and histopathologic remission of collagenous colitis (158). Collagenous colitis may rarely contribute to patient mortality (170).

STORAGE DISEASES

A number of forms of storage disease affect the gastrointestinal tract. These include lysosomal, glycogen, and lipid storage disorders.

Lysosomal Storage Diseases

Definition. *Lysosomal storage diseases* occur in patients with defectively functioning lysosomal enzymes. In these patients, the substrate of the defective enzyme is incompletely digested and accumulates within the lysosomes, leading to cellular dysfunction. Lysosomal storage diseases are classified into three categories: 1) sphingolipidoses (Gaucher's disease); 2) mucopolysaccharidoses (Hurler's and Hunter's diseases); and 3) glycogen storage disease, such as Pompe's disease.

Etiology. Lysosomes contain various hydrolytic enzymes that function in the acid milieu present within lysosomes. These hydrolytic enzymes are synthesized in the endoplasmic reticulum and transported to the Golgi apparatus, where they undergo post-translational modifications. They are then transported into lysosomes where they function to hydrolyze various macromolecules derived from the outside environment or from other intracellular organelles.

The lysosomal storage disorders result from various enzymatic defects, which include the absence of an enzyme activator or a protective protein, lack of a substrate activator protein, lack of a transport protein required for egress from the lysosome, defects in post-translational processing, or synthesis of catalytically inactive proteins (185). The sites where the lysosomal storage disorders become manifest represent those sites where the material that needs degradation occurs.

Special Techniques. The lysosomal disorders are usually diagnosed by enzymatic assay of white blood cells or fibroblasts or by rectal biopsy. Acid phosphatase stains highlight the cellular inclusions present in lysosomal storage diseases. The tissues may also be examined by PAS, Luxol fast blue, and Sudan black stains; for acid phosphatase activity; and under ultraviolet light to show the accumulation of autofluorescent material. The use of both histologic and ultrastructural examination to demonstrate the disease is advocated. Because the stored substances are often lipids, frozen sections may be necessary to demonstrate their accumulation. Thus, when a lysosomal storage disorder is suspected, a piece of unfixed tissue must be snap-frozen for further analysis. Ultrastructural examination confirms the histologic changes and demonstrates the characteristic ultrastructural features for each group of diseases.

Glycogen Storage Diseases

Etiology. *Glycogen storage disease 1A* (GSD1A) results from a deficiency of the microsomal enzyme glucose-6-phosphatase in liver, kidney, and intestinal mucosa. Its activity is normal in *glycogen storage disease 1B*, but cytoplasmic glucose-6-phosphatase is not transported to the endoplasmic reticulum by the glucose-6-phosphate translocase T1.

Clinical Features. Impaired gluconeogenesis, fasting hypoglycemia, hepatomegaly, lactic acidosis, hyperlipidemia, hyperuricemia, impaired platelet function, and bleeding diathesis are common to both glycogen storage diseases 1A and 1B (174). Glycogen storage disease 1B is additionally complicated by recurrent pyogenic infections caused by apparent neutropenia and neutrophil dysfunction not observed in glycogen storage disease 1A (183).

Pathologic Findings. The gross and histologic features of glycogen storage disease 1B are indistinguishable from those of Crohn's disease, including ileal mucosal irregularities, colitis, stenosis involving the right side of the colon, and granulomatous inflammation (173, 184). This inflammatory bowel disease–like presentation may be the result of defective neutrophil function.

Hurler's and Hunter's Syndromes (Mucopolysaccharidoses)

Etiology. Patients with *mucopolysaccharidoses* have genetically determined deficiencies of the lysosomal enzymes involved in the degradation of mucopolysaccharides, which lead to their accumulation in the cell. Patients with *Hurler's syndrome* (*mucopolysaccharidosis I*) accumulate heparan sulfate and dermatan sulfate, as do patients with *Hunter's syndrome* (*mucopolysaccharidosis II*). Hurler's syndrome is inherited as an autosomal recessive disorder, whereas Hunter's is inherited as an X-linked recessive disorder. The mucopolysaccharides accumulate

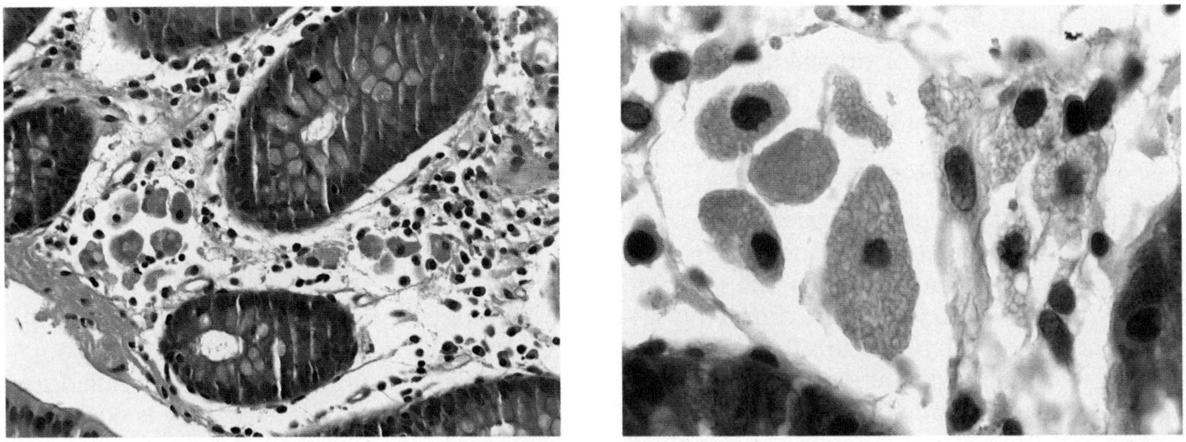

Figure 14-13

NIEMANN-PICK DISEASE

Left: Macrophages with vacuolated cytoplasm lie in the lamina propria of the colon.

Right: The macrophage cytoplasm is foamy with prominent round vacuoles containing sphingomyelin. (Courtesy of Dr. Lisa Yerian, Cleveland, OH.)

within the cells due to a failure to cleave the terminal sugar from the polysaccharide molecule.

Clinical Features. Patients with Hurler's and Hunter's syndromes present with involvement of many organs, including the gastrointestinal tract (178,181). The disease course is chronic and progressive, although the age of onset and the severity of the symptoms vary significantly (182).

Pathologic Findings. Fibroblasts, endothelial cells, and smooth muscle cells may appear vacuolated. Ultrastructurally, the intracellular, membrane-bound lysosomes contain variable amounts of opaque, flocculent lamellae representing mucopolysaccharides.

Niemann-Pick Disease

Etiology. *Niemann-Pick disease* results from absence of sphingomyelinase, so that sphingomyelin accumulates in many organs throughout the body, including the viscera.

Clinical Features. In severe cases, extreme visceral accumulations of sphingomyelin are present along with progressive wasting, and patients often die in the first few years of life.

Pathologic Findings. Macrophages accumulate sphingomyelin in many tissues, including the lamina propria of the gastrointestinal tract (fig. 14-13). Sphingomyelin can be highlighted with the use of special stains for lipids, including Sudan black and oil red-O. Ultrastructurally, the affected macrophages contain membranous cytoplasmic bodies that resemble concentric lamellated myelin figures. Parallel palisaded lamellae impart an appearance of zebra bodies (175).

Gangliosidoses

Etiology. *Tay-Sachs disease* is the prototype of the gangliosidoses. It results from a deficiency of the enzyme hexosaminidase A. This disease is particularly prevalent among Ashkenazi Jews. Hexosaminidase A catalyzes the degradation of GM2 ganglioside and because of the absence of the enzyme, this material accumulates within the cells, particularly of the nervous system.

Adult GM1 gangliosidosis is a recently identified rare form of hereditary neuronal storage disease.

Clinical Features. Hexosaminidase deficiency leads to lipid accumulation within cortical, cerebellar, and spinal tissue. Patients also develop diarrhea and autonomic dysfunction, including motility disturbances. Adult GM1 gangliosidosis has a benign clinical course with cerebral lesions restricted to the basal ganglia (179).

Pathologic Findings. Rectal biopsies play a role in the diagnosis of gangliosidosis by the demonstration of the characteristic changes in the autonomic neurons (172,176,177,180). The biopsies need to be deep enough to include the submucosal plexus. Ultrastructurally, ganglion, Schwann, perithelial, and endothelial cells, as well as histiocytes, all contain characteristic inclusions. The neural tissues contain electron-dense bodies, zebra bodies, and membranous cytoplasmic bodies. In patients with Tay-Sachs disease, these bodies are not found in other cell types. In contrast, patients with *Sandhoff's disease (hexosaminidase AB deficiency)* exhibit similar structures in nerves as well as mesenchymal tissues, such as endothelial cells and fibroblasts. Membrane-bound clear vacuoles are occasionally seen in the cytoplasm of rectal and cutaneous fibroblasts. The axons of the unmyelinated nerves appear normal.

Fabry's Disease

Etiology. *Fabry's disease*, an X-linked disorder of lipid metabolism, results from a deficiency of the enzyme alpha-galactosidase A that leads to accumulation of ceramide trihexosidase.

Clinical Features. Malabsorption sometimes affects patients with small intestinal involvement. Patients with Fabry's disease also present with enterovesical fistulas and lymphadenopathy.

Pathologic Findings. The neurons and nerve fibers of Meissner plexus, vascular endothelial cells, and histiocytes appear foamy and vacuolated. Their lipid content stains strongly with Sudan black, Luxol fast blue, PAS, and oil red-O stains on frozen sections. Ultrastructural examination shows the presence of zebra-like, lamellar, lysosomal inclusions.

Wolman's Disease

Etiology. *Wolman's disease (lysosomal acid esterase deficiency)* is a lethal heritable disorder affecting children.

Clinical Features. It is characterized clinically by hepatosplenomegaly and enlarged calcified adrenal glands. Patients develop persistent diarrhea and rarely survive for more than 1 year.

Pathologic Findings. Fat-laden histiocytes containing cholesterol and triglycerides infiltrate the superficial lamina propria. The mucosal accumulations are most marked in the jejunum.

Cholesterol Ester Storage Disease

Etiology. *Cholesterol ester storage disease* is a rare inherited disorder of lipid metabolism also due to a deficiency of lysosomal acid esterase, but it has a much more benign clinical course than Wolman's disease.

Pathologic Findings. The liver and spleen enlarge and serum cholesterol becomes elevated. Numerous foamy macrophages filled with cholesterol esters populate the muscularis mucosae and submucosa. Lipid droplets accumulate due to a block in the transport of cholesterol into lacteals. Lipid droplets are found in macrophages in the lamina propria of both the large and small intestine, alongside the lacteal endothelium, in the smooth muscle, and in vascular pericytes. The histiocytes that contain the cholesterol esters and carotenes impart an orange tinge to the mucosal surface. The myenteric plexus is vacuolated secondary to cholesterol ester deposits. The epithelium appears normal.

NEONATAL ENTEROPATHIES

Microvillus Inclusion Disease

Definition. *Microvillus inclusion disease* is a severe enteropathy resulting from a defect in microvillus formation. It is associated with watery diarrhea, and often presents on the first day of life. Synonyms include *congenital microvillus atrophy, familial microvillus atrophy*, and *Davidson's syndrome*.

Demography. Microvillus inclusion disease has been identified worldwide in infants from varying ethnic backgrounds. The disease may have a familial component as it sometimes occurs in multiple siblings (187). A genetic etiology is further supported by the observation that the disease appears to cluster in infants of Navajo descent (195,199).

Etiology. The mechanism by which microvillus inclusion disease develops is not known. The underlying defect is thought to be a genetic alteration that leads to abnormal trafficking of membrane proteins to the apical surface of differentiated epithelial cells (198).

Clinical Features. Infants with microvillus inclusion disease present with severe, watery diarrhea. In some cases, the diarrhea can be so watery that it can be mistaken for urine. The volume of stool output in this disease may exceed that seen in association with cholera (198). As a result, affected infants die of dehydration unless adequate fluid replacement is provided.

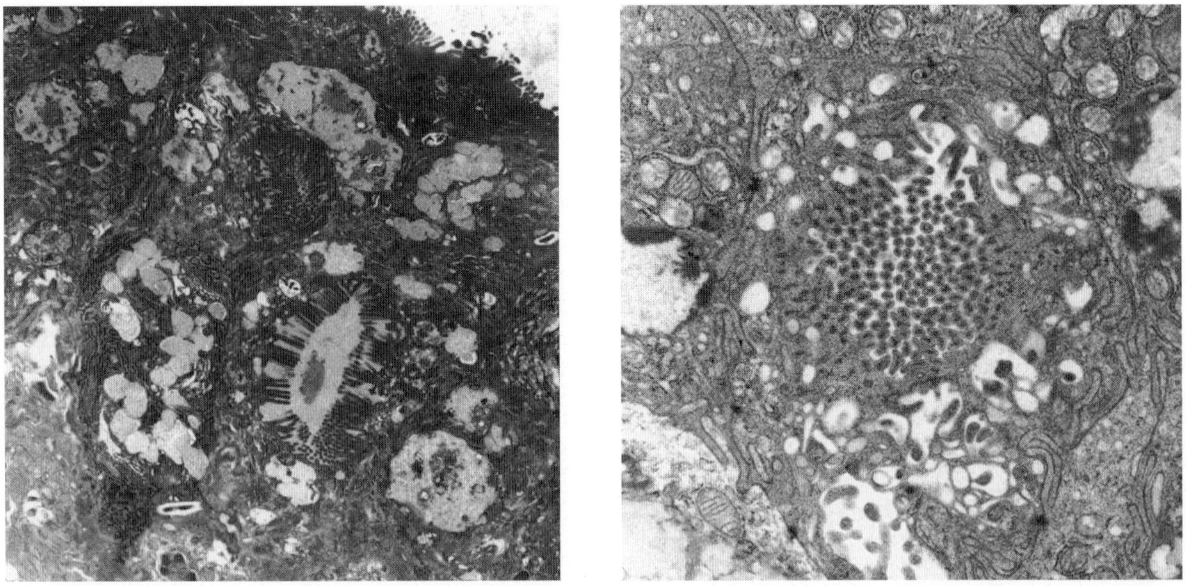

Figure 14-14

MICROVILLUS INCLUSION DISEASE

Left: Transmission electron micrograph shows typical inclusions lined by microvilli in the apical cytoplasm of the enterocytes.

Right: Higher-power view shows that the microvilli lining the inclusions contain all components normally present in brush border microvilli. (Courtesy of Dr. Margaret Collins, Cincinnati, OH.)

Pathologic Findings. Duodenal biopsies demonstrate the presence of villous atrophy, with little or no associated crypt hyperplasia. The lamina propria does not contain an increased number of inflammatory cells. The epithelium lining the villi appears disorganized, with focally piled up cells with vacuolated apical cytoplasm. The brush border focally appears poorly defined. PAS stains highlight the brush border loss, and also stain the apical cytoplasm of enterocytes, a finding not seen in normal duodenal mucosa (194). Immunostains for villin, carcinoembryonic antigen (polyclonal), or CD10 highlight the intracytoplasmic microvillus inclusions that characterize the disease (189,190). Microvillus inclusions are not present in every cell, and sometimes multiple levels on multiple blocks must be examined in order to make the diagnosis. Inclusions may be found not only in duodenal epithelial cells, but also in colonocytes, gastric epithelial cells, renal tubular cells, and gallbladder epithelial cells (187,192,197).

Special Techniques. Transmission electron microscopy demonstrates the diagnostic microvillus inclusions in surface epithelial cells (fig. 14-14). These inclusions are most commonly found in the apical cytoplasm, but may sometimes be seen in a more basal location. The inclusions are lined by a complete brush border that includes the microvillus membrane, microfilaments, the terminal web, and a surface filamentous coat. Another characteristic ultrastructural feature is the presence of apical secretory granules or vesicular bodies. These structures are membrane bound, and contain a mixture of amorphous granular material, small vesicles, and membrane fragments.

Treatment and Prognosis. Microvillus inclusion disease is a severe, intractable enteropathy requiring total parenteral nutrition and intravenous fluid support. The condition is inevitably fatal if these measures are not implemented. Small intestinal transplantation is often necessary. A less severe variant of the disease, which presents later and is associated with lesser symptoms and a better prognosis, may occur (193).

Tufting Enteropathy

Definition. *Tufting enteropathy,* also known as *intestinal epithelial dysplasia*, is a chronic watery diarrhea syndrome presenting in the first few months of life. The disorder is characterized by foci of clustered enterocytes with characteristic apical cytoplasmic projections.

Etiology. The etiology of this disorder is unknown. The disease is thought to have a genetic basis since it tends to cluster in certain families (188,196). Tufting enteropathy may develop secondary to abnormalities in the epithelial basement membrane or in expression of epithelial adhesion molecules (188,191).

Clinical Features. Most patients present with chronic watery diarrhea that begins shortly after birth. The disease may rarely develop in older patients (186).

Pathologic Findings. Jejunal biopsies demonstrate partial or total villous atrophy associated with crypt hyperplasia. There is no increase in inflammatory cells within the lamina propria. Intraepithelial lymphocytes are normal in number. The characteristic feature of the disease is the presence of focal epithelial "tufts" composed of clusters of closely packed enterocytes with rounded, tear-drop–shaped projections of their apical cytoplasm.

Treatment and Prognosis. The prognosis for patients with tufting enteropathy is variable. Most patients require total parenteral nutrition in order to remain adequately nourished for normal growth and development.

SMALL INTESTINAL TRANSPLANTATION

Demography. Intestinal transplantation is used to treat patients with irreversible intestinal failure and dependence on total parenteral nutrition (TPN). The introduction of TPN in the 1970s revolutionized the treatment of such patients, but some patients still experience life-threatening complications of TPN. Patients with TPN-associated liver disease, loss of vascular access, or recurrent sepsis are candidates for small intestinal transplantation.

Etiology. In pediatric patients, intestinal failure may occur in those who undergo extensive intestinal resections for necrotizing enterocolitis and intestinal congenital anomalies, including total aganglionosis, volvulus, gastroschisis, and atresia (203). Intestinal failure also occurs in children with functional disorders such as intestinal pseudoobstruction, microvillous inclusion disease, juvenile polyposis, and trauma (215). In adults, intestinal failure occurs most often secondary to resection for Crohn's disease, ischemia, desmoid tumors, trauma, or motility disorders (208).

Pathologic Findings. In preservation injury, the surface epithelium detaches from the underlying edematous lamina propria. No active inflammation is present (209). The degree of epithelial separation can be minimal to severe. When reperfusion is established, the crypt epithelium actively regenerates. Mild neutrophilic infiltrates may develop within 2 hours postperfusion.

Lymphatic regeneration needs to occur following the graft to establish the lymphatic drainage critical to the nutritional functions of the small bowel, including the absorption of chylomicrons. If this does not occur, lymphedema will develop. Impaired gut barrier function may eventually lead to sepsis and multiorgan failure.

Nerve regeneration also needs to occur. Within a year following surgery, ectopic large neurons gradually increase in number, not only in areas adjacent to the anastomoses but also in the remaining tissues up to 10 cm away from the lesion. Large ganglion neurons decrease. Outgrowth of neuron-specific enolase (NSE)-containing nerve fibers from the severed stumps, usually within a couple of weeks of transection, occurs. Weeks later, numerous bundles of fine nerve fibers interconnect the oral and anal ends of the cut myenteric plexus. The regenerating nerve fiber bundles initially lie among irregularly arranged smooth muscle cells. When failed grafts are evaluated, they demonstrate a lack of extrinsic adrenergic and perivascular fibers in all layers of the bowel wall but intrinsic peptidergic nerves and their receptors are retained following transplantation (201).

Detection of rejection after small intestinal transplantation is difficult and relies on histopathologic examination of the graft (209). Rejection represents a patchy, often ileal-centered process that progresses to mucosal ulceration and eventual fibrosis of the wall (212). A rejected graft demonstrates edema, cellular infiltration of the mucosa and submucosa, and epithelial damage. Early acute rejection usually occurs within 12 days, although it can occur later. Endothelial and crypt damage occurs within 3 days. Acute allograft rejection exhibits varying

Figure 14-15

MILD SMALL BOWEL TRANSPLANT REJECTION

A: The architecture of the small intestine is distorted by the loss of the normal villi. The lamina propria contains an increased number of mononuclear cells.

B: Numerous apoptotic bodies are in the bases of the crypts.

C: Neutrophils focally infiltrate the crypts.

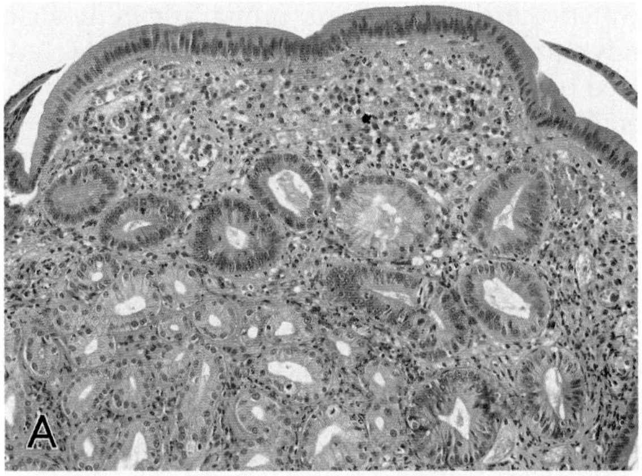

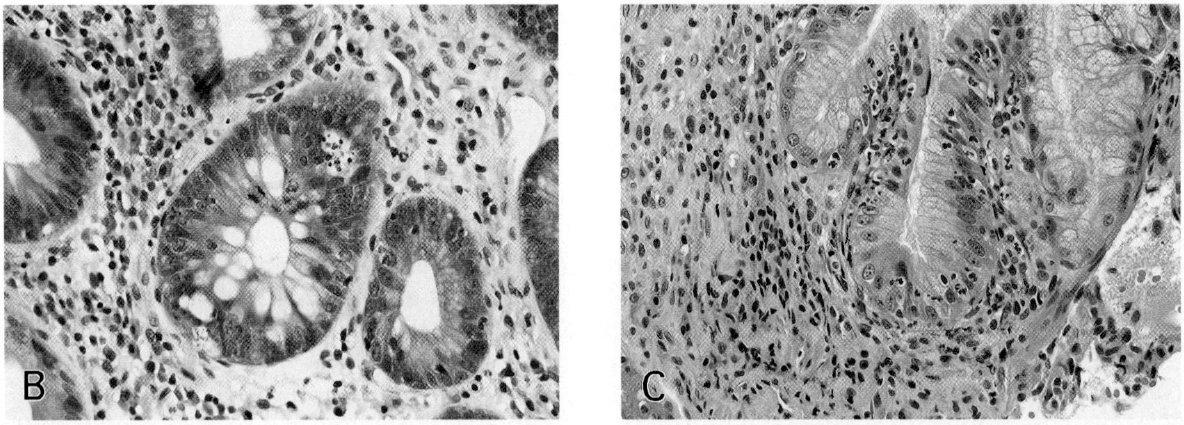

combinations of crypt injury, mucosal infiltration primarily by mononuclear cells, intraepithelial lymphocytes including blast-like lymphocytes, and increased crypt cell apoptoses (more than 2/10 crypts) (fig. 14-15). The lamina propria appears edematous. Cellular infiltrates can be present in the muscle and submucosa in the absence of mucosal changes.

In mild rejection, the inflammatory infiltrate surrounds small venules and capillaries in the deep mucosa at the crypt bases. These appear as early as 2 weeks and as late as 12 months after transplantation. The number of lymphocytes between the muscularis mucosae and crypts adjacent to the crypt epithelium is increased. Vessels between the crypts frequently appear reactive, with enlarged endothelial cells. Sometimes lymphocytes are seen in the vascular lumens. Other inflammatory cells are occasionally present, including plasma cells, eosinophils, and neutrophils (fig. 14-15).

With more substantial involvement, the inflammatory infiltrate becomes more widely dispersed in a patchy or coalescent distribution along with varying degrees of mucosal edema and lymphatic dilatation. Markedly enlarged Peyer patches, expanded by prominent accumulations of blastic lymphocytes, are found in the first month following transplant. This infiltrate consists predominantly of mononuclear cells admixed with lesser numbers of eosinophils and neutrophils. Pronounced mucosal eosinophilia may develop.

In severe rejection, allografts show unevenly distributed mucosal damage with an intact mucosa in the proximal and mid-jejunum, and flattening of the villi. Moderate glandular loss is seen in the distal jejunum and proximal ileum, with granulation tissue and regeneration, although the morphologic changes are distributed unevenly along the intestinal allograft (fig. 14-16).

Full-thickness biopsies may be helpful in diagnosing rejection, since sometimes the characteristic lesions are not seen in the mucosa, but only in the submucosa and muscularis, especially in patients on cyclosporine therapy

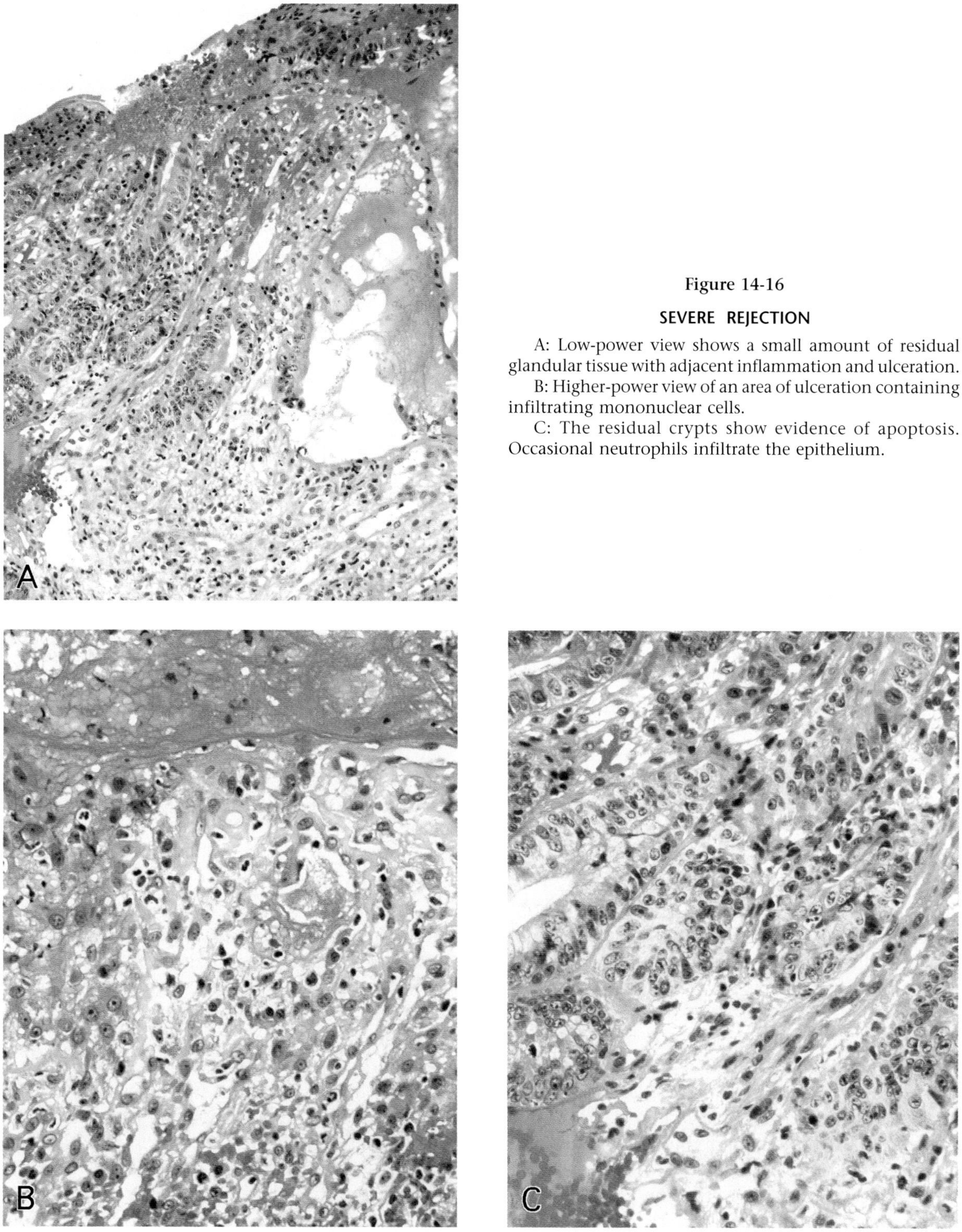

Figure 14-16

SEVERE REJECTION

A: Low-power view shows a small amount of residual glandular tissue with adjacent inflammation and ulceration.

B: Higher-power view of an area of ulceration containing infiltrating mononuclear cells.

C: The residual crypts show evidence of apoptosis. Occasional neutrophils infiltrate the epithelium.

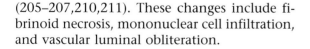

(205–207,210,211). These changes include fibrinoid necrosis, mononuclear cell infiltration, and vascular luminal obliteration.

If the patient survives the episodes of acute graft rejection, the patient becomes susceptible to the post-transplantation complications seen

Table 14-9

DISORDERS ASSOCIATED WITH INCREASED APOPTOSIS

Graft versus host disease
Drug therapy
Chemotherapy for malignancy
Radiation therapy
Transplant rejection
Zinc deficiency
Fasting
Inflammatory bowel disease
Acquired immunodeficiency syndrome (AIDS) enteropathy
Viral infections
Autoimmune enterocolitis

in other transplant patients. Chronic graft rejection is characterized histologically by villous atrophy and T-cell infiltration associated with obliterative arteriopathy and muscular fibrosis (200,204,209). The lamina propria is infiltrated by CD3-positive, CD25-positive lymphocytes and CD25-positive macrophages; there is abrasion of the cell surface epithelium and ultimately, mucosal sloughing (202,214). The obliterative arteriopathy primarily affects the large arteries of the serosa and mesentery, which show patchy luminal narrowing secondary to myointimal hyperplasia and subendothelial accumulation of foamy macrophages and scattered lymphocytes.

Crypt cell apoptosis is a variable but sometimes striking feature of intestinal rejection (fig. 14-15). Apoptotic bodies occur in the normal mucosa; the upper limit in native and normal allograft specimens is 2/10 consecutive crypts. Apoptotic cells are not specific for rejection, however, but may also be seen in other states (Table 14-9) (205,207,211).

Biopsies following treated rejection often demonstrate fibrosis with focal glandular loss, regenerative glands with reparative atypia, and atrophy with a thin mucosa and blunted villi. These changes occur more commonly following severe or persistent rejection, although they are not always present. Patients may develop moderate to severe eosinophilia.

When the bowel is successfully transplanted, the histologic features resemble those of the nontransplanted bowel at the anastomotic ends.

Table 14-10

COMPLICATIONS OF SMALL INTESTINAL TRANSPLANTATION

Preservation injury
Graft failure
Ischemic damage
Infection
Graft rejection
Graft versus host disease
Post-transplant lymphoproliferative disorders

Treatment and Prognosis. The use of intestinal transplantation can lead to long-term survival rates of 50 to 75 percent in some centers (216). The complications of transplantation are listed in Table 14-10.

Immunologic complications of transplantation include intestinal allograft rejection, post-transplant lymphoproliferative disease, cytomegalovirus infection, and graft versus host disease. Other complications include intestinal perforation, intestinal leaks, dehiscence with evisceration, bleeding, intraabdominal abscess, and ascites. Graft loss occurs as a result of rejection, infection, and technical complications, as well as the complications of TPN after graft removal (213).

A high incidence of infection complicates small bowel transplantation. Infections result both from excessive immunosuppression and compromised barrier function of the native or engrafted small bowel. Small bowel transplant patients who develop rejection or graft versus host disease may have shifts in the intestinal microflora toward potentially pathogenic organisms and bacterial translocation into recipient tissues. One may see massive bacterial overgrowth in the native intestine in patients with graft versus host disease.

Complicating cytomegalovirus infections occur as early as 2 days or up to years following transplantation (209) and the changes resemble those described in chapter 10. Many patients develop Epstein-Barr virus (EBV)-related post-transplant lymphoproliferative disorders (PTLD). PTLD may develop as early as 41 days after transplantation or may take years; the median time to the development of PTLD is 306 days (209). The tissues contain activated lymphocytes with crypt epithelial apoptosis and lymphoid tissue without apoptosis. The chief feature is a dense but heterogeneous lymphoid infiltrate comprised of small lymphocytes, plasma cells, and plasmacytoid lymphocytes. There are also large transformed lymphocytes typical of polymorphous PTLD. Eosinophilia may also be present. EBV in situ hybridization reactions help make the diagnosis.

REFERENCES

Food Allergy

1. Bender AE, Matthews DR. Adverse reactions to foods. Br J Nutr 1981;46:403–7.
2. Crowe SE, Perdue MH. Gastrointestinal food hypersensitivity: basic mechanisms of pathophysiology. Gastroenterology 1992;103:1075–95.
3. Sampson HA, Broadbent KR, Bernhisel-Broadbent J. Spontaneous release of histamine from basophils and histamine-releasing factor in patients with atopic dermatitis and food hypersensitivity. N Engl J Med 1989;321:228–32.
4. Sampson HA, Mendelson L, Rosen JP. Fatal and near-fatal anaphylactic reactions to food in children and adolescents. N Engl J Med 1992;327:380–4.
5. Sampson HA, Metcalfe DD. Food allergies. JAMA 1992;268:2840–4.

Cow's Milk Intolerance and Related Disorders

6. Host A. Frequency of cow's milk allergy in childhood. Ann Allergy Asthma Immunol 2002;89(Suppl 1):33–7.
7. Host A, Husby S, Osterballe O. A prospective study of cow's milk allergy in exclusively breast-fed infants. Incidence, pathogenetic role of early inadvertent exposure to cow's milk formula, and characterization of bovine milk protein in human milk. Acta Paediatr Scand 1988;77:663–70.
8. Maluenda C, Phillips AD, Briddon A, Walker-Smith JA. Quantitative analysis of small intestinal mucosa in cow's milk-sensitive enteropathy. J Pediatr Gastroenterol Nutr 1984;3:349–56.
9. Parker SL, Leznoff A, Sussman GL, Tarlo SM, Krondl M. Characteristics of patients with food-related complaints. J Allergy Clin Immunol 1990;86:503–11.
10. Phillips AD, Rice SJ, France NE, Walker-Smith JA. Small intestinal intraepithelial lymphocyte levels in cow's milk protein intolerance. Gut 1979;20:509–12.

10a. Sampson HA, Metcalfe DD. Food allergies. JAMA 1992;268:2840–4.

11. Waldmann T, Wochner R, Laster L, Gordon RS Jr. Allergic gastroenteropathy. A cause of excessive gastrointestinal protein loss. N Engl J Med 1967;276:762–9.
12. Walker-Smith J. Cow's milk allergy: a new understanding from immunology. Ann Allergy Asthma Immunol 2003;90(Suppl 3):81–3.

Allergic Proctocolitis

13. Goldman H, Proujansky R. Allergic proctitis and gastroenteritis in children. Clinical and mucosal features in 53 cases. Am J Surg Pathol 1986;10:75–86.
14. Jenkins HR, Pincott JR, Soothill JF, Milla PJ, Harries JT. Food allergy: the major cause of infantile colitis. Arch Dis Child 1984;59:326–9.
15. Lake AM, Whitington PF, Hamilton SR. Dietary protein-induced colitis in breast-fed infants. J Pediatrics 1982;101:906–10.
16. Levinson JD, Ramanathan VR, Nozick JH. Eosinophilic gastroenteritis with ascites and colon involvement. Am J Gastroenterol 1977;68:603–7.
17. Moore D, Lichtman S, Lentz J, Stringer D, Sherman P. Eosinophilic gastroenteritis presenting in an adolescent with isolated colonic involvement. Gut 1986;27:1219–22.
18. Naylor AR, Pollet JE. Eosinophilic colitis. Dis Colon Rectum 1985;28:615–8.
19. Odze RD, Bines J, Leichtner AM, Goldman H, Antonioli DA. Allergic proctocolitis in infants: a prospective clinicopathologic biopsy study. Hum Pathol 1993;24:668–74.
20. Odze RD, Wershil BK, Leichtner AM, Antonioli DA. Allergic colitis in infants. J Pediatr 1995;126:163–70.
21. Rosekrans PC, Meijer CJ, van der Wal AM, Lindeman J. Allergic proctitis, a clinical and immunopathological entity. Gut 1980;2:1017–23.
22. Winter HS, Antonioli DA, Fukagawa N, Marcial M, Goldman H. Allergy-related proctocolitis in infants: diagnostic usefulness of rectal biopsy. Mod Pathol 1990;3:5–10.

Eosinophilic Gastroenteritis

23. Bischoff SC. Mucosal allergy: role of mast cells and eosinophil granulocytes in the gut. Ballieres Clin Gastroenterol 1996;10:443–59.
24. Blackshaw AJ, Levinson DA. Eosinophilic infiltrates of the gastrointestinal tract. J Clin Pathol 1986;39:1–7.
25. Cello JP. Eosinophilic gastroenteritis—a complex disease entity. Am J Med 1979;67:1097–104.
26. Di Gioacchino MD, Pizzicannella G, Fini N, et al. Sodium cromoglycate in the treatment of eosinophilic gastroenteritis. Allergy 1990;45:161–6.
27. Felt-Bersma RJ, Meuwissen SG, Van Velzen D. Perforation of the small intestine due to eosinophilic gastroenteritis. Am J Gastroenterol 1984; 79:442–5.
28. Frigas E, Gleich GJ. The eosinophil and the pathophysiology of asthma. J Allergy Clin Immunol 1986;77:527–37.
29. Goldstein NA, Putnam PE, Dohar JE. Laryngeal cleft and eosinophilic gastroenteritis: report of 2 cases. Arch Otolaryngol Head Neck Surg 2000;126:227–30.
30. Justininch C, Katz A, Gurbindo C, et al. Elemental diet improves steroid-dependent eosinophilic gastroenteritis and reverses growth failure. J Pediatr Gastroenterol Nutr 1996;23:81–5.
31. Kaplan SM, Goldstein F, Kowlessar OD. Eosinophilic gastroenteritis. Report of a case with malabsorption and protein-losing enteropathy. Gastroenterology 1970;58:540–5.
32. Khan S, Orenstein SR. Eosinophilic gastroenteritis: epidemiology, diagnosis and management. Pediatr Drugs 2002;4:563–70.
33. Lee CM, Changchien CS, Chen PC, et al. Eosinophilic gastroenteritis: 10 years experience. Am J Gastroenterol 1993;88:70–4.
34. Lin HH, Wu CH, Wu LS, Shyu RY. Eosinophilic gastroenteritis presenting as relapsing severe abdominal pain and enteropathy with protein loss. Emerg Med J 2005;22:834–5.
35. Melamed I, Feanny SJ, Sherman PM, Roifman CM. Benefit of ketotifen in patients with eosinophilic gastroenteritis. Am J Med 1991;90:310–4.
36. Min KU, Metcalfe DD. Eosinophilic gastroenteritis. Immunol Allergy Clin North Am 1991; 11:799–813.
37. Naylor AR. Eosinophilic gastroenteritis. Scott Med J 1990;35:163–5.
38. Naylor AR, Pollet JE. Eosinophilic colitis. Dis Colon Rectum 1985;28:615–8.
39. Neustrom MR, Friesen C. Treatment of eosinophilic gastroenteritis with montelukast. J Allergy Clin Immunol 1999;104(Pt 1):506.
40. Park HS, Kim HS, Jang HJ. Eosinophilic gastroenteritis associated with food allergy and bronchial asthma. J Korean Med Soc 1995;10:216–9.
41. Perez-Millan A, Martin-Lorente JL, Lopez-Morante A, Yuguero L, Saez-Royuela F. Subserosal eosinophilic gastroenteritis treated efficaciously with sodium cromoglycate. Dig Dis Sci 1997;42:342–4.
42. Robert F, Omura E, Durant JR. Mucosal eosinophilic gastroenteritis with systemic involvement. Am J Med 1977;62:139–43.
43. Schwartz DA, Pardi DS, Murray JA. Use of montelukast as steroid sparing agent for recurrent eosinophilic gastroenteritis. Dig Dis Sci 2001;46:1787–90.
44. Shirai T, Hashimoto D, Suzuki K, et al. Successful treatment of eosinophilic gastroenteritis with suplatast tosilate. J Allergy Clin Immunol 2001;107:924–5.
45. Talley NJ, Shorter RG, Phillips SF, Zinsmeister AR. Eosinophilic gastroenteritis: a clinicopathological study of patients with disease of the mucosa, muscle layer, and subserosal tissues. Gut 1990;31:54–8.
46. Tedesco FJ, Huckaby CB, Hamby-Allen M, Ewing GC. Eosinophilic ileocolitis: expanding spectrum of eosinophilic gastroenteritis. Dig Dis Sci 1981;26:943–8.
47. Tytgat GN, Grijm R, Dekker W, den Hartog NA. Fatal eosinophilic enteritis. Gastroenterology 1976;71:479–83.
48. Weller PF. The immunobiology of eosinophils. N Engl J Med 1991;324:1110–8.
49. Whitington PF, Whitington GL. Eosinophilic gastroenteropathy in childhood. J Pediatr Gastroenterol Nutr 1988;7:379–85.

Inflammatory Fibroid Polyps

50. Balci NC, Radjazi S, Polat H. Adult intussusception secondary to inflammatory fibroid polyp: demonstration by MRI. Eur Radiology 2000;10:1708–10.
51. Bosch O, Gonzalez-Campos C, Jurado A, et al. Esophageal inflammatory fibroid polyp. Endoscopic and radiologic features. Dig Dis Sci 1994;39:2561–6.
52. Bradley B, Molloy PJ, Glick K, Kania RJ. Ileal intussusception and obstruction as presentation of inflammatory fibroid polyp. Dig Dis Sci 1995;40:812–3.
53. Costa PM, Marques A, Tavora I, Oliveira E, Diaz M. Inflammatory fibroid polyp of the esophagus. Dis Esophagus 2000;13:75–9.
54. Dabral C, Singh N, Singh PA, Misra V. Inflammatory fibroid polyp of small intestine in a child. Indian J Gastroenterol 2003;22:101.

55. Daum O, Hes O, Vanecek T, et al. Vanek's tumor (inflammatory fibroid polyp). Report of 18 cases and comparison with three cases of original Vanek's series. Ann Diagn Pathol 2003;7:337–47.
56. Gooszen AW, Tjon A Tham RT, Veselic M, Bolk JH, Lamers CB. Inflammatory fibroid polyp simulating malignant tumor of the colon in a patient with multiple hamartoma syndrome (Cowden's disease). AJR Am J Roentgenol 1995;165:1012–3.
57. Hizawa K, Iida S, Tada S, et al. Endoscopic evaluation of gastric inflammatory fibroid polyp. Surg Endosc 1995;9:397–400.
58. Hui YZ, Noffsinger AE, Yochman L, Hurtubise P, Fenoglio-Preiser CM. Delineation of the proliferative component of inflammatory fibroid polyps of the intestine. Int J Surg Pathol 1995;2:207–14.
59. Johnstone JM, Morson BC. Inflammatory fibroid polyp of the gastrointestinal tract. Histopathology 1978;2:349–61.
60. Kim MK, Higgins J, Cho EY, Ko YH, Oh YL. Expression of CD34, bcl-2, and kit in inflammatory fibroid polyps of the gastrointestinal tract. Appl Immunohistochem Mol Morphol 2000;8:147–53.
61. Kim YI, Kim WH. Inflammatory fibroid polyps of gastrointestinal tract. Evolution of histologic patterns. Am J Clin Pathol 1988;89:721–7.
62. LiVolsi VA, Perzin KH. Inflammatory pseudotumors (inflammatory fibroid polyps) of the small intestine: a clinicopathologic study. Am J Dig Dis 1975;20:325–6.
63. Makhlouf HR, Sobin LH. Inflammatory myofibroblastic tumor (inflammatory pseudotumors) of the gastrointestinal tract: how closely are they related to inflammatory fibroid polyps? Hum Pathol 2002;33:307–16.
64. Matsushita M, Hajiro K, Okazaki K, Takakuwa H. Endoscopic features of gastric inflammatory fibroid polyps. Am J Gastroenterol 1996;91:1595–8.
65. Maves CK, Johnson JF, Bove K, Malott RL. Gastric inflammatory pseudotumor in children. Radiology 1989;173:381–3.
66. Merkel IS, Rabinovitz M, Dekker A. Cecal inflammatory fibroid polyp presenting with chronic diarrhea. A case report and review of the literature. Dig Dis Sci 1992;37:133–6.
67. Miyata T, Yamamoto H, Kita H, et al. A case of inflammatory fibroid polyp causing small-bowel intussusception in which retrograde double-balloon enteroscopy was useful for the preoperative diagnosis. Endoscopy 2004;36:344–7.
68. Mori M, Tamura S, Enjoji M, Sugimachi K. Concomitant presence of inflammatory fibroid polyp and carcinoma or adenoma in the stomach. Arch Pathol Lab Med 1988;112:829–32.
69. Ormand JE, Talley NJ, Shorter RG, et al. Prevalence of *Helicobacter pylori* in specific forms of gastritis. Further evidence supporting a pathogenic role for H. pylori in chronic nonspecific gastritis. Dig Dis Sci 1991;36:142–5.
70. Sah SP, Agrawal CS, Rani S. Inflammatory fibroid polyp of the jejunum presenting as intussusception. Ind J Pathol Microbiol 2002;45:119–21.
71. Shalom A, Wasserman I, Segal M, Orda R. Inflammatory fibroid polyp and *Helicobacter pylori*. Aetiology or coincidence? Eur J Surg 2000;166:54–7.
72. Shigeno T, Fujimori K, Nakatsuji Y, Kaneko Y, Maejima T. Gastric inflammatory fibroid polyp manifesting massive bleeding and marked morphological changes for a short period. J Gastroenterol 2003;38:611–2.
73. Simmons MZ, Cho KC, Houghton JM, Levine CD, Javors BR. Inflammatory fibroid polyp of the esophagus in an HIV-infected individual: case study. Dysphagia 1995;10:59–61.
74. Stolte M, Finkenzeller G. Inflammatory fibroid polyp of the stomach. Endoscopy 1990;22:203–7.
75. Vanek J. Gastric submucosal granuloma with eosinophilic infiltration. Am J Pathol 1949;25:397–412.

Granulomatous and Xanthomatous Diseases

76. Abdou NI, NaPombejara C, Sagawa A, et al. Malakoplakia: evidence for monocyte lysosomal abnormality correctable by cholinergic agonist *in vitro* and *in vivo*. N Engl J Med 1977;297:1413–9.
77. Beniwal RS, Cummings OW, Cho WK. Symptomatic gastrointestinal sarcoidosis: case report and review of the literature. Dig Dis Sci 2003;48:174–8.
78. Bulger K, O'Riordan M, Purdy S, O'Brien M, Lennon J. Gastrointestinal sarcoidosis resembling Crohn's disease. Am J Gastroenterol 1988;83:1415–7.
79. Chaudhry AP, Saigal KP, Intengan M, Nickerson PA. Malakoplakia of the large intestine found incidentally at necropsy: light and electron microscopic features. Dis Colon Rectum 1979;22:73–81.
80. Clague RB. Sarcoidosis or Crohn's disease? Br Med J 1972;3:804.
81. Coletta U, Sturgill BC. Isolated xanthomatosis of the small bowel. Hum Pathol 1985;16:422–4.
82. Farman J, Ramirez G, Rybak B, Lebwohl O, Semrad C, Rotterdam H. Gastric sarcoidosis. Abdom Imaging 1997;22:248–52.
83. Fireman Z, Sternberg A, Yarchovsky Y, et al. Multiple antral ulcers in gastric sarcoid. J Clin Gastroenterol 1997;24:97–9.
84. Fleming RH, Nuzek M, McFadden DW. Small intestinal sarcoidosis with massive hemorrhage: report of a case. Surgery 1994;115:526–32.

85. Hayden AJ, Hardy DC, Jackson DE Jr. Malakoplakia of the colon. Mil Med 1986;151:567–9.
86. Hilzenrat N, Spanier A, Lamoureux E, Bloom C, Sherker A. Colonic obstruction secondary to sarcoidosis: nonsurgical diagnosis and management. Gastroenterology 1995;108:1156–9.
87. Kohn NN. Sarcoidosis of the colon. J Med Soc N J 1980;77:517–8.
88. Levinsky L, Cummiskey J, Romer FK, et al. Sarcoidosis in Europe: a cooperative study. Ann NY Acad Sci 1976;278:335–46.
89. Lewin KJ, Harell GS, Lee AS, Crowley LG. An electron-microscopic study: demonstration of bacilliform organisms in malacoplakic macrophages. Gastroenterology 1974;66:28–45.
90. Lewin KJ, Fair WR, Steigbiegel RT, Winberg CD, Droller MJ. Clinical and laboratory studies into the pathogenesis of malakoplakia. J Clin Pathol 1976;29:354–63.
91. Lindgren A, Engstrom CP, Nilsson O, Abrahamsson H. Protein-losing enteropathy in an unusual form of sarcoidosis. Eur J Gastroenterol Hepatol 1995;7:1005–7.
92. Long JP Jr, Althausen AF. Malakoplakia: a 25-year experience with a review of the literature. J Urol 1989;141:1328–31.
93. Lou TY, Teplitz C. Malakoplakia: pathogenesis and ultrastructural morphogenesis. A problem of altered macrophage (phagolysosomal) response. Hum Pathol 1974;5:191–207.
94. Lukens FJ, Machicao VI, Woodward TA, DeVault KR. Esophageal sarcoidosis: an unusual diagnosis. J Clin Gastroenterol 2002 34:54–6.
95. MacRury SM, McQuaker G, Morton R, Hume R. Sarcoidosis: association with small bowel disease and folate deficiency. J Clin Pathol 1992;45:823–5.
96. McClure J. Malacoplakia of the gastrointestinal tract. Postgrad Med J 1981;57:95–103.
97. Moran CA, West B, Schwartz IS. Malakoplakia of the colon in association with colonic adenocarcinoma. Am J Gastroenterol 1989;84:1580–2.
98. Neville E, Walker AN, James DG. Prognostic factors predicting the outcome of sarcoidosis: an analysis of 818 patients. Q J Med 1983;208:525–33.
99. Ng IO, Ng M. Colonic malacoplakia: unusual association with ulcerative colitis. J Gastroenterol Hepatol 1993;8:110–5.
100. Perez-Atayde AR, Lack EE, Katz AJ, Geha RS. Intestinal malakoplakia in childhood: case report and review of literature. Pediatr Pathol 1983;1:337–43.
101. Popovic OS, Brkic S, Bojic P, et al. Sarcoidosis and protein losing enteropathy. Gastroenterology 1980;78:119–25.
102. Radin DR, Chandrasoma P, Halls JM. Colonic malacoplakia. Gastrointest Radiol 1984;9:359–61.
103. Robert J, Lagace R, Delage C. Malakoplakia of the colon associated with a villous adenoma: report of a case. Dis Colon Rectum 1974;17:668–71.
104. Sanusi ID, Tio FO. Gastrointestinal malacoplakia. Report of a case and a review of the literature. Am J Gastroenterol 1974;62:356–66.
105. Sartwell PE. Racial differences in sarcoidosis. Ann NY Acad Sci 1976;278:368–70.
106. Satti MB, Abu-Melha A, Taha OM, Al-Idrissi HY. Colonic malacoplakia and abdominal tuberculosis in a child. Report of a case with review of the literature. Dis Colon Rectum 1985;28:353–7.
107. Scheiman J, Elta G, Colturi T, Nostrant T. Colonic xanthomatosis. Relationship to disordered motility and review of the literature. Dig Dis Sci 1988;33:1491–4.
108. Sprague R, Harper P, McClain S, Trainer T, Beeken W. Disseminated gastrointestinal sarcoidosis. Case report and review of the literature. Gastroenterology 1984;87:421–5,
109. Stampfl DA, Grimm IS, Barbot DJ, Rosato FE, Gordon SJ. Sarcoidosis causing duodenal obstruction. Case report and review of gastrointestinal manifestations. Dig Dis Sci 1990;35:526–32.
110. Veitch AM, Badger I. Sarcoidosis presenting as colonic polyposis: report of a case. Dis Colon Rectum 2004;47:937–9.
111. Yunis EJ, Estevez JM, Pinzon GJ, Moran TJ. Malacoplakia. Discussion of pathogenesis and report of three cases including one of fatal gastric and colonic involvement. Arch Pathol 1967;83:180–7.
112. Zurier RB, Weissmann G, Hoffstein S, Kammerman S, Tai HH. Mechanisms of lysosomal enzyme release from human leucocytes. II. Effects of cAMP and cGMP, autonomic agonists and agents which affect microtubule function. J Clin Invest 1974;53:297–309.

Autoimmune Enteropathy

113. Bousvaros A, Leichtner AM, Book L, et al. Treatment of pediatric autoimmune enteropathy with tacrolimus (FK506). Gastroenterology 1996;111:237–43.
114. Casis B, Fernandez-Vazquez I, Barnardos E, et al. Autoimmune enteropathy in an adult with autoimmune multisystemic involvement. Scand J Gastroenterol 2002;37:1012–6.
115. Colletti RB, Guillot AP, Rosen S, et al. Autoimmune enteropathy and nephropathy with circulating anti-epithelial cell antibodies. J Pediatr 1991;118:858–64.

116. Corazza GR, Biagi F, Volta U, Andreani ML, De Franceschi L, Gasbarrini G. Autoimmune enteropathy and villous atrophy in adults. Lancet 1997;350:106–9.
117. Cuenod B, Brousse N, Goulet O, et al. Classification of intractable diarrhea in infancy using clinical and immunohistological criteria. Gastroenterology 1990;99:1037–43.
118. Daum S, Sahin E, Jansen A, et al. Adult autoimmune enteropathy treated successfully with tacrolimus. Digestion 2003;68:86–90.
119. Ishikawa S, Kobayashi I, Hamada J, et al. Interaction of MCC2, a novel homologue of MCC tumor suppressor, with PDZ-domain protein AIE-75. Gene 2001;267:101–10.
120. Jenkins HR, Jewkes F, Vujanic GM. Systemic vasculitis complicating infantile autoimmune enteropathy. Arch Dis Child 1994;71:534–5.
121. Kobayashi I, Imamura K, Kubota M, et al. Identification of an autoimmune enteropathy-related 75-kilodalton antigen. Gastroenterology 1999;117:823–30.
122. Kobayashi I, Imamura K, Yamada M, et al. A 75-kD autoantigen recognized by sera from patients with X-linked autoimmune enteropathy associated nephropathy. Clin Exp Immunol 1998;111:527–31.
123. Martin-Villa JM, Regueiro JR, de Juan D, et al. T-lymphocyte dysfunctions occurring together with apical gut epithelial cell autoantibodies. Gastroenterology 1991;101:390–7.
124. Quiros-Tejeira RE, Ament ME, Vargas JH. Induction of remission in a child with autoimmune enteropathy using mycophenolate mofetil. J Pediatr Gastroenterol Nutr 2003;36: 482–5.

Lymphocytic Colitis

125. Agnarsdottir M, Gunnlaugsson O, Orvar KB, et al. Collagenous and lymphocytic colitis in Iceland. Dig Dis Sci 2002;47:1122–8.
126. Bogomoletz WV, Flejou JF. Newly recognized forms of colitis: collagenous colitis, microscopic (lymphocytic) colitis and lymphoid idiopathic proctitis. Semin Diagn Pathol 1991;8:178–89.
127. Bo-Linn GW, Vendrell DD, Lee E, Fordtran JS. An evaluation of the significance of microscopic colitis in patients with chronic diarrhea. J Clin Invest 1985;75:1559–69.
128. Bryant DA, Mintz ED, Puhr ND, Griffin PM, Petras RE. Colonic epithelial lymphocytosis associated with an epidemic of chronic diarrhea. Am J Surg Pathol 1996;20:1102–9.
129. DuBois RN, Lazenby AJ, Yardley JH, Hendrix TR, Bayless TM, Giardiello FM. Lymphocytic enterocolitis in patients with 'refractory sprue.' JAMA 1989;262:935–7.
130. Fernandez-Banares F, Salas A, Esteve M, Espinos J, Forne M, Viver JM. Collagenous and lymphocytic colitis: evaluation of clinical and histological features, response to treatment and long-term follow-up. Am J Gastroenterol 2003;98:340–7.
131. Fernandez-Banares F, Salas A, Forne M, Esteve M, Espinos J, Viver JM. Incidence of collagenous and lymphocytic colitis: a 5-year population-based study. Am J Gastroenterol 1999;94:418–23.
132. Fine KD, Lee EL. Efficacy of open-label bismuth subsalicylate for the treatment of microscopic colitis. Gastroenterology 1998;114:29–36.
133. Giardiello FM, Lazenby AJ, Bayless TM, et al. Lymphocytic (microscopic) colitis. Clinicopathologic study of 18 patients and comparison to collagenous colitis. Dig Dis Sci 1989;34:1730–8.
134. Lazenby AJ, Yardley JH, Giardiello FM, Jessurun J, Bayless TM. Lymphocytic ("microscopic") colitis: a comparative histopathologic study with particular reference to collagenous colitis. Hum Pathol 1989;20:18–28.
135. Olesen M, Eriksson S, Bohr J, Jarnerot G, Tysk C. Lymphocytic colitis: a retrospective clinical study of 199 Swedish patients. Gut 2004;53: 536–41.
136. Olesen M, Eriksson S, Bohr J, Jarnerot G, Tysk C. Microscopic colitis: a common diarrhoeal disease. An epidemiologic study in Orebro, Sweden, 1993-1998. Gut 2004;53:346–50.
137. Osterholm MT, MacDonald KL, White KE, et al. An outbreak of a newly recognized chronic diarrhea syndrome associated with raw milk consumption. JAMA 1986;256:484–90.
138. Pardi DS. Microscopic colitis. Mayo Clinic Proc 2003;78:614–7.
139. Pardi DS, Ramnath VR, Loftus EV Jr, Tremaine WJ, Sandborn WJ. Lymphocytic colitis: clinical features, treatment and outcomes. Am J Gastroenterol 2002;97:2829–33.
140. Pardi DS, Smyrk TC, Tremaine WJ, Sandborn WJ. Microscopic colitis: a review. Am J Gastroenterol 2002;97:794–802.
141. Parsonnet J, Trock SC, Bopp CA, et al. Chronic diarrhea associated with drinking untreated water. Ann Intern Med 1989;110:985–91.
142. Read NW, Krejs GJ, Read MG, Santa Ana CA, Morawski SG, Fordtran JS. Chronic diarrhea of unknown origin. Gastroenterology 1980;78: 264–71.
143. Wolber R, Owen D, Freeman H. Colonic lymphocytosis in patients with celiac sprue. Hum Pathol 1990;21:1092–6.

Collagenous Colitis

144. Al-Ghamdi MY, Malatjalian DA, Veldhuyzen van Zanten S. Causation: recurrent collagenous colitis following repeated use of NSAIDs. Can J Gastroenterol 2002;16:861–2.
145. Baum CA, Bhatia P, Miner PB Jr. Increased colonic mucosal mast cells associated with severe watery diarrhea and microscopic colitis. Dig Dis Sci 1989;34:1462–5.
146. Berrebi D, Sautet A, Flejou JF, Dauge MC, Peuchmaur M, Potet F. Ticlopidine induced colitis: a histopathological study including apoptosis. J Clin Pathol 1998;51:280–3.
147. Bogomoletz WV. Collagenous, microscopic and lymphocytic colitis. An evolving concept. Virchows Arch A Pathol Anat 1994;424:573–9.
148. Castanet J, Lacour JP, Ortonne JP. Arthritis, collagenous colitis, and discoid lupus. Ann Intern Med 1994;120:89–90.
149. Farah DA, Mills PR, Lee FD, McLay A, Russell RI. Collagenous colitis: possible response to sulfasalazine and local steroid therapy. Gastroenterology 1985;88:792–7.
149a. Fernandez-Banares F, Salas A, Forne M, Esteve M, Espinos J, Viver JM. Incidence of collagenous and lymphocytic colitis: a 5-year population-based study. Am J Gastroenterol 1999;94:418–23.
150. Flejou JF, Grimaud JA, Molas G, Baviera E, Potet F. Collagenous colitis. Ultrastructural study and collagen immunotyping of four cases. Arch Pathol Lab Med 1984;108:977–82.
151. Gledhill A, Cole FM. Significance of basement membrane thickening in the human colon. Gut 1984;25:1085–8.
152. Giardiello FM, Hansen FC 3rd, Lazenby AJ, et al. Collagenous colitis in setting of nonsteroidal antiinflammatory drugs and antibiotics. Dig Dis Sci 1990;35:257–60.
153. Gran JT, Husby G. Joint manifestations in gastrointestinal diseases. 2. Whipple's disease, enteric infections, intestinal bypass operations, gluten-sensitive enteropathy, pseudomembranous colitis and collagenous colitis. Dig Dis 1992;10:295–312.
154. Greenson JK, Giardiello FM, Lazenby AJ, Pena SA, Bayless TM, Yardley JH. Antireticulin antibodies in collagenous and lymphocytic (microscopic) colitis. Mod Pathol 1990;3:259–60.
155. Gremse DA, Boudreaux CW, Manci EA. Collagenous colitis in children. Gastroenterology 1993;104:906–9.
156. Grouls V, Vogel J, Sorger M. Collagenous colitis. Endoscopy 1982;14:31–3.
157. Jarnerot G, Hertervig E, Granno C, et al. Familial occurrence of microscopic colitis: a report on five families. Scand J Gastroenterol 2001;36:959–62.
158. Jarnerot G, Tysk C, Bohr J, Eriksson S. Collagenous colitis and fecal stream diversion. Gastroenterology 1995;109:449–55.
159. Jessurun J, Yardley JH, Giadiello FM, Hamilton SR, Bayless TM. Chronic colitis with thickening of the subepithelial collagen layer (collagenous colitis): histopathologic findings in 15 patients. Hum Pathol 1987;18:839–48.
160. Kakar S, Pardi DS, Burgart LJ. Colonic ulcers accompanying collagenous colitis: implication of nonsteroidal anti-inflammatory drugs. Am J Gastroenterol 2003;98:1834–7.
161. Kenesi-Laurent M, Chapelon-Abric C, Fattah ZA, Naudin G, Godeau P. The first case of CRST syndrome associated with collagenous colitis. J Rheumatol 1991;18:1765–7.
162. Lindstrom CG. 'Collagenous colitis' with watery diarrhoea—a new entity? Pathol Eur 1976; 11:87–9.
163. Loftus EV Jr. Microscopic colitis: epidemiology and treatment. Am J Gastroenterol 2003;98: S31–6.
164. Molas GJ, Flejou JF, Potet F. Microscopic colitis, collagenous colitis and mast cells. Dig Dis Sci 1990;35:920–1.
164a. Pardi DS, Ramnath VR, Loftus EV Jr, Tremaine WJ, Sandborn WJ. Lymphocytic colitis: clinical features, treatment and outcomes. Am J Gastroenterol 2002;97:2829–33.
164b. Pardi DS, Smyrk TC, Tremaine WJ, Sandborn WJ. Microscopic colitis: a review. Am J Gastroenterol 2002;97:794–802.
165. Rampton DS, Baithun SI. Is microscopic colitis due to bile-salt malabsorption? Dis Colon Rectum 1987;30:950–2.
166. Riddell RH, Tanaka M, Mazzoleni G. Non-steroidal anti-inflammatory drugs as a possible cause of collagenous colitis: a case-control study. Gut 1992;33:683–6.
167. Thomson RD, Lestina LS, Bensen SP, Toor A, Maheshwari Y, Ratcliffe NR. Lansoprazole-associated microscopic colitis: a case series. Am J Gastroenterol 2002;97:2908–13.
168. Van Tilburg AJ, Lam HG, Seldenrijk CA, et al. Familial occurrence of collagenous colitis. A report of two families. J Clin Gastroenterol 1990;12:279–85.
169. Wengrower D, Pollak A, Okon E, Stalnikowicz R. Collagenous colitis and rheumatoid arthritis with response to sulfasalazine. A case report and review of the literature. J Clin Gastroenterol 1987;9:456–60.
170. Widgren S, MacGee W. Collagenous colitis with protracted course and fatal evolution. Report of a case. Pathol Res Pract 1990;186:303–6.
171. Wilcox GM, Mattia A. Collagenous colitis associated with lansoprazole. J Clin Gastroenterol 2002;34:164–6.

Storage Diseases

172. Adachi M, Volk BW, Schneck L, Torii J. Fine structure of myenteric plexus in various lipidoses. Arch Pathol 1969;87:228–41.
173. Couper R, Kapelushnik J, Griffiths AM. Neutrophil dysfunction in glycogen storage disease Ib: association with Crohn's-like colitis. Gastroenterology 1991;100:549–54.
174. Czapek EE, Deykin D, Salzman EW. Platelet dysfunction in glycogen storage disease type 1. Blood 1973;41:235–47.
175. da Silva V, Vassella F, Bischoff A, Spycher M, Wiesmann UN, Herschkowitz N. Niemann-Pick's disease. Clinical, biochemical and ultrastructural findings in a case of the infantile form. J Neurol 1975;211:61–8.
176. Derry DM, Fawcett JS, Andermann F, Wolfe LS. Late infantile systemic lipidosis. Major monosialogangliosidosis, delineation of two phenotypes. Neurology 1968;18:340–8.
177. Federico A, Palmeri S, Malandrini A, Fabrizi G, Mondelli M, Guazzi GC. The clinical aspects of adult hexosaminidase deficiencies. Dev Neurosci 1991;13:280–7.
178. Glew RH, Basu A, Prence EM, Remaley AT. Lysosomal storage diseases. Lab Invest 1985;53: 250–69.
179. Goldman JE, Katz D, Rapin I, Purpura DP, Suzuki K. Chronic GM1 gangliosidosis presenting as dystonia: I. Clinical and pathological features. Ann Neurol 1981;9:465–75.
180. Ikeda S, Ushiyama M, Nakano T, Kikkawa T, Kondo K, Yanagisawa N. Ultrastructural findings of rectal and skin biopsies in adult GM1-gangliosidosis. Acta Pathol Jpn 1986;36:1823–31.
181. Muenzer J. Mucopolysaccharidoses. Adv Pediatrics 1986;33:269–302.
182. Muenzer J. The mucopolysaccharidoses: a heterogeneous group of disorders with variable pediatric presentations. J Pediatr 2004;44:S27–34.
183. Narisawa K, Igarashi Y, Otomo H, Tada K. A new variant of glycogen storage disease type I probably due to a defect in the glucose-6-phosphate transport system. Biochem Biophys Res Commun 1978;83:1360–4.
184. Roe TF, Thomas DW, Gilsanz V, Isaacs H Jr, Atkinson JB. Inflammatory bowel disease in glycogen storage disease type Ib. J Pediatrics 1986;109:55–9.
185. Tager JM. Inborn errors of cellular organelles: an overview. J Inherit Metab Dis 1987;10:3–10.

Neonatal Enteropathies

186. Cameron DJ, Barnes GL. Successful pregnancy outcome in tufting enteropathy. J Pediatr Gastroenterol Nutr 2003;36:158.
187. Cutz E, Sherman PM, Davidson GP. Enteropathies associated with protracted diarrhea of infancy: clinicopathological features, cellular and molecular mechanisms. Pediatr Pathol Lab Med 1997;17:335–68.
188. Goulet O, Kedinger M, Brousse N, et al. Intractable diarrhea of infancy with epithelial and basement membrane abnormalities. J Pediatr 1995;127:212–9.
189. Groisman GM, Amar M, Livne E. CD10: a valuable tool for the light microscopic diagnosis of microvillous inclusion disease (familial microvillous atrophy). Am J Surg Pathol 2002;26:902–7.
190. Groisman GM, Ben-Izhak O, Schwersenz A, Berant M, Fyfe B. The value of polyclonal carcinoembryonic antigen immunostaining in the diagnosis of microvillus inclusion disease. Hum Pathol 1993;24:1232–7.
191. Patey N, Scoazec JY, Cuenod-Jabri B, et al. Distribution of cell adhesion molecules in infants with intestinal epithelial dysplasia (tufting enteropathy). Gastroenterology 1997;113:833–43.
192. Phillips AD, Jenkins P, Raafat F, Walker-Smith JA. Congenital microvillous atrophy: specific diagnostic features. Arch Dis Child 1985;60: 135–40.
193. Phillips AD, Schmitz J. Familial microvillus atrophy: a clinicopathological survey of 23 cases. J Pediatr Gastroenterol Nutr 1992;14:380–96.
194. Phillips AD, Szafranski M, Man LY, Wall WJ. Periodic acid–Schiff staining abnormality in microvillous atrophy: photometric and ultrastructural studies. J Pediatr Gastroenterol Nutr 2000;30:34–42.
195. Pohl JF, Shub MD, Trevelline EE, et al. A cluster of microvillus inclusion disease in the Navajo population. J Pediatr 1999;134:103–6.
196. Reifen RM, Cutz E, Griffiths AM, Ngan BY, Sherman PM. Tufting enteropathy: a newly recognized clinicopathological entity associated with refractory diarrhea in infants. J Pediatr Gastroenterology Nutr 1994;18:379–85.
197. Rhoads JM, Vogler RC, Lacey SR, et al. Microvillus inclusion disease. In vitro jejunal electrolyte transport. Gastroenterology 1991;100:811–7.
198. Sherman PM, Mitchell DJ, Cutz E. Neonatal enteropathies: defining the causes of protracted diarrhea of infancy. J Pediatr Gastroenterol Nutr 2004;38:16–26.
199. Schofield DE, Agostini RM Jr, Yunis EJ. Gastrointestinal microvillus inclusion disease. Am J Clin Pathol 1992;98:119–24.

Intestinal Transplantation

200. Banner B, Dean P, Williams J. Morphologic features of rejection in long-surviving canine small bowel transplants. Transplantation 1988;46:665–9.
201. Bass BL, Sayadi H, Harmon JW, Wall S, Korman LY. VIP receptors and content after bowel transplantation. J Surg Res 1989;46:431–8.
202. Brousse N, Canioni D, Rambaud C, et al. Intestinal transplantation in children: contribution of immunohistochemistry. Transplant Proc 1990;22:2495–6.
203. Caniano DA, Beaver BL. Meconium ileus: a fifteen-year experience with forty-two neonates. Surgery 1987;102:699–702.
204. Diliz-Perez HS, McClure J, Bedetti C, et al. Successful small bowel allotransplantation in dogs with cyclosporine and prednisone. Transplantation 1984;37:126–9.
205. Elmes ME. Apoptosis in the small intestine of zinc-deficient and fasted rats. J Pathol 1977;123:219–23.
206. Grover R, Lear PA, Ingham Clark CL, Pockley AG, Wood RF. Method for diagnosing rejection in small bowel transplantation. Br J Surg 1993;80:1024–6.
207. Ijiri K. Apoptosis (cell death) induced in mouse bowel by 1,2-dimethylhydrazine, methylazoxymethanol acetate, and gamma-rays. Cancer Res 1989;49:6342–6.
208. Langnas AN. Advances in small-intestine transplantation. Transplantation 2004;77:S75–8.
209. Lee R, Nakamura K, Tsamandas A, et al. Pathology of human intestinal transplantation. Gastroenterology 1996;110:1820–34.
210. Millard PR, Dennison A, Hughes DA, Collin J, Morris PJ. Morphology of intestinal allograft rejection and the inadequacy of mucosal biopsy in its recognition. Br J Exp Pathol 1986;67:687–98.
211. Monchik GJ, Russell PS. Transplantation of small bowel in the rat: technical and immunological considerations. Surgery 1971;70:693–702.
212. Oberhuber G, Schmid T, Thaler W, Luze T, Klima G, Margreiter R. Increased number of intraepithelial lymphocytes in rejected small-bowel allografts: an analysis of subpopulations involved. Transplant Proc 1990;22:2454–5.
213. Reyes J, Bueno J, Kocoshis S, et al. Current status of intestinal transplantation in children. J Pediatr Surg 1998;33:243–54.
214. Sugitani A, Reynolds JC, Todo S. Immunohistochemical study of enteric nervous system after small bowel transplantation in humans. Dig Dis Sci 1994;39:2448–56.
215. Todo S, Reyes J, Furukawa H, et al. Outcome analysis of 71 clinical intestinal transplantations. Ann Surg 1995;222:270–80.
216. Vanderhoof JA. Short bowel syndrome in children and small intestinal transplantation. Pediatr Clin North Am 1996;43:533–50.

15 INFLAMMATORY BOWEL DISEASE

Idiopathic inflammatory bowel disease (IBD) includes two chronic gastrointestinal disorders of unknown etiology: ulcerative colitis (UC) and Crohn's disease (CD). The natural history of IBD differs from patient to patient, and depends on which disease is present. Disease severity at the onset, disease extent, and patient age at the time of diagnosis, along with other patient variables, determine overall disease severity and the likelihood of subsequent morbidity and mortality. Once established, IBD patients suffer episodic acute flares and relapses that become superimposed on chronic disease. As a result, the patient is likely to suffer from disabling disease for decades.

DEMOGRAPHY

Both CD and UC are predominantly diseases of young adults, occurring with a peak incidence between 15 and 30 years of age. After age 10, there is a rapid incidence increase for both diseases. Age-specific incidence rates are slightly greater for males with UC and for females with CD (2). Both diseases show three peak incidence rates: the first and highest occurs between ages 20 and 24 years, the second at ages 40 to 44 years, and the third at ages 60 to 64. In females, the first peak appears at ages 15 to 19, 5 years younger than in males (10,11). By age 60, the incidence of UC exceeds that of CD.

Epidemiologic studies show that the incidence and prevalence of IBD vary significantly depending on the patient's geographic location and racial or ethnic background. There has been an increase in the incidence of CD in the past several decades in Western countries; the incidence of UC has also increased somewhat. In addition, the mean age at diagnosis of patients with CD has decreased in recent times (5). The annual incidence of IBD in the United States is estimated at approximately 6/100,000 population (5). Incidence rates for both diseases are higher in urban than in rural areas, and in industrialized than nonindustrialized countries (7).

IBD occurs worldwide: the incidence is relatively low in Asian, Mediterranean, and Middle Eastern countries (3), and higher in European countries, the United States, Canada, Australia, and New Zealand. This may reflect racial, ethnic, and genetic factors. Prevalence rates for IBD among non-Caucasians in the United States are lower than rates for Caucasians. In one study, the prevalence rates for CD were 43.6/100,000 for Caucasians, 29.8/100,000 for African-Americans, 4.1/100,000 for Hispanics, and 5.6/100,000 for Asians (4). A study of African-American children reported a CD incidence rate of 7 to 12/100,000 (6). Among ethnic groups, Jews in the United States have a greater risk for developing IBD than non-Jewish Caucasians (8). The incidence rate is 2 to 4 times greater and the prevalence 2 to 9 times greater in this group. Ashkenazi Jews exhibit a particularly high IBD risk (1), especially those originating in Middle Europe, Poland, or Russia (8,9).

ETIOLOGY

The pathophysiology of IBD involves complex interactions between genetic, environmental, and immunologic factors (fig. 15-1).

Genetic Factors

There is considerable evidence that the development of both CD and UC is determined, at least in part, by genetic factors. Overwhelming evidence shows that IBD clusters within families. This finding is true for both UC and CD. In population-based studies, 5 to 10 percent of individuals with IBD have an affected family member (22,37,47). In fact, having a family member with IBD represents the greatest risk factor for developing the disease. Individuals with a first-degree relative with IBD have a 10- to 15-fold increased risk of also developing the disease compared with those without an affected family member (42,43,48). Approximately 75 percent of families with multiple affected members show concordance for disease

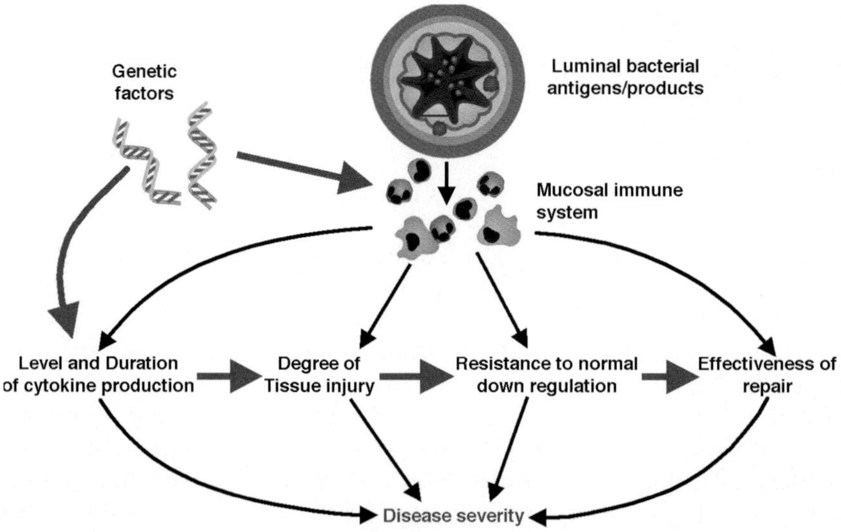

Figure 15-1

INFLAMMATORY BOWEL DISEASE

Inflammatory bowel disease (IBD) likely results from a combination of genetic predisposition, cellular alterations, and altered immunity. The genetic influences affect both the predisposition to injury and the nature of the response to the injury.

type (i.e., all affected family members have CD or all have UC). In the remaining 25 percent, some members have CD while others have UC (16). This finding suggests that UC and CD may have some common, as well as distinct, susceptibility genes. Twin studies show that monozygotic twin concordance for CD ranges from 42 to 58 percent (51–53). Monozygotic twin concordance for UC is significantly lower, ranging from 6 to 17 percent. These findings suggest that although there is a strong genetic component that determines susceptibility to IBD, environmental factors also play an important role in disease development.

Genetic linkage studies have identified a number of potential genetic susceptibility loci for IBD. These are listed in Table 15-1.

IBD1. The *IBD1* locus is located in the pericentromeric region of chromosome 16, and was originally described by Hugot et al. (29). This locus is linked only to CD, not UC. The locus contains the gene *NOD2/CARD15*, which has now been definitively identified as responsible for disease linkage to this chromosomal region (39).

The family of Nod proteins includes NOD2/CARD15 as well as several additional regulatory proteins. The Nod proteins contain a central nucleotide-binding domain and an N-terminal caspase recruitment domain (30). In addition, they possess a C-terminal leucine-rich repeat (LRR) region that has a high degree of homology with plant genes known to be involved in disease resistance (14,54). This finding suggests that Nod proteins may play a similar role in mammals (30).

NOD2 protein is expressed in monocytes (31, 41), intestinal epithelial cells, and intestinal Paneth cells (27,33). The protein recognizes and binds bacterial peptidoglycan, resulting in activation of the proinflammatory cytokine, NF-κB (23). It is the LRR region of the protein that functions in peptidoglycan recognition. Human mutations in *NOD2* occur in both the LRR region and in the central nucleotide-binding domain. Three major mutations have been described in the LRR region, all of which are associated with CD (13,19,21,24,28,57,58). Interestingly, these mutations occur predominantly in Caucasian populations and are extremely rare in Asian and African-American populations (18,32,34,59). Mutations in the nucleotide-binding domain result in Blau's syndrome, a rare disease characterized by early-onset granulomatous arthritis, uveitis, and skin rash (36).

Patients who have one defective copy of *NOD2* have a 2- to 4-fold increased risk for the development of CD, while homozygous mutants show a 20- to 40-fold increased risk (21, 28,55). Approximately 8 to 17 percent of CD patients carry two mutant *NOD2* alleles. *NOD2* mutations are associated with disease located in the small intestine, as well as stricturing and fistulizing forms of the disease (12,13,21,26,35, 44,57,58). CD-associated mutations in the LRR of *NOD2* result in inactivation of the protein and a resultant defect in the cellular response to

Table 15-1

MAJOR SUSCEPTIBILITY LOCI FOR INFLAMMATORY BOWEL DISEASE

Locus Designation	Chromosomal Location	IBD[a] Type	Candidate Genes
IBD1	16q12	CD	*NOD2*
IBD2	12q13	UC	*VDR, IFN-γ*[b]
IBD3	6p13	CD, UC	*MHC I, MHC 2, TNF-α*
IBD4	14q11	CD	TCR α/γ complex
IBD5	5q31-33	CD	*IL3, IL4, IL5, IL13, CSF-2*
IBD6	19p13	CD, UC	*ICAM-1, C3, TBXA2R, LTB4H*
Other	1p36	CD, UC	*TNF-R* family, *CASP9*
Other	3p	CD, UC	*HGFR, EGFR, GNAI2*
Other	7q	CD, UC	*MUC-3*

[a]IBD = Inflammatory bowel disease; CD = Crohn's disease; UC = ulcerative colitis.

[b]VDR = vitamin D receptor; IFN-γ = interferon-gamma; MHC = major histocompatibility complex; TNF-α = tumor necrosis factor-alpha; TCR = T-cell receptor; IL = interleukin; CSF = colony-stimulating factor; ICAM = intercellular adhesion molecule; HGFR = hepatocyte growth factor receptor; EGFR = epidermal growth factor receptor.

peptidoglycan (18). This abnormality in monocytes could result in an inability of the innate immune system to recognize bacterial products, and a subsequent overreaction to bacteria by the adaptive immune system (40). In addition, defective NOD2 protein function in intestinal epithelial and Paneth cells may result in an abnormal immunologic response to normal commensal bacteria within the gastrointestinal tract.

A genetic test for *NOD2/CARD15* is not available commercially at this time. Testing family members of patients with CD for alterations in this gene is not recommended given the overall prevalence of the disease, and therefore, the probability of an asymptomatic, gene-positive individual developing the disease. A lack of interventional strategies for gene-positive patients also argues against gene testing at the present time.

IBD2. The *IBD2* gene locus lies on chromosome 12, and appears to be more closely linked to the development of UC than CD (15). A number of possible candidate genes are located in this region, but investigation of several of these has yielded negative results (50,56).

IBD3. Several studies have linked the *IBD3* locus, located on chromosome 6, to both UC and CD (15,25,45,49,60). This region contains the major histocompatability complex (*MHC*), as well as the tumor necrosis factor (*TNF*) gene. Several human leukocyte antigen (HLA) associations with IBD are well known. Among Caucasians, susceptibility to UC has been convincingly linked to the HLADRB1*0103 allele. In addition, this allele is associated with severe colitis and extraintestinal manifestations of UC (20,41). In Japanese and Jewish populations, susceptibility to UC has been linked to the HLADRB1*1052 allele. Polymorphisms in TNF-α and their relationship to the risk of CD are also under current investigation (38).

IBD5. The *IBD5* locus resides on chromosome 5q31-q33. It was identified by a genome-wide scan of Canadian families with early onset CD. Heterozygous carriage of the risk alleles increased the risk for developing CD 2-fold, while homozygous carriage increases this risk 6-fold (46). The specific causative gene has not yet been identified. This region does, however, contain a number of genes that encode immunoregulatory cytokines including interleukins (IL)3, IL4, IL5, and IL14. This locus also contains genes for colony-stimulating factor isoform 2 and interferon regulatory factor isoform 1 (17).

Environmental Factors

Numerous data suggest that environmental factors play a role in the development and progression of both forms of IBD. Susceptibility genes for IBD demonstrate only incomplete penetrance, and, as noted earlier, concordance rates for monozygotic twins are 48 to 52 percent for CD and only 6 to 17 percent for UC (96a,101a,102a). Factors other than genotype must be involved in the pathogenesis of IBD. In addition, the incidence of IBD has increased in the developed parts of the world over that last 50 years, and is now becoming increasingly common in less-developed countries as they become more industrialized and the standard of living improves. Environmental changes that might affect the development of the mucosal immune system or the indigenous enteric flora include improved hygiene, consumption of sterile or at least noncontaminated foods, childhood vaccinations, and increased age at first exposure to a variety of intestinal pathogens (95).

Food Antigens. Numerous studies have demonstrated that exposure to food-associated antigens plays an important role in the gastrointestinal inflammation that occurs in patients with CD. Patients treated with simplified or elemental diets containing proteins in the form of amino acids or small peptide fragments improve symptomatically and show decreased inflammation as determined endoscopically and through serum marker studies (72,86). In one study, rectal exposure of CD patients to a series of food antigens resulted in increased rectal blood flow and lymphocyte proliferation in comparison to control patients (103), a finding that suggests patients with CD show gut-specific sensitization to food antigens. Reactions were seen with antigens to yeast and to citrus, although individual patients also reacted to other antigen groups. Although it is possible that sensitivity to food antigens is merely a reflection of exposure to antigens through mucosal defects, the absence of similar sensitivities in patients with UC makes this possibility unlikely.

It is not likely, however, that exposure to food-associated antigens represents the primary abnormality in patients with CD. Instead, exposure to food in the proximal gastrointestinal tract may lead to sensitization and stimulation of the immune system in genetically susceptible individuals.

Infectious Agents. For many years investigators have been suspicious that IBD may have an infectious etiology. These suspicions are based on several observations. First, CD patients have an increased incidence of childhood infections including pharyngitis, tonsilitis, and rhinitis (104, 106). In addition, gastroenteritis in early infancy has been linked to later development of CD (90). Studies have shown that patients with CD tend to have increased serum levels of antibodies directed against nonpathogenic as well as pathogenic enteric organisms (61,75). Many studies have attempted to link IBD to infections with *Mycobacteria*, *Yersinia*, and several viruses (66–69,71,79,81,93,97,98); however, no definitive link with any one infectious agent has ever been made (64,73,77,82,88,89,92,105).

Current evidence, instead, suggests that the resident bacterial flora of the gut may be a factor in initiating and propagating the inflammation in IBD (96). In CD patients, T lymphocytes are hyperreactive to bacterial antigens, a factor that suggests that local bacterial tolerance mechanisms are abnormal in these individuals (91). Patients with both UC and CD show higher numbers of bacteria attached to their intestinal mucosa than do unaffected individuals (100). In addition, bacterial invasion of the mucosa has been reported in both UC and CD patients (78). IBD patients also have increased mucosal production of immunoglobulin (Ig)G antibodies directed against a wide range of commensal organisms (83). The clinical observation that, in some patients, disease flares may be ameliorated by antibiotic administration is supportive of a bacterial role. Finally, recent evidence suggests that the *NOD2* CD susceptibility gene is involved in regulation of host responses to bacterial organisms (73a). Overall, many view IBD as a disease initiated by a general loss of tolerance for the commensal bacteria of the gastrointestinal tract.

Tobacco Use and Exposure. The association between tobacco use and the development of IBD is well established. Smoking decreases the risk for the development of UC, but exacerbates and aggravates CD (62,63,65,76,99,102). Former smokers have a lower risk of UC than do those who never smoked. Exposure to passive smoke also appears to confer a lessened risk of developing UC relative to nonexposed nonsmokers (94). Interestingly, nicotine has been shown to have an inhibitory effect on Th2 lymphocyte function, the type of cell most implicated in UC (85). Indeed, nicotine-based enemas have been shown to be beneficial in patients with milder forms of distal colitis. Nicotine has no effect on the Th1 cells characteristic of the CD inflammatory response.

Other Environmental Factors. Epidemiologic data suggest that use of nonsteroidal anti-inflammatory drugs (NSAIDs) can exacerbate existing UC, and may even induce it de novo (70). This effect was initially attributed to the cyclooxygenase (COX)-1 inhibitory effect of the drugs, but recent reports suggest that even COX-2–specific inhibitors demonstrate this effect (87). Possible mechanisms by which NSAIDs exert these effects include inhibition of protective mucosal prostaglandin production and increased leukocyte migration and adherence. It has been estimated that NSAID use increases the risk of IBD by as much as 30 percent.

As many as 40 percent of UC patients report that psychological stress represents a trigger for their disease (80,101). There is evidence to link psychological stress with increased susceptibility to infection and illness through stress-related impairment of the immune system (74). Some animal models suggest that stress may play a role in the development of colitis. Cotton-top tamarins, primates that spontaneously develop colitis and serve as a model for human IBD, develop colitis only during long-term captivity (84).

Host Factors

Intestinal Permeability. Increased intestinal permeability may play a role in the pathogenesis of CD. Increased permeability not only occurs in the intestines of patients affected by the disease, but also in their unaffected first-degree relatives (111). It has been suggested that this increased permeability may represent a predisposing factor to the development of CD because a leaky intestinal barrier intensifies antigen absorption, leading to exaggerated systemic immune stimulation (110).

Appendectomy. Appendectomy early in life (before the age of 20) has been shown in several studies to decrease the risk of developing UC (107,112,113). Interestingly, the risk for UC is reduced only in patients who undergo appendectomy for acute appendicitis, and not in those whose appendices are removed because of nonspecific abdominal pain or incidentally during surgery for other causes (107). This finding suggests that the appendicitis that results in appendectomy, rather than appendectomy itself, is protective. Alternatively, there may be other factors among patients destined to develop UC that prevent those individuals from developing appendicitis (109). A recent report suggests that the risk for CD may also be decreased in patients who have undergone appendectomy (108).

Immunologic Factors

Both CD and UC are, at least in part, disorders of immunity. It is currently believed that the main abnormality responsible for the development of inflammation in these disorders is an exaggerated T-cell response to commensal bacteria or other pathogens (123,143). CD4-positive T lymphocytes act as immune regulators, controlling the activities of other components of the immune system through the production and secretion of a variety of cytokines. In recent years, two functionally different populations of CD4-positive T cells have been recognized. The T-helper 1 (T_H1) subset orchestrates cell-mediated immune responses, and synthesizes and secretes IL2, IL12, and interferon-gamma (IFN-γ). T-helper 2 (T_H2) cells mediate humoral responses, and produce IL4, IL5, IL10, and IL13. These two subsets of CD4-positive T cells regulate each other reciprocally through key cytokines. For example, IFN-γ, secreted by T_H1 cells, suppresses the development of the T_H2 response, while IL4, IL10, and IL13 secreted by T_H2 cells, inhibits T_H1 (122,123a).

CD is associated with T_H1 cytokine production (134,136). UC, on the other hand, does not fit clearly into either the T_H1 or T_H2 category, although a modified T_H2 response seems to occur in established UC (123–124). Although the types of cytokines produced in UC and CD differ somewhat, both diseases are associated with abnormal immune responses to nonpathogenic commensal bacteria within the gut. Cross-reactivity of peripheral blood and colonic lamina propria CD4-positive T cells with indigenous flora in patients with UC and CD suggests that abnormal T-cell–specific immune responses to the normal flora of the host are important in the pathogenesis of both diseases (120).

Activated T lymphocytes are regulated by both effector and regulator T-cell subpopulations in healthy gut mucosa. Effector T cells are capable of inducing intestinal inflammation, while regulator T cells are able to control or prevent inflammation. The immunosuppressive function of the regulator cells is mediated through the production of IL10 and transforming growth factor-beta (TGF-β). These regulator cells are thought to play pivotal roles in mediating tolerance toward luminal antigens (125,129). Genetically engineered IL10 deficient mice develop severe transmural inflammation of the small and large intestine, reminiscent of CD (128). Studies suggest that defects in the IL10 and TGF-β regulatory signaling pathways may exist in humans with UC (131,135).

Activation of effector cytotoxic T cells and release of cytokines result in the generation of activated matrix metalloproteinases, enzymes that are mediators of tissue destruction. Cytokines act directly on the microvasculature, upregulate adhesion molecules, and enhance recruitment of additional effector cells including neutrophils and macrophages; the latter amplify and perpetuate the inflammatory response and contribute to additional tissue injury.

Autoantibodies. Numbers of mucosal B cells and plasma cells increase in UC, a finding that initially suggested that the disease was antibody mediated and complement dependent (126). Patients with UC also have circulating autoantibodies, including those directed against human intestinal tropomyosin isoform (130,138) as well as anticolonocyte antibodies (132). The production of antiself antibodies is now thought to represent a phenomenon that is a secondary protective response aimed at clearing apoptotic cells (133).

Patients with UC commonly have circulating antineutrophil antibodies (ANCAs) (119, 130,132,137,140,148). ANCAs were initially described as sensitive and specific markers for active Wegener's granulomatosis but are now known to occur in a wide range of diseases. The prevalence of a positive perinuclear (p) ANCA in UC patients ranges from 49 to 86 percent (121,139). The pANCA pattern is 93 to 97 percent specific (146,148), but only 46 to 60 percent sensitive for the diagnosis (118). pANCAs are also found in up to 25 percent of patients with CD (121,141,144,145). The titers of these antibodies, however, do not correlate with the degree of severity of the associated colitis, and although they may serve as a convenient clinical marker for UC, their role in the pathogenesis of the disease is unclear (114,142). A recent report suggests that pANCA in UC may represent a cross-reacting antibody to an antigenic target on *Escherichia coli* and *Bacteroides* bacterial strains (117).

Apoptosis. In normal mucosa, the inflammatory response is terminated by induction of apoptosis in activated T cells once the pathogen has been eliminated. In CD, however, mucosal T lymphocytes are resistant to apoptosis, leading to their accumulation and the persistence of the inflammatory response (115,127). In UC patients, T cells are more susceptible to Fas-mediated apoptosis (116). The Fas ligand is strongly expressed by T cells in active UC, but not in CD, suggesting that Fas-Fas ligand–induced apoptosis contributes to mucosal damage in UC (147,149).

CROHN'S DISEASE

Definition. *Crohn's disease* is an idiopathic chronic inflammatory disease that most commonly affects the terminal ileum and cecal region, but may affect any portion of the gastrointestinal tract from the mouth to the anus. Diseased segments are frequently separated by intervening "skip areas" of essentially endoscopically normal gut. Inflammation in CD may be transmural, resulting in stenosis, peri-intestinal abscesses, or fistulas. Dividing CD into inflammatory, stricturing, and perforating subtypes has provided a useful classification to predict response to interventions and outcomes.

Demography. As noted previously, there has been a steady rise in the incidence and prevalence of CD in Western Europe, Canada, and the United States over the past several decades (152,171a,174,191,192). The incidence of CD ranges from 3.4 to 14.6/100,000 in differing Western countries (152,171a,174,198, 199). CD affects all ages and both sexes, but its incidence peaks in the 2nd and 3rd decades of life. A second minor peak in incidence occurs in the 4th and 5th decades. CD is more common among Caucasians than other racial groups (169a, 176a), and is more common in Jewish than non-Jewish populations (186a).

Clinical Features. The signs and symptoms of CD are often subtle, frequently resulting in a delay in diagnosis until months, or sometimes, years after symptom onset. The presentation of a patient with CD depends in large part on the location, extent, and severity of the gastrointestinal involvement. CD most frequently affects the ileocecal region, followed (in decreasing order of frequency) by the terminal ileum alone, diffuse involvement of the small bowel, and isolated colonic disease (166).

Patients with ileocolonic disease experience intermittent episodes of crampy, often postprandial, abdominal pain. Pain may be referred to the periumbilical region, especially in children (166). The abdominal discomfort may be accompanied by loose stools. Stools are small, frequent at night, loose to watery, but not usually overtly bloody. Such symptoms are often attributed to dietary factors or irritable bowel disease. The past history commonly includes perirectal or perianal abscesses and fistulas. Physical examination may localize tenderness to the right lower quadrant. Occasionally, an inflammatory mass is palpable.

Patients with diffuse, small intestinal CD present with diffuse abdominal pain, diarrhea, anorexia, and weight loss. Malabsorption may also occur. These patients demonstrate diffuse abdominal tenderness on physical examination.

Colonic CD may mimic UC. Patients complain of diarrhea often containing blood and/or mucus, and crampy lower abdominal pain that may be relieved with defecation.

Growth retardation occurs in many pediatric patients with CD (167,173), and may occur before other signs or symptoms develop. The growth failure and malnutrition result from inadequate dietary intake, malabsorption, increased nutritional requirements, and in treated patients, from drug therapy, particularly corticosteroid use.

Progressive transmural inflammation with scarring and deep ulceration may ultimately lead to symptoms associated with intestinal obstruction, perforation, bleeding, or fistula formation. When obstruction develops, it usually does so in the distal ileum. Extensive mucosal ulceration predisposes the patient to bacterial translocation with all of its complications (170), including a predisposition to bacterial endocarditis (169). There is altered small intestinal motility with abnormal receptor-mediated small intestinal contraction (202). Deep linear ulcers or fistulas sometimes give rise to profound lower gastrointestinal bleeding (151,177).

Anorectal complications are common in patients with CD, and in some, may be the most troubling aspect of their disease. Approximately one quarter of patients with CD involving the small bowel and three quarters of individuals with colonic CD will have an anal lesion sometime during the course of their disease (193). Anorectal complications are more likely to occur during severe attacks, when the colon is extensively involved. Perianal involvement may predate, postdate, or develop concurrently with primary intestinal CD. Lesions in this area consist of perianal abscesses, ulcers, fissures, fistulas, and strictures of the anal canal.

Esophageal involvement occurs in as many as 6 percent of CD patients (171). Esophageal lesions include esophagitis, aphthous ulcers, strictures, and granulomas (189). Gastric CD typically involves the distal stomach, and results in thickening and sometimes granulomatous inflammation of the gastric wall. In some patients, this distal inflammation results in pyloric obstruction. Patients with gastric CD often have concomitant duodenal involvement. Gastric CD may, however, antedate small bowel involvement, and some of the reported cases of isolated granulomatous gastritis may actually represent early gastric CD. Patients with gastroduodenal involvement present with early satiety, nausea, vomiting, and epigastric pain.

A sudden worsening of clinical symptoms or an unusual disease presentation should alert one to the possibility of ischemia or viral infection superimposed on preexisting CD. Ischemia may develop secondarily to vasculitis, or may occur because of endothelialitis resulting from infection with cytomegalovirus, particularly if immunosuppressive therapy has been utilized.

Gross Findings. CD classically involves the distal 15 to 25 cm of the terminal ileum, often in association with disease involving the right colon, but any part of the gastrointestinal tract may be involved. Transition from involved to uninvolved areas is usually abrupt in the small bowel, but is less well defined in the large intestine.

The external surface of the involved bowel appears hyperemic and may be covered with a serosal exudate (fig. 15-2). Areas of serositis are rough and nodular, and may coexist with dense fibrous adhesions between bowel loops or between the bowel and other abdominal or pelvic organs or the abdominal wall. Fat encircles the antimesenteric serosal surface, producing a pattern known as "creeping fat" (fig. 15-3). Miliary serosal lesions, the macroscopic equivalent of granulomas, may be seen. The miliary lesions are multiple, minute, whitish nodules on the serosal surface. They are usually distributed along the serosal lymphatics and seen on the surface of the adjacent mesentery and peritoneum. They grossly resemble peritoneal seeding by carcinoma or serosal involvement by miliary tuberculosis.

Initially, the intestinal wall remains pliable, even though it may appear slightly thickened,

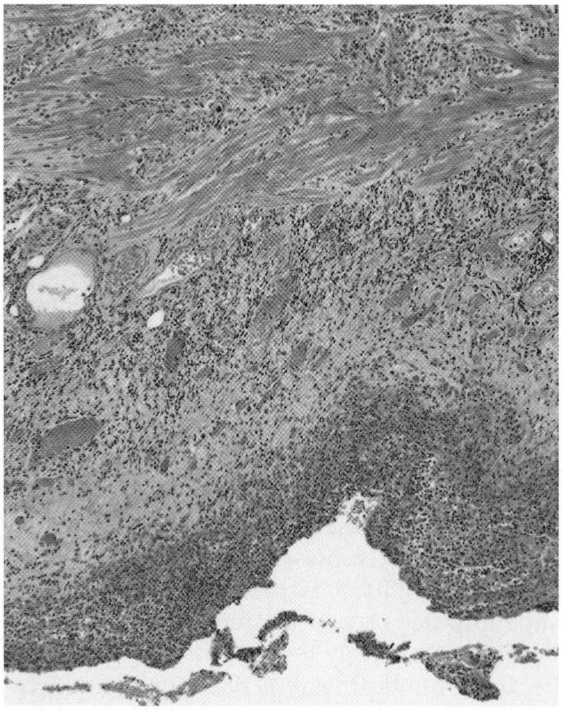

Figure 15-2

SEROSAL SURFACE APPEARANCE IN CROHN'S DISEASE

The marked acute serositis corresponds to the portions of the serosal surface covered by exudate.

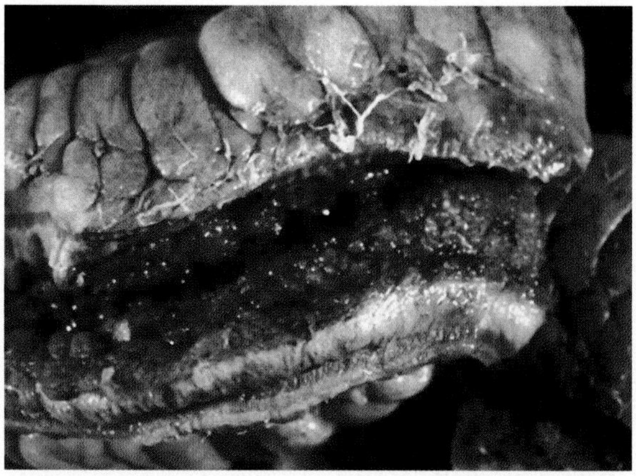

Figure 15-3

CREEPING FAT IN A PATIENT WITH CROHN'S DISEASE

The overlying serosa appears dull and fibrous adhesions can be seen. (Courtesy of the Division of Gastrointestinal Pathology, Armed Forces Institute of Pathology, Washington, DC.)

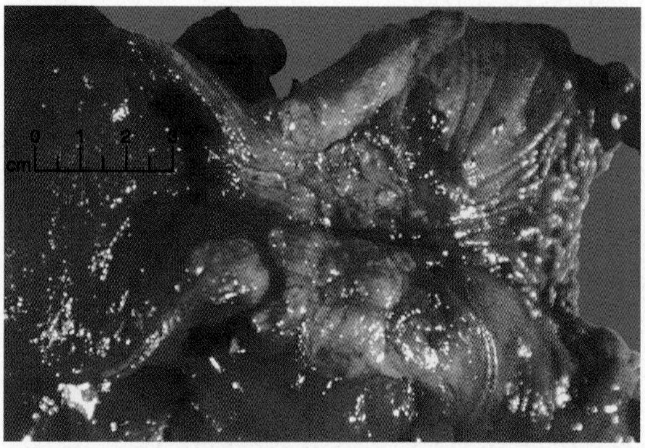

Figure 15-4

CROHN'S STRICTURE

The terminal ileum is markedly narrowed just proximal to the ileocecal valve. The mucosa is extensively ulcerated, showing a cobblestone pattern.

but with disease progression, the bowel becomes increasingly fibrotic and rigid. Eventually, a stricture may develop, resulting in obstruction (fig. 15-4). This usually occurs in the area of the distal ileum near the ileocecal valve. Large inflammatory pseudotumors may form at this site, simulating carcinoma. Granulomas within the lymph nodes may be grossly visible as tiny gray-white specks.

The earliest grossly visible mucosal change is the formation of an aphthous ulcer. As these ulcers enlarge, they may develop a hemorrhagic rim, which makes them visible. In their early stages, aphthous ulcers are most easily seen in the colon because villi tend to obscure their presence in the small intestine. Aphthous ulcers are not specific for CD, but also occur in other conditions including infectious enterocolitis. In addition, aphthous type ulcers may be transiently found following use of phosphate-based bowel preparations. In some patients, these tiny ulcers are the only or predominant sign of the disease, whereas in other patients, they are associated with more severe changes elsewhere in the bowel. Recognition of discrete ulcers in areas of otherwise normal mucosa may precede the development of more flagrant changes of CD by weeks or years.

Aphthous ulcers eventually enlarge into discontinuous, serpiginous or linear ulcers. At this stage, the mucosa appears reddened and swollen. Islands of nonulcerated mucosa are

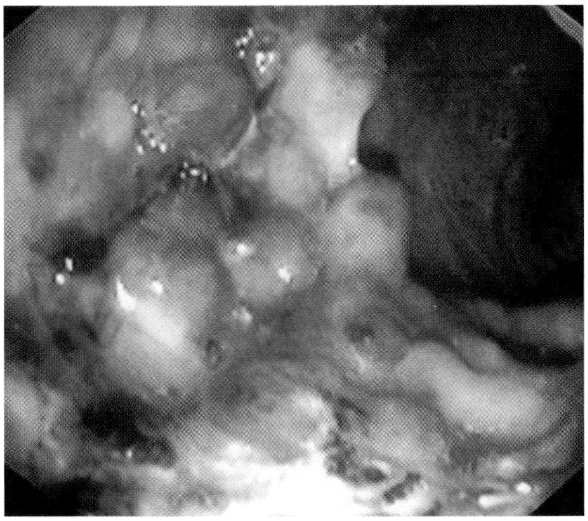

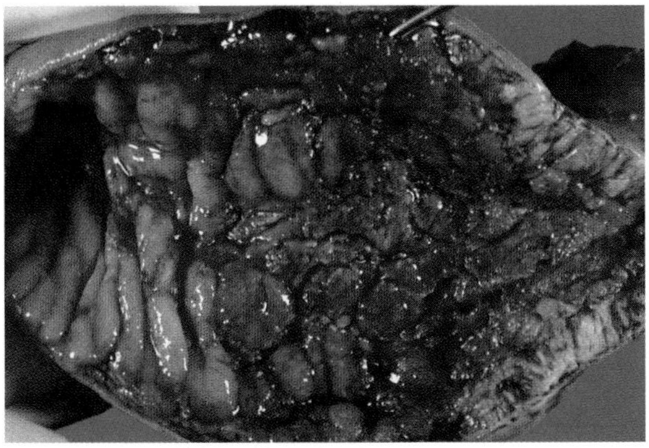

Figure 15-5

MUCOSAL COBBLESTONING IN CROHN'S DISEASE

Top: Endoscopic view of the ileal mucosa shows narrow ulcers running in different directions, giving the mucosal surface a cobblestone-like appearance.

Bottom: Numerous linear ulcers criss-cross the mucosa of the terminal ileum, giving it a cobblestone appearance.

interspersed among ulcerated areas, producing a cobblestoned appearance (fig. 15-5). Intervening "normal" bowel separates diseased bowel segments, creating skip areas (fig. 15-6). This patchy pattern of inflammation contrasts with the continuous pattern of inflammation and prominent rectal involvement seen in UC.

When the linear ulcers heal, long "railroad track" scars remain. With disease progression, the cut surface of the bowel demonstrates full-thickness inflammation, scarring, and fibrosis of the submucosa, muscularis propria, and serosa. The mucosa may ultimately become atrophic in long-standing disease.

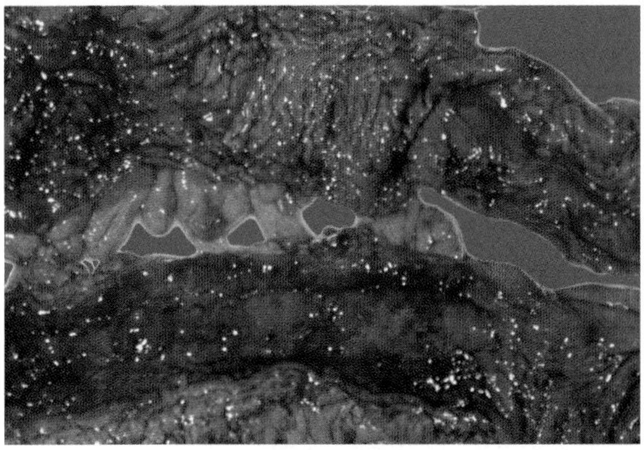

Figure 15-6

CROHN'S DISEASE

There are areas of colonic mucosal flattening, ulceration, and cobblestoning. More normal-appearing colonic mucosa intervene between areas that are actively inflamed and ulcerated.

Inflammatory polyps and pseudopolyps develop in association with CD (fig. 15-7). The former consist of inflamed mucosa, whereas the latter are residual mucosal islands between areas of ulceration. Inflammatory polyps may on occasion become quite large, measuring several centimeters in maximum dimension; however, they are rarely large enough to precipitate bowel obstruction. In addition to the presence of bulky, lobulated polyps, narrow, tall, filiform postinflammatory polyps may be seen, the result of abnormally healed mucosal remnants after ulceration. Inflammatory polyps may bleed, and may also aggravate colonic protein loss.

Fistulas and adhesions occur less commonly in patients with colonic involvement than in those with small intestinal disease. Fistulas often develop spontaneously, but occur more frequently in patients who have had previous surgery and who have residual diseased bowel. If the process remains localized, an abscess forms.

Perforation of the intestine is uncommon, affecting 1.5 percent of CD patients (164). The reason for this is that penetration of the tissues by the inflammatory process occurs slowly, causing loops of inflamed bowel to adhere to one another, thereby walling off any free perforation that might occur. Occasionally, a mass may be palpable as a consequence. Perforations result from deep penetration of fissures or fistulas through the bowel wall, or from complicating ischemia.

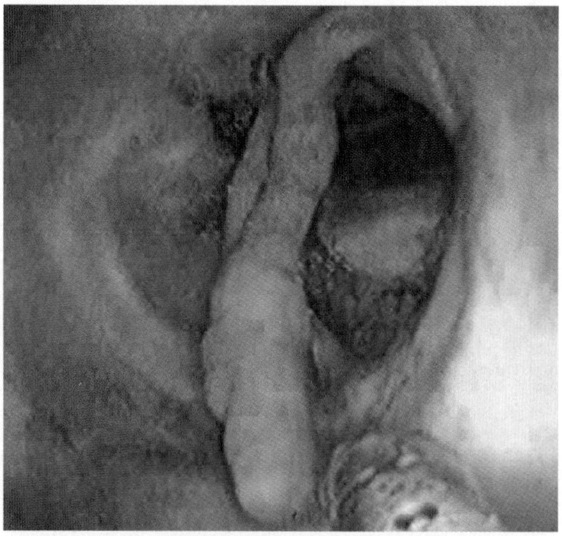

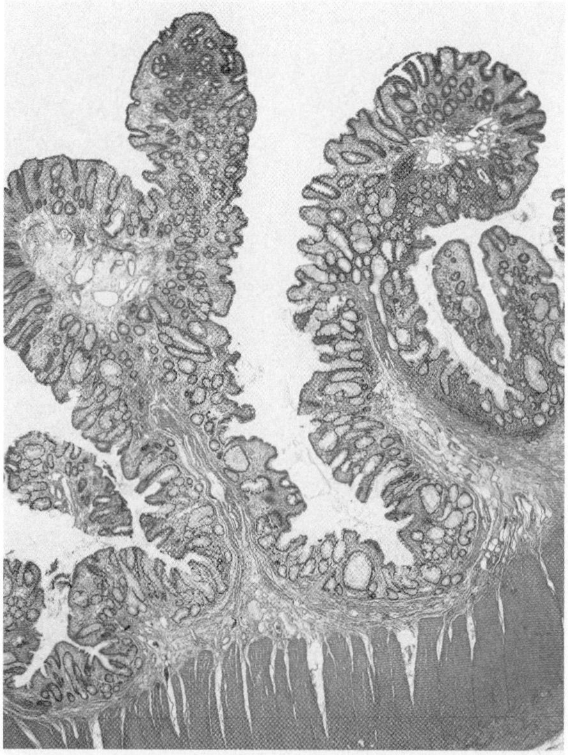

Figure 15-7

FILIFORM POLYPS IN CROHN'S DISEASE

Above: Endoscopic view of a long finger-like post-inflammatory polyp in a strictured area of the ileum.

Right: Low-power view shows the mucosa thrown into elongated, finger-like, filiform polyps.

CD is frequently complicated by strictures in the small and large intestine. These strictures lead to partial, intermittent obstruction. Strictures and fistulas are more common with ileitis, ileocolitis, and perianal disease than with disease predominating in the colon. Strictures may be multiple. They result from transmural inflammation, fibrosis, scarring, and fibromuscular proliferation. Malignant change may also lead to strictures and bowel obstruction.

Microscopic Findings. The ease of making the diagnosis of CD depends on whether a biopsy or resection specimen is examined. Resection specimens are more likely to exhibit all of the classic changes of CD, especially those that typically affect the deeper layers of the bowel wall. The biopsy diagnosis of CD remains more problematic because all the characteristic histologic features, including granulomas, are nonspecific, especially when only the mucosa and superficial submucosa are available for examination. The pattern and distribution of changes in biopsies are frequently characteristic enough to suggest that CD is present or to enable the exclusion of other entities in the differential diagnosis.

Architectural Changes. The patchy distribution of CD results in an epithelium that exhibits a range of changes, depending on whether or not the tissues are examined early or late in the course of the disease and whether the tissues come from more normal or more diseased parts of the bowel. The epithelium ranges from completely normal, to acutely damaged, chronically damaged, or regenerative. In areas affected by active disease, the normal architecture of crypts and villi is distorted (fig. 15-8). This architectural distortion is characterized by glandular irregularity and branching as well as glandular shortening in which the bases of the crypts no longer reach the muscularis mucosae. These architectural changes are appreciated best in sections of crypts cut in a plane perpendicular to the muscularis mucosae. In tangentially cut sections, the distorted crypts are recognized by the presence of cross sections of glands that show variable diameters (fig. 15-9). The epithelium lining the distorted glands often appears hyperplastic. In the small intestine, villi become distorted or atrophic. Pyloric metaplasia is frequently seen (see below). The presence of distorted villi and/or crypts, areas of pyloric metaplasia, or increased numbers of Paneth cells, especially in the left colon, indicates that the disease is chronic.

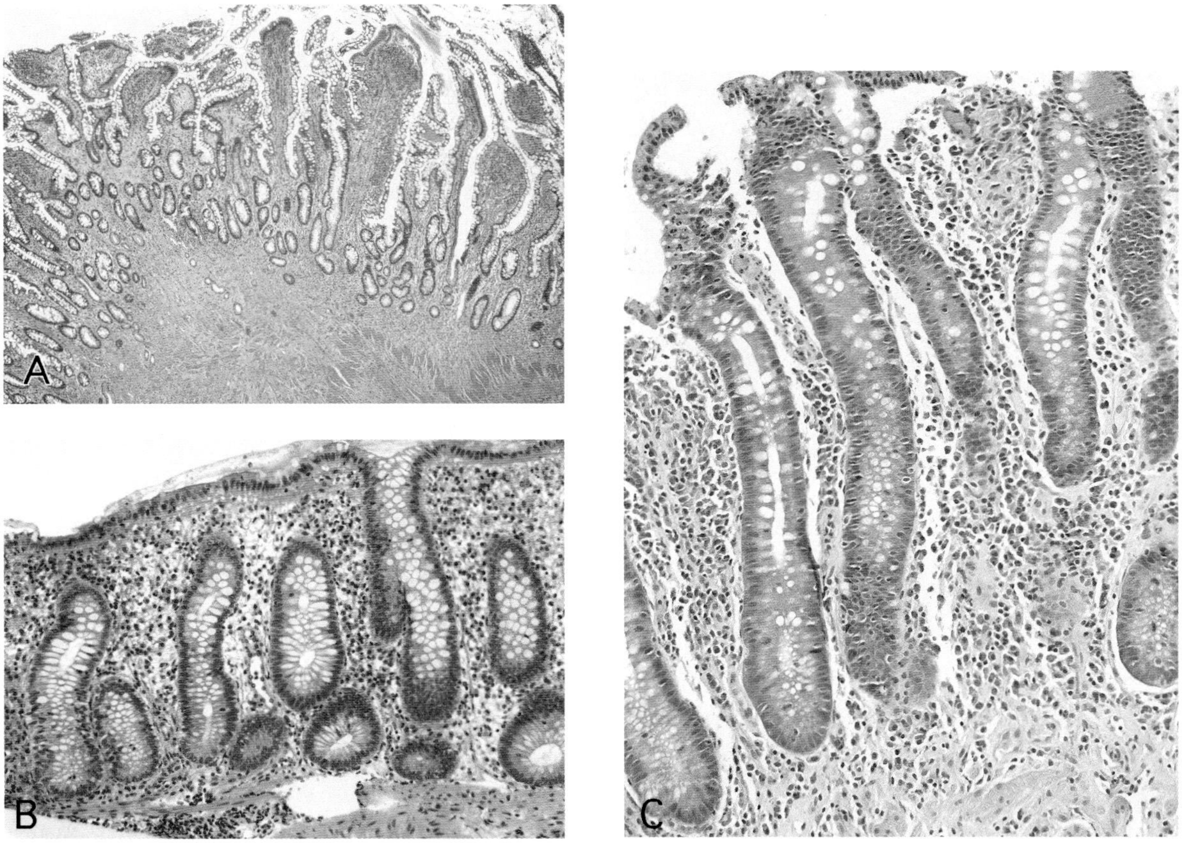

Figure 15-8

ARCHITECTURAL ALTERATIONS IN CROHN'S DISEASE

A: In the ileum, the villi appear blunted and irregular. The crypts are elongated and branched in many areas. The glands no longer rest on the muscularis mucosae, but are separated from it by fibrous tissue.

B: Some architectural abnormalities are present even in areas of inactive disease. This photograph shows a branched colonic crypt, but no significant inflammation.

C: The colonic crypts are elongated and irregular, but the architecture is not as severely altered as is often seen in ulcerative colitis.

Mucosal Inflammatory Infiltrate. Early in the course of CD, increased numbers of mucosal plasma cells, lymphocytes, macrophages, mast cells, eosinophils, and neutrophils can be seen in nearly all layers of the bowel wall. A basal lymphoplasmacytic infiltrate occupies the lower part of the mucosa (fig. 15-10). In active disease, neutrophils emigrate from the circulation into the mucosa, infiltrating the intestinal epithelium, and forming the lesion known as cryptitis (fig. 15-11). Collections of neutrophils within the crypt lumens are called crypt abscesses (fig. 15-11). Variable edema or fibrosis is present, depending on the stage of the disease. The inflammatory infiltrate often surrounds submucosal and serosal lymphatics and blood vessels where they penetrate the muscularis propria. Denser lymphocytic aggregates also lie in the submucosa away from the lymphatics or are scattered throughout all layers of the bowel wall (fig. 15-12).

An early but nonspecific finding of CD is an increased number of eosinophils and macrophages in the lamina propria beneath the surface epithelium (fig. 15-13). Mucosal and submucosal mast cell hyperplasia and degranulation are constant features of both UC and CD. Dendritic cells lie adjacent to granulomas and fissures. They are arranged in band-like zones at the bottom of ulcers or fissures, perhaps playing a scavenging role directed against microbial

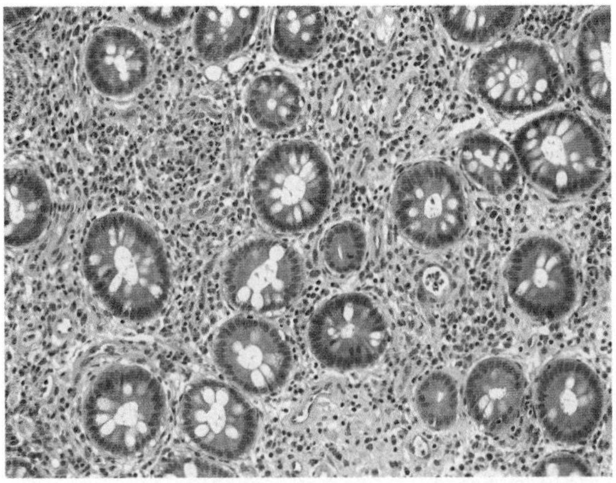

Figure 15-9

ACTIVE CROHN'S COLITIS

Architectural distortion is present in this tangential section. The crypts are no longer evenly spaced, nor are they of similar size and shape. Crypt abscesses are present, an indicator of active disease.

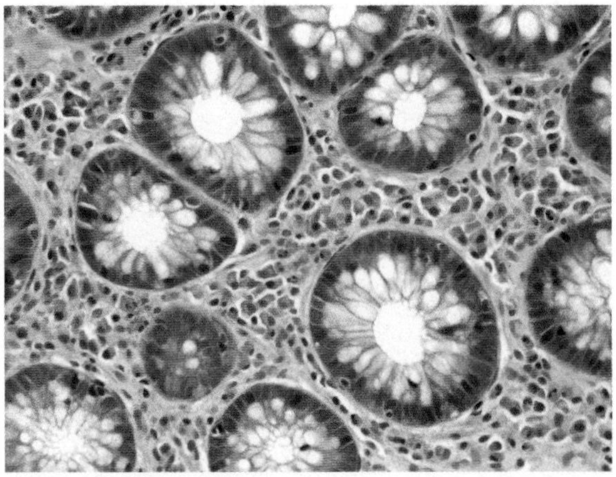

Figure 15-10

CROHN'S DISEASE

The lamina propria contains a dense mixed inflammatory infiltrate composed of lymphocytes, plasma cells, and numerous eosinophils. No active inflammation is present in this microscopic field.

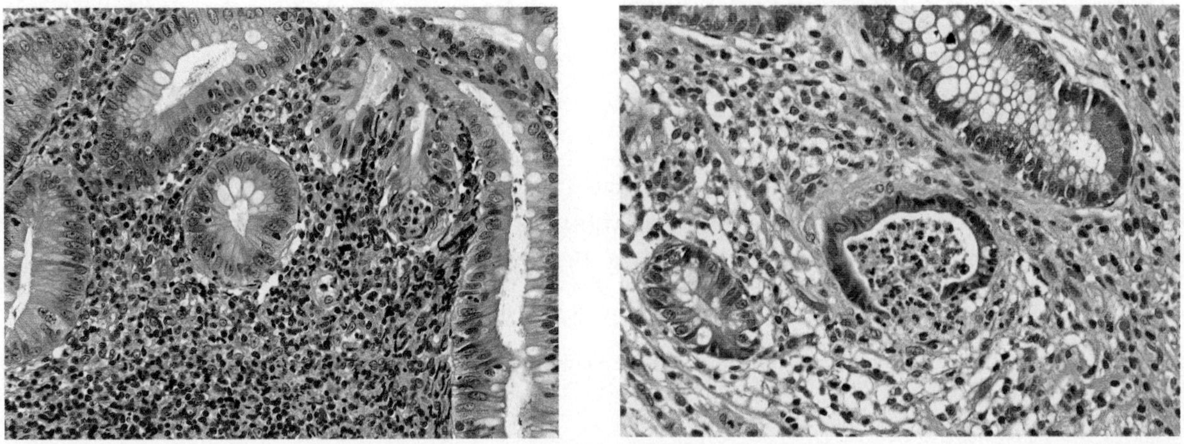

Figure 15-11

ACTIVE INFLAMMATION IN CROHN'S DISEASE

Left: The lamina propria contains a dense infiltrate of chronic inflammatory cells. In addition, focal cryptitis is present in which neutrophils infiltrate the colonic epithelium individually and in small groups.

Right: A cluster of neutrophils forms a crypt abscess with rupture as neutrophils spill into the surrounding lamina propria.

agents or dietary substances penetrating the gastrointestinal wall through the mucosal defects. Aggregates of macrophages lead to the formation of noncaseating granulomas.

Aphthous and Other Ulcers. Two distinctive types of ulceration affect the small and large intestines in CD. The first is the histologic equivalent of the grossly evident aphthous ulcer. This lesion develops even before inflammatory cells diffusely infiltrate the lamina propria.

Aphthous ulcers initially develop in areas overlying lymphoid follicles (fig. 15-14). Antigen entry into M cells located in these areas may lead to the proliferation of antigen-sensitized cells and granuloma formation. As the lesion progresses, it superficially ulcerates, obliterating

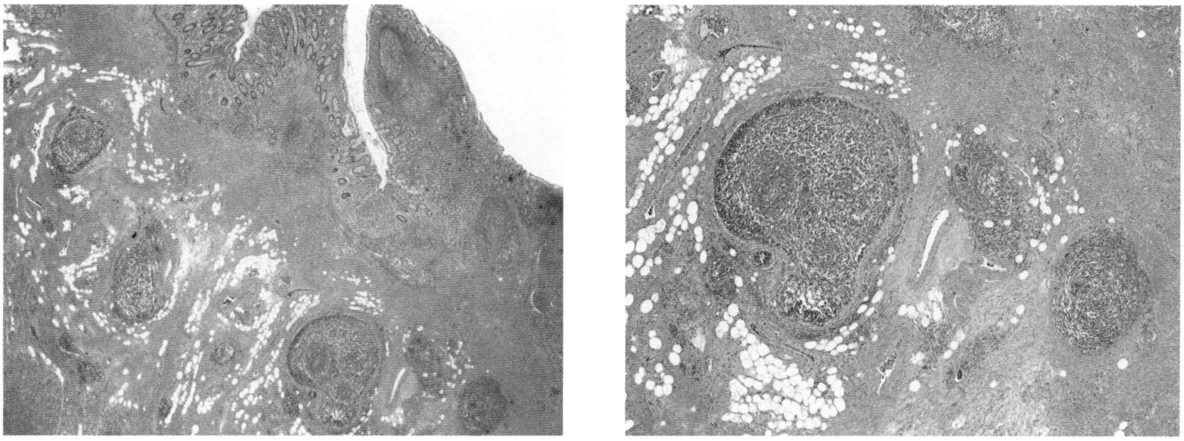

Figure 15-12

LYMPHOID AGGREGATES IN CROHN'S DISEASE

Left: Many round lymphoid aggregates are in the colonic wall.
Right: In some foci, germinal centers are within the nodular mural collections of lymphocytes.

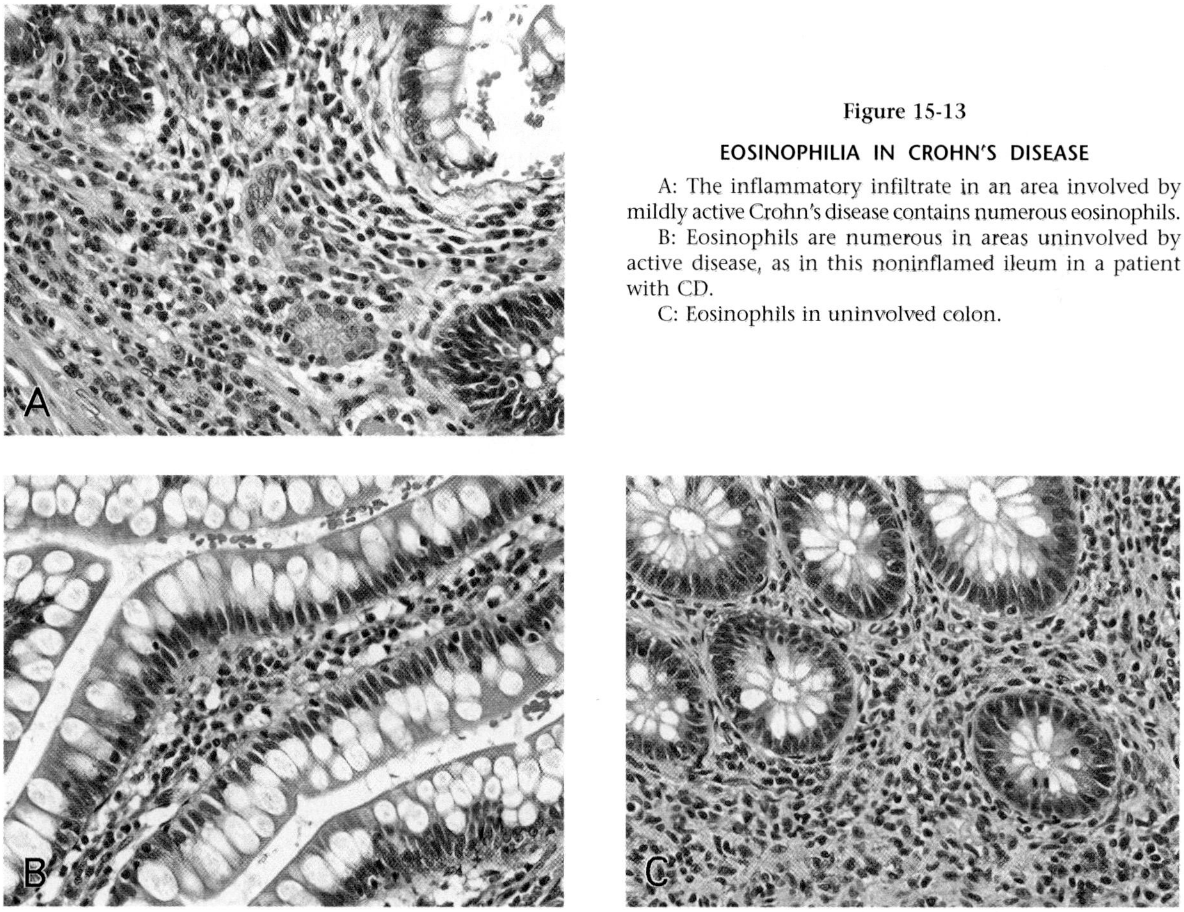

Figure 15-13

EOSINOPHILIA IN CROHN'S DISEASE

A: The inflammatory infiltrate in an area involved by mildly active Crohn's disease contains numerous eosinophils.

B: Eosinophils are numerous in areas uninvolved by active disease, as in this noninflamed ileum in a patient with CD.

C: Eosinophils in uninvolved colon.

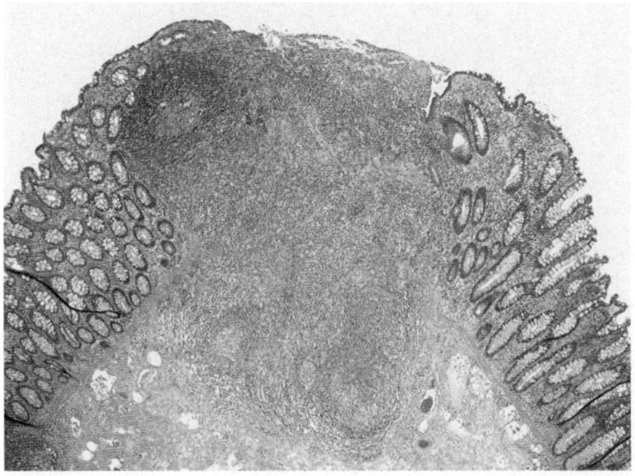

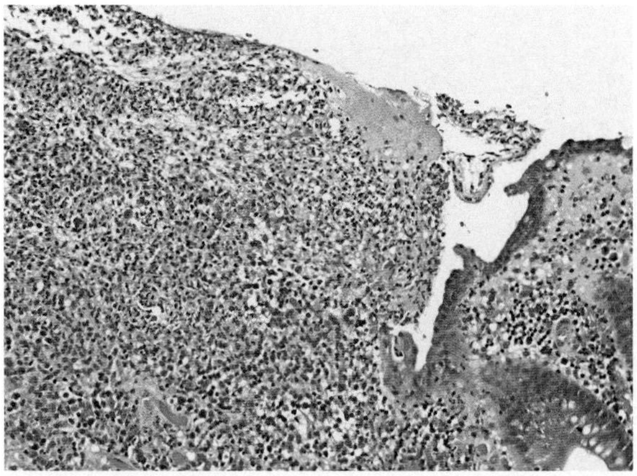

Figure 15-14

EARLY APHTHOUS ULCER FORMATION

Left: There is neutrophilic infiltration of the surface epithelium overlying this lymphoid aggregate and superficial erosion of the epithelium. Scattered crypts showed evidence of cryptitis.

Right: Higher-power view of the edge of the ulcer overlying the lymphoid follicle has scattered neutrophils admixed with lymphocytes.

its associated lymphoid follicle. A thin stream of mucus, neutrophils, and inflammatory debris enters from the ulcer mouth and empties into the bowel lumen. The ulcers progressively enlarge, forming a continuum with the larger ulcers normally seen in CD.

Knife-like, fissuring ulcers are typical of CD. They are deep, narrow, and oriented at right angles to the long axis of the bowel (fig. 15-15). Deep fissures may extend through the bowel wall and are the basis for fistula formation. Fissures contain acute inflammatory cells and a granulation tissue lining with conspicuous pale, plump histiocytic cells. The latter resemble the epithelioid histiocytes seen in granulomas. Giant cells may also be present.

Healed ulcers result in architectural distortion and a thickened or duplicated muscularis mucosae often associated with marked dense submucosal fibrosis (fig. 15-16). As a result, it is often impossible to distinguish the muscularis mucosae from the submucosa or underlying muscularis propria. These structures fuse with one another and may be replaced with dense fibrous tissue. The areas of fibrosis show proliferation of fibroblasts and myofibroblasts, usually with accompanying chronic inflammatory cells. Fibrosis extends from the bowel wall to involve adjacent structures and traps within it lobules of fat that may demonstrate variable degrees of necrosis. Ulcer healing may also entrap glandular epithelium within the submucosa or deeper tissues, a finding sometimes referred to as *enteritis cystica profunda*. These glands can sometimes be difficult to differentiate from invasive carcinoma (see below).

Mucosal Metaplasia. Patients with chronic disease often develop pyloric metaplasia, especially in the ileum (fig. 15-17). These metaplastic cells are sometimes also referred to as "ulcer-associated cell lineage cells." The pyloric-like glands usually occur singly or in clusters in the mucosa adjacent to ulcer margins. They are also found in areas of healed ulceration, away from actively inflamed mucosa. Metaplastic cells share many features of pyloric and Brunner glands, although they do not extend deeper than the muscularis mucosae, a feature that distinguishes them from Brunner glands. The cells appear clear or pale-staining and have a columnar shape. Their cytoplasm contains indistinct neutral mucin granules. The nuclei are round to oval and are located near the base of the cell.

These pyloric-like glands develop from the base of intestinal crypts where they extrude and proliferate downward, ramifying in the lamina propria to form a new gland. The gland then generates a duct that penetrates the surface, where it carries out secretions and also supplies cells to cover the surface (186).

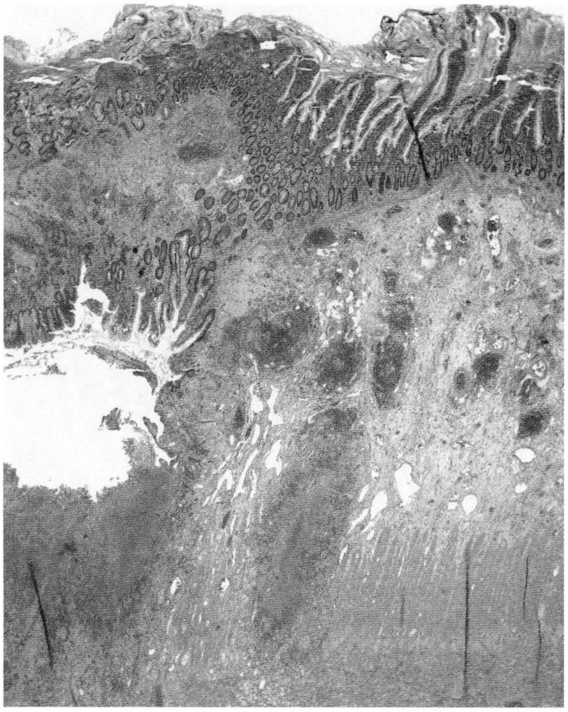

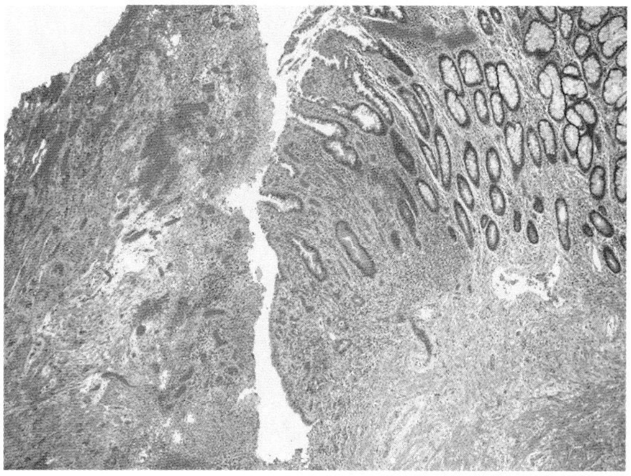

Figure 15-15

FISSURE IN CROHN'S DISEASE

Left: Low-power view of transmural inflammation in the terminal ileum. A deep knife-like fissure extends through the submucosa into the underlying muscularis propria. To the left, an abscess is forming.

Above: A mucosal fissure in another CD patient. The ulcer is deep and oriented perpendicular to the muscularis mucosae.

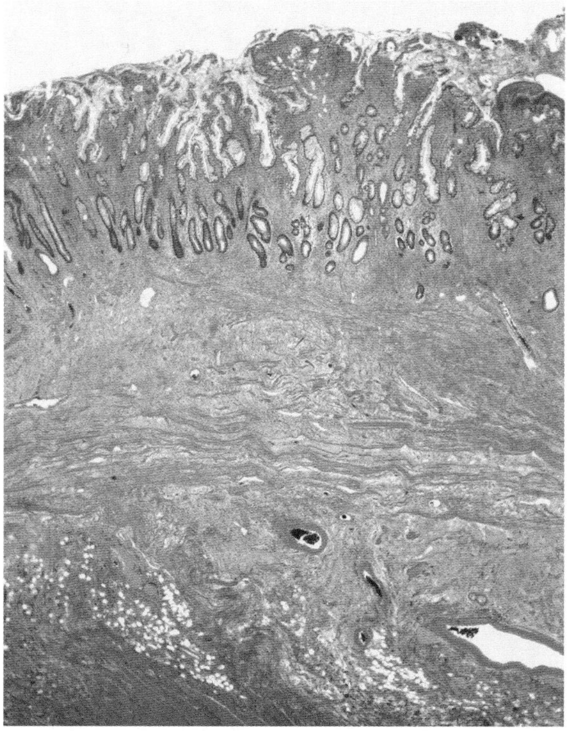

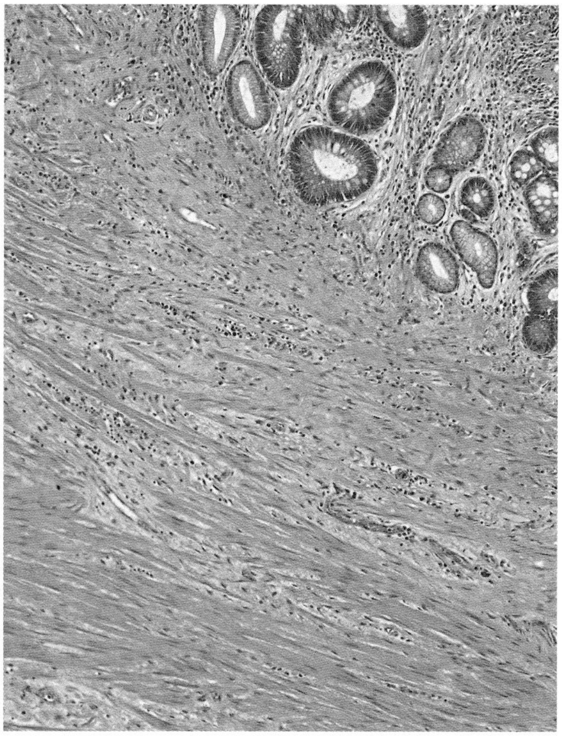

Figure 15-16

CROHN'S DISEASE

Left: There is poor distinction between the muscularis mucosae and the underlying submucosa.
Right: Higher-power view demonstrates marked thickening, duplication, and fragmentation of the muscularis mucosae.

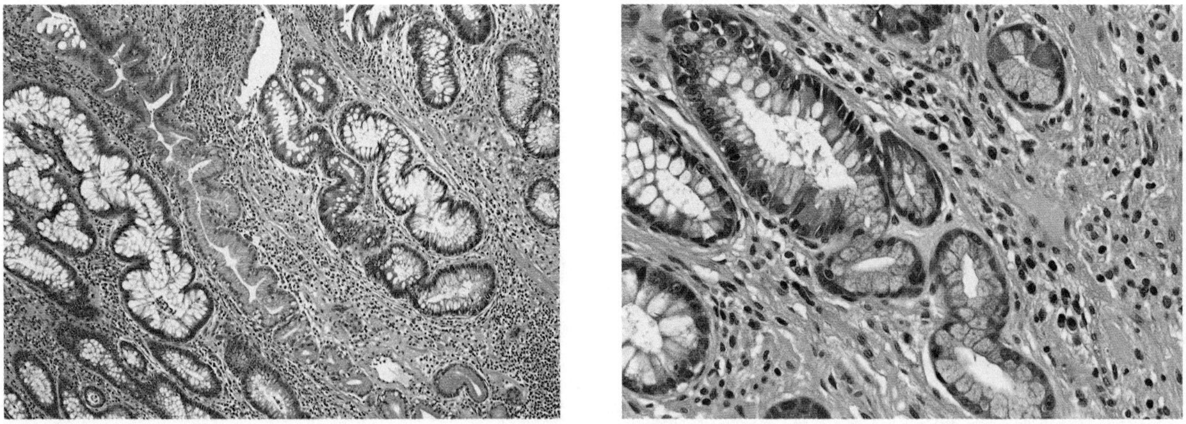

Figure 15-17

PYLORIC METAPLASIA

Left: Low-power view of the terminal ileum in a patient with active CD. The gland in the center appears more eosinophilic than its neighbors on either side.

Right: Higher-power view shows replacement of the normal enterocytes and goblet cells by cells with eosinophilic, vacuolated cytoplasm, resembling those seen in pyloric glands of the stomach. In addition, a few eosinophilic Paneth cells lie scattered in the crypt bases.

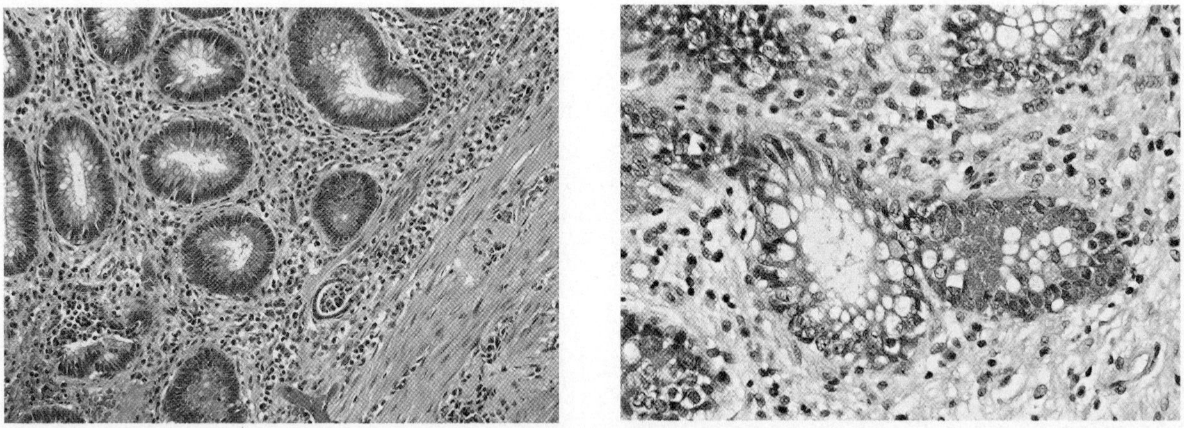

Figure 15-18

PANETH CELL METAPLASIA

Left: Paneth cells are present in the bases of the glands in this section taken from the sigmoid colon of a patient with IBD. Paneth cells are not normally present on the left side of the colon, and should therefore be regarded as metaplastic, and an indicator of chronic injury.

Right: Paneth cells with coarse eosinophilic granules.

Paneth cell metaplasia often develops in the large intestine of patients with CD (fig. 15-18). The number of Paneth cells in the small bowel may increase; however, these cells do not represent a form of metaplasia since Paneth cells are normally present in this location. It is important to note that Paneth cell metaplasia is not specific for CD, but can be seen in any chronic ulcerating disease process involving the colon.

Lymphoid Aggregates. Lymphoid aggregates, which may contain germinal centers, generally lie at the mucosal-submucosal junction as well as within deeper layers of the bowel wall, including the subserosal adipose tissue layer (see fig.

15-13). Lymphoid aggregates form even in the absence of granulomas, and may be more helpful than granulomas in establishing the diagnosis of CD. Lymphoid aggregates are not specific for CD since they can also be found in patients with UC. Their presence in the submucosa or deeper portions of the bowel wall, however, separated from the muscularis mucosae, and associated with submucosal edema or fibrosis in the presence of an intact mucosa, suggests the diagnosis of CD. Lymphoid hyperplasia within the terminal ileum in CD patients may additionally present as multiple lymphoid polyps.

Granulomas. The presence of small, compact, sarcoid-like granulomas is the sine qua non for the diagnosis of CD and, when present, is a reliable histopathologic criterion for differentiating CD from UC. Granulomas assume particular diagnostic significance only when they are seen in tissues remote from areas of ulceration in situations where foreign body or mucin granulomas are unlikely. Although the presence of granulomas represents a useful diagnostic feature for CD, they can be seen in numerous other conditions (Table 15-2).

The reported frequency with which granulomas are identified in CD varies markedly between studies. Possible explanations for this include the criteria used to diagnose granulomas; whether or not isolated giant cells are included among granulomas; the number of biopsies obtained; and the number of sections examined. Granulomas are found in the bowel wall in 50 to 87 percent of colectomy specimens (187,195) and in 15 to 36 percent of colonoscopic biopsies (179, 180). Upper gastrointestinal biopsies may also show granulomas in a small percentage of cases (205). Granulomas may additionally be found in regional lymph nodes, usually in association with granulomas elsewhere in the bowel wall.

Fewer granulomas occur in the ileum than in the colon in patients with CD. Granulomas progressively increase in number from the ileum to a maximum number in the rectum (155). Granulomas also occur in various other tissues and organs, including lymph nodes, pancreas, mesentery, peritoneum, liver, lung, kidney, and, occasionally, bones, joints, and skeletal muscle. The presence of granulomas does not indicate disease activity, nor does it affect the postoperative recurrence rate (184).

Table 15-2

CONDITIONS ASSOCIATED WITH INTESTINAL GRANULOMAS

Infection
Bacterial infection
Mycobacterium
Yersinia
Campylobacter
Salmonella
Shigella
Escherichia coli
Neisseria gonorrhoeae
Clostridium difficile
Treponema pallidum
Fungal infection
Chlamydial infection
Parasitic infection
Diversion Colitis
Sarcoidosis
Foreign Bodies
Chronic Granulomatous Disease of Childhood
Diverticular Disease–Associated Colitis

The granulomas consist of small, localized, well-formed, loose or more compact aggregates of epithelioid histiocytes, with or without Langerhans giant cells, and are often surrounded by a cuff of lymphocytes (fig. 15-19). Older lesions may show varying degrees of hyalinization and fibrosis. Granulomas that have definite foci of necrosis or suppuration, or are restricted to the edges of ruptured crypts, are not specific for CD (159,183). In addition, isolated pericryptal clusters of histiocytes as well as Langerhans type giant cells may be seen in patients with UC (172), most likely as a result of crypt rupture or herniation (fig. 15-20).

Vascular Lesions. Vascular lesions affect approximately 5 percent of CD patients. Obliterative changes include intimal proliferation, subintimal fibrosis, medial hypertrophy, medial fibrosis, and adventitial fibrosis, all without a significant inflammatory cell component. Degenerative arterial lesions may narrow the vascular lumen due to duplication of the internal elastic lamina with medial hypertrophy. Venous lesions feature an irregular vascular sclerosis with thickening of the wall due to hyperplasia of fibrous, elastic, and muscular tissues. Inflammatory vascular lesions consist of perivascular inflammation and chronic inflammatory and/

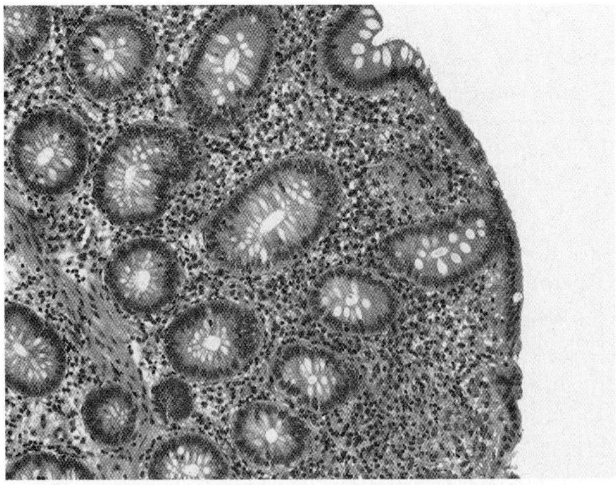

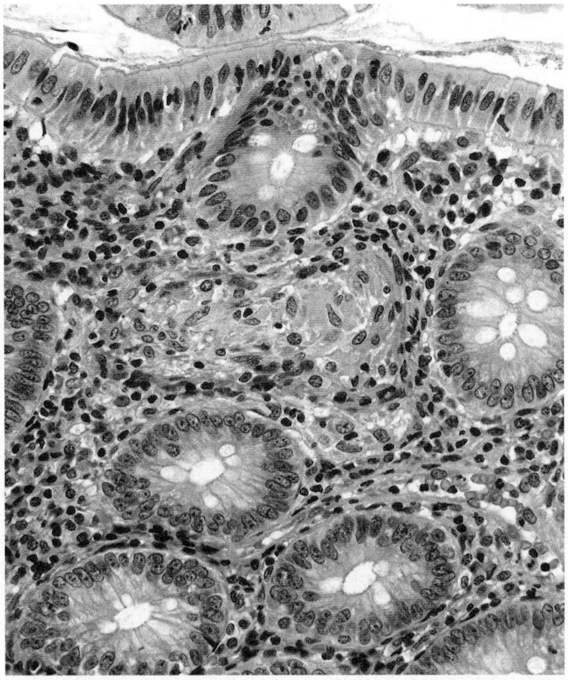

Figure 15-19

GRANULOMAS IN CROHN'S DISEASE

Above: A small compact granuloma in the upper portion of the mucosa is not associated with a damaged crypt.

Right: Higher-power view shows a compact collection of histiocytes without evidence of necrosis.

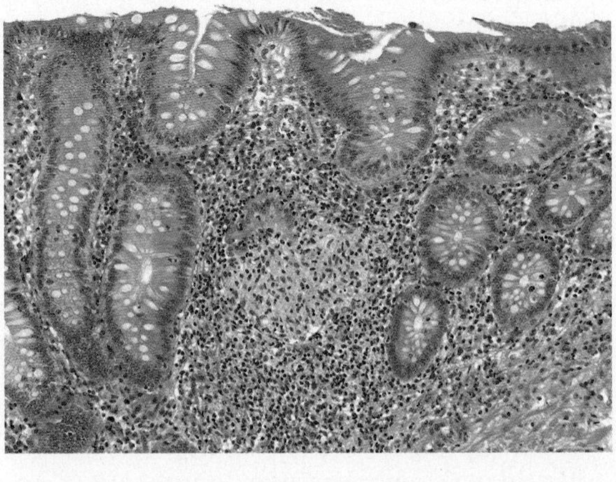

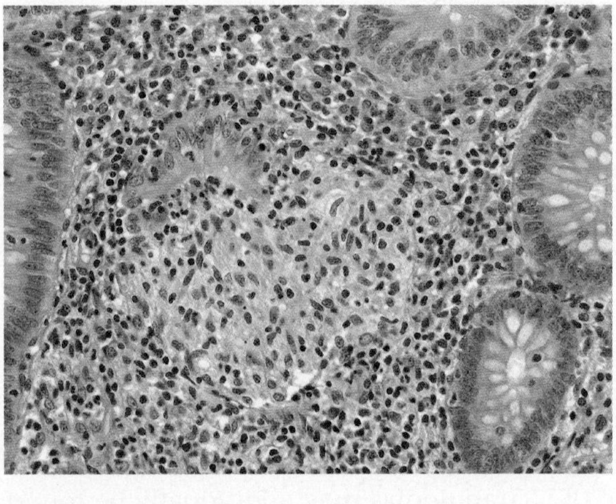

Figure 15-20

GRANULOMA ASSOCIATED WITH CRYPT RUPTURE

Left: A cluster of histiocytes (center) forms a small granuloma.

Right: On higher power, this focus of granulomatous inflammation is clearly associated with a partially destroyed colonic crypt. This biopsy was taken from a patient with UC, not CD.

or granulomatous cell infiltrates associated with an obliterative vasculopathy (fig. 15-21). Lymphocytes and plasma cells infiltrate one or more layers of small arteries or arterioles, interrupting the internal elastic fibers. The vascular changes seen in CD must be distinguished from primary systemic vasculitis involving the gastrointestinal tract. When primary vasculitis affects a patient with CD, extraintestinal manifestations of the disorder are usually evident.

Another notable feature of CD is submucosal lymphatic dilatation, which commonly coexists with edema and lymphoid hyperplasia (fig. 15-22). Plasma cells, eosinophils, and neutrophils

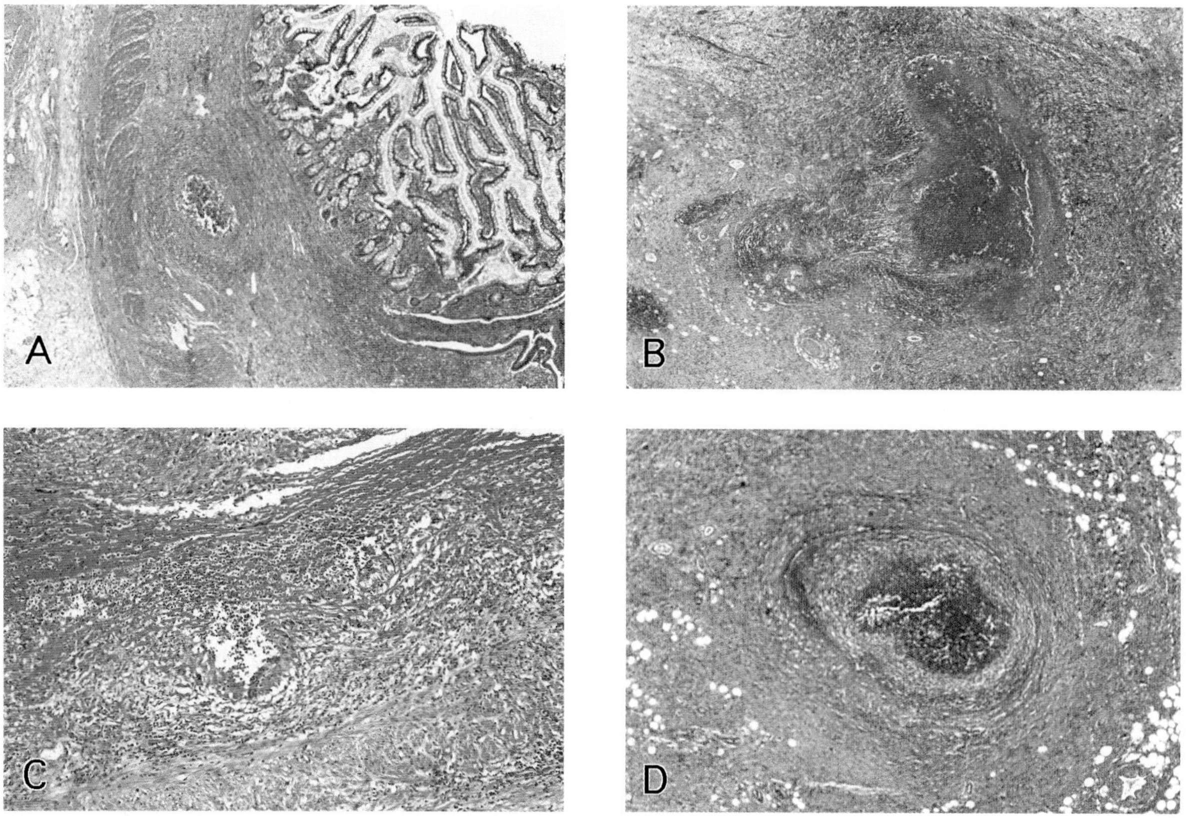

Figure 15-21

VASCULITIS IN CROHN'S DISEASE

A: A markedly inflamed submucosal vessel.

B: Higher-power view shows infiltration of the vessel wall by inflammatory cells with thrombosis. In some areas, the wall of the vessel demonstrates fibrinoid necrosis.

C: Higher-power view of the inflamed, necrotic vessel wall.

D: A Verhoeff stain shows the damage to the wall of another vessel. There is prominent intimal fibrosis with near complete occlusion of the vascular lumen.

may infiltrate along the dilated vessels. In more advanced stages of the disease, fibrous tissue replaces the edema.

Neural Changes. The autonomic neural plexuses often appear hypertrophic in CD (fig. 15-23). Large, irregular, fusiform nerve bundles are present throughout the submucosa and muscularis propria. These often contain increased numbers of ganglion cells. Occasionally, striking plexiform neuromatous proliferations are seen in association with tortuous thick-walled arterioles. They express MHC class II antigens (163) and thus the abnormal nerves become infiltrated with mast cells, lymphocytes, and plasma cells. The nerves also show evidence of extensive axonal and dendritic swelling and degeneration (194).

Displaced Epithelium. It is not uncommon to encounter displaced epithelium in resection specimens from CD patients (fig. 15-24). This is referred to as *enteritis cystica profunda* and *colitis cystica profunda* when it affects the small bowel and colon, respectively. Displaced epithelium results from epithelial implantation into the submucosa, muscularis propria, or serosa following mucosal ulceration or the formation of mucosal microdiverticula, a common event in CD patients. Mucosal repair following regeneration of an ulcer leaves the detached epithelium buried in the submucosa. It eventually becomes covered by intact mucosa. Displaced epithelium also results from epithelialization of fissures or fistulous tracts. The displaced epithelium often

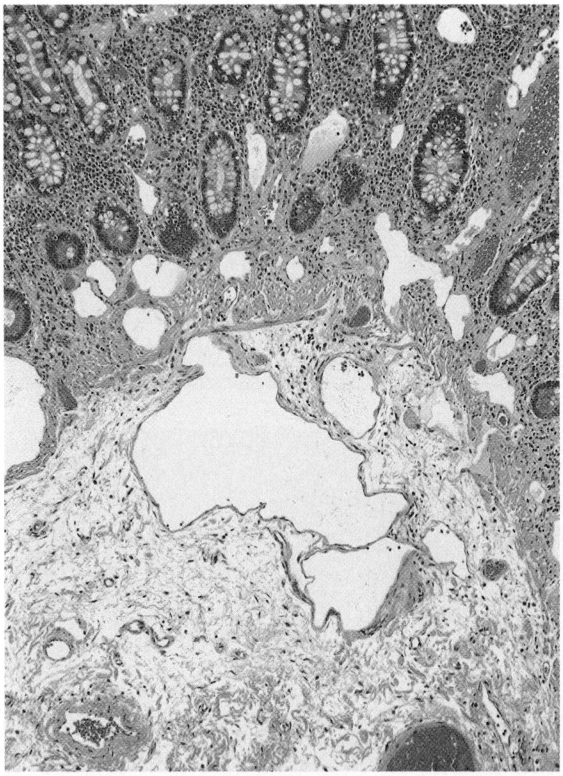

Figure 15-22

LYMPHANGIECTASIA IN CROHN'S DISEASE

The submucosal and mucosal lymphatic channels of the ileum are prominently dilated.

becomes cystically dilated, and contains large accumulations of mucin.

Grossly, the bowel wall containing displaced epithelium appears thickened. The cut surface demonstrates numerous cystic submucosal spaces that may contain mucin. The mucosa overlying such lesions usually shows histologic evidence of active or healed CD. Histologically, mucus-filled cysts are seen in the submucosa, muscularis propria, and serosa. These are lined by cuboidal to columnar epithelium containing numerous goblet cells, enterocytes, and Paneth cells, all supported by a normal lamina propria. Sometimes the cyst lining disappears due to pressure atrophy.

It is sometimes difficult to determine whether the displaced epithelium represents invasive mucinous carcinoma or merely displaced epithelium, especially when the lamina propria does not surround the glands or when the benign epithelium produces excessive amounts of mucin, resulting in large mucinous cysts containing scant epithelial elements (fig. 15-25). Features that help to rule out malignancy include the absence of desmoplasia, the presence of surrounding lamina propria, and an absence of cytologic atypia within the displaced glands. In some cases, however, it is impossible to determine whether one is dealing with displaced epithelium or invasive cancer, especially in cases where the overlying surface epithelium appears dysplastic.

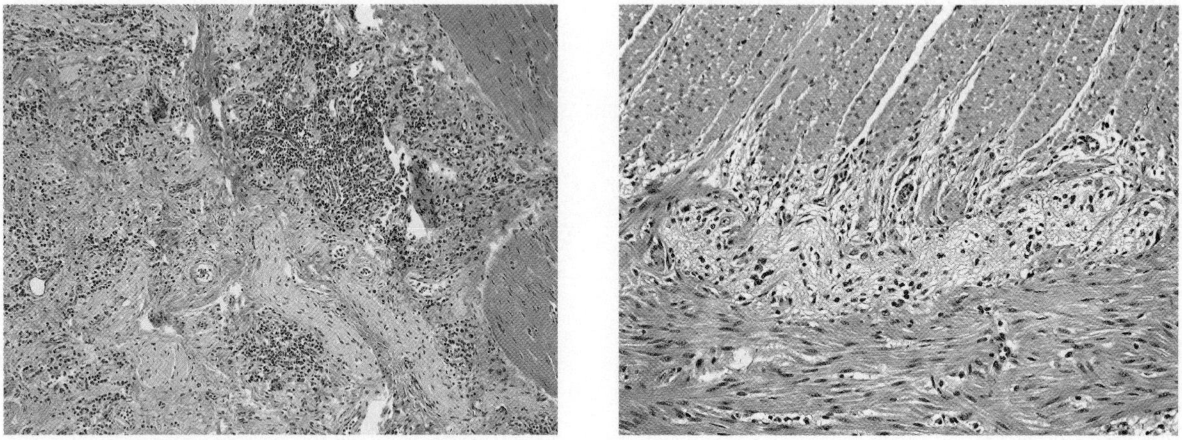

Figure 15-23

NEURAL HYPERPLASIA

Left: Disordered aggregates of large nerve fibers are in the submucosa.
Right: Hypertrophic nerve fibers are also seen in the myenteric plexus.

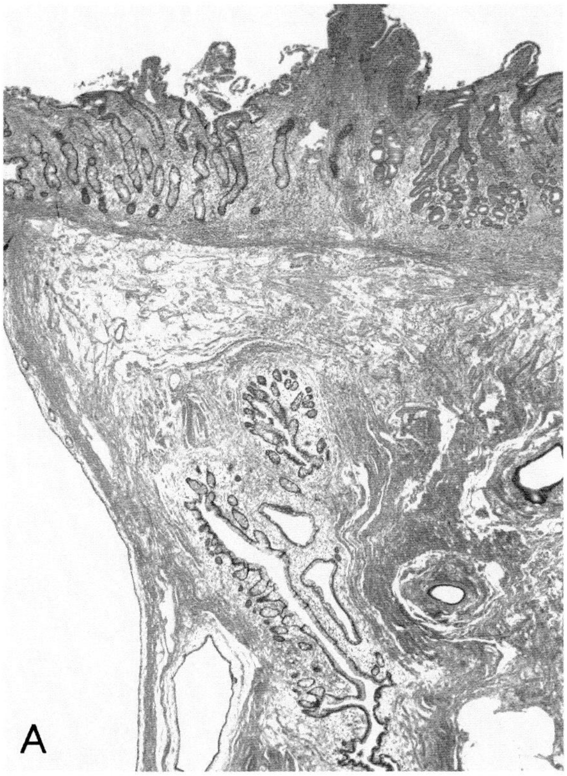

Figure 15-24

ENTERITIS CYSTICA PROFUNDA

A: Glands are deep within the submucosa of the ileum.

B: Cystically dilated gland within the submucosa.

C: These glandular elements are surrounded by normal-appearing lamina propria. In addition, the cells are basally arranged without evidence of cytologic atypia.

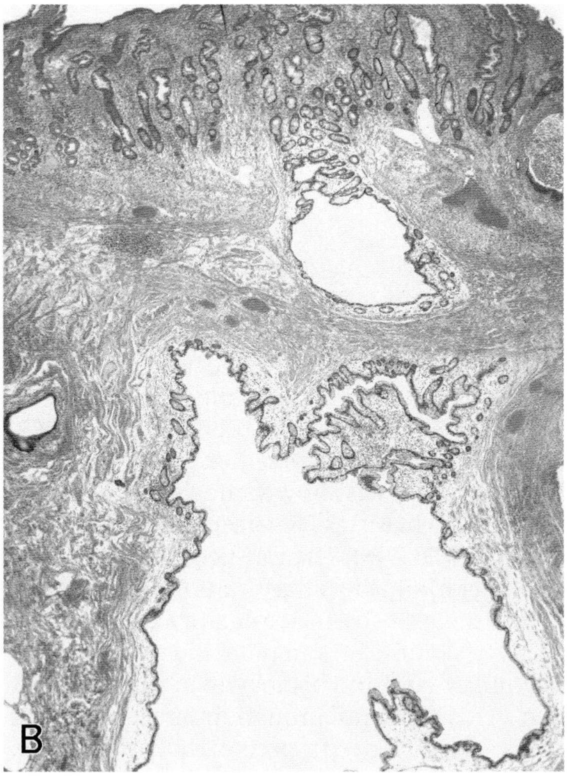

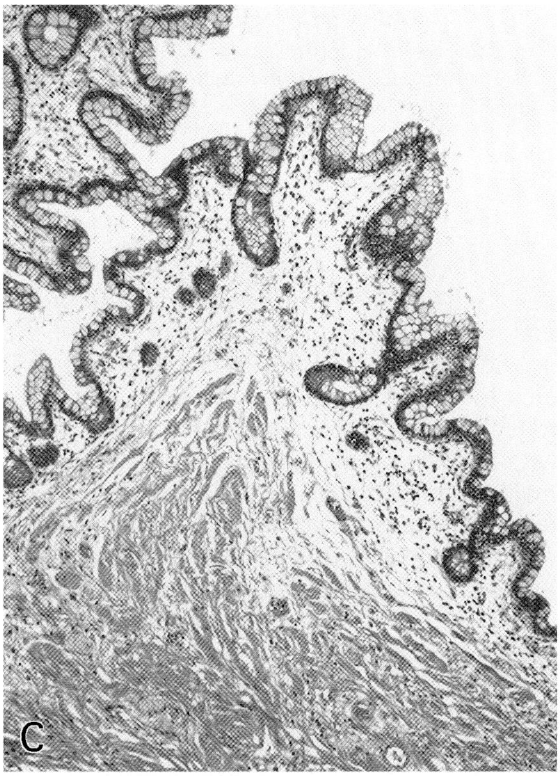

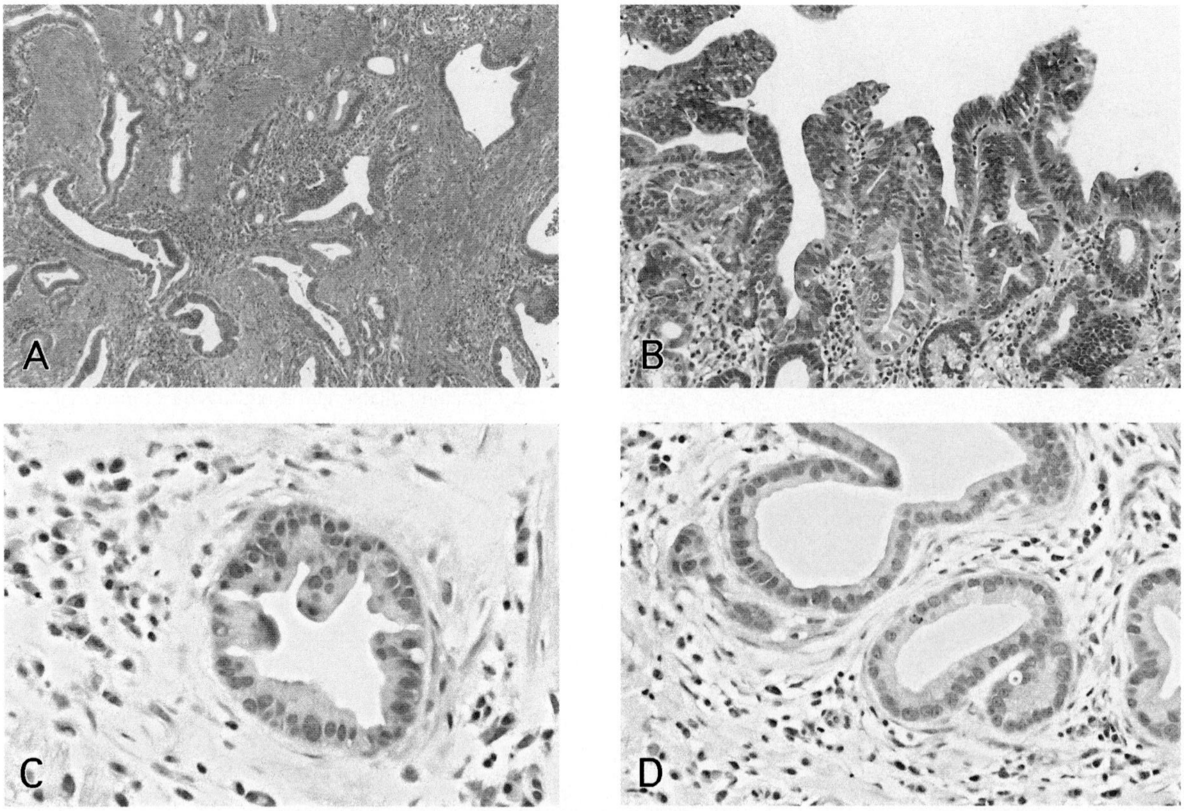

Figure 15-25

CROHN'S DISEASE, ENTERITIS CYSTICA PROFUNDA, AND INVASIVE ADENOCARCINOMA

A: Low-power view of an area of enteritis cystica profunda. The glands are surrounded by lamina propria.

B: The surface epithelium in this portion of the ileum shows evidence of dysplasia. The nuclei are large and atypical, and have lost their normal polarity.

C: Invasive well-differentiated adenocarcinoma: a gland with cytologic atypia, no surrounding lamina propria, and instead, a desmoplastic type stroma.

D: A few single invading cells lie within the desmoplastic stroma.

Histologic Features of Proximal Gastrointestinal Lesions. The villous architecture in the proximal small intestine may appear normal or the mucosa may be completely flattened and covered by an abnormal surface epithelium infiltrated by large numbers of neutrophils. Such areas of flattening may lie adjacent to more normal-appearing tissues. In the nonileal small intestine, the most severe damage occurs proximal to the ligament of Treitz. The mucosa may show histologic changes similar to those seen in the ileum (fig. 15-26). Erosions, increased numbers of lamina propria plasma cells and neutrophils, crypt abscesses, and pyloric gland metaplasia, often in the absence of granulomas, are seen. Surface epithelial cells vary from normal, to cuboidal, to completely flattened. Some appear vacuolated and others are frankly megaloblastic, presumably due to coexisting vitamin deficiencies. Very few intraepithelial lymphocytes are seen, but neutrophils are common. A normal biopsy does not exclude the diagnosis of CD because duodenal involvement may be patchy.

Gastric biopsies show some degree of abnormality in as many as 75 percent of patients with CD (175,176,205). The most commonly identified alteration is focal infiltration of the gastric pits and glands by inflammatory cells (fig. 15-27). These infiltrates may include neutrophils, T lymphocytes, and histiocytes in variable numbers. This focal inflammation affects both the neck region and deep aspects of the gastric glands,

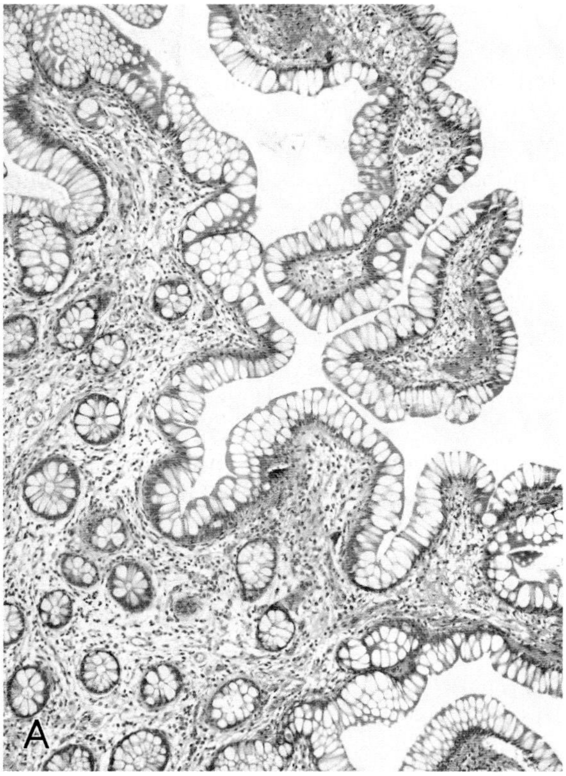

Figure 15-26

DUODENAL CROHN'S DISEASE

A: The duodenal architecture is distorted, and the lamina propria is edematous. There is no active inflammation in this tissue fragment.

B: Another tissue fragment from the same biopsy specimen shows dense inflammation within the lamina propria.

C: A crypt abscess is present.

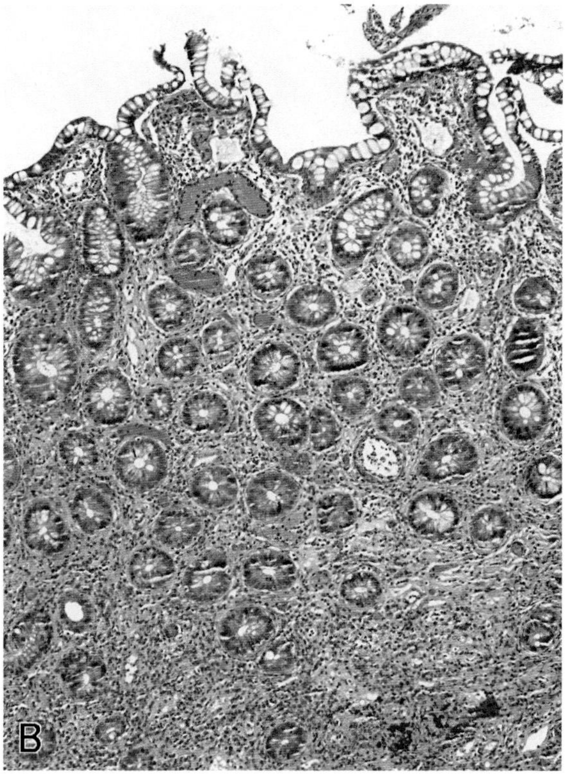

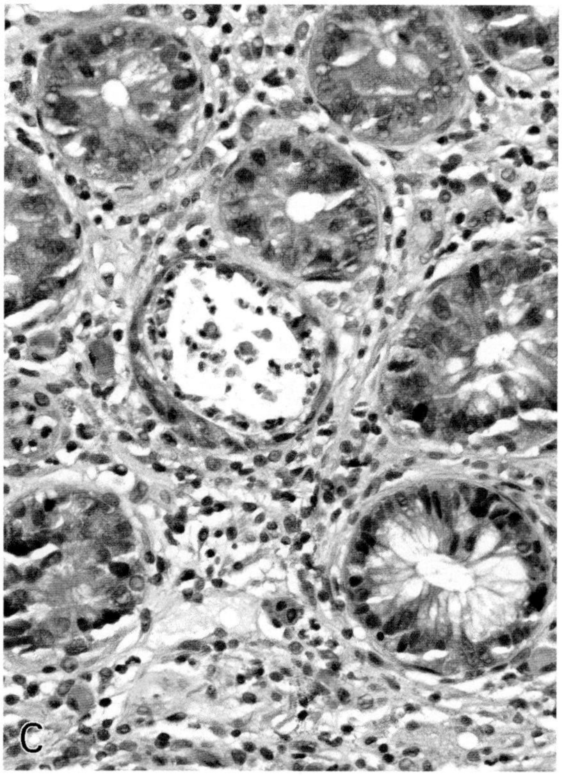

and is more commonly seen in the antrum than in the body of the stomach (175,176). Granulomas are seen in 9 to 16 percent of patients (fig. 15-28) (162,175,176,194,205). Granulomas are almost always associated with focal active gastritis. The major differential diagnosis is with *Helicobacter pylori* gastritis. *H. pylori* gastritis may also demonstrate chronic active inflammation, but the infiltrates are almost entirely neutrophilic, and localize to the neck region of the glands. The presence of deep active inflammation should alert the pathologist to the possibility of CD. *H. pylori* infection should be ruled out with the use of special stains in all patients with any form of chronic active gastritis. It is important to note that some patients with CD may have superimposed *H. pylori* infection (175,176,205).

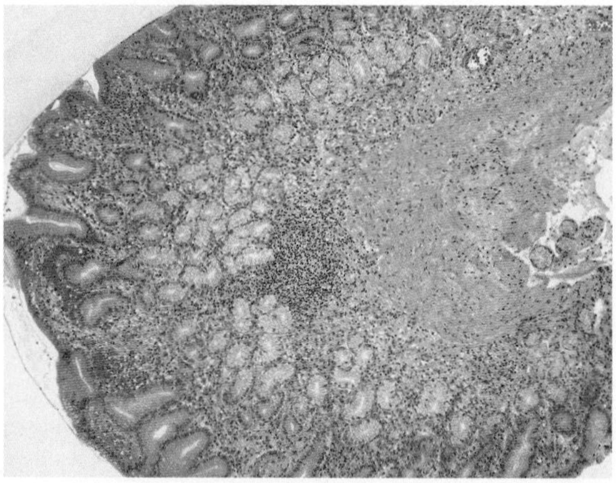

Figure 15-27

GASTRIC CROHN'S DISEASE

The antral biopsy shows patchy inflammation. A cluster of lymphocytes is in the deep mucosa. Less well-defined lymphocytic infiltrates are in other areas of the biopsy.

CD may affect the esophagus and when it does, it may be difficult to distinguish from other forms of granulomatous esophagitis, especially if a history of CD is not known. Clinically, severe forms of esophageal CD may simulate carcinoma because of the presence of an irregular, stenotic esophageal segment. Radiographic studies may demonstrate the presence of one or more aphthous ulcers, inflammation, fistulas, and strictures.

Crohn's Disease of the Head and Neck Region. Lesions may develop on the lips, epiglottis, and aryepiglottic folds of patients with CD (153,154, 204). Oral vesicular lesions and aphthous ulcers affect many patients. Typical CD is usually present in the gastrointestinal tract of these individuals, but occasionally the disease presents first in the oropharynx. Oral lesions appear grossly nodular and firm. Biopsy demonstrates the presence of chronic inflammatory cells and granulation tissue. Well-formed, noncaseating granulomas may also be present.

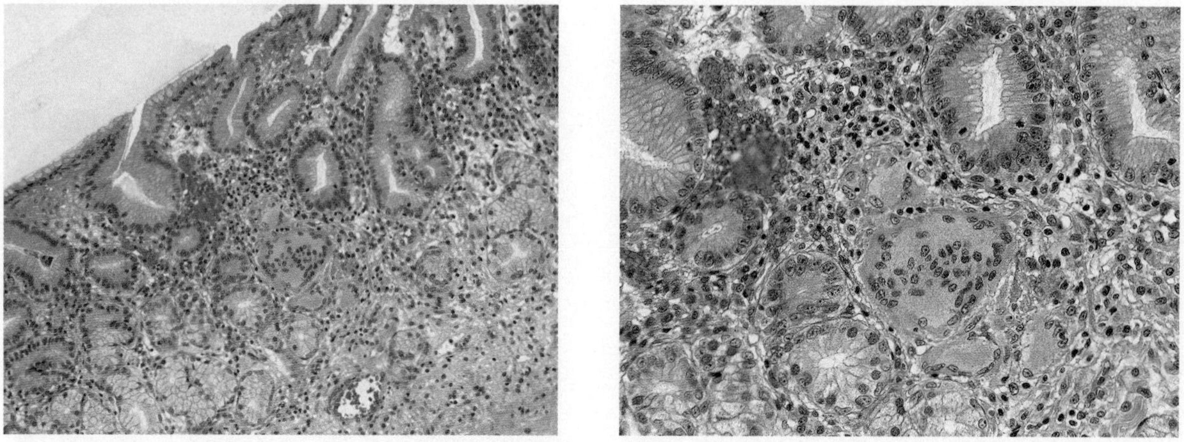

Figure 15-28

GRANULOMATOUS GASTRITIS IN CROHN'S DISEASE

Left: A small cluster of histiocytes is in the lamina propria.

Right: Higher-power view shows a compact aggregate of histiocytes and multinucleated giant cells. This granuloma is not associated with damaged gastric glands.

Differential Diagnosis. The differential diagnosis of CD includes UC (see below), other forms of active enterocolitis, and granulomatous enterocolitis. Differentiating IBD from acute infectious enterocolitis is sometimes difficult. Infectious enterocolitis generally lacks the architectural distortion and metaplastic changes commonly seen with IBD. In addition, the inflammation in infectious enterocolitis is often superficial. The inflammation within the lamina propria often contains numerous neutrophils, and edema is prominent in acute self-limited enterocolitis. The basal plasmacytosis characteristic of IBD is not seen. Cryptitis occurs commonly, and crypt abscesses are sometimes seen, but are not as prominent a feature as they are in IBD.

There are numerous causes of granulomatous enterocolitis, all of which enter into the differential diagnosis of CD. These are listed in Table 15-2. The granulomas seen in granulomatous enterocolitis with an infectious etiology frequently show evidence of necrosis, a finding that is almost never seen in CD-associated granulomas. In addition, acid-fast or Grocott stains may demonstrate the presence of mycobacterial or fungal organisms. Parasitic organisms may be identified on routine hematoxylin and eosin (H&E)-stained sections. Sarcoidosis is associated with the presence of compact granulomas similar to those seen in association with CD, but the other inflammatory changes that characterize IBD are absent.

Diverticular disease–associated colitis or isolated sigmoiditis may appear histologically identical to CD. Differentiation between these diseases requires knowledge of the distribution of the inflammation, and the presence or absence of diverticula.

Treatment. The medical treatment of CD is individualized based on the severity of symptoms and sites of involvement in each patient. Treatment options include steroids, anti-inflammatory agents, immunosuppressive agents, antibiotics, and the new biologic agents. Other forms of therapy include nutritional or dietary treatment and administration of probiotics.

Corticosteroids. Corticosteroids are effective in decreasing disease activity and inducing remission in most CD patients. Due to systemic side effects, however, long-term use of steroids is avoided. Newer agents, such as budesonide, that act only on the gastrointestinal mucosa and have fewer systemic effects are also useful, although many patients experience adverse reactions. Corticosteroid treatment has not been demonstrated to maintain remission.

Antiinflammatory Agents. Antiinflammatory agents such as sulfasalazine and mesalazine are used to treat mild to moderately active CD, or as maintenance medication in patients who have achieved remission of their disease through the use of steroids. These medications have significant side effects including headaches, nausea, pancreatitis, anemia, and dermatitis. Preparations that are released in the small intestine may be of value in enteric forms of the disorder. In general, patients with CD require higher doses of mesalamine than are traditionally used for patients with UC.

Immunosuppressive Agents. Azathioprine and 6-mercaptopurine are indicated in patients with steroid-dependent CD, extensive small intestinal disease, gastroduodenal disease, recurrent disease following prior bowel resection, and perianal fistulas refractory to other therapies. Methotrexate is used for long-term maintenance in adults with CD who are intolerant of the former preparations. Cyclosporine use in CD has been disappointing. Side effects of immunosuppressive agents include hypersensitivity reactions, bone marrow suppression, pancreatitis, and infectious complications.

Antibiotics. The antibiotics metronidazole and ciprofloxacin have been used with some success in treating patients with mild to moderate CD, especially when the disease involves the colon. Some success has been achieved using these preparations as maintenance therapies, but established, controlled data are lacking.

Biologic Agents. Infliximab (Remicade), the first biologic agent effective in the treatment of CD, revolutionized the treatment of this disease. Infliximab is a monoclonal, chimeric anti-TNF-α antibody that acts both through neutralization of free TNF-α as well as through induction of apoptosis by binding membrane-bound TNF-α on cytotoxic T lymphocytes (197, 200). Infliximab is effective in treating CD patients with disease that remains refractory to conventional therapies (196). It is also effective for the maintenance of remission in these patients (188). This drug is also used to treat fistulizing forms of CD (150,182).

Infliximab appears to be safe for short-term therapy; the effects of its long-term use are not yet known. Patients treated with infliximab may develop human antichimeric antibodies directed against the anti-TNF-α antibody itself, or may develop autoantibodies including antinuclear antibodies and antidouble stranded DNA antibodies (157,201). Some patients develop drug-induced lupus erythematosus (160). The formation of autoantibodies can be prevented by simultaneous administration of immunosuppressive agents (190). Patients also have infusion reactions and increased infections, especially those of the upper respiratory tract. An additional complication of infliximab treatment is reactivation of latent tuberculosis. Therefore, it is recommended that patients be tuberculin tested prior to the start of treatment. There is concern that long-term therapy with the drug could increase the risk for immunoproliferative disorders, but this has not yet been established.

Nutritional Therapy. Complete bowel rest and concomitant parenteral nutrition can result in clinical remission in many patients with CD, including those with steroid refractory disease (161). Subsequent studies have demonstrated that similar results may be achieved with elemental diets, oligomeric and other predigested feeds, as well as polymeric liquid formula diets, especially in pediatric patients with short segment ileal disease (165,168,185). Nutritional intervention is especially important in the treatment of pediatric CD patients in whom growth retardation is a major problem. Aggressive nutritional support is indicated in patients with malabsorption, blind loops, and short bowel syndrome since numerous vitamin and trace element deficiencies may occur in these patients.

Surgery. The majority of patients with CD require surgery at some time during their lives. In general, radical resection does not decrease the recurrence rate of the disease, and repeated resections place patients at risk for the development of short bowel syndrome (181). Therefore, conservative surgical techniques have evolved in recent times to treat patients with CD-associated complications not amenable or responsive to medical therapy. Surgery in CD patients is indicated for treatment of abdominal abscesses, internal or external fistulas, bleeding, bowel obstruction secondary to strictures, and medically intractable disease. Many patients experience recurrence of their disease (181), but many also report an overall improvement in their quality of life following surgery (156).

Prognosis. CD is a chronic illness, with the majority of patients experiencing recurrent disease. Nearly all patients have a recurrence within 10 years of their initial diagnosis. Recurrence occurs more often in patients with ileocecal disease (53 percent) than with isolated colonic disease (45 percent) or isolated small bowel disease (44 percent) (203). Patients who have undergone surgical procedures are also prone to disease recurrence (178).

Patients with CD may develop numerous complications of their disease, some of which impact patient survival (Table 15-3). Patient survival is not influenced by disease extent at the time of diagnosis. Community- and population-based studies demonstrate that the survival rate of patients with CD is similar to, or slightly less than, that observed in the non-IBD population. There are more severe forms of the disease that tend to be included in statistics from tertiary referral centers where morbidity, surgical rates, and mortality are greater. Patients with CD die of their underlying IBD, as well as from associated diseases, including gastrointestinal cancer, respiratory diseases, and other gastrointestinal diseases (158).

ULCERATIVE COLITIS

Definition. *Ulcerative colitis* is a chronic IBD in which the inflammation remains confined to the colon. The rectum is involved in 95 percent of patients. The more proximal portions of the colon demonstrate variable degrees of involvement. The inflammation is diffuse and continuous, and is for the most part, confined to the mucosa.

Demography. In recent decades, the incidence of UC in the United States, Canada, and Europe has risen (219a,250a,267,277a). This increase in UC incidence may be related to improved diagnosis due mainly to the increased use of sigmoidoscopy and fecal occult blood testing in the community. UC mostly affects young white people, but there is an increasing recognition that the disease affects many ages and many ethnic groups (219a,242). The incidence of

Table 15-3

COMPLICATIONS OF CROHN'S DISEASE

Local Gastrointestinal
Perforation
Hemorrhage
Fistulas to adjacent bowel
Fistulas to urinary bladder
Fistulas to vagina
Intestinal obstruction
Enterolith production
Malabsorption
Lactose deficiency
Zinc deficiency
Psoas abscesses
Extraintestinal Manifestations
Bronchitis
Emphysema
Asthma
Amyloidosis
Neoplasms
Small bowel carcinoma
Large intestinal carcinoma
Cholangiocarcinoma
Lymphoma
Squamous cell carcinomas, anus and vagina

UC inversely correlates with smoking, and clinical relapses have been associated with smoking cessation (243,273).

Clinical Features. There is a wide range of clinical features affecting all age groups. Diarrhea and urgency of defecation, bloody diarrhea, attacks of crampy abdominal pain, and perianal soreness are common in the early stages of the disease. The most consistent feature of UC is the presence of blood and mucus in the stool. Patients complain of crampy abdominal pain that is worst at the time of defecation. Abdominal pain is usually less severe than in CD. The location of pain within the abdomen depends on the extent of the disease. Patients with left-sided colitis complain of lower abdominal discomfort, while pancolitis is associated with diffuse abdominal pain. In children, growth failure, characterized by decreased linear growth and delayed sexual maturation, may occur, although less commonly than in CD patients (265).

Approximately 30 percent of patients have an abrupt onset of disease, occasionally mimicking an infectious or dysenteric illness. The disease may be explosive, with the sudden onset of bloody diarrhea, continuous abdominal pain, anorexia, weight loss, iron deficiency anemia, and persistent fever. Acute problems include bleeding, fulminant disease, and toxic megacolon. Acute and massive rectal bleeding affects up to 3 percent of patients (220). The bleeding originates from widespread ulceration of the mucosa overlying telangiectatic vessels of the lamina propria.

Characteristically, UC is a chronic mucosal disease with relapses and spontaneous remissions. Relapses are relatively unpredictable except that the disease activity in foregoing years indicates a 70 to 80 percent probability that the disease will continue the following year (242). UC progresses to a more serious form in approximately 54 percent of patients. Factors associated with disease progression include the extent of disease at diagnosis, the presence of joint symptoms, younger age at diagnosis, and severe bleeding (220). Various infections (cytomegalovirus, *Salmonella*, and *Clostridium difficile*), medications, and intervening ischemic disease may also complicate or exacerbate UC.

Gross Findings. Disease extent and involvement vary with the clinical severity. The distal bowel is always involved, with variable proximal continuous extension (fig. 15-29). Some patients show evidence of pancolitis with diffuse involvement of the entire colon. The ileum is generally not involved except to a minor degree by "backwash ileitis." In rare instances, the rectum is spared. This occurs mainly in patients who have been treated prior to resection or biopsy with enema preparations (210,236,237,255).

Since UC is primarily characterized by inflammation that remains limited to the mucosa, the external surface of the colon usually appears normal, except that in chronic UC, the overall length of the colon may be shortened. This is not true in cases in which carcinoma or toxic megacolon have developed. In the case of toxic megacolon, the colon appears massively dilated and the wall is paper-thin (fig. 15-30). Frequently, fibrinous or fibrinopurulent exudates are seen on the peritoneal surfaces. The descending and sigmoid colon usually show the most severe involvement. Edema widely separates the fibers of the muscularis propria, sometimes leading to perforation.

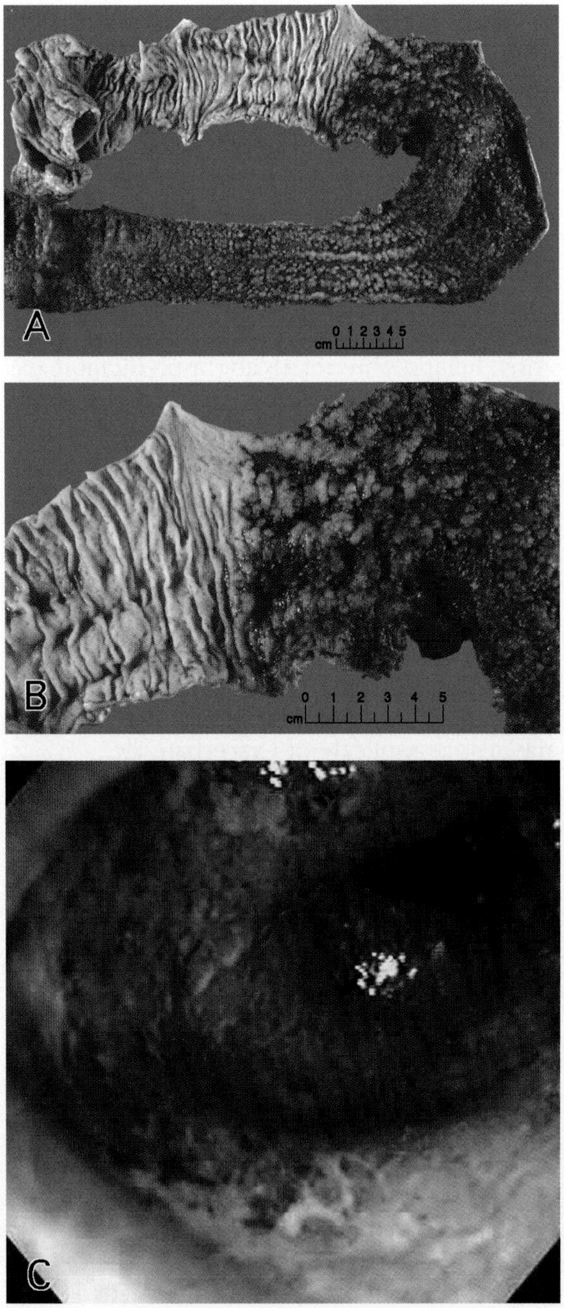

Figure 15-29

GROSS APPEARANCE OF THE COLON IN ULCERATIVE COLITIS

A: The distal two thirds of the colon shows extensive ulceration and pseudopolyp formation. Note the diffuse, continuous involvement of the diseased segment of colon. The proximal one third is essentially normal in appearance.

B: The transition from the inflamed colon to normal-appearing colon is abrupt.

C: Endoscopically, the mucosa is markedly erythematous with foci of erosion and ulceration.

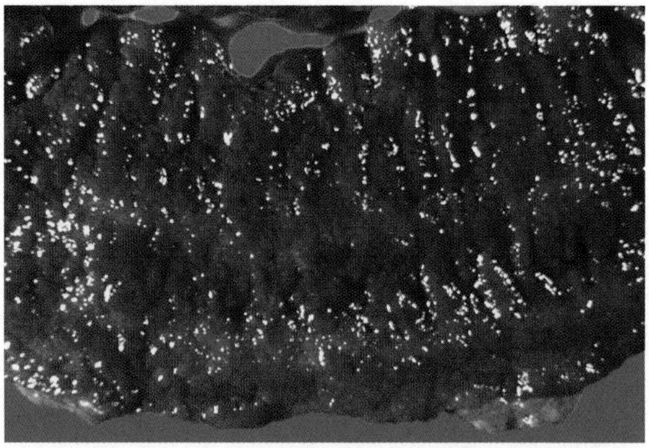

Figure 15-30

FULMINANT ULCERATIVE COLITIS

The colonic mucosa appears ulcerated and diffusely hemorrhagic.

Typically, when one opens a colon resected for active UC, blood oozes diffusely from the congested vasculature of the mucosal surface. The disease usually involves the rectum and extends for a variable distance proximally in a continuous fashion. The transition from diseased to uninvolved mucosa is often abrupt. Variations in the intensity of inflammation may give a false impression of discontinuous focal or skip lesions, particularly in acute UC with patchy full-thickness mucosal loss. Ulcerated areas may have intervening mucosa that looks macroscopically normal. Additionally, treatment with steroid enemas and mucosal healing may lead to the gross impression of rectal sparing. Grossly apparent skip areas or areas of rectal sparing, however, generally show histologic evidence of the architectural abnormalities characteristic of healed colitis.

In active UC, the mucosa acquires a diffuse, uniformly granular and erythematous, hemorrhagic appearance. Ulcers undermine adjacent intact mucosa to form polypoid mucosal tags or pseudopolyps (figs. 15-31, 15-32). Inflammatory polyps are discrete areas of mucosal inflammation and regeneration. These polyps do not correlate with disease severity, although they occur most commonly in patients with severe chronic disease. Their distribution depends on the extent of the colitis. Both localized and diffuse forms of inflammatory polyposis complicate UC; however, polyps are numerous only in a minority of cases. Inflammatory polyps are

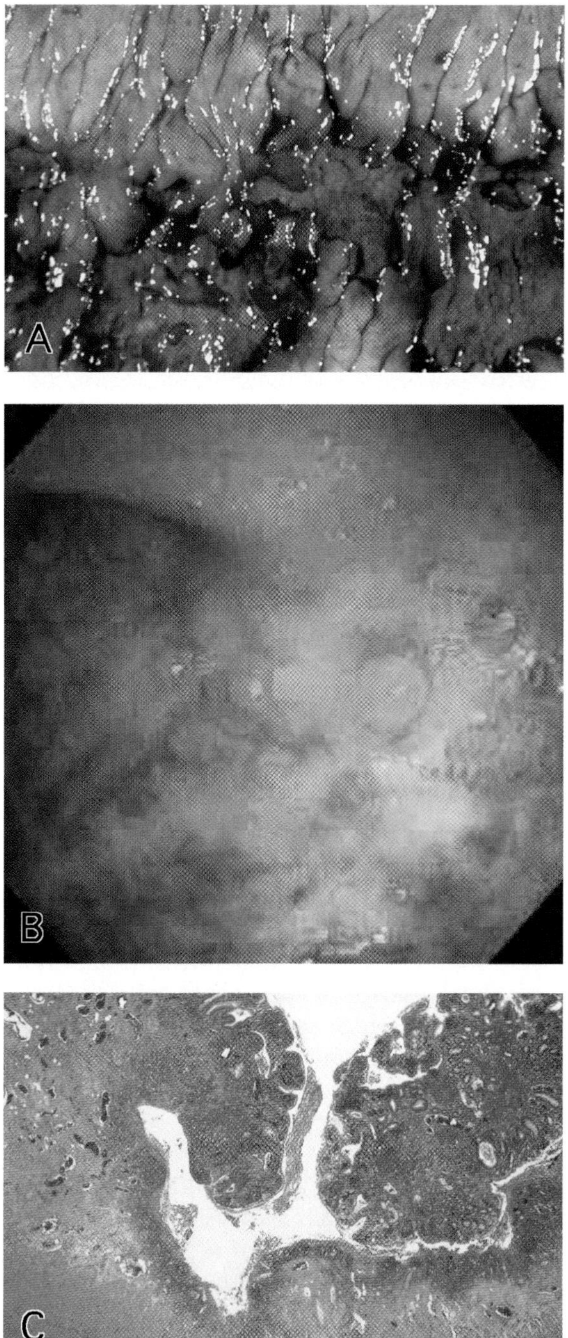

Figure 15-31

PSEUDOPOLYPS IN ULCERATIVE COLITIS

A: Large ulcers have intervening areas of mucosal regeneration. These regenerative islands appear as polyps raised above the ulcerated areas.

B: Endoscopic view of scattered pseudopolyps.

C: Low-power photomicrograph shows an area of undermining ulceration flanked by polypoid regenerative islands of mucosa.

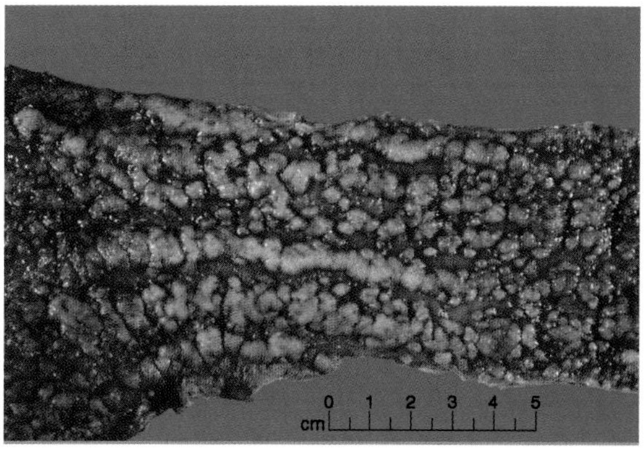

Figure 15-32

ULCERATIVE COLITIS

There is widespread ulceration of the colon. The remaining nonulcerated mucosa appears as multiple pseudopolyps.

typically short, measuring less than 1.5 cm in height. There are also unusual inflammatory polyps that attain a large size or have a bizarre architecture. Such large postinflammatory polyps may produce acute intestinal obstruction (224) and intussusception (223), or mimic carcinomas (228). In addition, they may bleed or aggravate protein loss from the colon.

Once formed, postinflammatory polyps tend to persist and may serve as an indicator of previous episodes of colitis. They are more prominent in the colon than in the rectum and can completely spare the distal large bowel. Fused polyps create a labyrinthine appearance and mucosal bridging. Polyp fusion results from the approximation of two adjacent polyps that become superficially ulcerated. Fibroblasts grow into the granulation tissue between the polyp surfaces.

The presence of broad areas of superficial ulceration that are covered by an overlying mucopurulent exudate results in partial or complete loss of the mucosa in some areas. The ulcers exhibit a linear distribution, particularly in relation to the attachment of the taeniae coli. Deep ulceration, with exposure of the underlying muscularis propria or penetration of it, is seen only in fulminant UC. Extensive longitudinal ulcers, especially if connected by transverse ulcers, are not a feature of UC but are more characteristic of CD.

The terminal ileum becomes involved only in continuity with active pancolitis. This occurs

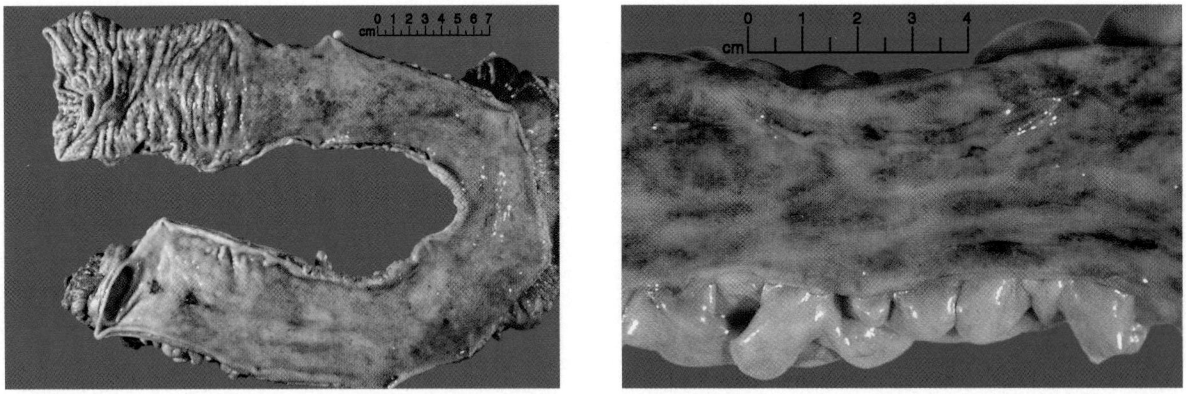

Figure 15-33

MUCOSAL ATROPHY IN LONG-STANDING ULCERATIVE COLITIS

Left: The distal three quarters of the colon shows diffuse loss of the normal pattern of folding. The uninvolved proximal colon appears essentially normal.

Right: Higher-power view shows a flattened, thinned mucosa.

in 10 to 20 percent of patients. The ileal inflammation, known as backwash ileitis, is thought to result from incompetence of the ileocecal valve and reflux of intestinal contents across it. Grossly, the ileal mucosa appears diffusely abnormal, contrasting with the aphthous ulcers and discontinuous and serpiginous ulcerations of CD. The involved ileum shows inflammation, erosions, and sometimes ulcerations. The ileitis usually resolves following colectomy.

In chronic quiescent UC, the mucosa appears granular, with or without postinflammatory polyps, and the hemorrhagic component is muted or absent. When UC goes into remission it is possible for the mucosa to return to a normal gross appearance, or appear smooth and atrophic with a loss of the normal pattern of folding (fig. 15-33). Sometimes the most striking gross feature is intestinal shortening with loss of the haustral folds, which produces an appearance of a contracted, stiff, thickened bowel. This shortening results from muscular abnormalities and is best seen in the distal colon and rectum.

Microscopic Findings. UC is characterized by inflammation restricted primarily to the mucosa, but sometimes involving the submucosa (fig. 15-34). Varying degrees of active (neutrophilic) inflammation are superimposed on chronic changes. The chronic changes include architectural abnormalities such as crypt branching and widening of the distance between the bases of the glands and the muscularis mucosae. Metaplastic changes such as Paneth cell metaplasia are also common.

Active Colitis. The hallmark of activity in UC is the presence of neutrophils, with the level of activity more or less correlating with the number of acute inflammatory cells in the lamina propria. In active UC, there is an intense inflammatory cell infiltrate within the lamina propria, neutrophilic infiltration of the glandular epithelium, mucin depletion, and surface ulceration. The term *chronic active colitis* indicates the presence of such acute inflammatory activity superimposed on a background of chronic damage. The degree of activity can be further characterized by subjective estimations of the amount of inflammation, such as mild, moderate, or severe.

An early feature of active colitis is the formation of cryptitis, which evolves to the formation of crypt abscesses and crypt ulcers (fig. 15-35). As in CD, cryptitis reflects the migration of neutrophils into the crypt epithelium. A collection of neutrophils in the crypt lumen is a crypt abscess. Although crypt abscesses are characteristic of active UC, basing the diagnosis of this disease on their identification is probably not prudent since crypt abscesses occur as part of acute inflammation associated with many disorders, including CD and acute self-limited colitis. Crypt ulcers are areas of crypt destruction from the inflammation. Once the crypt ruptures, a process sometimes referred to as crypt

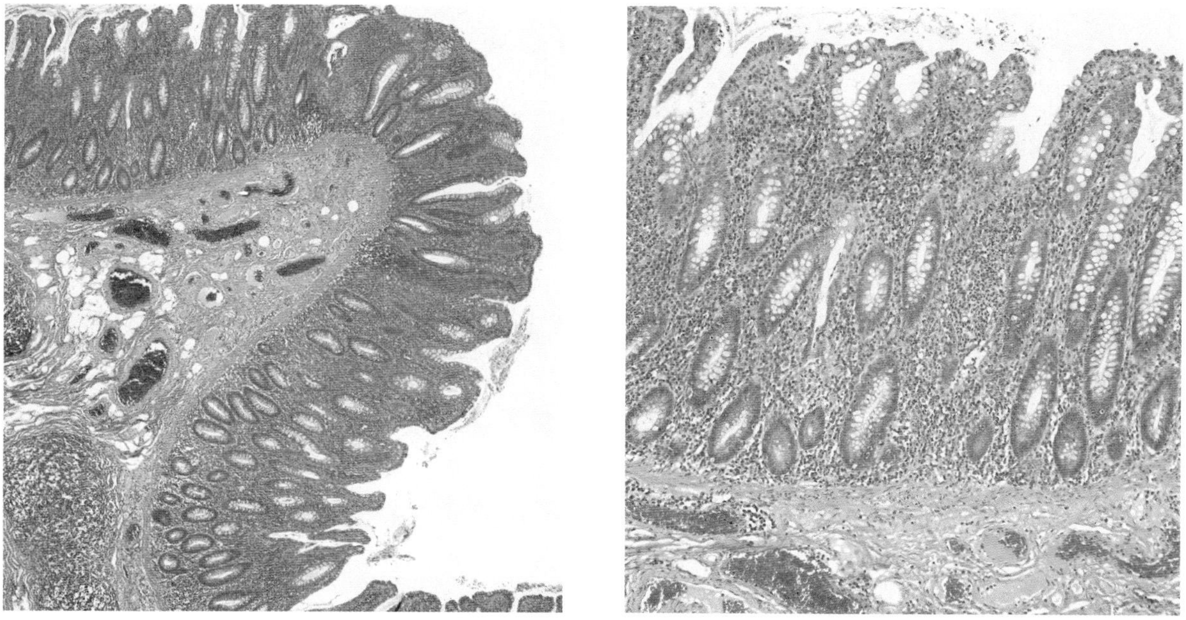

Figure 15-34

ULCERATIVE COLITIS

Left: Dense chronic active inflammation in the colon of a patient with pancolitis. The inflammation is limited to the mucosa.

Right: Higher-power view of a dense chronic inflammatory infiltrate within the lamina propria. Scattered foci of active inflammation are present. The inflammation does not bridge the muscularis mucosae.

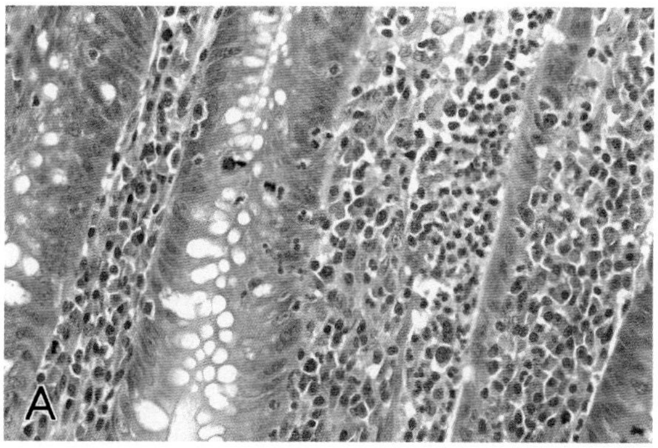

Figure 15-35

ACTIVE INFLAMMATION IN ULCERATIVE COLITIS

A: The crypt in the middle of the photograph contains infiltrating neutrophils. The epithelium is regenerative in appearance. The adjacent crypt on the right has more extensive inflammation with formation of a crypt abscess.

B: Neutrophils are present within the lumens of the two crypts in the center. Such collections are referred to as crypt abscesses.

C: Neutrophils have accumulated in the crypt lumen, and the epithelium has been damaged to the extent that the crypt is partially destroyed. Neutrophils spill out into the surrounding lamina propria.

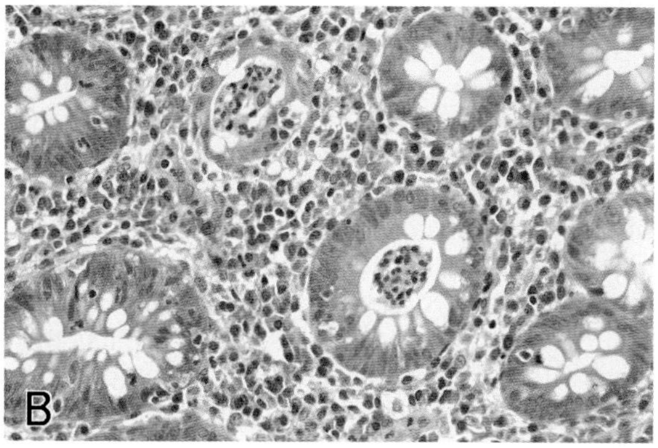

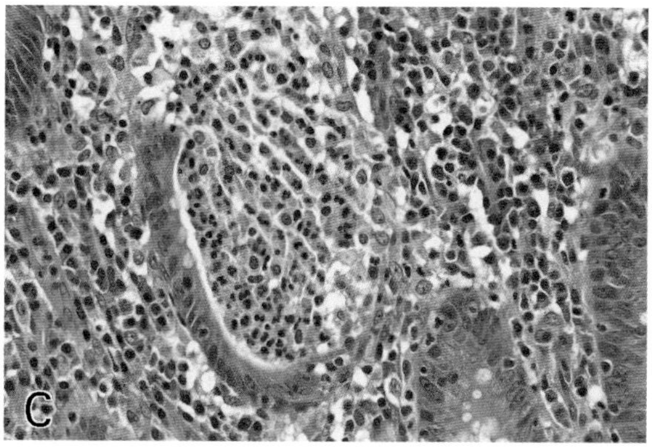

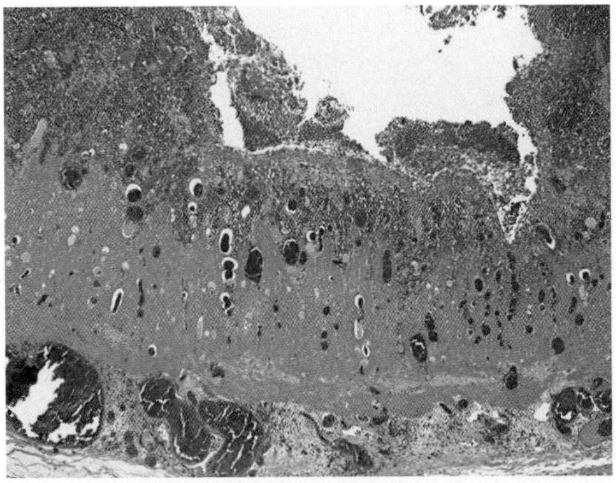

Figure 15-36

SEVERELY ACTIVE ULCERATIVE COLITIS

An area of deep ulceration is present in this case of fulminant UC. The inflammation in this area extends to the muscularis propria.

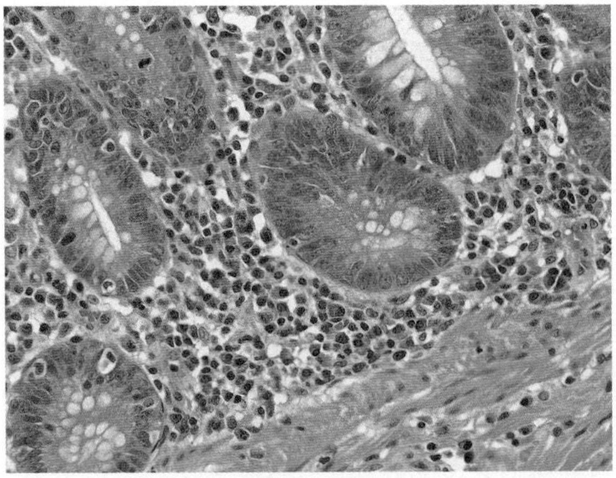

Figure 15-37

BASAL PLASMACYTOSIS IN ULCERATIVE COLITIS

Examination of the deep aspect of the lamina propria in a colon involved by UC shows a dense infiltrate of plasma cells extending down to the muscularis mucosae. This distribution of inflammation is referred to as basal plasmacytosis.

herniation, the luminal contents and mucus escape into the surrounding lamina propria, sometimes eliciting a histiocytic response. Such histiocytic collections may simulate the granulomas seen in CD. The presence of acute inflammation, primarily based in the epithelium rather than the lamina propria, distinguishes UC from acute self-limited colitis.

Crypt abscesses play a role in the generation of areas of mucosal ulceration because, when they lead to crypt rupture, the inflammation spreads laterally beneath the mucosa, causing it to slough and leaving an ulcer. Ulcers may also spread into the submucosa and undermine adjacent, relatively intact mucosa. The ulcers associated with UC tend to be small and generally shallow, but in severe UC, they may extend to the muscularis propria (fig. 15-36). Deep penetration of the muscular layer or serosa, however, only occurs in toxic megacolon.

The acute inflammatory changes of active UC are superimposed on chronic inflammatory changes within the colonic mucosa. Basal accumulations of lymphocytes and plasma cells (referred to as basal lymphoplasmacytosis), together with hyperplasia of lymphoid tissue, probably represent an early immunologic manifestation of the underlying disease process (fig. 15-37). Hyperplastic mucosal lymphoid follicles may be quite prominent, especially in the rectum. The inflammation remains superficial and primarily mucosal. Occasionally, this inflammation extends into the superficial submucosa. The lamina propria contains a dense infiltrate of lymphocytes and plasma cells. Eosinophils may be present in variable numbers. As the intensity of inflammation increases, the mucosa becomes extensively superficially ulcerated.

Resolving Colitis. Active disease resolves spontaneously or in response to therapy. Initially, there is a reduction in vascular dilatation and disappearance of the acute inflammation. During the healing phase, the epithelium actively regenerates, epithelial continuity is restored, and the inflammatory infiltrate and abscesses begin to resolve. Epithelial regeneration extends from the base of the crypts and from the edge of the ulcers. As the cells regenerate, they may show a syncytial-like appearance with large amounts of cytoplasm (fig. 15-38). They may appear flattened at first, but gradually increase in height, first becoming cuboidal and then eventually columnar in shape. During this regeneration, the epithelium appears mucin depleted (fig. 15-38). As it matures and the inflammation subsides, however, the epithelial mucin content is restored. The regenerated crypts may appear branched (fig. 15-38).

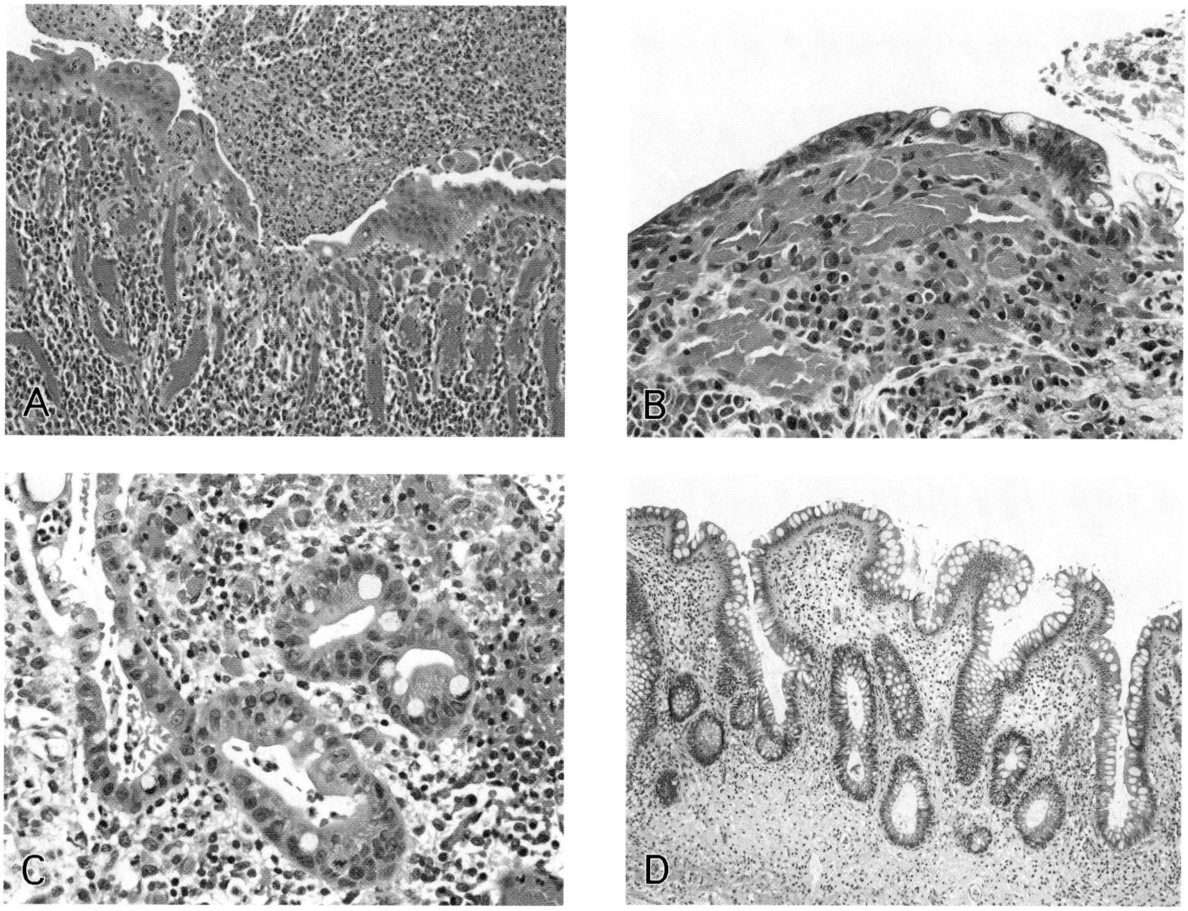

Figure 15-38

EPITHELIAL REGENERATION IN ULCERATIVE COLITIS

A: The cells attempting to reepithelialize this area of ulceration have enlarged nuclei, prominent nucleoli, and abundant eosinophilic cytoplasm. The cell borders are indistinct, giving them a syncytial appearance.

B: Reepithelialized ulcer with regenerative, cuboidal epithelial cells.

C: These regenerative glands have evidence of mucin depletion. Only a few goblet cells are seen in the crypts.

D: Regeneration may result in branching of the glands and other architectural abnormalities, as seen here.

Lymphocytes and plasma cells decrease in number and tend to become more focal as the inflammation subsides. Variable numbers of acute and chronic inflammatory cells and Paneth cells are present during this phase. Resolution of the chronic inflammation may produce a patchy infiltrate that can resemble CD in biopsy specimens.

It takes weeks to months for active disease to become quiescent. If the resolution is complete and if the initial damage was minimal, complete architectural restoration can occur. More commonly, however, permanent architectural abnormalities, such as distorted crypts, persist. These represent useful histologically identifiable signs of former active disease.

Fulminant Colitis. Patients with fulminant colitis usually have pancolitis. Microscopic examination shows mucosal denudation and replacement by highly vascular granulation tissue. There is intense infiltration of the mucosa by histiocytes, plasma cells, lymphocytes, and neutrophils. Marked submucosal edema may accompany the inflammation. The inflammatory changes in fulminant colitis may extend to the circular and longitudinal layers of the muscularis propria, with varying degrees of muscle degeneration and necrosis. Often, individual

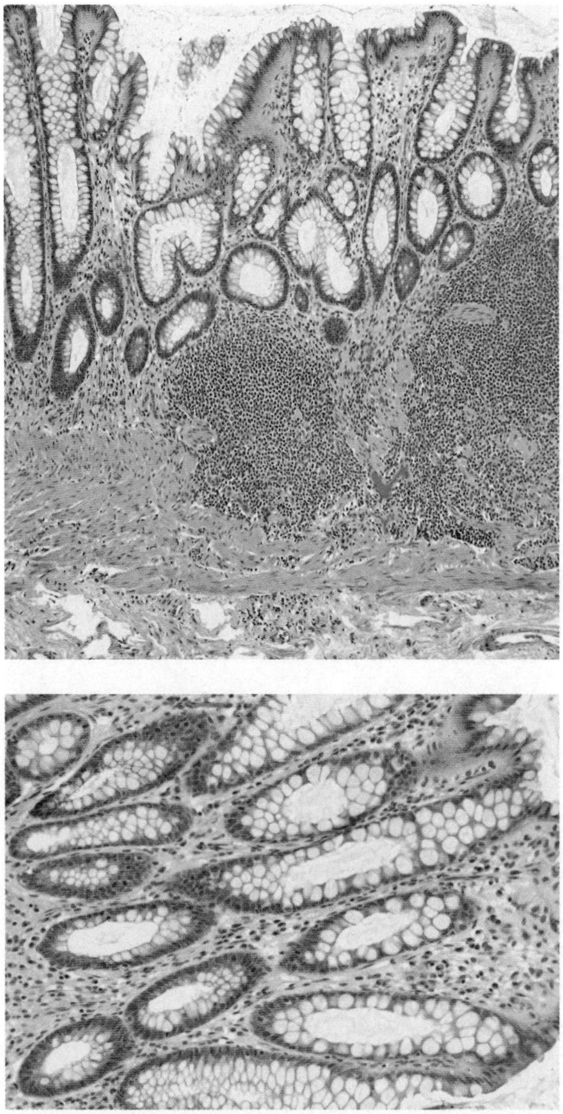

Figure 15-39

QUIESCENT ULCERATIVE COLITIS

Top: There is mild residual architectural distortion of the crypts, but the lamina propria is normocellular.

Bottom: Normal cellularity of the lamina propria is associated with an essentially normal glandular epithelium. No active inflammation is present.

muscle fibers appear shortened and rounded; aggregates of eosinophilic-staining cytoplasm are within the myofibrils. The bowel wall, however, lacks the fibrosis or the prominent lymphocytic aggregates seen in CD. Prominent lymphoid follicles are present in the submucosa in fulminant UC but they should not be present in areas away from the ulceration.

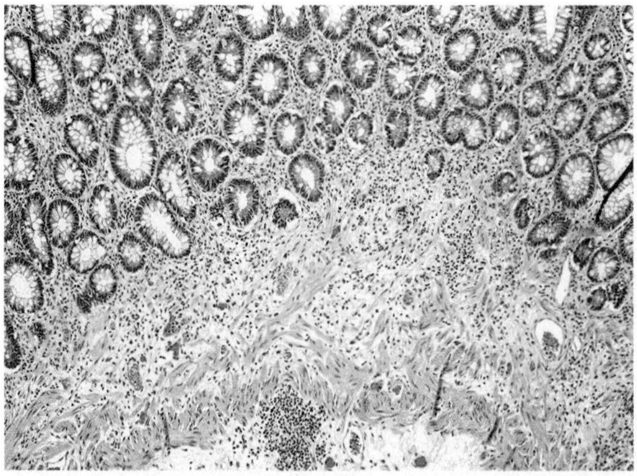

Figure 15-40

ULCERATIVE COLITIS ARCHITECTURAL ABNORMALITIES

In addition to branched and irregular crypts, crypt shortening occurs in UC. In this example, the glands do not rest on the muscularis mucosae as occurs in the normal colon. The intervening lamina propria is mildly fibrotic and contains an inflammatory infiltrate composed of lymphocytes, plasma cells, and eosinophils.

Quiescent Colitis. In quiescent UC, the mucosa may appear normal or diffusely atrophic with architectural changes resulting from the damage that occurred during active disease (fig. 15-39). Mucosal atrophy takes the form of loss of crypt parallelism with branching or a severe reduction in the number of crypts per unit area. The crypts characteristically shorten and the space between the base of the crypts and the muscularis mucosae widens (gland shortfall) (fig. 15-40). The muscularis mucosae may appear thickened and frayed due to previous ulceration and muscular regeneration. Paneth cell metaplasia distal to the hepatic flexure, pyloric metaplasia, and endocrine cell hyperplasia often indicate a long history of colitis.

Ileitis. Backwash ileitis affects a proportion of patients with severe pancolitis. Inflammation of the distal ileum is thought to occur in these patients secondary to reflux of colonic contents into the ileum through an incompetent ileocecal valve. Histologically, the ileal mucosa shows evidence of active inflammation (fig. 15-41). Neutrophilic infiltrates are present, sometimes including crypt abscesses. Features of chronic injury, such as architectural distortion or pyloric metaplasia, should not be seen, and when present, should raise the possibility of CD.

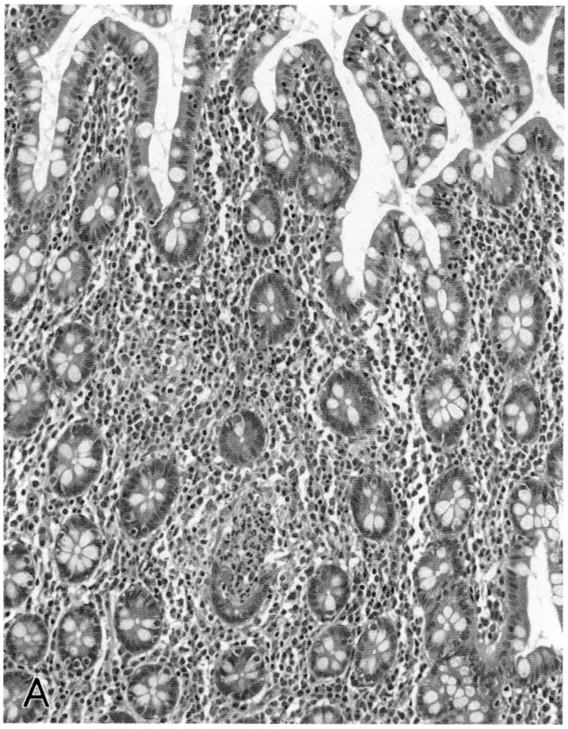

Figure 15-41

BACKWASH ILEITIS

A: The ileal mucosal architecture is relatively preserved, and does not show the chronic changes seen in CD. The lamina propria contains scattered neutrophils, and a crypt abscess is present.

B: Higher-power view demonstrates ileal crypt abscesses associated with backwash ileitis.

C: The colon shows diffuse pancolitis. The inflammation is limited to the mucosa, and has the diffuse distribution characteristic of UC.

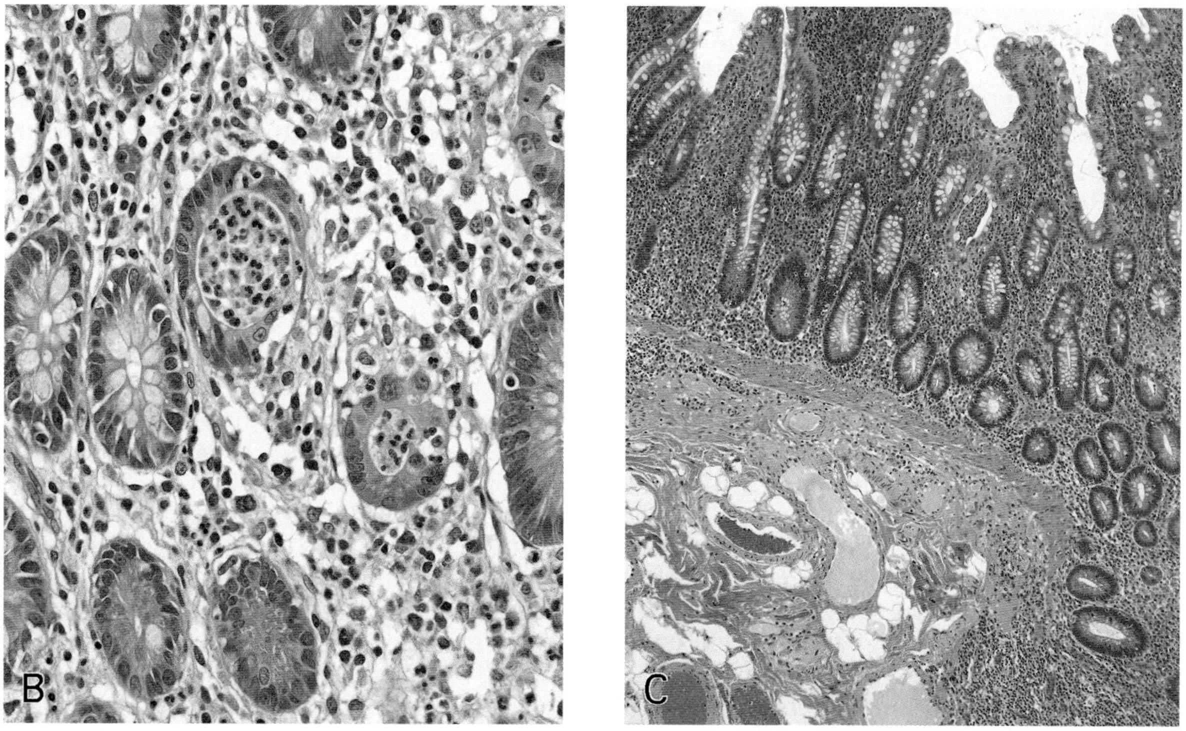

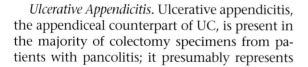

Ulcerative Appendicitis. Ulcerative appendicitis, the appendiceal counterpart of UC, is present in the majority of colectomy specimens from patients with pancolitis; it presumably represents part of the continuous inflammatory process that characterizes UC (fig. 15-42). Appendiceal involvement, however, may also be seen in a proportion of patients without pancolitis (214,

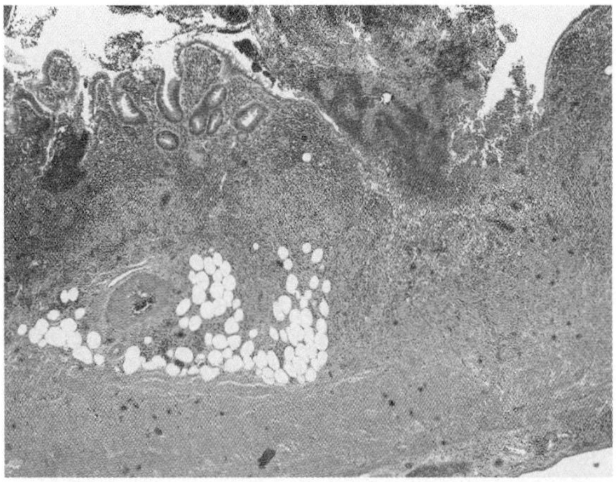

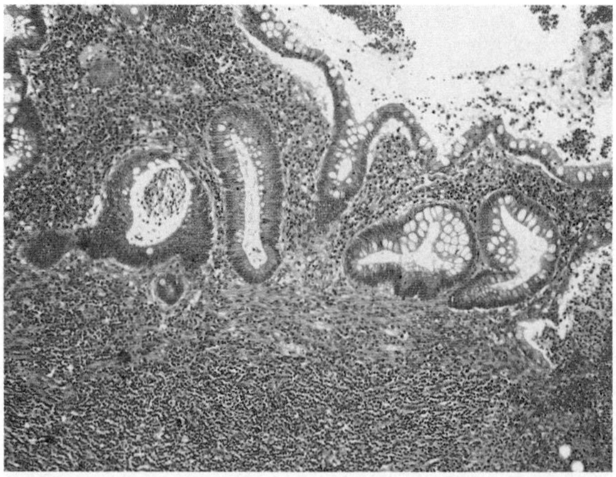

Figure 15-42

ULCERATIVE APPENDICITIS

Left: Patchy ulceration of the appendiceal mucosa.

Right: On higher power, features typical of UC elsewhere in the colon are present. There is distortion of the crypt architecture, and areas of active inflammation with crypt abscess formation.

227,230,240). Additionally, some patients demonstrate patchy cecal inflammation or appendiceal orifice inflammation associated with left-sided colitis (215,256,281). Studies suggest that such "skip lesions" are of no clinical significance, and should not be misinterpreted as features of CD in patients with otherwise typical UC.

Upper Gastrointestinal Involvement. Rare cases of chronic active duodenal or gastric inflammation have been reported in association with UC (250,271,278). It is as yet unclear whether these cases represent an unusual manifestation of UC or a separate associated disorder. Longer follow-up of the reported cases is required before such a determination can be made.

Strictures. Disagreement exists concerning the frequency of benign strictures in chronic UC. Strictures develop as a result of muscular hypertrophy and thickening of the muscularis mucosae and muscularis propria rather than from fibrosis as occurs in CD. The hypertrophic muscle remains in a spastic or contracted state, resulting in intestinal hypomotility. In addition, there are secondary changes that occur in the muscle that lead to motility abnormalities, shortening and contraction of the large intestine, and loss of the haustral folds (238,274). These changes are thought to occur secondary to the long-standing effects of cytokines on the colonic smooth muscle cells (279).

Sometimes strictures form on an ischemic basis in patients with UC. Ischemic strictures show extensive fibrosis, and the mucosa and submucosa become replaced by granulation tissue. Ischemia often complicates concurrent infection with cytomegalovirus (fig. 15-43). When fibrosis does develop in the setting of UC, it never develops to the same extent as seen in CD, even when there is deep ulceration with destruction of the muscularis mucosae. The diagnosis of a complicating malignancy must be seriously entertained in patients with long-standing UC who have a colon stricture.

Differential Diagnosis. Approximately 5 percent of IBD patients exhibit overlapping features of both UC and CD, and thus fall into the category of "indeterminate" colitis (221,248,254, 282). The term indeterminate colitis is used because of inadequate clinical information on the extent and distribution of the disease, or because of inadequate information from radiographic or endoscopic studies. Indeterminate colitis does not represent a disease entity itself, and should only be used as a provisional diagnosis pending the availability of additional information. In most cases, a definitive diagnosis of either UC or CD can be made within a few years of the initial diagnosis of indeterminate colitis (249).

Establishing the diagnosis of IBD is often not difficult in endoscopic biopsy material, but

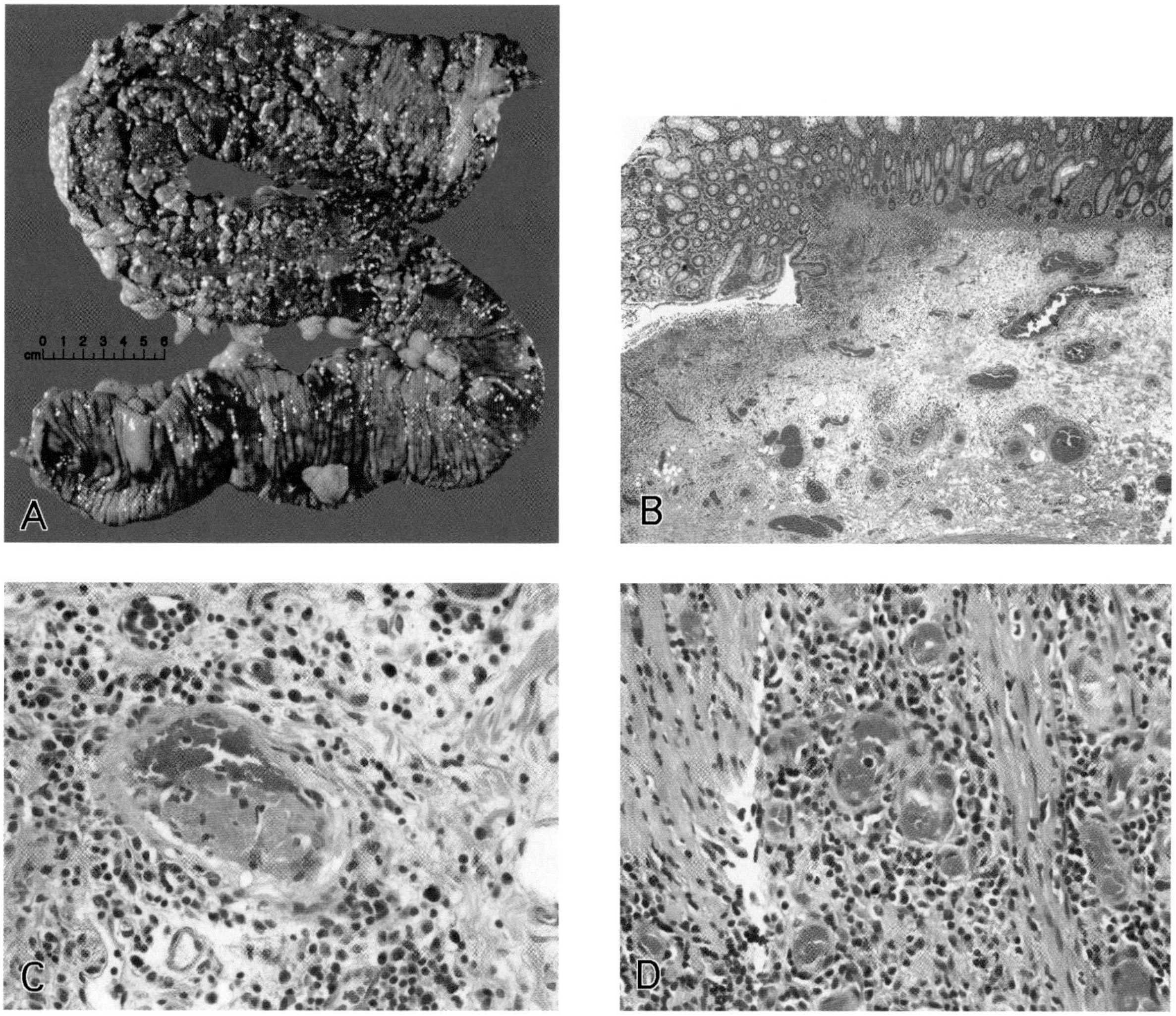

Figure 15-43

CYTOMEGALOVIRUS INFECTION IN ULCERATIVE COLITIS

A: There is widespread ulceration, typical of active UC. Edema and hemorrhage are present in the proximal colon; these represent ischemia superimposed on the patient's underlying UC.

B: Low-power view of apparent active IBD with extensive ulceration. A submucosal vessel contains a fibrin thrombus.

C: Higher-power view of the thrombosed submucosal vessel.

D: A typical cytomegalovirus inclusion in an endothelial cell underlying an area of ulceration.

differentiating between UC and CD often is. IBD is best distinguished from the other forms of colitis by the use a systematic approach when evaluating biopsy material (Table 15-4). Such a systematic approach involves evaluation of several parameters, including epithelial alterations (whether acute or chronic), changes in the lamina propria, vascular changes, and changes in the muscularis mucosae. Signs of chronicity include architectural alterations with prominent crypt branching or atrophy, a villiform structure, Paneth cell or pyloric metaplasia, lymphoid follicles, or prominent plasma cells above the muscularis mucosae. The diagnosis of different forms of colitis does not rely solely on the histologic features that are present. Knowledge of the endoscopic appearance, the clinical features, and the disease distribution are essential. Such a diagnostic approach facilitates the distinction of UC from the diseases that mimic it (Table 15-5).

Table 15-4

FEATURES TO BE EVALUATED IN BIOPSIES FOR INFLAMMATORY BOWEL DISEASE

Architectural Changes
- Crypt orientation (distortion)
- Crypt length
- Distance of crypt bases from muscularis mucosae
- Intercryptal distance
- Crypt branching
- Villiform transformation of crypt surface

Epithelial Changes
- Mucus content
- Presence of Paneth or pyloric cells
- Presence or absence of intraepithelial lymphocytes or eosinophils
- Cryptitis

Lamina Propria Changes
- Presence or absence of inflammation
- Nature of inflammation: acute or chronic

Distribution of Inflammatory Changes
- Focal or diffuse
- Superficial or basal
- Within crypts or in lamina propria
- Mucosal or extension beyond mucosa

Other Features
- Presence or absence of specific microorganisms
- Presence or absence of fibrosis
- Presence or absence of granulomas

Table 15-5

DISEASES THAT MAY MIMIC INFLAMMATORY BOWEL DISEASE CLINICALLY

Bacterial Infection
- *Escherichia coli* O157
- *Salmonella*
- *Shigella*
- Tuberculosis
- *Clostridium*
- *Campylobacter*
- *Staphylococcal* enteritis
- *Yersinia*

Other Infections
- Lymphogranuloma venereum
- Histoplasmosis
- Chlamydial colitis-proctitis
- Cytomegalovirus colitis
- Amebiasis
- Schistosomiasis
- Anisakiasis

Ischemic Colitis

Eosinophilic Gastroenteritis

Behcet's Disease

Uremic Colitis

Radiation Colitis

Diverticulitis

Drug-Induced Colitis

Colitis in Graft Versus Host Disease

Table 15-6

GROSS FEATURES OF CROHN'S DISEASE VERSUS ULCERATIVE COLITIS

Feature	Crohn's Disease	Ulcerative Colitis
Distribution	Segmental, 50% have normal rectum	Diffuse, circumferential continuous with rectum[a]
Terminal ileum	Often thickened, ulcerated and stenosed, creeping mesenteric fat, terminal 15–25 cm	Involved 10%, short segment, backwash ileitis
Colonic involvement	Predominantly right-sided, granulomas	Usually left-sided and continuous to right
Rectal involvement	+	+++
Anal disease	+++	+
Mucosal surface	Aphthous ulcers, linear ulcers, cobblestone appearance, fissures	Granular, ulcers
Mucosal atrophy	Minimal	Marked
Serosa	Inflamed, creeping fat, adhesions	Usually normal
Colon shortening	Due to fibrosis	Due to muscle hypertrophy
Strictures	Common	Rare
Fistulas	10% with enteroenteric or enterocutaneous	Rare
Free perforation	Very rare	Occurs with toxic megacolon
Pseudopolyps	Occur	Common

[a]The appendix may be involved in the absence of right-sided disease.

Table 15-7

MICROSCOPIC FEATURES OF CROHN'S COLITIS VERSUS ULCERATIVE COLITIS

Feature	Crohn's Colitis	Ulcerative Colitis
Distribution of the inflammation	Skip lesions, transmural	Diffuse, mucosal and submucosal, transmural in toxic megacolon
Crypt architectural distortion	Minimal	Marked
Paneth cell metaplasia	Occurs	Common
Cytoplasmic mucin	Slightly reduced	Mucin depleted, greatly reduced
Vascular telangiectasia	Seldom prominent	Prominent
Edema	Marked	Minimal
Lymphoid hyperplasia	Common, separated from muscularis mucosae, transmural and pericolonic tissue, associated with submucosal edema, fibrosis	Rare, mucosa and submucosa, not associated with edema and fibrosis
Crypt abscesses	Present, often few in number	Common
Granulomas (sarcoid-like)	Common	Absent
Aphthous ulcers	Common	Rare
Fissures and sinuses	Common	Absent
Submucosa	Normal, inflamed or reduced width	Normal or reduced width
Focal lymphoid aggregates in submucosa	Presence suggests CD[a] especially when deep	Usually absent
Neural hyperplasia	Common	Rare
Inflammatory and pseudopolyps	Less common than in UC	Common
Filiform polyposis, giant polyps, postinflammatory polyps	Occurs	Occurs
Ileal inflammation	Common	Minimal, not more than 10 cm involved
Anal involvement	Granulomas	Nonspecific
Lymph nodes	Granulomas	Reactive hyperplasia

[a]CD = Crohn's disease; UC = ulcerative colitis.

Patients with UC and CD share many similarities, but there are also significant differences that create the need to distinguish between them (Tables 15-6 and 15-7). Different surgical approaches are used to treat IBD patients depending on the nature of the underlying disease. Surgical techniques for continent ileostomy or ileoanal anastomosis with construction of a pouch reservoir allows one to avoid an ileostomy following colectomy. The operation is designed to improve the quality of life in UC patients by preserving fecal continence. This procedure, however, is generally not used to treat CD patients (218). Total proctocolectomy in a UC patient with backwash ileitis allows the ileum to heal, but the same operation in a patient with CD ileocolitis may leave residual disease or may be followed by a high incidence of stomal dysfunction and recurrent ileitis. A misdiagnosis is particularly hazardous to the patient with CD who undergoes a colectomy with construction of an ileal pouch reservoir because a significant number of these patients develop recurrent CD in the pouch, resulting in chronic inflammation and pouch failure (235,239). As a result, pathologists are under great pressure to distinguish UC from CD on biopsies before the patient undergoes surgical intervention.

When the diseases are well developed, UC and CD have unique and distinguishing features that allow their separation. Since no single feature is invariably present, however, and because all of the features change with time, all of the pathologic features need to be assessed in aggregate.

The presence of a villous mucosal surface, basal lymphoid aggregates, crypt atrophy, and surface erosions all favor the diagnosis of UC, whereas the presence of granulomas favors the diagnosis of CD. Because CD is a focal disease, a patient with CD may have biopsy specimens that show a completely normal mucosa, focal or diffuse colitis, or granulomas.

Preservation of colonic mucin is a common feature of CD, but it may only represent a manifestation of an essentially focal disorder, and it may not distinguish CD from UC. Its main value is to distinguish a normal biopsy from specimens showing IBD. The presence of any significant ileal disease establishes the diagnosis of CD rather than UC with backwash ileitis. Ileocecal valve incompetence in UC can produce ileal changes (backwash ileitis), but the involved ileal segment should be short and the bowel should lack other characteristic features of CD.

Treatment. *Antiinflammatory Agents.* Antiinflammatory agents such as sulfasalazine, as well as the newer 5-aminosalicylic acid medications, are a mainstay in treating patients with mild to moderate UC. These agents are useful for both inducing disease remission and for maintenance therapy. They may be administered orally, or in patients with disease limited to the left colon, administered topically in enema preparations.

Corticosteroids. Intravenous corticosteroids may be required in the treatment of patients with moderate or severe UC. Topical steroid enemas are used in patients with left-sided colitis, or to "cool down" the rectum of patients with more extensive disease prior to surgery. Corticosteroids have no role in maintenance once remission has been achieved.

Immunosuppressive Therapy. Azathioprine and 6-mercaptopurine are used in the treatment of UC due to their steroid-sparing effects. These drugs have a delayed onset of action, however, and are therefore not useful for treating acute fulminant disease. Cyclosporine and tacrolimus have also been used to treat patients with steroid refractory UC (216) and have a more rapid onset of action than other immunosuppressive agents.

Biological Agents. The anti-TNF-α antibody, infliximab, is extremely useful for treating patients with CD. Several reports, mainly uncontrolled data, suggest that this agent may also be of benefit in the treatment of patients with severe UC (206,213,276). Large, long-term studies are still needed for a complete assessment of the efficacy and safety of this drug in patients with UC.

A recent report suggests that topical treatment of the rectal mucosa with epidermal growth factor may be an effective treatment for left-sided UC. Epidermal growth factor is a potent mitogenic peptide that has been shown to stimulate healing when applied topically to skin wounds (211), and is beneficial in the treatment of necrotizing enterocolitis in newborns (277).

Probiotics. The use of probiotics has been successful in the treatment of some patients with UC (241,264). Probiotics are live microbial food ingredients that alter the enteric flora and are thought to have a favorable effect on health. Probiotic activity has most commonly been associated with lactobacilli and bifidobacteria, but other nonpathogenic bacterial strains, including certain *Escherichia coli* and enterococci, as well as nonbacterial organisms such as *Saccharomyces boulardii* have been used. The mechanisms by which these probiotics function include production of antimicrobials, competitive metabolic interaction with proinflammatory organisms, and inhibition of adherence and translocation of pathogens (209,219,272). Probiotics may also influence mucosal defenses of the mucosal immune system and epithelial function through their impact on intercellular signaling (229,232,272).

Effects of Therapy on Histology. Various therapies used to treat IBD, whether local instillation of corticosteroid enemas or systemically administered anti-inflammatory agents, may suppress some of the more classic gross or histologic features associated with the diagnosis of UC. Suppression of rectal inflammation can lead to the false impression of rectal sparing. Therapy may also predispose the intestine to develop secondary complicating features, such as cytomegalovirus infection, with or without secondary endothelialitis, and ischemia. In addition, *C. difficile* infection may occur in patients on immunosuppression.

Surgery. Surgical therapy for UC is used either for emergencies or as elective treatment. Indications for urgent surgery, in decreasing order of frequency, include failed medical treatment in patients with acute severe colitis, toxic megacolon, perforation, or severe bleeding (252). There are essentially three indications for elective colectomy for UC. These include failed medical treatment, growth retardation in a child with UC, and the development, or concern for, neoplastic transformation in a patient with long-standing disease. Failed medical treatment includes chronic disease, recurrent acute exacerbations, severe symptoms in an otherwise systemically well patient, suboptimal quality of life, steroid dependence, or extraintestinal manifestations of the disease.

In patients undergoing emergency surgery, the most common procedure is colectomy with ileostomy and preservation of the rectosigmoid stump. Under the conditions of elective surgery, several surgical options exist including conventional proctocolectomy, colectomy with ileorectal anastomosis, and restorative proctocolectomy with ileal reservoir (253).

Histologic Features of the Ileal Pouch. Three basic patterns of mucosal change may be seen in pelvic ileal pouches: 1) normal mucosa or mild villous atrophy with absent or mild inflammation; 2) transient atrophy with temporary moderate or severe villous atrophy, followed by normalization of architecture; and 3) constant atrophy with permanent subtotal or total villous atrophy and severe pouchitis (see below) (fig. 15-44). The pouch develops colonic metaplasia; pouchitis most commonly affects those in whom metaplasia has developed (246).

Pouchitis. Restorative proctocolectomy with ileal pouch-anal anastomosis has become the surgical treatment of choice for most patients with medically refractory UC. This procedure removes all of the diseased mucosa while maintaining fecal continence and transanal defecation. The most common long-term complication of this procedure is nonspecific inflammation of the ileal reservoir, commonly known as pouchitis (231,245,257,263,269). This complication affects 14 to 47 percent of patients (225, 245,253,257,259,270) and becomes chronic in 5 percent (246).

Clinical symptoms of pouchitis include diarrhea, rectal bleeding, abdominal cramps, urgency, tenesmus, and malaise. In severe cases, these symptoms are accompanied by incontinence and fever (270). Endoscopic findings include edema, mucosal erythema, granularity, friability, bleeding, loss of the vascular pattern, and the presence of a mucus exudate and small superficial areas of ulceration (figs. 15-44, 15-45) (217,247). Generally, a significant relationship exists between the endoscopic and the histologic features.

Bacterial overgrowth resulting from stasis is thought to play a major role in the development of pouchitis (251,268). Anaerobic bacterial concentrations in ileal pouchitis correlate with the presence of nonspecific histologic changes, including villous atrophy and chronic inflammation. Fecal stasis and aerobic and anaerobic bacterial overgrowth may contribute to the development of colonic metaplasia (266). Other factors that may play a role in the development of pouchitis include the presence of volatile fatty acids, fecal bile acids, oxygen free radicals, ischemia, platelet-activating factor, and hormonal factors (208,212,226,244,245,251,268).

Patients with pouchitis have a pattern of mucosal inflammation similar to that seen in UC (figs. 15-46, 15-47). Early changes consist of neutrophilic and eosinophilic inflammation with architectural distortion, Paneth cell metaplasia, a partial transition to the colonic mucinous phenotype, and an increased proliferative index (207). Refractory chronic pouchitis may resemble CD. Review of the colectomy specimen usually shows unequivocal UC, however, and the patients do not have any other clinical, radiologic, or pathologic evidence to support a diagnosis of CD. Because of the histologic resemblance to CD, the presence of transmural inflammation, granulomas, fibrosis, or strictures in areas distant from the anastomosis should be excluded. Review of previous biopsy material also proves helpful in delineating the true nature of the inflammatory process.

Prognosis. Since the introduction of effective medical and surgical treatments in the early 1960s, patients with UC have a surprisingly low mortality rate. Patients have a normal life expectancy compared with persons in the general population (219a,222,258,262,275). Severe acute attacks, usually occurring during the first 2 years of disease, are the major killer, especially in patients over 50 years of age (280). Patients with long-standing extensive disease have an increased risk for the development of dysplasia or colorectal carcinoma (260).

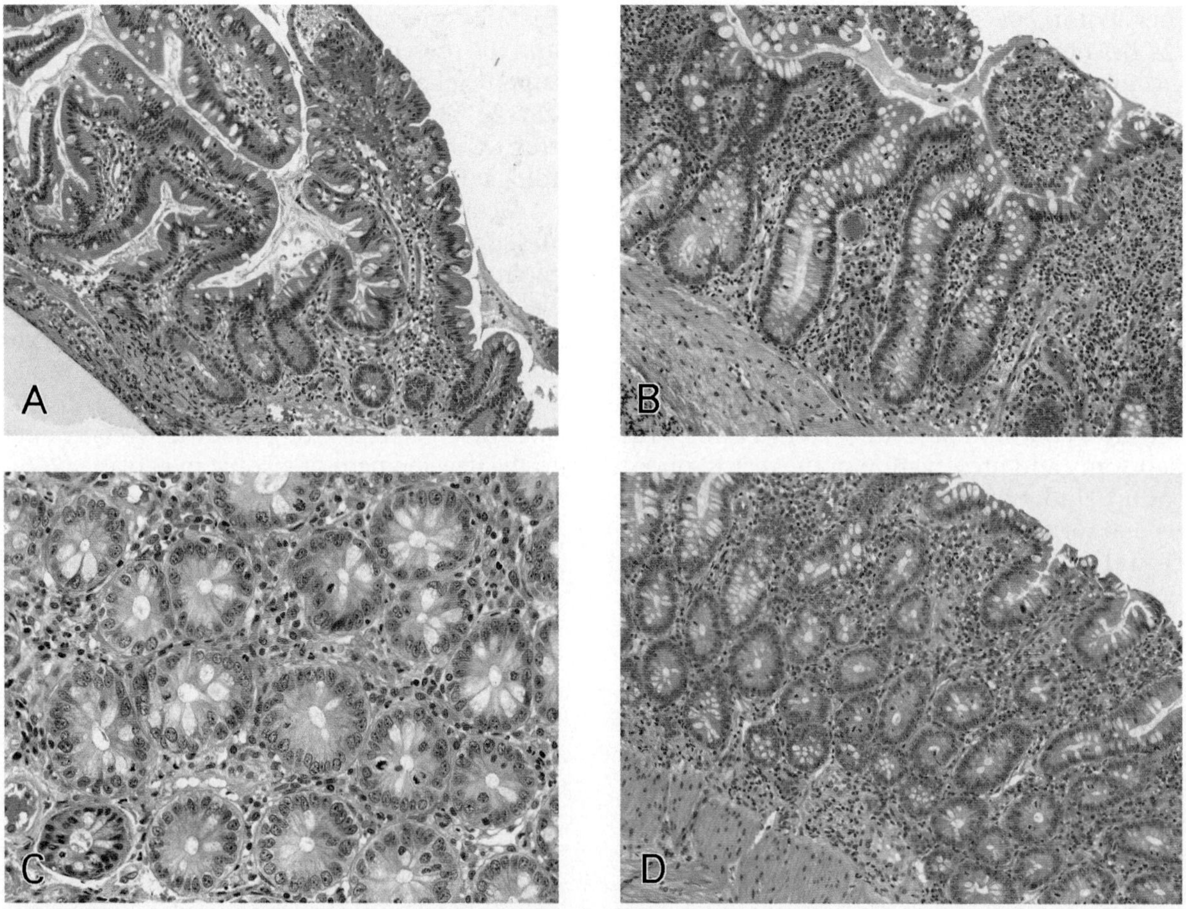

Figure 15-44

HISTOLOGIC CHANGES IN THE ILEAL POUCH

A: The ileum leading into the ileal pouch is essentially normal in appearance. The villi are long and slender. No inflammatory infiltrates are present.

B: Mild architectural changes in an ileal pouch. The villi are somewhat blunted and the crypts are irregular. The lamina propria contains an increased number of inflammatory cells.

C: Higher-power view of the lamina propria infiltrate shows occasional neutrophils.

D: Ileal pouch with more extensive architectural alterations. The villi are completely flattened and the mucosa now resembles that of the colon.

Animal Models. Numerous animal models exist for the study of IBD (reviewed in 233,234, 261). These animal models may be divided into four basic categories: 1) spontaneous colitis models; 2) inducible colitis models in mice with normal immune systems; 3) adoptive transfer models in immunocompromised animals; and 4) genetically engineered models. The most commonly studied animal models for IBD are summarized in Table 15-8.

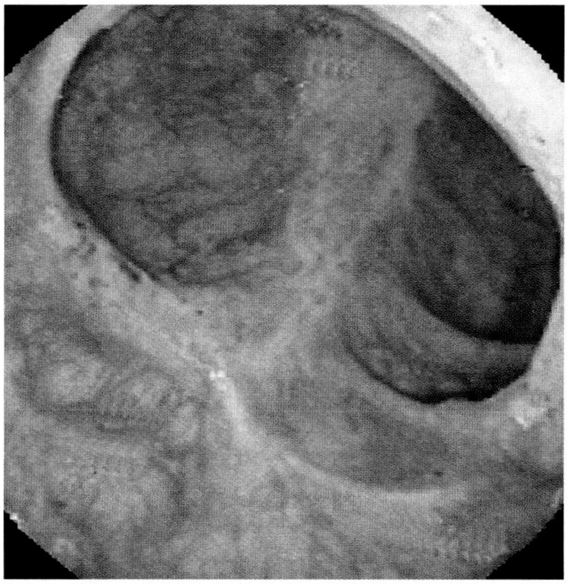

Figure 15-45

POUCHITIS

Severe diffuse pouchitis with an edematous, granular, ulcerated mucosa that is friable and bleeds spontaneously. The appearance is identical to that of active IBD.

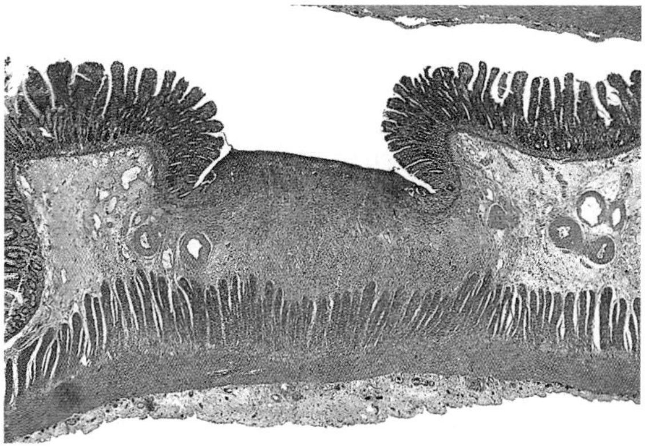

Figure 15-46

POUCHITIS

Shallow linear ulcerations along an anastomotic line within an ileoanal J-pouch.

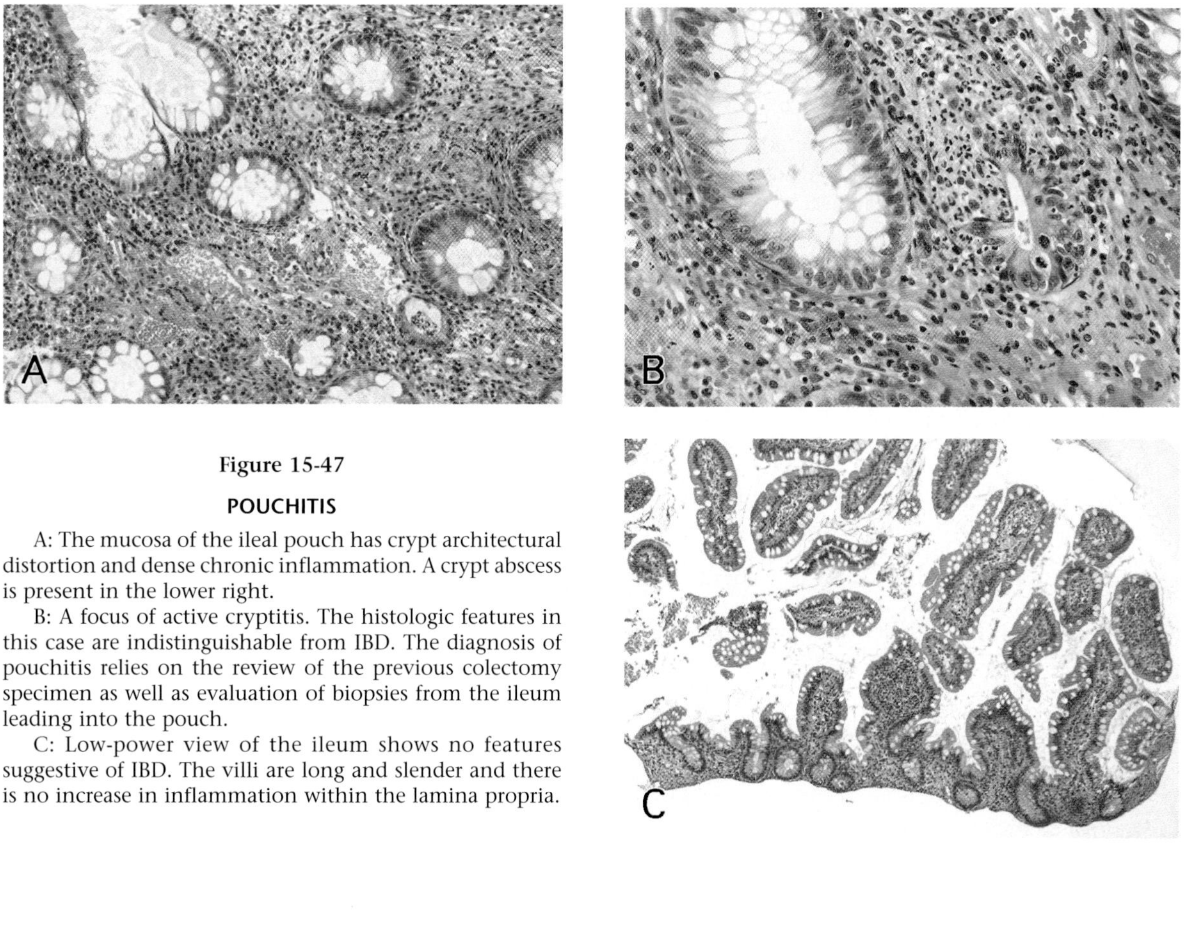

Figure 15-47

POUCHITIS

A: The mucosa of the ileal pouch has crypt architectural distortion and dense chronic inflammation. A crypt abscess is present in the lower right.

B: A focus of active cryptitis. The histologic features in this case are indistinguishable from IBD. The diagnosis of pouchitis relies on the review of the previous colectomy specimen as well as evaluation of biopsies from the ileum leading into the pouch.

C: Low-power view of the ileum shows no features suggestive of IBD. The villi are long and slender and there is no increase in inflammation within the lamina propria.

Table 15-8

ANIMAL MODELS OF INFLAMMATORY BOWEL DISEASE

Spontaneous Colitis Models	**Genetically Engineered Models**
Cotton-topped tamarin	IL2 knockout/IL2 R knockout mice
C3H/HeJBir mice	IL10 knockout mice
SAMP/Yit mice	STAT3 knockout mice
	T-cell receptor mutant mice
Inducible Colitis Models	TNF-3' UTR knockout mice
Trinitrobenzene sulfonic acid-induced colitis	Trefoil factor-deficient mice
Oxazolone colitis	IL7 transgenic mice
Dextran sulfate sodium colitis	STAT-4 transgenic mice
Carrageenan colitis	HLA B27 transgenic rats
Peptidoglycan-polysaccharide colitis	
Adoptive Transfer Models	
CD4+/CD45Rb^{high} T-cell transfer colitis	
Colitis induced by transfer of hsp60-specific CD8 T cells	

REFERENCES

Demography

1. Bennett RA, Rubin PH, Present DH. Frequency of inflammatory bowel disease in offspring of couples both presenting with inflammatory bowel disease. Gastroenterology 1991;100:1638–43.
2. Ekbom A, Helmick C, Zack M, Adami HO. The epidemiology of inflammatory bowel disease: a large, population-based study in Sweden. Gastroenterology 1991;100:350–8.
3. Hiwatashi N, Yamazaki H, Kimura M, Morimoto T, Watanabe H, Toyota T. Clinical course and long-term prognosis of Japanese patients with ulcerative colitis. Gastroenterol Jpn 1991;26: 312–8.
4. Kurata JH, Kantor-Fish S, Frankl H, Godby P, Vadheim CM. Crohn 's disease among ethnic groups in a large health maintenance organization. Gastroenterology 1992;102:1940–8.
5. Loftus EV Jr, Silverstein MD, Sandborn WJ, Tremaine WJ, Harmsen WS, Zinsmeister AR. Crohn's disease in Olmsted County, Minnesota,1940-1993: incidence, prevalence, and survival. Gastroenterology 1998;114:1161–8.
6. Ogunbi SO, Ransom JA, Sullivan K, Schoen BT, Gold BD. Inflammatory bowel disease in African-American children living in Georgia. Pediatrics 1998;133:103–7.
7. Oliva-Hemker M, Fiocchi C. Etiopathogenesis of inflammatory bowel disease: the importance of the pediatric perspective. Inflamm Bowel Dis 2002;8:112–28.
8. Roth M, Peterson G, McElree C, Feldman E, Rotter JI. Geographic origins of Jewish patients with inflammatory bowel disease. Gastroenterology 1989:97:900–4.
9. Roth MP, Petersen GM, McElree C, Vadheim CM, Panish JF, Rotter JI. Familial empiric risk estimates of inflammatory bowel disease in Ashkenazi Jews. Gastroenterology 1989;96:1016–20.
10. Taylor KB. Ulcerative colitis and Crohn's disease of the colon: symptoms, signs, and laboratory aspects. In: Kirsner JB, Shorter RG, eds. Inflammatory bowel disease, 2nd ed. Philadelphia: Lea and Febiger; 1980:141.
11. Yoshida Y, Murata Y. Inflammatory bowel disease in Japan: studies of epidemiology and etiopathogenesis. Med Clin North Am 1990;74:67–90.

Genetic Factors

12. Abreu MT, Taylor KD, Lin YC, et al. Mutations in NOD2 are associated with fibrostenosing disease in patients with Crohn's disease. Gastroenterology 2002;123:679–88.
13. Ahmad T, Armuzzi A, Bunce M, et al. The molecular classification of the clinical manifestations of Crohn's disease. Gastroenterology 2002;122:854–66.
14. Aravind L, Dixit VM, Koonin EV. The domains of death: evolution of the apoptosis machinery. Trends Biochem Sci 1999;24:47–53.
15. Barmada MM, Brant SR, Nicolae DL, et al. A genome scan in 260 inflammatory bowel disease-affected relative pairs. Inflamm Bowel Dis 2004;10:15–22.
16. Binder V. Genetic epidemiology in inflammatory bowel disease. Dig Dis 1998;16:351–5.
17. Bonen DK, Cho JH. The genetics of inflammatory bowel disease. Gastroenterology 2003;124: 521–36.

18. Bonen DK, Nicolae DL, Moran T, et al. Racial differences in NOD2 variation: characterization of NOD2 in African-Americans with Crohn's disease. Gastroenterology 2002;122:A29.
19. Bonen DK, Ogura Y, Nicolae DL, et al. Crohn's disease associated NOD2 variants share a signaling defect in response to lipopolysaccharide and peptidoglycan. Gastroenterology 2003;124: 140–7.
20. Brophy S, Pavy S, Lewis P, et al. Inflammatory eye, skin, and bowel disease in spondyloarthritis: genetic, phenotypic, and environmental factors. J Rheumatol 2001;28:2667–73.
21. Cuthbert AP, Fisher SA, Mirza MM, et al. The contribution of NOD2 gene mutations to the risk and site of disease in inflammatory bowel disease. Gastroenterology 2002;122:867–74.
22. Farmer RG, Michener WM, Mortimer EA. Studies of family history among patients with inflammatory bowel disease. Clin Gastroenterol 1980;9:271–7.
23. Girardin SE, Boneca IG, Viala J, et al. Nod2 is a general sensor of peptidoglycan through muramyl dipeptide (MDP) detection. J Biol Chem 2003:278:8869–72.
24. Hampe J, Cuthbert A, Croucher PJ, et al. Association between insertion mutation in NOD2 gene and Crohn's disease in German and British populations. Lancet 2001;357:1925–8.
25. Hampe J, Schreiber S, Shaw SH, et al. A genomewide analysis provides evidence for novel linkages in inflammatory bowel disease in a large European cohort. Am J Hum Genet 1999;64:808–16.
26. Helio T, Halme L, Lappalainen M, et al. CARD15/NOD2 gene variants are associated with familially occurring and complicated forms of Crohn's disease. Gut 2003;52:558–62.
27. Hisamatsu T, Suzuki M, Reinecker HC, et al. CARD15/NOD2 functions as an antibacterial factor in human intestinal epithelial cells. Gastroenterology 2003;124:993–1000.
28. Hugot JP, Chamaillard M, Zouali H, et al. Association of NOD2 leucine-rich repeat variants with susceptibility to Crohn's disease. Nature 2001;411:599–603.
29. Hugot JP, Laurent-Puig P, Gower-Rousseau, et al. Mapping of a susceptibility locus for Crohn's disease on chromosome 16. Nature 1996;379: 821–3.
30. Inohara N, Nunez G. The NOD: a signaling module that regulates apoptosis and host defense against pathogens. Oncogene 2001;20: 6473–81.
31. Inohara N, Ogura Y, Nunez G. Nods: a family of cytosolic proteins that regulate the host response to pathogens. Curr Opin Microbiol 2002;5:76–80.
32. Inoue N, Tamura K, Kinouchi Y, et al. Lack of common NOD2 variants in Japanese patients with Crohn's disease. Gastroenterology 2002;123:86–91.
33. Lala S, Ogura Y, Osborne C, et al. Crohn's disease and the NOD2 gene: a role for Paneth cells. Gastroenterology 2003;125:47–57.
34. Leong RW, Armuzzi A, Ahmad T, et al. NOD2/ CARD15 gene polymorphisms and Crohn's disease in the Chinese population. Aliment Pharmacol Ther 2003;17:1465–70.
35. Lesage S, Zouali H, Cezard JP, et al. CARD15/ NOD2 mutational analysis and genotype-phenotype correlation in 612 patients with inflammatory bowel disease. Am J Hum Genet 2002; 70:845–57.
36. Miceli-Richard C, Lesage S, Prieur AM, et al. CARD15 mutations in Blau syndrome. Nature Gen 2001;29:19–20.
37. Monsen U, Bernell O, Johansson C, Hellers G. Prevalence of inflammatory bowel disease among relatives of patients with Crohn's disease. Scand J Gastroenterol 1991;26:302–6.
38. Negoro K, Kinouchi Y, Hiwatashi N, et al. Crohn's disease is associated with novel polymorphisms in the 5′ flanking region of the tumor necrosis gene. Gastroenterology 1999;117: 1062–8.
39. Ogura Y, Bonen DK, Inohara N, et al. A frameshift mutation in NOD2 associated with susceptibility to Crohn's disease. Nature 2001;411: 603–6.
40. Ogura Y, Inohara N, Benito A, et al. Nod2, a Nod1/Apaf-1 family member that is restricted to monocytes and activates NF-kappaB. J Biol Chem 2001;276:4812–8.
41. Orchard T, Thiyagaraja S, Welsh K, Wordsworth BP, Hill-Gaston JS, Jewell DP. Clinical phenotype is related to HLA genotype in the peripheral arthropathies of inflammatory bowel disease. Gastroenterology 2000;118:274–8.
42. Orholm M, Munkholm P, Langholz E, Nielsen OH, Sorensen IA, Binder V. Familial occurrence of inflammatory bowel disease. N Engl J Med 1991;324:84–8.
43. Peeters M, Nevens H, Baert F, et al. Familial aggregation in Crohn's disease: increased age-adjusted risk and concordance in clinical characteristics. Gastroenterology 1996;111:597–603.
44. Radlmayr M, Torok HP, Martin K, Folwaczny C. The c-insertion mutation of the NOD2 gene is associated with fistulizing and fibrosteniotc phenotypes in Crohn's disease. Gastroenterology 2002;122:2091–2.
45. Rioux JD, Daly MJ, Silverberg MS, et al. Genetic variation in the 5q31 cytokine gene cluster confers susceptibility to Crohn disease. Nat Genet 2001;29:223–8.

46. Rioux JD, Silverberg MS, Daly MJ, et al. Genomewide search in Canadian families with inflammatory bowel disease reveals two novel susceptibility loci. Am J Hum Genet 2000;66:1863–70.
47. Russell MG, Pastoor CJ, Janssen KM, et al. Familial aggregation of inflammatory bowel disease: a population-based study in South Limburg, The Netherlands. The South Limburg IBD Study Group. Scand J Gastroenterol Suppl 1997;223:88–91.
48. Satsangi J, Rosenberg WM, Jewell DP. The prevalence of inflammatory bowel disease in relatives of patients with Crohn's disease. Eur J Gastroenterol Hepatol 1994;6:413–6.
49. Satsangi J, Welsh KI, Bunce M, et al. Contribution of genes of the major histocompatibility complex to susceptibility and disease phenotype in inflammatory bowel disease. Lancet 1996; 347:1212–7.
50. Stokkers PC, Huibregtse K Jr, Leegwater AC, et al. Analysis of a positional candidate gene for inflammatory bowel disease: NRAMP2. Inflamm Bowel Dis 2000;6:92–8.
51. Subhani J, Montgomery SM, Pounder RE, Wakefield AJ. Concordance rates of twins and siblings in inflammatory bowel disease. Gut 1998;42:A40.
52. Thompson NP, Driscoll R, Pounder RE, Wakefield AJ. Genetics versus environment in inflammatory bowel disease: results of a British twin study. BMJ 1996;312:95–6.
53. Tysk C, Lindberg E, Jarnerot G, Floderus-Myrhed B. Ulcerative colitis and Crohn's disease in an unselected population of monozygotic and dizygotic twins. A study of heritability and the influence of smoking. Gut 1988;29:990–6.
54. van der Biezen EA, Jones JD. The NB-ARC domain: a novel signaling motif shared by plant resistance gene products and regulators of cell death in animals. Curr Biol 1998;8:R226–7.
55. van der Linde K, Boor PP, Houwing-Duistermaat JJ, et al. CARD15 and Crohn's disease: healthy homozygous carriers of the 3020insC frameshift mutation. Am J Gastroenterol 2003; 98:613–7.
56. van Heel DA, Carey AH, Jewell DP. Identification of novel polymorphisms in the beta7 integrin gene: family-based association studies in inflammatory bowel disease. Genes Immun 2001;2:455–60.
57. Vavassori P, Borgiani P, D'Apice MR, et al. 3020insC mutation within the NOD2 gene in Crohn's disease: frequency and association with clinical pattern in an Italian population. Dig Liver Dis 2002;34:153.
58. Vermiere S, Wild G, Kocher K, et al. CARD15 genetic variation in a Quebec population: prevalence, genotype-phenotype relationship, and haplotype structure. Am J Hum Genet 2002;71:74–83.
59. Yamazaki K, Takazoe M, Tanaka T, et al. Absence of mutation in the NOD2/CARD 15 gene among 483 Japanese patients with Crohn's disease. J Hum Genet 2002;478:469–72.
60. Yang H, Plevy SE, Taylor K, et al. Linkage of Crohn's disease to the major histocompatibility complex region is detected by multiple nonparametric analyses. Gut 1999;44:519–26.

Environmental Factors

61. Blaser MJ, Miller RA, Lacher J, Singleton JW. Patients with active Crohn's disease have elevated serum antibodies to antigens of seven enteric bacterial pathogens. Gastroenterology 1984;87:888–94.
62. Boyko EJ, Koepsell TD, Perera DR, Inui TS. Risk of ulcerative colitis among former and current cigarette smokers. N Engl J Med 1987;316:707–10.
63. Calkins BM. A meta-analysis of the role of smoking in inflammatory bowel disease. Dig Dis Sci 1989;34:1841–54.
64. Chiba M, Fukushima T, Horie Y, Iizuka M, Masamune O. No *Mycobacterium paratuberculosis* detected in intestinal tissue, including Peyer's patches and lymph follicles, of Crohn's disease. J Gastroenterol 1998;33:482–7.
65. Cottone M, Rosselli M, Orlando A, et al. Smoking habits and recurrence in Crohn's disease. Gastroenterology 1994;106:643–8.
66. Daszak P, Purcell M, Lewin J, Dhillon AP, Pounder RE, Wakefield AJ. Detection and comparative analysis of persistent measles virus infection in Crohn's disease by immunogold electron microscopy. J Clin Pathol 1997;50:229–304.
67. Dell'Isola B, Poyart C, Goulet O, et al. Detection of *M. paratuberculosis* by polymerase chain reaction in children with Crohn's disease. J Infect Dis 1994;169:449–51.
68. Ekbom A, Daszak P, Kraaz W, Wakefield AJ. Crohn's disease after in-utero measles virus exposure. Lancet 1996;348:515–7.
69. Ekbom A, Wakefield AJ, Zack M, Adami HO. Perinatal measles infection and subsequent Crohn's disease. Lancet 1994;344:508–10.
70. Evans JM, McMahon AD, Murray FE, McDevit DG, MacDonald TM. Non-steroidal anti-inflammatory drugs are associated with emergency admission to hospital for colitis due to inflammatory bowel disease. Gut 1997;40:619–20.
71. Fidler HM, Thurrell W, Johnson NM, Rok GA, McFadden JJ. Specific detection of *Mycobacterium paratuberculosis* DNA associated with granulomatous tissue in Crohn's disease. Gut 1994;35:506–10.
72. Greenberg GR. Nutritional support in inflammatory bowel disease: current status and future directions. Scand J Gastroenterol Suppl 1992;192:117–22.

73. Haga Y, Funakoshi O, Kuroe K, et al. Absence of measles viral genomic sequence in intestinal tissues from Crohn's disease by nested polymerase chain reaction. Gut 1996;38:211–5.
73a. Hampe J, Cuthbert A, Croucher PJ, et al. Association between insertion mutation in NOD2 gene and Crohn's disease in German and British populations. Lancet 2001;357:1925–8.
74. Herbert TB, Cohen S. Stress and immunity in humans: a meta-analytic review. Psychosom Med 1993;55:364–79.
75. Ibbotson JP, Pease PE, Allan RN. Serological studies in Crohn's disease. Eur J Clin Microbiol 1987;6:286–90.
76. Jick H, Walker AM. Cigarette smoking and ulcerative colitis. N Engl J Med 1983;308:261–3.
77. Kanazawa K, Haga Y, Funakoshi O, et al. Absence of *Mycobacterium paratuberculosis* DNA in intestinal tissues from Crohn's disease by nested polymerase chain reaction. J Gastroenterol 1999;34:200–6.
78. Kleessen B, Kroesen AJ, Buhr HJ, Blaut M. Mucosal and invading bacteria in patients with inflammatory bowel disease compared with controls. Scand J Gastroenterol 2002;37:1034–41.
79. Lamps LW, Madhusudhan KT, Havens JM, et al. Pathogenic *Yersinia* DNA is detected in bowel and mesenteric lymph nodes from patients with Crohn's disease. Am J Surg Pathol 2003;27:220–7.
80. Levenstein S, Prantera C, Varvo V. Stress and exacerbation in ulcerative colitis: a prospective study of patients enrolled in remission. Am J Gastroenterol 2000;95:1213–20.
81. Lisby G, Andersen J, Engbaek K, Binder V. *Mycobacterium paratuberculosis* in intestinal tissue from patients with Crohn's disease by a nested primer polymerase chain reaction. Scand J Gastroenterol 1994;29:923–6.
82. Liu Y, van Kruiningen HJ, West AB, Cartun RW, Cortot A, Colombel JF. Immunocytochemical evidence of *Listeria, Escherichia coli,* and *Streptococcus* antigens in Crohn's disease. Gastroenterology 1995;108:1396–404.
83. Macpherson A, Khoo UY, Forgacs I, Philpott-Howard J, Bjarnason I. Mucosal antibodies in inflammatory bowel disease are directed against intestinal bacteria. Gut 1996;38:365–75.
84. Madara JL, Podolsky DK, King NW, Sehgal PK, Moore R, Winter HS. Characterization of spontaneous colitis in cotton-top tamarins (*Sanguinus oedipus*) and its response to sulfasalazine. Gastroenterology 1985;88:13–9.
85. Madretsma S, Wolters LM, van Dijk JP. In-vivo effect of nicotine on cytokine production by human non-adherent mononuclear cells. Eur J Gastroenterol Hepatol 1996;8:1017–20.
86. Mansfield JC, Giaffer MH, Holdsworth CD. Controlled trial of oligopeptide versus amino acid diet in treatment of active Crohn's disease. Gut 1995;36:60–6.
87. McCartney SA, Mitchell JA, Fairclough PD, Farthing JM, Warner TD. Selective COX-2 inhibitors and human inflammatory bowel disease. Aliment Pharmacol Ther 1999;13:1115–7.
88. Nielsen LL, Nielsen NM, Melbye M, Sodermann M, Jacobsen M, Aaby P. Exposure to measles in utero and Crohn's disease: Danish register study. Br Med J 1998;316:196–7.
89. Pardi DS, Tremaine WJ, Sandborn WJ, Loftus EV Jr, Poland GA, Melton LJ 3rd. Perinatal exposure to measles virus is not associated with the development of inflammatory bowel disease. Inflamm Bowel Dis 1999;5:104–6.
90. Persson PG, Leijonmarck CE, Bernell O, Hellers G, Ahlbom A. Risk indicators for inflammatory bowel disease. Int J Epidemiol 1993;22:268–72.
91. Pirzer U, Schonhaar A, Fleischer B, Hermann I, Meyer zum Buschenfelde KH. Reactivity of infiltrating T lymphocytes with microbial antigens in Crohn's disease. Lancet 1991;338:1238–9.
92. Rowbotham DS, Mapstone NP, Trejdosiewicz LK, Howdle PD, Quirke P. *Mycobacterium paratuberculosis* DNA not detected in Crohn's disease tissue by fluorescent polymerase chain reaction. Gut 1995;37:660–7.
93. Sanderson JD, Moss MT, Tizard ML, Hermon-Taylor J. *M. paratuberculosis* DNA in Crohn's disease tissue. Gut 1992;33:890–6.
94. Sandler RS, Sandler DP, McDonnell CW, Wurzelmann JI. Childhood exposure to environmental tobacco smoke and the risk of ulcerative colitis. Am J Epidemiol 1992;135:603–8.
95. Shanahan F. Crohn's disease. Lancet 2002;359: 62–9.
96. Shanahan F. Inflammatory bowel disease: immunodiagnostics, immunotherapeutics, and ecotherapeutics. Gastroenterology 2001;120: 622–35.
96a. Subhani J, Montgomery SM, Pounder RE, Wakefield AJ. Concordance rates of twins and siblings in inflammatory bowel disease. Gut 1998;42:A40.
97. Suenaga K, Yokoyama Y, Nishimori I, et al. Serum antibodies to *Mycobacterium paratuberculosis* in patients with Crohn's disease. Dig Dis Sci 1999;44:1202–7.
98. Suenaga K, Yokoyama Y, Okazaki K, Yamamoto Y. Mycobacteria in the intestine of Japanese patients with inflammatory bowel disease. Am J Gastroenterol 1995;90:76–80.
99. Sutherland LR, Ramcharan S, Bryant H, Fick G. Effect of cigarette smoking on recurrence of Crohn's disease. Gastroenterology 1990;98: 1123–8.
100. Swidsinski A, Ladhoff A, Pernthaler A, et al. Mucosal flora in inflammatory bowel disease. Gastroenterology 2002;122:44–54.

101. Theis MK, Boyko EJ. Patients perception of causes of inflammatory bowel disease. Am J Gastroenterol 1994;89:397–404.

101a. Thompson NP, Driscoll R, Pounder RE, Wakefield AJ. Genetics versus environment in inflammatory bowel disease: results of a British twin study. BMJ 1996;312:95–6.

102. Tysk C, Jarnerot G. Has smoking changed the epidemiology of ulcerative colitis? Scand J Gastroenterol 1992;27:508–12.

102a. Tysk C, Lindberg E, Jarnerot G, Floderus-Myrhed B. Ulcerative colitis and Crohn's disease in an unselected population of monozygotic and dizygotic twins. A study of heritability and the influence of smoking. Gut 1988;29:990–6.

103. van den Bogaerde J, Cahill J, Emmanuel AV, et al. Gut mucosal response to food antigens in Crohn's disease. Aliment Pharmacol Ther 2003;16:1903–15.

104. Whorlwell PJ, Holdstock G, Whorwell GM, Wright R. Bottle feeding, early gastroenteritis, and inflammatory bowel disease. Br Med J 1979;1:382.

105. Wu SW, Pao CC, Chan J, Yen TS. Lack of mycobacterial DNA in Crohn's disease tissue. Lancet 1991;337:174–5.

106. Wurzelman JI, Lyles CM, Sandler RS. Childhood infection and the risk of inflammatory bowel disease. Dig Dis Sci 1994;39:555–60.

Host Factors

107. Anderson RE, Olaison G, Tysk C, Ekbom A. Appendicectomy and protection against ulcerative colitis. N Engl J Med 2001;344:808–14.

108. Anderson RE, Olaison G, Tysk C, Ekbom A. Appendectomy is followed by increased risk of Crohn's disease. Gastroenterology 2003; 124:40–6.

109. Ardizzone S, Bianchi Porro G. Inflammatory bowel disease: new insights into the pathogenesis and treatment. J Intern Med 2002;252:475–96.

110. Fiocchi C. Inflammatory bowel disease: etiology and pathogenesis. Gastroenterology 1998: 115:182–205.

111. Hollander D, Vadheim C, Brettholz E, Petersen GM, Delahunty T, Rotter JI. Increased intestinal permeability in patients with Crohn's disease and their relatives: a possible etiologic factor. Ann Intern Med 1986;105:883–5.

112. Koutroubakis IE, Blachonikolis IG. Appendectomy and the development of ulcerative colitis: results of a metaanalysis of published case-control studies. Am J Gastroenterol 2000;95:171–6.

113. Rutgeerts P, D'Haens G, Hiele M, Geboes K, Vantrappen G. Appendectomy protects against ulcerative colitis. Gastroenterology 1994;106: 1251–3.

Immunologic Factors

114. Bartunkova J, Kolarova I, Sediva A, Holzelova E. Antineutrophil cytoplasmic antibodies, anti-*Saccharomyces cerevisiae* antibodies, and specific IgE to food allergens in children with inflammatory bowel diseases. Clin Immunol 2002;102:162–8.

115. Boirivant M, Marini M, Di Felice G, et al. Lamina propria T cells in Crohn's disease and other gastrointestinal inflammation show defective CD2 pathway-induced apoptosis. Gastroenterology 1999;116:557–65.

116. Boirivant M, Pica R, De Maria R, et al. Stimulated human lamina propria T cells manifest enhanced Fas-mediated apoptosis. J Clin Invest 1996;98:2616–22.

117. Cohavy O, Bruckner D, Cordon LK, et al. Colonic bacteria express an ulcerative colitis pANCA-related protein epitope. Inf Immun 2000;68:1542–8.

118. Colombel JF, Reumaux D, Duthilleul P, et al. Antineutrophil cytoplasmic autoantibodies in inflammatory bowel diseases. Gastroenterol Clin Biol 1992;16:656–60.

119. Das KM. Relationship of extraintestinal involvement in inflammatory bowel disease: new insights into autoimmune pathogenesis. Dig Dis Sci 1999;44:1–13.

120. Duchmann R, May E, Heike M, Knolle P, Neurath M, Meyer zum Buschenfelde KH. T cell specificity and cross reactivity towards enterobacteria, bacteroides, bifidobacterium, and antigens from resident intestinal flora in humans. Gut 1999;44:812–8.

121. Duerr RH, Targan SR, Landers CJ, Sutherland LR, Shanahan F. Anti-neutrophil cytoplasmic antibodies in ulcerative colitis: comparison with other colitides/diarrheal illnesses. Gastroenterology 1991;100:1590–6.

122. Elson CO. Commensal bacteria as targets in Crohn's disease. Gastroenterology 2000;119: 254–7.

123. Farrell JR, Peppercorn MA. Ulcerative colitis. Lancet 2002:359:331–40.

123a. Fiocchi C. Inflammatory bowel disease: etiology and pathogenesis. Gastroenterology 1998: 115:182–205.

124. Fuss IJ, Neurath M, Boirivant M, et al. Disparate CD4+ lamina propria (LP) lymphokine secretion profiles in inflammatory bowel disease. Crohn's disease LP cells manifest increased secretion of IFN-gamma, whereas ulcerative colitis LP cells manifest increased secretion of IL-5. J Immunol 1996;157:1261–70.

125. Groux H, O'Garra A, Bigler M, et al. A CD4+ T-cell subset inhibits antigen-specific T-cell responses and prevents colitis. Nature 1997;389: 737–42.

126. Halstenson TS, Brandtzaeg P. Local complement activation in inflammatory bowel disease. Immunol Res 1991;10:485–92.
127. Ina K, Itoh J, Fukushima K, et al. Resistance of Crohn's disease T cells to multiple apoptosis signals is associated with a Bcl-2/Bax mucosal imbalance. J Immunol 1999;163:1081–90.
128. Kuhn R, Lohler J, Rennick D, Rajewsky K, Miller W. Interleukin-10-deficient mice develop chronic enterocolitis. Cell 1993:75:263–74.
129. Liu Z, Geboes K, Colpaert S, et al. Prevention of experimental colitis in SCID mice reconstituted with CD45Rbhigh CD4+ T cells by blocking the CD40-CD154 interactions. J Immunol 2000;164:6005–14.
130. MacDonald TT, Monteleone G, Pender DL. Recent developments in the immunology of inflammatory bowel disease. Scand J Immunol 2000;51:2–9.
131. Melgar S, Yeung MM, Bas A, et al. Over-expression of interleukin 10 in mucosal T cells of patients with active ulcerative colitis. Clin Exp Immunol 2003;134:127–37.
132. Merger M, Croitoru K. Infections in the immunopathogenesis of chronic inflammatory bowel disease. Semin Immunol 1998;10:69–78.
133. Mizoguchi A, Mizoguchi E, Chiba C, et al. Cytokine imbalance and autoantibody production in T cell receptor-alpha mutant mice with inflammatory bowel disease. J Exp Med 1996;183:847–56.
134. Mullin GE, Lazenby AJ, Harris ML, Mayless TM, James SP. Increased interleukin-2 messenger RNA in the intestinal mucosal lesions of Crohn's disease but not ulcerative colitis. Gastroenterology 1992;102:1620–7.
135. Nielsen OH, Koppen T, Tudiger N, Horn T, Eriksen J, Kirman I. Involvement of interleukin-4 and -10 in inflammatory bowel disease. Dig Dis Sci 1996;41:1766–93.
136. Niessner M, Volk BA. Altered Th1/Th2 cytokine profiles in the intestinal mucosa of patients with inflammatory bowel disease as assessed by quantitative reverse transcribed polymerase chain reaction (RT-PCR). Clin Exp Immunol 1995;101:428–35.
137. Olives JP, Breton A, Hugot JP, et al. Antineutrophil cytoplasmic antibodies in children with inflammatory bowel disease. J Pediatr Gastroenterol Nutr 1997;25:142–8.
138. Onuma EK, Amenta PS, Ramaswamy K, Lin JJ, Das KM. Autoimmunity in ulcerative colitis (UC): a predominant colonic mucosal B cell response against human tropomyosin isoform 5. Clin Exp Immunol 2000;121:466–71.
139. Oudkerk-Pool M, Ellerbroek PM, Ridwan BU, et al. Serum antineutrophil cytoplasmic autoantibodies in inflammatory bowel disease are mainly associated with ulcerative colitis: a correlation study between perinuclear antineutrophil cytoplasmic autoantibodies and clinical parameters, medical and surgical treatment. Gut 1993;34:46–50.
140. Proujansky R, Fawcett PT, Gibney KM, Treem WR, Hyams JS. Examination of anti-neutrophil cytoplasmic antibodies in childhood inflammatory bowel disease. J Pediatr Gastroenterol Nutr 1993;2:193–7.
141. Reumaux D, Meziere C, Colombel JF, Duthilleul P, Muller S. Distinct production of autoantibodies to nuclear components in ulcerative colitis and in Crohn's disease. Clin Immunol Immunopathol 1995;77:349–57.
142. Roozendaal C, Pogany K, Hummel EJ, et al. Titres of anti-neutrophil cytoplasmic antibodies in inflammatory bowel disease are not related to disease activity. Q J Med 1999;92:651–8.
143. Sartor RB. Pathogenesis and immune mechanisms of chronic inflammatory bowel diseases. Am J Gastroenterol 1997;92(Suppl):S5-11.
144. Satsangi J, Landers CJ, Welsh KI, Koss K, Targan S, Jewell DP. The presence of anti-neutrophil antibodies reflects clinical and genetic heterogeneity within inflammatory bowel disease. Inflamm Bowel Dis 1998;4:18–26.
145. Saxon A, Shanahan F, Lander C, Ganz T, Targan SR. A distinct subset of antineutrophil cytoplasmic antibodies is associated with inflammatory bowel disease. J Allergy Clin Immunol 1990;86: 202–10.
146. Sung JY, Chan FKL, Lawton J, et al. Anti-neutrophil cytoplasmic antibodies (ANCA) and inflammatory bowel diseases in Chinese. Dig Dis Sci 1994;39:886–92.
147. Ueyama H, Kiyohara T, Sawada N, et al. High Fas ligand expression on lymphocytes in lesions of ulcerative colitis. Gut 1998;43:48–55.
148. Winter HS, Landers CJ, Winkelstein A, Vidrich A, Targan SR. Anti-neutrophil cytoplasmic antibodies in children with ulcerative colitis. J Pediatr 1994;5:707–11.
149. Yukawa M, Iizuka M, Horie Y, et al. Systemic and local evidence of increased Fas-mediated apoptosis in ulcerative colitis. In J Colorectal Dis 2002;17:70–6.

Crohn's Disease

150. Agnholt J, Dahlerup JF, Buntzen S, Tottrup A, Nielsen SL, Lundorf E. Response, relapse and mucosal immune regulation after infliximab treatment in fistulizing Crohn's disease. Aliment Pharmacol Ther 2003;17:703–10.
151. Belaiche J, Louis E, D'Haens G, et al. Acute lower gastrointestinal bleeding in Crohn's disease: characteristics of a unique series of 34 patients. Am J Gastroenterol 1999;94:2177–81.

152. Bernstein CN, Blanchard JF, Rawsthorne P, Wajda A. Epidemiology of Crohn's disease and ulcerative colitis in a central Canadian province: a population-based study. Am J Epidemiol 1999;149:916–24.
153. Bishop RP, Brewster AC, Antonioli DA. Crohn's disease of the mouth. Gastroenterology 1972;62:302–6.
154. Burgdorf W. Cutaneous manifestations of Crohn's disease. J Am Acad Dermatol 1981;5: 689–95.
155. Chambers TJ, Morson BC. Large bowel biopsy in the differential diagnosis of inflammatory bowel disease. Invest Cell Pathol 1980;3:159–73.
156. Delaney CP, Kiran RP, Senagore AJ, et al. Quality of life improves within 30 days of surgery for Crohn's disease. J Am Coll Surg 2003; 196:714–21.
157. De Rycke L, Kruithof E, Van Damme N, et al. Antinuclear antibodies following infliximab treatment in patients with rheumatoid arthritis or spondylarthropathy. Arthritis Rheum 2003;48:1015–23.
158. Ekbom A, Helmick CG, Zack M, Holmberg L, Adami HO. Survival and causes of death in patients with inflammatory bowel disease: a population-based study. Gastroenterology 1992;103:954–60.
159. El Maraghi NR, Mair NS. The histopathology of enteric infection with Yersinia pseudotuberculosis. Am J Clin Pathol 1979;71:631–9.
160. Favalli EG, Sinigaglia L, Varenna M, Arnoldi C. Drug-induced lupus following treatment with infliximab in rheumatoid arthritis. Lupus 2002;11:753–5.
161. Forbes A. Review article: Crohn's disease—the role of nutritional therapy. Aliment Pharmacol Ther 2002;16(Suppl 4):48–52.
162. Gad A. The diagnosis of gastroduodenal Crohn's disease by endoscopic biopsy. Scand J Gastroenterol Suppl 1989;24:23–8.
163. Geboes K, Rutgeerts P, Ectors N, et al. Major histocompatibility class II expression on the small intestinal nervous system in Crohn's disease. Gastroenterology 1992;103:439–47.
164. Greenstein AJ, Sachar DB, Mann D, Lachman P, Heimann T, Aufses AH Jr. Spontaneous free perforation and perforated abscess in 30 patients with Crohn's disease. Ann Surg 1987;205: 72–6.
165. Griffiths AM, Ohlsson A, Sherman PM, Sutherland LR. Meta-analysis of enteral nutrition as a primary treatment of active Crohn's disease. Gastroenterology 1995;108:1056–67.
166. Hendrickson BA, Gokhale R, Cho JH. Clinical aspects and pathophysiology of inflammatory bowel disease. Clin Microbiol Rev 2002;15:79–94.
167. Kirschner BS. Permanent growth failure in pediatric inflammatory bowel disease. J Pediatr Gastroenterol Nutr 1993;16:368–72.
168. Kobayashi K, Katsumata T, Yokoyama K, Takahashi H, Igarashi M, Saigenji K. A randomized controlled trial of total parenteral nutrition and enteral nutrition by elemental and polymeric diet as primary therapy in active phase of Crohn's disease. Jap J Gastroenterol 1998;95:1212–21.
169. Kreuzpaintner G, Horstkotte D, Heyll A, Losse B, Strohmeyer G. Increased risk of bacterial endocarditis in inflammatory bowel disease. Am J Med 1992;92:391–5.
169a. Kurata JH, Kantor-Fish S, Frankl H, Godby P, Vadheim CM. Crohn 's disease among ethnic groups in a large health maintenance organization. Gastroenterology 1992;102:1940–8.
170. Laffineur G, Lescut D, Vincent P, Quandalle P, Wurtz A, Colombel JF. Bacterial translocation in Crohn's disease. Gastroenterol Clin Biol 1992;16:777–81.
171. Lenaerts C, Roy CC, Vaillancourt M, Weber AM, Morin CL, Seidman E. High incidence of upper gastrointestinal tract involvement in children with Crohn's disease. Pediatrics 1989;83: 777–81.
171a. Loftus EV Jr, Silverstein MD, Sandborn WJ, Tremaine WJ, Harmsen WS, Zinsmeister AR. Crohn's disease in Olmsted County, Minnesota,1940-1993: incidence, prevalence, and survival. Gastroenterology 1998;114:1161–8.
172. Mahadeva U, Martin JP, Patel NK, Price AB. Granulomatous ulcerative colitis: a reappraisal of the mucosal granuloma in the distinction of Crohn's disease from ulcerative colitis. Histopathology 2002;41:50–5.
173. Markowitz J, Grancher K, Rosa J, Aiges H, Daum F. Growth failure in pediatric inflammatory bowel disease. J Pediatr Gastroenterol Nutr 1993;16:373–80.
174. Munkholm P, Langholz E, Nielsen OH, Kreiner S, Binder V. Incidence and prevalence of Crohn's disease in the county of Copenhagen, 1962-1987: a sixfold increase in incidence. Scand J Gastroenterol 1992;27:609–14.
175. Oberhuber G, Hirsch M, Stolte M. High incidence of upper gastrointestinal tract involvement in Crohn's disease. Virchows Arch 1998;432:49–52.
176. Oberhuber G, Puspok A, Oesterreicher C, et al. Focally enhanced gastritis: a frequent type of gastritis in patients with Crohn's disease. Gastroenterology 1997;112:698–706.

176a. Ogunbi SO, Ransom JA, Sullivan K, Schoen BT, Gold BD. Inflammatory bowel disease in African-American children living in Georgia. Pediatrics 1998;133:103–7.
177. Pardi DS, Loftus EV Jr, Tremaine WJ, et al. Acute major gastrointestinal hemorrhage in inflammatory bowel disease. Gastrointest Endosc 1999;49:153–7.
178. Pennington L, Hamilton SR, Bayless TM, Cameron JL. Surgical management of Crohn's disease: influence of disease at margin of resection. Ann Surg 1980;192:311–8.
179. Petri M, Poulsen SS, Christensen K, Jarnum S. The incidence of granulomas in serial sections of rectal biopsies from patients with Crohn's disease. Acta Pathol Microbiol Immunol Scand [A] 1982;90:145–7.
180. Podolsky DK. Inflammatory bowel disease. N Engl J Med 1991;325:928–37.
181. Poggioli G, Pierangeli F, Laureti S, Ugolini F. Review article: indication and type of surgery in Crohn's disease. Aliment Pharmacol Ther 2002;16(Suppl 4):59–64.
182. Present DH, Rutgeerts P, Targan SR, et al. Infliximab for the treatment of fistulas in patients with Crohn's disease. N Engl J Med 1999: 340:1398–405.
183. Pulimood AB, Ramakrishna BS, Kurian G, et al. Endoscopic mucosal biopsies are useful in distinguishing granulomatous colitis due to Crohn's disease from tuberculosis. Gut 1999; 45:537–41.
184. Ramzan NN, Leighton JA, Heigh FI, Shapiro MS. Clinical significance of granuloma in Crohn's disease. Inflamm Bowel Dis 2002;8:168–73.
185. Riordan AM, Ruxton CH, Hunter JO. A review of associations between Crohn's disease and consumption of sugars. Eur J Clin Nutr 1998;52:229–38.
186. Roberts IS, Stoddart RW. Ulcer-associated cell lineage ("pyloric metaplasia") in Crohn's disease: a lectin histochemical study. J Pathol 1993;171:13–9.
186a. Roth M, Peterson G, McElree C, Feldman E, Rotter JI. Geographic origins of Jewish patients with inflammatory bowel disease. Gastroenterology 1989:97:900–4.
187. Rotterdam H, Korelitz BI, Sommers SC. Microgranulomas in grossly normal rectal mucosa in Crohn's disease. Am J Clin Pathol 1977;67:550–4.
188. Rutgeerts P, D'Haens G, Targan SR, et al. Efficacy and safety of retreatment with anti-tumor necrosis factor antibody to maintain remission in Crohn's disease. Gastroenterology 1999;117: 761–9.
189. Ruuska T, Vaajalahti P, Arajarvi P, Maki M. Prospective evaluation of upper gastrointestinal mucosal lesions in children with ulcerative colitis and Crohn's disease. J Pediatr Gastroenterol Nutr 1994;19:181–6.
190. Sandborn WJ, Hanauer SB. Infliximab in the treatment of Crohn's disease: a user's guide for clinicians. Am J Gastroenterol 2002;97:2962–72.
191. Sedlack RE, Whisnanat J, Elveback LR, Kurland LT. Incidence of Crohn's disease in Olmsted County, Minnesota, 1935-1975. Am J Epidemiol 1980;112:759–63.
192. Shivananda S, Lennard-Jones J, Logan R, et al. Incidence of inflammatory bowel disease across Europe: is there a difference between north and south? Results of the European Collaborative Study on Inflammatory Bowel Disease (EC-IBD). Gut 1996;39:690–7.
193. Statter MB, Hirschl RB, Coran AC. Inflammatory bowel disease. Pediatr Surg 1993;40:1213–31.
194. Steinhoff MM, Kodner IJ, DeSchryver-Kecskemeti K. Axonal degeneration/necrosis: a possible ultrastructural marker for Crohn's disease. Mod Pathol 1988;1:182–7.
195. Surawicz CM, Meisel JL, Ylvisaker T, Saunders DR, Rubin CE. Rectal biopsy in the diagnosis of Crohn's disease: value of multiple biopsies and serial sectioning. Gastroenterology 1981;81:66–71.
196. Targan SR, Hanauer SB, Van Deventer SJ, et al. A short-term study of chimeric monoclonal antibody cA2 to tumor necrosis factor-alpha for Crohn's disease. N Engl J Med 1997; 337:1029–35.
197. Ten Hove T, van Montfrans C, Peppelenbosch MP, Van Deventer SJ. Infliximab treatment induces apoptosis of activated lamina propria T-lymphocytes in Crohn's disease. Gut 2002;50: 206–11.
198. Thomas GA, Millar-Jones D, Rhodes J, Roberts GM, Williams GT, Mayberry JF. Incidence of Crohn's disease in Cardiff over 60 years: 1986-1990 an update. Eur J Gastroenterol Hepatol 1995;7:401–5.
199. Trallori G, Palli D, Saieva C, et al. A population-based study of inflammatory bowel disease in Florence over 15 years (1978-92). Scand J Gastroenterol 1996;31:892–9.
200. Van Deventer SJ. Transmembrane TNF-alpha, induction of apoptosis, and the efficacy of TNF-targeting therapies in Crohn's disease. Gastroenterology 2001;121:1242–6.
201. Vermeier S, Norman M, Van Assche G, et al. Autoimmunity associated with anti-tumor necrosis factor alpha treatment in Crohn's disease: a prospective cohort study. Gastroenterology 2003;125:32–9.

202. Vermillion DL, Huizinga JD, Riddell RH, Collins SM. Altered small intestinal smooth muscle function in Crohn's disease. Gastroenterology 1993;104:1692–9.
203. Whelan G, Farmer RG, Fazio VW, Goormastic M. Recurrence after surgery in Crohn's disease. Relationship to location of disease (clinical pattern) and surgical indication. Gastroenterology 1985;88:1826–33.
204. Wilder WM, Slagle GW, Hand AM, Watkins WJ. Crohn's disease of the epiglottis, aryepiglottic folds, anus, and rectum. J Clin Gastroenterol 1980;2:87–91.
205. Wright CL, Riddell RH. Histology of the stomach and duodenum in Crohn's disease. Am J Surg Pathol 1998;22:383–90.

Ulcerative Colitis

206. Actis GC, Bruno M, Pinna-Pintor M, Rossini FP, Rizzetto M. Infliximab for treatment of steroid-refractory ulcerative colitis. Digest Liver Dis 2002;34:631–4.
207. Apel R, Cohen Z, Andrews CW Jr, McLeod R, Steinhart H, Odze RD. Prospective evaluation of early morphological changes in pelvic ileal pouches. Gastroenterology 1994;107:435–43.
208. Armstrong DN, Ballentyne GH, Adrain TE, Bilchik AJ, McMillen MA, Modlin IM. Adaptive increase in peptide YY and enteroglucagon after proctocolectomy and pelvic ileal reservoir construction. Dis Colon Rectum 1991;34:119–25.
209. Bengmark S. Ecological control of the gastrointestinal tract. The role of probiotic flora. Gut 1998;42:2–7.
210. Bernstein CN, Shanahan F, Anton PA, Weinstein WM. Patchiness of mucosal inflammation in treated ulcerative colitis: a prospective study. Gastrointest Endosc 1995;42:232–7.
211. Brown GL, Nanney LB, Griffen J, et al. Enhancement of wound healing by topical treatment with epidermal growth factor. N Engl J Med 1989;321:76–9.
212. Chaussade S, Denizot Y, Valleur P, et al. Presence of PAF-acether in stool of patients with pouch ileoanal anastomosis and pouchitis. Gastroenterology 1991;100:1509–14.
213. Chey W. Infliximab for patients with refractory ulcerative colitis. Inflamm Bowel Dis 2001; 1(Suppl):S30–3.
214. Davidson AM, Dixon MF. The appendix as a "skip lesion" in ulcerative colitis. Histopathology 1990;16:93–5.
215. D'Haens G, Geboes K, Peeters M, et al. Patchy cecal inflammation associated with distal ulcerative colitis: a prospective endoscopic study. Am J Gastroenterol 1997;92:1275–9.
216. D'Haens G, Lemmens L, Geboes K, et al. Intravenous cyclosporine versus intravenous corticosteroids as single therapy for severe attacks of ulcerative colitis. Gastroenterology 2001;120:1323–9.
217. Di Fibo G, Miglioli M, Lauri A, et al. Endoscopic assessment of acute inflammation of the reservoir after restorative proctocolectomy with ileoanal reservoir. Gastrointest Endosc 1990;36:6–9.
218. Dozois RR, Kelly KA, Welling DR, et al. Ileal pouch-anal anastomosis: comparison of results in familial adenomatous polyposis and chronic ulcerative colitis. Ann Surg 1989;210:268–71.
219. Dugas B, Mercenier A, Lenoir-Wijnkoop I, Arnaud C, Dugas N, Postaire E. Immunity and probiotics. Immunol Today 1999;20:387–90.
219a. Ekbom A, Helmick C, Zack M, Adami HO. The epidemiology of inflammatory bowel disease: a large, population-based study in Sweden. Gastroenterology 1991;100:350–8.
220. Farmer M, Petras RE, Hunt LE, Janosky JE, Galandiuk S. The importance of diagnostic accuracy in colonic inflammatory bowel disease. Am J Gastroenterol 2000;95:3184–8.
221. Farmer RG, Easley KA, Rankin GB. Clinical patterns, natural history, and progression of ulcerative colitis: a long-term follow-up of 1116 patients. Dig Dis Sci 1993;38:1137–46.
222. Farrokhyar F, Swarbrick ET, Crace RH, Hellier MD, Gent AE, Irvine EJ. Low mortality in ulcerative colitis and Crohn's disease in three regional centers in England. Am J Gastroenterol 2001;96:501–7.
223. Forde KA, Gold RP, Holck S, Goldberg MD, Kaim PS. Giant pseudopolyposis in colitis with colonic intussusception. Gastroenterology 1978;75:1142–6.
224. Forde KA, Gold RP, Weber C. Giant pseudopolyposis and antegrade colonic obstruction: report of a case. Dis Colon Rectum 1980;23: 583–6.
225. Gemlo BT, Wong WD, Rothenberger DA, Goldberg SM. Ileal pouch-anal anastomosis: patterns of failure. Arch Surg 1992;127:784–6.
226. Gertner DJ, Rampton DS, Madden MV, Talbot IC, Nicholls RJ, Lennard-Jones JE. Increased leukotriene B-4 release from ileal pouch mucosa in ulcerative colitis compared with familial adenomatous polyposis. Gut 1994;35:1429–32.
227. Goldblum JR, Appelman HD. Appendiceal involvement in ulcerative colitis. Mod Pathol 1992;5:607–10.
228. Goldenberg B, Mori K, Friedman IH, Shinya H, Buchwald RP. Fused inflammatory polyps simulating carcinoma in ulcerative colitis. Am J Gastroenterol 1980;73:441–4.

229. Gordon JI, Hooper LV, McNevin SM, Wong M, Bry L. Epithelial cell growth and differentiation III. Promoting diversity in the intestine: conversations between the microflora, epithelium, and diffuse GALT. Am J Physiol 1997;273:G565–70.
230. Groisman GM, George J, Harpaz N. Ulcerative appendicitis in universal and nonuniversal ulcerative colitis. Mod Pathol 1994;7:322–5.
231. Gustavsson S, Weiland LH, Kelly KA. Relationship of backwash ileitis to ileal pouchitis after ileal pouch-anal anastomosis. Dis Colon Rectum 1987;30:25–8.
232. Haller D, Bode C, Hammes WP, Pfeifer AM, Schiffrin EJ, Blum S. Non-pathogenic bacteria elicit a differential cytokine response by intestinal epithelial cell/leucocyte co-cultures. Gut 2000;47:79–87.
233. Hibi T, Ogata H, Sakuraba A. Animal models of inflammatory bowel disease. J Gastroenterol 2002;37:409–17.
234. Hoffmann JC, Pawlowski NN, Kuhl AA, Hohne W, Zeitz M. Animal models of inflammatory bowel disease: an overview. Pathobiology 2002;70:121–30.
235. Hyman NH, Fazio WW, Tuckson WB, Lavery IC. Consequences of ileal pouch-anal anastomosis for Crohn's colitis. Dis Colon Rectum 1991;34:653–7.
236. Kim B, Barnett JL, Kleer CG, Appelman HD. Endoscopic and histological patchiness in treated ulcerative colitis. Am J Gastroenterol 1999;94:3259–62.
237. Kleer CG, Appelman HD. Ulcerative colitis: patterns of involvement in colorectal biopsies and changes with time. Am J Surg Pathol 1998; 22:983–9.
238. Koch TR, Carney JA, Go VL, Szurszewski JH. Spontaneous contractions and some electrophysiologic properties of circular muscle from normal sigmoid colon and ulcerative colitis. Gastroenterology 1988;95:77–84.
239. Koltun WA, Schoetz DJ, Roberts PL Jr, Murray JJ, Coller JA, Veidenheimer MC. Indeterminate colitis prediposes to perineal complications after ileal pouch-anal anastomosis. Dis Colon Rectum 1991;34:857–60.
240. Kroft SH, Stryker SJ, Rao MS. Appendiceal involvement as a skip lesion in ulcerative colitis. Mod Pathol1994;7:912–4.
241. Kruis W, Schutz E, Fric P, Fixa B, Judmaier G, Stolte M. Double-blind comparison of an oral Escherichia coli preparation and mesalazine in maintaining remission of ulcerative colitis. Aliment Pharmacol Ther 1997;11:853–8.
242. Langholz E, Munkholm P, Davidsen M, Binder V. Course of ulcerative colitis: analysis of changes in disease activity over years. Gastroenterology 1994;107:3–11.
243. Lashner BA, Hanauer SB, Silverstein MD. Testing nicotine gum for ulcerative colitis patients: experience with single-patient trials. Dig Dis Sci 1990;35:827–32.
244. Levin KE, Pemberton JH, Phillips SF, Zinsmeister AR, Pezim ME. Role of oxygen free radicals in the etiology of pouchitis. Dis Colon Rectum 1992;35:452–6.
245. Lohmuller JL, Pemberton JH, Dozois RR, Ilstrup D, Van Heerden J. Pouchitis and extraintestinal manifestations of inflammatory bowel disease after ileal pouch-anal anastomosis. Ann Surg 1990;211:622–9.
246. Luukkonen P, Jarvinen H, Tanskanen M, Kahri A. Pouchitis—recurrence of the inflammatory bowel disease? Gut 1994;35:243–6.
247. Madden MV, Farthing MJ, Nicholls RJ. Inflammation in the ileal reservoir: pouchitis. Gut 1990;31:247–9.
248. Marcello PW, Schoetz DJ Jr, Roberts PL, et al. Evolutionary changes in the pathologic diagnosis after the ileoanal pouch procedure. Dis Colon Rectum 1997;40:263–9.
249. Meucci G, Bortoli A, Riccioli FA, et al. Frequency and clinical evolution of indeterminate colitis: a retrospective multi-centre study in northern Italy. Eur J Gastroenterol Hepatol 1999;11:909–13.
250. Mitomi H, Atari E, Uesugi H, et al. Distinctive diffuse duodenitis associated with ulcerative colitis. Dig Dis Sci 1997;42:684–93.
250a. Munkholm P, Langholz E, Nielsen OH, Kreiner S, Binder V. Incidence and prevalence of Crohn's disease in the county of Copenhagen, 1962-1987: a sixfold increase in incidence. Scand J Gastroenterol 1992;27:609–14.
251. Nasmyth DG, Godwin PGR, Dixon MF, Williams NS, Johnston D. Ileal ecology after pouch-anal anastomosis or ileostomy: a study of mucosal morphology, fecal bacteriology, fecal volatile fatty acids, and their interrelationship. Gastroenterology 1989;96:817–24.
252. Nicholls RJ. Review article: ulcerative colitis—surgical indications and treatment. Aliment Pharmacol Ther 2002;16(Suppl 4):25–8.
253. Nicholls RJ, Moskowitz RL, Shepherd NA. Restorative proctocolectomy with ileal reservoir. Br J Surg 1985;72(Suppl):S76–9.
254. Nicholls RJ, Wells AD. Indeterminate colitis. Bailliere's Clin Gastroenterol 1992;6:105–12.
255. Odze R, Antonioli D, Peppercorn M, Goldman H. Effect of topical 5-aminosalicylic acid (5-ASA) therapy on rectal mucosal biopsy morphology in ulcerative colitis. Am J Surg Pathol 1993;17:869–75.

256. Okawa K, Aoki T, Sano K, Harihara S, Kitano A, Kuroki T. Ulcerative colitis with skip lesions at the mouth of the appendix: a clinical study. Am J Gastroenterol 1998;93:2405–10.
257. Oresland T, Fasth S, Nordgren S, Hulte L. The clinical and functional outcome after restorative proctocolectomy: a prospective study in 100 patients. Int J Colorectal Dis 1989;4:50–6.
258. Palli D, Trallori G, Saieva C, et al. General and cancer specific mortality of a population based cohort of patients with inflammatory bowel disease: the Florence study. Gut 1998;42:175–9.
259. Pemberton JH, Kelly KA, Beart RW, Dozois RR, Wolff BG, Ilstrup DM. Ileal pouch-anal anastomosis for chronic ulcerative colitis: long-term results. Ann Surg 1987;206:504–13.
260. Persson PG, Bernell O, Leijonmarck CE, Farahmand BY, Hellers G, Ahlbom A. Survival and cause-specific mortality in inflammatory bowel disease: a population-based cohort study. Gastroenterology 1996;110:1339–45.
261. Pizarro TT, Arseneau KO, Bamias G, Cominelli F. Mouse models for the study of Crohn's disease. Trends Mol Med 2003;9:218–22.
262. Probert CS, Jayanthi V, Wicks AC, Mayberry JF. Mortality in patients with ulcerative colitis in Leicestershire, 1972-1989. An epidemiological study. Dig Dis Sci 1993;38:538–41.
263. Rauh SM, Schoetz DJ Jr, Roberts PL, Murray JJ, Coller JA, Veidenheimer MC. Pouchitis—is it a wastebasket diagnosis? Dis Colon Rectum 1991;34:685–9.
264. Rembacken BJ, Snelling AM, Hawkey PM, Chalmers DM, Axon AT. Non-pathogenic *Escherichia coli* versus mesalazine for the treatment of ulcerative colitis: a randomised trial. Lancet 1999;354:635–9.
265. Rosenthal SR, Snyder JD, Hendricks KM, Walker WA. Growth failure and inflammatory bowel disease: approach to treatment of a complicated adolescent problem. Pediatrics 1983;72:481–90.
266. Rothenberger DA. Pouchitis and empiricism: can we progress? Mayo Clin Proc 1994;69:491–2.
267. Rubin GP, Hungin AP, Kelly PJ, Ling J. Inflammatory bowel disease: epidemiology and management in an English general practice population. Aliment Pharmacol Ther 2000;14:1553–9.
268. Ruseler-van Embden JG, Schouten WR, van Lieshout LM. Pouchitis: result of microbial imbalance? Gut 1994;35:658–64.
269. Sandborn WJ. Pouchitis following ileal pouch-anal anastomosis: definition, pathogenesis and treatment. Gastroenterology 1994;107:1856–60.
270. Sandborn WJ, Tremaine WJ, Batts KP, Pemberton JH, Phillips SF. Pouchitis after ileal pouch-anal anastomosis: a pouchitis disease activity index. Mayo Clin Proc 1994;69:409–15.
271. Sasaki M, Okada K, Koyama S, et al. Ulcerative colitis complicated by gastroduodenal lesions. J Gastroenterol 1996;31:585–9.
272. Shanahan F. Probiotics and inflammatory bowel disease: is there a scientific rationale? Inflamm Bowel Dis 2000;6:107–15.
273. Smith MB, Lashner BA, Hanauer SB. Smoking and inflammatory bowel disease in families. Am J Gastroenterol 1988;83:407–9.
274. Snape WJ, Williams R, Hyman PE. Defect in colonic smooth muscle contraction in patients with ulcerative colitis. Am J Physiol 1991;261: G987–91.
275. Stonnington CM, Phillips SF, Zinsmeister AR, Melton LJ 3rd. Prognosis of chronic ulcerative colitis in a community. Gut 1987;28:1261–6.
276. Su C, Salzberg BA, Lewis JD, et al. Efficacy of anti-tumor necrosis factor therapy in patients with ulcerative colitis. Am J Gastroenterol 2002;97:2577–84.
277. Sullivan PB, Brueton MJ, Tabara ZB, Goodlad RA, Lee CY, Wright NA. Epidermal growth factor in necrotising enteritis. Lancet 1991;338;53–4.
277a. Tysk C, Jarnerot G. Has smoking changed the epidemiology of ulcerative colitis? Scand J Gastroenterol 1992;27:508-12.
278. Valdez R, Appelman HD, Bronner MP, Greenson JK. Diffuse duodenitis associated with ulcerative colitis. Am J Surg Pathol 2000;24: 1407–13.
279. Vrees MD, Pricolo VE, Potenti FM, Cao W. Abnormal motility in patients with ulcerative colitis: the role of inflammatory cytokines. Arch Surg 2002;137:439–46.
280. Winther KV, Jess T, Langholz E, Munkholm P, Binder V. Survival and cause-specific mortality in ulcerative colitis: follow-up of a population-based cohort in Copenhagen County. Gastroenterology 2003;125:1576–82.
281. Yang SK, Jung HY, Kang GH, et al. Appendiceal orifice inflammation as a skip lesion in ulcerative colitis: an analysis in relation to medical therapy and disease extent. Gastrointest Endosc 1999;49:743–7.
282. Yu CS, Pemberton JH, Larson D. Ileal pouch-anal anastomosis in patients with indeterminate colitis. Dis Colon Rectum 2000;43:1487–96.

16 NON-NEOPLASTIC POLYPOSIS SYNDROMES

The inherited non-neoplastic (hamartoma) syndromes have gastrointestinal polyposis as a component feature, but the extent and type of polyps vary significantly from one syndrome to the next. Hamartomatous gastrointestinal polyps are found in Bannayan-Riley-Ruvalcaba syndrome, Cowden's syndrome, juvenile polyposis syndrome, and Peutz-Jeghers syndrome. Patients may develop multiple gastrointestinal mucosal polyps, as well as numerous extraintestinal lesions.

The most common polyposis syndromes involve neoplastic intestinal adenomas; these are covered in the Fascicle on intestinal neoplasms (3). The less common non-neoplastic (hamartomatous) polyposis syndromes are described in this chapter. Patients with these syndromes are at increased risk for tumor development. A knowledge of the number of polyps present, their location, the patient age, the family history, the presence of extraintestinal manifestations, and the underlying genetic alterations helps classify the specific syndrome (Table 16-1). *PTEN* mutations are found in 80 percent of patients with Cowden's syndrome and 60 percent of patients with Bannayan-Riley-Ruvalcaba syndrome (1,2). Because *PTEN* mutations underlie the changes in both diseases, some suggest that they belong to a single genetic entity termed the PTEN-hamartoma tumor syndrome (1,2).

PEUTZ-JEGHERS SYNDROME

Definition. *Peutz-Jeghers syndrome* (PJS) is an autosomal dominant disorder characterized by: 1) mucocutaneous melanin pigmentation; 2) hamartomatous intestinal polyposis preferentially affecting the small intestine; and 3) an elevated risk for the development of malignancies. Associated extraintestinal neoplasms include ovarian, cervical, testicular, pancreatic, and breast tumors. The following criteria are used to diagnose PJS: 1) three or more histologically confirmed Peutz-Jeghers polyps, or 2) any number of Peutz-Jeghers polyps with a family history of PJS, or 3) characteristic prominent mucocutaneous pigmentation with a family history of PJS, or 4) any number of Peutz-Jeghers polyps and characteristic prominent mucocutaneous pigmentation (4).

Demography. PJS has an estimated incidence of 1/120,000 births (27). Approximately 50 percent of cases are familial and 50 percent are sporadic with new mutations. Based on the number of families registered in the Finnish Polyposis Registry, the incidence of PJS is roughly one tenth that of familial adenomatous polyposis (4). PJS has been diagnosed in an individual as young as 15 days; males and females are equally affected.

Etiology. Germline mutations or loss of heterozygosity (LOH) in the *STK11* gene located at 19p13.3 accounts for most PJS cases (7,13,16, 20). PJS kindreds inherit mutations in the *STK11* gene as a single hit on one allele, corresponding to the autosomal dominant inheritance pattern. The second hit then occurs in affected PJS tissues (9,10,23). Germline mutations are usually truncating, but missense mutations also occur (9,15,17,20). Approximately 70 percent of familial PJS patients have *STK11* mutations and 30 to 70 percent of patients with sporadic disease also have these mutations (23).

STK11, which encodes a novel serine-threonine kinase, consists of nine exons and is ubiquitously expressed in adults (9,10,13,15,17). Codons 50-337 encode the catalytic kinase

Table 16-1

NON-NEOPLASTIC POLYPOSIS SYNDROMES

Hereditary Syndromes
Peutz-Jeghers syndrome (*STK11* mutation)
Juvenile polyposis (*SMAD4* or *BMPRIA* mutation)
Cowden's disease (*PTEN* mutation)
Bannayan-Riley-Ruvalcaba syndrome (*PTEN* mutation)
Familial hyperplastic gastric polyposis
Nonhereditary Syndromes
Cronkhite-Canada syndrome
Lymphoid polyposis

domain of the gene. The STK11 gene product localizes to both the nucleus and the cytoplasm (18) and is a substrate of the cyclic adenosine monophosphate (AMP)-dependent protein kinase (7). Identification of the PJS gene makes genetic screening possible for affected families. Mutation testing is done by utilizing full gene sequencing of the 23-Kb gene containing the nine exons. Patients with neoplastic transformation of their hamartomas exhibit LOH on 19p in addition to *β-catenin* gene mutations, or mutations or LOH at the *p53* locus. These findings suggest that mutations of the *β-catenin* gene or *p53* may help convert hamartomatous polyps into adenomas and carcinomas (16).

Clinical Features. Most patients present with mucosal pigmentation and intestinal polyposis (12). Polyps may occasionally be absent; conversely, some patients have only intestinal polyps. The hyperpigmentation commonly emerges in infancy or in childhood and consists of greenish black to brown melanin deposits on the lips, buccal mucosa, periorbital area, nose, hands, feet, and occasionally, the genital or perianal skin (14). Over 95 percent of patients have melanin spots, most commonly on lips (95 percent) and buccal mucosa (66 to 83 percent). Pigmented lesions of the lips and oral cavity generally develop by 2 years of age. Pigmented lesions tend to fade by puberty, except for the buccal lesions (25).

Most PJS patients develop gastrointestinal symptoms during adolescence or young adulthood. A third of the patients have symptoms before age 10; half have symptoms before age 20 (24). Diffuse gastrointestinal polyposis causes intussusception (28) or obstruction presenting as recurrent attacks of crampy abdominal pain (24). The polyps preferentially develop in the small intestine (64 to 67 percent of cases), especially in the jejunum, although they may arise throughout the entire gastrointestinal tract. Polyps that autoamputate, twist, intussuscept, or prolapse become ischemic and cause bleeding, anemia, or massive hemorrhage. The polyposis may progress, with intermittent polyp growth and the appearance of new "crops" of polyps that may appear simultaneously in different parts of the bowel.

PJS polyps should be removed because they are prone to mechanical injury and they may contain areas of dysplasia or invasive cancer. Because rectal polyps occur in less than one third of patients, sigmoidoscopy is generally less useful for screening than it is in familial adenomatous polyposis.

Radiologic Findings. Radiologic examination using ultrasound, computerized tomography (CT) scan, upper gastrointestinal examination, and barium enema detects polyps in various regions of the gastrointestinal tract (21). The distribution of the lesions suggests the diagnosis.

Gross Findings. The polyps of PJS arise throughout the gastrointestinal tract to affect the jejunum, ileum, colon, stomach, duodenum, and appendix in decreasing order of frequency. Rare polyps develop in the esophagus, nasopharynx, and urinary tract. Gastric PJS polyps occur less commonly in Western populations than in the Japanese (16,18). Large sessile polyps may develop in the stomach; gastric polyps are usually larger than the polyps seen in juvenile polyposis, Canada-Cronkhite syndrome, and Cowden's disease. Most gastric lesions arise in the antrum (19).

Intestinal polyps usually number in the dozens. They are sessile or pedunculated, with coarsely lobulated, dark heads resembling adenomas (fig. 16-1). They range in size from a few millimeters to over 7 cm; most measure 0.5 to 3.0 cm in diameter. Grossly, they resemble other gastrointestinal polyps. Clusters of polyps lying adjacent to one another can resemble one large polyp (fig. 16-2). When epithelial islands lie deep in the intestinal wall or on the serosa, intramural nodules may be present.

Microscopic Findings. PJS polyps have a distinctive histologic appearance. They consist of gastrointestinal epithelium indigenous to the site of origin arranged on an arborizing muscular framework. The muscle fibers extend out from the center of the lesion like the branches of a tree, becoming progressively thinner as they reach the polyp surface (fig. 16-3). These muscle bundles appear relatively hypovascular. Even when intussusception occurs with secondary infarction of the polyp, ghosts of the prominent muscle fibers remain visible (fig. 16-4).

In the small intestine, cells of the normal small bowel mucosa, including goblet, absorptive, endocrine, and Paneth cells, line the crypts and villi (fig. 16-3). The goblet cells may appear hypermucinous. Duodenal lesions may

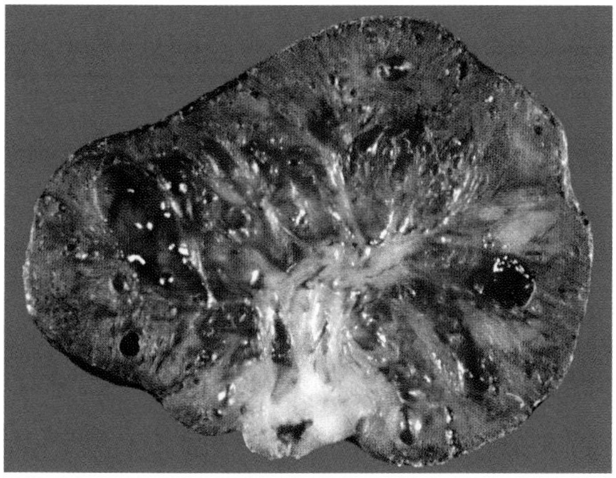

Figure 16-1

PEUTZ-JEGHERS POLYP

The polypoid appearance and the central muscular core are seen in a bisected polyp.

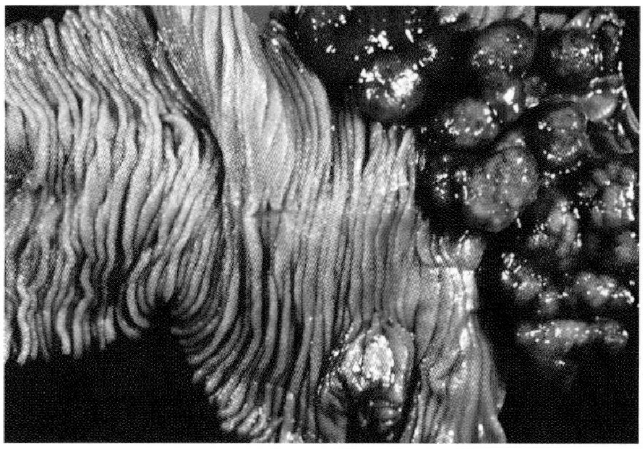

Figure 16-2

PEUTZ-JEGHERS POLYP

Clusters of Peutz-Jeghers polyps in the small intestine appear as one large polyp.

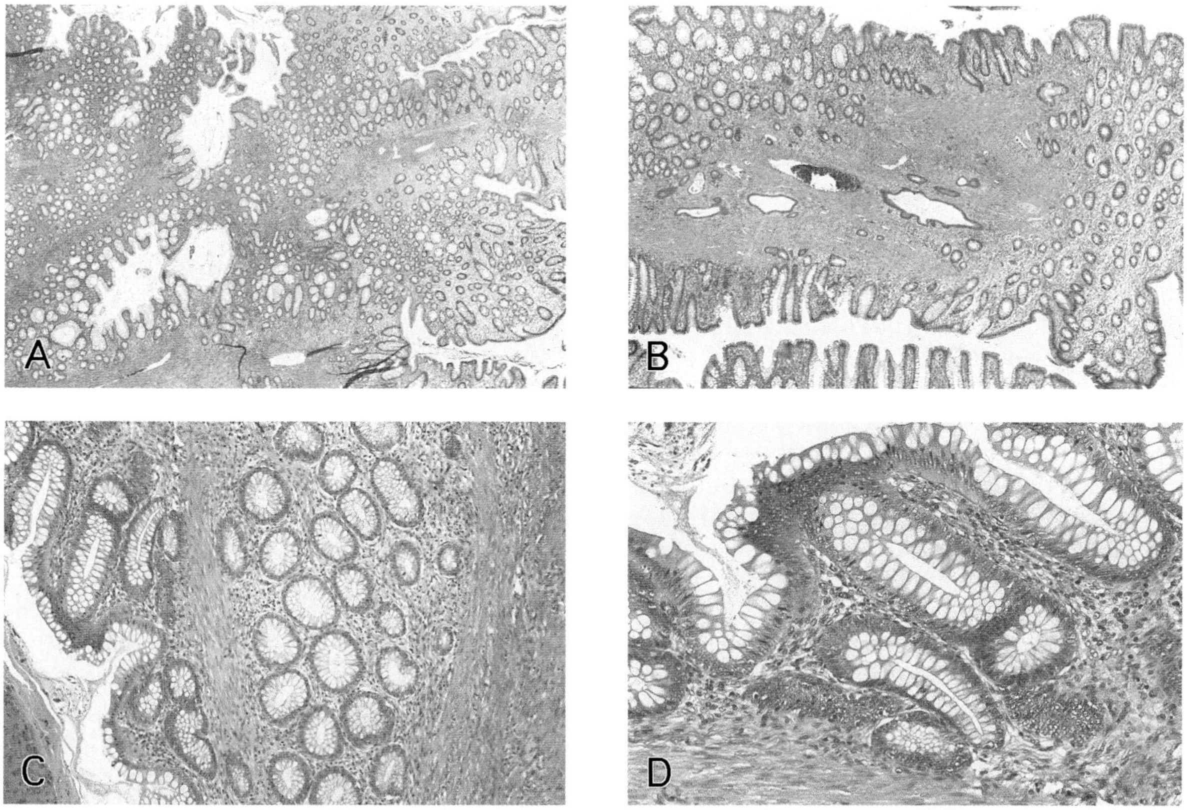

Figure 16-3

HISTOLOGIC FEATURES OF PEUTZ-JEGHERS POLYPS

A,B: Low- and higher-magnification views of the prominent muscular component which lines the various fronds of the polyp. It is covered on both sides by mucosa.

C: The prominent muscular bands separate intestinal mucosa.

D: There are numerous goblet cells and lamina propria covering the muscular core.

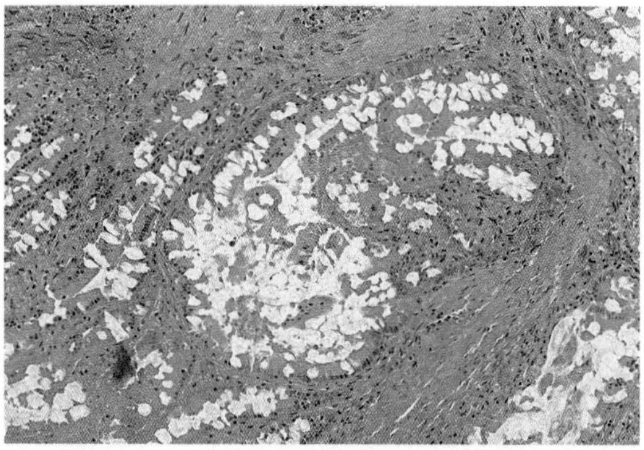

Figure 16-4

INFARCTED PEUTZ-JEGHERS POLYP

The polyp was at the lead point of an intussusception in a 10-year-old. Much of the epithelium is degenerated and necrotic. The prominent smooth muscle bands remain.

contain Brunner glands. The epithelial cells usually retain their normal relationship with one another: columnar and goblet cells may predominate in the surface portion whereas Paneth and endocrine cells lie at the crypt bases next to the muscular framework.

PJS polyps in the colon contain colonic mucosa. The replication zone at the crypt base is usually relatively short, and mature cells line the elongated, often branched glands. The epithelium includes absorptive and goblet cells, with goblet cells predominating in most cases. The surface may have a villous architecture. Colonic PJS polyps contain arborizing bands of smooth muscle, but these may be less prominent than the smooth muscle bands found in small intestinal polyps; the muscle bands may be absent in small colonic polyps. Unlike juvenile polyps, the lamina propria of PJS polyps appears normal.

Gastric polyps show prominent foveolar hyperplasia, pit epithelium, and variable numbers of deep glands. The most diagnostic feature of gastric polyps is a central core of finely arborizing smooth muscle branches originating from the muscularis mucosae. Gastric PJS polyps frequently lack the smooth muscle bundles, however, and resemble the more common gastric hyperplastic polyps.

The surfaces of polyps often become superficially eroded and acutely inflamed. As a result, abnormally long rows of darkly staining regen-

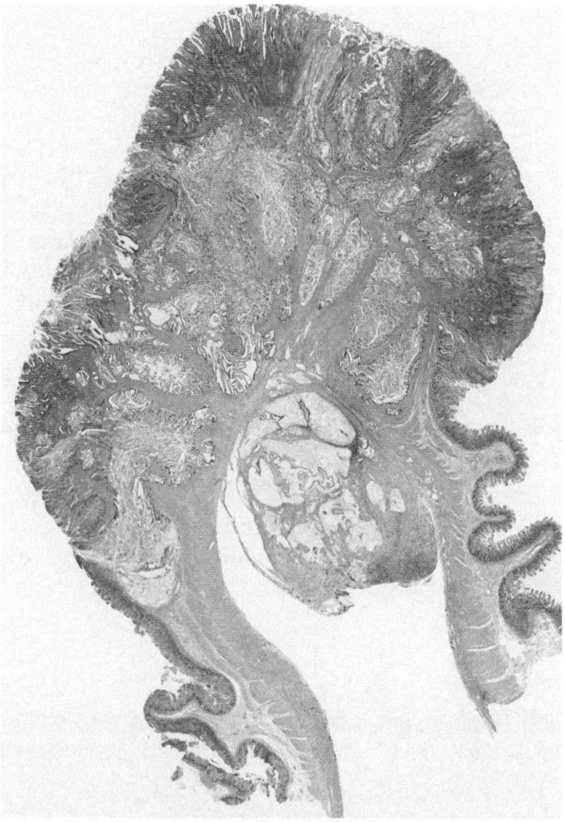

Figure 16-5

EPITHELIAL DISPLACEMENT IN A PEUTZ-JEGHERS POLYP

Numerous glands are displaced into the submucosa and even onto the serosal surface. At low power they appear as mucinous pools. Higher magnification of the lesion disclosed that they were benign.

erative cells may line elongated crypts and glands. The regenerative epithelium appears immature and contains numerous mitoses. Some glands become cystically dilated. Hyperplastic areas show intraluminal papillary projections, producing a serrated pattern reminiscent of that found in hyperplastic polyps or serrated adenomas. PJS polyps lack the prominent edematous stroma seen in juvenile polyps. Inflammation is usually not prominent. Hemosiderin deposits indicate previous mucosal erosion (22).

Benign glands and mucinous cysts may lie in the submucosa (fig. 16-5), muscularis propria, or even in the serosa in 10 percent of polyps involving the small intestine (22). This finding is unusual in gastric or large intestinal lesions (22). The cysts result from one of two processes: as a part of hamartomatous intestinal lesions or from glandular entrapment secondary to trauma, intussusception, or surface erosion. Sometimes the deep glands connect with the superficial glands; in other cases they lack continuity with the overlying mucosa. Rarely, glands are found deep in the bowel wall or in the serosa, in the absence of a surface polyp. Such lesions have prominent intramural mucinous cysts partially or totally lined by normal goblet cells, absorptive cells, endocrine cells, and/or Paneth cells. Infoldings of columnar epithelium and dystrophic calcification are seen in the mucinous pools. The benign appearance of the displaced epithelium differentiates these areas from invasive mucinous carcinoma (22). Deep mucinous cysts may lack an epithelial lining.

Microscopic Variants. Rare polyps contain areas of osseous metaplasia (17).

Differential Diagnosis. Two major differential diagnostic problems exist with respect to PJS polyps: 1) the polyp type and 2) whether or not the lesion contains invasive cancer. Because gastric PJS polyps often resemble the more common gastric hyperplastic polyps, as well as the polyps occurring in the stomach of patients with juvenile polyposis or Cronkhite-Canada syndrome, it is important to correlate the biopsy findings with the clinical history and other features characteristic of each syndrome in order to establish the correct diagnosis. Gastric hyperplastic polyps seldom, if ever, contain the arborizing smooth muscle bundles characteristic of classic PJS polyps. In the colon, PJS polyps with extensive hyperplasia may superficially resemble a large hyperplastic polyp. The latter, however, typically contains large numbers of glands and lacks arborizing muscle bundles. Juvenile polyps contain numerous small cysts filled with mucus and inflammatory cells, and contain a disproportionately large amount of stroma when compared with the glands.

It is also possible to over-read epithelial misplacement as invasive malignancy. Cells appearing histologically and cytologically benign, with a brush border and lack of cellular atypia, help distinguish PJS polyps from carcinoma. Circumscribed foci of signet ring cells may occur in PJS polyps as a result of gland degeneration from intestinal intussusception, polyp stretching, or torsion. These events cause focal mucosal ischemia and epithelial sloughing. The sloughed epithelial cells assume a rounded shape and signet ring-like appearance; however, they lack the usual cytologic features necessary to make a diagnosis of signet ring cell carcinoma. In addition, these cells are usually E-cadherin positive, while true signet rings cells are not.

Treatment and Prognosis. It is recommended that individuals suspected of having PJS undergo regular upper gastrointestinal endoscopy, colonoscopy, and small bowel studies, since intestinal, gastric, and colonic lesions are found in 88 to 100 percent, 24 to 49 percent, and 60 percent of patients, respectively. These polyps, especially when they occur in the jejunum and ileum, can lead to intussusception (26).

Carcinoma of the intestinal tract is a frequent complication of PJS. There are well-documented reports of carcinoma arising in PJS and in some cases, associated adenomatous or dysplastic changes are observed within the hamartomatous polyp (5,8,11,14). For these reasons, PJS is also now considered to be among the gastrointestinal cancer syndromes. The carcinoma risk is 15 times greater for patients with PJS than for the general population. The frequency of neoplasia ranges between 3 and 6 percent. When neoplasms develop, 73 percent arise in the gastrointestinal tract, and include large intestinal, gastric, pancreatic, small intestinal, and gallbladder carcinomas (figs. 16-6, 16-7), as well as gastrointestinal stromal tumors. Adenocarcinoma is most common in the duodenum and stomach, occurring in up to 3 percent of patients. Cancer usually doesn't develop until after age 30, with a mean age of 43 years. By age 65, there is a 93 percent rate of developing cancer, whether it is gastrointestinal or extragastrointestinal in location (6). An excess of extragastrointestinal malignancies (breast, cervix, ovarian, testicular) also occurs.

Because of the increased risk for cancer, it is recommended that patients undergo screening. The screening recommendations for gastrointestinal malignancies include colonoscopy beginning with symptoms or in the late teens if no symptoms occur. The interval between examinations is determined by the number of polyps, but it should be at least every 3 years once it begins. Screening for pancreatic cancer involves endoscopic or abdominal ultrasound

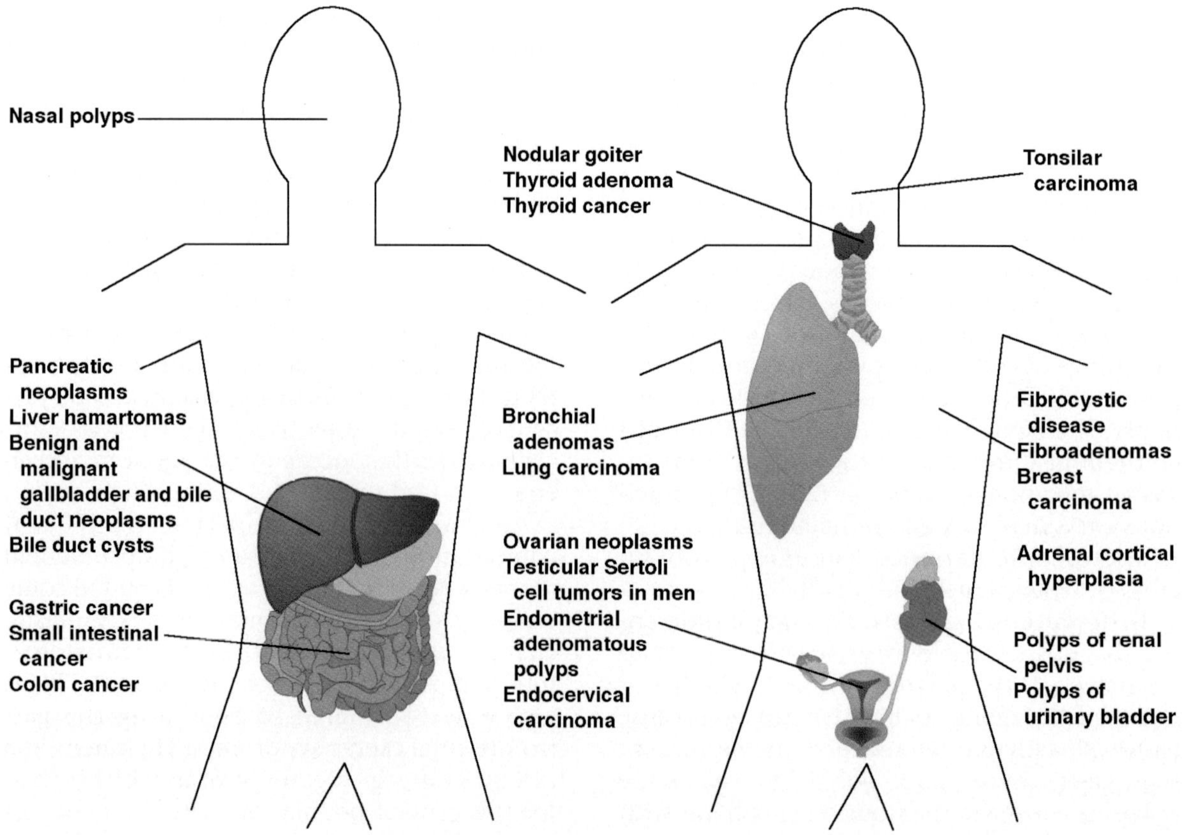

Figure 16-6

DIAGRAMMATIC REPRESENTATION OF THE NEOPLASMS ASSOCIATED WITH PEUTZ-JEGHERS SYNDROME

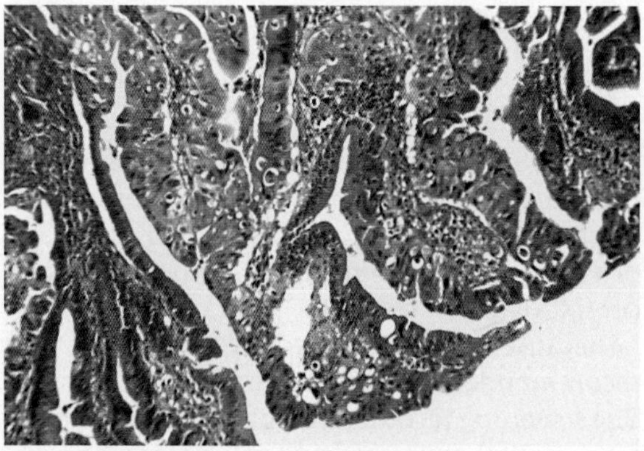

Figure 16-7

INTRAEPITHELIAL NEOPLASIA DEVELOPING IN A PEUTZ-JEGHERS POLYP

The cells lining the glands of this polyp have been replaced by cells with an increased nuclear to cytoplasmic ratio and cytologic atypia.

every 1 to 2 years after age 30. Screening for gastric neoplasia consists of upper gastrointestinal endoscopy every 2 years starting at age 10. Screening for small bowel neoplasms occurs via annual hemoglobin and small bowel X ray every 2 years beginning at age 10. Screening for breast carcinoma involves an annual breast exam and mammography every 2 to 3 years beginning at age 25. Screening for gynecologic neoplasms involves annual pelvic exam with Papanicolaou (PAP) smear beginning around age 20. Screening for testicular tumors begins at age 10.

JUVENILE POLYPOSIS SYNDROME

Definition. *Juvenile polyposis syndrome* (JPS) is an autosomal dominant syndrome characterized by multiple gastrointestinal hamartomatous polyps in the absence of the extraintestinal features classic for other hamartomatous polyposis syndromes, such as Bannayan-Riley-Ruvalcaba syndrome and Cowden's disease. The following diagnostic criteria have been established for the diagnosis of JPS: 1) five or more juvenile polyps of the colorectum, or 2) extracolonic juvenile polyps, or 3) any number of juvenile polyps in a patient with a family history of JPS (29,54). There are many other terms for JPS: *generalized juvenile polyposis, juvenile polyposis coli, juvenile polyposis of infancy, gastric juvenile polyposis, juvenile polyposis of the stomach, familial juvenile polyposis, hamartomatous gastrointestinal polyposis, hyperplastic inflammatory polyps,* and *retention polyps.*

Demography. JPS is 10 times less common than familial adenomatous polyposis (46), with an incidence of 0.6 to 1.0 cases/100,000 in Western populations. Juvenile polyps, however, are the most common pediatric polyps, affecting an estimated 1 percent of children and adolescents (49). JPS occurs in both sporadic and familial forms (58); approximately 20 to 50 percent of suspected individuals have the familial form. The age of onset, number of polyps, polyp location, and the development of further polyps vary. Patients range in age from 10 to 63 years, however, patients in the first two decades of life (mean age at diagnosis of 18.5 years) are most commonly affected. The disorder affects both sexes (35).

Etiology. JPS is an autosomal dominant disorder with mutations in either the *SMAD4* tumor suppressor gene (36,43–45,50,53) located at 18q21.1 or in the bone morphogenic protein receptor 1A (*BMPR1A*) gene. Both of these genes are involved in transforming growth factor-beta (TGF-β) signaling (48,61a,62,63). Genetic testing is available for both of these known genetic mutations.

Juvenile polyps have been described in the stomach, small bowel, and colon in infants and an autosomal recessive inheritance has been suggested for some kindreds (56).

Clinical Features. The clinical course depends on patient age, polyp number, polyp location, and the form of JPS present. Most patients present in childhood; only 15 percent present as adults (35). Infants with JPS are likely to have more severe symptoms and complications (51) than older individuals. Patients with JPS of infancy develop diarrhea, protein-losing enteropathy, intussusception, gastrointestinal bleeding, and rectal prolapse (35). Other clinical manifestations of JPS include polyp prolapse, hypokalemia, cachexia, anemia, malnutrition, and abdominal pain (52). Bleeding affects 84 to 95 percent of patients (51) and occurs more commonly in children; intussusception tends to affect infants. Autoamputation, resulting in the passage of tissue, also occurs (51). The number of new polyps decreases as the patient ages (42). Gastric polyps affect the antrum and extend to the fundus, eventually becoming more numerous, larger, and pedunculated. Gastric polyps are present either as part of a generalized polyposis syndrome or as part of familial gastric polyposis, and are associated with gastric hyperplastic and adenomatous polyps.

Radiologic Findings. Radiographic examination delineates the distribution of the polyps as follows: colorectal, 98 percent; gastric, 3.6 percent; duodenal, 2.3 percent; and jejunal and ileal, 6.3 percent (35).

Gross Findings. Patients with JPS usually have 10 to hundreds of polyps (46). Most polyps are located in the rectosigmoid. Juvenile polyps are usually small, round, smooth-surfaced lesions, ranging in size from less than 1 mm to 5 cm; most measure from less than 1 to 2 cm in diameter (figs. 16-8–16-10). Patients presenting in late childhood or adulthood usually have completely normal-appearing intervening mucosa. Larger polyps tend to be pedunculated, with a short stalk; only about 25 percent are sessile. Larger lesions are grayish pink-red, spherical, mushroom-like, cerebriform, often ulcerated, and covered by an inflammatory exudate. The cut surface displays variably sized mucus-containing cysts embedded in a gray fibrous stroma. Pedunculated polyps may twist, causing ischemia and hemorrhage, and resulting in autoamputation.

Microscopic Findings. Typical juvenile polyps consist of gastrointestinal glands indigenous to the site of origin, surrounded by an increased amount of edematous, often inflamed stroma. The stromal-epithelial ratio is disproportionately larger than normal. Stroma widely separates branched, sometimes cystic, variably sized tortuous glands. The polyps often appear more disorderly than other polyps due to the cystically dilated glands and large stromal content (fig. 16-11). The glands are lined by columnar, cuboidal, or flattened epithelium. The lining may appear hyperplastic, with a serrated

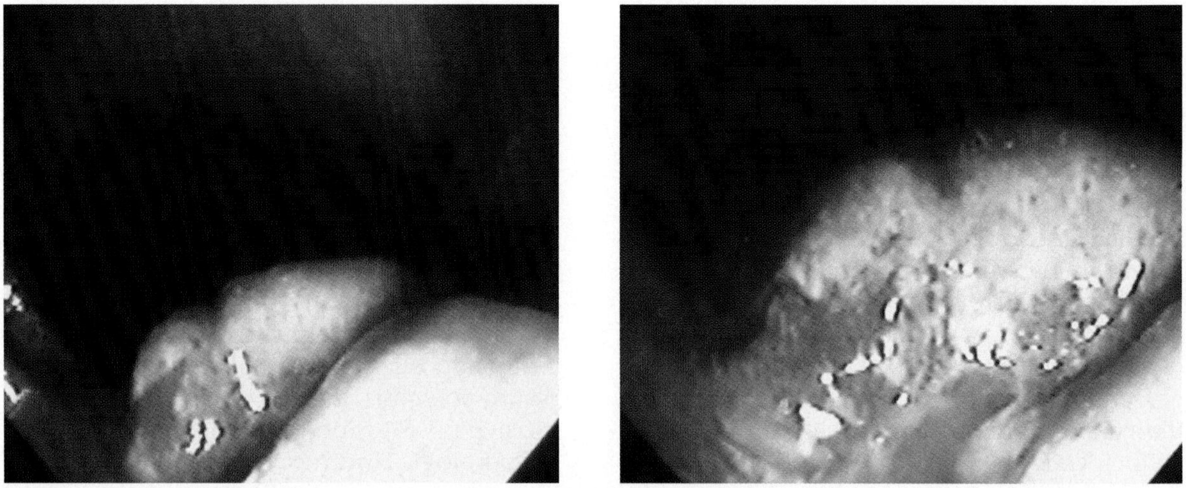

Figure 16-8

JUVENILE POLYPOSIS SYNDROME

Left: Endoscopic appearance of an irregular polyp within the mucosa.
Right: Higher-magnification view.

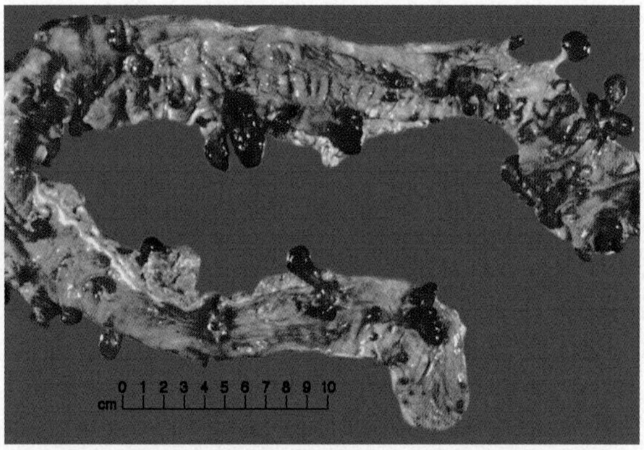

Figure 16-9

JUVENILE POLYPOSIS SYNDROME

Resected specimen shows the presence of multiple pedunculated, reddish, juvenile polyps distributed throughout the large bowel.

pattern resembling that seen in hyperplastic polyps or serrated adenomas. Polyp surfaces are covered by a single layer of cuboidal or columnar epithelial cells, often with interspersed goblet cells (fig. 16-11). The cysts contain either mucus or inflammatory debris (fig. 16-11). When the glands rupture, mucus, inflammatory cells, and cellular debris extend into the surrounding lamina propria. Sometimes the epithelial lining completely disappears. Repeated torsion may cause stromal hemorrhage, surface ulceration, and inflammation. Eroded polyps develop a granulation tissue cap. Regenerative atypia is common below eroded areas and may simulate dysplasia.

The stroma often contains dilated vessels, areas of hemorrhage or hemosiderin, and variable numbers of lymphocytes, plasma cells, neutrophils, and eosinophils (fig. 16-11). Neutrophils surround eroded or ulcerated areas. The stroma may also contain prominent lymphoid follicles. Smooth muscle fibers are usually absent except in the center of pedunculated polyps. These are arranged less densely than in PJS polyps.

Disease Variants. Several variants of JPS exist: 1) *infantile juvenile polyposis*, transmitted as a non–sex-linked recessive trait, with a tendency toward death before age 2 years (37); 2) *familial juvenile polyposis coli* (51), the most common form, which remains limited to the colon and is inherited as an autosomal dominant trait with high penetrance (38,56); 3) *familial juvenile gastric polyposis*; and 4) *generalized juvenile polyposis*, characterized by the development of numerous juvenile polyps in the stomach, small intestine, colon, and rectum, in various combinations (29–32,40,45,48).

Generalized gastrointestinal JPS affects all ages; a positive family history is present in 20 to 50 percent of patients (35). Several families

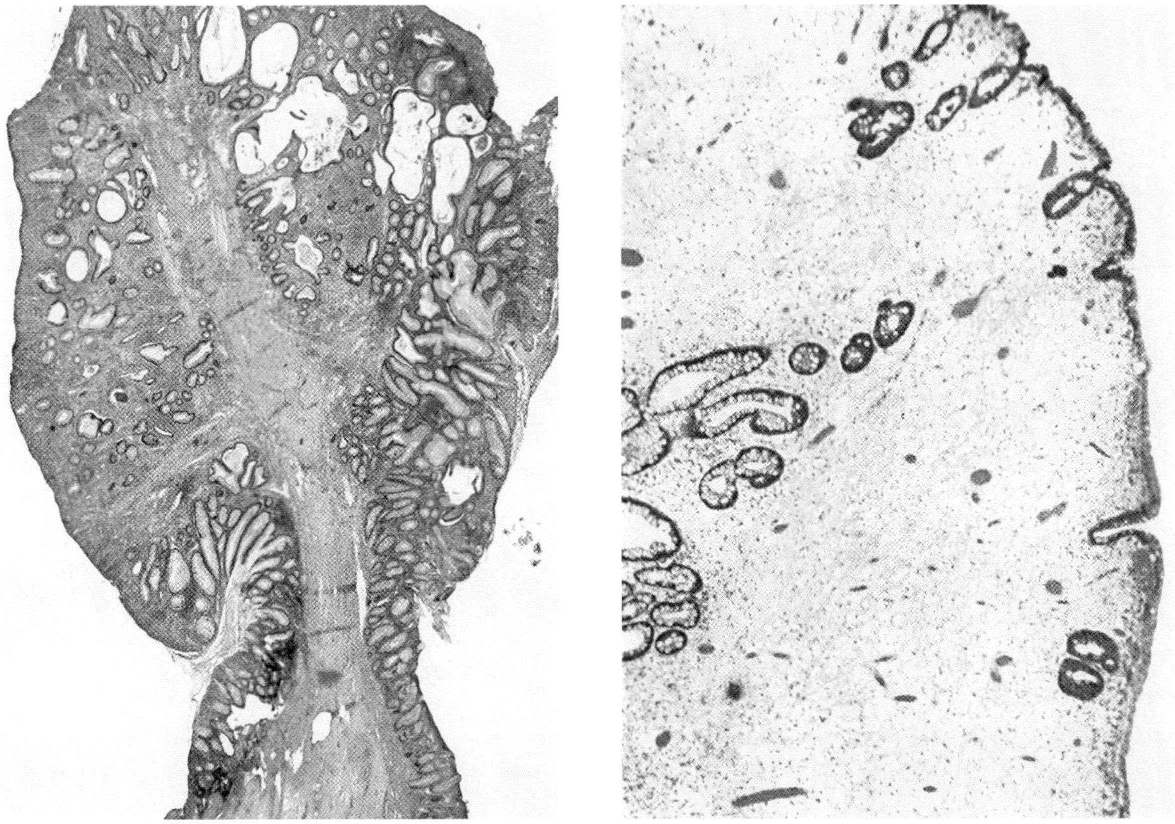

Figure 16-10

JUVENILE POLYPOSIS SYNDROME

Left: Whole mount section shows a juvenile polyp with a central stalk containing normal mucosa and submucosa. The head of the polyp consists of a proliferation of glands and a disproportionate amount of stroma.

Right: A different lesion shows a large amount of edematous stroma.

with autosomal dominant JPS display extraintestinal manifestations, including pulmonary and/or cerebral arteriovenous malformations, cutaneous telangiectasia, subarachnoid hemorrhage, hypertrophic pulmonary osteoarthropathy, and digital clubbing (30,34,38). Such patients often present in childhood and adolescence with polyps occurring in the large and small bowel, sometimes associated with grossly visible foci of lymphoid hyperplasia (30,32, 33,57). It is currently unclear whether this form of disease is due to a single gene abnormality distinct from juvenile polyposis or represents cases of coincidental juvenile intestinal polyposis and Osler-Rendu-Weber disease. This entity has been described under OMIM entry 175050 and also as hereditary hemorrhagic telangiectasia with juvenile polyposis coli (55).

The histologic features of JPS vary widely and are mimicked by a number of other disorders (see Differential Diagnosis).

Atypical Juvenile Polyps. Atypical juvenile polyps have the characteristic gross appearance of a multilobulated mass containing a number of closely packed polyps attached to a single stalk. Such lesions contain less stroma and more epithelium than the typical juvenile polyp, and they often acquire a villous or papillary architecture. Atypical juvenile polyps account for approximately 16 percent of all juvenile polyps, and may be more prone to dysplasia than are the usual juvenile polyps.

Osseous Metaplasia in Juvenile Polyps. Rare juvenile polyps contain areas of osseous metaplasia. These areas are usually located superficially in the polyps and presumably result from

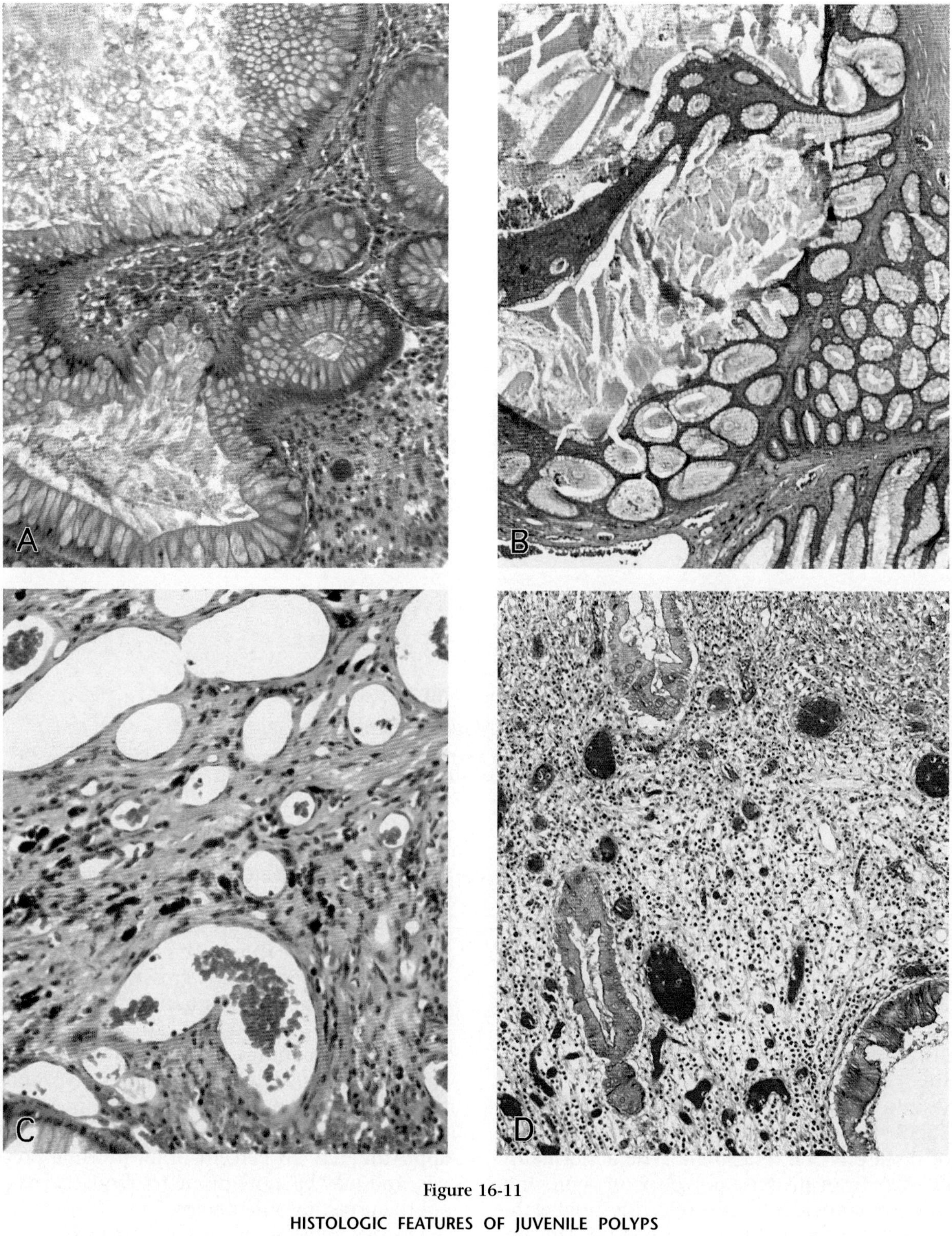

Figure 16-11

HISTOLOGIC FEATURES OF JUVENILE POLYPS

A: Portion of a juvenile polyp shows regeneration within the colonic glands.
B: The large cystic spaces within juvenile polyps often contain inspissated debris and mucus, as shown here.
C: Dilated vessels and stromal hemosiderin are indicative of previous erosion.
D: Erosion of the surface of the polyp leads to chronic inflammation and congestion of the lamina propria.

metaplasia of reparative lesions, perhaps in the area of previous surface granulation tissue caps (fig. 16-12).

Differential Diagnosis. Some juvenile polyps consist of very hyperplastic glands resembling the more common hyperplastic polyps or even adenomas, but the edematous stroma with inflammatory cells serves to differentiate these entities. Juvenile polyps also closely resemble the polyps seen in the Cronkhite-Canada syndrome. On a histologic basis, it is difficult, if not impossible, to differentiate juvenile polyps from hyperplastic polyps or polyps of the Cronkhite-Canada syndrome. Knowledge of the patient's age and symptoms, and the distribution and number of polyps is required.

Treatment and Prognosis. Patients with large polyps tend to develop local mechanical problems. Those with a particularly extensive polyp burden may have anemia and malnutrition secondary to diarrhea and protein loss. Repeated colonoscopic clearance of polyps reverses the malnutrition and growth retardation seen in severe cases. Large polyps with broad stalks may be difficult to remove endoscopically because they contain prominent vasculature and require greater degrees of electrocautery for their excision (49). Surgery may be required for patients with uncontrolled symptoms, malignancy, or when endoscopic clearance is not possible. Despite a report of the possible benefit from omeprazole therapy (52), in general, the results of pharmacologic treatments have been disappointing.

JPS patients have an increased risk for tumor development in the colon, stomach, duodenum, biliary tree, and pancreas, ranging from 20 to 70 percent. Cancer risk increases with age, not with polyp size and number (31,32,35,46,59,61). Dysplasia and carcinoma develop within both gastric and colonic juvenile polyps (fig. 16-13) (39). The dysplasia is usually graded as low grade, although occasionally it is more severe (61). Recently, Coburn (31) summarized reports in the English literature on the occurrence and prognosis of gastrointestinal carcinomas developing in patients with JPS. Of 218 patients with JPS who developed cancer, a family history of polyps was present in 50 percent, and 15 percent had associated congenital malformations. The mean age at diagnosis of carcinoma was 35.5 years, with a range of 4 to 60 years. Most malignancies arose in the distal colon and rectum, with isolated cancers in the stomach or duodenum. Tumor stage at diagnosis was usually advanced, with poor patient survival.

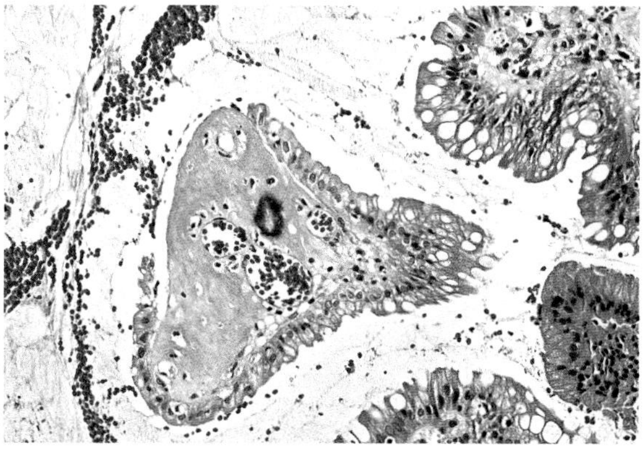

Figure 16-12

JUVENILE POLYP WITH OSSEOUS METAPLASIA

A focus of bone formation is in this polyp. This likely represents a reaction to previous erosion or ulceration.

The screening of families includes a careful clinical history, colonoscopy of potentially affected members, and surveillance colonoscopy of members in whom polyps have been identified and removed. Once removed, the polyps must be examined for the presence of adenomatous foci.

Animal Models. SMAD4 knockout mice develop a syndrome resembling JPS (60). Transgenic expression of noggin inhibits BMP signaling, which leads to a condition mimicking JPS in the transgenic mice (41).

COWDEN'S SYNDROME (MULTIPLE HAMARTOMA SYNDROME)

Definition. *Cowden's syndrome* (CS) is an autosomal dominant, multiple hamartoma syndrome characterized by a high risk of breast, thyroid, and endometrial cancers. It is caused by germline mutations in *PTEN*, which is a tumor suppressor gene located on 10q23 (75). The International Cowden Consortium developed a set of consensus diagnostic criteria (Table 16-2) (65).

Demography. The estimated incidence of CS is 1/200,000 (74–76); 10 to 50 percent of cases are familial (73). More than 90 percent of individuals affected by CS are believed to manifest the phenotype by age 20 (71). By age 30, 99

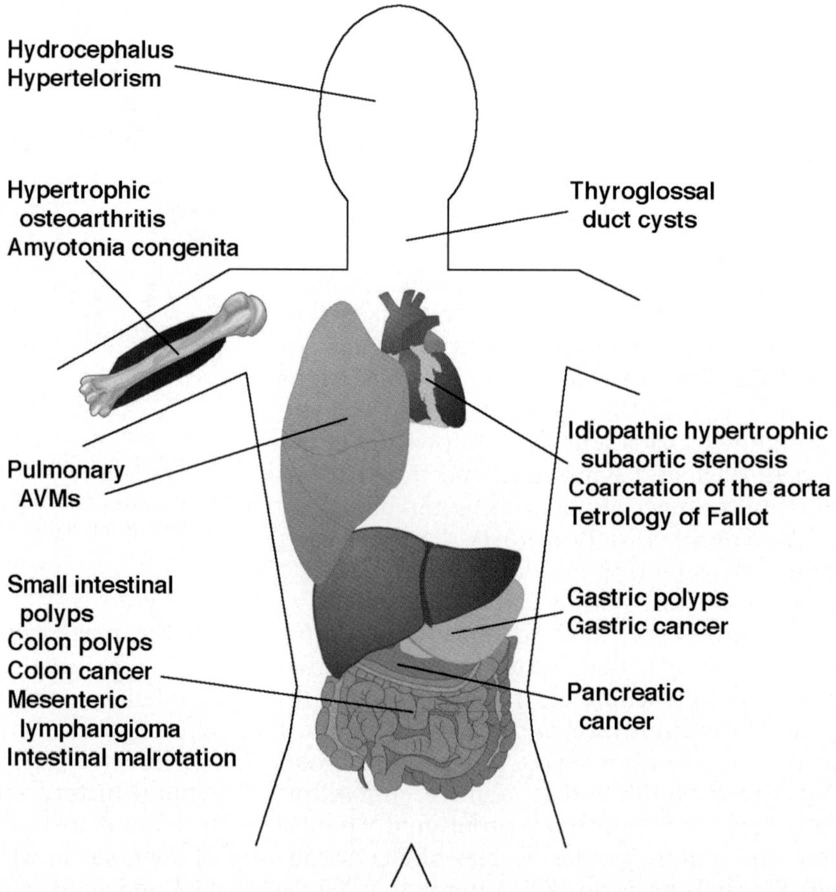

Figure 16-13

DIAGRAMMATIC REPRESENTATION OF SOME OF THE LESIONS ASSOCIATED WITH JUVENILE POLYPOSIS SYNDROME

Table 16-2

INTERNATIONAL COWDEN'S SYNDROME CONSORTIUM OPERATIONAL CRITERIA FOR THE DIAGNOSIS OF COWDEN'S SYNDROME

Pathognomonic Criteria
- Mucocutaneous lesions:
  - Facial tricholemmomas
  - Acral keratoses
  - Papillomatous papules
  - Mucosal lesions

Major Criteria
- Breast carcinoma
- Thyroid carcinoma, especially follicular thyroid carcinoma
- Macrocephaly (megalencephaly)(95%)
- Lhermitte-Duclos disease
- Endometrial carcinoma

Minor Criteria
- Other thyroid lesions (e.g., adenoma or multinodular goiter)
- Mental retardation (IQ ≤ 75)
- Gastrointestinal hamartomas
- Fibrocystic disease of the breast
- Lipomas
- Fibromas
- Genitourinary tumors (renal cell carcinoma or uterine fibroids) or malformations

Operational Diagnosis in an Individual
- Mucocutaneous lesions alone if: there are ≥6 facial papules, of which 3 or more must be trichilemmoma, or cutaneous facial papules and oral mucosal papillomatosis, or oral mucosal papillomatosis and acral keratoses, or palmoplantar keratoses, ≥6
- Two major criteria but one must include macrocephaly or Lhermitte-Duclos disease
- One major and three minor criteria
- Four minor criteria

Operational Diagnosis in a Family Where One Individual is Diagnostic for Cowden's Syndrome
- The pathognomonic criterion
- Any one major criterion with or without minor criteria
- Two minor criteria

percent develop at least the mucocutaneous signs of the syndrome, although any of the other clinical features can also be present. The most common manifestations are mucocutaneous lesions, thyroid abnormalities, fibrocystic disease and carcinoma of the breast, multiple early-onset uterine leiomyomas, and macrocephaly (69,71a,72,79). CS is associated with Lhermitte-Duclos disease (craniomegaly, choroidal hamartoma, and conjunctival papilloma); males and females are equally affected. Patients range in age from 4 to 75 years, with a median of 39 years.

Etiology. CS results from *PTEN* gene mutations. *PTEN* encodes a dual specificity phosphatase, a substrate of which is phosphatidylinositol 3,4,5,5-triphosphate, a phospholipid in the phosphatidylinositol-3-kinase pathway. PTEN affects apoptosis and inhibits cell spreading via the focal adhesion kinase pathway. Mutations include missense and nonsense point mutations, deletions, insertions, and splice site mutations. They are scattered over the entire length of the *PTEN* gene, with the exception of the first, fourth, and last exons (82). Approximately two thirds of mutations are found in exons 5, 7, and 8; 40 percent lie in exon 5. Mutations within the phosphatase core motif of the gene and 5′ of it appear to be associated with the involvement of five or more organs. Identification of such mutations represents a surrogate marker for the severity of disease (72). Polymorphisms are also found in the gene (82).

Some CS patients may also have a duplication of 15q11-q13 (80). This chromosomal locus is deleted in the Prader-Willi/Angelman syndrome and is a hot spot of chromosomal duplication (80). Additionally, CS patients sometimes have associated neurofibromatosis.

It is unclear whether a mutation in the *BMPR1A* gene, which encodes a bone morphogenic protein receptor belonging to the TGF-β-receptor superfamily, is a rare susceptibility gene for CS (83a). *BMPR1A* is also a susceptibility gene for JPS.

Clinical Features. Facial tricholemmomas are considered to be a pathognomonic feature of the syndrome (65). Other common manifestations include papillomatous papules, acral keratoses, thyroid abnormalities (50 to 70 percent; goiter, adenoma, and carcinoma), breast lesions (75 to 100 percent; fibroadenomas, fibrocystic disease, and adenocarcinoma) (fig. 16-14) (77, 83), gastrointestinal hamartomas (60 to 80 percent), macrocephaly (40 percent), and genitourinary abnormalities, including endometrial cancers (40 to 50 percent) and uterine leiomyomas (65). Patients present with a number of facial abnormalities including a beaked nose; mandibular, maxillary, and soft palate hypoplasia; and a high arched palate. They also have cafe-au-lait spots, papillomatosis of the lips and oropharynx, multiple ocular lesions including retinal gliomas (66), odontitis, dental caries, adenoid facies, kyphoscoliosis, pectus excavatum, and mental retardation (79). Some patients develop parathyroid adenomas. Skeletal abnormalities, including bone cysts, syndactyly, and other digit abnormalities, affect 33 percent of patients (66).

Up to 80 percent of patients who undergo endoscopy have gastrointestinal polyps (fig. 16-15) (68,71). Polyps develop in the esophagus, stomach, duodenum, terminal ileum, distal colon, and rectum; patients may develop gastric carcinoma (72). The polyps usually do not cause symptoms. The most common gastrointestinal lesions are esophageal glycogen acanthosis (fig. 16-16), numerous gastric hyperplastic polyps, and multiple hamartomatous polyps in the rectosigmoid (69,81). Patients may also have coexisting intestinal ganglioneuromatosis (71). CS and Bannayan-Riley-Ruvalcaba syndrome share overlapping features (Table 16-3). Because the clinical literature on CS consists mostly of reports of the most florid cases, and unusual family or individual case reports, the entire spectrum of the component manifestations may be unknown (65).

Gross Findings. The distal large intestine is preferentially affected in CS. Grossly, the lesions resemble hyperplastic polyps. The lesions are usually small (less than or equal to 6 mm in diameter) and not well visualized on barium enema studies but are easily seen endoscopically. The majority lie distal to the hepatic flexure. Glycogen acanthosis is seen in the esophagus. Polyps are seen in the stomach and duodenum as well. Here they tend to be sessile lesions measuring a few millimeters in diameter.

Microscopic Findings. Hamartomas involve organs derived from all three germ layers. The classic hamartoma associated with CS is the

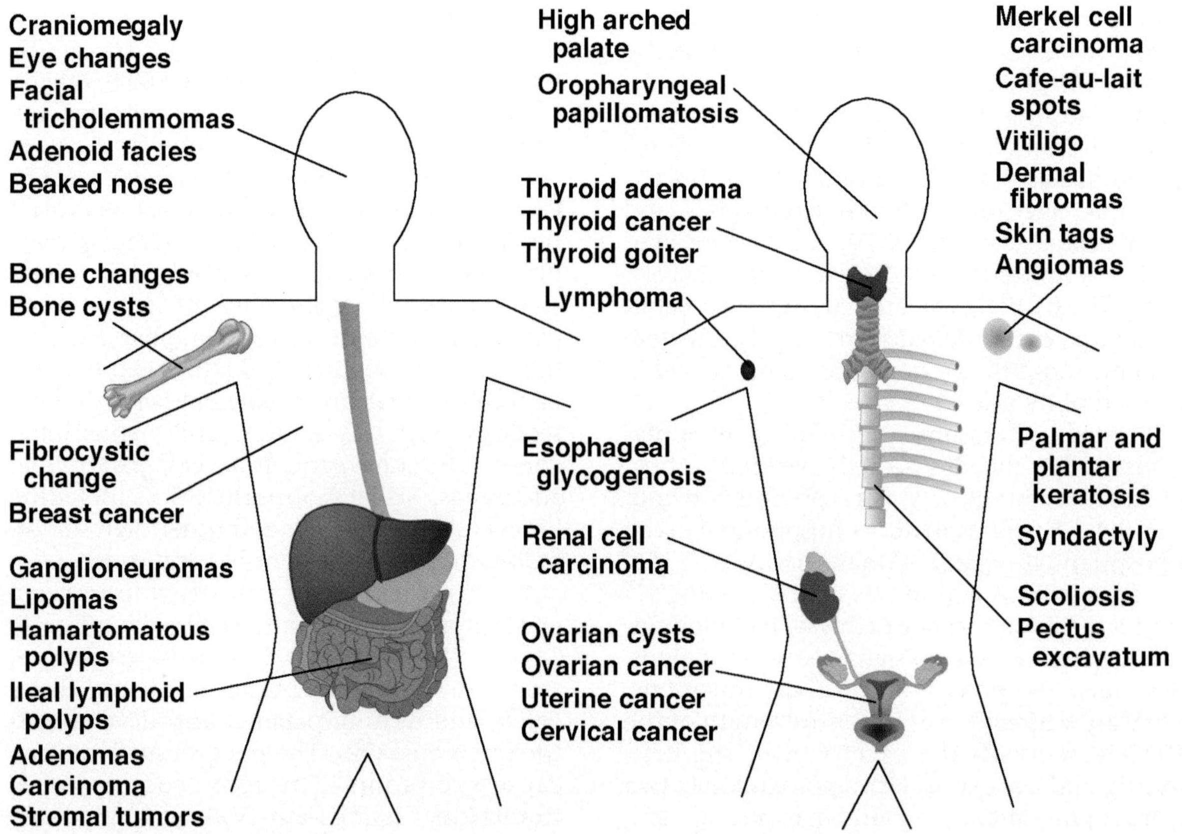

Figure 16-14

DIAGRAMMATIC REPRESENTATION OF MAJOR LESIONS DEVELOPING IN COWDEN'S SYNDROME

Table 16-3

COMPARISON OF COWDEN'S SYNDROME (CS) AND BANNAYAN-RILEY-RUVALCABA SYNDROME (BRRS)

	CS	BRRS
PTEN mutations	+	+
Multiple lipomas	+	+
Macrocephaly	+	+
Mucocutaneous lesions	+	–
Breast lesions	+	–
Thyroid lesions	+	+
Gastrointestinal lesions	+	+
Brain lesions	+	–
Facial abnormalities	+	–
Skeletal abnormalities	+	+
Mental retardation	+	+
Penile pigmented macules	–	+
Delayed motor development	–	+
Cancer development	+	?

tricholemmoma which affects 99 percent of CS patients. Patients develop mucocutaneous lesions (facial tricholemmomas, oral papillomas, and acral keratoses), breast lesions (fibrocystic disease and carcinoma), thyroid abnormalities (multinodular goiter and carcinoma), and gastrointestinal abnormalities (65,67).

Histologically, a diverse group of polypoid lesions can develop anywhere in the gastrointestinal tract. Colonic polyps include inflammatory polyps, lipomas, adenomas, hamartomatous polyps, juvenile polyps, hyperplastic polyps (fig. 16-17), fibromas, nodular lymphoid hyperplasia, ganglioneuromas (fig. 16-18), lymphoid polyps, and epithelioid leiomyomas (64,66, 70,71,77). There may be a mixture of cell types, including fibroblasts and adipose tissue. The usual CS colonic polyp contains an elongated, irregular, regenerative-appearing crypt epithelium with cystic dilatation, mild edema, inflammation, and variable fibrosis. Cellular pleomorphism and

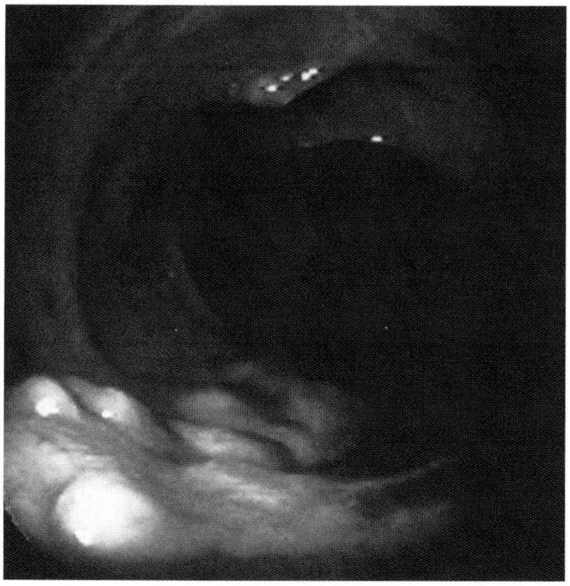

Figure 16-15

COWDEN'S SYNDROME

Gastrointestinal endoscopy shows the presence of numerous gastrointestinal polyps. (Figs. 16-15–16-18 are from the same patient.)

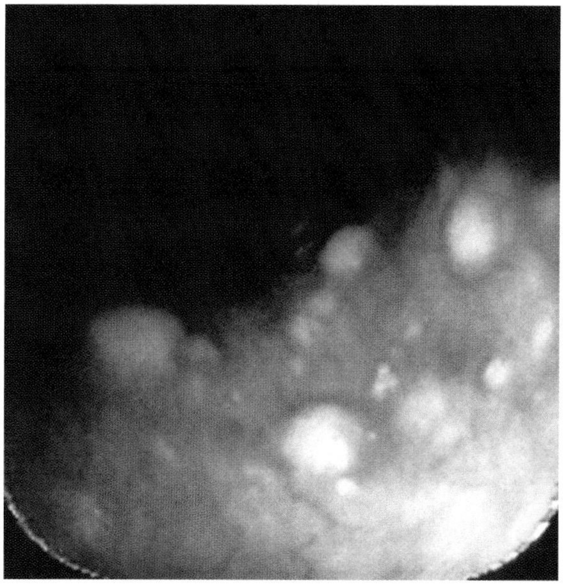

Figure 16-16

GLYCOGEN ACANTHOSIS IN COWDEN'S SYNDROME

The esophagus is lined by numerous spherical nodules that represent hyperglycogenated epithelium.

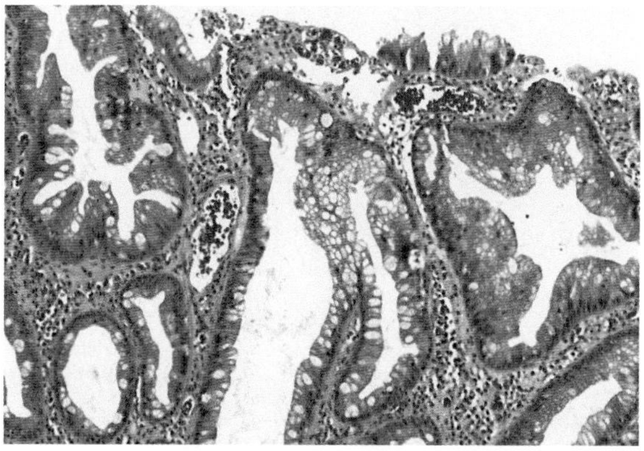

Figure 16-17

HYPERPLASTIC POLYP IN COWDEN'S SYNDROME

If the full history of the patient was not known it might be difficult to recognize this as being part of Cowden's disease.

atypia are absent. The collagen table underlying the luminal surface may be thickened as is seen in patients with hyperplastic polyps or collagenous colitis. Biopsies of the polyps may show only mild glandular architectural distortion with variable fibrosis and inflammation of the lamina propria, predominantly consisting of plasma cells, lymphocytes, and eosinophils (fig. 16-18). Fat cells may be present in the lamina propria. Dysplasia and adenomas are rare.

Most gastric polyps are hyperplastic, with elongated, cystically dilated, foveolar epithelium; lamina propria edema; and inflammation similar to that seen in sporadic hyperplastic polyps. The polyps may contain neural elements (fig. 16-19). The surface epithelium usually appears completely normal, unless erosion with regeneration has occurred. Patients also develop duodenal lymphangiectasia, duodenal lymphoid polyps, or jejunal lymphangiomas.

Differential Diagnosis. The diagnosis is made when there are appropriate clinical features, including multiple tricholemmomas or a history of thyroid or breast abnormalities. Without this clinical information, the disorder is difficult to differentiate from other polyposis syndromes, including neurofibromatosis, basal cell nevus syndrome, proteus syndrome, and the Bannayan-Riley-Ruvalcaba syndrome. There may also be overlap between these syndromes. PJS is initially considered in the differential diagnosis but pigmentation of the perioral region, pathognomonic for PJS, is absent. Additionally, PJS hamartomas

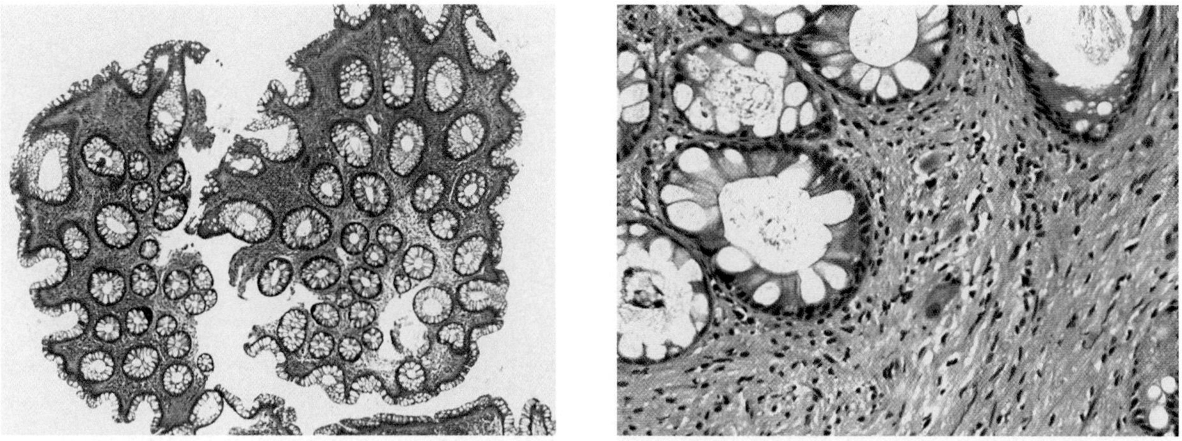

Figure 16-18

COWDEN'S SYNDROME

Left: The histologic features of the colonic polyps differ but generally show regenerative mucosa.
Right: A careful search disclosed a proliferation of spindle cells within the lamina propria, which also contained ganglion cells.

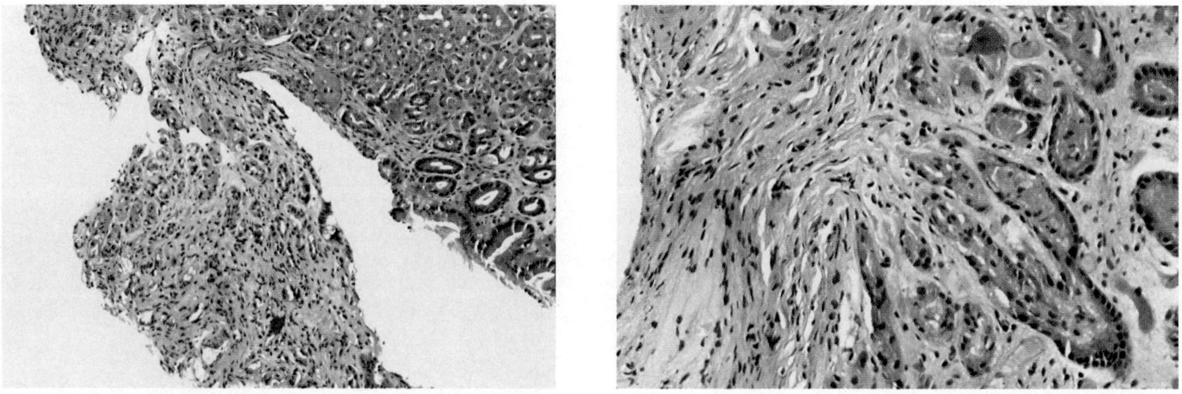

Figure 16-19

COWDEN'S SYNDROME: GASTRIC BIOPSY

Left: At low-power magnification, a portion of the gastric mucosa from one of the numerous polyps present within the stomach shows glandular distortion, which at first glance appears to be the result of mucosal fibrosis. Immunostains for neural markers were positive.

Right: At higher magnification, the spindle cell proliferation is seen partly destroying the glands. Reactive changes are present in the superficial gastric mucosa.

occur more often in the small intestine and show a well-organized, tree-like, smooth muscle architecture supporting normal-appearing epithelium. JPS can be considered, particularly in patients with predominantly colorectal polyps. Juvenile polyps, however, typically have an inflammatory appearance and patients lack the clinical stigmata of CS. The differential diagnosis also includes those disorders in which ganglion cells are present within the lamina propria. Ganglion cells are found in patients with ganglioneuromas, multiple endocrine neoplasia, and neurofibromatosis.

Treatment and Prognosis. Patients with CS do not appear to have a significantly increased risk of developing gastrointestinal cancer and many believe that gastrointestinal examinations are unnecessary unless gastrointestinal symptoms are present. Screening strategies for extraintestinal tumors are more appropriate. Seventy-four percent of patients develop extraintestinal malignant disease; the majority are invasive ductal breast carcinomas and thyroid tumors. The risk for breast cancer is estimated to range from 25 to 50 percent (69,71,79). The mean age of diagnosis is likely to be 10 years earlier than for breast cancer occurring in the general population. Men also develop breast cancer. The risk of thyroid cancer (predominantly follicular carcinoma) may be as high as 10 percent (78,79). The malignancies often cause patient death. Patients also have an increased risk of endometrial cancer.

Other tumors that develop in patients with CS include glioblastoma multiforme, cerebellar dysplastic gangliocytoma, mucocutaneous basal cell and squamous cell carcinomas, malignant melanoma, lymphoma, Merkel cell carcinoma, nonsmall cell lung cancer, uterine and ovarian cancers, renal cell carcinoma, urothelial carcinomas of the bladder, osteosarcomas, and, more rarely, several gastrointestinal cancers, including gastric (79), colorectal, hepatocellular, and pancreatic carcinomas.

Animal Models. Heterozygous *PTEN* knockout mice show pathologic characteristics similar to those in human CS and its related syndromes.

BANNAYAN-RILEY-RUVALCABA SYNDROME

Definition. *Bannayan-Riley-Ruvalcaba syndrome* (BRRS) is a rare autosomal dominant congenital disorder characterized by macrocephaly, lipomatosis, hemangiomatosis, and speckled penis (87). Synonyms include *Riley-Smith syndrome, Bannayan-Zonana syndrome, Soto's syndrome, Ruvalcaba-Myhre-Smith syndrome, macrocephaly, multiple lipomas*, and *hemangiomata syndrome*.

Demography. This rare syndrome (85,90) is inherited as an autosomal dominant disorder (90) and mainly affects men. By 1988, 12 patients with the syndrome had been identified (89a).

Etiology. Patients with the BRRS share a disease susceptibility locus with CS: 60 percent of BRRS patients have germline *PTEN* mutations (89,89a,90,90a,91,92). A significant difference in mutation status is found in familial versus sporadic cases of BRRS (88a). In contrast to CS, none of the mutations are in the phosphatase core motif. Since CS and BRRS share overlapping clinical features, including hamartomas, lipomatosis, and overlapping *PTEN* mutations, it has been proposed that CS and BRRS belong to a single genetic entity termed the "*PTEN* hamartoma tumor syndrome" (85a). In BRRS, 60 percent of *PTEN* mutations occur within exons 6 to 9 contrasting with CS in which 65 percent of *PTEN* mutations occur in the first five exons or the promoter regions. Some BRRS patients have *PTEN* gene deletions (90b,90c).

Clinical Features. BRRS is noted at birth or shortly thereafter and is characterized by delayed psychomotor development, ileal and colonic juvenile polyps, lingual lesions, subcutaneous and visceral lipomas and hemangiomas, multiple variable congenital anomalies, macrocephaly, mental retardation, central nervous system vascular malformations, ocular abnormalities, skeletal abnormalities including lipid storage myopathy (86), thyroid tumors, and pigmented penile macules. Patients may also exhibit widespread verrucous changes of the lips (86) and Hashimoto's disease (90).

Microscopic Findings. The intestinal polyps are histologically identical to juvenile polyps.

Treatment and Prognosis. Due to the overlapping features of BRRS and CS, it is unclear whether there is an increased incidence of gastrointestinal cancer. Some recommend that affected patients undergo screening similar to that performed for patients with CS (88).

CRONKHITE-CANADA SYNDROME

Definition. *Cronkhite-Canada syndrome* (CCS) is a nonhereditary, adult gastrointestinal polyposis syndrome associated with alopecia, skin hyperpigmentation, onychodystrophy, patchy vitiligo, marked edema, tetany, glossitis, cataracts, and intestinal polyposis (fig. 16-20) (93,95,96).

Demography. The disorder occurs worldwide and affects both sexes equally. Patients range in age from 31 to 83 years, contrasting with JPS in which patients range in age from 7 to 28 years (99). Eighty percent of patients present after age 50.

Etiology. All cases are sporadic and CCS is not a genetic disease. Proposed etiologic theories include nutritional deficiency states, an acquired disaccharidase deficiency accompanied by a bacterial overgrowth disorder, an infectious disorder, a disturbance in intestinal mucin secretion, or a nonspecific immune disorder (92,93, 95,96). Others suggest that epithelial damage,

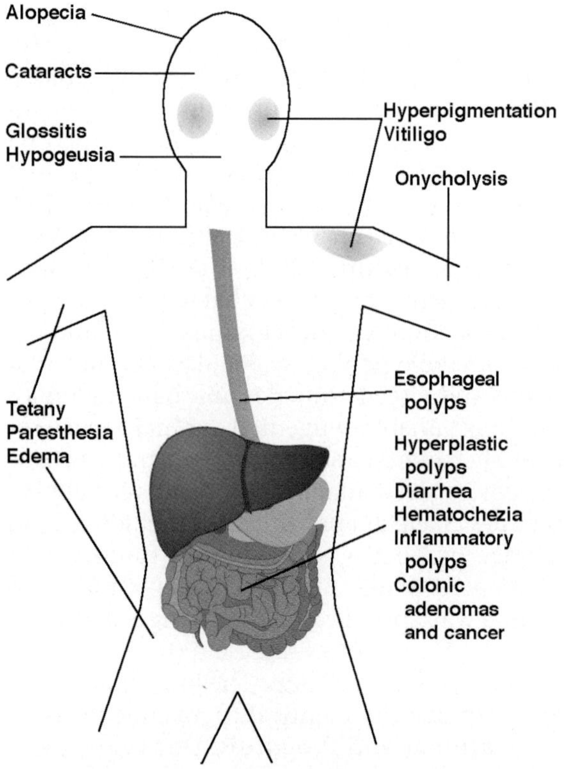

Figure 16-20

DIAGRAMMATIC SUMMARY OF SOME OF THE LESIONS ASSOCIATED WITH CRONKHITE-CANADA SYNDROME

followed by a secondary failure to synthesize or release growth factors, plays a role in the development of the lesions (93,97).

Clinical Features. The usual manifestations are chronic diarrhea, protein-losing enteropathy, weight loss, abdominal pain, anorexia, weakness, hematochezia, vomiting, paresthesias, and xerostomia. The diarrhea usually consists of loose, watery bowel movements occurring 5 to 7 times per day. These may be grossly bloody and the blood loss may be significant enough to require transfusions. The malabsorption syndrome that invariably develops in these patients is attributable to diffuse small intestinal mucosal injury.

Characteristic physical findings include nail changes (dystrophy, thinning, splitting), hair loss, and dermal hyperpigmentation. Complete loss of all fingernails and toenails occurs in some patients. Partial or total regeneration of nails occurs spontaneously, despite active disease. When new nail growth occurs, the distal end of the new nail continues to exhibit an irregular, ragged appearance. Cronkhite and Canada (93) interpreted the nail changes as resulting from vitamin deficiencies secondary to malabsorption, whereas Jarnum and Jensen (97) believe them to be an inherent part of the syndrome. Hair loss is rapid, occurring in the first few weeks, and it affects the entire body.

Laboratory findings include hypoproteinemia, particularly hypoalbuminemia, anemia, blood in the stool, and deficiencies in electrolytes (K^+ and Ca^{++}), vitamins (vitamin B12), and minerals (zinc and magnesium).

Radiologic Findings. Radiographic studies of the gastrointestinal tract show multiple nodular or polypoid filling defects in the stomach and colon. Intestinal lesions range from a few millimeters to 3 cm in diameter. Gastric lesions are seen on a background of thickened rugal folds. Small intestinal radiographs show diffuse coarsening of the mucosal pattern (94).

Gross Findings. Multiple (5 to 10) polyps develop in the stomach, small intestine, colon, and rectum, sometimes occupying the entire mucosal surface of these sites. Polyp density is greatest in the stomach and colon, followed by the duodenum, ileum, and jejunum (93,95). The polyps vary in color from red to bluish, sometimes demonstrating areas of surface ulceration and hemorrhage. Most polyps are sessile although they may be pedunculated. The gross appearance of the polyps varies from diffuse mucosal micronodularity or granularity, to gelatinous-appearing pedunculated polyps. Gastric polyps tend to grow in the antrum and form hyperplastic gastric folds, mimicking Menetrier's disease. Gastric and intestinal lesions can spontaneously regress.

Microscopic Findings. Polyp morphology reflects the site of origin. The gastric mucosa undergoes a transformation that results in alternating relatively atrophic and polypoid areas. The multiple, sessile, broad-based polyps consist of dilated, irregular foveolar glands and mucin-filled cysts lined by simple mucinous epithelium without evidence of metaplasia or atypia. The lamina propria becomes edematous and is focally infiltrated by plasma cells, eosinophils, and neutrophils. Smooth muscle fibers extend up into the mucosa. The lesions resemble gastric

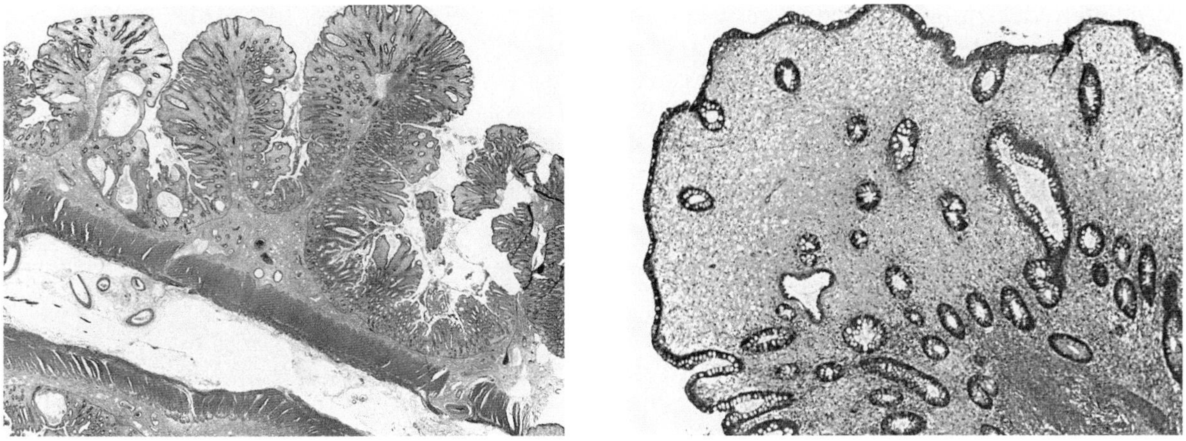

Figure 16-21

CRONKHITE-CANADA SYNDROME

Left: The colonic mucosa appears polypoid and the lamina propria is edematous.

Right: Marked lamina propria edema distorts the mucosal architecture. There is minimal associated inflammation. (Fig. 2-48 from Atlas of Tumor Pathology, Fascicle 32, Third Series.)

hyperplastic polyps. The nonpolypoid intervening mucosa contains cystically dilated glands, in contrast to the normal intervening mucosa seen in JPS. There may be glandular atrophy with pseudopyloric metaplasia in the body. The glands develop a corkscrew shape, become cystic, and are lined by hypertrophic, bizarre mucous cells. A secondary histiocytic infiltrate may surround glands that rupture. Cysts may also occur in the submucosa. There may be a relationship with Menetrier's disease, since both disorders share clinical and histologic similarities and both are reversible. Adenomatous changes can be present, as can coexisting colorectal carcinomas (98).

Intestinal lesions are essentially similar to those arising in the stomach, appearing as irregular nodules and foci of mucosal atrophy. Both the polyps and the intervening mucosa may show prominent edema, variable inflammation, and dilated cysts (fig. 16-21). The degree of inflammation and edema tends to be greater than in the stomach and the lesions tend to involve the entire thickness of the bowel wall. Villi and crypts decrease in number. Goblet cells increase in the remaining crypts. The epithelium may appear normal, atrophic, degenerative, or regenerative (93).

Differential Diagnosis. The differential diagnosis often includes gastrointestinal inflammatory conditions. In biopsy specimens of CCS polyps, only areas of edema and inflammation may be seen. With superficial biopsies, CCS may be indistinguishable from inflammatory polyps. Biopsies may also demonstrate what appears to be an area of gastritis. Gastric lesions share features with JPS and Menetrier's disease (92). In this situation, the diagnosis is only possible if one is aware of the other features of the clinical syndrome. The only reliable distinction between CCS and colonic JPS is the pedunculated growth of the polyps in the latter. Pedunculation is not always present in juvenile polyps; however, CCS tends to affect older individuals as compared with JPS. In CCS, the nonpolypoid intervening mucosa may contain cystically dilated glands, a feature lacking in JPS.

Treatment and Prognosis. Symptom onset may be acute and the course rapidly progressive. The major clinical problem is protein loss from the damaged mucosa and variable malabsorption. Profound malnutrition may occur and is a major cause of morbidity and mortality. Aggressive supportive therapy with nutritional supplementation, fluid and electrolyte replacement, and transfusion of blood components is warranted to correct the existing or impending deficiencies. The use of total parenteral nutrition is successful in some patients. The mortality rate is 50 to 60 percent.

While spontaneous remissions occur, survival beyond 2 years for symptomatic patients is uncommon. Other therapies have included corticosteroids, antibiotics, and surgery, but results are unpredictable. Since as many as 20 percent of CCS patients develop adenoma or carcinoma, colonoscopic surveillance is indicated (99–101). The neoplasms develop primarily in the colon and less often in the stomach (99–101). Colon lesions tend to be proximally located. Surgery is recommended when complications such as bleeding, intussusception, bowel obstruction, malignancy, or prolapse develop.

FAMILIAL HYPERPLASTIC GASTRIC POLYPOSIS

Definition. The term *familial hyperplastic gastric polyposis* is applied to patients who have more than 50 genetically acquired gastric hyperplastic polyps (102,103).

Demography. To date, only a single large kindred has been studied.

Etiology. Familial hyperplastic gastric polyposis may represent a new syndrome with an autosomal dominant mode of inheritance (102,103). Gastric polyps develop in 34 to 60 percent of affected patients.

Clinical Features. Psoriasis affects a third of the family members (102,103). The polyps tend to remain asymptomatic and there is a slightly increased risk for the development of gastric cancer over that seen in the general population.

Gross Findings. The polyps average 1 cm in size, and most are smaller than 1.5 cm. They generally are uniform in shape and size, are scattered throughout the gastric fundus and body, and are less frequent in the cardia and antrum.

Microscopic Findings. Histologically, the polyps resemble ordinary hyperplastic polyps. The hyperplastic foveolar epithelium lining the polyps develops a papillary or villous configuration, sometimes with atypia. Chronic gastritis is seen in the surrounding mucosa.

Differential Diagnosis. The differential diagnosis includes isolated hyperplastic polyps, juvenile polyposis, and the CCS. These disorders can be separated from one another by knowledge of the clinical features of the patient. Familial hyperplastic gastric polyposis differs from the other syndromes in that the patients have familial aggregation, the disorder affects young individuals of several generations, and the patients exhibit marked foveolar hyperplasia (102,103).

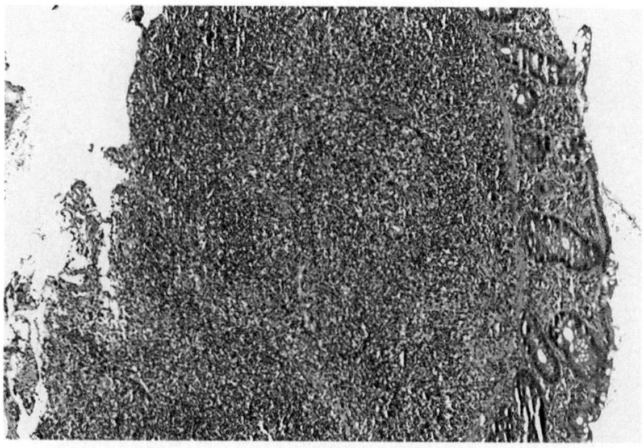

Figure 16-22

LYMPHOID POLYPOSIS

Typical lymphoid polyps have prominent lymphoid tissue with discernible germinal centers surrounded by a collar of normal small lymphocytes.

Treatment and Prognosis. Patients have an increased incidence of gastric cancer, which is both intestinal and diffuse in type. The foveolar hyperplasia and hyperplastic polyps play a key role in the development of diffuse carcinoma in patients with familial hyperplastic gastric polyposis syndrome (102,103). The foveolar cells in some patients display prominent globoid features.

LYMPHOID POLYPOSIS

Definition. *Lymphoid polyposis*, also known as *nodular lymphoid hyperplasia*, is characterized by the presence of multiple lymphoid polyps.

Demography. There are three forms of lymphoid polyposis: idiopathic, reactive, and associated with hypogammaglobulinemia. The idiopathic type is the most common and involves lesions in the small intestine or colon. This form occurs in children usually as an incidental finding, as well as in individuals undergoing resection for appendicitis, inflammatory bowel disease, and familial polyposis. In the latter condition, the lymphoid polyps grossly resemble small adenomas. Some patients with hypogammaglobulinemia and lymphoid polyposis have coexisting giardiasis.

Clinical Features. Lymphoid polyposis is usually an incidental finding at endoscopy or during examination of resected specimens.

Gross Findings. Lymphoid polyposis appears as several round, pale nodules measuring 3 to 5 mm. It affects any part of the intestine but is particularly common in the ileum.

Microscopic Findings. Histologically, lymphoid polyps consist of normal lymphoid tissue with prominent germinal centers located mainly at the junction of the mucosa and the submucosa (fig. 16-22).

Differential Diagnosis. The major entity in the differential diagnosis is lymphomatous polyposis. The major distinction between the two lesions is that one is histologically benign and the other is malignant. The usual techniques that separate benign from malignant lymphoid proliferations can be used to separate histologically equivocal cases.

Treatment and Prognosis. Lymphoid polyposis is a self-limited condition with no serious consequences.

REFERENCES

General

Bussey HJ. Gastrointestinal polyposis syndrome. In: Anthony PP, MacSween SN, eds. Recent advances in histopathology. Gastrointestinal pathology. Edinburgh: Churchill Livingstone; 1984:169.

Bussey HJ. Polyposis syndromes of the gastrointestinal tract. In: Sherlock P, Morson BC, Barbara L, Veronesi U, eds. Precancerous lesions of the gastrointestinal tract. New York: Raven Press; 1983:43.

Erbe RW. Inherited gastrointestinal-polyposis syndromes. N Engl J Med 1976;294:1101–4.

Fenoglio-Preiser CM. Histological features of polyposis syndromes in colonic polyposes. In: Watne AE, ed. Problems in general surgery. Philadelphia: Lippincott; 1993:707–23.

Fenoglio-Preiser CM, Noffsinger, AE, Stemmermann GN, Lantz PE, Listrom MB, Rilke FO. Gastrointestinal pathology: an atlas and text. Philadelphia: Lippincott Raven; 1999.

Haggitt RC, Reid BJ. Hereditary gastrointestinal polyposis syndromes. Am J Surg Pathol 1986;12: 871–87.

Hamilton SR, Aaltonen LA. Pathology and genetic tumours of the digestive system. WHO classification of tumors. Lyons, France: IARC Press; 2000.

Radi MJ, Fenoglio-Preiser CM. Polyps of the colon and the polyposis syndromes. In: Shorter RG, Kirschner JB, eds. Diseases of the colon, rectum, and anal canal. Baltimore: Williams & Wilkins; 1988:417–30.

Rustgi AK. Hereditary gastrointestinal polyposis and nonpolyposis syndromes. N Engl J Med 1994;331: 1694–702.

Sachatello CR, Griffen WO Jr. Hereditary polypoid diseases of the gastrointestinal tract. A working classification. Am J Surg 1975:129;198–203.

Introduction

1. Fenoglio-Preiser CM, Pascal RR, Perzin KH. Tumors of the intestines. Atlas of Tumor Pathology, 2nd Series, Fascicle 27. Washington, DC: Armed Forces Institute of Pathology; 1990.
2. Marsh DJ, Coulon V, Lunetta KL, et al. Mutation spectrum and genotype analyses in Cowden disease and Bannayan-Zonana syndrome in two hamartoma syndromes with germline *PTEN* mutation. Hum Mol Genet 1998;7:507–15.
3. Marsh DJ, Kum JB, Lunetta KL, et al. *PTEN* mutation spectrum and genotype-phenotype correlations in Bannayan-Riley-Ruvalcaba syndrome suggest a single entity with Cowden syndrome. Hum Mol Genet 1999;8:1461–72.

Peutz-Jeghers Syndrome

4. Aaltonen LA, Jarvinen H, Gruber SB, Billaud M, Jass R. Peutz-Jeghers syndrome. In: Hamilton SR, Aaltonen LA, eds. Pathology and genetics of tumours of the digestive system, 3rd ed. WHO International Classification of Tumors, Berlin: Springer-Verlag; 2000:74–6.
5. Boardman LA, Thibodeau SN, Schaid DJ, et al. Increased risk for cancer in patients with the Peutz-Jeghers syndrome. Ann Intern Med 1998; 128:896–9.
6. Burt RW, Jacobi RF. Polyposis syndromes In: Yamada T ed. Textbook of gastroenterology, 4th ed. Philadelphia:Lippincott Williams & Wilkins; 2003:1914–39.
7. Collins SP, Reoma JL, Gamm DM, Ohler MD. LKB1, a novel serine/threonine protein kinase and potential tumour suppressor, is phosphorylated by cAMP-dependent protein kinase (PKA) and prenylated in vivo. Biochemistry 2000;345: 673–80.
8. Giardiello FM, Brensinger JD, Tersmette AC, et al. Very high risk of cancer in familial Peutz-Jeghers syndrome. Gastroenterology 2000;119: 1447–53.
9. Hemminki A, Markie D, Tomlinson I, et al. A serine/ threonine kinase gene defective in Peutz-Jeghers syndrome. Nature 1998;391:184–7.

10. Hemminki A, Tomlinson I, Markie D, et al. Localization of a susceptibility locus for Peutz-Jeghers syndrome to 19p using comparative genomic hybridization and targeted linkage analysis. Nat Genet 1997:15:87–90.
11. Hizawa K, Iida M, Matsumoto T, et al. Cancer in Peutz-Jeghers syndrome. Cancer 1993;72:2777–81.
12. Jeghers H, McKusick VA, Katz KH. Generalized intestinal polyposis and melanin spots on the oral mucosa, lips and digits: a syndrome of diagnostic significance. N Engl J Med 1949;241: 1031–6.
13. Jenne DE, Riemann H, Nezu J, et al. Peutz-Jeghers syndrome is caused by mutations in a novel serine threonine kinase. Nat Genet 1998;18:38–43.
14. McGarrity TJ, Kulin HE, Zaino RJ. Peutz-Jeghers syndrome. Am J Gastroenterol 2000;95:596–604.
15. Mehenni H, Blouin JL, Radhakrishna U, et al. Peutz-Jeghers syndrome: confirmation of linkage to chromosome 19p13.3 and identification of a potential second locus, on 19q13.4. Am J Hum Genet 1997;61:1327–34.
16. Miyaki M, Iijima T, Hosono K, et al. Somatic mutations of *LKB1* and *beta-catenin* genes in gastrointestinal polyps from patients with Peutz-Jeghers syndrome. Cancer Res 2000;60:6311–3.
17. Narita T, Ohnuma H, Yokoyama S. Peutz-Jeghers syndrome with osseous metaplasia of the intestinal polyps. Pathol Int 1995;45:388–92.
18. Nezu J, Oku A, Shimane M. Loss of cytoplasmic retention ability of mutant LKB1 found in Peutz-Jeghers syndrome patients. Biochem Biophys Res Commun 1999;261:750–5.
19. Reid JD. Intestinal carcinoma in the Peutz-Jeghers syndrome. JAMA 1974;229:833–4.
20. Resta N, Simone C, Mareni C, et al. STK11 mutations in Peutz-Jeghers syndrome and sporadic colon cancer. Cancer Res 1998;58:4799–801.
21. Sener RN, Kumcuoglu Z, Elmas N, Oyar O, Tugran C. Peutz-Jeghers syndrome: CT and US demonstration of small bowel polyps. Gastrointest Radiol 1991;16:21–3.
22. Shepherd NA, Bussey HJ, Jass JR. Epithelial misplacement in Peutz-Jeghers polyps. A diagnostic pitfall. Am J Surg Pathol 1987;11:743–9.
23. Trojan J, Brieger A, Raedle J, Roth WK, Zeuzem S. Peutz-Jeghers syndrome: molecular analysis of a three-generation kindred with a novel defect in the serine threonine kinase gene STK11. Am J Gastroenterol 1999;94: 257–61.
24. Utsunomiya J, Gocho H, Miyanga T, Hamaguchi E, Kashimure A. Peutz-Jeghers syndrome: its natural course and management. Johns Hopkins Med J 1975;136:71–82.
25. Wennstrom J, Pierce ER, McKusick VA. Hereditary benign and malignant lesions of the large bowel. Cancer 1984;34:850–7.
26. Westerman AM, Entius MM, de Baar E, et al. Peutz-Jeghers syndrome: 78-year follow-up of the original family. Lancet 1999;353:1211–5.
27. Wirtzfeld DA, Petrelli NJ, Rodriguez-Bigas MA. Hamartomatous polyposis syndromes: molecular genetics, neoplastic risk, and surveillance recommendations. Ann Surg Oncol 2001;8:319–27.
28. Wu YK, Tsai CH, Yang JC, Hwang MH. Gastroduodenal intussusception due to Peutz-Jeghers syndrome. A case report. Gastroenterology 1994;41:134–6.

Juvenile Polyposis

29. Aaltonen LA, Jass JR, Howe JR. Juvenile polyposis. In: Hamilton SR, Aaltonen LA, eds. WHO international classification of tumors: pathology and genetics of tumours of the digestive system, 3rd ed. Berlin: Springer-Verlag; 2000:130–2.
30. Baert AL, Casteels-Van Daele M, Broeckx J, Wijndaele L, Wilms G, Eggermont E. Generalized juvenile polyposis with pulmonary arteriovenous malformations and hypertrophic osteoarthropathy. AJR Am J Roentgenol 1983;141: 661–2.
31. Coburn MC, Pricolo VE, DeLuca FG, Bland RI. Malignant potential in intestinal juvenile polyposis syndromes. Ann Surg Oncol 1995;2:386–91.
32. Coffin CM, Dehner LP. What is a juvenile polyp? An analysis based on 21 patients with solitary and multiple polyps. Arch Pathol Lab Med 1996;120:1032–8.
33. Conte WJ, Rotter JL. Hereditary generalized juvenile polyposis, arteriovenous malformations and colonic carcinoma. Clin Res 1982;30: 93A.
34. Cox KL, Frates RC Jr, Wong A, Gandhi G. Hereditary generalized juvenile polyposis associated with pulmonary arteriovenous malformation. Gastroenterology 1980;78:1566–70.
35. Desai DC, Neale KF, Talbot IC, Hodgson SV, Phillips RK. Juvenile polyposis. Br J Surg 1995;82:14–7.
36. Friedl W, Kruse R, Uhlhaas S, et al. Frequent 4-bp deletion in exon 9 of the SMAD4/MADH4 gene in familial juvenile polyposis patients. Genes Chromosomes Cancer 1999;25:403–6.
37. Gilinsky N, Elliot MS, Price SK, Wright JP. The nutritional consequences and neoplastic potential of juvenile polyposis coli. Dis Colon Rectum 1986;29:417–20.
38. Goodman ZD, Yardley JH, Melligan FD. Pathogenesis of colonic polyps in multiple juvenile polyposis. Report of a case associated with gastric polyps and carcinoma of rectum. Cancer 1979;43:1906–13.
39. Grotsky HW, Rickert RR, Smith WD, Newsome JF. Familial juvenile polyposis coli. A clinical and pathologic study of a large kindred. Gastroenterology 1982;82:494–501.
40. Haggitt RC, Pitcock JA. Familial juvenile polyposis of the colon. Cancer 1970;26:1232–6.

41. Haramis AP, Begthel H, van den Born M, et al. De novo crypt formation and juvenile polyosis on BMP inhibition in mouse intestine. Science 2004;303:1684–6.
42. Hofting I, Pott G, Schrameyer B, Stolte M. Familiäre juvenile polyposis mit vorwiegender Magenbeteiligung. Z Gastroenterol 1993;31:480–3.
43. Houlston R, Bevan S, Williams A, et al. Mutations in DPC4 (SMAD4) cause juvenile polyposis syndrome, but only account for a minority of cases. Hum Mol Genet 1998;7:1907–12.
44. Howe JR, Ringold JC, Summers RW, Mitros FA, Nishimura DY, Stone EM. A gene for familial juvenile polyposis maps to chromosome 18q21.1. Am J Hum Genet 1998;62:1129–36.
45. Howe JR, Roth S, Ringold JC, et al. Mutations in the SMAD4/DPC4 gene in juvenile polyposis. Science 1998;280:1086–8.
46. Jass JR. Juvenile polyposis. In: Phillips RK, Spigelman AD, Thomson JP, eds. Familial adenomatous polyposis and other polyposis syndromes. London: Edward-Arnold; 1994.
47. Jass JR, Burt R. Hyperplastic polyposis. In: Hamilton SR, Aaltonen LA, eds. WHO international classification of tumors, 3rd ed. Pathology and genetics of tumours of the digestive system. Berlin: Springer-Verlag; 2000:135–6.
48. Longy M, Lacomb D. Cowden disease. Report of a family and review. Ann Genet 1996;39:35–42.
49. Lowichik A, Jackson WD, Coffin CM. Gastrointestinal polyposis in childhood: clinicopathologic and genetic features. Pediatr Dev Pathol 2003;6:371–91.
50. Marsh DJ, Roth S, Lunetta KL, et al. Exclusion of PTEN/MMAC1/TEP1 and 10q22-24 as the susceptibility locus for juvenile polyposis syndrome (JPS). Cancer Res 1997;57:5017–20.
51. Mazier WP, Bowman HE, Sun KM, Muldoon JP. Juvenile polyps of the colon and rectum. Dis Colon Rectum 1974;17:523–7.
52. Nicholls S, Smith V, Davies R, Doig C, Thomas A, Miller V. Diffuse juvenile non-adenomatous polyposis: a rare cause of severe hypoalbuminaemia in childhood. Acta Paediatr 1995;84:1447–8.
53. Olschwang S, Serova SO, Lenoir PP, Muleris M, Parc R, Thomas G. PTEN germ-line mutations in juvenile polyposis coli. Nat Genet 1998;18:12–4.
54. Online Mendelian Inheritance in Man, OMIM™ Johns Hopkins University, Baltimore MD. MIM #174900 (1/12/2002): www.ncbi.nlm.nih.gov/omim.
55. Online Mendelian Inheritance in Man, OMIM™ Johns Hopkins University, Baltimore MD. MIM #175050. (6/20/1997): www.ncbi.nlm.nih.gov/omim.
56. Scharf GM, Becker JH, Laage NJ. Juvenile gastrointestinal polyposis or the infantile Cronkhite-Canada syndrome. J Pediatr Surg 1986;21:953–4.
57. Simpson EL, Dalinka MK. Association of hypertrophic osteo-arthropathy with gastrointestinal polyposis. AJR Am J Roentgenol 1985;144:983–4.
58. Smilow PC, Pryor CA, Swinton NW. Juvenile polyposis coli. A report of three patients in three generations of one family. Dis Colon Rectum 1966;9:248–54.
59. Subramony C, Scott-Conner CE, Skelton D, Hall TJ. Familial juvenile polyposis. Study of a kindred: evolution of polyps and relationship to gastrointestinal carcinoma. Am J Clin Pathol 1994;102:91–7.
60. Takaku K, Miyoshi H, Matsunuga A, Oshima M, Sasaki N, Taketo MM. Gastric and duodenal polyps in Smad4 (Dpc4) knockout mice. Cancer Res 1999;59:6113–7.
61. Vaiphei K, Thapa BR. Juvenile polyposis (coli)—high incidence of dysplastic epithelium. J Pediatr Surg 1997;32:1287–90.
61a. Wirtzfeld DA, Petrelli NJ, Rodriguez-Bigas MA. Hamartomatous polyposis syndromes: molecular genetics, neoplastic risk, and surveillance recommendations. Ann Surg Oncol 2001;8:319–27.
62. Zhou XP, Waite KA, Pilarski R, et al. Germline PTEN promoter mutations and deletions in Cowden/Bannayan-Riley-Ruvalcaba syndrome result in aberrant PTEN protein and dysregulation of the phosphoinositol-3-kinase/Akt pathway. Am J Hum Genet 2003;73:404–11.
63. Zhou XP, Woodford-Richens K, Lehtonen R, et al. Germline mutations in BMPR1A/ALK3 cause a subset of cases of juvenile polyposis syndrome and of Cowden and Bannayan-Riley-Ruvalcaba syndromes. Am J Hum Genet 2001;69:704–11.

Cowden's Syndrome

64. Carlson GJ, Nivatvongs S, Snover DC. Colorectal polyps in Cowden's disease (multiple hamartoma syndrome). Am J Surg Pathol 1984;8:763–70.
65. Eng C. PTEN: one gene, many syndromes. Hum Mutat 2003;22:183–98.
66. Gentry WC, Reed WB, Siegal JM. Cowden disease. Birth Defects 1975;11:137–41.
67. Gorensek M, Matko I, Skralovnik A, Rode M, Satler J, Jutersek A. Disseminated hereditary gastrointestinal polyposis with orocutaneous hamartomatosis (Cowden's disease). Endoscopy 1984;16:59–63.
68. Haibach H, Burns TW, Carlson HE, Burman KD, Deftos LJ. Multiple hamartoma syndrome (Cowden's disease) associated with renal cell carcinoma and primary neuroendocrine carcinoma of the skin (Merkel cell carcinoma). Am J Clin Pathol 1992;97:705–12.
69. Hanssen AM, Fryns JP. Cowden syndrome. J Med Genet1995;32:117–9.
70. Hizawa K, Iida M, Matsumoto T, et al. Gastrointestinal manifestations of Cowden's disease. Report of four cases. J Clin Gastroenterol 1994;18:13–8.
71. Lashner BA, Riddell RH, Winans CS. Ganglioneuromatosis of the colon and extensive glycogenic acanthosis in Cowden's disease. Dig Dis Sci 1986;31:213–6.

71a. Longy M, Lacomb D. Cowden disease. Report of a family and review. Ann Genet 1996;39:35–42.
72. Mallory SB. Cowden syndrome (multiple hamartoma syndrome). Dermatol Clin 1995;13:27–31.
73. Marsh DJ, Kum JB, Lunetta KL, et al. PTEN mutation spectrum and genotype-phenotype correlations in Bannayan-Riley-Ruvalcaba syndrome suggest a single entity with Cowden syndrome. Hum Mol Genet 1999;8:1461–72.
74. Nelen MR, Kremer H, Konings IB, et al. Novel PTEN mutations in patients with Cowden disease: absence of clear genotype-phenotype correlations. Eur J Hum Genet 1999;7:267–73.
75. Nelen MR, Padberg GW, Peeters EA, et al. Localization of the gene for Cowden disease to chromosome 10q22-23. Nat Genet 1996;13:114–6.
76. Nelen MR, van Staveren WC, Peeters EA, et al. Germline mutations in the PTEN/MMAC1 gene in patients with Cowden disease. Hum Mol Genet 1997;6:1383–7.
77. Schrager CA, Schneider D, Bruener A, Tsou HC, Peacocke M. Clinical and pathological features of breast disease in Cowden's syndrome: an underrecognized syndrome with an increased risk of breast cancer. Hum Pathol 1998;29:47–53.
78. Starink TM. Cowden's disease: analysis of fourteen new cases. J Am Acad Dermatol 1985;11: 1127–32.
79. Starink TM, van der Veen JP, Arwert F, et al. The Cowden syndrome: a clinical and genetic study in 21 patients. Clin Genet 1986;29:222–33.
80. Suzuki T, Ichinose M, Matsubara Y, et al. Cowden's disease with a defined genetic alteration—chromosomal duplication at 15q11-q13. J Gastroenterol 1997;32:696–9.
81. Taylor AJ, Dodds WJ, Stewart ET. Alimentary tract lesions in Cowden's disease. Br J Radiol 1989;62:890–2.
82. Tsou HC, Ping XL, Xie XX, et al. The genetic basis of Cowden's syndrome: three novel mutations in PTEN/MMAC1/TEP1. Hum Genet 1998; 102:467–73.
83. Tsubosa Y, Fukutomi T, Tsuda H, et al. Breast cancer in Cowden's disease: a case report with review of the literature. Jpn J Clin Oncol 1998;28:42–6.
83a. Zhou XP, Woodford-Richens K, Lehtonen R, et al. Germline mutations in BMPR1A/ALK3 cause a subset of cases of juvenile polyposis syndrome and of Cowden and Bannayan-Riley-Ruvalcaba syndromes. Am J Hum Genet 2001;69:704–11.

Bannayan-Riley-Ruvalcaba Syndrome

84. Arch EM, Goodman BK, Van Wesep RA, et al. Deletion of PTEN in a patient with Bannayan-Riley-Ruvalcaba syndrome suggests allelism with Cowden disease. Am J Med Genet 1997;71:489–93.
85. DiLiberti JH, Weleber RG, Budden S. Ruvalcaba-Myhre-Smith syndrome: a case with probable autosomal-dominant inheritance and additional manifestations. Am J Med Genet 1983;15:491–5.
85a. Eng C. PTEN: one gene, many syndromes. Hum Mutat 2003;22:183–98.
86. Fargnoli MC, Orlow SJ, Semel-Concepcion J, Bolognia JL. Clinicopathologic findings in the Bannayan-Riley-Ruvalcaba syndrome. Arch Dermatol 1996;132:1214–8.
87. Gorlin RJ, Cohen MM Jr, Condon LM, Burke BA. Bannayan-Riley-Ruvalcaba syndrome. Am J Med Genet 1992;44:307–14.
88. Hendriks YM, Verhallen JT, van der Smagt JJ, et al. Bannayan-Riley-Ruvalcaba syndrome: further delineation of the pheonotype and management of PTEN mutation-positive cases. Fam Cancer 2003;2:79-85.
88a. Marsh DJ, Coulon V, Lunetta KL, et al. Mutation spectrum and genotype analyses in Cowden disease and Bannayan-Zonana syndrome in two hamartoma syndromes with germline *PTEN* mutation. Hum Mol Genet 1998;7:507–15.
89. Marsh DJ, Dahia PL, Zheng Z, et al. Germline mutations in PTEN are present in Bannayan-Zonana syndrome. Nat Genet 1997;16:333–4.
89a. Marsh DJ, Kum JB, Lunetta KL, et al. PTEN mutation spectrum and genotype-phenotype correlations in Bannayan-Riley-Ruvalcaba syndrome suggest a single entity with Cowden syndrome. Hum Mol Genet 1999;8:1461–72.
90. Ruvalcaba RH, Myhre S, Smith DW. Sotos syndrome with intestinal polyposis and pigmentary changes of the genitalia. Clin Genet 1980;18: 413–6.
90a. Starink TM, van der Veen JP, Arwert F, et al. The Cowden syndrome: a clinical and genetic study in 21 patients. Clin Genet 1986;29:222–33.
90b. Zhou XP, Waite KA, Pilarski R, et al. Germline PTEN promoter mutations and deletions in Cowden/Bannayan-Riley-Ruvalcaba syndrome result in aberrant PTEN protein and dysregulation of the phosphoinositol-3-kinase/Akt pathway. Am J Hum Genet 2003;73:404–11.
90c. Zhou XP, Woodford-Richens K, Lehtonen R, et al. Germline mutations in BMPR1A/ALK3 cause a subset of cases of juvenile polyposis syndrome and of Cowden and Bannayan-Riley-Ruvalcaba syndromes. Am J Hum Genet 2001;69:704–11.
91. Zigman AF, Lavine JE, Jones MC, Boland CR, Carethers JM. Localization of the Bannayan-Riley-Ruvalcaba syndrome gene to chromosome 10q23. Gastroenterology 1997;113:1433–7.

Cronkhite-Canada Syndrome

92. Burke A, Sobin L. The pathology of Cronkhite-Canada polyps. A comparison to juvenile polyposis. Am J Surg Pathol 1989;13:940–6.
93. Cronkhite LW, Canada WJ. Generalized gastrointestinal polyposis. An unusual syndrome of polyposis, pigmentation, alopecia and onychotrophia. N Engl J Med 1955;252:1011–15.
94. Dachman AH, Buck JL, Burke AP, Sobin LH. Cronkhite-Canada syndrome: radiologic features. Gastrointest Radiol 1989;14:285–90.
95. Daniel ES, Ludwig SL, Lewin KJ, et al. The Cronkhite-Canada syndrome: an analysis of clinical and pathologic features and therapy in 55 patients. Medicine 1982;61:293–309.
96. Finan MC, Ray MK. Gastrointestinal polyposis syndromes: Cronkhite Canada syndrome. Dermatol Clin 1989;7:419–34.
97. Jarnum S, Jensen H. Diffuse gastrointestinal polyposis with ectodermal changes. A case with severe malabsorption and enteric loss of plasma proteins and electrolytes. Gastroenterology 1966;50:107–13.
98. Johnson GK, Soergel KH, Hensley GT, Dodds WJ, Hogan WJ. Cronkhite-Canada syndrome: gastrointestinal pathology and morphology. Gastroenterology 1972;63:140–51.
99. Katayama Y, Kimura M, Konn M. Cronkhite-Canada syndrome associated with a rectal cancer and adenomatous changes in colonic polyps. Am J Surg Pathol 1985;9:65–71.
100. Nonomura A, Ohta G, Ibata T, et al. Cronkhite-Canada syndrome associated with sigmoid cancer. Case report and review of 54 cases with the syndrome. Acta Pathol Jpn 1980;30:825–45.
101. Yokoyama S, Yamashita H, Moriuchi A, et al. Cronkhite-Canada syndrome associated with adenosquamous carcinoma in gastric polyps. Report of an autopsy case. Stomach Intest 1983;18:981–90.

Gastric Hyperplastic Polyposis

102. Carneiro F, David L, Seruca L, Castedo S, Nesland JM, Sobrinho-Simoes M. Hyperplastic polyposis and diffuse carcinoma of the stomach. A study of a family. Cancer 1993;72:323–9.
103. Seruca R, Carneiro F, Castedo S, David L, Lopes C, Sobrinho-Simoes M. Familial gastric polyposis revisited. Autosomal dominant inheritance confirmed. Cancer Genet Cytogenet 1991;53:97–100.

17 MOTILITY DISORDERS

INTRODUCTION

Normal gastrointestinal motility depends on intact neuromuscular function. Extrinsic control of peristalsis includes the sympathetic (thoracolumbar) and parasympathetic (vagal) innervation in the ganglionated plexuses. Intrinsic control includes the enteric nervous system, smooth muscle cells, and interstitial cells of Cajal, with the latter serving both as pacemaker cells and as intermediaries of enteric innervation (1–3,6).

Gastrointestinal motility diseases constitute a complex array of clinical and pathologic disorders. They result from neural, muscular, or neuromuscular diseases (Table 17-1), and they occur at any age. The diseases may be primary motility disorders or they may complicate systemic diseases. Primary motility diseases more typically affect children than adults. Conversely, secondary conditions, such as scleroderma-associated myopathy, diabetic neuropathy, drug-induced damage, or viral infections more frequently affect adults. Primary motility disorders may be familial or sporadic. They may remain limited to the gut, as in Hirschsprung's disease, or they may be part of a generalized peripheral autonomic neuropathy, as in familial visceral neuropathy. Familial disorders are inherited as both autosomal recessive and autosomal dominant diseases.

The clinical and pathologic findings of gastrointestinal motility disorders may be subtle or dramatic. They can present as dysphagia, gastroparesis, intestinal pseudoobstruction, constipation, or intestinal diverticulosis. A consensus group of pediatric and adult gastroenterologists defined intestinal pseudoobstruction as "a rare, severe disabling disorder characterized by repetitive episodes or continuous symptoms and signs of bowel obstruction, including radiographic documentation of a dilated bowel with air-fluid levels in the absence of a fixed, lumen-occluding lesion" (5). *Ogilvie's syndrome* is a term used synonymously with acute colonic pseudoobstruction. Megaesophagus, megaduodenum, megajejunum, megacolon, and megarectum describe visceral enlargement of each of these anatomic sites. There is no

Table 17-1

GASTROINTESTINAL NEUROMUSCULAR DISORDERS

Neural Disorders
Neural developmental abnormalities
Hirschsprung's disease and its variants
Intestinal internal sphincter achalasia
Maturational arrest
Intestinal neuronal dysplasia
Megacystis-microcolon and intestinal hypoperistalsis
Severe idiopathic constipation
Absent enteric nervous system
Visceral neuropathies
Sporadic
Familial
Paraneoplastic pseudoobstruction
Infections
Herpes zoster
Cytomegalovirus
Epstein-Barr virus
Bacterial
Chagas' disease
Idiopathic ganglionitis
Autoimmune autonomic neuropathies
Achalasia
Allgrove's syndrome
Slow transit constipation
Complications of systemic neurologic disorders
Parkinson's disease
Wallenberg's syndrome
Amyotrophic lateral sclerosis
Muscle Disorders
Visceral myopathies
Sporadic
Familial
Mitochondrial myopathies
Autoimmune enteral leiomyositis
Diffuse leiomyomatosis
Neuromuscular Disorders
Infiltrative diseases
Scleroderma
Amyloidosis
Diabetic neuropathy
Toxic neuromuscular disorders
Drug induced
Radiation induced
Amanita poisoning

agreement on the criteria for the minimum diameters of the dilated gastrointestinal segments.

General Clinical Features

Patients present with a wide array of poorly defined gastrointestinal complaints, including abdominal distension, nausea, vomiting, constipation, diffuse esophageal spasm, delayed gastric emptying, and early satiety. Small intestinal pseudoobstruction leads to diarrhea, malabsorption, and steatorrhea secondary to slowed intestinal transit times, which also allows for secondary bacterial overgrowth. Some patients become malnourished with extreme weight loss. Recurrent postprandial upper abdominal pain, associated with bloating, nausea, and vomiting, indicates that combined gastric and small intestinal disease is present.

Extraintestinal manifestations depend on the nature of the underlying disease; these help define some syndromes. Features suggesting autonomic dysfunction include postural dizziness, difficulties in visual accommodation to bright light, and sweating abnormalities. Recurrent urinary infections and difficulty emptying the urinary bladder suggest a general visceral neuromyopathic disorder. Patients should be questioned about drug use. Patients bedridden for prolonged periods of time, such as those with dementia, stroke, and spinal cord injuries, are particularly prone to developing megacolon and chronic pseudoobstruction.

Pathologic Features

Radiologic Findings. Radiologic examination may show ileus, massive bowel dilatation, and slowed gastrointestinal transit times. Poor peristalsis leads to stasis with air-fluid levels. A microcolon may develop. Other radiologic features include esophageal dilatation with aperistalsis, gastric dilatation and delayed emptying, megaduodenum with segmental dilatation of the jejunum and ileum, and diverticulosis.

Microscopic Findings. Even though the clinical or gross findings may be dramatic, the histologic features are often inconspicuous, and they also overlap with the nonspecific neural or muscular histologic abnormalities accompanying other conditions, such as carcinoma or previous surgery. Additionally, there are patients who present with clinically evident motility disorders, who have histologic abnormalities that have not been well described or placed into specific syndromes.

Histologic examination using conventional hematoxylin and eosin (H&E) stains may have limited usefulness in evaluating many neuromuscular disorders. Special stains or ultrastructural examination, techniques not typically used in the evaluation of other gastrointestinal disorders, may be required. These include silver stains, assessment of acetylcholinesterase activity, and immunohistochemical staining for c-kit, neurofilament protein, PGP 9.5, S-100 protein, glial fibrillary acidic protein (GFAP), neural cell adhesion molecule (NCAM), and ret or nerve growth factor receptor (NGFR). Whole mount preparations can also be very helpful because they allow the visualization of the two-dimensional plexuses lying within the layers of the intestinal wall. They can be used to define the number of ganglion cells and neurons per surface area. This approach is most typically used for research purposes rather than for clinical diagnosis (7). Some histologic changes are so subtle that they require neuronal counting to document their presence. This is fraught with problems since the number of nerves and ganglia vary with age and with other disease processes.

Diagnostic Workup. Multiple modalities are used to diagnose motility disorders. They are clinically diagnosed using specific physiologic measurements of gastrointestinal motor function, including scintigraphy, gastroduodenojejunal manometry, and surface electrogastrography. The clinician should seek the pathologist's assistance to rule out the presence of infiltrative lesions, such as amyloidosis or connective tissue diseases, or to document the presence of neuromuscular abnormalities.

Treatment

Treatment of motility disorders ranges from dietary changes to surgery to intestinal transplantation in severe cases. Dietary measures, including frequent small meals low in fat and fiber, help some patients with gastroparesis. Prokinetic drugs such as cisapride, metoclopramide, erythromycin, domperidone, leuprolide, misoprostol, and octreotide acetate are beneficial in some cases. Octreotide exerts its effects mainly on the small bowel, and is particularly helpful in scleroderma. Patients who have acute colonic pseudoobstruction, such as following surgery or severe illness, may benefit from treatment with neostigmine, which rapidly decompresses the colon (4). In patients with irreversibly dilated bowels, no drug improves motility.

Bowel decompression through gastrostomy and jejunostomy may be beneficial in patients with pseudoobstruction. Small bowel transplantation is the only definitive cure for patients with chronic pseudoobstruction. Candidates for transplantation include those receiving total parenteral nutrition with frequent episodes of sepsis, limited intravenous access to nutritional support, or impending liver failure. Small bowel transplantation tends to be challenging in this clinical setting.

DEVELOPMENT OF THE ENTERIC NERVOUS SYSTEM

The enteric nervous system, a distinct division of the autonomic nervous system, is relatively independent of the central nervous system (18). It consists of a collection of autonomic ganglion-associated neural connections within the bowel wall. The intrinsic innervation of the gut wall consists of two interconnected ganglionated nerve plexuses, the myenteric plexus located between the longitudinal and circular muscle coats and the submucosal plexus. These plexuses extend in an uninterrupted fashion from the esophagus to the anus. The intrinsic plexuses collectively innervate the gastrointestinal mucosa, muscle layers, and blood vessels, and they contain reflex pathways that mediate activities such as peristalsis. The extrinsic innervation consists of parasympathetic and sensory nerves; disruption of this system produces little or no functional motor impairment (11,16,18).

Enteric neurons originate from the neural crest (16) in the dorsal neural tube. Here, the neural crest stem cells divide, giving rise to multipotential progenitors that divide further to give rise to differentiated cells. The differentiation process is influenced by: 1) the site of origin in the neural tube; 2) the environment into which the multipotential stem cells migrate; and 3) the responsivity of multiple lineages of precursor cells to the neurotrophic factors. Enteric neural crest cells originate from two distinct levels of the neural tube: the vagal and sacral regions (10). A dual developmental gradient leads to a cranial-caudal migration in the preumbilical gut and a caudal-cranial migration in the postumbilical gut (12) as shown by the fact that colonic and gastric ganglia appear before ileal ganglia. The neural crest–derived precursors migrate along defined pathways to colonize the bowel wall.

Enteric neuronal migration and differentiation involve a complex interaction of lineage-determined microenvironmental elements, including a number of transcription factors, tyrosine kinase receptors and their ligands, the extracellular matrix, and specific adhesion molecules (12–17,21). The transgenic and knockout technologies that allow genetic manipulation of the mouse embryo have led to the identification of a number of genes that are critical to the development of the enteric nervous system (9,12–15,17,19). Table 17-2 lists some of the known factors controlling neuronal development and differentiation.

By birth, normal enteric ganglia contain both mature and immature neurons. Premature infants have more immature neurons than term infants. Mature neurons are larger than immature neurons and have a distinct cell membrane, a vesicular nucleus, and a large amount of basophilic cytoplasm. Immature neurons are small cells with dark nuclei, clumped chromatin, and scant cytoplasm (fig. 17-1). Neural stains highlight immature neurons. The normal mature colon contains 7.0 ganglion cells/mm of myenteric plexus, 3.6/mm in the jejunum, and 4.3/mm in the ileum in 3-μm sections (20). Ganglion cells lie approximately 1 mm apart; they may occur in clusters of from 1 to 5 cells in normal adults (8). Normal neonates often have plentiful, prominent ganglion cells, but they appear small when they are immature (20).

NEURAL DISORDERS

Developmental gastrointestinal neural abnormalities result from failed neural migration or failed neural differentiation. Developmental neural diseases occur alone or they coexist with systemic disorders such as neurofibromatosis. Most congenital myenteric plexus abnormalities fall into one of five categories: aganglionosis,

Table 17-2

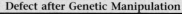

FACTORS INVOLVED IN THE DEVELOPMENT OF THE ENTERIC NERVOUS SYSTEM

Gene	Defect after Genetic Manipulation
RET/GDNF/GFRD1 Encodes ret, a receptor tyrosine kinase expressed by neural crest-derived cells that colonize the gut. Ret is the functional receptor for GDNF[a]	Knockout leads to complete failure of enteric neurons and glia to develop in the entire bowel below the foregut
Mash1 Encodes a transcription factor required for development of the autonomic nervous system	Knockout leads to aganglionosis of the esophagus and gastric cardia; absence of early lineage of enteric neurons in the rest of the bowel
Sox10 Encodes a transcription factor expressed by ENS[b] precursors before and after colonization of gut mesenchyme	Sox transgenics develop distal intestinal aganglionosis and die shortly after birth
Phox2 Homeodomain-containing transcription factor expressed by neural crest cells as they invade foregut mesenchyme	*Phox2* knockout mice die in utero; there is an absence of foregut and midgut ENS
EDNRB (endothelin receptor B) Growth factor receptor	Neural crest cells in *EDNRB* knockouts fail to colonize the hindgut
NCX1 Homeobox transcription factor expressed by ENS after midgestation in the distal gut	Homozygous targeted disruption animals show neural hyperplasia and hyperganglionosis
HOX4 Homeobox transcription factor expressed in foregut	Transgenic animals show abnormal ganglia in colon and short segment hypoganglionosis in distal colon

[a]GDNF = glial cell-derived neurotropic factor.
[b]ENS = enteric nervous system.

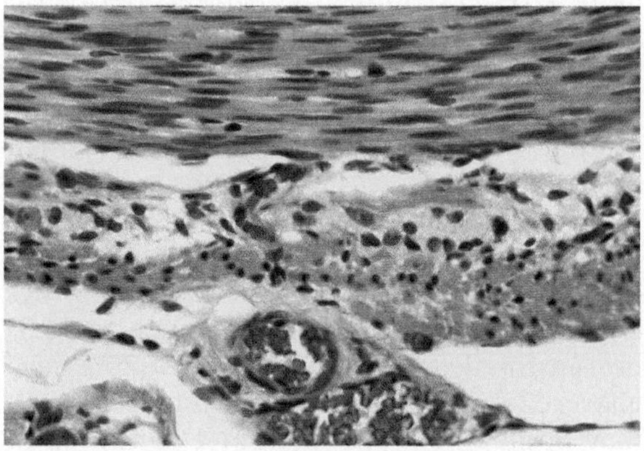

Figure 17-1

MYENTERIC PLEXUS OF A PREMATURE BABY

Immature ganglion cells are lined up along the edge of the myenteric plexus. These cells are small and dark, and recognized with difficulty by those unfamiliar with their appearance.

hypoganglionosis, hyperganglionosis, ganglionic immaturity, and poorly classified abnormalities. The pathogenesis of developmental disorders of the enteric nervous system results from genetic defects, anoxia, or inflammation.

Hirschsprung's Disease

Definition. *Hirschsprung's disease* (HD) is a congenital disorder characterized by intestinal megacolon, neural hyperplasia, and absent gastrointestinal ganglia. Several forms of HD are defined below. The disorder previously known as ultrashort HD is now referred to as achalasia of the internal sphincter; it is discussed in a later section.

Classic HD. The aganglionic segment begins in the distal colorectum and extends proximally for variable distances into the adjoining proximally dilated bowel.

Short Segment HD. The aganglionic segment involves several centimeters of the rectum and rectosigmoid.

Long Segment HD. The aganglionic segment involves most or all of the large bowel and it may extend into the small bowel (43).

Zonal Colonic Aganglionosis (Skip Segment HD). A short bowel segment is involved in this form of HD. Ganglion cells are present both proximal and distal to the aganglionic segment.

Aganglionic megacolon, congenital megacolon, and *aganglionosis* are synonyms of HD.

Demography. HD affects 1/5,000 to 30,000 live births; 80 percent of patients are male (70). Approximately 4 to 6 percent of cases are familial (70,73). The disease is likely to be familial when the megacolon extends to the cecum. Mothers with HD are more likely to have affected children than are fathers with HD. Five percent of patients have an affected sibling (73).

Nine percent of patients have total colonic aganglionosis (70). Zonal segmental aganglionosis is rare (76,89).

Etiology. HD is a heterogeneous genetic disorder with autosomal dominant, autosomal recessive, and polygenic forms of inheritance. Current etiologic hypotheses revolve around two schools of thought: arrested neuroblast migration and intestinal microenvironmental abnormalities causing failed neuronal differentiation. This condition is linked to specific genetic mutations in about 50 percent of cases.

There are four susceptibility genes for HD: the *RET* protooncogene on 10q11 (23–25,39, 40,50,72); its ligand, the glial cell line-derived neurotropic factor (*GDNF*) gene family; the endothelin B receptor (*EDNRB*) gene on 13q22 (35); and its ligand, the endothelin 3 (*EDN3*) gene (46,60) or neurturin, a *RET* ligand (Table 17-3) (38). An as yet unidentified gene located on chromosome 21q22 may also be involved (66). Modifier genes may also play a role in the pathogenesis of familial HD (75).

The ret protein is a tyrosine kinase receptor with extracellular cadherin-like and cysteine-rich domains, a transmembrane domain, and an intracellular tyrosine kinase domain (77,80). Point mutations in the *RET* gene give rise to HD, multiple endocrine neoplasia (MEN) types 2A and 2B, and familial medullary thyroid carcinoma (Table 17-4) (72). In the case of MEN2, the *RET* mutations are activating, i.e., they enhance the function of the encoded protein, whereas in HD, the mutations are inactivating and lead to loss of function (41).

Evidence pointing to the role of *RET* in the causation of some cases of HD include: 1) gross deletions encompassing the region of the *RET* gene in patients with HD (44,61); 2) genetic analyses of familial HD demonstrating linkage to the chromosomal region containing *RET* (26, 62); 3) *RET* expression in enteric ganglia and their precursors in fetal mice (67); and 4) mice with knockout of the *RET* gene developing HD (78). More than 50 mutations, including missense, nonsense, deletion, and insertion mutations,

Table 17-3

MUTATIONS IN HIRSCHSPRUNG'S DISEASE

Mutated Gene	Function	Disease
RET (intracellular tyrosine kinase domain)	Tyrosine kinase receptor	Short segment HD[a] Long segment HD
RET (extracellular domain)	Tyrosine kinase receptor	Long segment HD
EDNRB	Growth factor receptor	Short segment HD
EDN3	Ligand for EDNRB	Shah-Waardenburg syndrome

[a]HD = Hirschsprung's disease.

Table 17-4

DISEASE-RELATED *RET* GENE MUTATIONS

	HD[a]	PTC	MEN2A	FMTC	MEN2B	Sporadic MTC
Mutations	Various mutations through the gene (see text)	Gene rearrangements *RET/PTC1* *RET/PTC2* *RET/PTC3*	Missense mutations at cysteine residues: 609 611 618 620 634 (most common)	Missense mutations at cysteine residues: 609 611 618 620	A missense mutation at codon 918 (Met → Thr)	A missense mutation at codon 918 (Met → Thr)

[a]HD = Hirschsprung's disease; PTC = papillary thyroid carcinoma; MEN = multiple endocrine neoplasia; FMTC = familial medullary thyroid carcinoma.

have been described in HD. These mutations occur throughout the gene, without any mutational hot spots (28,88). The mutations can be placed loosely into two groups: frame shift or missense mutations that disrupt the structure of the intracellular tyrosine kinase domains (64), or missense mutations in exons 2, 3, 5, or 6 of the extracellular domain (40). Patients with mutations of the intracellular domain have either short segment or long segment HD, whereas those with mutations in the extracellular domain of *RET* have long segment HD. *RET* mutations are more common in familial cases (50 percent) than in sporadic cases (15 to 33 percent) (28,72).

EDNRB mutations are associated with short segment HD (69). Homozygosity for *EDN3* mutations causes the Shah-Waardenburg syndrome, a combination of HD with Waardenburg's syndrome. Several genes may modify severity of the HD phenotype in patients with or without coexisting intestinal neuronal dysplasia type B. The first is illustrated by a large Mennonite HD pedigree that showed a segregated missense mutation in the *EDNRB* gene (69). This family had marker alleles at 21q22 that were highly suggestive of an HD genetic modifier linked to this chromosomal region (47). This mutation may account for the prevalence of HD among trisomy 21 patients (47). Another HD modifier is exemplified by genes encoding glial cell derived neurotrophic factor (GDNF) (74,75,84) and more recently, neurturin (34), two highly homologous natural ligands of the ret tyrosine kinase receptor.

The finding of cytomegalovirus (CMV) genetic material in 8.8 percent of cases of HD suggests a role for antenatal CMV infection as an etiologic factor in some patients (80). Zonal HD is thought to have an ischemic etiology.

Pathophysiology. Alterations in intrinsic gastrointestinal innervation contribute to the clinical and pathologic features of HD. Vasoactive intestinal polypeptide and nitric oxide (59), components of the nonadrenergic, noncholinergic system (85) that relaxes smooth muscle and forms part of the inhibitory component of the peristaltic reflex, are absent (57). Extrinsic parasympathetic, cholinergic, and sympathetic adrenergic innervations persist, however. As a result, the distal aganglionic bowel is under constant, unopposed extramural stimulation so that it becomes narrowed, spastic, and unable to support peristalsis. There is constant internal sphincter muscular contraction. Carbon monoxide–producing neurons may also be abnormal in these patients (30).

The pathogenesis of the enterocolitis, which affects some patients, is not well understood. Enterocolitis is likely a consequence of the toxemia resulting from stasis and bacterial proliferation in the dilated colonic lumen. Patients who develop enterocolitis have abnormal mucosal immune defenses (27,51). Risk factors for enterocolitis include a delayed diagnosis of HD, long segment disease, family history of HD, female gender, and trisomy 21 (81).

Clinical Features. HD is the most common form of congenital intestinal obstruction. It often presents within the first 24 to 48 hours of life in infants who cannot spontaneously pass meconium. As many as 80 percent of cases are diagnosed during the first year of life. Most of the remaining 20 percent are diagnosed in early childhood; about 10 percent of HD cases present in adults.

Some patients appear perfectly normal at birth but they develop abdominal distension, vomiting, and obstipation during the first day or two of life. The lack of propulsive movements and of inhibitory reflexes in an intestinal segment leads to severe constipation and marked dilatation of the proximal ganglionic segment. Patients develop abdominal distension, repeated intestinal obstructions, enterocolitis, and meconium plug syndrome. Infants with obstruction but without megacolon should be suspected of having HD involving the entire colon.

The diagnosis of HD usually requires a combination of presenting clinical symptoms, radiologic findings, rectal manometry, and histologic or histochemical features. Failure of the internal sphincter to relax following intrarectal balloon distension highly suggests the diagnosis.

In young children, vomiting and progressive abdominal distension develop secondarily to dilatation and hypertrophy of the colon proximal to the narrowed segment. Constipation may alternate with diarrhea. Reduced food intake and malabsorption result in failure to thrive. As the nutritional status deteriorates, infections may worsen the underlying motility problem. Some patients develop a mucosal prolapse at the junction of the ganglionic and

Table 17-5

ABNORMALITIES ASSOCIATED WITH HIRSCHSPRUNG'S DISEASE

Genetic Abnormalities
Down's syndrome
Tetrasomy 9p
Tetrasomy 9q
Congenital Abnormalities
Deafness
Intestinal malrotation
Esophageal and intestinal atresia
Hypothalamic hamartoblastoma
Cartilage-hair hypoplasia
Dandy-Walker cysts
Brachydactyly
Tetraamelic postaxial polydactyly
Congenital hypoventilation (Ondine's curse)
Bilateral discolored irides
Holoprosencephaly
Polydactyly
Imperforate anus
Congenital muscular dystrophy
Infantile osteopetrosis
Tumors
Neuroblastoma
Neurofibromatosis
Medullary carcinoma of the thyroid
Pheochromocytoma
Other Syndromes
Jaw winking syndrome
Hadad's syndrome
Goldberg-Shprintzen syndrome
Achalasia

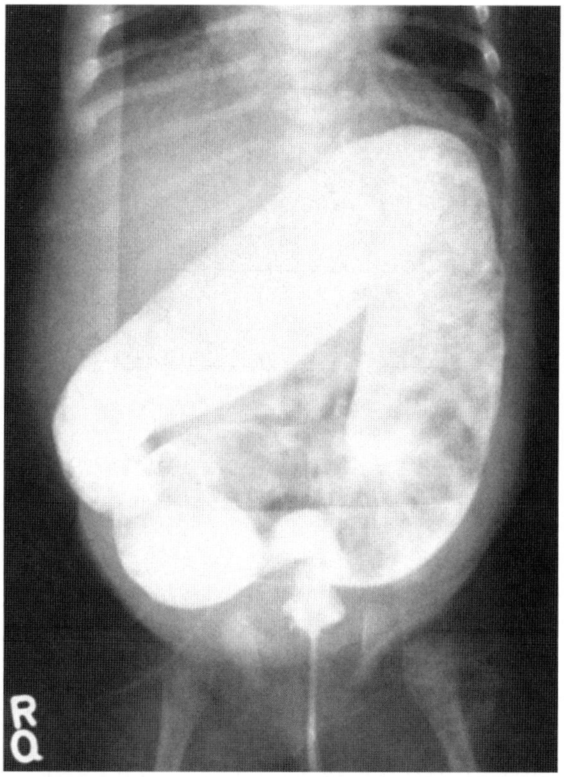

Figure 17-2

HIRSCHSPRUNG'S DISEASE

Barium enema in an infant with Hirschsprung's disease shows massive proximal dilatation of the large intestine. The distal large bowel appears stenotic.

aganglionic bowel due to different luminal pressures in these bowel segments. Mucosal prolapse is more prominent in older patients and correlates with disease duration (31).

HD patients may also present in the neonatal period with perforation due to coexisting necrotizing enterocolitis or volvulus (79). Enterocolitis, a major source of morbidity and mortality, both before and after definitive surgical treatment, is preventable by early diagnosis and colostomy (58). Major presenting features of enterocolitis include abdominal distension, explosive diarrhea, vomiting, fever, lethargy, rectal bleeding, sepsis, toxemia, mucosal ulceration, and colonic perforation.

Associated congenital anomalies or other diseases are seen in 10 to 15 percent of patients (Table 17-5) (33,37,42,45,52–55,64,68,71). Ten percent of patients have Down's syndrome; 5 percent have other serious neurologic abnormalities (29).

Gross Findings. The widely dilated, fluid-filled, hypertrophic colon empties into a funnel-shaped transitional zone that extends to the anus (figs. 17-2, 17-3). Plain abdominal films may show air-fluid levels. In adults, an abrupt, smooth rectal transition zone with proximal colonic dilatation, in the setting of an appropriate clinical history, suggests the diagnosis (65). The anal canal and rectum are small and empty, and the anal sphincter is tight.

Microscopic Findings. The typical features of HD include an absence of ganglion cells (fig. 17-4) and increased numbers of hypertrophic, nonmyelinated, cholinergic nerves (part of the extrinsic parasympathetic innervation) in the submucosa and myenteric plexus (fig. 17-4). A good correlation exists between the density of cholinergic innervation and the severity of the clinical symptoms. Normally, ganglion cells are distributed at intervals of approximately 1 mm

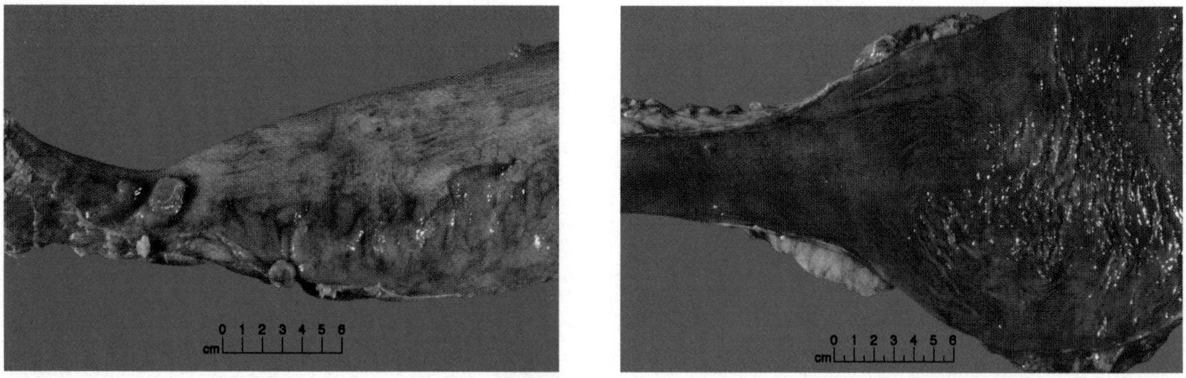

Figure 17-3

HIRSCHSPRUNG'S DISEASE

Left: Unopened bowel has a proximal area of dilatation tapering into an area of narrowing.
Right: Opened bowel shows its internal features.

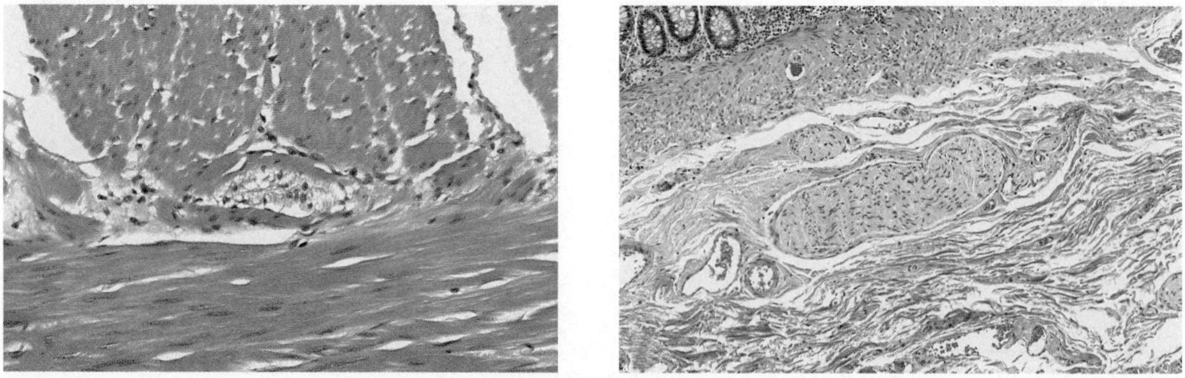

Figure 17-4

HIRSCHSPRUNG'S DISEASE

Left: There is an absence of ganglion cells in the myenteric plexus.
Right: Large hypertrophic nerve trunks are evident.

with clusters of 1 to 5 cells and a density of 17 cells/mm^2. In HD, ganglion cells are absent from both plexuses in the distal narrowed bowel segment and are decreased in number in the first few centimeters of the funnel-shaped transitional region.

Determining whether ganglion cells are present in premature infants may be difficult due to the sparse cytoplasm and inconspicuous nuclei of immature ganglion cells (fig. 17-1). Immature ganglion cells form rosette-like structures arranged around a central neuropil-type matrix, producing a horseshoe-like structure. Because immature ganglia are less distinctive than mature ones, they may mimic macrophages, smooth muscle cells, and Schwann cells. Ganglia can be stained with special stains to highlight their presence (see Special Techniques).

Patients with HD have an abnormal synapse distribution. There are fewer synaptophysin-positive synapses within the circular and longitudinal muscle layers in the transitional segments and in aganglionic segments (56). The adrenergic innervation of an aganglionic gut is also abnormal: there are alterations in numbers of adrenergic and peptidergic nerves (vasoactive intestinal polypeptide, substance P, serotonin, calcitonin gene–related peptide, and neuropeptide Y–containing nerve fibers). Patients with HD also have a relative loss of interstitial cells of Cajal (86,87).

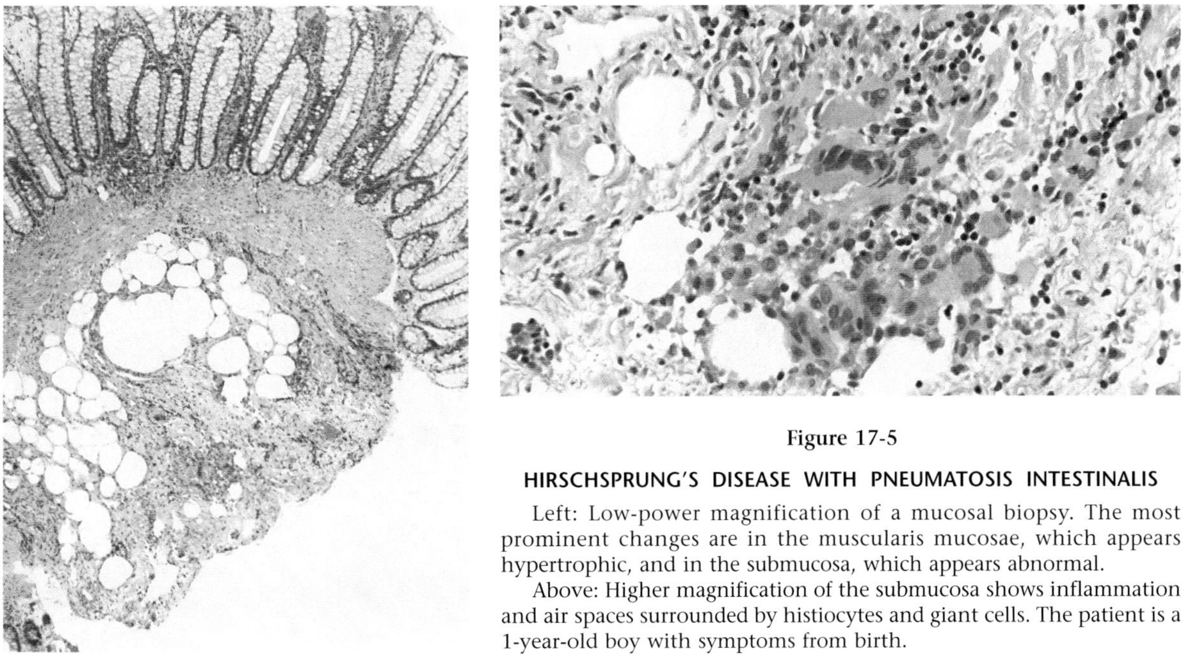

Figure 17-5

HIRSCHSPRUNG'S DISEASE WITH PNEUMATOSIS INTESTINALIS

Left: Low-power magnification of a mucosal biopsy. The most prominent changes are in the muscularis mucosae, which appears hypertrophic, and in the submucosa, which appears abnormal.

Above: Higher magnification of the submucosa shows inflammation and air spaces surrounded by histiocytes and giant cells. The patient is a 1-year-old boy with symptoms from birth.

Increased numbers of mast cells are seen in all of the bowel layers in the aganglionic portions of HD. These produce nerve growth factor, which stimulates neural growth. Sometimes the mast cells are in direct contact with the hypertrophic nerves.

The bowel wall proximal to the aganglionic segment is often biopsied for frozen section analysis during surgical resections to ensure that the proximal resection margin is normal. Submucosal nerve trunks over 40 µm in diameter strongly correlate with abnormal innervation and aganglionosis (fig. 17-4) (66). Ganglionated segments never show nerve trunks larger than this. If hypertrophic nerve trunks or abnormal ganglion cells are present in frozen sections, the surgeon should extend the resection proximally and monitor it with additional frozen sections to identify a region that contains completely normal neural structures. This helps prevent recurrent disease.

While it may be commonplace to use frozen sections in the context of monitoring resection margins, they have also been used to make the initial diagnosis. This practice is not recommended because there is a high rate of incorrect frozen diagnoses (63).

Once resection specimens are received, the extent of the aganglionosis should be determined and the status of the proximal margin ascertained, if this was not done intraoperatively. A progressive increase in the number of ganglion cells occurs as one progresses proximally in the funnel-shaped transitional zone located between the aganglionic and normally innervated bowel. The transitional zone usually occurs over a short distance in which ganglia appear almost simultaneously in both the myenteric and submucosal plexuses. The transitional zone may contain abnormally shaped ganglia. Some patients have longer transitional zones than others; prominent nerve trunks may be present for several centimeters. Some transition zones show features of colonic neuronal dysplasia (see below). Patients who develop postoperative symptoms may have either a retained portion of the transitional zone with neuronal dysplasia or an aganglionic segment, or they may have developed an acquired hypoganglionosis (34) secondary to postoperative ischemia or infection.

If enterocolitis develops, the histology may include crypt dilatation with mucin depletion, cryptitis, crypt abscesses, mucosal ulcers, transmucosal necrosis, and perforation. Enterocolitis affects both ganglionic and aganglionic intestinal segments, and resembles other forms of enterocolitis. Pneumatosis intestinalis may be present (fig. 17-5).

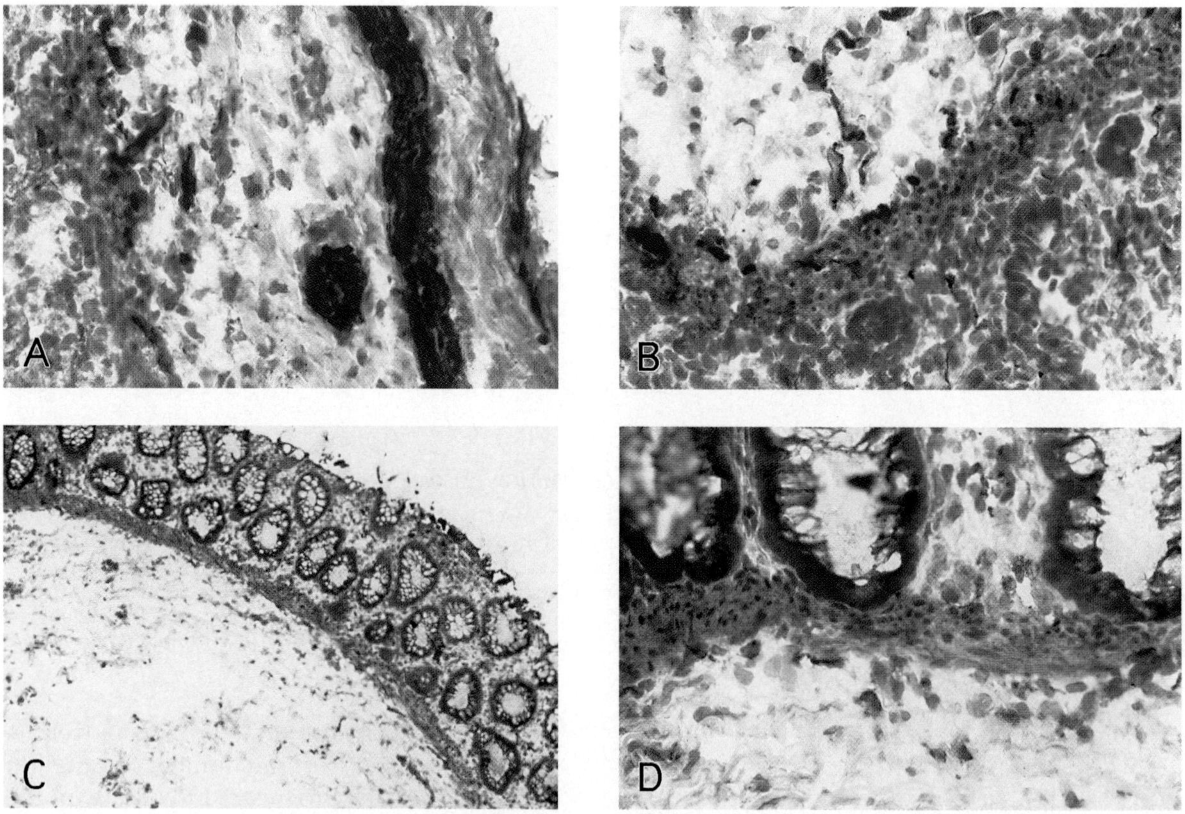

Figure 17-6

HIRSCHSPRUNG'S DISEASE SPECIMEN STAINED FOR ACETYLCHOLINESTERASE

A: Staining of the aganglionic segment shows the presence of very thick nerve trunks and thick cholinergic nerve twigs.

B: These thickened, irregular cholinergic nerve fibers are also seen in the area of the muscularis mucosae.

C: In the transitional zone of the same resection specimen, the large neural trunks and the finer cholinergic nerve fibers around the muscularis mucosae are absent.

D: Higher magnification of the thin fibers in the muscularis mucosae.

Histologic Variants. There are several histologic variants of HD. One is associated with *intestinal neuronal dysplasia* (IND). Generally, there is a hypoganglionic transitional zone at the cranial end of the aganglionic segment but hyperganglionic segments can also be found and qualify for diagnosis of HD-associated IND.

Total colonic aganglionosis can be divided into two groups based on the histologic findings. Some cases are histologically similar to short segment and long segment disease, whereas in others, the bowel is aganglionic, but there is little or no neural hyperplasia. The latter finding can lead to a false negative diagnosis.

Special Techniques. Acetylcholinesterase (ACE) enzymatic staining is a very reliable method for diagnosing HD (fig. 17-6). This technique demonstrates an increased network of coarse, thickened, irregular cholinergic nerve fibers within the muscularis mucosae and lower mucosa. The lamina propria fibers travel in a plane parallel to the mucosal surface. Increased ACE nerve fibers are consistently present in short and long segment HD but they may be absent in total colonic aganglionosis, as noted above. ACE staining patterns are less dramatic in neonates than in older individuals, possibly leading to a false negative diagnosis (32).

Antibodies to PGP 9.5, S-100 protein, neuropeptide Y, neuron specific enolase (NSE), neurofilament protein (40,49,63), or the microtubule-associated protein (MAP)5, all highlight nerve fibers. NSE or ret antibodies (fig. 17-7) intensely stain ganglion cells, facilitating recognition of small immature ganglion cells.

Differential Diagnosis. A number of congenital disorders are associated with megacolon (Table 17-6). Disorders in the differential diagnosis of neural hyperplasia include neurofibromatosis, MEN2b, Crohn's disease, and neuronal dysplasia.

Treatment and Prognosis. Surgery is invariably necessary for the treatment of symptomatic HD. Operations vary, depending on the extent of the aganglionosis. Surgery is also used to treat the enterocolitis, especially in the face of an impending perforation. The traditional management of HD involves the creation of a proximal diverting ostomy. This is followed by a second operation in which a definitive pull-through procedure is performed after the intestine has decompressed and the infant has had a chance to grow. With the advent of improved perioperative patient care, laparoscopy, and managed care-directed pressure to reduce hospital costs, other surgical management options have been explored. Common themes embraced by these newer approaches include definitive surgery

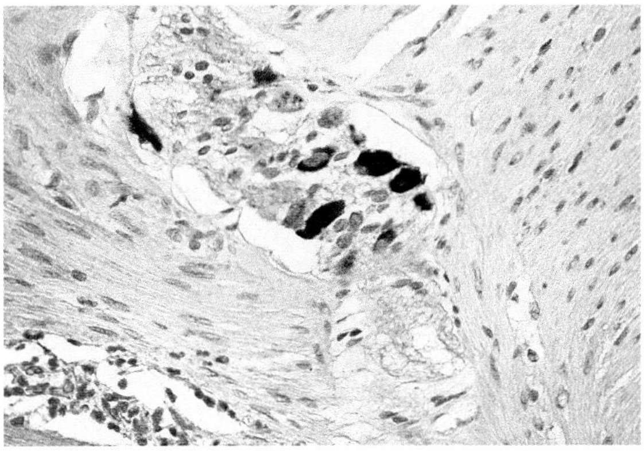

Figure 17-7

RET IMMUNOSTAINING OF A NORMAL GANGLION

The ganglion cells are clearly stained.

Table 17-6

CONGENITAL CONDITIONS ASSOCIATED WITH MEGACOLON

Condition	Prominent Features	Inheritance
Cartilage-hair hypoplasia	Short stature with metaphyseal dysplasia, sparse and fine hair, immunodeficiency; HD[a] is uncommon	AR[b]
Down's syndrome	Short stature, brachycephaly, upward-slanting palpebral fissures, small mouth, heart defects, joint hypermobility, mental retardation	Trisomy 21
Hirschsprung brachydactyly	Broad distal phalanges, nail hypoplasia of thumbs and halluces	? XLR
Hirschsprung cleft palate	Microcephaly, prominent nose with hypertelorism, synophrys, submucous cleft palate, sparse hair, mental retardation	? AR
Hirschsprung coloboma	Microcephaly, iris colobomas, hypertelorism, bulbous nose, mental retardation	AR
Hirschsprung digit hypoplasia	Upward-slanting palpebral fissures, micrognathia, hypoplastic distal digits and nails, growth and mental retardation	AR
Lesch-Nyhan syndrome	Mental retardation, self-mutilation, choreoathetosis, hyperuricemia; HD is uncommon	XLR
Multiple endocrine neoplasia, type 3	Marfanoid habitus, thick lips, nodules of tongue and lips, endocrine neoplasms	AD
Pallister-Hall syndrome	Prenatal growth deficiency, hypothalamic hamartoblastoma, laryngeal cleft, postaxial polydactyly, imperforate anus, heart defects, lethal (similar to severe Smith-Lemli-Opitz syndrome)	Sporadic
Riley-Day syndrome	Absent tearing, corneal ulceration, decreased pain sensation, smooth tongue with decreased taste, vomiting, fever, mental impairment	AR
Smith-Lemli-Opitz syndrome	Microcephaly, bitemporal narrowing, ptosis, nostril anteversion, hypotonia, incomplete genital development in males, mental retardation	AR
Waardenburg-Shah syndrome	Telecanthus, white forelock or piebaldism, deafness; HD uncommon	AD

[a]HD = Hirschsprung's disease.
[b]AR = autosomal recessive; XLR = X-linked recessive; AD = autosomal dominant.

without the need for stomas, operative correction in the newborn period, the use of laparoscopy to make smaller incisions (48), and the avoidance of an incision altogether, using a complete transanal colon resection (22). One-stage procedures are especially attractive in infants without enterocolitis (82); however, a single stage operation may carry with it a higher risk of enterocolitis than a two-stage operation (82).

Patients who have associated IND tend to have delayed restoration of normal defecation following treatment. Persistent constipation is the most important long-term problem in patients operated on for HD. Inadequate resection, anastomotic strictures, coexisting IND, and achalasia of the internal anal sphincter also cause persistent constipation (53). Constipation persists in 10 to 27 percent of patients and in up to 40 percent of patients with disseminated IND associated with HD. As many as 79 percent of patients may have associated IND (50).

Animal Models. Animal models have played an important role in unraveling the neural abnormalities present in HD. *Hox-4* transgenic mice and *RET* knockout mice develop congenital megacolon. The latter develop total gastrointestinal aganglionosis (69,78). Mutations of the *EDNRB* gene produce megacolon, spotty coat color, and aganglionosis confined to the rectosigmoid in piebald lethal mice. This suggests different functions for *RET*-mediated and *EDNRB*-mediated signaling pathways in the establishment of the enteric nervous system. *C-erbB2* knockout mice also develop megacolon (36). HD animal models are described in detail in references 35, 54, and 83.

Intestinal Neuronal Dysplasia

Definition. Patients with IND have defective gastrointestinal neuromuscular innervation. IND occurs in two forms: type A is characterized by decreased gastrointestinal sympathetic innervation, and type B is characterized by increased numbers of ganglion cells, a dysplastic submucosal plexus, and defective neuronal nerve fiber differentiation (97,108). These diseases are very controversial and poorly understood, and consensus definitions for each entity are not available. This group of diseases requires more study.

IND type A is also known as *hypoganglionosis*. *IND type B* is also known as *hyperganglionosis*. The entity known as *oligoneuronal disease*, which is sometimes called the *hypogenetic type of dysganglionosis* (134), may also be a form of IND type A.

Table 17-7

CAUSES OF ACQUIRED INTESTINAL NEURONAL DYSPLASIA TYPE A

Infections
Drugs
Inflammatory bowel disease
Other intestinal inflammatory conditions
Necrotizing enterocolitis
Status postsurgery
Status postradiotherapy
Prenatal ischemic events

Demography. IND type A is relatively rare, and probably accounts for only 5 percent of congenital gastrointestinal neuronal defects. The frequency of isolated IND type B varies from 0.3 to 40 percent of all rectal suction biopsies (132). IND occurs as an isolated disorder (135) or it coexists with neurofibromatosis, MEN2b, HD, intestinal malrotation (102), or short bowel syndrome. Some suggest that 25 to 79 percent of patients with HD have associated IND type B (132). Others, however, rarely encounter HD-associated IND. These incidence differences result from variable diagnostic criteria, biopsy procedures, staining techniques, and patient age. In HD, IND lies within, or just proximal to, the aganglionic transitional zone (100,108,129,130,135,137). Patients have also been described with aganglionosis involving the entire colon and terminal ileum, and coexisting jejunal and gastric IND. IND accounts for residual symptoms in HD patients following pull-through operations (109). IND affects both children and adults (114–117,119).

Etiology. IND is both a congenital and an acquired disease. IND type A may result from a developmental hypoplasia of the myenteric plexus (134), possibly due to abnormal expression of neurotrophic factors. Table 17-7 lists causes of acquired IND type A. Pediatric patients with MEN2b and IND type B have symptoms suggesting that both disorders result from mutations in the same domain of the *RET* protooncogene. In some cases, IND and neurofibromatosis are familial and associated with tandem duplication

Table 17-8

CONDITIONS ASSOCIATED WITH INTESTINAL NEURONAL DYSPLASIA

Tumors
Carcinoid tumors
Familial gastrointestinal stromal tumors
Lipoblastomatosis
Medullary carcinoma of the thyroid
Neurofibromatosis
Pheochromocytoma
Paraneoplastic Syndromes
Cystic Fibrosis
Other Gastrointestinal Abnormalities
Anal atresia
Choledochal cyst
Congenital hyperplasia of the interstitial cells of Cajal
Esophageal atresia
Hirschsprung's disease
Intestinal duplication
Microvillous atrophy
Persistent urachus
Pyloric stenosis
Rectal or sigmoid stenosis
Extraabdominal Malformations
Aortic stenosis
Congenital diaphragmatic hernia
Vertebral body malformations

in the *NF1* gene and a reciprocal translocation (t15;16)(q26.3;q12.1) (91). IND may also be one component of a complex malformation pattern, since it can coexist with extraintestinal and nonobstructive intestinal malformations (Table 17-8) (92,98,103,105,121,122,130,131). IND is also associated with intestinal microvillus atrophy (130) and lipoblastomatosis.

Pathophysiology. Patients with IND type A lack the normal number of ganglion cells, leading to motility abnormalities. IND type B is characterized by a malformation of the parasympathetic submucosal plexus. Disturbed innervation of the nonadrenergic, noncholinergic excitatory nerves contribute to abnormal motility patterns (119).

Clinical Features. The symptoms caused by IND type A resemble those seen in HD. In newborns, there may be delayed meconium discharge; infants and small children show rare bowel evacuations that respond to enemas. With increasing age, fecal masses can be palpated through the abdominal wall. The colon becomes dilated and contains fecalomas. Distension causes intermittent colicky pain, often relieved by massive flatulence. Some children experience overflow discharge of stool. The diagnosis of IND type A is usually difficult to establish. X-ray studies, determination of transit times, and anorectal manometry are not reliable indicators of the disease (135). IND type A is encountered in three forms: 1) an isolated form occurring as a segmental or even disseminated disease; 2) hypoganglionosis of variable length adjacent to aganglionic HD; and 3) hypoganglionosis in combination with IND type B in a proximal segment.

IND type B also clinically both mimics and complicates HD. HD-associated IND is a disseminated process in one third of patients and localized in the remaining. Patients present with constipation, intestinal obstruction, intussusception, or volvulus (112,120). Gastrointestinal symptoms include nausea/vomiting, diarrhea, constipation, and fecal incontinence. Symptoms develop insidiously, with progressive development of severe constipation that results in overflow incontinence (132). The mean age at diagnosis is 1.5 years. Many patients eventually spontaneously develop normal colonic motility (132). IND type B is thought to have an unfavorable course if the condition is associated with ganglionic heterotopia in the mucosa or if there are large numbers of immature ganglia.

A significant number of patients develop severe intraabdominal complications during the perinatal period, including necrotizing enterocolitis, meconium ileus, or bowel perforation especially in premature neonates. Conditions associated with IND are listed in Table 17-8.

Gross Findings. IND can be diffuse, involving both the small and large intestine, or it may remain confined to a single intestinal segment. Extensive disease may involve the stomach and esophagus (125,131,138). The bowel grossly appears either normal or variably dilated.

Microscopic Findings. *IND Type A.* Mucosal biopsies with histochemical analyses are usually not helpful in diagnosing IND type A because the disease is only reliably detected in the parasympathetic system of the myenteric plexus. Therefore, full-thickness biopsies are essential for the diagnosis (132). Patients with IND type A have a reduced number of myenteric ganglia and myenteric plexus neurons, no

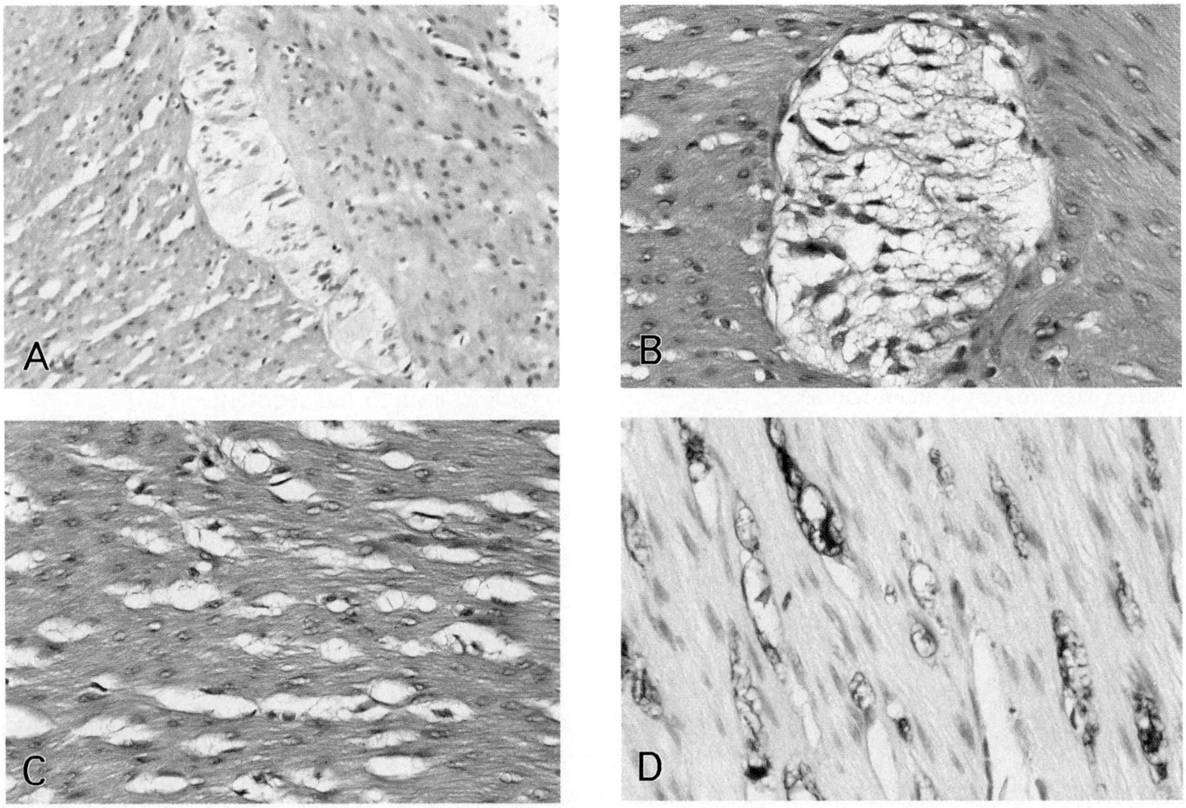

Figure 17-8

INTESTINAL NEURONAL DYSPLASIA TYPE A

A: Small submucosal and myenteric ganglia with immature neuroblast-like cells.

B: Higher magnification of one of the ganglia shows the immature, small, shriveled ganglion cells and swelling of the surrounding neural structures.

C: The swollen nerves are seen passing through the muscularis propria.

D: S-100 protein immunostain of the muscularis propria highlights the swollen nerve fibers.

or low colonic mucosal ACE levels, and hypertrophy of the muscularis mucosae and the circular muscle of the muscularis propria (120, 128). Absent or small submucosal and myenteric ganglia containing only one or two ganglion cells and immature neuroblast-like cells extend throughout the affected parts of the gastrointestinal tract (fig. 17-8) (96,119). Patients with IND type A may also have a reduction in the interstitial cells of Cajal, perhaps contributing to the dysmotility. Some patients have irreversible neuronal degeneration (fig. 17-8).

There is no consensus as to how few ganglion cells there should be to make a diagnosis of IND type A. Meier-Ruge (117) suggests that a 10-fold decrease in the number of ganglion cells per centimeter of bowel as compared to normal bowel is diagnostic. The distance between the ganglia in IND type A is nearly double that of the normal bowel; the average cell size is slightly greater than normal (135).

IND Type B. Controversy also exists over the diagnostic criteria for IND type B. Criteria for IND B include: 1) hyperplasia of the parasympathetic myenteric and submucosal plexuses characterized by increased numbers of neurons and ganglia (fig. 17-9) (93,110); 2) giant submucosal ganglia containing 7 to 15 ganglion cells (93, 113,116,117); 3) hypertrophic nerve bundles containing an increased number of thickened, beaded and disorganized axons (fig. 17-10); 4) increased ACE activity in the nerves of the mucosa, submucosa, and arterial adventitia (93,116); and 5) a proliferation of fine nerve fibers in the

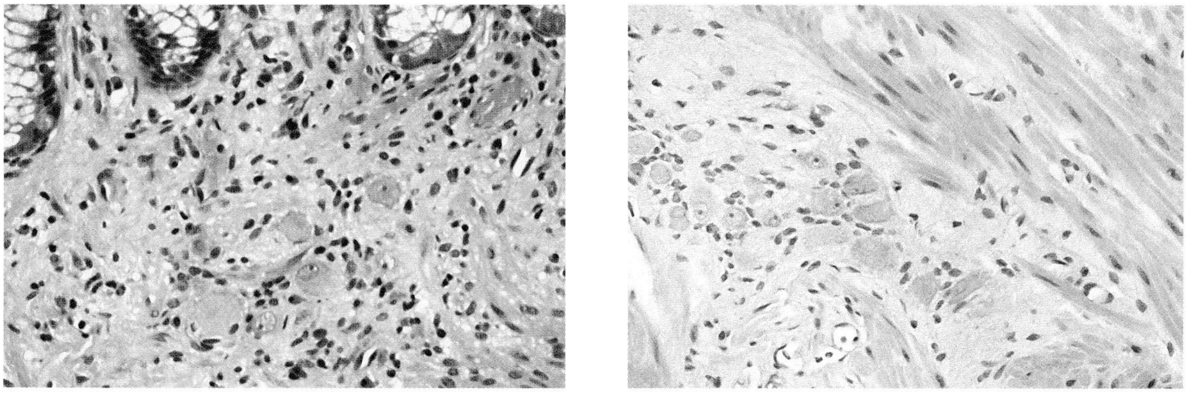

Figure 17-9

INTESTINAL NEURONAL DYSPLASIA TYPE B

Left: A large collection of ganglion cells is evident in the mucosa. The distance from the base of the crypts to the muscularis mucosae is widened and contains numerous ganglion cells.

Right: The myenteric plexus shows unusually large collections of ganglion cells.

lamina propria and circular muscle (133). The diagnostic controversy is best exemplified by a study in which three pathologists agreed on the diagnosis in only 14 percent of children without aganglionosis (112). Smith (136) also found that according to the criteria described by Borchard, only 11 percent of patients with megacolon had the obligatory criteria (hyperplasia of the submucosal plexus, an increase in ACE-positive nerve fibers around submucosal blood vessels, and ACE activity in the lamina propria).

These discrepancies reflect the fact that cases diagnosed as IND may be heterogeneous in nature, and the fact that there are no accepted criteria that cover all the histologic features that are seen. Furthermore, the suggested criteria are not universally accepted. The diagnosis of IND type B is further complicated by the fact that the density of ganglion cells in the myenteric plexus decreases significantly with age during the first 3 to 4 years of life. Finally, estimates of nerve cell density are influenced by section thickness (139).

In some of cases of IND type B, there are increased nerve cells per ganglion (approximately 10 cells per ganglion versus 4 per ganglion in normal children). The individual nerve cells are reduced in size (20 percent smaller) when compared with normal mature ganglion cells. These nerves show an increase in the number of ACE-positive nerve fibers and an absence of NCAM and nicotinamide adenine dinucleated phosphate (NADPH) diaphorase activity (106). The giant ganglia, hyperganglionosis, and increased numbers of nerves are demonstrable in the muscularis propria and the myenteric plexus (the motor division of the enteric nervous system) as well as in the mucosa and submucosal plexus (secretory and sensory division) (95,112,135).

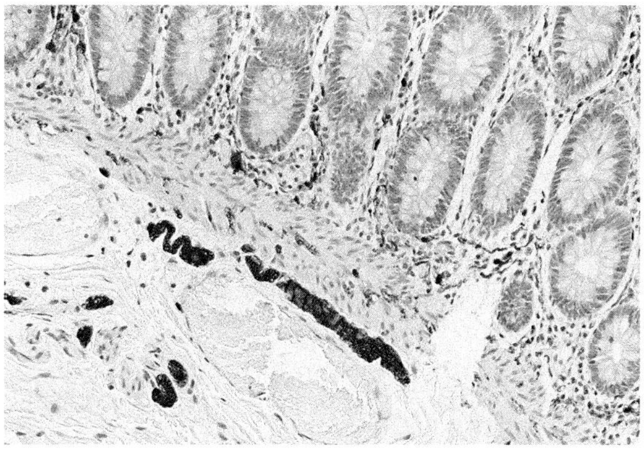

Figure 17-10

INTESTINAL NEURONAL DYSPLASIA TYPE B

S-100 protein immunostain highlights the thickened nerves in the superficial submucosa.

The diagnostic criteria relating to nerve cell density may overlap with age-related changes (116). The morphology of the myenteric plexus also varies at different levels of the gut. The density of the neural meshwork increases in the distal direction and is highest in the sigmoid colon and proximal rectum. In the lower parts of the rectum, the meshwork is less compact, and small ganglia and fibers extend in longitudinal directions. Many neurons contain bizarre nuclei and a poorly defined cytoplasm.

Giant ganglia are thought to result from the premature expression of laminin and other trophic factors during embryologic life, blocking neuroblast migration into the submucosa and myenteric plexus (123,124,125,133). Only about 5 percent of the ganglia in IND are giant ganglia (115). The specificity of giant ganglia as a marker for IND type B has been questioned, since occasional giant ganglia can be found in individuals without a history of constipation. Furthermore, the presence of giant ganglia may be age independent, whereas hyperplasia of the submucosal plexus and increases in ACE activity in the nerve fibers of the lamina propria appear to be age-dependent findings that disappear with maturation of the enteric nervous system (115). Therefore, neural hyperplasia is significantly more common in neonates than in older individuals (95).

Patients with IND type B may also have hyperplasia of the interstitial cells of Cajal. This can be visible grossly as a thick, white, fibrous band between the inner circular and outer longitudinal muscle layers throughout the full length of the resected bowel. Microscopically, this bandlike layer consists of haphazardly arranged spindle- to oval-shaped cells. The nuclei are long and oval, with slightly tapered ends, and possess hyperchromatic or clumped chromatin and occasional small nucleoli. The cells have a moderate amount of eosinophilic cytoplasm; mitotic figures are rare. The muscle layers are partially replaced by these hyperplastic spindle cells and focally the full thickness of the inner muscular layer can be involved. Residual myenteric plexus can be identified in the midst of the hyperplastic cells.

Patients with IND type B often have large numbers of mast cells in the bowel wall compared to normal. Mast cells produce nerve growth factors that support the development and functional maintenance of the sympathetic and cholinergic neurons, and they may be important in the neuronal hyperplasia seen in this condition (111). We have also seen endocrine cell hyperplasia associated with hyperganglionosis in the neonate.

Individuals with IND type B often have secondary changes in the muscularis propria. There may be areas of significant muscle atrophy in one or another layer of the muscularis propria; alternatively, there may be hyperplasia of either the circular or longitudinal layer of the muscularis propria; or these two changes may both be present. These secondary changes undoubtedly reflect abnormal innervation of the muscle layers and the neuromuscular junction (107).

Overall, it would be desirable to have better quantitative diagnostic criteria for IND type B to distinguish normal variants from pathologic conditions, particularly in very young children. Moore et al. (118) introduced a morphologic scoring system based on the finding of hyperganglionosis, giant ganglia, neuronal maturity, heterotopic neuronal cells, and ACE activity in the lamina propria, muscularis mucosae, or adventitia of submucosal blood vessels. Hyperganglionosis and increased ACE activity of nerve fibers in the lamina propria had major importance in this scoring system. The best diagnostic indicator of IND in adults may be the detection of 6 to 10 giant ganglia with more than seven nerve cells in 15 biopsy sections (90). Some suggest that to make a reliable diagnosis of IND type B, at least 30 serial sections must be examined and that they need to contain a minimum of four giant ganglion cross sections (117). It is further suggested that the nerve cell profiles be stained by an enzyme histochemical reaction specific for nerves (117).

Given all the confusion surrounding the diagnosis of IND type B, the question arises how to best diagnose the changes present. Our current practice is to be descriptive. We state that hyperganglionosis is present and state the number of ganglion cells/ganglia. We also state whether neuronal hyperplasia is present or not. If tissue was received for ACE staining, we describe whether ACE staining in nerves is increased and whether there is neural hyperplasia on the H&E or other stained sections. We also describe whether the neurons and ganglion cells appear histologically normal. If only large ganglia are present, we suggest that the change may be age-related and may resolve with time, requiring no therapy.

Histologic Variants. A variant of IND affects older patients who present with chronic diarrhea, pseudoobstruction, and multiple polyps, which contain prominent ganglioneuromatous proliferations within the lamina propria. The submucosal ganglia and myenteric plexus become infiltrated with chronic inflammatory cells.

Special Techniques. ACE histochemistry is a widely accepted technique for diagnosing enteric neuronal disorders, particularly HD and IND type B. The rapid ACE technique may be of great value in determining the extent of IND intraoperatively. A slight or moderate increase in ACE activity in the parasympathetic nerve fibers in the lamina propria and around submucosal vessels is present in approximately 60 percent of cases (111). The number of NCAM-positive nerve growth factor receptor (NGFR) fibers in the lamina propria and muscularis mucosae is also markedly decreased in IND (111). This finding is considered to be helpful, especially in diagnosing IND in neonatal cases where hyperganglionosis may be a normal finding. Newer neuronal markers, such as NADPH diaphorase histochemistry and immunohistochemistry, lactate dehydrogenase (LDH) histochemistry, and succinate dehydrogenase histochemistry may be used (93,101,115,129). An increased number of giant ganglia with more than seven LDH-positive nerve cells is suggested to be typical for IND type B. Abnormal neural proliferations can be highlighted by silver stains or antibodies to S-100 protein, NSE, PGP 9.5, neuropeptide Y, or neurofilament protein. Recently, Cuprolinic blue has been proposed as the method that stains the largest number of ganglion cells. This stain only stains cell bodies and not the axons, which makes distinguishing individual cells relatively easy. We have also used ret immunostains to highlight the ganglion cells.

Hutson et al. (104) performed immunofluorescence for the presence of neurotransmitters associated with excitatory nerves (substance P [SP]) and those associated with inhibitory nerves (vasoactive intestinal polypeptide [VIP]) (104). These two peptides represent functional markers for the colonic contraction (SP) and relaxation (VIP) necessary for forward propulsion (99). The authors found two variants of IND: one with an isolated deficiency of SP labeling in colonic nerves and a second group with deficient staining for both SP and VIP (104). Interstitial cells of Cajal are diffusely immunoreactive for c-kit, CD34, and vimentin but nonreactive for S-100 protein, smooth muscle actin, desmin, neurofilament, and NSE.

Differential Diagnosis. Clinically, IND mimics HD but the histologic features distinguish the two disorders, except in those situations where IND coexists with HD. The presence of giant ganglia, immature ganglia, and heterotopic nerve cells aids in the diagnosis of IND. The lesions differ from the neurofibromas of neurofibromatosis by the diffuse exaggeration of normal neural tissue, contrasting with the tumor formation seen in neurofibromas (94, 137). Overlap may exist between the two conditions. IND type A can also be seen in other settings (see Table 17-7).

Treatment and Prognosis. Some patients, especially those with IND type B, outgrow their disease as the enteric nervous system matures. Patients with persistent symptoms are managed medically with prokinetic agents, colonic irrigations, and cathartics. If bowel symptoms persist after 6 months of conservative treatment, internal sphincter myotomy should be considered (134). Resection and pull-through operations may be indicated for extensive IND (127). The decision to treat with surgery is usually based on the patient's clinical symptoms. Individuals who develop ileus may require resection (138). Patients with both aganglionosis and IND have a worse prognosis than those with only one or the other disease.

Animal Models. *Hox11L1* is a homeobox gene involved in peripheral nervous system development as confirmed by knockout mice exhibiting megacolon. This gene localizes to human chromosome 2p13.1->p12 at a 14cr interval between WI5987 (D2STO88N) and GCT1B4 (B2S4797) (126).

Neuronal Maturational Arrest

Definition. *Neuronal maturational arrest syndromes* are characterized by the failure of neural elements to mature properly. Synonyms include *neuronal immaturity* and *ganglionic immaturity*.

Etiology. The underlying cause(s) of failed neuronal maturation is unknown. Pathogenetic mechanisms may include: 1) failure of normal numbers of neural crest cells to migrate into the gut; 2) inadequate neural proliferation in the gut; or 3) death of neuroblasts once they arrive in the gut. The lesion may result from failure of the local microenvironment to support normal neuronal development during fetal life. There have also been reports of delayed maturation of the interstitial cells of Cajal, contributing to pseudoobstruction in neonates.

Clinical Features. Children present with poorly defined motility disorders, including intestinal pseudoobstruction or chronic constipation.

Microscopic Findings. The histologic features differ depending on the stage at which myenteric plexus development ceased. Patients exhibit several major histologic abnormalities: 1) no myenteric plexus seen in either H&E-stained or specially stained sections; 2) small numbers of neuronal structures (ganglia and nerve trunks) are present; however, the neurons are small and have only one or two processes, and the ganglia lack the nerve tracts and mesh-like structures that characterize the normal myenteric plexus; or 3) an apparently normal myenteric plexus is seen on H&E-stained sections but there is a deficiency of neurons as seen by silver or immunohistochemical staining. These neurons lack neurofilaments, further confirming their immaturity. The ganglion cells may also line up at the periphery of the ganglia as occurs in premature infants (see fig. 17-1). There is no inflammation or neural degeneration. These findings contrast with those seen in patients with HD or IND type B in that there is no neural hyperplasia.

Special Techniques. Silver stains, enzymatic stains, or immunostains facilitate the diagnosis. We utilize immunostaining for the ret protein in order to highlight the presence of ganglion cells, which may be small, to distinguish them from the nerve-supporting enteric glia. A number of immunostains can be used to highlight the neurons.

Differential Diagnosis. Other motility disorders.

Treatment. Neuronal immaturity often spontaneously improves with conservative therapy and the normal development of the child.

Internal Anal Sphincter Achalasia

Definition. *Internal anal sphincter achalasia* is the failure of relaxation of the internal anal sphincter in the presence of ganglion cells as seen in rectal suction biopsies (142,144,145). This abnormality is also known as the *utrashort form of HD*.

Pathophysiology. Achalasia results from abnormal innervation of the internal anal sphincter. Normal relaxation of the internal anal sphincter occurs by the activation of intramural nonadrenergic, noncholinergic (NANC) nerves (146–148) via nitric oxide (NO), the transmitter in NANC signaling (140). In achalasia, there are abnormalities in NO synthase and NADPH diaphorase. The latter mediates internal anal sphincter relaxation in the absence of NO synthase innervation.

Clinical Features. Anal achalasia is a disorder that only affects the internal anal sphincter. This disorder presents in a manner similar to that of HD, but there are ganglion cells on rectal biopsy (141). Anorectal manometry demonstrates the absence of rectosphincteric reflex during rectal balloon inflation (143).

Microscopic Findings. Rectal biopsies have ganglion cells and normal ACE activity (142, 144,145).

Treatment. Patients are treated by internal sphincter myotomy.

Absent Enteric Nervous System

Definition. An *absent enteric nervous system* means an absence of nerves and ganglia from the stomach to the colon.

Clinical Features. A unique case report described a full-term infant who developed severe perinatal pseudoobstruction in the absence of gastrointestinal neurons and ganglia (149).

Microscopic Findings. In the above case, no nerves or ganglia were present in the Auerbach plexus, within the muscularis propria or myenteric plexus area. S-100 protein and ACE staining confirmed the absence of neural structures. Sporadic PGP 9.5 positivity identified extrinsic nerves associated with the submucosal blood vessels and within the area of the Auerbach plexus. Electron microscopy failed to show enteric nerve fibers and neuronal cell bodies and their associated Schwann cells within Auerbach plexus. Extrinsic nerve fibers were sparse. Interstitial cells of Cajal in Auerbach plexus (ICC-AP) were quite prominent in the area between the circular and longitudinal muscle layers and their distribution resembled that seen in normal human tissues. The ICC-AP processes were in close apposition with each other and with nearby smooth muscle cells, but no gap junctions were found.

No close contacts were found between the ICC-AP and extrinsic nerves.

In the inner third of the circular muscles, no normal interstitial cells of Cajal were detected. Interstitial cells of Cajal of the deep muscle plexus, located between the inner and outer division of the circular muscle layers in the zone of connective tissue, were in various stages of injury. They were characterized by partial or complete destruction of their organellar contents. Their long thin processes frequently contacted adjacent circular muscle cells. The normal distribution of the ICC-AP and their normal close contacts with smooth muscle cells appeared to be sufficient for the generation of regular rhythmic slow wave activities, even in the absence of interstitial cells of Cajal in the deep muscle plexus.

Treatment and Prognosis. The child received enteral feedings, but the infant's feeding tolerance was limited by his impaired gastric emptying and he eventually died of hepatic failure.

Familial Visceral Neuropathies

Definition. *Hereditary familial visceral neuropathies* are a group of genetic diseases characterized by pseudoobstruction (fig. 17-11), myenteric plexus abnormalities, variable inheritance patterns, and characteristic extraintestinal manifestations (Table 17-9).

Demography. These diseases are rare.

Clinical Features. The clinical findings of each syndrome are listed in Table 17-9.

Microscopic Findings. These are listed in Table 17-9. The nerves often appear vacuolated (fig. 17-12). Silver stains or immunostains highlight both the number and the shape of the neurons and nerve fibers of the myenteric plexus.

Special Studies. Ultrastructural examination of the autosomal recessive visceral neuropathy with intranuclear inclusions form of the disease shows intranuclear neuronal inclusions consisting of a random array of straight or slightly curving filaments. These filaments have a characteristic beaded pattern with a periodicity of 15 to 30 nm. They measure 17 to 27 nm in diameter.

Paraneoplastic Pseudoobstruction

Definition. *Paraneoplastic pseudoobstruction* develops in patients with neuroendocrine or neural neoplasms caused by the production of neuronal autoantibodies that cross-react with neural tissues, destroying them (151,152,158).

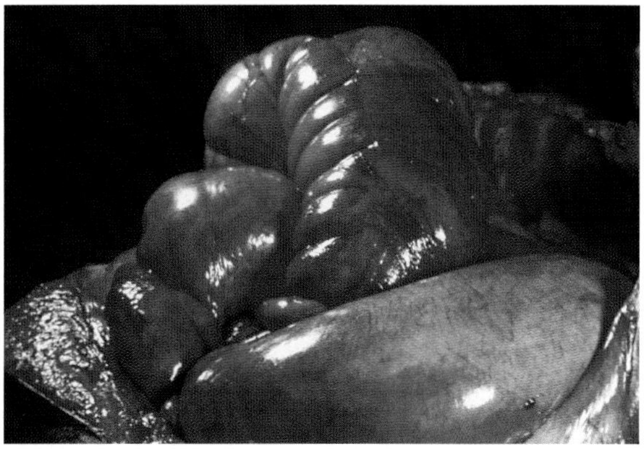

Figure 17-11

MEGACOLON

The body of this patient with intestinal pseudoobstruction has been opened and the dilated stomach and colon bulge out of the abdominal cavity. A feature such as this can be seen in patients with primary neuropathies or primary myopathies.

Demography. Patients with small cell carcinoma of the lung (150), carcinoid tumors, medulloblastomas, and oligodendrogliomas (150,155) develop the disease.

Pathophysiology. Some patients with neural and neuroendocrine tumors develop distinctive antineuronal autoantibodies (151,154,158), including type 1 antineuronal nuclear antibodies, also defined as anti-anti Hu on the basis of their molecular target, type 2 antineuronal nuclear antibodies (or anti-Ri), anti-Purkinje cell cytoplasmic antibodies (anti-yo), N-type voltage-gated calcium channel antibodies, P/Q type calcium channel antibodies, and ganglionic and muscle type nicotinic acetylcholine receptor antibodies (156,159,160). The most commonly identified antineuronal antibody is anti-HU, an immunoglobulin G. It recognizes a group of proteins with molecular weights in the range of 35 to 40 kDa that are expressed by both neurons and neoplastic cells. Hu antigens include four nervous system–specific RNA-binding proteins (identified as HuD, HuC, HuR, and Hel-N1). These share sequence homology with the embryonic lethal abnormal vision-binding protein of Drosophila. The anti-HuD antibodies evoke neuronal apoptosis that may contribute to impairment of the enteric nervous system (153).

Table 17-9

FINDINGS IN VISCERAL NEUROPATHIES

Disease and Genetic Transmission	Clinical Findings	Gastrointestinal Lesions	Microscopic Lesions	Silver Stains	Extraintestinal Lesions
Familial Forms					
Autosomal recessive with mental retardation, basal ganglia calcification	CIIP[a] Mental retardation	Megaduodenum, generalized dilation of small intestine, redundant colon	Atrophy of smooth muscle in all gastrointestinal tissues	Argyrophilic neurons decrease in number, remaining neurons appear misshapen and pyknotic	Extensive focal calcification of basal ganglia and subcortical white matter
Autosomal recessive neuronal intranuclear inclusion disease	CIIP Diffuse neurologic abnormalities, mild autonomic insufficiency, denervation hypersensitivity of pupillary and esophageal smooth muscle, progressive spasticity, ataxia, absent deep tendon reflexes, dysarthria, gastroparesis, neurogenic bladder	Dilation and nonperistaltic hypoactivity involving the esophagus, stomach, and small intestine; extensive colonic diverticulosis	Reduction and degeneration of myenteric plexus neurons, eosinophilic neurofilament containing intranuclear inclusions in myenteric and submucosal plexus neurons	Decreased neurons in myenteric plexus, remaining argyrophilic neurons are misshapen with only a few processes	Neural inclusions in central and peripheral nervous systems
Autosomal dominant visceral neuropathy	Predominantly present with intestinal pseudoobstruction, symptom onset at any age, postprandial abdominal pain, distension, diarrhea, constipation	Abnormal gastric emptying, dominant segmental dilation of jejunum and ileum, small intestinal diverticulosis, proximal small intestine always involved	Hypertrophy of smooth muscle, reduction and degeneration of myenteric plexus, argyrophilic neurons	Decreased number of degenerated neurons with poorly defined cell borders and decreased silver staining, some neurons appear vacuolated or beaded	None
Autosomal recessive visceral neuropathy type II	Symptoms start in infancy	Hypertrophic pyloric stenosis, short dilated small intestine, intestinal malrotation	Neural abnormalities, neuroblasts present, hypertrophy of muscularis propria, no muscle degeneration	Deficiency of argyrophilic cells, no visible intrinsic neurons or processes	CNS malformations with heterotopia and absence of operculum temporale, patent ductus arteriosus
Sporadic Visceral Neuropathy					
Type I sporadic	Similar to other forms of CIIP	Affects both the large and small intestine	Reduced myenteric neurons, no inflammation, neuronal swelling, gliosis, no inclusions	Neuronal swelling, fragmentation and dropout, eventually neurons disappear	None
Type II sporadic	Similar to other forms of CIIP	Affects both the large and small intestine	Degenerated argyphilic and argyrophobic neurons, loss of antral staining producing signet ring cell appearance, no inflammation	Axonal disorganization and degeneration	None

[a]CIIP = chronic idiopathic intestinal pseudoobstruction; CNS = central nervous system.

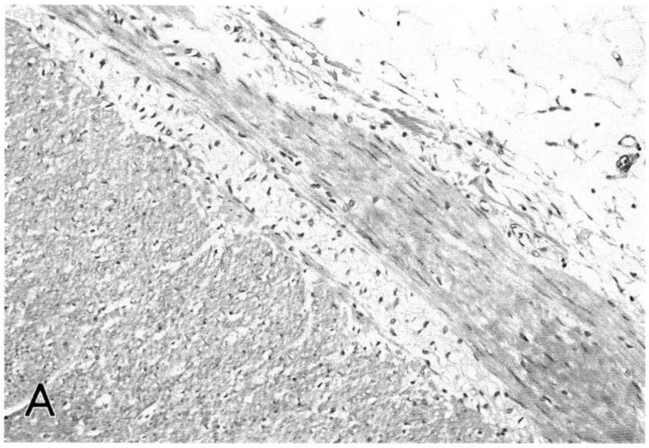

Figure 17-12

PRIMARY NEUROPATHY

This patient had massive dilation of the colon.

A: Medium magnification shows an area of the myenteric plexus that appears vacuolated.

B: Abnormal-looking ganglia are present.

C: An antibody to S-100 protein highlights the vacuolization of the nerves.

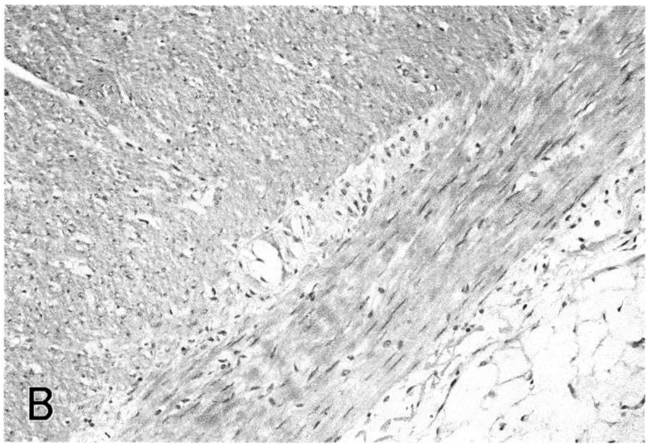

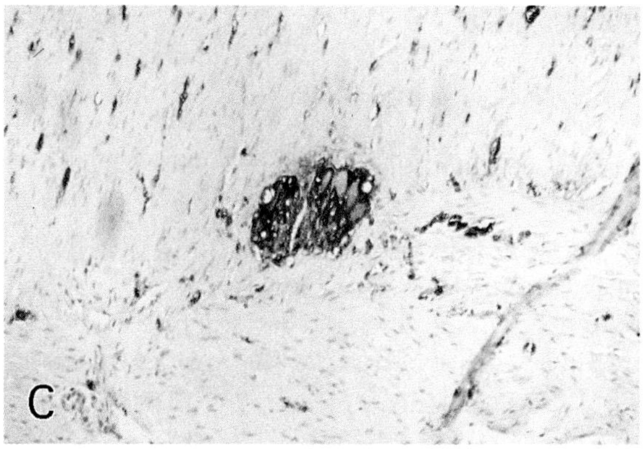

Clinical Features. Patients present with gastrointestinal dysmotility and autonomic dysfunction, often before the underlying malignancy is diagnosed. They experience weight loss, pseudoobstruction, constipation, gastroparesis, gastroesophageal reflux, esophageal dysmotility suggestive of spasm or achalasia, intractable dysphagia, postprandial fullness, nausea, vomiting, diarrhea, fecal incontinence, and bloating (150,154,158). They also develop associated peripheral, sensory, and motor neuropathies; neurogenic bladders; ataxia; encephalopathy; orthostatic hypotension; and decreased deep tendon reflexes (150,154,156,157), giving a clue to the likely etiology of this motility disorder.

Gross Findings. Pseudoobstruction results in dilatation of the stomach, small intestine, and colon.

Microscopic Findings. Myenteric neurons, from the esophagus to the colon, are reduced in number and the myenteric plexus is infiltrated with plasma cells, lymphocytes, and eosinophils (fig. 17-13). Remaining neurons appear vacuolated and display cytoplasmic irregularities and decreased cellular processes. Axons swell, become fragmented, and drop out. The damage leads to gliosis, sometimes completely replacing the nerve tracts. Only a few normal-appearing neurons remain. The key finding suggesting the diagnosis is the presence of lymphoid cells and plasma cells within the myenteric plexus.

Special Techniques. Serologic testing for the Hu antibody offers a simple means of distinguishing those patients with paraneoplastic gastrointestinal tract dysmotility syndromes (151). Rarer autoantibodies can also be evaluated.

Differential Diagnosis. The differential diagnosis includes toxic neural damage from drugs, infection, or an autoimmune neuropathy, as well as aganglionosis in the absence of a tumor.

Treatment and Prognosis. The treatment of the underlying tumor may not necessarily reverse the intestinal manifestations, which require symptomatic and supportive therapy.

INFECTIOUS CAUSES OF MOTILITY DISORDERS

Demography. Some patients with viral infections and many patients with Chagas' disease develop gastrointestinal motility disorders. Herpes zoster and cytomegalovirus (CMV) damage

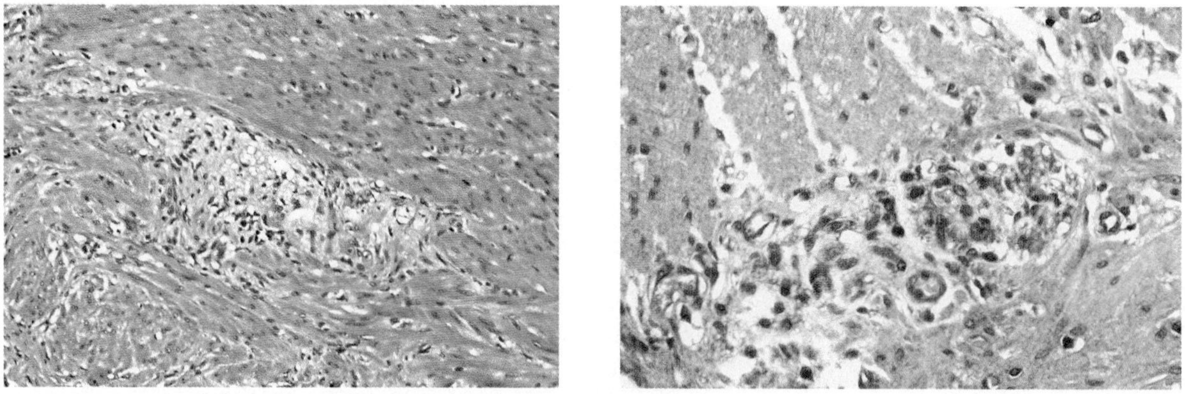

Figure 17-13

PARANEOPLASTIC PSEUDOOBSTRUCTION

The patient had a carcinoid tumor of the ovary.
Left: Hematoxylin and eosin (H&E) stain highlights the increased cellularity of the myenteric plexus.
Right: Many of the cells are small lymphocytes (leukocyte common antigen immunostain).

the myenteric plexus, leading to the development of pseudoobstruction in immunocompromised patients. Some bacterial infections also result in motility disorders or irritable bowel syndrome.

Etiology. Secondary gastrointestinal neuropathies can be caused by neurotropic viruses, including herpes zoster (162), Epstein-Barr (EBV) virus (169) and CMV (161). Other infections result in autoimmune attacks on neural structures due to the presence of cross-reacting antigens, such as those present in some *Campylobacter* infections. Chagas' disease is discussed in chapter 10.

Clinical Features. Delayed gastric emptying occurs as a consequence of acute viral gastroenteritis, due to CMV (163,164,166,168), rotavirus (161), or Norwalk or Hawaii virus infections (167). Generally, if there is a delay in gastric emptying, it is transient and returns to normal after the patient recovers from the viral infection (161,165). Patients may also develop tachygastria (an accelerated gastric rhythm), causing nausea and vomiting (168). In some patients, symptoms persist following treatment (166). Some patients present with pseudoobstruction and abdominal pain (167). Autonomic neuropathies may also be seen in patients with neurotropic viral infections (170).

Gross Findings. In patients with viral infections, especially CMV and, to a lesser extent, herpes simplex virus (HSV), the various gastrointestinal surfaces may appear normal or there may be erosion or ulcers anywhere from the esophagus to the rectum. The gastrointestinal tract may also show any of the features seen with any other pseudoobstruction syndrome.

Microscopic Findings. Patients with infectious causes of motility disorders may show any of the features discussed in chapter 10. Here, the focus is on those that relate to the motility disorders. In CMV or HSV infection, viral inclusions may be identified, or not. The diagnosis can be made by demonstrating CMV or HSV intranuclear inclusions in the myenteric plexus neurons or in the muscle fibers. The typical mucosal effects of viral gastroenteritis may also be present, or the patient may have healed viral gastroenteritis with little inflammatory injury to the gastrointestinal mucosa. In patients without obvious inclusions, the enteric nerves may harbor either latent virus or residual inflammation without significant mucosal alterations.

Special Techniques. Gastrointestinal motility abnormalities may be documented utilizing gastric emptying scintiscans to demonstrate delayed gastric or intestinal transit. Bacteria or viruses can often be cultured directly from the tissues (166). In patients without obvious inclusions, ultrastructural examination, immunohistochemistry, or *in situ* hybridization demonstrates the presence of the virus.

Differential Diagnosis. Other causes of gastrointestinal motility disorder.

Treatment. The beginning of this chapter discusses general approaches to the treatment of motility disorders. Treatment of specific infections is discussed in chapter 10.

IDIOPATHIC GANGLIONITIS

Definition. *Idiopathic ganglionitis* is a motility disorder associated with chronic inflammation that affects the ganglia, in the absence of a known cause for the inflammation. Synonyms include *acquired intestinal aganglionosis* and *acquired megacolon-megarectum.*

Demography. The disorder often affects young women of an average age of 25 years (171).

Etiology. The etiology of idiopathic ganglionitis is poorly understood. Most cases are due to autoimmune circulating enteric neuronal antibodies in the absence of cancer (173,175).

Pathophysiology. In some patients, the development of idiopathic ganglionitis correlates with abnormalities in the concentration of enteric neurotransmitters and enzyme activity. There is a significant decrease in VIP concentration and ACE activity in the nerves of the muscularis propria and in the nerve cell bodies in the myenteric plexus.

Clinical Features. Patients present with severe constipation and abdominal pain late in childhood. Some have associated mental retardation or psychiatric disorders. Initially, the motility disorder remains limited to the colon; later it involves the entire gastrointestinal tract. There may be abdominal pain, nausea, vomiting, malnutrition, diarrhea, and weight loss due to extreme inanition and hypergammaglobulinemia (173).

Gross Findings. The rectum tends to be full of stool; fecal impaction is not unusual. A rectal diameter over 6.5 cm at the pelvic brim on lateral radiographic view is common, as is a cecal diameter in excess of 12 cm.

Microscopic Findings. Patients without cancer and without central nervous system involvement may show extensive ganglionitis with neuronal vacuolization and loss. A diffuse lymphoplasmacytic infiltrate may affect all layers of the intestinal wall. The infiltrate also extensively damages the submucosal and myenteric nerve plexuses, resulting in a marked reduction in the number of myenteric nerve fibers. CD3- and CD4-positive T lymphocytes surround the altered nerves. The histology of the musculature varies, appearing hypertrophic or atrophic, probably secondary to the neural abnormalities (173,175).

Differential Diagnosis. The differential diagnosis includes paraneoplastic ganglionitis and Chagas' disease (172,174).

ACHALASIA

Definition. *Achalasia* is a rare disorder of unknown etiology associated with neuronal degeneration that results in esophageal aperistalsis, impaired esophageal motility, and failed relaxation of the lower esophageal sphincter. Achalasia is also known as *cardiospasm* and *megaesophagus.*

Demography. Achalasia affects about 7 to 13/100,000 in Europe and the United States (196, 205). The disorder typically affects adults between the ages of 21 and 60 years (180,185), affecting both sexes equally. Approximately one third of patients are newly diagnosed after age 60 (192). The disease is rare in children (179,222,224). Some cases are sporadic; others are familial (188, 209,210,221), with the latter often inherited as an autosomal recessive trait (204,220). Familial forms of the disease occur alone or in the presence of multisystem disease. One form of familial disease combines achalasia and adrenocorticotropin unresponsiveness (206). Another consists of microcephaly, optic atrophy, ataxia, mental retardation or developmental delay, and achalasia (195,207,221). Familial cases account for less than 2 percent of the total (187,224).

Etiology. Achalasia probably results from a combination of genetic, autoimmune, and infectious factors (176). Familial achalasia may result from a common exposure to an infection or environmental toxin or it may represent a genetically transmitted disease. Implicated environmental factors include bacteria, viruses (184,202,213), toxic agents such as combat gas, and esophageal trauma; fetal ischemic esophageal damage results from gastrointestinal malrotations (177,181).

An autoimmune etiology is suspected because of the association of achalasia with the class II human leukocyte antigen (HLA) DQw1, and evidence of circulating antibodies against the myenteric plexus (200). A significant association exists between idiopathic achalasia and the DQB1*0602 allele and the DRB1*15 allele in white patients. In blacks, there is no association between these two alleles and achalasia but a trend is present with DRB1*12, suggesting that

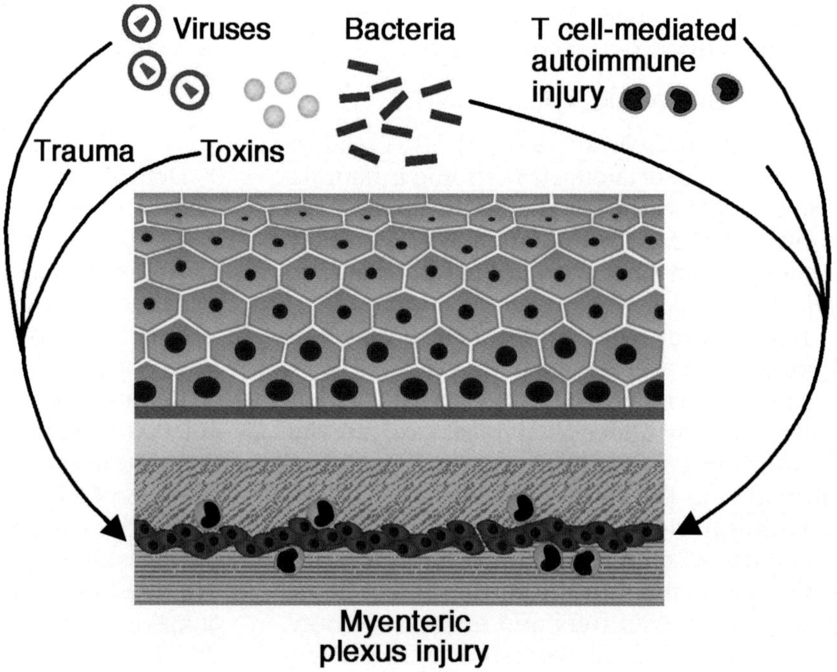

Figure 17-14

DIAGRAM OF THE PATHOGENESIS OF ACHALASIA

idiopathic achalasia is associated with HLA alleles in a race-specific manner (223). The expression of HLA antigens on ganglion cells could initiate their autoimmune destruction by T lymphocytes (198). The ganglia of 80 percent of achalasia patients express one of these histocompatibility antigens.

Some postulate that an unknown factor triggers the expression of the DQw1 class II HLA antigen on myenteric ganglia. This antigen is then recognized as foreign by T lymphocytes, which initiate an autoimmune process, destroying neurons and ganglion cells (217,222).

A final theory suggests that achalasia complicates neurologic and psychiatric diseases, including Parkinson's disease, depression (215), hereditary cerebellar ataxia, and neurofibromatosis (208,212). The various theories are combined in figure 17-14.

Pathophysiology. Achalasia is the best-characterized esophageal motility disorder. Patients with achalasia exhibit defective intrinsic and extrinsic esophageal innervation (194). The degenerative process preferentially affects NO-producing inhibitory neurons that affect the relaxation of the esophageal smooth muscle. There is also loss of inhibitory, nonadrenergic, noncholinergic vagal nerve fibers and VIP-containing nerve fibers that results in a hypertonic lower esophageal sphincter due to its failure to fully relax.

Clinical Features. Since the esophagus never completely empties, a column of swallowed food builds up within it (193). This presents clinically as recurrent, progressive dysphagia, pain, regurgitation, dyspepsia, retrosternal fullness, aspiration syndromes, and weight loss (178,183). Aspiration pneumonia occurs when the retained esophageal contents harbor bacteria (203). As the esophagus dilates, it may compress the bronchi. Although most patients are symptomatic for years before seeking medical attention, some severely symptomatic patients present early. Regurgitation may cause nocturnal coughing and aspiration. Erosive esophagitis complicates achalasia when acid reflux develops, but may also occur secondary to bacterial fermentation in a stagnant esophageal pool.

Radiologic Findings. Chest radiographs show a dilated esophagus with an air-fluid level due to retained food and saliva. Early, the esophagus appears minimally to moderately dilated and the lower esophageal sphincter remains contracted. Over time, the esophagus progressively dilates and all esophageal motility ceases. The sphincter remains closed except for occasional brief periods of relaxation, and acquires a "bird's beak" appearance due to the

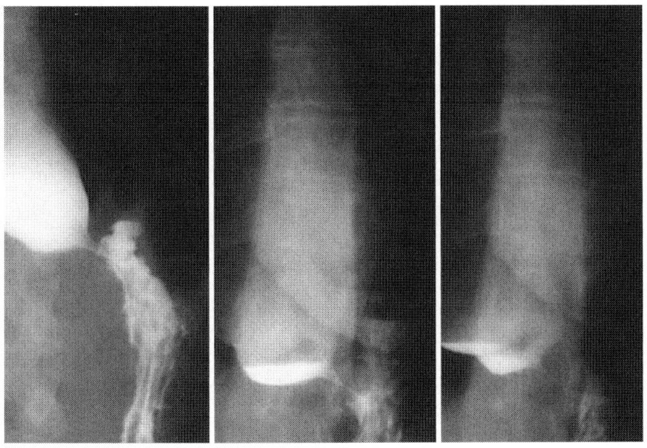

Figure 17-15

ACHALASIA

The characteristic "birds-beak" pattern of achalasia is seen on upper gastrointestinal examination.

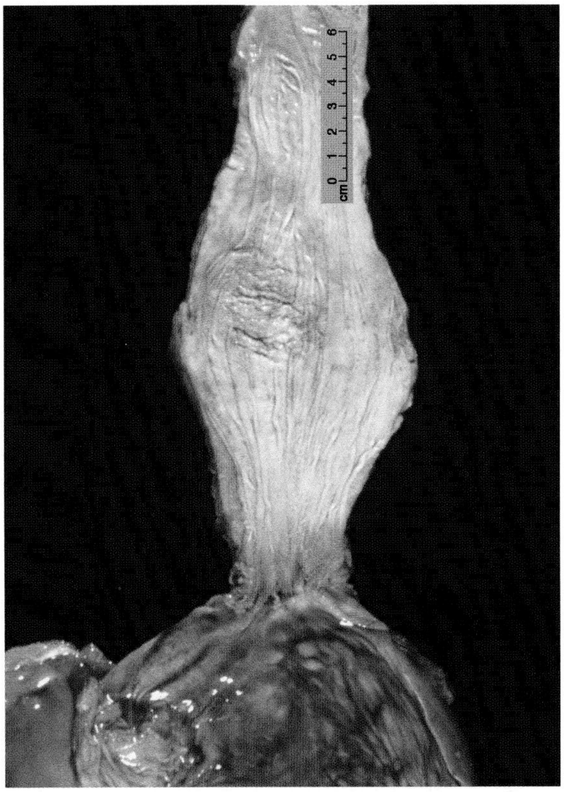

Figure 17-16

GROSS APPEARANCE OF THE ESOPHAGUS IN ACHALASIA

The distal esophagus is dilated in comparison with the more proximal esophagus.

presence of a shortened, angulated, narrowed distal esophagus (fig. 17-15).

Gross Findings. The characteristic gross features of achalasia consist of an enormously dilated, lengthened esophagus that tapers into a shortened narrowed tube at the esophagogastric junction (fig. 17-16). In advanced disease, diverticula form, sometimes attaining a diameter of 10 cm or more. Some patients develop esophagobronchial fistulas.

Microscopic Findings. Histologic abnormalities affect the esophageal myenteric plexus, dorsal vagal nucleus, and vagal trunks. The earliest changes consist of myenteric inflammation with injury to, and subsequent loss of, neurons and ganglia and subsequent fibrosis of the myenteric plexus (186,189,198,199). Ganglionitis develops consisting of a mixture of lymphocytes and eosinophils with a less conspicuous population of plasma cells and mast cells. The majority of the myenteric lymphocytes are CD3-, CD8-positive T cells. The lymphocytes express T-cell intracytoplasmic antigen (TIA-1), indicating that they are either resting or activated cytotoxic T cells. The TIA-1 cells appear to decrease in number as the disease progresses (190).

In late-stage disease, the infiltrate becomes more patchy and localized in and around myenteric nerves (fig. 17-17). Occasionally, there is marked eosinophilia of the muscularis propria. Auerbach plexus widens as scar tissue and small infiltrating inflammatory cells replace dying neurons (fig. 17-18) (191,199,214). Satellite cells increase in number and may be difficult to distinguish from the lymphocytes (214). Lewy bodies, identical to those seen in Parkinson's disease, may be found in the ganglion cells in the myenteric plexus.

Patients with disease severe enough to necessitate esophageal resection may completely lack myenteric ganglia, especially in the dilated segment (199). Some patients have residual ganglion cells in the proximal esophagus and a few randomly distributed ganglion cells in the mid- and distal esophagus. There may also be reduced numbers of ganglion cells in the proximal stomach. In most severe cases, an almost total loss of the myenteric ganglion cells affects the distal third of the esophagus. The remaining ganglion cells appear degenerated. The muscularis propria appears atrophic, hypertrophic (182, 199), or normal depending on disease severity; the changes tend to preferentially involve the

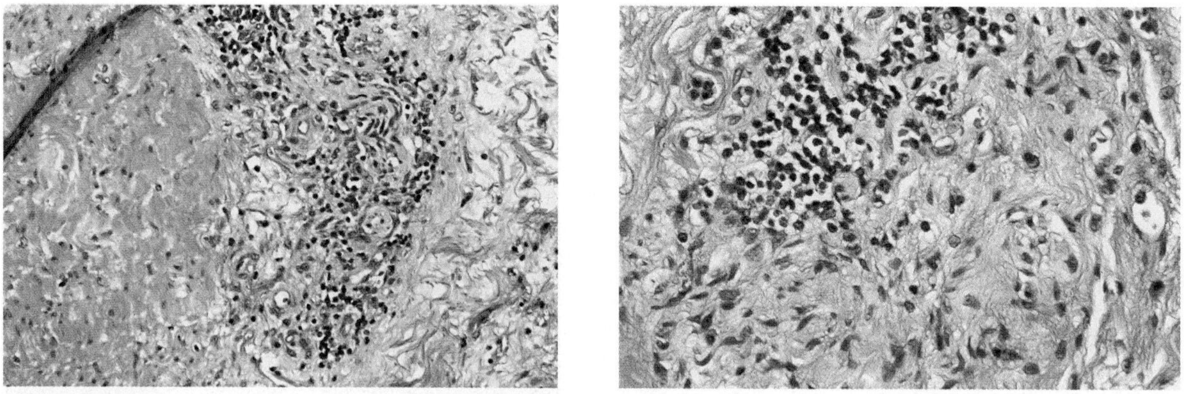

Figure 17-17

ACHALASIA

Medium- (left) and high-power (right) views of a patchy infiltrate that surrounds the nerves and myenteric ganglia.

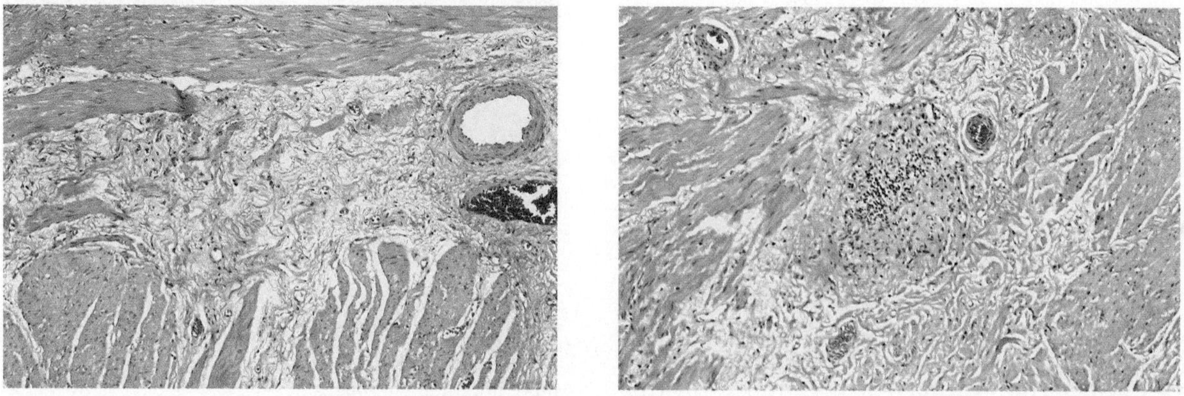

Figure 17-18

ACHALASIA

The area of the myenteric plexus (left) widens due to the presence of fibrosis. Inflammation is also present (right).

inner circular layer, especially distally (197). These changes are secondary to the neural and ganglionic alterations.

Nonspecific mucosal abnormalities include diffuse squamous hyperplasia and lymphocytic esophagitis. The lymphocytes infiltrate the lamina propria and submucosa surrounding submucosal ducts and glands and form prominent germinal centers. With the passage of time, chronic inflammation and ulceration result in fibrosis and stricture formation.

Special Techniques. Manometry is often the diagnostic modality used to diagnose achalasia, particularly in patients with early stage disease with minimal endoscopic or radiographic abnormalities (200). Resting lower esophageal sphincter pressure is elevated in 90 percent of patients. In achalasia, the sphincter relaxes by only 30 percent, contrasting with 100 percent relaxation in normal individuals (193).

Differential Diagnosis. The clinical features are mimicked by Chagas' disease and by diffuse esophageal leiomyomatosis. The histologic features are mimicked by Chagas' disease, autoimmune ganglionitis, and paraneoplastic pseudoobstruction.

Treatment and Prognosis. No therapy can reverse or halt the enteric neuronal degeneration. Therefore, treatment of the disease is aimed at decreasing the resting pressure in the

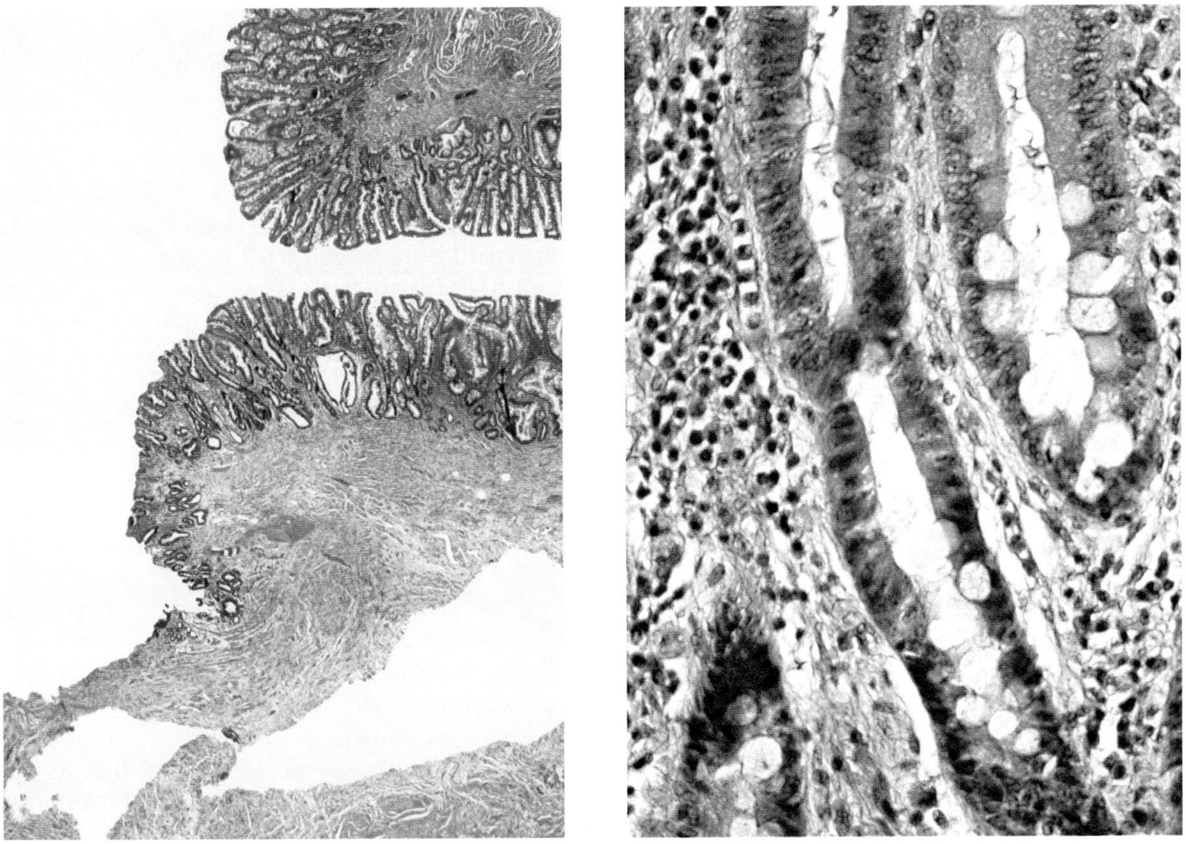

Figure 17-19

BARRETT ESOPHAGUS

The patient developed Barrett esophagus after treatment by sphincterotomy for achalasia.
Left: Low-power magnification.
Right: Area of Barrett esophagus. Dysplasia is present as well.

lower esophageal sphincter by pharmacological or mechanical means to the point that the sphincter no longer poses a substantial barrier to the passage of ingested material. Esophagomyotomy and pneumatic dilatation remain the major treatment modalities (216). Patients who are poor operative risks can be given a trial of medical therapy with nitrates or calcium channel blockers (201). These agents have been used with variable success (186,218,219). Intrasphincteric injection with botulinum toxin is gaining widespread use, particularly in the elderly (201). The botulinum toxin induces immediate symptomatic improvement that lasts for approximately 6 months in approximately two thirds of patients. Most patients need repeated injections to maintain remission. Unfortunately, botulinum toxin therapy is expensive (189).

Other experimental therapies have been proposed for the treatment of achalasia, including endoscopic myotomy of the lower esophageal sphincter or endoscopic injection of ethanolamine into the sphincter (206).

Carcinomas may develop in long-standing achalasia. This risk is estimated to be 33-fold normal in patients who have had the disease for decades (205,217). The tumors, which are usually squamous cell in type, can arise at all levels of the esophagus but they are most common in its middle third (210).

Patients who have undergone a previous esophagomyotomy and who experience esophageal reflux show all the changes and complications associated with reflux disease (see chapter 3), including Barrett esophagus (fig. 17-19) and adenocarcinomas (198,199).

ACHALASIA OF THE CARDIA IN ALLGROVE'S SYNDROME

Definition. *Allgrove's syndrome*, which features achalasia, addisonianism (adrenocorticotropin hormone [ACTH] insensitivity), and alacrima (lack of tears), is an autosomal recessive disorder recently associated with the *AAAS* gene encoding the Aladin protein.

Demography. Achalasia of the cardia associated with Allgrove's syndrome is a rare disorder in children characterized by defective relaxation of the cardia and aperistalsis in the esophageal body.

Etiology. The gene for Allgrove's syndrome has been linked to chromosome 12q13. Mutations of the *AAAS* gene lead to a presumptive lack of function of the encoded protein known as Aladin or Adracalin.

Clinical Features. Pediatric achalasia develops in the first 6 months of life and differs from the adult form of the disease in that the achalasia is part of a multisystemic disorder. Children often present with vomiting undigested food, failure to thrive, and recurrent chest infections. They also present with heaviness and pain in the chest, progressive dysphagia, nocturnal regurgitation, and weight loss. Associated abnormalities include alacrima, autonomic and motor neuropathy, short stature, microcephaly, and nerve deafness.

Pathologic Findings. All patients with Allgrove's syndrome show a striking widening of the myenteric plexus between the circular and longitudinal layer due to fibrosis. The fibrosis and necrosis of the muscle sometimes seen in esophageal achalasia are components of this disorder. Myenteric ganglia are absent or markedly decreased. Numerous CD3-positive lymphocytes surround the myenteric ganglia. The nerves fail to stain for neuronal NO synthase; however, thick inducible nitric oxide synthase (iNOS) nerve bundles are present in the intermuscular plane in all cases.

AUTOIMMUNE AUTONOMIC NEUROPATHY

Definition. *Idiopathic autonomic neuropathy* results in severe panautonomic failure. Sympathetic failure manifests as severe orthostatic hypotension and anhidrosis. Parasympathetic failure includes dry mouth, sexual dysfunction, impaired pupillary response to light and accommodation, and a fixed heart rate. Many patients have gastrointestinal dysmotility and present with anorexia, early satiety, abdominal pain, vomiting after eating, and constipation or diarrhea. Motor and sensory neural abnormalities are minimal or absent.

Pathophysiology. As in myasthenia gravis, autoantibodies specific for neuronal nicotinic acetylcholine receptors in autonomic ganglia (ganglionic receptors) may disrupt cholinergic synaptic transmission and lead to autonomic failure.

Clinical Features. Panautonomic failure develops in a subacute manner (over a period of days or weeks) (225,226). The course of the disease is generally slow and recovery is incomplete (225). The clinical findings are listed above in the disease definition.

Gross Findings. The gross features are similar to those of many pseudoobstruction syndromes.

Microscopic Findings. The histologic features are identical to those seen in paraneoplastic neuropathy.

Special Techniques. Serologic studies to detect ganglionic receptor antibodies establish the diagnosis.

Differential Diagnosis. An identical syndrome develops in patients with paraneoplastic neuropathy.

CHRONIC SEVERE IDIOPATHIC CONSTIPATION

Definition. *Chronic severe idiopathic constipation* in adults is a distinctive clinical syndrome without an obvious cause, but with subtle neural abnormalities. Synonyms include *idiopathic chronic constipation*, *colonic inertia*, and *slow transit constipation*.

Demography. The disease typically affects two major groups of patients: adult women who have severe chronic constipation and children with a similar presentation. Children range in age from 0.25 to 10 years, with a mean of 4.5 years.

Etiology. The etiology of idiopathic constipation is poorly understood. Many adults use antidepressants and narcotics for abdominal pain and related disorders, making it unclear whether the disease is a primary myenteric plexus disorder or the result of long-term cathartic, antidepressant, or narcotic use (abuse) (227). If there is any history of the use of these drugs, the case should be classified as a drug-induced motility disorder and not an idiopathic disorder. Some postulate that the abnormalities are developmental in origin, rather than an acquired destructive lesion, since frank axonal degeneration, Schwann cell hyperplasia, and inflammation are absent (227).

Pathophysiology. The pathogenetic mechanisms are poorly understood and believed to be multifactorial in nature (228). Abnormalities of the enteric nervous system or the interstitial cells of Cajal are thought to cause the disease (232,233).

Clinical Features. Patients present with chronic constipation. Symptoms vary in their severity. Adults with severe disease may have no more than one bowel movement per week, despite laxative use. Patients may also develop abdominal pain, bloating, and nausea, and may require manual disimpaction. Rarely, marked ileus and large intestinal pseudoobstruction develop (227). Other complications include stercoral ulceration, intestinal ischemia, gastrointestinal bleeding, bowel perforation, and peritonitis. Patients may also exhibit abnormal gastric emptying and gastroparesis.

Gross Findings. Despite the fact that patients experience severe constipation, the degree of intestinal dilatation is seldom sufficient to warrant a diagnosis of megacolon or megarectum. If the bowel is resected, the intestinal wall may appear contracted, thickened, and markedly stenotic. Alternatively, the bowel may appear dilated and thinned. Stercoral ulcers may be present. Polyps may appear to be present, however, they represent areas of mucosal prolapse.

Microscopic Findings. The histologic features of this entity are usually not seen unless the pseudoobstruction or stercoral ulcers are severe enough to warrant a resection. Myenteric plexus abnormalities are usually present. These include decreased, small, irregular neurons; decreased neuronal processes; and clusters of variably sized intraganglionic nuclei, which represent glia (fig. 17-20), Schwann cells, or immature neurons (227,231–233). There is also a notable decrease in ganglionic density and size. The changes are significantly greater in the ascending and descending colon. In other patients, there may be an increase in neuronal supporting tissues demonstrable by staining for S-100 protein. There are also increased numbers of PGP 9.5-immunoreactive nerve fibers in the muscularis propria (227). The ratio of the thickness of the circular to longitudinal muscle is significantly lower in the left colon of constipated subjects than in normal individuals (229). Melanosis coli is frequently present.

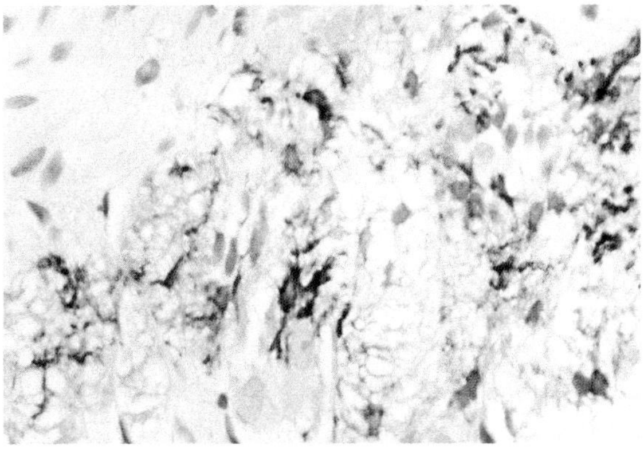

Figure 17-20

GLIOSIS IN A PATIENT WITH CHRONIC CONSTIPATION

Many dendritically-shaped glial cells are in the myenteric plexus (glial fibrillary acidic protein [GFAP] immunostain).

The topographic organization of the interstitial cells of Cajal resembles that of control populations, but there can be a significant reduction of these cells in all layers except for the outer longitudinal muscle layer.

Differential Diagnosis. Other motility disorders.

Prognosis and Treatment. Surgical intervention is considered a therapeutic option (230).

MUSCLE DISORDERS

Intestinal muscle diseases occur either as a primary disorder or secondary to muscular dystrophy, progressive systemic sclerosis, Ehlers-Danlos syndrome, dermatomyositis, and systemic lupus erythematosus. Adults commonly have systemic manifestations of the underlying disease; few patients have only gastrointestinal disease. In contrast, children rarely have gastrointestinal smooth muscle disease as part of a systemic disorder.

Megacystis-Microcolon and Intestinal Hypoperistalsis Syndrome

Definition. *Megacystis-microcolon and intestinal hypoperistalsis syndrome* (MMIHS) is a rare, generally fatal, congenital disorder affecting newborns. It is characterized by intestinal and urinary bladder distension; an atonic, short, dilated small intestine; a displaced or malrotated microcolon; and widespread gastrointestinal hypoperistalsis, hydronephrosis, and hydroureters (237,240,242). The entity is also known as *neonatal small left colon syndrome, adynamic bowel disease, non-Hirschsprung's megacolon*, and *neonatal hollow visceral myopathy. Prune belly syndrome* may be the male equivalent.

Demography. Less than 100 cases have been reported. MMIHS predominantly affects girls (female to male ratio, 4 to 1) (237,240,242). An autosomal recessive mode of inheritance is present (236,237). More than 50 percent of patients are born to diabetic mothers.

Etiology. Although it has been suggested that this condition may result from neuronal maturational arrest (242) or a primary cellular defect of contractile fiber synthesis (236), more recent evidence suggests that it results from the absence of the alpha-3 nicotinic acetylcholine receptor subunit (241).

Clinical Features. MMIHS invariably presents during the first week of infancy. All patients develop vomiting and abdominal distension due to intestinal pseudoobstruction, as well as distended urinary bladder due to bladder pseudoobstruction. Other features include lax abdominal musculature, incomplete intestinal rotation, a short bowel, microcolon and microileum, and decreased or absent intestinal peristalsis. Patients often have associated central and peripheral neurologic disturbances. A megaesophagus resembling achalasia may develop. Other changes are listed in Table 17-10 (237).

Table 17-10

MEGACYSTIS-MICROCOLON–ASSOCIATED CONDITIONS

Gastrointestinal Abnormalities
Anal atresia
Colonic atresia
Esophageal atresia
Imperforate anus
Intestinal malrotation
Intestinal stenosis
Mesenteric anomalies
Omphalocele
Pyloric hypertrophy
Neural Changes
Abnormal motor development
Blindness
Failed spontaneous respiration at birth
Mental retardation
Partial deafness
Seizures
Genitourinary Abnormalities
Cryptorchidism
Distended cloaca-bladder
Hydronephrosis
Hydroureter
Hydrourethra
Megacystis
Penile hypoplasia
Renal dysplasia
Urachal remnant
Other Changes
Cardiomyopathy
Cleft palate
Limb malformations
Syndromic facies

Gross Findings. Prenatal sonography at 18 to 20 weeks shows the characteristic changes. After the birth, the most common gross abnormalities are megacystis, bilateral hydronephrosis, megaureters, short bowel, microileum, microcolon, and intestinal malrotation with malfixation (235). Plain films show either dilated small bowel loops or a gasless abdomen with an evident gastric bubble. A large urinary bladder is present in all patients. Ganglioneuromas may be found in the uterus.

Microscopic Findings. The major pathologic abnormalities involve the intestinal musculature. The longitudinal muscle coat is thinned, and abundant connective tissue lies between the muscle fibers. There is also vacuolization and degeneration of the smooth muscle cells of the bowel and bladder (234,240). Ultrastructurally, the smooth muscle cells show disorganization of the myofilaments, degeneration of the cytoplasmic central core, and abundant proliferation of interstitial connective tissue. Excessive intracytoplasmic smooth muscle cell glycogen displaces contractile fibers to the cellular periphery, suggesting a fundamental defect of glycogen energy utilization (236). These changes affect the smooth muscle of the intestine and bladder (240). Most cases fail to show any neural or ganglionic abnormalities (234).

Special Studies. Ultrastructural studies show the vacuolar degeneration of smooth muscle cells, abundant connective tissue between the muscle cells, and myofiber disorganization (238,240).

Treatment and Prognosis. Patient prognosis is generally poor. Most patients die in the

Table 17-11

CLASSIFICATION OF FAMILIAL VISCERAL MYOPATHIES

	Type I	Type II	Type III	Type IV
Genetic transmission	Autosomal dominant	Autosomal recessive	Autosomal recessive	Autosomal recessive? Consanguineous marriage
Age at onset	After first decade of life	Teenagers	Middle age	Childhood
Percent symptomatic	<50%	>75%	100%	Unknown
Symptoms	Varies from dysphagia and constipation to intestinal pseudo-obstruction	Severe abdominal pain, intestinal pseudo-obstruction	Intestinal pseudoobstruction	Intestinal pseudoobstruction
Extragastro-intestinal manifestations	Megacystis, uterine inertia, mydriasis	Ptosis and external ophthalmoplegia, mild degeneration of striated muscle	None	Unknown
Gross findings	Esophageal dilation, megaduodenum, redundant colon, and megalocystis	Gastric dilation, slight dilation of entire SI,[a] SI diverticulosis	Marked dilation of the entire GI tract from the esophagus to the rectum	Gastroparesis, tubular SI without diverticula, normal colon, normal esophagus
Microscopic findings	Degeneration and fibrosis of both muscle layers of digestive tract	Resembles type I	Resembles type I	Severe vacuolar degeneration and atrophy of the SI longitudinal muscle, marked hypertrophy of the circular muscle

[a]SI = small intestine; GI = gastrointestinal.

first few days of life from intestinal pseudoobstruction and sepsis (239); occasional patients live up to 4 years. Those patients who survive usually need to be maintained on total parenteral nutrition. They may also require renal transplantation for renal failure. Some cases are diagnosed in utero and mothers may elect to terminate these pregnancies.

Animal Models. Transgenic mice lacking nicotinic acetylcholine receptors show some of the phenotypic features of MMIHS.

Hollow Visceral Myopathies

Definition. *Hollow visceral myopathies* are muscle disorders that affect all the hollow viscera, including the entire gastrointestinal tract, urinary tract, and gallbladder.

Demography. Hollow visceral myopathies affect both children and adults, and are the most common causes of chronic primary intestinal pseudoobstruction (252–259). Seventy-five percent of symptomatic patients are females.

Etiology. The genetic mode of transmission differs (Table 17-11) (246). Some cases are sporadic, others are familial. Other cases have a relationship with glycogenosis type IV (257) or polysaccharidosis (250,251).

Clinical Features. Symptoms often appear in the second decade of life, usually after menarche, and persist with recurrences of varying intensity and chronicity (244,245,253). Other forms only become evident in middle age. Many patients with sporadic visceral myopathy go unrecognized clinically. Symptoms include dysphagia, heartburn, bloating, postprandial right upper quadrant abdominal pain, distension, nausea, vomiting, constipation, and alternating diarrhea and constipation. Patients are usually short, underweight, and malnourished, and have postprandial abdominal pain, leading to decreased food intake. Sigmoid or cecal volvulus results from a redundant colon (246). Patients with bacterial overgrowth in a dilated duodenum develop malabsorption and diarrhea. Antibiotics may improve the diarrhea (243). Severe constipation may occur during pregnancy. In some women, spontaneous labor does not occur and may need to be induced. Mydriasis affects 50 percent of patients but it does not affect vision. Dysplastic nevus syndrome may be associated with the disorder (249).

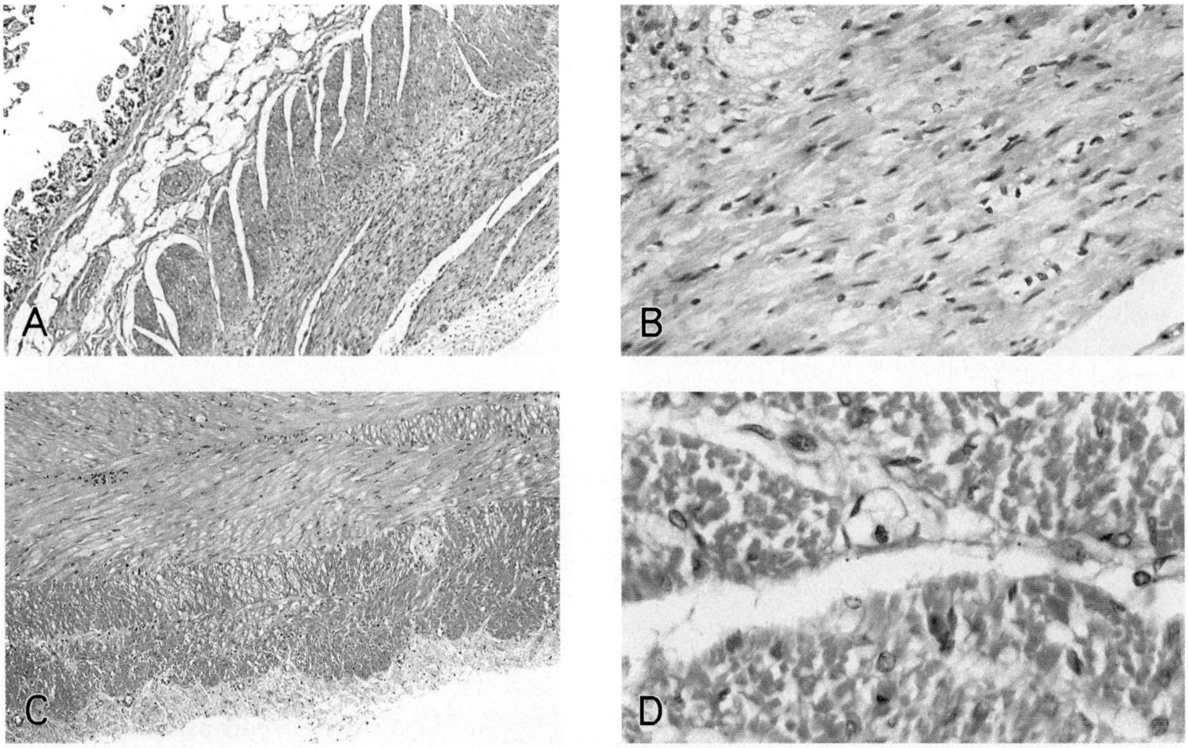

Figure 17-21

PRIMARY MYOPATHY

A: Low-power view of the small intestine shows irregular staining in the outer layer of the muscularis propria.
B: Higher magnification shows atrophic muscle fibers surrounded by fibrous tissue.
C: The muscle has a moth-eaten appearance. (Figures C and D are from a different patient.)
D: Higher magnification shows the smudgy, atrophic smooth muscle cells.

Intestinal pseudoobstruction develops in most symptomatic cases. It is characterized by gastric and small intestinal dilatation and diffuse small intestinal diverticulosis (253,254). Perforation of small intestinal diverticula, with peritonitis and intraabdominal abscesses can occur (244,252). Extragastrointestinal manifestations include megacystis and microscopic hematuria.

Gross Findings. Typically, patients develop an atonic dilated esophagus, megaduodenum, redundant colon, and megacystis. Megaduodenum is usually detected during early teenage years. The stomach and distal small intestine usually appear normal, although the jejunum may become distended. Pathologists examine the gastrointestinal tract either following surgical resection or at autopsy. Typically what is seen is segmental dilatation and thinning of the alimentary tract with gradual tapering into a more normal diameter. Areas of dilatation vary considerably in length. Megaduodenum is particularly common. Multiple diverticula are usually seen (256).

Microscopic Findings. The morphologic abnormalities in all of the familial myopathies resemble one another. The myopathic changes may be more pronounced in either the longitudinal or circular layer of the muscularis propria (256,257). Some patients have abnormalities in both layers (243,260). Changes may also be present in smooth muscle cells in the muscularis mucosae and in the blood vessels. The characteristic lesions involve muscle cell degeneration, muscle cell loss, and fibrosis of the muscularis propria. Many smooth muscle fibers appear swollen, with clear cytoplasm (figs. 17-21, 17-22). The cytoplasm of smooth muscle cells commonly appears rarified or vacuolated and the cells may have indistinct boundaries. Many muscle fibers appear densely eosinophilic and

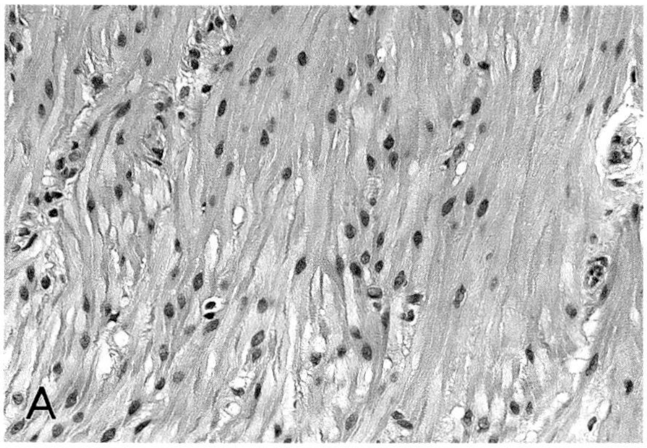

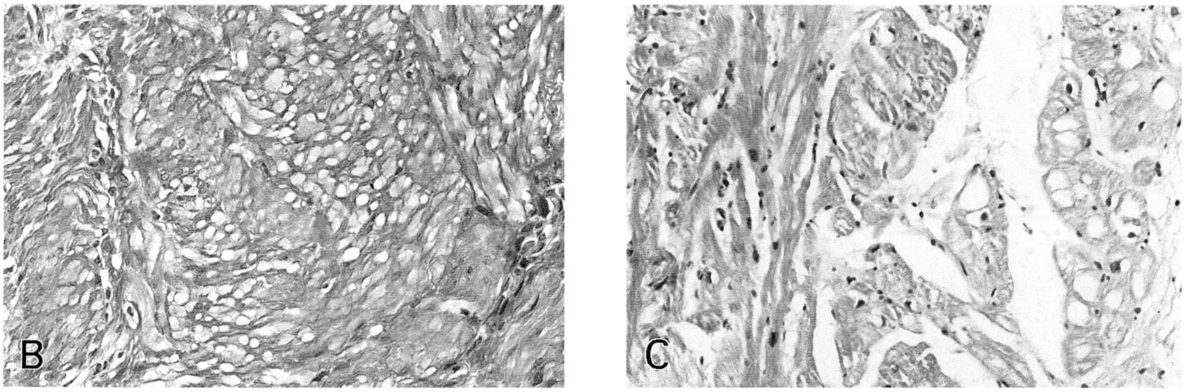

Figure 17-22

SPORADIC VISCERAL MYOPATHY

A: This area of the bowel shows prominent vacuolization but not much inflammation.

B: Prominent vacuolization of the smooth muscle fibers is highlighted by the red trichrome stain. Some fibrosis is present, as shown by the blue staining.

C: There is prominent cytoplasmic vacuolization of the smooth muscle fibers.

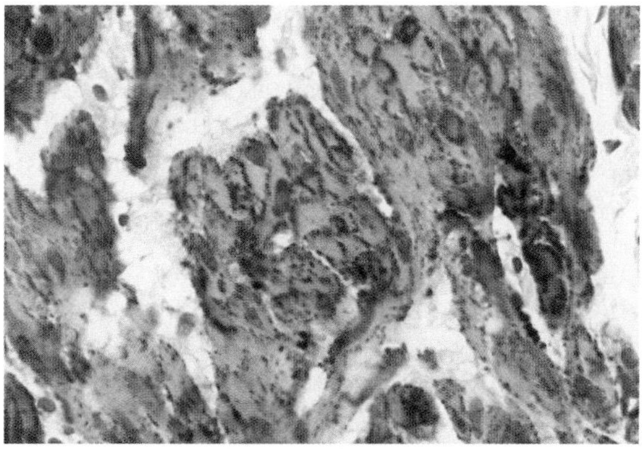

Figure 17-23

VISCERAL MYOPATHY

Alpha-actin stain shows the presence of prominent "peripheralization." The central portion of the muscle fibers is relatively devoid of staining.

others appear fragmented and thread-like. The muscle cells may have a smudgy appearance, with indistinct cell boundaries, fragmentation, and cellular dropout. This creates spaces apparently containing cellular debris.

The muscle cells of the muscularis propria and muscularis mucosae may contain numerous ovoid, translucent gray, cytoplasmic inclusions (248), which may be easily visualized in routine H&E-stained sections, but are enhanced by their strong positivity for periodic acid–Schiff (PAS) (248). Some inclusions stain at the periphery with antibodies to muscle-specific actin (fig. 17-23).

Ultrastructurally, the muscle cells appear very abnormal (fig. 17-24). The muscularis propria may show marked nuclear enlargement and hyperchromasia. Muscle hypertrophy may occur in early stages of familial visceral myopathy. The hypertrophy is most marked in the muscularis mucosae and may represent a compensatory response to the degeneration of the muscularis propria.

In late-stage disease, a severe reduction in cell numbers is accompanied by extensive patchy fibrosis, a change easily highlighted with trichrome stains. Collagen is sometimes deposited around degenerating muscle cells, producing a honeycombed appearance. In the most advanced stages, the muscle layers are completely replaced by collagen and the intestinal wall is extremely thinned (246,247,249). The myenteric plexus,

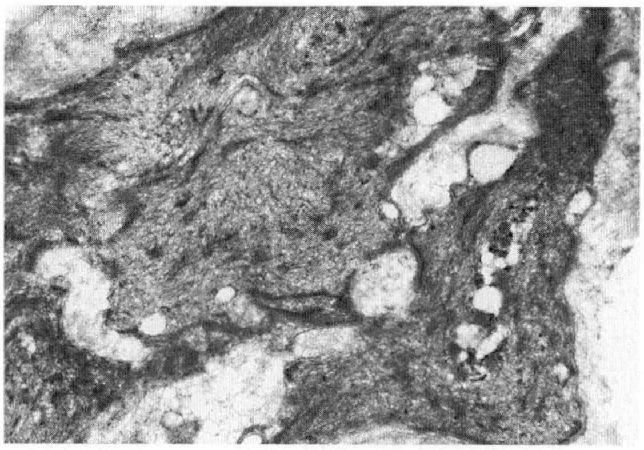

Figure 17-24

ULTRASTRUCTURAL APPEARANCE OF THE MUSCLE CELLS IN PRIMARY MYOPATHY

The individual cells appear abnormal, with the dense bodies and actin filaments arranged in a haphazard architectural pattern.

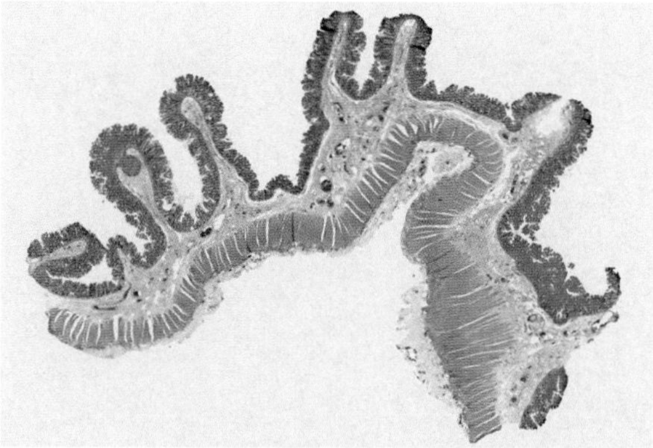

Figure 17-25

PRIMARY MYOPATHY

The architecture of the bowel wall is distinctly abnormal. The mucosa is thrown up into long polypoid structures. The "polyps" are extensions of the submucosa covered by normal-appearing mucosa. The muscle abnormalities are not visible at this power.

neurons, nerve processes, and nerve terminals all appear normal. No acute inflammatory cells, lymphocytes, or plasma cells are seen in the muscle layer. Vasculitis is absent.

Patients with a malabsorption syndrome due to luminal stasis develop a chronic mucosal inflammatory cell infiltrate in the superficial lamina propria, which tends to be patchy (256). A myopathy may be suspected when the bowel appears polypoid due to mucosal prolapse (fig. 17-25).

Differential Diagnosis. The clinical differential diagnosis includes other causes of megacolon, including metabolic causes such as hypothyroidism and hypercalcemia, and systemic disorders such as amyloidosis, progressive systemic sclerosis, and diabetes. In late-stage disease, the muscle lesions mimic those seen in scleroderma or diabetes, but these two disorders can be distinguished clinically.

Treatment. Mild to moderate constipation is managed by milk of magnesia or bulk-forming laxatives. Malabsorption from bacterial overgrowth in diverticula is treated with antibiotics. Severe diverticulosis may need to be resected. Patients who present with postprandial pain, distension, and weight loss due to a megaduodenum may benefit from an end-to-side duodenojejunostomy. Sigmoid or cecal volvulus may require emergency resection.

Nonfamilial Primary Myopathies

Definition. *Nonfamilial myopathies* are gastrointestinal myopathies that affect patients who do not have a family history of the disease.

Etiology. Unknown.

Clinical Features. Patients present at all ages. Infants in the first few months of life present with pseudoobstruction and total gastrointestinal involvement. Adults experience recurrent or persistent bowel obstruction, dysphagia, nausea, vomiting, postprandial abdominal pain, and bloating. Bowel habits are erratic and alternate between constipation and diarrhea. Less severe symptoms are vague and nonspecific. Sometimes the diagnosis is not made until a complication, such as pseudoobstruction, volvulus, stercoral ulceration, or perforation, results. The perforation usually results from ischemia secondary to vascular obstruction during volvulus, torsion, or intussusception.

Gross Findings. The gross features resemble those of other forms of chronic intestinal pseudoobstruction.

Microscopic Findings. The histologic abnormalities primarily involve the smooth muscle. The changes are most severe in the muscularis propria but similar abnormalities affect the muscularis mucosae and vascular smooth muscles. Changes include smooth muscle

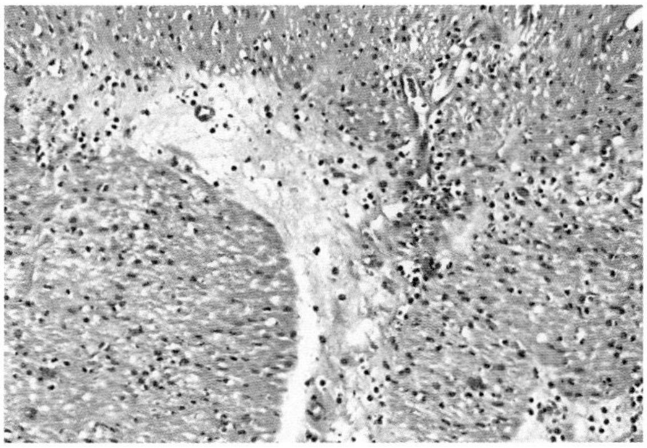

Figure 17-26

PRIMARY MYOPATHY

Primary myopathies usually involve the smooth muscle of the intestinal wall. There may be a variable diffuse, mixed acute and chronic inflammatory cell infiltrate with interstitial fibrosis and perinuclear cytoplasmic vacuolization.

edema, fragmentation, and fiber degeneration involving both layers of the muscularis propria.

The changes may be associated with a variable, diffuse, mixed acute and chronic inflammatory cell infiltrate; marked nuclear enlargement and irregularity; interstitial fibrosis; and perinuclear cytoplasmic vacuolization (fig. 17-26). The inflammation is scattered throughout both muscle layers. Fibrosis replaces the muscularis propria in advanced stages, causing thinning of the intestinal wall. Focal secondary smooth muscle hypertrophy leads to increased thickness of the muscle layers. The presence of the inflammatory infiltrate and the lack of a family history distinguish this disorder from the familial visceral myopathies (fig. 17-26).

The mucosa sometimes exhibits the polypoid projections typical of the redundant mucosal folds that can be present in any motility disorder. These folds consist of upward submucosal extensions covered by an essentially normal mucosa.

Treatment. The treatment is the same as for the familial form of the disease.

Mitochondrial Myopathies

Definition. *Mitochondrial myopathies* are a group of diseases characterized by the presence of defective mitochondrial DNA and various neuromuscular abnormalities. The mitochondrial encephalomyopathy syndromes are shown in Table 17-12 (265,266,275,278).

Table 17-12

MITOCHONDRIAL MYOPATHIES

Kearns-Sayre syndrome
OGIMD syndrome (oculo-gastrointestinal muscular dystrophy)
MNGIE syndrome (mitochondrial neurogastrointestinal encephalomyopathy)
MELAS syndrome (mitochondrial myopathy, encephalomyopathy, lactic acidosis, stroke-like episodes)
MEPOPL syndrome (mitochondrial encephalopathy, sensorimotor polyneuropathy, ophthalmoplegia, pseudoobstruction)
POLIP syndrome (polyneuropathy, ophthalmoplegia, leukoencephalopathy, intestinal pseudoobstruction)
Myoclonic epilepsy with ragged red fibers

Etiology. Mitochondrial myopathies are a heterogeneous group of disorders resulting from structural, biochemical, or genetic mitochondrial derangements. Mitochondria contain DNA known as mitochondrial DNA, or mtDNA (267), which contains 37 genes (263). It differs from nuclear DNA in that it is maternally inherited, demonstrates DNA heteroplasmy and mitotic segregation, and is more susceptible to mutation than nuclear DNA (263,270,281). (Heteroplasmy refers to the fact that cells and tissue harbor both wild type and mutant mtDNA.) Point mutations in mitochondrial structural genes result in impaired mitochondrial protein synthesis (262) and disruption of oxidative phosphorylation and the respiratory chain (272,274). There is no relationship between the site of mutation and the clinical phenotype (263). Additionally, the presence of heteroplasmy allows different tissues harboring the same mtDNA mutation to be affected to different degrees, thus resulting in tremendous symptom variation.

Mitochondrial neurogastrointestinal encephalomyopathy (MNGIE) is an autosomal recessive disease associated with multiple deletions of mtDNA. Some patients have homozygous or compound heterozygous mutations in the gene encoding thymidine phosphorylase (*TP*) located on chromosome 22q13.32-qter, which results in a markedly increased concentration of thymine in the blood (276). Thymidine phosphorylase is not a mitochondrial protein, but it appears to have a selective effect on the mitochondrial nucleotide pools required for maintaining the integrity and abundance of mtDNA.

Kearns-Sayre syndrome is a sporadic condition almost invariably associated with large-scale rearrangements (deletions and more rarely duplications) in the mitochondrial genome (264). A deletion of 4,977 base pairs flanked by a 13-bp direct repeat is the usual molecular defect in Kearns-Sayer syndrome (273). Other large deletions may be identified as well.

Clinical Features. Mitochondrial myopathies should always be considered when there is an unexplained association of neuromuscular, gastrointestinal, and non-neuromuscular symptoms. These disorders are usually maternally inherited. Several mitochondrial myopathies have characteristic gastrointestinal as well as multisystem alterations: gastrointestinal dysmotility with pseudoobstruction, abdominal pain and persistent vomiting, gastric and duodenal dilatation, duodenal diverticulosis (277), ophthalmoparesis (271), ptosis, peripheral neuropathy, lactic acidosis, leukodystrophy as determined by magnetic resonance imaging of the brain, increased cerebrospinal fluid protein, and muscle wasting; esophageal motility is variably affected.

The gastrointestinal and hepatic manifestations of mitochondrial myopathies present at any age: in the neonate with hepatomegaly or hepatic failure, in infancy with failure to thrive and diarrhea, and in childhood and early adulthood with hepatic failure and chronic intestinal pseudoobstruction. Patients may appear chronically malnourished and exhibit severe growth failure. There may be obvious muscle wasting and patients may complain of severe burning pain and paresthesias of the feet (277). Some of the mitochondrial myopathies, particularly those with *oculogastrointestinal muscular dystrophy,* which includes ptosis, diplopia, and intestinal pseudoobstruction, are sometimes included under the *familial visceral myopathies type II* (chronic intestinal pseudoobstruction with ophthalmoplegia).

Microscopic Findings. The external layer of the muscularis propria becomes atrophic, and there are increased numbers of abnormal-appearing mitochondria in ganglia and smooth muscle cells. Megamitochondria manifest as cytoplasmic inclusions in submucosal ganglion cells. They are round, brightly eosinophilic, and refractile, and demonstrable in rectal suction biopsies (277). Microvesicular steatosis affects the liver, skeletal and gastrointestinal smooth muscle, and Schwann cells of the peripheral nerves. Skeletal muscle fibers may show a massive mitochondrial proliferation, resulting in ragged red fibers histologically (261,263,269,279).

Special Studies. Mitochondrial myopathies can be diagnosed based on biochemical respiratory chain analysis or by mitochondrial DNA analysis. Ultrastructural examination of the eosinophilic inclusions discloses the megamitochondria. There are increased numbers of mitochondria within endothelial and vascular smooth muscle cells (268,280). Mitochondrial enzyme analysis of fresh frozen skeletal muscle reveals a respiratory chain defect.

Differential Diagnosis. The differential diagnosis includes other gastrointestinal neuromuscular disorders. The clinical features distinguish this group of lesions from other neuromuscular disorders. Biochemical, ultrastructural, and genetic studies document the mitochondrial myopathy. The consistent and early involvement of the gastrointestinal tract distinguishes MNGIE from other mitochondrial disorders with ragged red fibers, such as Kearns-Sayre syndrome.

Treatment and Prognosis. Therapy is largely supportive, including total parenteral nutrition and treatment of complications, including perforated diverticula and bacterial overgrowth. The prognosis of patients with MNGIE is poor and prior to the availability of long-term parenteral nutrition, the average patient died at around age 30 (269). General recommendations include avoidance of extremes in temperatures, prompt treatment of fever and infections, and avoidance of overexercise. Drugs known to interfere with mitochondrial function, such as phenytoin, chloramphenicol, and tetracycline, are to be avoided. Therapy with coenzyme Q, riboflavin, and other vitamins, cofactors, and oxygen scavengers may be useful (266,272,274, 278). They are used with the aim of mitigating, postponing, or preventing damage to the respiratory chain (263).

Autoimmune Enteric Myositis

Definition. *Autoimmune enteric myositis* combines intestinal pseudoobstruction with a diffuse transmural lymphoid infiltrate in the absence of neural damage.

Demography. Autoimmune enteric myositis is very rare (283–287).

Etiology. The disorder may follow a typical attack of acute gastroenteritis (287). One patient had a history of chronic active hepatitis. This is of interest because immune responses to hepatitis viruses may result in the production of smooth muscle antibodies through molecular mimicry (282). Hepatitis B virus shows sequence homology with myosin and caldesmon and hepatitis C virus shares sequence homologies with vimentin and myosin, but to a different sequence of myosin than hepatitis B virus. Thus different viruses induce autoimmune reactivity to different smooth muscle proteins and to different parts of the same protein.

Pathophysiology. Autoantibodies can be detected in patients with the disorder. These include antineutrophil cytoplasmic antibody (ANCA), antinuclear antibodies, anti-DNA antibodies, and antismooth muscle antibodies, supporting an autoimmune etiology. The myositis results in a severe T-cell–mediated inflammatory disorder involving the intestinal muscularis propria. The autoimmune injury appears to be clinically limited to the muscularis propria, particularly the circular muscle layer. Other sites, such as the bladder, are not involved, as is seen in visceral myopathies (287). The lymphoid infiltrate causes myonecrosis and smooth muscle cell dropout. The lymphocytes also secrete cytokines that inhibit smooth muscle contractility.

Clinical Features. Patients present in the same way as other patients with chronic intestinal pseudoobstruction due to other causes.

Gross Findings. The gross features of the bowel resemble those of other causes of pseudoobstruction.

Microscopic Findings. The ileum and colon have normal architecture and normal enteric ganglia. There is a modest increase in the cellularity of the lamina propria and a profound and florid lymphocytic infiltrate involving the muscularis propria. This infiltrate is especially dense around blood vessels and the circular muscle. The infiltration of the muscularis propria can be intense enough to obscure the circular muscle coat. The infiltrate is largely CD3- and CD8-positive with some CD3-negative and CD4-positive cells and occasional B cells. Smooth muscle actin immunoreactivity is lost in the inner circular muscle.

As the disease progresses, myonecrosis occurs in the circular muscle layer. Lymphoid cells infiltrate the lamina propria, submucosa, muscularis propria, and serosa of the ileum and colon. Although there are scattered lymphocytes in the myenteric plexus, there are no neural abnormalities. Both layers of the muscularis propria become thickened secondary to muscular hyperplasia, hypertrophy, and collagen deposition. Following treatment with immunosuppressive agents, the infiltrates decrease, although some lymphocytic infiltrates may remain.

Treatment and Prognosis. Treatment with immunosuppressive drugs may alleviate the pseudoobstruction. Some patients, however, require parenteral nutrition (287).

Diffuse Leiomyomatosis

Definition. *Diffuse (esophageal) leiomyomatosis* is benign pseudomuscular hypertrophy of the esophageal wall, predominantly involving its lower third (288,289).

Demography. Diffuse leiomyomatosis is a rare condition with approximately only 40 cases reported to date.

Etiology. Sporadic and hereditary cases have been described. Genetic analyses have demonstrated a relationship with a large deletion in the COL-A4, A5, A6 locus, which includes genes encoding the αV and αVI chains of collagen IV. (288,289,293,294). Close segregation of diffuse leiomyomatosis and sex-linked Alport's syndrome has been documented in most males with the disease (288,289).

Clinical Features. Initial symptoms usually appear during childhood or adolescence. The usual age of onset is 6 years in males and 10 years in females. Clinical manifestations include dysphagia, postprandial vomiting, and substernal or epigastric pain. Patients with rectal involvement may develop symptoms resembling Hirschsprung's disease, with chronic constipation and rectal dilatation as well as the lack of a rectal anal inhibitory reflex during repeated anorectal manometries.

Gross Findings. Leiomyomatosis involves the esophagus as well as extraesophageal organs such the female genital tract and the tracheobronchial tract (290,295,297). It can also involve the periurethral and perirectal areas, and the clitoris and vulva. If rectal involvement is present, the walls of the rectum and anal canal are markedly thickened and the rectum markedly dilated (291,292,297). The involved tissue contains a thickened muscular wall. Examination of the esophagus shows dilatation of the proximal lumen and variable degrees of segmental stenosis at the lower end (296,297). These features may lead to a mistaken diagnosis of achalasia, especially since esophageal manometry may show similar abnormalities (296a).

Microscopic Findings. Biopsies of the thickened muscular layer usually show diffuse benign muscular hypertrophy that infiltrates the enteric plexuses. There is extensive replacement of the normal fiber pattern by irregular plexiform fibers in the thickened esophageal muscular layer. The process may affect either one or both of the circular and longitudinal muscle layers, but the muscularis mucosae is minimally involved. Usually only minimal atypia without mitoses is seen (288,289). The muscular hypertrophy predominates in the lower third of the esophagus, but it may involve the entire length of the organ as well as the adjacent proximal stomach. The nerve strands are thin and only rare ganglion cells are seen. The esophageal mucosa is typically normal, but there may be associated esophagitis or Barrett esophagus, or even complications of Barrett esophagus.

Treatment and Prognosis. Because of the severe pain, patients with diffuse leiomyomatosis undergo partial or subtotal esophagectomy with proximal gastrectomy (290, 291,295).

MOTILITY DISORDERS ACCOMPANYING CONNECTIVE TISSUE DISEASES

Scleroderma

Definition. *Scleroderma* is a generalized autoimmune connective tissue disorder characterized by fibrosis and degenerative changes of the skin and multiple internal organs, including the gastrointestinal tract. By definition, esophageal scleroderma is part of the CREST syndrome (calcinosis cutis, Raynaud's phenomenon, esophageal sclerosis, sclerodactyly, and telangiectasia). Scleroderma is also known as *progressive systemic sclerosis*.

Demography. Scleroderma has a worldwide distribution. It occurs four to six times more frequently in women than in men, usually affecting women in the 3rd to 5th decades. Scleroderma is the most common systemic disease causing generalized gastrointestinal dysmotility. Ethnic origin plays a role in disease susceptibility. The disease is significantly more likely in black than white women.

Etiology. Scleroderma is an autoimmune connective tissue disorder that is associated with an increased frequency of class I and class II MHC alleles. Autoantibody associations divide patients into two groups: those with anticentromere antibodies (ACA) have limited scleroderma, and those with antitopoisomerase-1 (SCL-70) antibodies have the diffuse form of the disease. In some patients, antibodies specifically inhibiting M3-muscarinic receptor–mediated enteric cholinergic neurotransmission may provide a pathogenetic mechanism for the gastrointestinal dysfunction seen with this disease.

Pathophysiology. The pathogenesis of scleroderma involves vascular, immunologic, and fibrotic processes. Progressive fibrosis of various internal organs, including the gastrointestinal tract, is the pathologic hallmark of scleroderma, and the extent and rate of progression of the fibrosing process are major factors in determining the course and prognosis in patients with this disorder (fig. 17-27). This fibrosing process results in disruption of the normal architecture of the affected organs, ultimately leading to their dysfunction and failure. Fibrosis of the walls of medium-sized and small arterioles also plays a critical role in causing many manifestations of the disease.

Mast cells and eosinophils may also play a critical role in these fibrosing processes. Heparin-binding growth factors may provide the link between activation of both endothelial cells and fibroblasts. Endothelial cells are targets of the immune activity, but they may also act as immune co-stimulators. The cytokines produced by many cells are bound, protected, and enhanced by heparin, which is produced by activated mast cells. These factors may cause

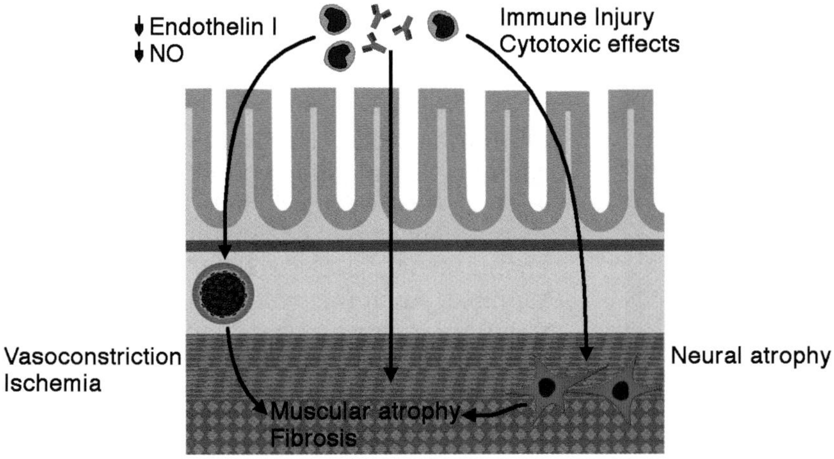

Figure 17-27

DIAGRAM OF THE PATHOGENESIS OF THE CHANGES PRESENT IN SCLERODERMA

endothelial cell proliferation and excess collagen production by fibroblasts. The microvascular system is one of the first targets involved (312,313), resulting in damage to the capillaries and the induction of perivascular infiltrates.

The excessive tissue fibrosis is due to expansion of fibrogenic clones of tissue fibroblasts. Persistent activation of genes encoding multiple extracellular matrix proteins in scleroderma fibroblasts distinguishes the controlled repair that occurs during normal wound healing from the uncontrolled connective tissue deposition that results in the fibrosis characteristic of scleroderma (306). Subpopulations of fibroblasts also demonstrate disturbed regulation of collagen turnover by transforming growth factor-beta (TGF-β) and collagen receptors (305).

Vasoconstriction secondary to increased levels of the vasoconstrictor endothelin 1 and decreased NO results in ischemia (298). Neural and muscular dysfunction follow (301,315,319). Neural dysfunction due to neural atrophy and collagen deposition occurs before smooth muscle contractility is impaired (316). Complete denervation releases the intestinal smooth muscle from its customary inhibitory factors, resulting in loss of normal peristalsis. Motility disturbances develop prior to histologic evidence of smooth muscle atrophy. In the next stage, smooth muscle atrophy and fibrosis are superimposed on the preexisting neural damage.

Clinical Features. Visceral disease often dominates the clinical picture, sometimes preceding the development of skin changes. The esophagus, small intestine, colon, and stomach are affected in decreasing order of frequency (300,313,317,319). Gastrointestinal symptoms include heartburn, nausea, vomiting, dysphagia, diarrhea, constipation, and fecal incontinence. There is a particularly high incidence of esophageal involvement in patients with Raynaud's phenomenon.

Smooth muscle atrophy leads to loss of esophageal peristalsis, dysphagia, and a defective lower esophageal sphincter. These changes predispose the patient to develop heartburn, nocturnal cough, recurrent pulmonary infections, and asthma secondary to severe reflux esophagitis. Patients with scleroderma also develop dysphagia from lower esophageal rings. The rings develop at the esophagogastric junction, generally affecting patients over age 30 (309). All of the complications of gastroesophageal reflux disease discussed in chapter 3 affect scleroderma patients.

Gastric dysmotility and delayed gastric emptying affect more than 50 percent of patients (319). Gastroparesis and antral distension cause dyspepsia. Gastric involvement may cause bleeding secondary to the development of vascular abnormalities, including gastric antral vascular ectasia (310).

Patients may also have severe intestinal motility disturbances and pseudoobstruction. Forty percent of patients with generalized scleroderma develop intestinal symptoms in the 4th to 6th decades of life (317). Small intestinal and colonic involvement may lead to life-threatening complications. Patients with small intestinal

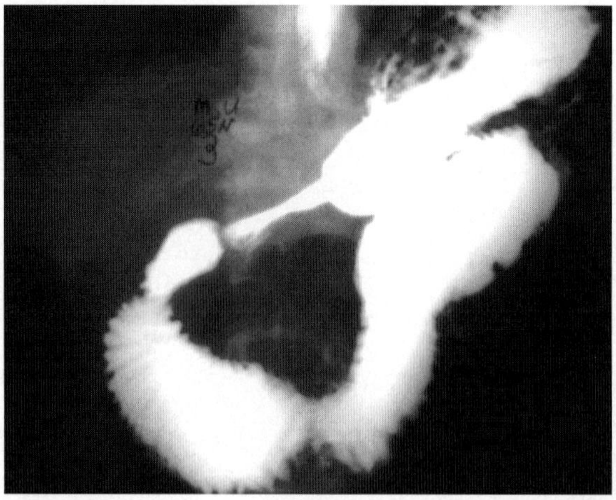

Figure 17-28

SCLERODERMA

The small bowel appears dilated and the valvulae conniventes are especially prominent. (Courtesy of Dr. Joel Lichtenstein, Seattle, WA.)

involvement have anorexia, early satiety, halitosis, nausea, vomiting, intestinal pseudoobstruction and distension, abdominal pain, weight loss, impaired motility, malabsorption, steatorrhea, diarrhea, constipation, and intestinal perforation (299,302,304,307). They also develop multiple diverticula, which may contribute to the malabsorption (312).

Colonic involvement affects 10 to 50 percent of patients (300). Patients with large intestinal disease develop colonic or rectal diverticula, pseudoobstruction, constipation, diarrhea, fecal incontinence, rectal prolapse, spontaneous perforation, and infarction. Anorectal involvement is almost as common as esophageal involvement. Disordered anorectal function occurs early in scleroderma, leading to fecal incontinence or rectal prolapse (308,317).

The extragastrointestinal features of scleroderma are associated with prominent, and often severe, microvascular alterations, frequently involving the hands and fingers.

Radiologic Findings. More than 50 percent of patients have radiologic evidence of dysmotility (fig. 17-28) (300). Ultrasonographic hyperechoic regions corresponding to fibrosis of the submucosa or muscularis propria predict esophageal functional abnormalities (311). There may also be associated esophagitis, mucosal rings, and stricture formation. The mucosal rings are fixed and symmetrical, measuring 2 to 4 mm in width. Other radiographic studies show small or large intestinal diverticulosis (303), absent peristalsis, or dilatation of any portion of the gastrointestinal tract. The small intestines may acquire a typical "hide-bound" appearance of closely packed valvulae conniventes.

Gross Findings. The gross features vary, depending on disease stage and the type of specimen examined. Anatomic studies show esophageal erosions or gastroesophageal reflux disease in 53 percent, strictures in 29 percent, and Barrett esophagus in 16 percent of patients. The esophagus appears variably dilated, often with concomitant distal esophagitis. Some patients develop gastric antral vascular ectasia or gastric thickening. Megaduodenum, small bowel dilatation, or diverticula are present in 42 percent and pneumatosis intestinalis in 8 percent. Eight percent of patients also have colonic dilatation or wide mouthed diverticula. The diseased intestines appear thickened, flaccid, atonic, and focally constricted, with loss of the colonic haustral pattern.

Microscopic Findings. The early changes of well-developed scleroderma are seldom seen because tissue is not removed until complications develop. Prominent but patchy smooth muscle atrophy affects the muscularis propria, particularly the inner circular layer (fig. 17-29). These changes are superimposed on neural damage. The muscle fibers appear fragmented and fibrotic, often disappearing completely (figs. 17-29, 17-30). The submucosa and muscularis propria become progressively atrophic and are replaced by fibrous tissue (315,318). Ceroid pigment granules may be deposited in degenerating muscle cells. Blood vessels may be markedly thickened with perivascular collagen deposition (fig. 17-31). Serosal fibrosis (where serosa is present) and submucosal fibrosis develop throughout the gut. Degranulating mast cells, macrophages, and activated lymphocytes infiltrate the perivascular tissue.

In uncomplicated cases, the mucosa appears normal. At most, there may be edema and a mild chronic inflammatory infiltrate in the lamina propria (307). Mucosal erosions and ulcerations may also develop, especially in patients with reflux esophagitis (fig. 17-32). Gastric alterations include gastric mucosal atrophy.

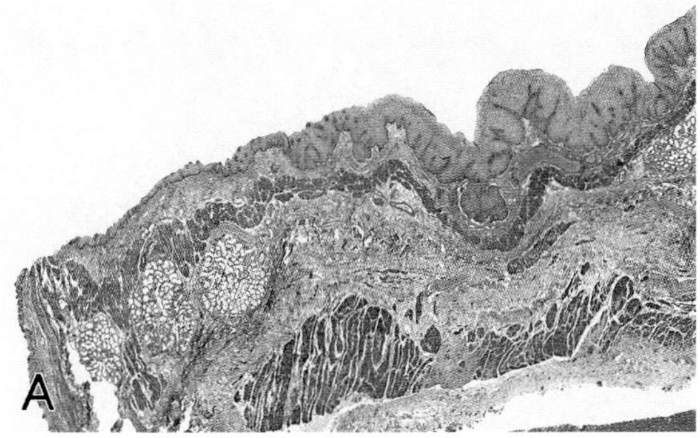

Figure 17-29

SCLERODERMA

A: Low magnification of the esophageal wall shows all of the layers. There is prominent submucosal fibrosis and atrophy of the muscularis propria.

B: Higher magnification shows the patchy myofiber dropout. It involves both the inner and outer muscular layers.

C: There is almost complete loss of the muscle fibers, with only occasional residual longitudinal muscle fibers evident.

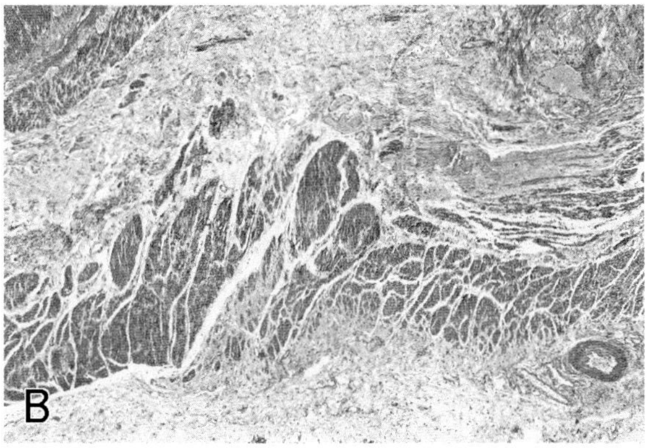

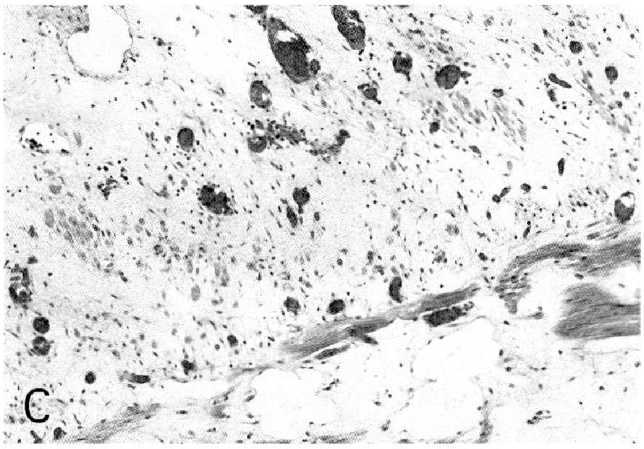

A

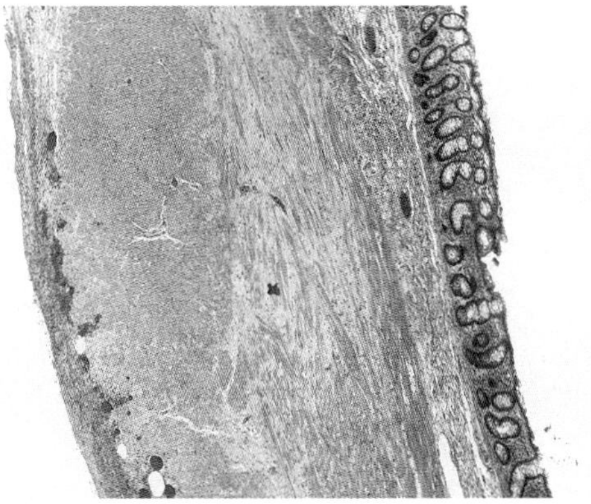

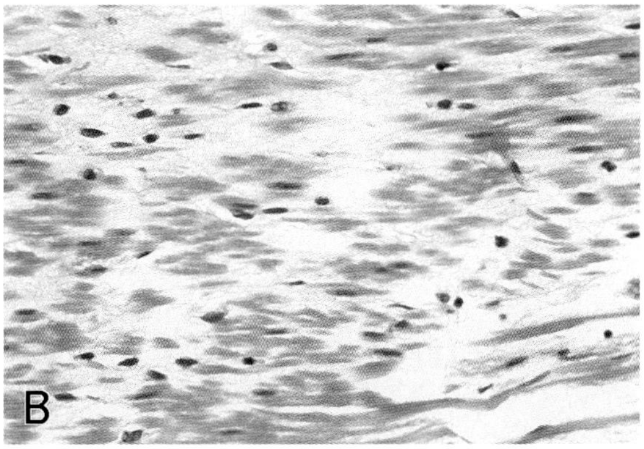

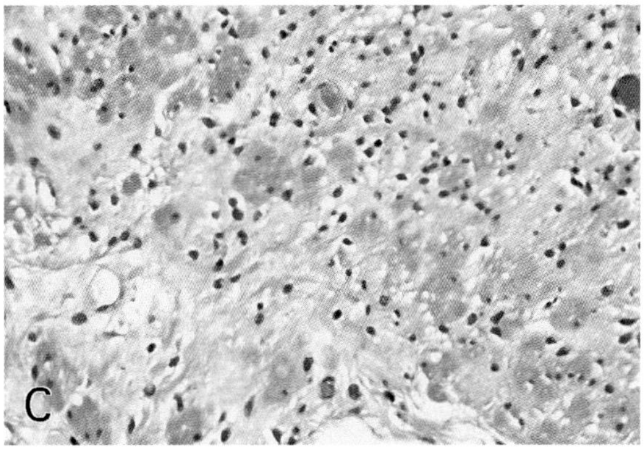

Figure 17-30

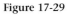

SCLERODERMA AFFECTING THE COLON

A: Low magnification of submucosal fibrosis. There is a serosal inflammatory infiltrate because diverticula were present, one of which ruptured.

B: Area of myofiber dropout.

C: Another area with muscle fiber degeneration, inflammation, and early fibrosis.

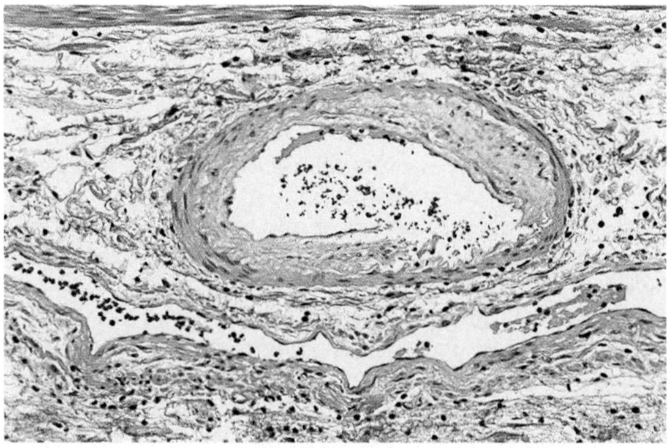

Figure 17-31

SCLERODERMA

A submucosal vessel is thickened and surrounded by a mild inflammatory infiltrate.

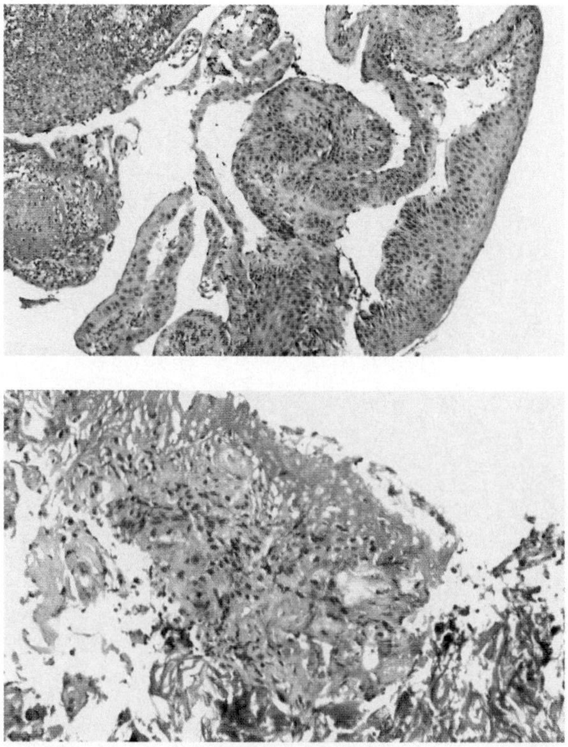

Figure 17-32

SCLERODERMA

Many patients with scleroderma develop severe reflux esophagitis, as is seen in this biopsy.

Top: Strips of esophageal mucosa with inflammatory exudates indicate the presence of erosions.

Bottom: Higher magnification shows the changes often present with reflux, including areas of fibrinopurulent exudate.

Duodenal Brunner glands may develop periglandular fibrosis (314). There may be a nonspecific increase in the mononuclear cells in the lamina propria of the intestine (fig. 17-33). This is often a manifestation of the decreased motility and a change in the bacterial flora. The fibrosis may mimic amyloidosis.

Patients with scleroderma may also develop eosinophilic gastroenteritis. The eosinophilic infiltrate often localizes in the basal mucosa and the muscularis propria, resulting in myonecrosis (fig. 17-34).

Special Studies. Specific serologic tests help identify the exact collagen vascular disease that is present. Antinuclear antibody (ANA) profiles are particularly helpful. ANAs are usually positive in scleroderma patients. Nuclear ribonucleoprotein (RNP) and centromere antibodies are more specific, but not as sensitive, markers. Patients with CREST have ANA restricted to the centromeric DNA. ANA with anti-SS-A/Ro specificity is associated with vasculitis and nephritis and ANA with anti-SS-dLA and anti-nRNP specificity is associated with milder clinical disease (304).

Differential Diagnosis. Early scleroderma can usually be differentiated from a visceral myopathy by the presence of fibrosis of the intestinal smooth muscle and the absence of a vacuolated honeycombed appearance. Remaining muscle cells appear normal or atrophic. The changes in scleroderma are patchier than those found in primary myopathies. In severe disease, it may be impossible to distinguish between a primary myopathy and scleroderma based solely on histologic examination. The clinical features, however, serve to separate the two disorders, as does serologic testing.

Treatment and Prognosis. Since there is no effective treatment for scleroderma, therapy is directed toward supportive symptomatic relief. Antireflux measures, including lifestyle changes and use of antacids, H2-receptor antagonists, and prokinetic agents, help alleviate the symptoms of reflux esophagitis and are important in preventing its complications, including peptic strictures and Barrett esophagus.

Early muscle dysfunction is partially reversible with prokinetic drugs. Prokinetic drugs also decrease the acidity of the refluxate, increase lower esophageal sphincter pressure, and increase gastric emptying. Prokinetic agents

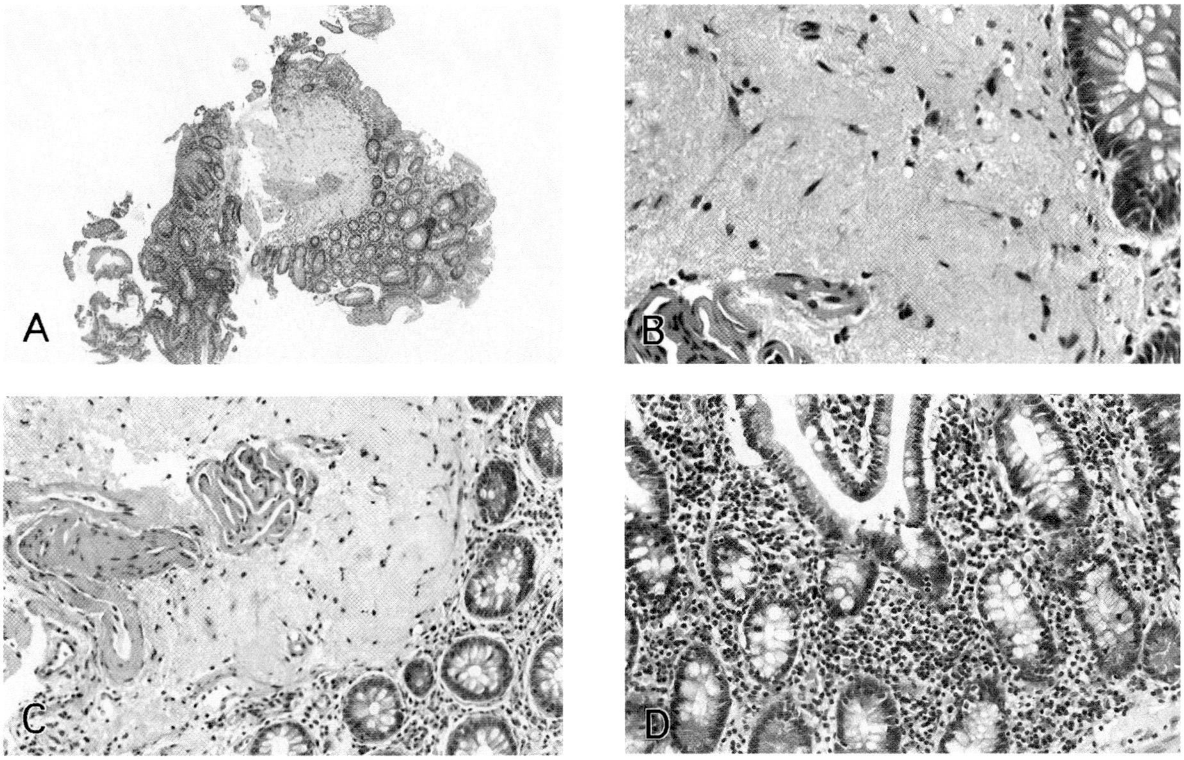

Figure 17-33

SCLERODERMA

Small intestinal biopsies sometimes show changes mimicking those found in amyloidosis due to the presence of marked submucosal fibrosis. These biopsies are not deep enough to indicate the muscular changes.

A: Low magnification view of such a biopsy.

B: Higher magnification shows the presence of acellular deposits involving the mucosa and submucosa. The deposits are negative with Congo red stains and blue with trichrome stains. The tissue is not as eosinophilic as in amyloidosis.

C: Vascular changes are sometimes seen in such biopsies.

D: There is a modest increase in the number of mononuclear cells in the lamina propria of the small intestine. Occasionally, regenerative features are seen in such tissues.

(metoclopramide, domperidone, cisapride, octreotide, and erythromycin) are also effective in treating pseudoobstruction.

Patients with end-stage disease characterized by severe muscle fibrosis are not amenable to pharmacologic functional restoration. The main therapeutic options for bacterial overgrowth are antibiotics and nutritional supplementation. Placement of enterostomy tubes for decompression and nutritional support may prove necessary in selected cases (317). Approximately 19 percent of patients require total parenteral or enteral nutrition.

Animal Models. Several animal models help elucidate the pathogenesis of scleroderma. A tight skin-2 mouse seems to be a promising model, since it shows enhanced collagen synthesis and deposition as well as mononuclear cell infiltrates.

Diabetes Mellitus

Definition. *Diabetic neuropathies* encompass a group of clinical syndromes affecting both somatic and autonomic peripheral nerves (321). The term *diabetic gastroenteropathy* describes a generalized gastrointestinal motility defect in the setting of diabetes. *Gastroparesis* is defined as delayed gastric emptying of either solids or liquids occurring in the absence of mechanical obstruction (331). *Diabetic gastropathy* is a term that encompasses a number of neuromuscular dysfunctions of the stomach, including abnormalities of gastric contractility and emptying, tone, and myoelectric activity in patients with diabetes.

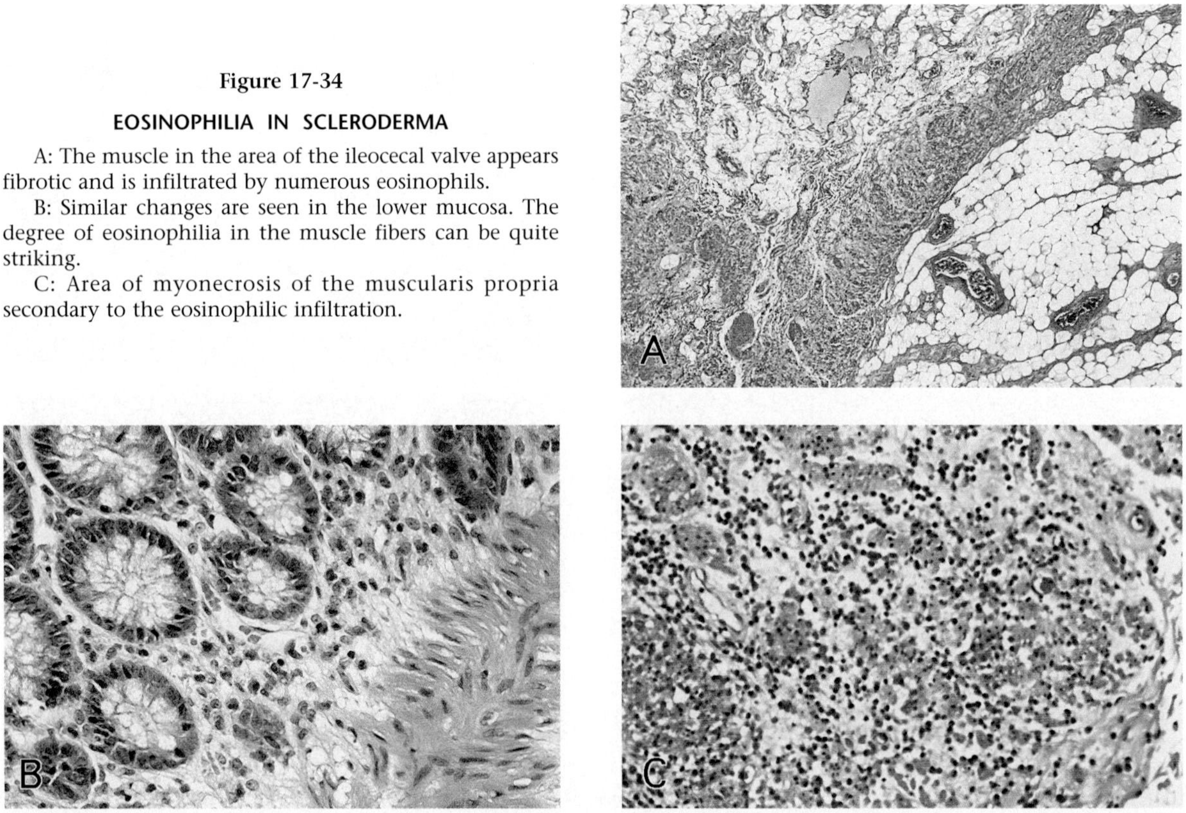

Figure 17-34

EOSINOPHILIA IN SCLERODERMA

A: The muscle in the area of the ileocecal valve appears fibrotic and is infiltrated by numerous eosinophils.

B: Similar changes are seen in the lower mucosa. The degree of eosinophilia in the muscle fibers can be quite striking.

C: Area of myonecrosis of the muscularis propria secondary to the eosinophilic infiltration.

Demography. Diabetes is the most common cause of chronic gastroparesis (322). It affects as many as 20 to 50 percent of diabetics, especially those with long-standing, poorly controlled disease.

Pathophysiology. Gastrointestinal diabetes-related alterations occur via six mechanisms: 1) a visceral neuropathy involving the parasympathetic or sympathetic nervous system; 2) a microangiopathy; 3) abnormal plasma glucose and electrolyte levels; 4) increased susceptibility to infections and bacterial overgrowth; 5) altered production of insulin, motilin, pancreatic polypeptide, somatostatin, gastrin, and glucagon; and 6) the effects of localized ischemia (330). The most important underlying condition appears to be the visceral autonomic neuropathy, which causes decreased motility, hypotonia, and possibly diminished secretions. Damage to enteric neurons or the interstitial cells of Cajal or subtle dysfunctions in these cells may also be responsible for the diabetic gastropathy (326).

Diabetic gastroparesis is characterized by difficulty in emptying solid foods into the duodenum. The delay results from food retention in the proximal stomach due to decreased motor activity and resulting in late antral filling. Hyperglycemia also delays gastric emptying, induces antral hypermotility, promotes pyloric contractions and gastric electrical dysrhythmias, and modulates esophageal and small intestinal motility (331). Diabetic gastroparesis may also contribute to inadequate glycemic control and impaired absorption of orally administered antidiabetic drugs. The predisposition to accelerated atherosclerosis is a risk factor for developing mesenteric ischemia and intestinal infarction.

Clinical Features. The gastrointestinal effects of diabetes are not commonly appreciated. Many diabetics, especially patients with type I diabetes, develop gastrointestinal problems, including gastroparesis, diarrhea, constipation, delayed esophageal and intestinal transit, megacolon, chronic nausea, weight loss, and fecal incontinence (322,324,328,329,333). Thirty to 50 percent of randomly selected patients with long-standing type I or type II diabetes exhibit delayed gastric emptying (322,323,325,332). An

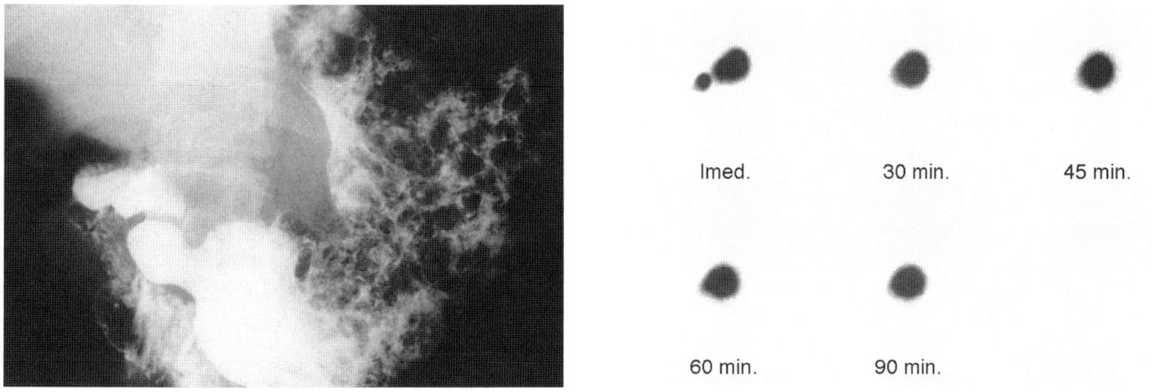

Figure 17-35

DIABETIC GASTROPARESIS

Left: The classic features of diabetic gastroparesis are seen. The stomach is enlarged and filled with a large amount of retained food.

Right: Technetium study shows retention of the gastric contents over time.

association exists between the onset of gastroparesis and other evidence of autonomic failure, including peripheral autonomic neuropathy, retinopathy, and nephropathy. Most commonly, gastroparesis manifests as postprandial fullness, vague epigastric pain, nausea, vomiting, heartburn, bloating, early satiety, excessive eructation, and anorexia. Symptom onset is usually insidious. Bezoar formation and pulmonary aspiration syndromes may be complications. Diabetic ketoacidosis and intragastric bezoars may cause severe pain.

Constipation affects approximately 60 percent of diabetics, alternating with diarrhea and mimicking irritable bowel syndrome. Additionally, small intestinal stasis and bacterial overgrowth result in bile salt deconjugation, defective micelle formation, fat malabsorption, steatorrhea, and diarrhea. Incontinence affects up to 24 percent of diabetics. The diarrhea and fecal incontinence mainly result from anorectal sphincter dysfunction, abnormal rectal sensation, rapid transit from uncoordinated small bowel motor activity, or absent myoelectric responses (331). Symptoms most commonly affect patients with poorly controlled disease.

Gross and Radiologic Findings. The stomach often appears massively dilated and the duodenal bulb may be dilated and atonic (fig. 17-35) (320). Other X-ray findings include prolonged gastrointestinal transit time, localized dilatation, and abnormal intestinal fold patterns. The radiologic criteria for gastroparesis are: 1) diminished gastric peristalsis with retention of barium contrast media at 30 minutes, without evidence of mechanical obstruction; 2) significant solid residue after an overnight fast; 3) elongated sausage-like configuration of the stomach, with only mild dilatation and without an air level; and 4) a dilated and/or atonic duodenal bulb.

Microscopic Findings. Glycosylation abnormalities result in abnormal collagen deposits, with resultant diffuse basement membrane thickening affecting vessels and nerves throughout the gastrointestinal tract. Capillary basement membranes become widened by a homogeneous, multilayered, eosinophilic substance. This thickening is most evident in the loose submucosal tissues. The mesenteric vessels develop accelerated atherosclerosis. The underlying vasculopathy causes variable degrees of ischemia. Similar basement membrane widening affects small nerve twigs (fig. 17-36). In end-stage disease, scattered necrobiotic smooth muscle cells appear as homogeneous, round eosinophilic bodies scattered among areas of smooth muscle atrophy and fibrosis (327).

Special Techniques. A practical approach to diagnosing diabetic gastropathies in patients with dyspepsia is to start with noninvasive gastric motility tests and to use invasive tests if further information is desired. The solid phase gastric emptying test and electrogastrography

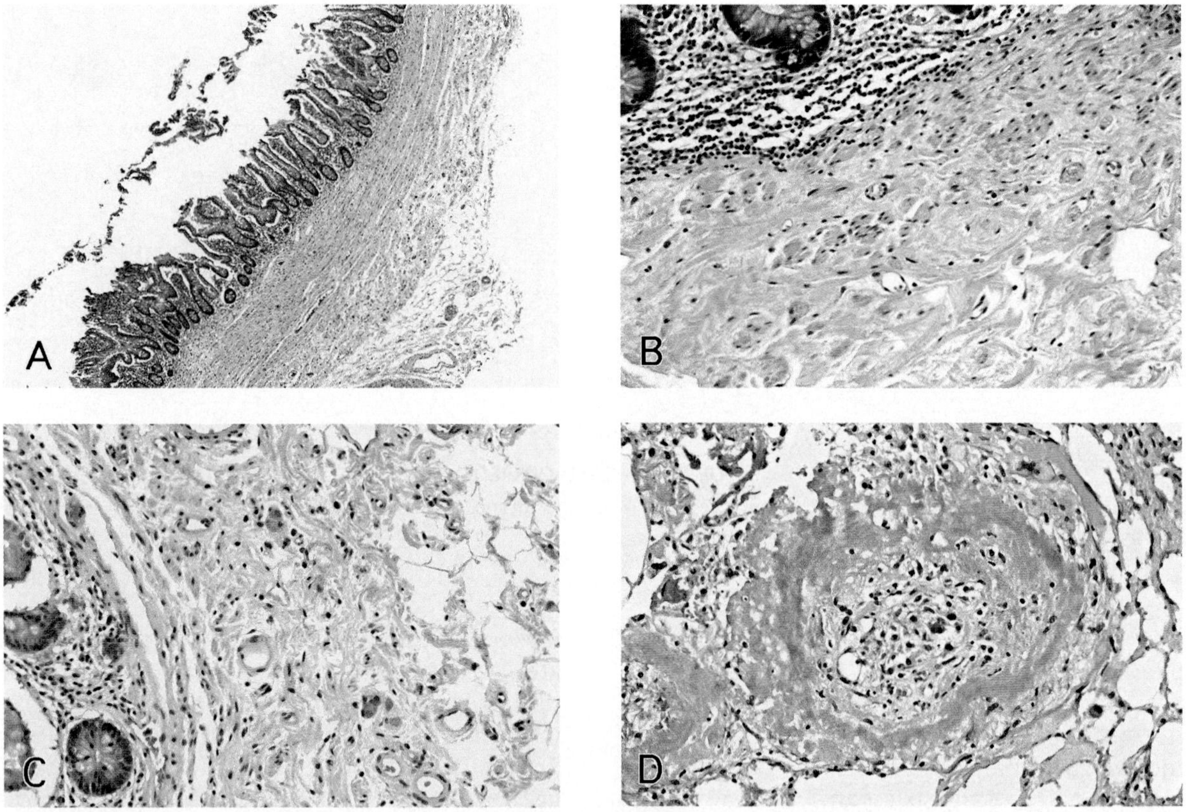

Figure 17-36

DIABETIC COLOPATHY

A: The muscularis mucosae is markedly thickened.
B: Higher magnification shows fibrosis between the muscle fibers.
C: Some of the changes center around the vessels.
D: The vessels in patients with diabetes often show other changes, including fibrinoid necrosis, as illustrated here.

reveal abnormalities in overall emptying and gastric myoelectric abnormalities, respectively (326). If further insights into gastric duodenal function are needed, then gastric ultrasound, antroduodenal manometry, and Barostat studies can be obtained (326).

Differential Diagnosis. Gastroparesis complicates other neuromuscular conditions besides diabetes. Acute gastroparesis may occur as part of acute gastroenteritis or secondary to drug administration. Metabolic disorders, including uremia, hypercalcemia, and hypokalemia, may also retard gastric emptying. The intestinal features of diabetes resemble other motility disorders, especially scleroderma.

Treatment and Prognosis. Treatment goals include reduction in upper gastrointestinal symptoms of nausea, vomiting, bloating, and early satiety and fullness as well as improvement in glycemic control. Normoglycemic control of the diabetes and prokinetic therapy, especially with cisapride, dramatically improves both the clinical and functional activity of patients with diabetic gastroparesis. Other useful prokinetic drugs include erythromycin and clonidine. In the most severe cases of diabetic gastroparesis, a gastrostomy may be indicated to vent the stomach and to prevent recurrent vomiting. (326). Rarely, invasive methods to provide nutritional support (jejunostomy) may be necessary if severe weight loss has occurred. Gastric emptying procedures are used (e.g., gastro-jejunostomy), but are seldom successful long term. Newer treatments try to augment NO signaling. There may also be a role for gastric pacing procedures. There is no evidence that either gastroparesis or delayed

Table 17-13

GASTROINTESTINAL AMYLOIDOSIS

Protein	Associated Disease	Forms of Amyloidosis
Immunoglobulin light chain (AL)	Multiple myeloma and other monoclonal B-cell and plasma cell proliferations	Primary amyloidosis: systemic disease associated with plasma cell dyscrasia (deposits in heart, kidney, gut, liver, and spleen), especially around blood vessels and sometimes between muscle fibers; massive submucosal gastrointestinal involvement is common
Serum amyloid-associated protein (AA)	Associated with chronic disease	Secondary amyloidosis: systemic chronic disease; amyloid deposits in blood vessels and in the mucosa; lamina propria deposits cause mucosal nodularity
Transthyretin, AA prealbumin (AF)	Hereditary amyloidosis	Hereditary familial amyloidosis: small intestine commonly involved; perireticular deposition throughout muscle fibers and in neural plexuses; single organ amyloid deposition
β2-microglobulin		Chronic renal disease

esophageal transit has any negative impact on the prognosis of patients with diabetes.

Amyloidosis

Definition. *Amyloidosis* consists of acellular eosinophilic proteinaceous tissue deposits. These proteins have a characteristic β-pleated structure, ultrastructural appearance, and tinctorial qualities.

Demography. The prevalence of amyloid deposits increases with age. In one autopsied patient population, amyloid was found in 36 percent (336).

Etiology. All known types of amyloid affect the gastrointestinal tract, including amyloid A (AA), amyloid of lambda or kappa light chain origin, transthyretin amyloid (ATTR), and β2-microglobulin (Aβ2M) (Table 17-13).

Pathophysiology. Two mechanisms explain the intestinal motor dysfunction present in patients with amyloidosis: 1) amyloid deposition in gastrointestinal smooth muscle, and 2) amyloid-induced damage to intrinsic or extrinsic nerves.

Clinical Features. Patients with primary and secondary amyloidosis have gastrointestinal involvement anywhere from the esophagus to the anus (334). In the esophagus, amyloid deposits in both striated and smooth muscles, leading to a weakening of both the proximal and distal esophageal sphincters (334). Esophageal involvement mimics achalasia. Patients with esophageal amyloidosis also develop esophageal aperistalsis due to muscular atrophy and neural abnormalities.

Intestinal pseudoobstruction develops as the result of either a myopathy or a neuropathy. Intestinal amyloid neuropathy leads to diarrhea, steatorrhea, or constipation (334,335).

Gastric amyloidosis presents as hematemesis or prolonged nausea and vomiting associated with weight loss, gastroparesis, gastric amyloid tumors, or gastric outlet obstruction. The chemical type of amyloid often determines the dominant clinical features (Table 17-13) (337).

Gross Findings. Grossly, the bowel may appear normal. Alternatively, intramural amyloid deposits cause mural rigidity. Bowels with Aβ2M amyloid deposits exhibit a distinctive rippled serosal appearance. Amyloid tumors produce firm, bulky, intramural masses. Endoscopic ultrasound may demonstrate thickening of the gastrointestinal wall with loss of the normal layered structure of the mucosa and submucosa.

Microscopic Findings. Eosinophilic, homogeneous, hyaline amyloid is deposited around the muscle fibers and blood vessels in the lamina propria and the myenteric plexus (fig. 17-37). The primary site of deposition varies with the type of amyloid present. Amyloid of light chains and Aβ2M are deposited throughout the gastrointestinal tract, especially the small intestine. Aβ2M preferentially deposits in the muscularis propria. The outline of the muscle layers is preserved but most muscle fibers are encircled by the amyloid deposits. They then become atrophic and disappear. Because the changes affect the deeper layers of the intestinal wall, they are hard to demonstrate on biopsy. The esophagus is less involved than the rest of the gastrointestinal

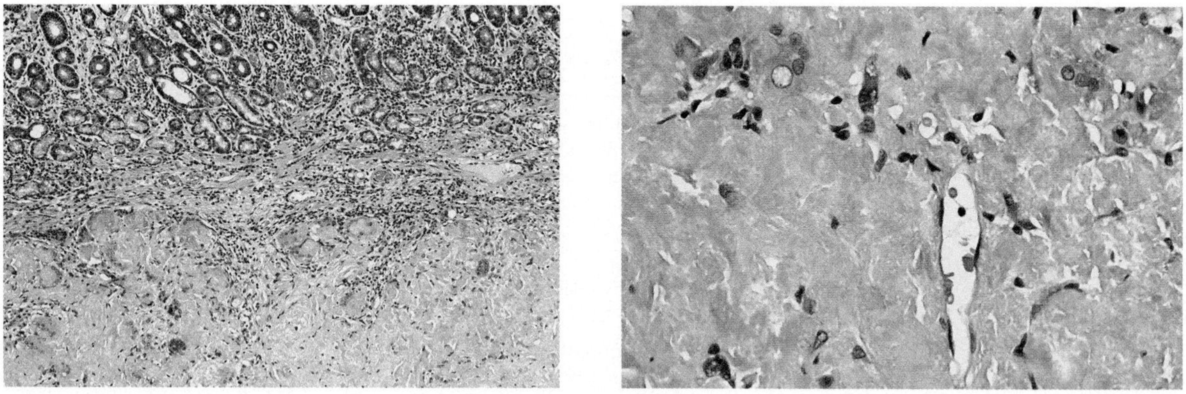

Figure 17-37

AMYLOIDOSIS

Left: Dense amyloid deposits involve the lower mucosa and muscularis mucosae as well as other layers of the gastric wall. Right: Higher magnification of the dense eosinophilic acellular deposits within the gastrointestinal wall.

tract in this form of amyloidosis. AA protein preferentially deposits in the myenteric plexus, without appreciable muscle infiltration. Patients with familial amyloidosis show a severe reduction in the number of ganglion cells or degeneration of ganglion cells without extensive deposition of amyloid in the enteric plexus.

Special Techniques. Amyloidosis is usually diagnosed on H&E-stained sections. Its presence is confirmed with a Congo red stain and the presence of a characteristic apple-green birefringence when examined under polarized light. It can also be confirmed ultrastructurally, in which case the amyloid fibers exhibit their characteristic periodicity. The different forms of amyloid are distinguished using immunostains for the specific protein.

Treatment and Prognosis. Therapy that reduces the supply of amyloid fiber precursor proteins improves patient prognosis; colchicine and chemotherapeutic modalities are used to treat patients with plasma cell dyscrasias. Other important therapeutic interventions include intensive nutritional support for malnourished patients, motility-enhancing drugs, octreotide therapy for motility disorders, and correction of clotting disorders in bleeding patients. The prognosis depends on the amyloid type, the nature of the underlying chronic inflammatory disorder (in secondary forms), and the status of other involved major organs, such as the heart or kidneys.

DRUG-INDUCED MOTILITY DISORDERS

A number of drugs are well known to affect gastrointestinal motility. Constipation secondary to drug ingestion occurs relatively frequently and must always be taken into account in evaluating patients for this complaint. Drug-induced constipation is also a well-known phenomenon accompanying the use of antidepressants. Sometimes these drugs lead to persistent constipation with frequent fecaloma formation. This is discussed in chapter 8.

REFERENCES

General References

Anuras S, Shaw A, Christensen J. The familial syndromes of intestinal pseudoobstruction. Am J Hum Genet 1981;33:584–91.

Fenoglio-Preiser CM, Noffsinger AE, Stemmermann GN, Lantz PE, Listrom MB, Rilke FO. Motility disorders. In: Fenoglio-Preiser CM, ed. Gastrointestinal pathology: an atlas and text, 2nd ed. Philadelphia: Lippicott-Raven; 1999:597–630.

Krishnamurthy S, Kelly MM, Rohrmann CA, Schuffler MD. Jejunal diverticulosis: a heterogeneous disorder caused by a variety of abnormalities of smooth muscle or myenteric plexus. Gastroenterology 1983;85:538–47.

Krishnamurthy S, Schuffler MD. Pathology of neuromuscular disorders of the small intestine and colon. Gastroenterology 1987;93:610–39.

Lake B. Hirschsprung's disease and related disorders. In: Whitehead R, ed. Gastrointestinal and oesophageal pathology. Edinburgh: Churchill Livingstone; 1995:327.

Mitros FA. Motor and mechanical disorders. In: Ming SC, Goldman H, eds. Pathology of the gastrointestinal tract, 2nd ed. Baltimore: Williams & Wilkins; 1998:241–66.

Schuffler MD. Neuromuscular abnormalities of small and large intestine. In: Whitehead R, ed. Gastrointestinal and oesophageal pathology, 2nd ed. Edinburgh: Churchill Livingstone; 1995:407.

Smith B. The neuropathology of the alimentary tract. London: Arnold; 1972:60.

Introduction

1. Costa M, Hennig GW, Brookes SJ. Intestinal peristalsis: a mammalian motor pattern controlled by enteric neural circuits. Ann NY Acad Sci 1998;860:464–6.
2. Coulie B, Camilleri M. Intestinal pseudo-obstruction. Annu Rev Med 1999;50:37–55.
3. Huizinga JD. Gastrointestinal peristalsis: joint action of enteric nerves, smooth muscle, and interstitial cells of Cajal. Microsc Res Tech 1999; 47:239–47.
4. Ponec RJ, Saunders MD, Kimmey MB. Neostigmine for the treatment of acute colonic pseudoobstruction. N Engl J Med 1999;341:37–41.
5. Rudolph CD, Hyman PE, Altschuler SM, et al. Diagnosis and treatment of chronic intestinal pseudo-obstruction in children: report of consensus workshop. J Pediatr Gastroenterol Nutr 1997;24:102–12.
6. Ward SM. Interstitial cells of Cajal in enteric neurotransmission. Gut 2000;47 (Suppl 4):40–3.
7. Wester T, O'Briain S, Puri P. Morphometric aspects of the submucous plexus in whole-mount preparations of normal human distal colon. J Pediatr Surg 1998;33:619–22.

Development of the Enteric Nervous System

8. Aldridge RT, Campbell PE. Ganglion cell distribution in the normal rectum and anal canal. A basis for the diagnosis of Hirschsprung's disease by anorectal biopsy. J Pediatr Surg 1968;3:475–90.
9. Baynash A, Hosoda K, Giaid A, et al. Integration of endothelin-3 with endothelin-B receptor is essential for development of epidermal melanocytes and enteric neurons. Cell 1994;179: 1277–85.
10. Meijers JH, Tibboel D, van der Kamp AW, van Haperen-Heuts IC, Molenaar JC. A model for aganglionosis in the chicken embryo. J Pediatr Surg 1989;6:557–61.
11. Furness JB, Costa M. The enteric nervous system. Edinburgh: Churchill Livingstone, 1987.
12. Gariepy CE. Intestinal motility disorders and development of the enteric nervous system. Pediatr Res 2001;49:605–13.
13. Gershon MD. Genes, lineages, and tissue interactions in the development of the enteric nervous system. Am J Physiol 1998;275:G869–73.
14. Gershon MD, Chalazonitis A, Rothman TP. From neural crest to bowel: development of the enteric nervous system. J Neurobiol 1993;24: 199–214.
15. Gershon MD, Tennyson VM. Microenvironmental factors in the normal and abnormal development of the enteric nervous system. Prog Clin Biol Res 1991;373:257–76.
16. Heaton ND, Garrett JR, Howard ER. The enteric nervous system: structure and pathology. In: Bannister R, ed. Anatomic failure. A textbook of clinical disorders of the autonomic nervous system, 2nd ed. Oxford: Oxford University Press; 1988:238–48.
17. Hosoda K, Hammer RE, Richardson JA, et al. Targeted and natural (piebald-lethal) mutations of endothelin-B receptor gene produce megacolon associated with spotted coat color in mice. Cell 1994;79:1267–76.
18. Langley JN. The autonomic nervous system, Part 1. Cambridge: Heffer; 1921.
19. Shirasawa S, Yunker AM, Roth KA, Brown GA, Horning S, Korsmeyer SJ. Enx (Hox11L1)-deficient mice develop myenteric neuronal hyperplasia and megacolon. Nat Med 1997;3:646–50.
20. Smith B. Pre- and post-natal development of the ganglion cells of the rectum and its surgical implications. J Pediatr Surg 1968;3:386–91.
21. Tsaur ML, Wan YC, Lai FP, Cheng HF. Expression of B-type endothelin receptor gene during neural development. FEBS Letters 1997;417: 208–12.

Hirschsprung's Disease

22. Albanese CT, Jennings RW, Smith B, Bratton B, Harrison MR. Perineal one-stage pull-through for Hirschsprung's disease. J Pediatr Surg 1999; 34:377–80.
23. Amiel J, Lyonnet S. Hirschsprung disease, associated syndromes, and genetics: a review. J Med Genet 2001;38:729–39.
24. Angrist M, Bolk S, Halushka M, Lapchak PA, Chakravarti A. Germline mutations in glial cell line-derived neurotrophic factor (GDNF) and RET in a Hirschsprung disease patient. Nat Genet 1996;14:341–4.
25. Angrist M, Bolk S, Thiel B, et al. Mutation analysis of the RET receptor tyrosine kinase in Hirschsprung disease. Hum Mol Genet 1995;4:821–30.
26. Angrist M, Kauffman E, Slaugenhaupt SA, et al. A gene for Hirschsprung disease (megacolon) in the pericentromeric region of human chromosome 10. Nat Genet 1993;4:351–6.
27. Aslam A, Spicer RD, Corfield AP. Children with Hirschsprung's disease have an abnormal colonic mucus defensive barrier independent of the bowel innervation status. J Pediatr Surg 1997;32:1206–10.
28. Attie T, Pelet A, Edery P, et al. Diversity of RET proto-oncogene mutations in familial and sporadic Hirschsprung disease. Hum Mol Genet 1995;4:1381–6.
29. Caniano DA, Teitelbaum DH, Qualman SJ. Management of Hirschsprung's disease in children with trisomy 21. Am J Surg 1990;159:402–4.
30. Chen Y, Lui VC, Sham MH, Tam PK. Distribution of carbon monoxide-producing neurons in human colon and in Hirschsprung's disease patients. Hum Pathol 2002;33:1030–6.
31. Chetty R, Govender D. Mucosal prolapse changes in Hirschsprung's disease. Histopathology 1997;30:324–7.
32. Chow CW, Chan WC, Yue PC. Histochemical criteria for the diagnosis of Hirschsprung's disease in rectal suction biopsies by acetylcholinesterase activity. J Pediatr Surg 1977;12:675–80.
33. Clausen N, Andersson P, Tommerup N. Familial occurrence of neuroblastoma, von Recklinghausen's neurofibromatosis, Hirschsprung's agangliosis and jaw-winking syndrome. Acta Pediatr Scand 1989;78:736–41.
34. Cohen MC, Moore SR, Noveling U, Kaschula RO. Acquired aganglionosis following surgery for Hirschsprung's disease. A report of five cases during a 33 year experience with pull-through procedures. Histopathology 1993;22:163–8.
35. Coventry S, Yost C, Palmiter RD, Kapur RP. Migration of ganglion cell precursors in the ileoceca of normal and lethal spotted embryos, a murine model for Hirschsprung disease. Lab Invest 1994;71:82–93.
36. Crone SA, Negro A, Trumpp A, Giovannini M, Lee KF. Colonic epithelial expression of ErbB2 is required for postnatal maintenance of the enteric nervous system. Neuron 2003;37:29–40.
37. Currie AB, Hemalatha AH, Doraiswamy NV, Cox SA. Colonic atresia associated with Hirschsprung's disease. J R Coll Surg Edinburg 1983;28: 31–4.
38. Doray B, Salomon R, Amiel J, et al. Mutation of the RET ligand, neurturin supports multigenic inheritance in Hirschsprung disease. Hum Mol Genet 1998;7:1449–52.
39. Edery P, Lyonnet S, Mulligan LM, et al. Mutations of the RET proto-oncogene in Hirschsprung's disease. Nature 1994;367:378–80.
40. Edery P, Pelet A, Mulligan LM, et al. Hirschsprung's disease: variable clinical expression at the RET locus. J Med Genet 1994;31:602–6.
41. Eng C. Seminars in medicine of the Beth Israel Hospital, Boston. The RET proto-oncogene in multiple endocrine neoplasia type 2 and Hirschsprung's disease. N Engl J Med 1996;335:943–51.
42. Farndon PA, Bianchi A. Waardenburg's syndrome associated with total aganglionosis. Arch Dis Child 1983;58:932–3.
43. Fekete CN, Ricour C, Martelli H, Jacob SL, Pellerin D. Total colonic aganglionosis (with or without ileal involvement). A review of 27 cases. J Pediatr Surg 1986;21:251–4.
44. Fewtrell MS, Tam PK, Thomson AH, et al. Hirschsprung's disease associated with a deletion of chromosome 10 (q11.2q21.2): a further link with the neurocristopathies? J Med Genet 1994;31:325–7.
45. Flageole H, Fecteau A, Laberge JM, Guttman FM. Hirschsprung's disease, imperforate anus, and Down's syndrome: a case report. J Pediatr Surg 1996;31:759–60.
46. Galvis DA, Yunis EJ. Comparison of neuropeptide y, protein gene product 9.5, and acetylcholinesterase in the diagnosis of Hirschprung's disease. Pediatr Pathol Lab Med 1997;17:413–25.
47. Garver KL, Law JC, Garber B. Hirschsprung disease: a genetic study. Clin Genet 1985;28:503–8.
48. Georgeson KE, Fuenfer MM, Hardin WD. Primary laparoscopic pull-through for Hirschsprung's disease in infants and children. J Pediatr Surg 1995;30:1017–21.
49. Hall CL, Lampert PW. Immunohistochemistry as an aid in the diagnosis of Hirschsprung's disease. Am J Clin Pathol 1985;83:177–81.
50. Heckenlauer K. Die neuronale intestinale dysplasie— eine literaturrecherche über die von 1971-1994 veröffentlichten Krankheitsfälle. Inaugural Dissertation, Universität München.
51. Imamura A, Puri P, Obriain DS, DJ Reen. Mucosal immune defense mechanisms in enterocolitis complicating Hirschsprung's disease. Gut 1992;33:801–6.
52. Janik JP, Wayne ER, Janik JS, Price MR. Ileal atresia with total colonic aganglionosis. J Pediatr Surg 1997;32:1502–3.

53. Joppich I. Late complications of Hirschsprung's disease. In: Holschneider AM, ed. Hirschsprung's disease. Stuttgart: Hippokrates; 1982:251–61.
54. Kapur RP, Yost C, Palmiter RD. A transgenic model for studying development of the enteric nervous system in normal and aganglionic mice. Development 1992;116:167–75.
55. Kelly JL, Mulcahy TM, O'Riordain DS, et al. Coexistent Hirschsprung's disease and eosphageal achalasia in male siblings. J Pediatr Surg 1997;32:1809–11.
56. Kobayashi H, Miyano T, Yamataka A, Lane GJ, Fujimoto T, Puri P. Use of synaptophysin polyclonal antibody for the rapid intra-operative immunohistochemical evaluation of functional bowel disorders. J Pediatr Surg 1997;32:38–40.
57. Koch T, Schulte-Bockholt A, Telford G, Otterson M, Murad TM, Stryker S. Acquired megacolon is associated with alteration of vasoactive intestinal peptide levels and acetylcholinesterase activity. Regul Pept 1993;48:309–19,
58. Kosloske AM, Goldthorn JF. Early diagnosis and treatment of Hirschsprung's disease in New Mexico. Surgery 1984;158:233–7.
59. Kusafuka T, Puri P. Altered mRNA expression of the neuronal nitric oxide synthase gene in Hirschsprung's disease. Pediatr Surg Intl 1997;32:1054–8.
60. Kusafuka T, Puri P. Mutations of the endothelin-B receptor and endothelin-3 genes in Hirschsprung's disease. Pediatr Surg Int 1997;12:19–23.
61. Luo Y, Ceccherini I, Pasini B, et al. Close linkage with the RET protooncogene and boundaries of deletion mutations in autosomal dominant Hirschsprung disease. Hum Mol Genet 1993;2:1803–8.
62. Lyonnet S, Bolino A, Pelet A, et al. A gene for Hirschsprung disease maps to the proximal long arm of chromosome 10. Nat Genet 1993;4:346–50.
63. Maia DM. The reliability of frozen-section diagnosis in the pathologic evaluation of Hirschsprung's disease. Am J Surg Pathol 2000;24:1675–7.
64. Melaragno MI, Brunoni D, Patricio FR, et al. A patient with tetrasomy 9p, Dandy-Walker cyst and Hirschsprung's disease. Ann Genet 1992;35: 79–84.
65. Mindelzun RE, Hicks SM. Adult Hirschsprung's disease: radiographic findings. Radiology 1986;160:623–5.
66. Monforte-Munoz H, Gonzalez-Gomez I, Rowland JM, Landing BH. Increased submucosal nerve trunk caliber in aganglionosis: a "positive" and objective finding in suction biopsies and segmental resections in Hirschsprung's disease. Arch Pathol Lab Med 1998;122:721–5.
67. Pachnis V, Mankoo B, Costantini F. Expression of the c-ret proto-oncogene during mouse embryogenesis. Development 1993;119:1005–17.
68. Poenaur D, Uroz-Tristan J, Leclerc S, Murphy S, Bensoussan AL. Imperforate anus, malrotation and Hirschsprung's disease: a rare association. Eur J Pediatr Surg 1995;5:187–9.
69. Puffenberger E, Hosoda K, Washington S, et al. A missense mutation of the endothelin-B receptor gene in multigenic Hirschsprung's disease. Cell 1994;79:1257–66.
70. Rescorla FJ, Morrison AM, Engles D, et al. Hirschsprung's disease: evaluation of mortality and long-term function in 260 cases. Arch Surg 1992;127:934–41.
71. Reynolds JF, Barber JC, Alford BA, et al. Familial Hirschsprung's disease and type d brachydactyly: a report of four affected males in two generations. Pediatrics 1983;71:246–9.
72. Romeo G, Ronchetto P, Luo Y, et al. Point mutations affecting the tyrosine kinase domain of the RET photo-oncogene in Hirschsprung's disease. Nature 1994;367:377–8.
73. Russell MB, Russell CA, Fenger K, Niebuhr E. Familial occurrence of Hirschsprung's disease. Clin Genet 1994;45:231–5.
74. Sakai T, Nirasawa Y, Itoh Y, Wakizaka A. Japanese patients with sporadic Hirschsprung: mutation analysis of the receptor tyrosine kinase protooncogene, endothelin-B receptor, endothelin-3, glial cell line-derived neurotrophic factor and neurturin genes: a comparison with similar studies. Eur J Pediatr 2000;159:160–7.
75. Salomon R, Attie T, Pelet A, et al. Germline mutations of the RET ligand GDNF are not sufficient to cause Hirschsprung disease. Nat Genet 1996;14:345–7.
76. Seldenrijk CA, van der Harten HJ, Kluck P, et al. Zonal aganglionosis: an enzyme and immunohistochemical study of two cases. Virchows Arch [A] 1986;410:75–81.
77. Schneider R. The human protooncogene ret: a communicative cadherin? Trends Biochem Sci 1992;17:468–9.
78. Schuchardt A, D'Agati V, Larsson-Blomberg L, Costantini F, Pachnis V. Defects in the kidney and enteric nervous system of mice lacking the tyrosine kinase receptor ret. Nature 1994;367:380–3.
79. Stringer MD, Drake DP. Hirschsprung's disease presenting as neonatal gastrointestinal perforation. Br J Surg 1991;78:188–9.
80. Tam PK, Quint WG, van Velzen D. Hirschsprung's disease: a viral etiology? Pediatr Pathol Lab Med 1992;12:807–10.
81. Teitelbaum DH, Caniano DA, Qualman SJ. The pathophysiology of Hirschsprung's associated enterocolitis: importance of histologic correlates. J Pediatr Surg 1989;24:1271–7.
82. Teitelbaum DH, Cilley RE, Sherman NJ, et al. A decade of experience with the primary pull-through for Hirschsprung disease in the newborn period: a multicenter analysis of outcomes. Ann Surg 2000;232:372–80.
83. Tennyson VM, Gershon MD, Sherman DL, et al. Structural abnormalities associated with congenital megacolon in transgenic mice that overexpress the *Hoxa-4* gene. Develop Dynam 1993;198:28–53.

84. Treanor J, Goodman L, de Sauvage F, et al. Characterization of a multicomponent receptor for GDNF. Nature 1996;382:80–3.
85. Tsuto T, Obata-Tsuto HL, Iwai N, Takahashi T, Ibata Y. Fine structure of neurons synthesizing vasoactive intestinal peptide in the human colon from patients with Hirschsprung's disease. Histochemistry 1989;93:1–8.
86. Vanderwinden JM, Rumessen JJ, Liu H, Descamps D, De Laet MH, Vanderhaeghen JJ. Interstitial cells of Cajal in human colon and in Hirschsprung's disease. Gastroenterology 1996;11:901–10.
87. Yamataka A, Kato Y, Tibboel D, et al. A lack of intestinal pacemaker (c-kit) in aganglionic bowel of patients with Hirschsprung's disease. J Pediatr Surg 1995;30:441–4.
88. Yin L, Barone V, Seri M, et al. Heterogeneity and low detection rate of RET mutations in Hirschsprung disease. Eur J Hum Genet 1994;2:272–80.
89. Yunis E, Sieber WK, Akers DR. Does zonal aganglionosis really exist? Report of a rare variety of Hirschsprung's disease and a review of the literature. Pediatr Pathol 1983;1:33–49.

Intestinal Neuronal Dysplasia

90. Ammann K, Stoss F, Meier-Ruge W. Intestinale neuronale Dysplasia des Erwachsenen als Ursache der chronischen Obstipation. Morphometrische Charakterisierung der Coloninnervation. Chirurg 1999;70:771–6.
91. Bahuau M, Laurendeau I, Pelet A, et al. Tandem duplication within the neurofibromatosis type I gene *(NF1)* and reciprocal t(15;16) (q26.3;q12.1) translocation in familial association of NF1 with intestinal neuronal dysplasia type B (IND B). J Med Genet 2000;37:146–50.
92. Berger S, Ziebell P, Offsler M, Hoffmann-von Kap-herr S. Congenital malformations and perinatal morbidity associated with intestinal neuronal dysplasia. Pediatr Surg 1998;13:474–9.
93. Borchard F, Meier-Ruge W, Wiebecke B, et al. Innervation Stoerungen des Dickdarms—Klassifikation und Diagnostik. Pathologe 1991; 12:171–4.
94. Carney JA, Go VL, Sizemore GW, Hayles AB. Alimentary tract ganglioneuromatosis: a major component of the syndrome of multiple endocrine neoplasia, type 2b. N Engl J Med 1976;295:1287–91.
95. Cord-Udy CL, Smith VV, Ahmed S, Risdon RA, Milla PJ. An evaluation of the role of suction rectal biopsy in the diagnosis of intestinal neuronal dysplasia. J Pediatr Gastroenterol Nutr 1997;24:1–6.
96. Erdohazi M. Retarded development of the enteric nerve cells. Dev Med Child Neurol 1974; 16:365–8.
97. Fadda B, Maier WA, Meier-Ruge W, et al. Neuronale intestinale Dysplasie: Eine Kritsche 10-Jahres-Analyse klinscher and bioptscher Diagnostik. Z Kinderchir 1983;38:305–11.
98. Feinstat T, Tesluk H, Schuffler MD, et al. Megacolon and neurofibromatosis; a neuronal intestinal dysplasia. Case report and review of the literature. Gastroenterology 1984;86:1573–9.
99. Furness JB, Young HM, Pompolo S, Bornstein JC, Kunze WA, McConalogue K. Plurichemical transmission and chemical coding of neurons in the digestive tract. Gastroenterology 1995;108:554–63.
100. Heitz PU, Komminoth P. Biopsy diagnosis of Hirschsprung's disease and related disorders. Curr Top Pathol 1990;81:257–75.
101. Holschneider AM. Clinical and electromanometric studies of postoperative continence in Hirschsprung's disease: relationship to the surgical procedure. In: Holschneider AM, ed. Hirschsprung's disease. Stuttgart: Hippokrates; 1982:221–42.
102. Holschneider AM, Meier-Ruge W, Ure BM. Hirschsprung's disease and allied disorders—a review. Eur J Pediatr Surg 1994;4:260–6.
103. Huang CC, Ko SF, Chuang JH, Chen WJ. Lipoblastomatosis combined with intestinal neuronal dysplasia. Arch Pathol Lab Med 1998;122:191–3.
104. Hutson JM, Chow CW, Borg J. Intractable constipation with a decrease in substance P-immunoreactive fibres: is it a variant of intestinal neuronal dysplasia? J Pediatr Surg 1996;31:580–3.
105. Karamanoglu T, Aygun B, Wade PR, et al. Regional differences in the number of neurons in the myenteric plexus of the guinea pig small intestine and colon: an evaluation of markers used to count neurons. Anat Rec 1996;244:470–80.
106. Kobayashi H, Hirakawa H, Puri P. Abnormal internal anal sphincter innervation in patients with Hirschsprung's disease and allied disorders. J Pediatr Surg 1996;31:794–9.
107. Kobayashi H, Hirakawa H, Puri P. Is intestinal neuronal dysplasia a disorder of the neuromuscular junction? J Pediatr Surg 1996;31:575–9.
108. Kobayashi H, Hirakawa H, Puri P. What are the diagnostic criteria for intestinal neuronal dysplasia? Pediatr Surg Int 1995;10:459–64.
109. Kobayashi H, Hirakawa H, Surana R, O'Briain DS, Puri P. Intestinal neuronal dysplasia is a possible cause of persistent bowel symptoms after pull-through operation for Hirschsprung's disease. J Pediatr Surg 1995;30:253–7.
110. Kobayashi H, O'Briain S, Hirakawa H, et al. A rapid technique for acetylcholinesterase staining. Arch Pathol Lab Med 1994;118:1127–9.
111. Kobayashi H, Yamataka A, Fujimoto T, Lane GJ, Miyano T. Mast cells and gut nerve development: implications for Hirschsprung's disease and intestinal neuronal dysplasia. J Pediatr Surg 1999;34:543–8.

112. Koletzko S, Ballauff A, Hadziselimovic F, Enck P. Is histological diagnosis of neuronal intestinal dysplasia related to clinical and manometric findings in constipated children? Results of a pilot study. J Pediatr Gastroenterol Nutr 1993;17:59–65.
113. Lumb PD, Moore L. Are giant ganglia a reliable marker of intestinal neuronal dysplasia type B (IND B)? Virchows Arch 1998;432:103–6.
114. Meier-Ruge W. Epidemiology of congenital innervation defects of the distal colon. Virchows Arch A Pathol Anat Histopathol 1992;420:171–7.
115. Meier-Ruge WA, Bronnimann PB, Gambazzi F, Schmid PC, Schmidt CP, Stoss F. Histopathological criteria for intestinal neuronal dysplasia of the submucosal plexus (type B). Virchows Arch 1995;426:549–56.
116. Meier-Ruge W, Gambazzi F, Käufeler RE, et al. The neuropathological diagnosis of neuronal intestinal dysplasia (NIB). Eur J Pediatr Surg 1994;4:267–73.
117. Meier-Ruge WA, Longo-Bauer CH. Morphometric determination of the methodological criteria for the diagnosis of intestinal neuronal dysplasia (IND B). Pathol Res Pract 1997;193: 465–9.
118. Moore SW, Laing D, Kaschula RO, et al. A histological grading system for the evaluation of co-existing NID with Hirschsprung's disease. Eur J Pediatr Surg 1994;4:293–7.
119. Munakata K, Okabe I, Morita K. Histologic studies of rectocolic aganglionosis and allied diseases. J Pediatr Surg 1978;13:67–75.
120. Navarro J, Sonsino E, Boige N, et al. Visceral neuropathies responsible for chronic intestinal pseudo-obstruction syndrome in pediatric practice: analysis of 26 cases. J Pediatr Gastroenterol Nutr 1990;11:179–95.
121. Nezelof C, Guy-Grand D, Thomine E. Les mégacolons avec hyperplasie des plexus myénteriques. Une entité anatomo-clinique, à propos de 3 cas. Presse Med 1970;78:1501–6.
122. O'Brien P, Kapusta L, Dardick I, Axler J, Gnidec A. Multiple familial gastrointestinal autonomic nerve tumors and small intestinal neuronal dysplasia. Am J Surg Pathol 1999;23:198–204.
123. Parikh DH, Tam PK, Lloyd DA, Van Velzen D, Edgar DH. Quantitative and qualitative analysis of the extracellular matrix protein, laminin, in Hirschsprung's disease. J Pediatr Surg 1992;27:991–6.
124. Parikh DH, Tam PK, Van Velzen D, Edgar D. Abnormalities in the distribution of laminin and collagen type IV in Hirschsprung's disease. Gastroenterology 1992;102:1236–41.
125. Phat VN, Sezeur A, Danne M, et al. Primary myenteric plexus alterations as a cause of megacolon in Von Recklinghausen's disease. Pathol Biol 1980;28:585–8.
126. Puliti A, Cinti R, Betsos N, Romeo G, Ceccherini I. HOX11L1, a gene involved in peripheral nervous system development, maps to human chromosome 2p13.1 —>p12 and mouse chromosome 6C3-D1. Cytogenet Cell Genet 1999; 84:115–7.
127. Puri P. Variant Hirschsprung's disease. J Pediatr Surg 1997;32:149–57.
128. Puri P, Fujimoto T. New observations on the pathogenesis of multiple intestinal atresias. J Pediatr Surg 1988;23:221–5.
129. Puri P, Lake BD, Nixon HH, Mishalany H, Claireaux AE. Neuronal colonic dysplasia: an unusual association of Hirschsprung's disease. J Pediatr Surg 1977;12:681–85.
130. Roggero P, Mazzola C, Fava G, Clerici-Bagozzi D, Martucciello G, Luzzani S. Intestinal microvillous atrophy and transient neuronal dysplasia. Transplant Proc 1997;29:1868–9.
131. Saul R, Sturner R, Burger P. Hyperplasia of the myenteric plexus. Its association with early infantile megacolon and neurofibromatosis. Am J Dis Child 1982;136:852–9.
132. Schärli AF. Neuronal intestinal dysplasia. Pediatr Surg Int 1992;7:2–7.
133. Schärli AF, Meier-Ruge W. Localized and disseminated forms of neuronal intestinal dysplasia mimicking Hirschsprung's disease. J Pediatr Surg 1981;16:164–70.
134. Schärli AF, Sossai R. Hypoganglionosis. Sem Pediatr Surg 1998;7:187–91.
135. Schofield DE, Yunis EJ. What is intestinal neuronal dysplasia? Pathol Ann 1992;1:249–62.
136. Smith VV. Isolated intestinal neuronal dysplasia: a descriptive pattern or a distinct clinicopathological entity? In: Hadziselimovic F, Herzog B, eds. Inflammatory bowel disease and morbus Hirschsprung. Dordrecht, The Netherlands: Kluwer Academic; 1992:203–14.
137. Spector B, Klintworth GK, Wells SA Jr. Histological study of the ocular lesions in multiple endocrine neoplasia syndrome type IIb. Am J Ophthalmol 1981;92:204–15.
138. Ure BM, Holschneider AM, Schulten D, Meier-Ruge W. Clinical impact of intestinal neuronal malformations: a prospective study in 141 patients. Pediatr Surg Intl 1997;12:377–82.
139. Wester T, O'Briain DS, Puri P. Notable postnatal alterations in the myenteric plexus of normal human bowel. Gut 1999;44:666–74.

Internal Anal Achalasia

140. Burleigh DE, D'Mello A. Neural and pharmacologic factors affecting motility of the internal anal sphincter. Gastroenterology 1983;84: 409–17.
141. Davidson M, Bauer CH. Studies of distal colonic motility in children. IV. Achalasia of the distal rectal segment despite presence of ganglia in the myenteric plexuses of this area. Pediatrics 1958;21:746–61.
142. Fujimoto T, Puri P, Miyano T. Abnormal peptidergic innervation in internal sphincter achalasia. Pediatr Surg Int 1992;7:12–7.

143. Holschneider AM. Internal sphincter achalasia. In: Holschneider AM, ed. Hirschprung's disease. New York: Verlag; 1982:203–18.
144. Lake BD, Puri P, Nixon HH, Claireaux AE. Hirschsprung's disease: an appraisal of histochemically demonstrated acetylcholinesterase activity in suction rectal biopsy specimens as an aid to diagnosis. Arch Pathol Lab Med 1978;102:244–7.
145. Neilson IR, Yazbeck S. Ultrashort Hirschsprung's disease: myth or reality. J Pediatr Surg 1990;25:1135–8.
146. O'Kelly T, Brading A, Mortensen N. Nerve mediated relaxation of the human internal anal sphincter: the role of nitric oxide. Gut 1993;34:689–93.
147. Rattan S, Chakder S. Role of nitric oxide as a mediator of internal anal sphincter relaxation. Am J Physiol 1992;262:G107–12.
148. Tottrup A, Glavind EB, Svane D. Involvement of the L-arginine-nitric oxide pathway in internal anal sphincter relaxation. Gastroenterology 1992;102:409–15.

Absent Enteric Nervous System

149. Huizinga JD, Thuneberg L, Kluppel M, Malysz J, Mikkelsen HB, Bernstein A. W/kit gene required for interstitial cells of Cajal and for intestinal pacemaker activity. Nature 1995;373:347–9.

Paraneoplastic Pseudoobstruction

150. Chinn JS, Schuffler MD. Paraneoplastic visceral neuropathy as a cause of severe gastrointestinal motor dysfunction. Gastroenterology 1988;95:1279–86.
151. Condom E, Vidal A, Rota R, Graus F, Dalmau J, Ferrer I. Paraneoplastic intestinal pseudo-obstruction associated with high titres of Hu autoantibodies. Virchows Archiv A Pathol Anat 1993;423:507–11.
152. Dalmau J, Furneaux H, Gralla R, et al. Detection of the anti-Hu antibody in the serum of patients with small cell lung cancer—a quantitative Western blot analysis. Ann Neurol 1990; 27:544–52.
153. De Giorgio R, Bovara M, Barbara G, et al. Anti-HuD-induced neuronal apoptosis underlying paraneoplastic gut dysmotility. Gastroenterology 2003;125:70–9.
154. Gerl A, Storck M, Schalhorn A, et al. Paraneoplastic chronic intestinal pseudoobstruction as a rare complication of bronchial carcinoid. Gut 1992;33:1000–3.
155. Gultekin SH, Dalmau J, Graus Y, Posner JB, Rosenblum MK. Anti-Hu immunolabeling as an index of neuronal differentiation in human brain tumors. Am J Surg Pathol 1998;22:195–200.
156. Kiers L, Altermatt HJ, Lennon VA. Paraneoplastic antineuronal nuclear IgG autoantibodies (type I) localize antigen in small cell lung carcinoma. Mayo Clin Proc 1991;66:1209–16.
157. Kimmel DW, O'Neill BP, Lennon VA. Subacute sensory neuronopathy associated with small cell carcinoma: diagnosis aided by autoimmune serology. Mayo Clin Proc 1988;63:29–32.
158. Lennon VA, Sas DF, Busk MF, et al. Enteric neuronal autoantibodies in pseudoobstruction with small-cell lung carcinoma. Gastroenterology 1991;100:137–42.
159. Posner JB, Dalmau JO. Paraneoplastic syndromes affecting the central nervous system. Annu Rev Med 1997;48:157–66.
160. Sutton I, Winer JB. The immunopathogenesis of paraneoplastic neurological syndromes. Clin Sci (Lond) 2002;102:475–86.

Infectious Causes of Motility Disorders

161. Bardhan PK, Salam MA, Molla AM. Gastric emptying of liquid in children suffering from acute rotaviral gastroenteritis. Gut 1992;3:26–9.
162. Kebede D, Barthel JS, Singh A. Transient gastroparesis associated with cutaneous herpes zoster. Dig Dis Sci 1987;32:318–22.
163. Koch KL. Stomach. In: Schuster MM, ed. Atlas of gastrointestinal motility in health and disease. Baltimore: Williams & Wilkins; 1993;158–76.
164. Mathias JR, Baskin GS, Reeves-Darby VG, Clench MH, Smith LL, Calhoon JH. Chronic intestinal pseudoobstruction in a patient with heart-lung transplant. Therapeutic effect of leuprolide acetate. Dig Dis Sci 1992;37:1761–8.
165. Meeroff JC, Schreiber DS, Trier JS, Blacklow NR. Abnormal gastric motor function in viral gastroenteritis. Ann Intern Med 1980;92:370–3.
166. Nowak TV, Goddard M, Batteiger B, Cummings OW. Evolution of acute cytomegalovirus gastritis to chronic gastrointestinal dysmotility in a nonimmunocompromised adult. Gastroenterology 1999;116:953–8.
167. Sonsino E, Mouy R, Foucaud P, et al. Intestinal pseudoobstruction related to cytomegalovirus infection of myenteric plexus. N Engl J Med 1984;311:196–7.
168. Van Thiel DH, Gavaler JS, Schade RR, Chien MC, Starzl TE. Cytomegalovirus infection and gastric emptying. Transplantation 1992;54:70–3.
169. Vassallo M, Camilleri M, Caron BL, Low PA. Gastrointestinal motor dysfunction in acquired selective cholinergic dysautonomia associated with infectious mononucleosis. Gastroenterology 1991;100:252–8.
170. Yahr MD, Frontera AT. Acute autonomic neuropathy. Its occurrence in infectious mononucleosis. Arch Neurol 1975;32:132–3.

Idiopathic Ganglionitis

171. Arista-Nasr J, Gonzàlez-Romo, Keirns C, Larriva-Sahd J. Diffuse lymphoplasmacytic infiltration of the small intestine with damage to nerve plexus. Arch Pathol Lab Med 1993;117:812–9.

172. Goin JC, Sterin-Borda L, Bilder CR, et al. Functional implications of circulating muscarinic cholinergic receptor autoantibodies in chagasic patients with achalasia. Gastroenterology 1999;117:798–805.
173. Horoupian DS, Kim Y. Encephalomyeloneuropathy with ganglionitis of the myenteric plexus in the absence of cancer. Ann Neurol 1982;11:628–32.
174. Singaram C, Koch J, Gaumnitz EA, et al. Nature of neuronal loss in human achalasia. Gastroenterology 1996;110:A259
175. Smith V, Gregson N, Foggensteiner L, Neale G, Milla P. Acquired intestinal aganglionosis and circulating autoantibodies without neoplasia or other neural involvement. Gastroenterology 1997;112:1366–71.

Achalasia

176. Adams CW, Brain RH, Ellis FG, Kaunteze R, Trounce JR. Achalasia of the cardia. Guy's Hosp Rep 1961;110:191–236.
177. Adams CW, Brain RH, Trounce JR. Ganglion cells in achalasia of the cardia. Virchows Arch 1976;372:75–9.
178. Ali GN, Hunt DR, Jorgensen JO, deCarle DJ, Cook IJ. Esophageal achalasia and coexistent upper esophageal sphincter relaxation disorder presenting with airway obstruction. Gastroenterology 1995;109:1328–32.
179. Arber N, Grossman A, Lurie B, et al. Epidemiology of achalasia in central Israel. Rarity of esophageal cancer. Dig Dis Sci 1993;38:1920–5.
180. Atkinson M. Antecedents of achalasia. Gut 1994;35:861–2.
181. Barrett NR. Achalasia of the cardia. Reflections on a clinical study of over 100 cases. Br Med J 1964;i:1135–9.
182. Becker DJ, Castell DO. Acute airway obstruction in achalasia: possible role of defective belch reflex. Gastroenterology 1989;97:1323–6.
183. Benini L, Sembenini C, Bulighin GM, et al. Achalasia. A possible late cause of postpolio dysphagia. Dig Dis Sci 1996;41:516–8.
184. Berquist WE, Byrne WJ, Ament ME. Achalasia: diagnosis, management, and clinical course in 16 children. Pediatrics 1983;71:798–805.
185. Bolivar JC, Herendeen TL. Carcinoma of the esophagus and achalasia. Ann Thorc Surg 1970;10:81–9.
186. Bortolotti M, Labo G. Clinical and manometric effects of nifedipine in patients with esophageal achalasia. Gastroenterology 1981;80:39–44.
187. Bosher P, Shaw A. Achalasia in siblings. Clinical and genetic aspects. Am J Dis Child 1981;135:709–10.
188. Cassella RR, Brown AL, Sayre GP. Achalasia of the esophagus: pathology and etiological considerations. Ann Surg 1964;160:470–4.
189. Castell DO, Katzka DA. Botulinum toxin for achalasia: to be or not to be? Gastroenterology 1996;110:1650–2.
190. Clark SB, Rice TW, Tubbs RR, Richter JE, Goldblum JR. The nature of the myenteric infiltrate in achalasia: an immunohistochemical analysis. Am J Surg Pathol 2000;24:1153–8.
191. Clouse RE, Abramson BK, Todorczuk JR. Achalasia in the elderly. Effects of aging on clinical presentation and outcome. Dig Dis Sci 1991;36:225–8.
192. Cohen S, Lipshutz W. Lower esophageal sphincter dysfunction in achalasia. Gastroenterology 1971;61:814–20.
193. Couturier D, Samama J. Clinical aspects and manometric criteria in achalasia. Hepatogastroenterology 1991;38:481–7.
194. Dumars KW, Williams JJ, Steele-Sandlin C. Achalasia and microcephaly. Am J Med Gen 1980;6:309–14.
195. Earlam RJ, Ellis FH Jr, Nobrega FT. Achalasia of the esophagus in a small urban community. Mayo Clin Proc 1969;44:478–83.
196. Ehrich E, Aranoff G, Johnson WG. Familial achalasia associated with adrenocortical insufficiency, alacrima, and neurological abnormalities. Am J Med 1987;26:637–44.
197. Goldblum JR, Rice TW, Richter JE. Histopathologic features in esophagomyotomy specimens from patients with achalasia. Gastroenterology 1996;111:648–54.
198. Goldblum JR, Whyte RI, Orringer MB, et al. Achalasia: a morphologic study of 42 resected specimens. Am J Surg Pathol 1994;18:327–37.
199. Hirano I, Tatum RP, Shi G, Sang Q, Joehl RJ, Kahrilas PJ. Manometric heterogeneity in patients with idiopathic achalasia. Gastroenterology 2001;120:789–98.
200. Jamieson GG. Gastro-esophageal reflux following myotomy for achalasia. Hepatogastroenterology 1991;38:506–9.
201. Jones DB, Mayberry JF, Rhodes J, Munro J. Preliminary report of an association between measles virus and achalasia. J Clin Pathol 1983; 36:655–7.
202. Karsell PR. Achalasia, aspiration, and atypical mycobacteria. Mayo Clin Proc 1993;68:1025–6.
203. Marshall JB, Diaz-Arias AA, Bochna GS, Vogele KA. Achalasia due to diffuse esophageal leiomyomatosis and inherited as an autosomal dominant disorder. Report of a family study. Gastroenterology 1990;98:1358–65.
204. Mayberry JF, Rhodes J. Achalasia in the city of Cardiff from 1926 to 1977. Digestion 1980;20: 248–52.
205. Meijssen MA, Tilanus HW, van Blankenstein M, et al. Achalasia complicated by oesophageal squamous cell carcinoma: a prospective study in 195 patients. Gut 1992;33:155–8.

206. Moreto M, Ojembarrena E, Rodriguez ML. Endoscopic injection of ethanolamine as a treatment for achalasia: a first report. Endoscopy 1996;28:539–45.
207. Murphy MS, Gardner-Medwin D, Eastham EJ. Achalasia of the cardia associated with hereditary cerebellar ataxia. Am J Gastroenterol 1989;84:1329–30.
208. Nagler RW, Schwartz RD, Stahl WN. Achalasia in fraternal twins. Ann Intern Med 1963;59: 906–9.
209. Nihoul-Fekete C, Bawab F, Lortat-Jacob S, Arhan P. Achalasia of the esophagus in childhood. Surgical treatment in 35 cases, with special reference to familial cases and glucocorticoid deficiency association. Hepatogastroenterology 1991;38:510–3.
210. Procter DD, Faser JL, Mangano MM, Calkins DR, Rosenberg SJ. Small cell carcinoma of the esophagus in a patient with longstanding primary achalasia. Am J Gastroenterol 1992;87: 664–7.
211. Qualman SJ, Hupt HM, Yang P, Hamilton SR. Esophageal Lewy bodies associated with ganglion cell loss in achalasia. Similarity to Parkinson's disease. Gastroenterology 1984;87: 848–56.
212. Robertson CS, Martin BA, Atkinson M. Varicella-zoster virus DNA in the oesophageal myenteric plexus in achalasia. Gut 1993;34:299–302.
213. Smith B. The neurologic lesion in achalasia of the cardia. Gut 1970;11:388–91.
214. Sonnenberg A, Massey BT, McCarty DJ, Jacobsen SJ. Epidemiology of hospitalization for achalasia in the United States. Dig Dis Sci 1993;38:233–44.
215. Spiess AE, Kahritas PJ. Treating achalasia: from whalebone to laprascope. JAMA 1998;280:638–42.
216. Storch WB, Eckardt VF, Weinbeck KM, et al. Autoantibodies to Auerbach's plexus in achalasia. Cell Mol Biol 1995;41:1033–8.
217. Streitz JM, Ellis FH, Gibb SP, Heatley GM. Achalasia and squamous cell carcinoma of the esophagus: analysis of 241 patients. Ann Thorac Surg 1995;59:1604–9.
218. Traube M, Dubovik S, Lange RC, McCallum RW. The role of nifedipine therapy in achalasia: results of a randomized, double-blind, placebo-controlled study. Am J Gastroenterol 1989;84:1259–62.
219. Triadafilopoulos G, Aaronson M, Sackel S, Burakoff R. Medical treatment of esophageal achalasia. Double-blind crossover study with oral nifedipine, verapamil, and placebo. Dig Dis Sci 1991;36:260–7.
220. Tyce FA, Brough W. The appearance of an undescribed syndrome and the inheritance of multiple diseases in three generations of a family. Psych Res Rep Am Psych Assoc 1962;15:73–5.
221. Verne GN, Hahn AB, Pineau BC, Hoffman BJ, Wojciechowski BW, Wu WC. Association of HLA-DR and -DG alleles with idiopathic achalasia. Gastroenterology 1999;117:26–31.
222. Wong RK, Johnson LF. Achalasia. In: Esophageal function in health and disease. Castle D, Johnston L, eds. New York: Elsevier Biomedical; 1983:99.
223. Wong RK, Maydonovitch CL, Metz SJ, Baker JR Jr. Significant DQw1 association in achalasia. Dig Dis Sci 1989;34:349–52.
224. Zimmerman FH, Rosensweig NS. Achalasia in a father and son. Am J Gastroenterol 1984;79: 506–8.

Autoimmune Autonomic Neuropathies

225. Suarez GA, Fealey RD, Camilleri M, Low PA. Idiopathic autonomic neuropathy: clinical, neurophysiologic, and follow-up studies on 27 patients. Neurology 1994;44:1675–82.
226. Young RR, Asbury AK, Corbett JL, Adams RD. Pure pan-dysautonomia with recovery: description and discussion of diagnostic criteria. Brain 1975;98:613–36.

Chronic Severe Idiopathic Constipation

227. Krishnamurthy S, Heng Y, Schuffler MD. Chronic intestinal pseudo-obstruction in infants and children caused by diverse abnormalities of the myenteric plexus. Gastroenterology 1993;104:1398–408.
228. McIntyre PB, Pemberton JH. Pathophysiology of colonic motility disorders. Surg Clin North Am 1993;73:1225–43.
229. Murray RD, Qualman SJ, Powers P, et al. Rectal myopathy in chronically constipated children. Pediatr Pathol 1992;12:787–98.
230. Nyam DC, Pemberton JH, Ilstrup DM, Rath DM. Long-term results of surgery for chronic constipation. Dis Colon Rectum 1997;40:273–9.
231. Park HJ, Kamm MA, Abbasi AM, Talbot TC. Immunohistochemical study of the colonic muscle and innervation in idiopathic chronic constipation. Dis Colon Rectum 1995;38:509–13.
232. Wedel T, Roblick UJ, Ott V, et al. Oligoneuronal hypoganglionosis in patients with idiopathic slow-transit constipation. Dis Colon Rectum 2002;45:54–62.
233. Wedel T, Spiegler J, Soellner S, et al. Enteric nerves and interstitial cells of Cajal are altered in patients with slow-transit constipation and megacolon. Gastroenterology 2002;123:1459–67.

Megacystis-Microcolon

234. Anneren G, Meurling S, Olsen L. Megacystis microcolon intestinal hypoperistalsis syndrome (MMIHS), an autosomal recessive disorder: clinical reports and review of the literature. Am J Med Genet 1991;41:251–4.

235. Chen CP, Wang TY, Chuang CY. Sonographic findings in a fetus with megacystis-microcolon-intestinal hyperperistalsis syndrome. J Clin Ultra 1998;26:217–20.
236. Ciftci AO, Cook RC, van Velzen D. Megacystis microcolon intestinal hypoperistalsis syndrome: evidence of a primary myocellular defect of contractile fiber synthesis. J Pediatr Surg 1996;31:1706–11.
237. Granata C, Puri P. Megacystis-microcolon-intestinal hypoperistalsis syndrome. J Pediatr Gastroenterol Nutr 1997;25:12–9.
238. Kubota M, Ikeda K, Ito Y. Autonomic innervation of the intestine from a baby with megacystis microcolon intestinal hypoperistalsis syndrome. II. Electro-physiological study. J Pediatr Surg 1989;24:1267–70.
239. Kupferman JC, Stewart CL, Schapfel DM, Kaskel FJ, Fine RN. Megacystis-microcolon-intestinal hypoperistalsis syndrome. Pediatr Nephrol 1995;9:626–7.
240. Puri P, Lake BD, Gorman F, et al. Megacystis-microcolon-hyoperistalsis syndrome: a visceral myopathy. J Pediatr Surg 1983;18:64–9.
241. Richardson CE, Morgan JM, Jasani B, et al. Megacystis-microcolon-intestinal hypoperistalsis syndrome and the absence of the alpha3 nicotinic acetylcholine receptor subunit. Gastroenterology 2001;121:350–7.
242. Tanner MS, Smith B, Lloyd JK. Functional intestinal obstruction due to deficiency of argyrophilic neurons in the myenteric plexus. Familial syndrome presenting with short small bowel, malrotation, and pyloric hypertrophy. Arch Dis Child 1976;51:837–41.

Hollow Visceral Myopathies

243. Alstead EM, Murphy MN, Flanagan AM, Bishop AE, Hodgson JH. Familial autonomic visceral myopathy with degeneration of muscularis mucosae. J Clin Pathol 1988;41:424–9.
244. Anuras S. Intestinal pseudoobstruction syndrome. Ann Rev Med 1988;30:1–15.
245. Anuras S, Mitros FA, Milano A, et al. Familial visceral myopathy with external ophthalmoplegia and autosomal recessive transmission. Gastroenterology 1983;84:346–53.
246. Faulk DL, Anuras S, Gardner GD, Mitros FA, Summers RW, Christensen J. A familial visceral myopathy. Ann Intern Med 1978;89:600–6.
247. Fitzgibbons PL, Chandrasoma PT. Familial visceral myopathy: evidence of diffuse involvement of intestinal smooth muscle. Am J Surg Pathol 1987;11:846–54.
248. Fogel S, DeTar M, Shimada H, Chandrasoma P. Sporadic visceral myopathy with inclusion bodies. A light-microscopic and ultrastructural study. Am J Surg Pathol 1993;17:473–81.
249. Foucar E, Lindholm J, Anuras S, et al. A kindred with dysplastic nevus syndrome associated with visceral myopathy and multiple basal cell carcinomas. Lab Invest 1985;52:32A.
250. Goebel HH, Shin YS, Gullotta F, et al. Adult polyglycosan body myopathy. J Neuropathol Exp Neurol 1992;51:24–35.
251. Greene GM, Weldon DC, Ferrans VJ, et al. Juvenile polysaccharidosis with cardioskeletal myopathy. Arch Pathol Lab Med 1987;111: 977–82.
252. Igarashi M, MacRae D, O-Uchi T, Alford BR. Cochleo-saccular degeneration in one of three sisters with hereditary deafness, absent gastric motility, small bowel diverticulosis and progressive sensory neuropathy. Ann Otol Rhinol Laryngol 1981;43:4–16.
253. Ionasescu V, Thompson SH, Ionasescu R, et al. Inherited ophthalmoplegia with intestinal pseudo-obstruction. J Neurol Sci 1983;59:215–28.
254. Jones SC, Dixon MF, Lintott DJ, Axon AT. Familial visceral myopathy: a family with involvement of four generations. Dig Dis Sci 1992;37: 464–9.
255. McMaster KR, Powers JM, Hennigar GR Jr, Wohltmann HJ, Farr GH Jr. Nervous system involvement in type IV glycogenosis. Arch Pathol Lab Med 1979;103:105–11.
256. Mitros FA, Schuffler MD, Teja K, Anuras S. Pathologic features of familial visceral myopathy. Hum Pathol 1982;13:825–33.
257. Nonaka M, Goulet O, Arahan P, et al. Primary intestinal myopathy, a cause of chronic idiopathic intestinal pseudo-obstruction syndrome (CIPS): clinicopathological studies of seven cases in children. Pediatr Pathol 1989;9:409–24.
258. Rodrigues CA, Shepherd NA, Lennard-Jones JE, et al. Familial visceral myopathy: a family with at least 6 involved members. Gut 1989;30: 1285–92.
259. Schuffler MD, Lowe MC, Bill AH. Studies of idiopathic intestinal pseudoobstruction. I. Hereditary hollow visceral myopathy: clinical and pathological studies. Gastroenterology 1977;73:327–38.
260. Smout AJ, deWilde K, Kooyman CD, Ten Thije OJ. Chronic idiopathic intestinal pseudo-obstruction. Coexistence of smooth muscle and neuronal abnormalities. Dig Dis Sci 1985;30: 282–7.

Mitochondrial Encephalomyopathies

261. Bardosi A, Creutzfeldt W, DiMauro S, et al. Myoneuro-gastrointestinal encephalopathy (MNGIE syndrome) due to partial deficiency of cytochrome c oxidase: a new mitochondrial multisystem disorder. Acta Neuropathol 1987; 74:248–58.
262. DiMauro S, Moraes CT. Mitochondrial encephalomyopathies. Arch Neurol 1993;50:1197–208.
263. DiMauro S, Schon EA. Mitochondrial respiratory-chain diseases. N Engl J Med 2003;348: 2656–68.

264. Fromenty B, Carrozzo R, Shanske S, Schon EA. High proportions of mtDNA duplications in patients with Kearns-Sayre syndrome occur in the heart. Am J Med Genet 1997;71:443–52.
265. Fukuhara N, Tokiguchi S, Shirakawa K, Tsubaki T. Myoclonus epilepsy associated with ragged-red fibers (mitochondrial abnormalities): disease entity or a syndrome? Light and electron microscopic studies of two cases and review of literature. J Neurol Sci 1980;47:117–33.
266. Gold R, Seibel P, Reinelt G, et al. Phosphorus magnetic resonance spectroscopy in the evaluation of mitochondrial myopathies: results of a 6-month therapy study with coenzyme Q. Eur J Neurol 1996;36:191–6.
267. Grossman LI, Shoubridge EA. Mitochondrial genetics and human disease. Bioessays 1996;18:983–91.
268. Hasegawa H, Matusoka T, Goto YI, Nanoka I. Strongly succinate dehydrogenase-reactive blood vessels in muscles from patients with mitochondrial myopathy, encephalopathy, lactic acidosis, and stroke-like episodes. Ann Neurol 1991;29:610–5.
269. Hirano M, Silvestri G, Blake DM, et al. Mitochondrial neurogastrointestinal encephalomyopathy (MNGIE): clinical, biochemical, and genetic features of an autosomal recessive mitochondrial disorder. Neurology 1994;44:721–7.
270. Johns DR. Mitochondrial DNA and disease. N Eng J Med 1995;333:638–44.
271. Kearns TP, Sayre GP. Retinitis pigmentosa, external ophthalmoplegia and complete heart block. Arch Ophthalmol 1958;60:280–7.
272. Moraes CT. Mitochondrial disorders. Curr Opin Neurol 1996;9:369–74.
273. Moraes CT, DiMauro S, Zeviani M, et al. Mitochondrial DNA deletions in progressive external ophthalmoplegia and Kearns-Sayre syndrome. N Engl J Med 1989;320:1293–9.
274. Moraes CT, Ricci E, Petruzzella V, et al. Molecular analysis of the muscle pathology associated with mitochondrial DNA deletion. Nat Genet 1991;1:359–67.
275. Mueller LA, Camilleri M, Emslie-Smith AM. Mitochondrial neurogastrointestinal encephalopathy: manometric and diagnostic features. Gastroenterology 1999;116:959–63.
276. Nishino I, Spinazzola A, Hirano M. Thymidine phosphorylase gene mutations in MNGIE, a human mitochondrial disorder. Science 1999;283:689–92.
277. Perez-Atayde AR, Fox V, Teitelbaum JE, et al. Mitochondrial neurogastrointestinal encephalomyopathy. Diagnosis by rectal biopsy. Am J Surg Pathol 1998;22:1141–7.
278. Peterson PL. The treatment of mitochondrial myopathies and encephalomyopathies. Biochim Biophys Acta 1995;1271:275–80.
279. Sabatelli M, Servedei S, Ricci E, et al. Myoneuro-intestinal disease and encephalopathy (MNGIE syndrome): a patient with multiple deletions of mitochondrial DNA (abstract). Neurology 1992;42:418.
280. Sakuta R, Nonaka I. Vascular involvement in mitochondrial myopathy. Ann Neurol 1989;25:594–601.
281. Sherratt EJ, Thomas AW, Alcolado JC. Mitochondrial DNA defects: a widening clinical spectrum of disorders. Clin Sci 1997;92:225–35.

Autoimmune Enteric Myositis

282. Bogdanos DP, Choudhuri K, Vergani D. Molecular mimicry and autoimmune liver disease: virtuous intentions, malign consequences. Liver 2001;21:225–32.
283. Mann SD, Debinski HS, Kamm MA. Clinical characteristics of chronic idiopathic intestinal pseudo-obstruction in adults. Gut 1997;41: 675–81.
284. McDonald GB, Schuffler MD, Kadin ME, Tytgat GN. Intestinal pseudoobstruction caused by diffuse lymphoid infiltration of the small intestine. Gastroenterology 1985;89:882–9.
285. Nezelof C, Vivien E, Bigel P, et al. Idiopathic myositis of the small intestine. An unusual cause of chronic intestinal pseudo-obstruction in children. Arch Fr Pediatr 1985;42:823–8.
286. Rigby SP, Schott JM, Bliss P, Higgens CS, Kamm MA. Dilated stomach and weak muscles. Lancet 2000;356:1898.
287. Ruuska TH, Karikoski R, Smith VV, Milla PJ. Acquired myopathic intestinal pseudo-obstruction may be due to autoimmune enteric leiomyositis. Gastroenterology 2002;122:1133–9.

Diffuse Leiomyomatosis

288. Antignac C, Heidet L. Mutations in Alport syndrome associated with diffuse esophageal leiomyomatosis. Contrib Nephrol 1996;117:172–82.
289. Antignac C, Zhou J, Sanak M, et al. Alport syndrome and diffuse leiomyomatosis: deletions in the 5' end of the COL4A5 collagen gene. Kidney Int 1992;42:1178–83.
290. Cochat P, Guibaud P, Garcia Torres R, Roussel B, Guarner V, Larbre F. Diffuse leiomyomatosis in Alport syndrome. J Pediatr 1988;113:339–43.
291. Federici S, Ceccarelli PL, Bernardi F, et al. Esophageal leiomyomatosis in children: report of a case and review of the literature. Eur J Pediatr Surg 1998;8:358–63.
292. Guillem P, Delcambre F, Cohen-Solal L, et al. Diffuse esophageal leiomyomatosis with perirectal involvement mimicking Hirschsprung disease. Gastroenterology 2001;120:216–20.
293. Heidet L, Cohen-Solal L, Boye E, et al. Novel COL4A5/COL4A6 deletions and further characterization of the diffuse leiomyomatosis-Alport syndrome (DL-AS) locus define the DL critical region. Cytogenet Cell Genet 1997;78:240–6.

294. Heidet L, Dahan K, Zhou J, et al. Deletions of both alpha 5(IV) and alpha 6(IV) collagen genes in Alport syndrome and in Alport syndrome associated with smooth muscle tumours. Hum Mol Genet 1995;4:99–108.
295. Leborgne J, Le Neel JC, Heloury Y, et al. Diffuse esophageal leiomyomatosis. Apropos of 5 cases with 2 familial cases. Chirurgie 1989;115:277–85.
296. Levine MS, Buck JL, Pantongrag-Brown L, Buetow PC, Hallman JR, Sobin LH. Leiomyosarcoma of the esophagus: radiographic findings in 10 patients. AJR Am J Roentgenol 1996;167:27–32.
296a. Marshall JB, Diaz-Arias AA, Bochna GS, Vogele KA. Achalasia due to diffuse esophageal leiomyomatosis and inherited as an autosomal dominant disorder. Report of a family study. Gastroenterology 1990;98:1358–65.
297. Schapiro RL, Sandrock AR. Esophagogastric and vulvar leiomyomatosis: a new radiologic syndrome. J Can Assoc Radiol 1973;24:184–7.

Scleroderma

298. Bedarida GV, Kim D, Blaschke TF, Hoffman BB. Venodilation in Raynaud's disease. Lancet 1993;342:1451–4.
299. Bortolotti M, Turba E, Tosti A, et al. Gastric emptying and interdigestive antroduodenal motility in patients with esophageal scleroderma. Am J Gastroenterol 1991;86:743–7.
300. Cohen S, Fisher R, Lipshutz W, Turner R, Myers A, Schumacher R. The pathogenesis of esophageal dysfunction in scleroderma and Raynaud's disease. J Clin Invest 1972;51:2663–8.
301. D'Angelo WA, Fries JF, Masai AT, Shulman LE. Pathologic observations in systemic sclerosis (scleroderma). A study of fifty-eight autopsy cases and fifty-eight matched controls. Am J Med 1969;46:428–40.
302. Ebert EC, Ruggiero FM, Seibold JR. Intestinal perforation. A common complication of scleroderma. Dig Dis Sci 1997;42:549–53.
303. Govoni M, Muccinelli M, Panicali P, et al. Colonic involvement in systemic sclerosis: clinical-radiological correlations. Clin Rheumatol 1996;15:271–6.
304. Hang LM, Nakamura RM. Current concepts and advances in clinical laboratory testing for autoimmune diseases. Crit Rev Clin Lab Sci 1997;34:275–311.
305. Haustein UF, Herrmann K. Environmental scleroderma. Clin Dermatol 1994;12:467–73.
306. Jimenez SA, Saitta B. Alterations in the regulation of expression of the alpha 1(I) collagen gene (COL1A1) in systemic sclerosis (scleroderma). Semin Immunopathol 1999;21:397–414.
307. Kahn IJ, Geffries GH, Sleisinger MH. Malabsorption in scleroderma: correction by antibiotics. N Engl J Med 1966;274:1339–44.
308. Lock G, Holstege A, Lang B, Scholmerich J. Gastrointestinal manifestations of progressive systemic sclerosis. Am J Gastroenterol 1997;92:763–71.
309. Lovy MR, Levine JS, Steigerald JC. Lower esophageal rings as a cause of dysphagia in progressive systemic sclerosis—coincidence or consequence? Dig Dis Sci 1983;28:780–3.
310. Manolios N, Eliades C, Duncombe V, Spencer D. Scleroderma and watermelon stomach. J Rheumatol 1996;23:776–8.
311. Miller LS, Liu JB, Klenn PJ, et al. Endoluminal ultrasonography of the distal esophagus in systemic sclerosis. Gastroenterology 1993;105:31–9.
312. Pearson JD. The endothelium: its role in scleroderma. Ann Rheum Dis 1991;50:866–71.
313. Rodnan GP, Medsger TA Jr, Buckingham RB. Progressive systemic sclerosis-CREST syndrome: observations on natural history and late complications in 90 patients. Arthritis Rheum 1975;18:423–8.
314. Rosson RS, Yesner R. Peroral duodenal biopsy in progressive systemic sclerosis. N Engl J Med 1965;272:391–4.
315. Russell ML, Friesen D, Henderson RD, Hanna WM. Ultrastructure of the esophagus in scleroderma. Arthritis Rheum 1982;25:1117–23.
316. Seibold JR. Critical tissue ischaemia in scleroderma: a note of caution. Ann Rheum Dis 1994;53:289–90.
317. Sjogren RW. Gastrointestinal features of scleroderma. Curr Opin Rheumatol 1996;8:569–75.
318. Stafford-Brad FJ, Kahn HJ, Ross TM, Russell ML. Advanced scleroderma bowel: complications and management. J Rheumatol 1988;15:869–74.
319. Wegener M, Adamek RJ, Wedmann, Jergas M, Altmeyer P. Gastrointestinal transit through esophagus, stomach, small and large intestine in patients with progressive systemic sclerosis. Dig Dis Sci 1994;39:2209–15.

Diabetes

320. Cho S, Turner M, Henry D. Gastroparesis diabeticorum. J Can Assoc Radiol 1983;34:32–5.
321. Greene DA, Sima AA, Albers JW, Pfeifer M. Diabetic neuropathy. In: Rifkin H, Porte D. Ellenberg and Rifkin diabetes mellitus. New York: Elsevier; 1989:710.
322. Horowitz M, Fraser R. Disordered gastric motor function in diabetes mellitus. Diabetologia 1994;37:543–51.
323. Jones KL, Horowitz M, Wishart JM, Maddox AF, Harding PE, Chatterton BE. Relationships between gastric emptying, intragastric meal distribution and blood glucose concentrations in diabetes mellitus. J Nucl Med 1995;36:2220–8.
324. Katz LA, Spiro H. Gastrointestinal manifestation of diabetes. N Engl J Med 1966;275:1350–61.
325. Keshavarzian A, Iber FL, Vaeth J. Gastric emptying in patients with insulin-requiring diabetes mellitus. Am J Gastroenterol 1987;82:29–35.

326. Koch KL. Diabetic gastropathy: gastric neuromuscular dysfunction in diabetes mellitus: a review of symptoms, pathophysiology, and treatment. Dig Dis Sci 1999;44:1061–75.
327. Kristensson K, Nordborg C, Olsson Y, Sourander P. Changes in the vagus nerve in diabetes mellitus. Acta Pathol Microbiol Scand 1971;79: 684–5.
328. Loo F, Dodds W, Soergel K, et al. Multipeaked esophageal peristaltic pressure waves in patients with diabetic neuropathy. Gastroenterology 1985;88:485–91.
329. Murray L, Lombard M, Aske J, et al. Esophageal function in diabetes mellitus with special reference to acid studies and relationship to peripheral neuropathy. Am J Gastroenterol 1987;82:840–3.
330. Nilsson PH. Diabetic gastroparesis: a review. J Diabetes Complications 1996;10:113–22.
331. Quigley EM. The pathophysiology of diabetic gastroenteropathy: more vague than vagal? Gastroenterology 1997;113:1790–2.
332. Urbina JA Payares G, Molina J, et al. Cure of short-term and long-term experimental Chagas' disease using DO870. Science 1996; 273:969–71.
333. Valdovinos MA, Camilleri M, Zimmerman BR. Chronic diarrhea in diabetes mellitus: mechanisms and an approach to diagnosis and treatment. Mayo Clin Proc 1993;68:691–702.

Amyloidosis

334. Gilat T, Spiro HM. Amyloidosis and the gut. Am J Dig Dis 1968;13:619–33.
335. Menke D, Kyle R, Fleming R, et al. Symptomatic gastric amyloidosis in patients with primary systemic amyloidosis. Mayo Clin Proc 1993;68:763–7.
336. Rocken S, Saeger W, Linke RP. Gastrointestinal amyloid deposits in old age. Report on 110 consecutive autopsical patients and 98 retrospective bioptic specimens. Pathol Res Pract 1994;190:641–9.
337. Tada S, Iida M, Yao T, Kitamoto T, Yao T, Fujishima M. Intestinal pseudo-obstruction in patients with amyloidosis: clinicopathologic differences between chemical types of amyloid protein. Gut 1993;34:1412–7.

Index*

*Numbers in boldface indicate table and figure pages.

B

C

F

G

I

N

O

P

T

U

V

W

X

Y

Z